T0251413

ION CHANNELS IN THE PULMONARY VASCULATURE

LUNG BIOLOGY IN HEALTH AND DISEASE

Executive Editor

Claude Lenfant
Former Director, National Heart, Lung, and Blood Institute
National Institutes of Health
Bethesda, Maryland

1. Immunologic and Infectious Reactions in the Lung, *edited by C. H. Kirkpatrick and H. Y. Reynolds*
2. The Biochemical Basis of Pulmonary Function, *edited by R. G. Crystal*
3. Bioengineering Aspects of the Lung, *edited by J. B. West*
4. Metabolic Functions of the Lung, *edited by Y. S. Bakhle and J. R. Vane*
5. Respiratory Defense Mechanisms (in two parts), *edited by J. D. Brain, D. F. Proctor, and L. M. Reid*
6. Development of the Lung, *edited by W. A. Hodson*
7. Lung Water and Solute Exchange, *edited by N. C. Staub*
8. Extrapulmonary Manifestations of Respiratory Disease, *edited by E. D. Robin*
9. Chronic Obstructive Pulmonary Disease, *edited by T. L. Petty*
10. Pathogenesis and Therapy of Lung Cancer, *edited by C. C. Harris*
11. Genetic Determinants of Pulmonary Disease, *edited by S. D. Litwin*
12. The Lung in the Transition Between Health and Disease, *edited by P. T. Macklem and S. Permutt*
13. Evolution of Respiratory Processes: A Comparative Approach, *edited by S. C. Wood and C. Lenfant*
14. Pulmonary Vascular Diseases, *edited by K. M. Moser*
15. Physiology and Pharmacology of the Airways, *edited by J. A. Nadel*
16. Diagnostic Techniques in Pulmonary Disease (in two parts), *edited by M. A. Sackner*
17. Regulation of Breathing (in two parts), *edited by T. F. Hornbein*
18. Occupational Lung Diseases: Research Approaches and Methods, *edited by H. Weill and M. Turner-Warwick*
19. Immunopharmacology of the Lung, *edited by H. H. Newball*
20. Sarcoidosis and Other Granulomatous Diseases of the Lung, *edited by B. L. Fanburg*

21. Sleep and Breathing, *edited by N. A. Saunders and C. E. Sullivan*
22. *Pneumocystis carinii* Pneumonia: Pathogenesis, Diagnosis, and Treatment, *edited by L. S. Young*
23. Pulmonary Nuclear Medicine: Techniques in Diagnosis of Lung Disease, *edited by H. L. Atkins*
24. Acute Respiratory Failure, *edited by W. M. Zapol and K. J. Falke*
25. Gas Mixing and Distribution in the Lung, *edited by L. A. Engel and M. Paiva*
26. High-Frequency Ventilation in Intensive Care and During Surgery, *edited by G. Carlon and W. S. Howland*
27. Pulmonary Development: Transition from Intrauterine to Extrauterine Life, *edited by G. H. Nelson*
28. Chronic Obstructive Pulmonary Disease: Second Edition, *edited by T. L. Petty*
29. The Thorax (in two parts), *edited by C. Roussos and P. T. Macklem*
30. The Pleura in Health and Disease, *edited by J. Chrétien, J. Bignon, and A. Hirsch*
31. Drug Therapy for Asthma: Research and Clinical Practice, *edited by J. W. Jenne and S. Murphy*
32. Pulmonary Endothelium in Health and Disease, *edited by U. S. Ryan*
33. The Airways: Neural Control in Health and Disease, *edited by M. A. Kaliner and P. J. Barnes*
34. Pathophysiology and Treatment of Inhalation Injuries, *edited by J. Loke*
35. Respiratory Function of the Upper Airway, *edited by O. P. Mathew and G. Sant'Ambrogio*
36. Chronic Obstructive Pulmonary Disease: A Behavioral Perspective, *edited by A. J. McSweeny and I. Grant*
37. Biology of Lung Cancer: Diagnosis and Treatment, *edited by S. T. Rosen, J. L. Mulshine, F. Cuttitta, and P. G. Abrams*
38. Pulmonary Vascular Physiology and Pathophysiology, *edited by E. K. Weir and J. T. Reeves*
39. Comparative Pulmonary Physiology: Current Concepts, *edited by S. C. Wood*
40. Respiratory Physiology: An Analytical Approach, *edited by H. K. Chang and M. Paiva*
41. Lung Cell Biology, *edited by D. Massaro*
42. Heart–Lung Interactions in Health and Disease, *edited by S. M. Scharf and S. S. Cassidy*
43. Clinical Epidemiology of Chronic Obstructive Pulmonary Disease, *edited by M. J. Hensley and N. A. Saunders*

44. Surgical Pathology of Lung Neoplasms, *edited by A. M. Marchevsky*
45. The Lung in Rheumatic Diseases, *edited by G. W. Cannon and G. A. Zimmerman*
46. Diagnostic Imaging of the Lung, *edited by C. E. Putman*
47. Models of Lung Disease: Microscopy and Structural Methods, *edited by J. Gil*
48. Electron Microscopy of the Lung, *edited by D. E. Schraufnagel*
49. Asthma: Its Pathology and Treatment, *edited by M. A. Kaliner, P. J. Barnes, and C. G. A. Persson*
50. Acute Respiratory Failure: Second Edition, *edited by W. M. Zapol and F. Lemaire*
51. Lung Disease in the Tropics, *edited by O. P. Sharma*
52. Exercise: Pulmonary Physiology and Pathophysiology, *edited by B. J. Whipp and K. Wasserman*
53. Developmental Neurobiology of Breathing, *edited by G. G. Haddad and J. P. Farber*
54. Mediators of Pulmonary Inflammation, *edited by M. A. Bray and W. H. Anderson*
55. The Airway Epithelium, *edited by S. G. Farmer and D. Hay*
56. Physiological Adaptations in Vertebrates: Respiration, Circulation, and Metabolism, *edited by S. C. Wood, R. E. Weber, A. R. Hargens, and R. W. Millard*
57. The Bronchial Circulation, *edited by J. Butler*
58. Lung Cancer Differentiation: Implications for Diagnosis and Treatment, *edited by S. D. Bernal and P. J. Hesketh*
59. Pulmonary Complications of Systemic Disease, *edited by J. F. Murray*
60. Lung Vascular Injury: Molecular and Cellular Response, *edited by A. Johnson and T. J. Ferro*
61. Cytokines of the Lung, *edited by J. Kelley*
62. The Mast Cell in Health and Disease, *edited by M. A. Kaliner and D. D. Metcalfe*
63. Pulmonary Disease in the Elderly Patient, *edited by D. A. Mahler*
64. Cystic Fibrosis, *edited by P. B. Davis*
65. Signal Transduction in Lung Cells, *edited by J. S. Brody, D. M. Center, and V. A. Tkachuk*
66. Tuberculosis: A Comprehensive International Approach, *edited by L. B. Reichman and E. S. Hershfield*
67. Pharmacology of the Respiratory Tract: Experimental and Clinical Research, *edited by K. F. Chung and P. J. Barnes*
68. Prevention of Respiratory Diseases, *edited by A. Hirsch, M. Goldberg, J.-P. Martin, and R. Masse*

69. *Pneumocystis carinii* Pneumonia: Second Edition, *edited by P. D. Walzer*
70. Fluid and Solute Transport in the Airspaces of the Lungs, *edited by R. M. Effros and H. K. Chang*
71. Sleep and Breathing: Second Edition, *edited by N. A. Saunders and C. E. Sullivan*
72. Airway Secretion: Physiological Bases for the Control of Mucous Hypersecretion, *edited by T. Takishima and S. Shimura*
73. Sarcoidosis and Other Granulomatous Disorders, *edited by D. G. James*
74. Epidemiology of Lung Cancer, *edited by J. M. Samet*
75. Pulmonary Embolism, *edited by M. Morpurgo*
76. Sports and Exercise Medicine, *edited by S. C. Wood and R. C. Roach*
77. Endotoxin and the Lungs, *edited by K. L. Brigham*
78. The Mesothelial Cell and Mesothelioma, *edited by M.-C. Jaurand and J. Bignon*
79. Regulation of Breathing: Second Edition, *edited by J. A. Dempsey and A. I. Pack*
80. Pulmonary Fibrosis, *edited by S. Hin. Phan and R. S. Thrall*
81. Long-Term Oxygen Therapy: Scientific Basis and Clinical Application, *edited by W. J. O'Donohue, Jr.*
82. Ventral Brainstem Mechanisms and Control of Respiration and Blood Pressure, *edited by C. O. Trouth, R. M. Millis, H. F. Kiwull-Schöne, and M. E. Schläfke*
83. A History of Breathing Physiology, *edited by D. F. Proctor*
84. Surfactant Therapy for Lung Disease, *edited by B. Robertson and H. W. Taeusch*
85. The Thorax: Second Edition, Revised and Expanded (in three parts), *edited by C. Roussos*
86. Severe Asthma: Pathogenesis and Clinical Management, *edited by S. J. Szefler and D. Y. M. Leung*
87. *Mycobacterium avium*–Complex Infection: Progress in Research and Treatment, *edited by J. A. Korvick and C. A. Benson*
88. Alpha 1–Antitrypsin Deficiency: Biology • Pathogenesis • Clinical Manifestations • Therapy, *edited by R. G. Crystal*
89. Adhesion Molecules and the Lung, *edited by P. A. Ward and J. C. Fantone*
90. Respiratory Sensation, *edited by L. Adams and A. Guz*
91. Pulmonary Rehabilitation, *edited by A. P. Fishman*
92. Acute Respiratory Failure in Chronic Obstructive Pulmonary Disease, *edited by J.-P. Derenne, W. A. Whitelaw, and T. Similowski*

93. Environmental Impact on the Airways: From Injury to Repair, *edited by J. Chrétien and D. Dusser*
94. Inhalation Aerosols: Physical and Biological Basis for Therapy, *edited by A. J. Hickey*
95. Tissue Oxygen Deprivation: From Molecular to Integrated Function, *edited by G. G. Haddad and G. Lister*
96. The Genetics of Asthma, *edited by S. B. Liggett and D. A. Meyers*
97. Inhaled Glucocorticoids in Asthma: Mechanisms and Clinical Actions, *edited by R. P. Schleimer, W. W. Busse, and P. M. O'Byrne*
98. Nitric Oxide and the Lung, *edited by W. M. Zapol and K. D. Bloch*
99. Primary Pulmonary Hypertension, *edited by L. J. Rubin and S. Rich*
100. Lung Growth and Development, *edited by J. A. McDonald*
101. Parasitic Lung Diseases, *edited by A. A. F. Mahmoud*
102. Lung Macrophages and Dendritic Cells in Health and Disease, *edited by M. F. Lipscomb and S. W. Russell*
103. Pulmonary and Cardiac Imaging, *edited by C. Chiles and C. E. Putman*
104. Gene Therapy for Diseases of the Lung, *edited by K. L. Brigham*
105. Oxygen, Gene Expression, and Cellular Function, *edited by L. Biadasz Clerch and D. J. Massaro*
106. $Beta_2$-Agonists in Asthma Treatment, *edited by R. Pauwels and P. M. O'Byrne*
107. Inhalation Delivery of Therapeutic Peptides and Proteins, *edited by A. L. Adjei and P. K. Gupta*
108. Asthma in the Elderly, *edited by R. A. Barbee and J. W. Bloom*
109. Treatment of the Hospitalized Cystic Fibrosis Patient, *edited by D. M. Orenstein and R. C. Stern*
110. Asthma and Immunological Diseases in Pregnancy and Early Infancy, *edited by M. Schatz, R. S. Zeiger, and H. N. Claman*
111. Dyspnea, *edited by D. A. Mahler*
112. Proinflammatory and Antiinflammatory Peptides, *edited by S. I. Said*
113. Self-Management of Asthma, *edited by H. Kotses and A. Harver*
114. Eicosanoids, Aspirin, and Asthma, *edited by A. Szczeklik, R. J. Gryglewski, and J. R. Vane*
115. Fatal Asthma, *edited by A. L. Sheffer*
116. Pulmonary Edema, *edited by M. A. Matthay and D. H. Ingbar*
117. Inflammatory Mechanisms in Asthma, *edited by S. T. Holgate and W. W. Busse*

118. Physiological Basis of Ventilatory Support, *edited by J. J. Marini and A. S. Slutsky*
119. Human Immunodeficiency Virus and the Lung, *edited by M. J. Rosen and J. M. Beck*
120. Five-Lipoxygenase Products in Asthma, *edited by J. M. Drazen, S.-E. Dahlén, and T. H. Lee*
121. Complexity in Structure and Function of the Lung, *edited by M. P. Hlastala and H. T. Robertson*
122. Biology of Lung Cancer, *edited by M. A. Kane and P. A. Bunn, Jr.*
123. Rhinitis: Mechanisms and Management, *edited by R. M. Naclerio, S. R. Durham, and N. Mygind*
124. Lung Tumors: Fundamental Biology and Clinical Management, *edited by C. Brambilla and E. Brambilla*
125. Interleukin-5: From Molecule to Drug Target for Asthma, *edited by C. J. Sanderson*
126. Pediatric Asthma, *edited by S. Murphy and H. W. Kelly*
127. Viral Infections of the Respiratory Tract, *edited by R. Dolin and P. F. Wright*
128. Air Pollutants and the Respiratory Tract, *edited by D. L. Swift and W. M. Foster*
129. Gastroesophageal Reflux Disease and Airway Disease, *edited by M. R. Stein*
130. Exercise-Induced Asthma, *edited by E. R. McFadden, Jr.*
131. LAM and Other Diseases Characterized by Smooth Muscle Proliferation, *edited by J. Moss*
132. The Lung at Depth, *edited by C. E. G. Lundgren and J. N. Miller*
133. Regulation of Sleep and Circadian Rhythms, *edited by F. W. Turek and P. C. Zee*
134. Anticholinergic Agents in the Upper and Lower Airways, *edited by S. L. Spector*
135. Control of Breathing in Health and Disease, *edited by M. D. Altose and Y. Kawakami*
136. Immunotherapy in Asthma, *edited by J. Bousquet and H. Yssel*
137. Chronic Lung Disease in Early Infancy, *edited by R. D. Bland and J. J. Coalson*
138. Asthma's Impact on Society: The Social and Economic Burden, *edited by K. B. Weiss, A. S. Buist, and S. D. Sullivan*
139. New and Exploratory Therapeutic Agents for Asthma, *edited by M. Yeadon and Z. Diamant*
140. Multimodality Treatment of Lung Cancer, *edited by A. T. Skarin*

141. Cytokines in Pulmonary Disease: Infection and Inflammation, *edited by S. Nelson and T. R. Martin*
142. Diagnostic Pulmonary Pathology, *edited by P. T. Cagle*
143. Particle–Lung Interactions, *edited by P. Gehr and J. Heyder*
144. Tuberculosis: A Comprehensive International Approach, Second Edition, Revised and Expanded, *edited by L. B. Reichman and E. S. Hershfield*
145. Combination Therapy for Asthma and Chronic Obstructive Pulmonary Disease, *edited by R. J. Martin and M. Kraft*
146. Sleep Apnea: Implications in Cardiovascular and Cerebrovascular Disease, *edited by T. D. Bradley and J. S. Floras*
147. Sleep and Breathing in Children: A Developmental Approach, *edited by G. M. Loughlin, J. L. Carroll, and C. L. Marcus*
148. Pulmonary and Peripheral Gas Exchange in Health and Disease, *edited by J. Roca, R. Rodriguez-Roisen, and P. D. Wagner*
149. Lung Surfactants: Basic Science and Clinical Applications, *R. H. Notter*
150. Nosocomial Pneumonia, *edited by W. R. Jarvis*
151. Fetal Origins of Cardiovascular and Lung Disease, *edited by David J. P. Barker*
152. Long-Term Mechanical Ventilation, *edited by N. S. Hill*
153. Environmental Asthma, *edited by R. K. Bush*
154. Asthma and Respiratory Infections, *edited by D. P. Skoner*
155. Airway Remodeling, *edited by P. H. Howarth, J. W. Wilson, J. Bousquet, S. Rak, and R. A. Pauwels*
156. Genetic Models in Cardiorespiratory Biology, *edited by G. G. Haddad and T. Xu*
157. Respiratory-Circulatory Interactions in Health and Disease, *edited by S. M. Scharf, M. R. Pinsky, and S. Magder*
158. Ventilator Management Strategies for Critical Care, *edited by N. S. Hill and M. M. Levy*
159. Severe Asthma: Pathogenesis and Clinical Management, Second Edition, Revised and Expanded, *edited by S. J. Szefler and D. Y. M. Leung*
160. Gravity and the Lung: Lessons from Microgravity, *edited by G. K. Prisk, M. Paiva, and J. B. West*
161. High Altitude: An Exploration of Human Adaptation, *edited by T. F. Hornbein and R. B. Schoene*
162. Drug Delivery to the Lung, *edited by H. Bisgaard, C. O'Callaghan, and G. C. Smaldone*
163. Inhaled Steroids in Asthma: Optimizing Effects in the Airways, *edited by R. P. Schleimer, P. M. O'Byrne, S. J. Szefler, and R. Brattsand*

164. IgE and Anti-IgE Therapy in Asthma and Allergic Disease, *edited by R. B. Fick, Jr., and P. M. Jardieu*
165. Clinical Management of Chronic Obstructive Pulmonary Disease, *edited by T. Similowski, W. A. Whitelaw, and J.-P. Derenne*
166. Sleep Apnea: Pathogenesis, Diagnosis, and Treatment, *edited by A. I. Pack*
167. Biotherapeutic Approaches to Asthma, *edited by J. Agosti and A. L. Sheffer*
168. Proteoglycans in Lung Disease, *edited by H. G. Garg, P. J. Roughley, and C. A. Hales*
169. Gene Therapy in Lung Disease, *edited by S. M. Albelda*
170. Disease Markers in Exhaled Breath, *edited by N. Marczin, S. A. Kharitonov, M. H. Yacoub, and P. J. Barnes*
171. Sleep-Related Breathing Disorders: Experimental Models and Therapeutic Potential, *edited by D. W. Carley and M. Radulovacki*
172. Chemokines in the Lung, *edited by R. M. Strieter, S. L. Kunkel, and T. J. Standiford*
173. Respiratory Control and Disorders in the Newborn, *edited by O. P. Mathew*
174. The Immunological Basis of Asthma, *edited by B. N. Lambrecht, H. C. Hoogsteden, and Z. Diamant*
175. Oxygen Sensing: Responses and Adaptation to Hypoxia, *edited by S. Lahiri, G. L. Semenza, and N. R. Prabhakar*
176. Non-Neoplastic Advanced Lung Disease, *edited by J. R. Maurer*
177. Therapeutic Targets in Airway Inflammation, *edited by N. T. Eissa and D. P. Huston*
178. Respiratory Infections in Allergy and Asthma, *edited by S. L. Johnston and N. G. Papadopoulos*
179. Acute Respiratory Distress Syndrome, *edited by M. A. Matthay*
180. Venous Thromboembolism, *edited by J. E. Dalen*
181. Upper and Lower Respiratory Disease, *edited by J. Corren, A. Togias, and J. Bousquet*
182. Pharmacotherapy in Chronic Obstructive Pulmonary Disease, *edited by B. R. Celli*
183. Acute Exacerbations of Chronic Obstructive Pulmonary Disease, *edited by N. M. Siafakas, N. R. Anthonisen, and D. Georgopoulos*
184. Lung Volume Reduction Surgery for Emphysema, *edited by H. E. Fessler, J. J. Reilly, Jr., and D. J. Sugarbaker*
185. Idiopathic Pulmonary Fibrosis, *edited by J. P. Lynch III*
186. Pleural Disease, *edited by D. Bouros*

187. Oxygen/Nitrogen Radicals: Lung Injury and Disease, *edited by V. Vallyathan, V. Castranova, and X. Shi*
188. Therapy for Mucus-Clearance Disorders, *edited by B. K. Rubin and C. P. van der Schans*
189. Interventional Pulmonary Medicine, *edited by J. F. Beamis, Jr., P. N. Mathur, and A. C. Mehta*
190. Lung Development and Regeneration, *edited by D. J. Massaro, G. Massaro, and P. Chambon*
191. Long-Term Intervention in Chronic Obstructive Pulmonary Disease, *edited by R. Pauwels, D. S. Postma, and S. T. Weiss*
192. Sleep Deprivation: Basic Science, Physiology, and Behavior, *edited by Clete A. Kushida*
193. Sleep Deprivation: Clinical Issues, Pharmacology, and Sleep Loss Effects, *edited by Clete A. Kushida*
194. Pneumocystis Pneumonia: Third Edition, Revised and Expanded, *edited by P. D. Walzer and M. Cushion*
195. Asthma Prevention, *edited by William W. Busse and Robert F. Lemanske, Jr.*
196. Lung Injury: Mechanisms, Pathophysiology, and Therapy, *edited by Robert H. Notter, Jacob N. Finkelstein, and Bruce A. Holm*
197. Ion Channels in the Pulmonary Vasculature, *edited by Jason X.-J. Yuan*

The opinions expressed in these volumes do not necessarily represent the views of the National Institutes of Health.

ION CHANNELS IN THE PULMONARY VASCULATURE

Edited by

Jason X.-J. Yuan

University of California, San Diego, California, U.S.A.

CRC Press
Taylor & Francis Group
Boca Raton London New York

CRC Press is an imprint of the
Taylor & Francis Group, an **informa** business

CRC Press
Taylor & Francis Group
6000 Broken Sound Parkway NW, Suite 300
Boca Raton, FL 33487-2742

© 2005 by Taylor & Francis Group, LLC
CRC Press is an imprint of Taylor & Francis Group, an Informa business

No claim to original U.S. Government works

This book contains information obtained from authentic and highly regarded sources. Reasonable efforts have been made to publish reliable data and information, but the author and publisher cannot assume responsibility for the validity of all materials or the consequences of their use. The authors and publishers have attempted to trace the copyright holders of all material reproduced in this publication and apologize to copyright holders if permission to publish in this form has not been obtained. If any copyright material has not been acknowledged please write and let us know so we may rectify in any future reprint.

Except as permitted under U.S. Copyright Law, no part of this book may be reprinted, reproduced, transmitted, or utilized in any form by any electronic, mechanical, or other means, now known or hereafter invented, including photocopying, microfilming, and recording, or in any information storage or retrieval system, without written permission from the publishers.

For permission to photocopy or use material electronically from this work, please access www.copyright.com (http://www.copyright.com/) or contact the Copyright Clearance Center, Inc. (CCC), 222 Rosewood Drive, Danvers, MA 01923, 978-750-8400. CCC is a not-for-profit organization that provides licenses and registration for a variety of users. For organizations that have been granted a photocopy license by the CCC, a separate system of payment has been arranged.

Trademark Notice: Product or corporate names may be trademarks or registered trademarks, and are used only for identification and explanation without intent to infringe.

Visit the Taylor & Francis Web site at
http://www.taylorandfrancis.com

and the CRC Press Web site at
http://www.crcpress.com

Introduction

Perhaps no field of modern biology has generated as much pioneering research work and scientific excitement as the biology of ion channels. About forty years ago it was recognized that ion channels are composed of proteins, or groups of proteins, embedded in the cell membrane. As well, it became clear that ion channels regulate transport of ions in and out of the cells.

Since, a significant amount of research has been conducted to uncover and purify ion channels and to determine their function and regulation. From this, the function of the cells themselves can be inferred and, as well, the function in health and disease of the organs where the cells are located.

For example, it is the movement of calcium into the cytoplasm through the calcium channel that triggers muscular contraction. Today, we know that nearly all cells are dependent on the actions of the ion channels to transfer ions needed by the cells for their various activities, or in some cases for the production of chemical energy (ATP). Knowledge of the normal function of ion channels will eventually lead to the development of compounds which can act on a specific disordered ion channel, or channels.

The pulmonary vasculature is an organ rich in ion channels which control and regulate vascular permeability and thus smooth muscle activity. This volume, titled *Ion Channels in the Pulmonary Vasculature*, edited by Dr. Jason X.-J. Yuan takes the reader through a unique and exciting journey. At the end, the reader will have an appreciation of what *may* cause dysfunction of the pulmonary vasculature leading, in turn, to vascular and lung tissue pathology.

Molecular biology which has flourished as a research tool during the last two decades is in full use by scientists studying ion channels. This volume opens the door to new research directions which should lead to even more novel therapeutic approaches.

When the series of monographs Lung Biology in Health and Disease was conceived, it was planned to bridge research with clinical needs and opportunities and ultimately to show how fundamental sciences can be translated to benefit patients. This monograph is a perfect paradigm of this concept. The pride that we have to present it to the readership is only equaled by the gratitude we have to the editor and to the extraordinary list of authors who contributed to this volume.

Claude Lenfant, MD
Gaithersburg, Maryland

Preface

The structure and function of the pulmonary vasculature are very different from those of the systemic (e.g., coronary, cerebral, renal, and mesenteric) vasculature. A typical example of functional differences between the pulmonary and systemic vasculatures is that hypoxia causes pulmonary vasoconstriction to maintain maximal oxygenation of the venous blood in the pulmonary artery, but causes systemic vasodilation to increase delivery of oxygen and nutrients to tissues and organs in need. The divergent vascular responses to hypoxia may relate to differential function and expression of ion channels in smooth muscle and endothelial cells of pulmonary and systemic arteries.

Electromechanical and pharmacomechanical coupling processes are two major excitation–contraction coupling mechanisms in pulmonary vascular smooth muscle. Electric excitability, which plays an important role in excitation–contraction coupling in the pulmonary vasculature, is mainly controlled by transmembrane ion flux in pulmonary artery smooth muscle cells. Indeed, many vasoactive substances regulate pulmonary vasomotor tone by altering membrane potential and ion (Na^+, K^+, Ca^{2+}, and Cl^-) channel activity in pulmonary vascular smooth muscle cells. Expression and functionality of ion channels in the plasma membrane not only regulate smooth muscle contractility, but also modulate cell motility, migration, proliferation, and apoptosis by governing cytoplasmic Ca^{2+} and K^+ concentrations. Furthermore, function and expression of ion channels in pulmonary vascular endothelial cells greatly contribute to the regulation of synthesis and secretion of endothelium-derived relaxing and constricting factors that play a pivotal role in pulmonary vasodilation and vasoconstriction. The ion channels in pulmonary vascular smooth muscle and endothelial cells are regulated not only by endogenous agonists (e.g., neurotransmitters, humoral vasoactive substances), but also by mitogens (e.g., growth factors, cytokines) to maintain normal pulmonary vascular function and structure. Defects in ion channel function and expression in the pulmonary vasculature are implicated in the development of pulmonary vascular diseases. Therefore, ion channels are also appropriate targets for developing novel therapeutic approaches for patients with pulmonary vascular diseases.

Over the last decade, considerable progress has been made in understanding the electrophysiological and pharmacological properties and molecular identity of ion channels in pulmonary vascular smooth muscle and endothelial cells, as well as the functional role of ion channels in the regulation of pulmonary vascular tone and remodeling. These significant findings provide a fundamental basis to specify the precise sequences of events involved in physiological regulation of pulmonary vascular function and structure, to identify the ion channels that play critical roles in the etiology and pathogenesis of pulmonary hypertension, and to develop new therapeutic approaches targeting on the ion channels for patients with pulmonary vascular diseases.

This book reviews the current knowledge on ion channels in the pulmonary vasculature and discusses the potential roles of ion channels in the pathogenesis and treatment of pulmonary vascular diseases. The book is divided into ten main sections. Chapters in each of the main sections address critical aspects (e.g., biophysical and pharmacological properties, molecular identification, pathogenic role) related to ion channels in the pulmonary vasculature under physiological and pathological conditions. *Section I: Cell Physiology* reviews the cellular mechanisms related to membrane potential, action potential, and excitation-contraction coupling in pulmonary vascular smooth muscle cells. The second section entitled *Ca^{2+}-Permeable Channels* is devoted to aspects of recent findings in the function and expression of three major plasmalemmal Ca^{2+} channels, voltage-dependent Ca^{2+} channels, receptor-operated Ca^{2+} channels, and store-operated Ca^{2+} channels, as well as the Ca^{2+} release channels in the intracellular organelles. *Section III: Na^+-Permeable Channels* highlights the functional role of the epithelial Na^+ channels in alveolar fluid absorption and discusses the electrophysiological properties, molecular identity and structure of voltage-gated Na^+ channels in pulmonary vascular smooth muscle cells. *Section IV: K^+-Permeable Channels* is designed to characterize the molecular identity and function of five classes of K^+ channels in pulmonary vascular smooth muscle and endothelial cells, voltage-gated K^+ channels, Ca^{2+}-activated K^+ channels, ATP-sensitive K^+ channels, inward rectifier K^+ channels, and tandem-pore and two transmembrane domain K^+ channels. The fifth section entitled *Cl^--Permeable Channels* highlights the recent findings of two important Cl^- channels, Ca^{2+}-activated Cl^-

channels and volume-sensitive Cl^- channels, along with their functions in regulating pulmonary vascular tone and cell volume control. The three chapters in *Section VI: O_2-Sensitive Ion Channels* discuss the molecular identification and electrophysiological characterization of the oxygen- or hypoxia-sensitive K^+ and Ca^{2+} channels, the transcriptional and functional regulation of these channels in pulmonary vascular smooth muscle and endothelial cells during hypoxia, and how ion channels in endothelial cells contribute to the regulation of smooth muscle contractility. A general description of structure, function, and regulation of the water channels, aquaporins, in the lung is given in *Section VII: Water Channels. Section VIII: Functional Roles of Cytoplasmic Ions and Ion Channels* emphasizes the roles of intracellular Ca^{2+} and K^+ ions as well as ion channel activity in the regulation of pulmonary vascular tone and vascular permeability, smooth muscle cell membrane potential, and programmed cell death. The next section (*Section IX: Role of Ion Channels in Pulmonary Vasculature Disease*) illustrates the pathogenic roles of ion channels (e.g., voltage-gated K^+ channels, two-pore domain K^+ channels, and transient receptor potential cation channels) in the development of pulmonary arterial hypertension. Finally, *Section X: Methodological Approaches* introduces the techniques commonly used for studying ion channel function and expression in the pulmonary vascular smooth muscle and endothelial cells, and provides practical instruction for the hands-on use of these techniques.

In summary, this book presents a global overview of the current state-of-the-art findings relevant to the normal function and molecular identity of ion channels expressed in the pulmonary vasculature, and the pathogenic role of ion channels in the regulation of pulmonary vascular tone and in pulmonary vascular remodeling processes associated with pulmonary vascular disease. The book provides a comprehensive review of the multiple families of ion channels that have been identified and characterized in pulmonary artery smooth muscle and endothelial cells from various species, as well as a useful and practical section outlining the different experimental tools available for studying ion channel physiology and molecular biology. A concerted effort has also been made to relate ion channel abnormalities to documented cases of pulmonary vascular disease. I sincerely hope that this book provides a timely and long-lasting guide for basic science investigators in the field of pulmonary vascular biology and electrophysiology, and for physician scientists whose research interest centers on vascular pathophysiology and pulmonary vascular diseases. I also hope that the book provides and lays down a research foundation for clinicians who are interested in translational research and subsequent applications in clinical practice.

The book could not have been completed without the support, encouragement, and love of my wife, Ayako Makino, Ph.D., to whom this book is dedicated. Compiling and organizing a book of this nature required tremendous time and effort of the contributors, publishers, colleagues, and assistants. I am especially grateful to Ms. Sandra Beberman and Dr. Claude Lenfant for their instruction and encouragement in compiling the volume, to Dr. Carmelle V. Remillard for her diligence in preparing the figures and revising the text, and to all the contributors for their patience and conscientiousness in preparing the manuscripts. Finally, I would like to take this opportunity to thank all my teachers, colleagues, and students from whom I continually learn.

Jason X.-J. Yuan

Contributors

Philip I. Aaronson Centre for Cardiovascular Biology and Medicine, King's College, London, U.K.

Abderrahmane Alioua Department of Anesthesiology, David Geffen School of Medicine at University of California Los Angeles, Los Angeles, California, U.S.A.

Stephen L. Archer University of Alberta, Edmonton, Alberta, Canada

Maninder Singh Bedi University of Pittsburgh, Pittsburgh, Pennsylvania, U.S.A.

Elena E. Brevnova Department of Medicine, University of California, San Diego, California, U.S.A.

Donna L. Cioffi University of South Alabama College of Medicine, Mobile, Alabama, U.S.A.

Lucie H. Clapp University College London, London, U.K.

Elizabeth A. Coppock Colorado State University, Fort Collins, Colorado, U.S.A.

David N. Cornfield University of Minnesota Medical School, Minneapolis, Minnesota, U.S.A.

Andrew R. L. Davies University of Bristol, Bristol, U.K.

Ian C. Davis University of Alabama at Birmingham, Birmingham, Alabama, U.S.A.

Steven M. Dudek Johns Hopkins University School of Medicine, Baltimore, Maryland, U.S.A.

Mansoureh Eghbali Department of Anesthesiology, David Geffen School of Medicine at University of California Los Angeles, Los Angeles, California, U.S.A.

Ivana Fantozzi Department of Medicine, University of California, San Diego, California, U.S.A.

Joe G. N. Garcia Johns Hopkins University School of Medicine, Baltimore, Maryland, U.S.A.

Jesus Garcia-Valdes Department of Anesthesiology, David Geffen School of Medicine at University of California Los Angeles, Los Angeles, California, U.S.A.

Iain A. Greenwood St. George's Hospital Medical School, London, U.K.

António Guia AVIVA Biosciences Corp., San Diego, California, U.S.A.

Christelle Guibert Institut National de la Santé et de la Recherche Médicale, and Université Victor Ségalen Bordeaux2, Bordeaux, France

Alison M. Gurney University of Strathclyde, Glasgow, Scotland, U.K.

Dayle S. Hogg University of Bristol, Bristol, U.K.

Eric Honoré Institut de Pharmacologie Moléculaire et Cellulaire, Sophia Antipolis, France

Yuji Imaizumi Nagoya City University, Nagoya, Japan

Luke J. Janssen Firestone Institute for Respiratory Health, St. Joseph's Hospital and McMaster University, Hamilton, Ontario, Canada

Steve H. Keller Department of Medicine, University of California, San Diego, California, U.S.A.

Landon S. King Johns Hopkins University School of Medicine, Baltimore, Maryland, U.S.A.

Kenji Kitamura Fukuoka Dental College, Seinan Jogakuin University, Fukuoka, Japan

Gregory A. Knock Centre for Cardiovascular Biology and Medicine, King's College, London, U.K.

Roland Z. Kozlowski University of Bristol, Bristol, U.K.

Hirosi Kuriyama Fukuoka Dental College, Seinan Jogakuin University, Fukuoka, Japan

William A. Large St. George's Hospital Medical School, London, U.K.

Normand Leblanc Center of Biomedical Research Excellence, University of Nevada School of Medicine, Reno, Nevada, U.S.A.

Mo-Jun Lin Johns Hopkins School of Medicine, Baltimore, Maryland, U.S.A.

Barry London University of Pittsburgh, Pittsburgh, Pennsylvania, U.S.A.

Rong Lu Department of Anesthesiology, David Geffen School of Medicine at University of California Los Angeles, Los Angeles, California, U.S.A.

Emi Maeno National Institute for Physiological Sciences, Okazaki, Japan

Mehran Mandegar Department of Medicine, University of California, San Diego, California, U.S.A.

Roger Marthan Institut National de la Santé et de la Recherche Médicale, and Université Victor Ségalen Bordeaux2, Bordeaux, France

Sadis Matalon University of Alabama at Birmingham, Birmingham, Alabama, U.S.A.

Sean McMurtry University of Alberta, Edmonton, Alberta, Canada

Bryan J. McVerry Johns Hopkins University School of Medicine, Baltimore, Maryland, U.S.A.

Dolly Mehta University of Illinois, Chicago, Illinois, U.S.A.

Evangelos D. Michelakis University of Alberta, Edmonton, Alberta, Canada

Shin-ichiro Mori National Institute for Physiological Sciences, Okazaki, Japan

Katsuhiko Muraki Nagoya City University, Nagoya, Japan

Takashi Nabekura National Institute for Physiological Sciences, Okazaki, Japan

Kazuhide Nishimaru[*] Department of Anesthesiology, David Geffen School of Medicine at University of California Los Angeles, Los Angeles, California, U.S.A.

Aaron Norris Colorado State University, Fort Collins, Colorado, U.S.A.

Kristen O'Connell Colorado State University, Fort Collins, Colorado, U.S.A.

Yasunobu Okada National Institute for Physiological Sciences, Okazaki, Japan

Bethany H. Parker Department of Medicine, University of California, San Diego, California, U.S.A.

Amanda J. Patel Institut de Pharmacologie Moléculaire et Cellulaire, Sophia Antipolis, France

Angela S. Piper St. George's Hospital Medical School, London, U.K.

Oleksandr Platoshyn Department of Medicine, University of California, San Diego, California, U.S.A.

Lawrence S. Prince University of Alabama at Birmingham, Birmingham, Alabama, U.S.A.

Carmelle V. Remillard Department of Medicine, University of California, San Diego, California, U.S.A.

Nancy J. Rusch Medical College of Wisconsin, Milwaukee, Wisconsin, U.S.A.

---

[*] *Current affiliation:* Department of Pharmacology, Yamagata University School of Medicine, Yamagata, Japan.

Amy Sanguinetti University of Nevada School of Medicine, Reno, Nevada, U.S.A.

Jean-Pierre Savineau Institut National de la Santé et de la Recherche Médicale, and Université Victor Ségalen Bordeaux2, Bordeaux, France

James S. K. Sham Johns Hopkins School of Medicine, Baltimore, Maryland, U.S.A.

Venkataramana Sidhaye Johns Hopkins University School of Medicine, Baltimore, Maryland, U.S.A.

Tiffany Sison University of California, San Diego, California, U.S.A.

Vladimir A. Snetkov Guy's King's and St. Thomas' School of Medicine, King's College, London, U.K.

Christopher Ian Spencer Johns Hopkins School of Medicine, Baltimore, Maryland, U.S.A.

Enrico Stefani Departments of Anesthesiology and Physiology, Brain Research Institute, David Geffen School of Medicine at University of California Los Angeles, Los Angeles, California, U.S.A.

Troy Stevens University of South Alabama College of Medicine, Mobile, Alabama, U.S.A.

Michael M. Tamkun Colorado State University, Fort Collins, Colorado, U.S.A.

Brian P. Tennant University College London, London, U.K.

Donna D. Tigno Department of Medicine, University of California, San Diego, California, U.S.A.

Ligia Toro Departments of Anesthesiology and Molecular & Medical Pharmacology, Brain Research Institute, David Geffen School of Medicine at University of California Los Angeles, Los Angeles, California, U.S.A.

Anita Umesh Johns Hopkins School of Medicine, Baltimore, Maryland, U.S.A.

Jeremy P. T. Ward Guy's King's and St. Thomas' School of Medicine, King's College, London, U.K.

Sean M. Wilson School of Pharmacy, Research Institute of Pharmaceutical Sciences (RIPS), University, Mississippi, U.S.A.

Songwei Wu University of South Alabama College of Medicine, Mobile, Alabama, U.S.A.

Jia Xu AVIVA Biosciences Corp., San Diego, California, U.S.A.

Xiao-Ru Yang Johns Hopkins School of Medicine, Baltimore, Maryland, U.S.A.

Ying Yu Department of Medicine, University of California, San Diego, California, U.S.A.

Jason X.-J. Yuan Department of Medicine, University of California, San Diego, California, U.S.A.

Masoud M. Zarei Center for Biomedical Studies, UTB/TSC, Brownsville, Texas, U.S.A.

Shen Zhang University of California, San Diego, California, U.S.A.

Contents

1

Membrane Electrical Properties of Vascular Smooth Muscle Cells of the Pulmonary Circulation

Sean M. Wilson
School of Pharmacy, Research Institute of Pharmaceutical Sciences (RIPS), University, Mississippi, U.S.A.

Normand Leblanc
Center of Biomedical Research Excellence, University of Nevada School of Medicine, Reno, Nevada, U.S.A.

I. INTRODUCTION

The pulmonary vasculature is a low-pressure, high-capacitance vascular bed that uniquely reacts to changes in O_2 tension in the perfusate. Unlike systemic arteries, which generally dilate in response to reduced Po_2, pulmonary arterial vessels constrict when the oxygen tension falls below a threshold of ~55 mmHg (1). The so-called hypoxic pulmonary vasoconstriction (HPV) has an absolute requirement for Ca^{2+} mobilization from the extracellular space and involves membrane depolarization of the pulmonary arterial smooth muscle cells. Until recently, our understanding of the ionic mechanisms acting not only in HPV but also in chronic hypoxia-induced alterations in pulmonary vasomotor tone and in primary and secondary forms of pulmonary hypertension was very limited.

During the past two decades, dispersion techniques were developed to isolate healthy pulmonary vascular smooth muscle cells from which membrane electrical properties could be studied at an unprecedented resolution with the patch clamp technique. In parallel, a panoply of molecular biological techniques were developed that permitted the identification, expression, and manipulation of genes encoding for distinct classes of ion channel proteins, transporters and, more recently, scaffolding proteins. Cell biological methods, in particular imaging techniques employing confocal microscopy and immunocytochemistry, provided more direct visualization of the spatial arrangement of membrane signaling proteins and how they regulate the function of smooth muscle cells.

This chapter reviews some of the biophysical principles that underlie the generation of transmembrane potentials in cells with emphasis on the electrical properties of pulmonary vascular myocytes. Section II first discusses the existence of ionic gradients across the cell membrane, particularly those of Na^+, K^+, and Cl^-, and then illustrates how they are maintained by ion transport systems. Section II. C introduces the notion of electrodiffusion at equilibrium and presents the Nernst and Goldman equations. Sections III and IV deal specifically with the electrical properties of pulmonary vascular smooth muscle cells studied at the multicellular level by intracellular recording techniques and at the single-cell level with the patch clamp technique. These two sections discuss in sequence the ionic basis of the resting membrane potential (E_m) of these cells, with special emphasis on the role of K^+ channels, and their excitability when activated by various stimuli.

II. ION DISTRIBUTION, PASSIVE ION FLUXES, AND IONIC EQUILIBRIA

A. Distribution of Na^+, K^+, and Cl^-

As in all other excitable cells, the generation of transmembrane potentials in smooth muscle cells, with the inside of the membrane exhibiting a negative potential relative to the outside or interstitial space, results from an asymmetrical distribution of ions across the membrane and the relative permeability of the membrane to different ions. Ionic gradients are maintained by active ion transporters (e.g., Na^+-K^+ pump, Ca^{2+}-ATPase), ion exchangers (e.g., Na^+-Ca^{2+} exchanger, HCO_3^-/Cl^- exchanger), or cotransporters (e.g., Na^+-K^+-Cl^- co-transporter). The establishment of such gradients allows for storage of potential wells that can be used as an excitatory mechanism to accomplish a specific function (contraction, secretion, adhesion, etc.) when the cell is stimulated. In this chapter we will limit our discussion to the cellular distribution of Na^+, K^+, and Cl^-, which have all been implicated in the excitability of pulmonary arterial smooth muscle cells. The distribution and role of Ca^{2+} as a second messenger is discussed at length in Chapter 2.

Few studies have determined the concentration of Na^+ and K^+ in pulmonary vascular myocytes, and information regarding the distribution of these ions arises mainly from investigations carried out in other smooth muscle cells. Spectrophotometric or radiolabeled isotope flux measurements in multicellular preparations all demonstrated that smooth muscle cells actively maintain an elevated K^+ concentration and a much lower Na^+ concentration in their cytoplasm, relative to the extracellular space. Maintenance of these asymmetrical gradients is primarily attributed to the activity of the ouabain-sensitive Na^+-K^+ pump, which extrudes 3 Na^+ out of the cell and carries 2 K^+ into the cell per cycle. Although these techniques consistently revealed, as in other cell types, the existence of asymmetrical gradients, the range of values for both internal Na^+ and K^+ concentrations varied considerably from study to study. Table 1 summarizes measurements of intracellular electrolyte concentrations obtained from vascular and nonvascular smooth muscles based on different techniques. Intracellular Na^+ ($[Na^+]_i$) and K^+ ($[K^+]_i$) concentrations ranged from 7.4 to 70 mM and from 88 to 165 mM, respectively. In rabbit pulmonary arteries, Casteels et al. (2) estimated $[Na^+]_i$ and $[K^+]_i$ to be 15 and 134 mM, respectively. A major problem associated with spectrophotometric and isotope flux studies is that

Table 1 Intracellular Electrolyte Concentrations Determined by Various Methods in Different Types of Smooth Muscles

Species	Smooth muscle type	$[Na^+]_i$ (mmol/L)	$[K^+]_i$ (mmol/L)	$[Cl^-]_i$ (mmol/L)	Method[a]	Ref.
	Nonvascular					
Guinea pig	Tenia coli	35	100	55	A	3
	Tenia coli	31	165	71	A	3
	Tenia coli	19	164	55	A	14
	Vas deferens	28	158	57	A	14
	Vas deferens			42	B	5
	Ureter	7.4			B	67
	Ureter	7–12			C	68
	Vascular					
Rat	Portal vein	45	138	86	A	3
	Aorta	74	110		A	69
	A7r5 cultures smooth muscle cells	4.4			C	70
	Mesenteric artery	11			A	71
Dog	Carotid artery	68	88	70	A	72
	aorta	70	129	54	A	73
Rabbit	Pulmonary artery	15	134	51	A	2

[a]Method of determination: A, Atomic absorption spectrophotometry and/or flux measurements using radioisotopes; B, use of ion-selective microelectrodes; C, use of ion-sensitive fluorescent indicator SFBI.

they rely on the accurate determination of the extracellular space (~35 mL/100 g_{ww}) (3) using an inert nonpermeable radiolabeled marker such as ^{14}C-inulin or ^{14}C-sorbitol and several assumptions about the number of compartments in which the ions are distributed. These techniques also cannot discriminate between bound and free ions. Early studies confirmed that K^+ displays an activity coefficient similar to that measured in the extracellular space (~0.75) (3). In contrast, a large fraction of intracellular Na^+ was considered to be bound and therefore non-ionized. Later estimates of $[Na^+]_i$ using Na^+-sensitive microelectrodes or the fluorescent Na^+ indicator SFBI, both of which sense free ionized ion concentration or activity, yielded a range of $[Na^+]_i$ that was much lower (4.4–12 mM) than that indicated by less sophisticated techniques (11–74 mM) (see Table 1).

Table 1 shows estimates of intracellular Cl^- concentration that were fairly similar in different types of smooth muscles, ranging from 42 to 86 mM, a concentration range generally higher than that measured in skeletal muscle cells (3) and that appeared to deviate from a purely passive distribution of internal Cl^- (4). Measurement of Cl^- activity in guinea pig ureter smooth muscle (~42 mM) with the aid of Cl^--sensitive microelectrodes confirmed that smooth muscle cells exhibit high internal Cl^- concentration, conferring an equilibrium for Cl^- ions that is more positive (~−24 mV) than the resting membrane potential of these cells (~−65 mV) (5). Moreover, the same study reported very good agreement between intracellular Cl^- measurements carried out using three distinct methods and suggested that the activity coefficient of Cl^- in the cytoplasm is similar to that in the extracellular space. Chlorine-36 efflux rate measurements in the rabbit pulmonary artery yielded similar estimates for intracellular Cl^- concentration (51mM) and equilibrium potential for Cl^- ($E_{Cl} = -26$ mV) (2). Later experiments confirmed that Cl^- is actively accumulated in smooth muscle cells by means of the Na, K, 2Cl cotransporter, Cl:HCO_3 exchanger, and a mechanism termed "pump III" (6).

B. Passive Ion Fluxes

Numerous earlier studies in multicellular smooth muscle preparations showed that these muscle cells display a unique resting permeability to ions. Ion flux rate measurements with radioisotopes under conditions in which ions were replaced in the extracellular solution allowed for absolute and relative unidirectional ion fluxes to be determined with the numerous caveats associated with this technique, including (1) uncertainty about the number of compartments in which the ion is distributed, (2) uncertainty about the membrane surfaces involved, and (3) the possibility that ion replacements might influence membrane permeability (7). Also, few studies have determined both passive influx and efflux rates for any given ion. Estimates of absolute and relative permeabilities thus rely on a number of assumptions. In spite of these limitations, these studies unequivocally showed that the permeability of the smooth muscle membrane to Na^+ (P_{Na}) and Cl^- (P_{Cl}) relative to K^+ (P_K) is elevated in comparison to that measured in nerve cells. In guineapig tenia coli, P_{Na}/P_K and P_{Cl}/P_K were respectively 0.16 and 0.61 (7) with absolute membrane permeabilities to Na^+, K^+, and Cl^- of 1.8×10^{-8}, 11×10^{-8}, and 6.7×10^{-8} cm/s, respectively. Consistent with the above study, Ohashi (8) determined the value $P_{Cl}/P_K = 0.4$ in the same preparation. Very similar determinations were made by Casteels et al. (2) in the rabbit pulmonary artery: P_{Na}/P_K and P_{Cl}/P_K of 0.22 and 0.63, respectively. As will be discussed in the next section, the high resting permeabilities to Na^+ and Cl^- relative to K^+ largely explains why the resting membrane potential of vascular smooth muscle cells is significantly less negative (~−40 to −60 mV) than the predicted equilibrium for K^+ ($E_K < -80$ mV).

C. Ionic Equilibria, Electrodiffusion, and Resting Membrane Potential

It is not within the scope of this chapter to elaborate in great detail about the fundamental biophysical principles associated with the generation of transmembrane potentials in cells. The interested reader is invited to consult more advanced textbooks on this topic (9,10). The following discussion provides background information to allow for a better understanding of specific aspects related to the development of the resting membrane potential of smooth muscle cells from pulmonary blood vessels. The foregoing sections have highlighted the asymmetrical distribution of ions across the cell membrane of smooth muscle cells including those of pulmonary arteries and the fact that the membrane displays some permeability at rest to Na^+, K^+, and Cl^-. Before the respective contributions of these ions to E_m can be considered, we must first understand their predicted equilibrium potential. This can be calculated using the Nernst equation,

$$E_{ion} = \frac{RT}{zF} \log \frac{[X]_o}{[X]_i}$$

where E_{ion} is the equilibrium potential of the ion X, R is the gas constant, T the temperature in Kelvin, z the valence of the ion, F the Faraday constant, and $[X]_o$ and $[X]_i$ the concentrations of the ion X in the extracellular space and cytoplasm, respectively. At 37°C, RT/zF is a constant that has a value of 60.8 mV, and E_{ion} depends only on the concentration gradient of the ion across the membrane. Because ions carry a net fixed charge in solution, any net flux across a membrane by simple diffusion will generate a transmembrane potential, which in turn influences the rate of diffusion of the ion by electrostatic interactions. This so-called electrodiffusion potential (E_{Diff}) is the basis for the development of membrane potential in cells. The equilibrium potential determines the value of the membrane potential at which no net flux of ions occurs. Of course, this equation assumes that the membrane must be permeable to a given ion for this ion to generate a transmembrane potential.

Figure 1 illustrates such concepts by using data reported by Casteels et al. (2) gathered from rabbit pulmonary arterial smooth muscle on the basis of ion flux measurements and electrophysiological recordings with microelectrodes. The resulting membrane potential was measured to be −57 mV by these authors, which is very similar to those reported in small (−51.5 mV) and large (−52.2 mV) rat pulmonary arteries (11) and small cat pulmonary arteries (−51 mV) at a Po_2 of 400 torr (12). In Fig. 1, the length and direction of the straight and wavy arrows, respectively, indicate the chemical forces (diffusion down their gradient) and electrical forces (due to charges) that act upon each ion. The arrow thickness is indicative of relative ion permeabilities across the membrane. As in other cell types, both

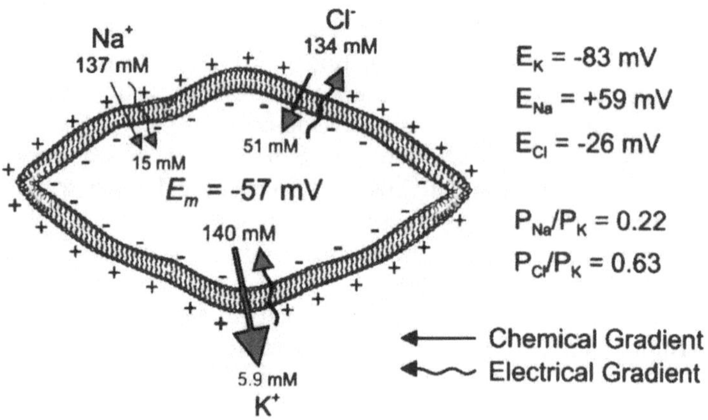

Figure 1 Schematic illustration of the transmembrane gradients of Na^+, K^+, and Cl^-, and the electrochemical forces acting upon these ions in the generation of the resting membrane potential of a pulmonary arterial smooth muscle cell. All values were derived from the study carried out in intact rabbit pulmonary arteries by Casteels et al. (2). As explained in the text, the length and direction of the arrows are representative of the relative inwardly vs. outwardly directed chemical (straight) or electrical (wavy) forces acting upon the ion. Arrow thickness is meant to illustrate the relative permeability of the membrane to the three ions. E_m is the resting membrane potential measured with microelectrodes; E_{Na}, E_K, and E_{Cl} are the calculated equilibrium potentials for Na^+, K^+ and Cl^-, respectively; P_{Na}/P_K and P_{Cl}/P_K reflect the permeability of the membrane to Na^+ and Cl^-, respectively, relative to K^+.

chemical and electrical forces promote net influx of Na^+. High K^+ permeability leads to net K^+ loss due to the predominance of the chemical gradient over the smaller electrostatic attraction favoring K^+ influx. Finally, net loss of Cl^- occurs at the resting membrane potential (RMP) due to a dominating electrical repulsion of the negative charge of this anion over its inwardly directed chemical gradient. In this particular example, if the membrane were solely permeable to K^+, E_m should be similar to E_K and would have a value more negative than $-80\,mV$. Because the measured E_m is $\sim 25\,mV$ more positive than E_K, other ionic conductances must contribute to the membrane potential at rest. In agreement with the contribution of other ions to the membrane potential is the deviation of the slope of the RMP vs. log $[K^+]_o$ relationship from a purely Nernstian behavior for K^+ ($\sim 61\,mV$/decade change in $[K^+]_o$): Suzuki and Twarog (11) measured a slope of 48 mV/decade change in $[K^+]_o$ in rat main pulmonary artery. As mentioned in the previous section, ion flux studies revealed a significant resting permeability to Na^+ and Cl^-. Figure 1 shows that the calculated E_{Na} and E_{Cl} are both more positive than E_m, which would make them candidate ions to participate in the generation of a transmembrane potential at rest. Consistent with a significant membrane permeability of Na^+ and Cl^- relative to K^+ measured in ion flux studies in smooth muscle, external Na^+ removal led to significant hyperpolarization of E_m in rabbit pulmonary arterial smooth muscle (2) and reduction of external Cl^- concentration hyperpolarized guineapig ureter (5) and guineapig tenia coli (13) smooth muscle. Quantitative analysis of the contribution of these three ions to the resting membrane potential (E_m) can be done using the constant-field Goldman equation,

$$E_m = \frac{RT}{zF}\log\frac{p_K[K]_o + P_{Na}[Na]_o + P_{Cl}[Cl]_i}{P_K[K]_i + P_{Na}[Na]_i + P_{Cl}[Cl]_o}$$

where P_K, P_{Na}, and P_{Cl} are the absolute membrane permeabilities to K^+, Na^+, and Cl^- in centimeters per second and $[X]_o$ and $[X]_i$ are the extracellular and intracellular concentrations of each ion in millimoles per liter. Unfortunately, and as briefly alluded to above, accurate determination of the absolute permeability of the membrane to a given ion-based flux measurement is very difficult and subject to cautious interpretation. A more useful variant of the Goldman equation described above is to express membrane potential as a function of the relative permeabilities. However, such a transformation of the equation becomes useful only when one of the ions is passively distributed or when the contribution of one of these ions is minimized by ion replacement with a nonpermeant ion. In smooth muscle, the latter strategy has to be followed because the three ions are not passively distributed and produce a significant flux at rest that contributes to E_m. Under conditions in which Cl^- is replaced by a less permeant anion such as isethionate or glutamate, the Goldman equation can be rearranged as

$$E_m = \frac{RT}{zF}\log\frac{[K]_o + (P_{Na}/P_K)[Na]_o}{[K]_i + (P_{Na}/P_K)[Na]_i}$$

Measurements of membrane potential in conditions of varied $[Na]_o$ and $[K]_o$ can provide an estimate of P_{Na}/P_K. In multicellular smooth muscle preparations, a valid estimation of relative permeabilities of the membrane using this approach relies on a number of assumptions: (1) Ion replacement of Na^+, K^+, or Cl^- with less permeant ions in the bathing medium does not influence P_{Na}, P_K, and/or P_{Cl}; (2) intracellular ion concentrations remain constant; and (3) there is no contribution from an electrogenic ion carrier system. In tenia coli, P_{Cl} is enhanced in $[K^+]_o$-free solution, whereas P_K is reduced by external replacement of Cl^- with nonpermeant anions (14) There is clear evidence for rapid shifts in intracellular Na^+ and Cl^- concentrations when the concentration of either one of these ions is diminished in the bathing medium (5,15). Finally, the active transport of Na^+ and K^+ by the Na^+-K^+-ATPase is electrogenic in smooth muscle cells. As in other cell types, the pump extrudes 3 Na^+ and accumulates 2 K^+ per cycle and thus leads to the extrusion of one net positive charge per cycle, which hyperpolarizes the cell. The Na^+-K^+ pump was shown to directly participate in determining E_m by as much as -10 to -20 mV in various cell types (3). In the rabbit pulmonary artery, blocking the pump by exposure to $[K]_o$-free solution or by the specific pump inhibitor ouabain depolarized the preparation by $\sim$8 mV (2), in agreement with the contribution of electrogenic Na^+ pumping to E_m. Consistent with the existence of such a transporter in vascular smooth muscle cells, Nakamura et al. (16) measured a ouabain-sensitive pump current of 1.2 pA/pF at +40 mV in whole-cell voltage-clamped guineapig mesenteric arterial smooth muscle cells dialyzed with 50 mM Na^+ and exposed to 10 mM $[K^+]_o$; under current-clamp conditions, the same group reported a 5 mV depolarization in response to 10 μM ouabain, suggesting a significant contribution of a pump potential (E_p) to E_m in these cells. Thus the equation of the resting membrane potential has to be modified to include a term accounting for the contribution of an Na^+-K^+ pump potential:

$$E_m = E_{Diff} + E_p$$

where E_p can be defined as

$$E_p = R_m i_p$$

where R_m is the membrane resistance in ohms per square centimeter and i_p is the current generated by the pump in microampere per square centimeter. The implication of such a contribution of the pump to E_m is that E_{Diff} has a more positive value than E_m, giving further support to the concept of high resting P_{Na} and P_{Cl} in smooth muscle cells, both of which display equilibrium potentials that are more positive than E_K (Table 1). In comparison to other excitable cells such as cardiac and skeletal muscle cells, and neurons, vascular smooth muscle cells exhibit a high R_m, which favors a larger contribution of E_p to E_m. Evaluation of the resting passive properties of multicellular (2,11) and single-cell (17) preparations of pulmonary arterial smooth muscle revealed strong outwardly rectifying properties. Consistent with the strong rectification of the membrane at rest, the input resistance (R_{inp}) measured from freshly dissociated pulmonary arterial myocytes from rabbit (18,19), rat (20), and human (21) ranged from 2 to 18 GΩ. This suggests that only a few ion channels are open at or near the resting membrane potential of these cells. This high R_m plus an Na^+-K^+ pump current density (16) that is of similar magnitude to that measured in cardiac muscle cells (22) are favorable conditions for a significant contribution of the Na^+-K^+ pump to E_m in nonstimulated myocytes. However, membrane depolarization triggered by constricting agonists, hypoxia, or other stimuli would tend to offset E_p due to marked reduction of R_m caused by the opening of numerous voltage-gated ion channels, yielding a resting membrane potential that is closer to E_{Diff}.

III. ION CHANNELS CONTRIBUTING TO THE RESTING MEMBRANE POTENTIAL OF PULMONARY ARTERY MYOCYTES

A. Role of K^+ Channels

The advent of cell isolation, patch clamp, and molecular biological techniques has allowed researchers to circumvent many of the major difficulties associated with the determination of ion permeabilities in multicellular preparations. These techniques have permitted the identification at the cellular and molecular levels of the transmembrane ion channel pores that are responsible for the ion fluxes measured with radioisotopes and other methods. Cell dialysis during whole-cell patch-clamp experiments, either under current-clamp mode to record membrane potential or under voltage-clamp conditions to record transmembrane macroscopic currents, allows for the precise control of the ionic composition of the intracellular milieu and the equilibrium potential of each of the ions of interest. Current-clamp experiments carried out in pulmonary arterial smooth muscle cells from various species yielded values of E_m that were similar to those determined in multicellular preparations using microelectrodes; Table 2 shows that E_m in pulmonary artery myocytes ranged from −38 to −58 mV. In spite of the high level of sophistication and accuracy of these techniques, it has been quite difficult to identify the channels responsible for determining the resting membrane potential of smooth muscle cells dispersed enzymatically from pulmonary vessels. Assessments of the contribution of the very small

Table 2 Passive Electrical Properties of Single Pulmonary Arterial Smooth Muscles Studied with the Patch-Clamp Technique in the Current-Clamp Whole-Cell Recording Mode[a]

Species	E_m (mV)	R_{inp} (GΩ)	C_m (pF)	Ref
Rat				
Freshly isolated cells	−38		~8–25	17
Freshly isolated cells	−54	5		20
Freshly isolated cells	−38			31
Freshly isolated cells	−54			40
Cultured cells	−41			26
Rabbit				
Freshly isolated cells with 1mM ATP	−55	17		18
Freshly isolated cells		18		19
Dog				
Freshly isolated cells	−58			
Human				
Cultured cells	−55	2.13	36.3	21

[a] E_m, resting membrane potential; R_{inp}, input resistance; C_m, cell capacitance.

currents measured around the RMP have often required the design of indirect strategies. This is because in some cases pharmacological tools are lacking and in others intracellular dialysis has resulted in current run down. For example, the biophysical and pharmacological characteristics of currents measured at positive potentials have often been extrapolated to the physiological range of membrane potentials. This can sometimes be misleading, because the action of many ion channel blockers is voltage-dependent (e.g., the block of delayed rectifier K^+ channels by 4-aminopyridine). Another strategy has been to use high extracellular $[K^+]_o$ to increase the driving force for K^+ within the physiological range of membrane potentials and thus allow the recording of measurable currents. One caveat of using this approach is that extracellular K^+ may directly influence gating of K^+ channels, which could result also in misinterpretation of the contribution of the K^+ channel under study.

Patch-clamp studies carried out in the 1990s identified four major classes of K^+ channels in vascular smooth muscle cells [for a review, consult Nelson and Quayle (23)]: (1) voltage-dependent K^+ channels (K_V), which can be subdivided into two classes: delayed rectifier (K_{dr}) and transient outward (*A*-like; I_{to}) K^+ channels; (2) large conductance Ca^{2+}-dependent K^+ channels (K_{Ca} or BK_{Ca}), which are both voltage-gated and activated by an elevation in intracellular Ca^{2+} concentration; (3) ATP-sensitive K^+ channels (K_{ATP}); and (4) inwardly rectifying K^+ channels (K_{ir}). In contrast to coronary and cerebral arterial smooth muscle cells, studies have generally failed to unequivocally identify Ba^{2+}-sensitive K_{ir} in pulmonary myocytes. Consistent with the possible lack of these channels or their minimal role in determining E_m in these cells, an increase in $[K]_o$ from 5 to 15 mM depolarized and contracted pulmonary arterial smooth muscle (11,24), an effect opposite the expected membrane hyperpolarization and vasorelaxation caused by K^+-induced activation of K_{ir} channels (23). Nevertheless, Chapter 13 provides a clearer view of the existence and role of these channels in the pulmonary vasculature. Although 4-AP-sensitive *A-like* transient outward K^+ currents have been described in pulmonary myocytes, it is thought that these channels would contribute little to resting E_m because their threshold for activation is more positive than E_m and they would be largely inactivated at the resting potential (25). K^+ channels that are modulated by intracellular ATP and nucleotide diphosphates have been described in pulmonary artery smooth muscle cells. However, it is thought that these channels play, at best, a minor role in generating E_m in "nonstimulated" cells, because the sulfonylurea compound glibenclamide (10 μM), a relatively specific inhibitor of K_{ATP}, did not affect E_m in rabbit (18) and rat (26) pulmonary myocytes dialyzed with a physiological concentration of ATP (3–5 mM) but significantly depolarized rabbit myocytes that had been hyperpolarized by the K_{ATP} channel agonist levcromakalim (27) or by cell dialysis with ATP-free pipette solution (18). Thus in the pulmonary vasculature, K_{ATP} channels appear to play a modulatory function under conditions of metabolic inhibition such as hypoxia (28) and hypertension (29).

Many studies have provided evidence for the expression of BK_{Ca} channels in the pulmonary vasculature. However, there is little evidence for an important role of these channels in determining E_m in resting nonstimulated adult myocytes when $[Ca^{2+}]_i$ is low (<150 nM). Indeed, low concentrations of tetraethylammonium chloride (TEA) (1–5 mM), which offer reasonable selectivity for inhibiting BK_{Ca} channels in vascular smooth muscle cells (23), or charybdotoxin (10–200 nM), a specific venom toxin inhibitor of these channels, did not influence E_m, $[Ca^{2+}]_i$, and/or tone in pulmonary myocytes or intact arteries (21,26,30,31). Consistent with these observations, BK_{Ca} channel inhibitors attenuated the noisy outward K^+ current at potentials more positive than ~−10 mV. There is also scarce evidence for a role of Ca^{2+} sparks in regulating the activity of BK_{Ca} channels in pulmonary myocytes. Spontaneous transient outward currents (STOCs) that result from the opening of clusters of BK_{Ca} channels by subsarcolemmal Ca^{2+} sparks [for a review, consult Jagger et al. (32)] were infrequently detected in rabbit (25) and rat (33) pulmonary myocytes, and only at positive potentials in rabbit myocytes (25) (see Chapter 24). Moreover, activation of Ca^{2+} sparks by caffeine led to membrane depolarization rather than hyperpolarization of rat myocytes as would be expected from the activation of BK_{Ca} channels (33). Although these channels appear to play a minor role, at best, in nonstimulated myocytes, they clearly serve an important role as a negative feedback mechanism to counteract the depolarizing action of constricting hormones that elevate $[Ca^{2+}]_i$. Endothelin-1 was shown to stimulate BK_{Ca} channels in rat pulmonary myocytes (34). Charybdotoxin potentiated the Ca^{2+} transient mediated by membrane depolarization induced by 4-AP, which specifically inhibits K_V (26). BK_{Ca} channels are also targeted by endothelium-derived nitric oxide (NO), which hyperpolarizes pulmonary arterial smooth muscle cells by a phosphorylation mechanism involving cGMP-dependent protein kinase (17,35), although a direct effect of NO on the channels themselves (36) cannot be excluded.

Convincing evidence from several laboratories has highlighted an important role for delayed rectifier K^+ channels in setting E_m in pulmonary arterial smooth muscle cells. As in other smooth muscle cell types, K_V channels in pulmonary artery smooth muscle cells are activated by membrane depolarization more positive than −50 mV, display relatively rapid activation and slow inactivation kinetics, and are sensitive to block by 4-AP (17,20,21,26,31,37,38). Current-clamp experiments have provided evidence that K_V channels represent the major K^+ conductance responsible for maintaining E_m. 4-Aminopyridine depolarizes pulmonary arterial myocytes (17,20,21,26,31,38), elevates the intracellular Ca^{2+} concentration that is in part sensitive to L-type Ca^{2+} channel blockade (26), and increases pulmonary arterial tone (26,30,39). Inhibition of K_V channels has been proposed to be responsible for the membrane depolarization associated with acute hypoxia (17,38,40) and suggested to play a major role in HPV (17,40), chronic hypoxia (20,39), and primary pulmonary hypertension (41,42). K_V channels are preferentially (relative to BK_{Ca} channels) expressed in cells from small pulmonary arteries, which are thought to be the main pulmonary arterial segment responsible for HPV (17). Developmental changes in the expression of these K^+ channels reveal a maturational shift from BK_{Ca} channels in the fetus toward K_V channels in the neonate, an observation that correlates well with the ability of the mature pulmonary vasculature to respond to a decrease in oxygen tension (43). Pulmonary myocytes express many members of the nine families of mammalian genes encoding for pore-forming α subunits of voltage-dependent K^+ channels, including Kv1.1, Kv1.2, Kv1.3, Kv1.4, Kv1.5, Kv1.6, Kv2.1, and Kv9.3 (40,44–47), and at least three ancillary β subunits (Kvβ1.1, Kvβ2, and Kvβ3) (46). On the basis of the biophysical and pharmacological characteristics of the K_v α subunits expressed in heterologous expression systems, investigators focused their attention on a few of these subunits and provided evidence that the basal K^+ conductance in pulmonary myocytes may result from homotetramers or heterotetramers formed by Kv1.2 and/or Kv1.5 and either Kv2.1 alone or coassembled with the electrically silent subunit Kv9.3 (40,45,46). Consistent with these suggestions, heterotetramers formed by cloned Kv1.2/Kv1.5 (47) and Kv2.1/Kv9.3 (40) were inhibited by acute hypoxia and were thus proposed to serve as O_2 sensors in HPV. Kv1.2 and Kv1.5 were both shown to be downregulated at both the mRNA and protein levels after chronic hypoxia (48), observations that correlated well with the associated membrane depolarization and elevated $[Ca^{2+}]_i$. Patients suffering from primary pulmonary hypertension exhibit reduced K_V current that is correlated with down regulation of Kv1.5 (42). The in vivo transfer of the Kv1.5 gene alleviated pulmonary hypertension, restored HPV in chronically hypoxemic rats, and O_2-sensitive K_V currents in pulmonary arterial myocytes (49).

Although much evidence pointed in the direction of K_V channels, one argument against the K_v channel hypothesis in setting E_m is that the channels suspected of participating in generating the resting potential activate at potentials more positive (~−40 mV) than E_m measured in pulmonary arterial smooth muscle cells (~−50 mV) (Table 2). Evans et al. (19) offered a novel perspective by providing evidence in favor of a sustained noninactivating voltage-dependent K^+ current called $I_{K(N)}$ that is active within the physiological range of membrane potentials and, like K_V channels, is also sensitive to block by 4-AP but at a concentration that is ~10-fold higher ($IC_{50} \approx 10$ mM). $I_{K(N)}$ activates very slowly with time ($\tau = 1.6$ s at −60 mV), and the threshold for activation was found to lie between −80 and −65 mV. Later experiments from the same group suggested that $I_{K(N)}$ is inhibited by hypoxia (50), is downregulated after chronic hypoxia (39), and is also the subject of maturational changes (51). More recently, Gurney et al. (52) reported the existence of TASK-1, a two-pore-domain K^+ channel, in rabbit pulmonary myocytes and showed that $I_{K(N)}$ shared many properties with those of TASK-1 expressed in mammalian cell lines: (1) sensitivity to extracellular pH; (2) low sensitivity to 4-AP; (3) block by Zn^{2+}; (4) stimulation in response to the volatile anesthetic halothane; and (5) block by the endocannabimoid anandamide. One caveat to this proposal is that $I_{K(N)}$ is voltage-activated (19) whereas TASK-1 lacks the voltage sensor present in the fourth transmembrane domain of all K_V channels. Whether TASK-1 is one component of the O_2-sensitive K^+ channel playing a role in HPV remains to be determined.

B. Is There Evidence for Na^+ and Cl^- Channels Open at Rest?

Because measured E_m is more positive than E_K by ~30 mV in pulmonary arterial smooth muscle cells, other ions must be participating in the electrodiffusion component of E_m. Ion concentration and flux measurements and electrophysiological experiments in intact pulmonary arterial smooth muscle showed that the membrane of these cells displays a significant permeability to both Na^+ and Cl^- at rest. Unfortunately, there is much work left to be done in this area before an accurate picture can be drawn. Tetrodotoxin (TTX)- and voltage-dependent Na^+ currents have been recorded from freshly isolated and cultured pulmonary myocytes (53,54). However, it is unknown whether the underlying channels produce a sustained inward window current near E_m. Another possibility is that the K^+ channels setting E_m may be imperfectly selective for K^+, exhibiting some permeability to Na^+. This appears unlikely, however, because the reversal potential of the time-dependent outward K^+ current recorded in rabbit pulmonary cells was unaffected by exposing the cells to Na^+-free medium (37). The low-threshold $I_{K(N)}$ was also shown to be very selective for K^+ (19). Finally, resting P_{Na} could arise from a yet unidentified background or leakage conductance (19), which is often dismissed on the basis that it is part of the seal resistance.

So far, two classes of Cl^- channels have been described in pulmonary arterial smooth muscle cells: (1) Ca^{2+}-activated Cl^- channels (Cl_{Ca}) (55–57) and (2) swelling- or volume-sensitive Cl^- channels (Cl_{Swell}) (58,59). It appears unlikely that Cl_{Ca} channels play a role in generating E_{ms} because the activation threshold for intracellular Ca^{2+} (~200 nM) (60) lies beyond the normal resting $[Ca^{2+}]_i$ (~100 nM). It is also uncertain whether Cl_{Swell} channels are open at rest, because their appearance is usually triggered by exposing the cell to hypotonic solution. It remains to be established whether a fraction of these channels are basally active in isotonic medium and might account for the high P_{Cl} measured at rest. Clearly, more experiments are needed to determine the nature of the channels responsible for the high resting Na^+ and Cl^- permeabilities in pulmonary arterial smooth muscle.

IV. THE ACTIVE STATE OF PULMONARY ARTERIAL SMOOTH MUSCLE CELLS

As for smooth muscle cells from many systemic arteries such as those of the coronary and cerebral vascular beds, pulmonary arterial smooth muscle cells do not normally fire action potentials under resting nonstimulated conditions (2,11). Graded membrane depolarization elicited by outward current pulses in field stimulation experiments did not evoke an action potential in rat pulmonary arteries (11). The same study showed that TEA (1–5 mM), a K^+ channel blocker, induced a sustained nonregenerative membrane depolarization that was associated with contraction. Electrical field stimulation, TEA (10 mM), and another nonspecific K^+ inhibitor, procaine (5 mM), produced similar effects on membrane potential recorded from rabbit pulmonary arteries (2). In contrast, other studies have provided evidence that pulmonary arterial smooth muscle cells can fire action potentials when stimulated. Figure 2 (12) shows the effects of hypoxia on membrane potential recorded continuously with a microelectrode from a small (<300 μm) pulmonary artery from the cat. Under well-oxygenated conditions, a stable E_m oscillating around −56 mV was recorded (A). When the Po_2 was reduced from 300 to 30 torr, E_m gradually depolarized to reach a level that triggered bursts of multiphasic action potentials (B and C) whose frequency increased with further membrane depolarization (D). Application of verapamil, a specific blocker of L-type Ca^{2+} channels, abolished action

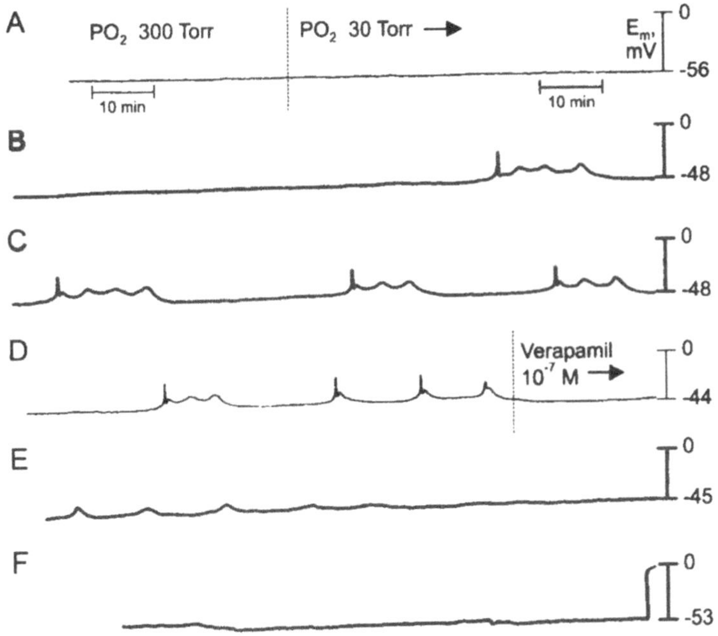

Figure 2 Hypoxia elicits Ca^{2+}-dependent action potentials in cat pulmonary arteries This is a chart recording of a continuous membrane potential (E_m) recording obtained with a microelectrode impaled in an intact small-caliber pulmonary artery from the cat. A–D show the effect of switching from a well-oxygenated control solution (partial oxygen pressure, Po_2, of 300 torr) to one in which the Po_2 was reduced ten-fold ($Po_2 = 30$ torr) as indicated by trace A. Note the gradual membrane depolarization in traces A and B, which resulted in the appearance of action potentials whose frequency increased with the extent of membrane depolarization in hypoxia. Trace D shows the effect of adding the Ca^{2+} channel blocker verapamil. Note that this compound abolished action generation and caused progressive repolarization of the membrane (E and F). (Reproduced from Ref. 12 with permission of the American Physiological Society.)

potentials (D and E) and led to progressive repolarization of the membrane (F). Action potential generation was insensitive to TTX, suggesting that the regenerative electrical responses did not originate from nerve terminals. The same study showed that the hypoxia-induced contraction increased with increasing $[Ca]_o$, and this contraction was abolished by verapamil.

Most patch-clamp studies in pulmonary arterial myocytes have failed to record all-or-none active regenerative responses. However, all have consistently reported that inhibition or downregulation of K_V channels (and perhaps $I_{K(N)}$) by 4-AP (17,20,26,39,45,50), hypoxia (17,26,38,39,45,50), or endothelin-1 (31) induces sustained membrane depolarization, elevation of intracellular Ca^{2+} levels comprising a transient and a maintained component, and contraction. One group was able to record action potentials in current clamped rat pulmonary myocytes (26). Figure 3 reproduces one figure from their study showing the effects of charybdotoxin (ChTX), glibenclamide (Gli), and 4-AP on E_m recorded in the absence or presence

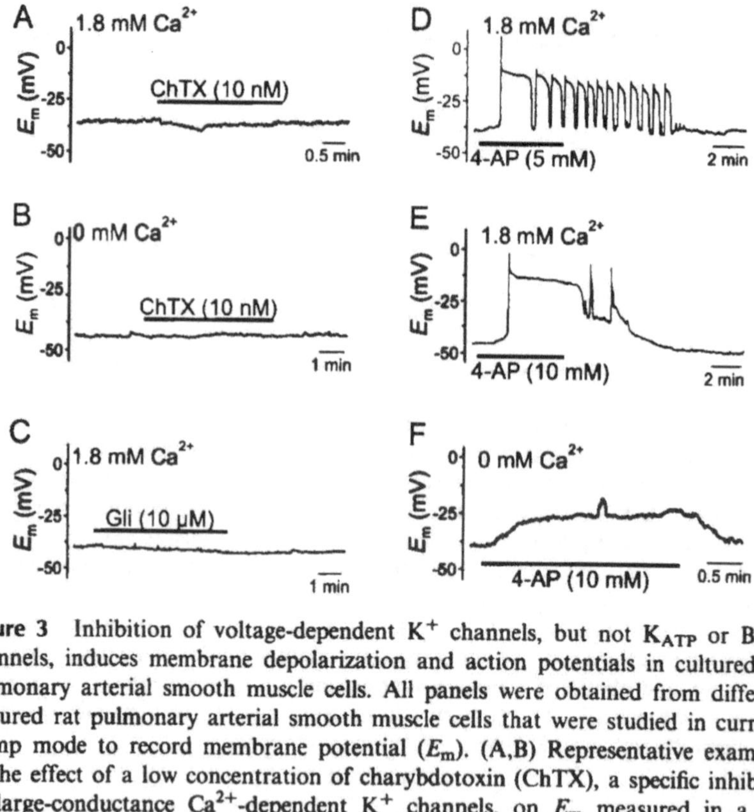

Figure 3 Inhibition of voltage-dependent K^+ channels, but not K_{ATP} or BK_{Ca} channels, induces membrane depolarization and action potentials in cultured rat pulmonary arterial smooth muscle cells. All panels were obtained from different cultured rat pulmonary arterial smooth muscle cells that were studied in current-clamp mode to record membrane potential (E_m). (A,B) Representative examples of the effect of a low concentration of charybdotoxin (ChTX), a specific inhibitor of large-conductance Ca^{2+}-dependent K^+ channels, on E_m measured in a cell exposed to 1.8 mM $[Ca]_o$ (A) or Ca^{2+}-free medium (B). (C). Effects of glibenclamide (Gli), a K_{ATP} channel antagonist, on E_m measured in the presence of extracellular Ca^{2+}. (D–F) Effects of 4-aminopyridine (4-AP), a blocker of voltage-dependent K^+ channels, on E_m measured in cells exposed to 1.8 mM $[Ca]_o$ (D and E) or Ca^{2+}-free medium (F). As explained in the text, 4-AP induced membrane depolarization and action potentials in myocytes exposed to 1.8 mM Ca^{2+} (D and E). The frequency and shape of the action potentials varied with the concentration of 4-AP (D and E). Panel F shows that although 4-AP was still able to cause membrane depolarization in the absence of extracellular Ca^{2+}, the blocker failed to evoke action potentials. (Reproduced from Ref. 26 with permission from the American Heart Association.)

of 1.8 mM Ca^{2+} in the bathing solution. As described in a previous section of this chapter, ChTx, with (Fig. 3A) or without (Fig. 3B) $[Ca]_o$, and glibenclamide (Fig. 3C) produced no effect on E_m consistent with a minor contribution of BK_{Ca} and K_{ATP} channels at rest. Figure 3D shows that 4-AP elicited membrane depolarization and spontaneous action potentials characterized by a Ca^{2+}-dependent upstroke, an initial rapid phase of repolarization followed by a long plateau that culminated in a final phase of repolarization that reached a negative but depolarized level of membrane potential. Another finding was that increasing the concentration of 4-AP from 5 to 10 mM enhanced the duration of the plateau of the action potential (Fig. 3E). Finally, action potential generation but not membrane depolarization in response to 4-AP was abolished by cell exposure to Ca^{2+}-free medium, consistent with the absolute requirement for Ca^{2+} entry from the extracellular space in evoking these responses. The same group also reported that hypoxia was also able to evoke action potentials (61).

Figure 4 summarizes schematically some of the basic concepts that are thought to be involved in electrogenesis during stimulation of pulmonary vascular smooth muscle cells. Inhibition of K_V or $I_{K(N)}$ channels by 4-AP, by hypoxia (through a redox and/or metabolic pathway), or through agonist-induced stimulation of a G-protein-coupled receptor that is coupled to phospholipase C causes membrane depolarization. This in turn increases the open probability of L-type Ca^{2+} channels (Ca_L), leading to Ca^{2+} entry, elevation of intracellular Ca^{2+}, and activation of the contractile machinery. Protein kinase C (PKC), which is stimulated by diacylglycerol (DAG) in receptor-mediated responses, may also directly stimulate Ca_L channels (62). Although the ionic nature of the conductance responsible for this initial membrane depolarization remains uncertain, we can speculate that in view of the high input resistance of these cells, opening of Ca_L channels may contribute to membrane depolarization and thus promote their gating. It is also possible that Ca^{2+} entry through Ca_L channels may raise $[Ca^{2+}]_i$ sufficiently to reach the threshold for activation of Ca^{2+}-activated Cl^- channels (~200 nM); activation of Cl_{Ca} would then induce Cl^- efflux (see Fig. 1), which would promote the opening of additional Ca_L channels. Opening of both Ca_L and Cl_{Ca} channels is therefore compatible with the observation that block of Ca_L channels by verapamil led to significant hyperpolarization of E_m in rat pulmonary arteries (12). Ca^{2+} release from the sarcoplasmic reticulum (SR), either through ryanodine receptors, which can be stimulated by hypoxia (38,63) and perhaps by Ca^{2+}-induced Ca^{2+} release, or by IP_3-sensitive Ca^{2+} release channels, would also play a role in elevating $[Ca^{2+}]_i$. In cells capable of generating action potentials, the initial depolarization may trigger an active all-or-none Ca_L-dependent action potential upstroke followed by an initial rapid repolarization phase that could result from several ionic mechanisms including activation of the transient K^+ current component of K_V (25) (I_A) (see inset in Fig. 4),

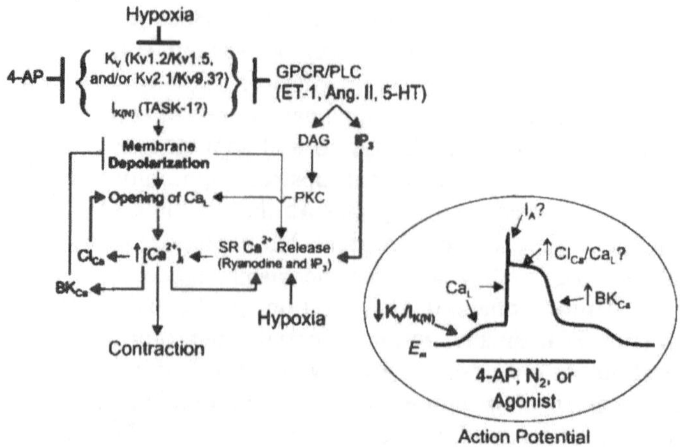

Figure 4 Hypothetical model illustrating the important role of ion channels in determining E_m, free intracellular Ca^{2+} concentration, and vascular tone in pulmonary arterial smooth muscle cells. This model highlights the central role of voltage-dependent K^+ channels (K_V and $I_{K(N)}$) in setting the negative resting membrane potential (E_m) measured in pulmonary myocytes, and how their inhibition by hypoxia or 4-aminopyridine (4-AP) or by the activation of G-protein-coupled receptor (GPCR) leads to membrane depolarization, activation of voltage-gated Ca^{2+} channels (Ca_L), elevation of intracellular Ca^{2+} concentration ($[Ca^{2+}]_i$), and cell contraction. Arrows indicate stimulation or production (e.g., DAG, IP_3). Lines ending with a cross bar indicate inhibition. The encircled inset illustrates hypothetical effects of 4-AP, hypoxia (N_2), or a constricting agonist (denoted by the thick bar below) on E_m and the ion conductances postulated to participate in the initial membrane depolarization and the different phases of the action potential. See text for detailed explanations. PLC, phopholipase C; Ang. II, angiotensin II; ET-1, endothelin-1; 5-HT, serotonin; DAG, diacylglycerol; PKC, protein kinase C; IP_3, inositol-trisphosphate; SR, sarcoplasmic reticulum; I_A, transient voltage-dependent component of K_V; Cl_{Ca}, Ca^{2+}-activated Cl channels; BK_{Ca} ; large conductance Ca^{2+}-dependent K^+ channels.

outward current caused by Cl^- influx through Cl_{Ca} channels at potentials beyond E_{Cl}, and partial inactivation of Ca_L channels. The long plateau of the action potential and the sustained phase of membrane depolarization in cells displaying tonic responses probably arise from the fine balance of inward and outward currents carried by Ca_L, Cl_{Ca}, BK_{Ca}, and uninhibited K_V and $I_{K(N)}$ channels. The final repolarization phase in cells generating action potentials is likely initiated by further inactivation of Ca_L channels (and deactivation of Cl_{Ca} channels) combined with the maintained activation of K_V and BK_{Ca} channels under conditions in which $[Ca^{2+}]_i$ remains elevated. Although very simplistic, this model nevertheless provides a useful framework to allow for understanding the important role of membrane potential in determining pulmonary vascular tone at rest and during physiologically relevant stimulations.

The reader should be aware that other important ionic mechanisms outside the scope of this chapter have received attention recently. Capacitative Ca^{2+} entry (CCE), a voltage-independent Ca^{2+} entry pathway triggered by SR Ca^{2+} store depletion, has been demonstrated in pulmonary arterial smooth muscle cells. Such a mechanism was shown to elevate $[Ca^{2+}]_i$ and induce vasoconstriction (64–66) and has been proposed as a major pathway for Ca^{2+} entry during HPV (66) (see Chapter. 25). Consistent with this hypothesis, there is evidence for the expression of several members of the "transient receptor potential" (TRP) family of genes in pulmonary smooth muscle cells (64,65). These genes are thought to encode for nonselective cation channels that are activated by a receptor, Ca^{2+} store depletion, or mechanical forces (see Chapters 5, 6, 21, and 27).

V. SUMMARY AND CONCLUDING REMARKS

Studies of the past 40 years have allowed for the identification at the cellular and molecular levels of many ion channel pathways that are involved inthe control of membrane potential of pulmonary arterial smooth muscle cells at rest and during stimulation. There is clear evidence supporting the notion that membrane depolarization is the key event leading to elevation of intracellular Ca^{2+} levels and increases in pulmonary arterial smooth muscle tone. Experiments in intact pulmonary arteries have shown that the restingmembrane potential of these cells may be the sum of an electrodiffusion potential created by passive diffusion of ions down their electrochemical gradient and the relative ion permeability of the membrane and a potential generated by electrogenic Na^+ pumping, although a contribution of thelatter to E_m has not been confirmed in isolated pulmonary arterial smooth muscle cells (19). Early studies showed that the membranes of pulmonary vascular smooth muscle cells exhibit a high permeability to Na^+ and Cl^- relative to K^+, and this property may be responsible for the deviation of E_m (~ -50 mV) from the measured equilibrium potential for K^+ (< -80 mV). Although the nature of the Na^+ and Cl^- conductances determining E_m at rest still remains elusive, patch clamp studies in freshly isolated or cultured pulmonary arterial smooth muscle have highlighted a unique role for 4-aminopyridine-sensitive voltage-dependent K^+ channels (K_V, $I_{K(N)}$) in setting E_m in these cells and most likely serving as one of possibly many O_2 sensors playing a role in hypoxic pulmonary vasoconstriction. Resting pulmonary vascular smooth muscle cells do not exhibit spontaneous action potentials. However, some but not all studies have demonstrated the ability of pulmonary vascular smooth muscle cells to fire L-type Ca^{2+} channel-dependent action potentials, which were detected in response to the depolarization mediated by hypoxia or inhibition of voltage-dependent K^+ channels by 4-AP.

Although significant advances have been made recently, the molecular mechanisms involved in the modulation of K^+ channel activity by low O_2 is still unclear. What are the relative contributions of K_V and $I_{K(N)}$ in generating E_m? Can a resting permeability to Na^+ and Cl^- be identified at the cellular and molecular levels? What are the reasons for the ability of certain pulmonary vascular smooth muscle cells (blood vessel caliber, species, age, gender, technical differences, etc.) to elicit action potentials whereas others seem to respond only by graded membrane depolarization? How is CCE intertwined with membrane-potential-dependent mechanisms of vasoconstriction? These and many other questions should be the subject of future investigations.

ACKNOWLEDCMENTS

This work was supported by grants from the Canadian Institutes of Health Research (NL; CIHR MOP-10863), National Institutes of Health (NL: NIH NCRR 5 P2015581; SW: NIH 1R03AI55642), and the Western Affiliate of the American Heart Association (NL: 0355060Y).

REFERENCES

1. Archer SL, Weir EK, McMurtry IF. Mechanisms of acute hypoxic and hyperoxic changes in pulmonary vascular reactivity. In: Weir EK, Reeves JT, eds. Pulmonary Vascular Physiology and Pathophysiology. New York: Marcel Dekker, 89:241–290.
2. Casteels R, Kitamura K, Kuriyama H, Suzuki H. The membrane properties of the smooth muscle cells of the rabbit main pulmonary artery. J Physiol 1977; 271:41–61.
3. Prosser CL. Smooth muscle. Annu Rev Physiol 1974; 36:503–535.
4. Casteels R, Kuriyama H. Membrane potential and ion content in the smooth muscle of the guinea-pig's taenia coli at different external potassium concentrations. J Physiol 1966; 184:120–130.
5. Aickin CC, Brading AF. Measurement of intracellular chloride in guinea-pig vas deferens by ion analysis, chloride efflux and micro-electrodes. J Physiol 1982; 326:139–154.
6. Chipperfield AR, Harper AA. Chloride in smooth muscle. Progr Biophys Mol Biol 2000; 74:175–221.
7. Droogmans G, Casteels R. Membrane potential and ion transport in smooth muscle cells. In: Bülbring E, Shuba MF, eds. Physiology of Smooth Muscle. New York: Raven, 1976:11–18.
8. Ohashi, H. The relative contribution of K and Cl to the total increase of membrane conductance produced by adrenaline on the smooth muscle of guinea-pig taenia coli. J Physiol 1971; 212:561–575.
9. Hille B. Ion Channels of Excitable Membranes. 3rd ed. Sunderland, MA: Sinauer Associates, 2001.
10. Plonsey R, Barr RC. Bioelectricity: A Quantitative Approach. New York: Plenum Press, 1988.

11. Suzuki H, Twarog BM. Membrane properties of smooth muscle cells in pulmonary arteries of the rat. Am J Physiol 1982; 242:H900–H906.
12. Harder DR, Madden JA, Dawson C. Hypoxic induction of Ca^{2+}-dependent action potentials in small pulmonary arteries of the cat. J Appl Physiol 1985; 59:1389–1393.
13. Kuriyama H. The influence of potassium, sodium and chloride on the membrane potential of the smooth muscle of taenia coli. J Physiol 1963; 166:15–28.
14. Casteels R. The relation between the membrane potential and the ion distribution in smooth muscle cells. In: Bülbring E, Brading AF, Jones AW, Tomita T, eds. Smooth Muscle. Baltimore: Williams & Wilkins, 1970:70–99.
15. Aickin CC, Brading AF. Advances in the understanding of transmembrane ionic gradients and permeabilities in smooth muscle obtained by using ion-selective micro-electrodes. Experientia 1985; 41:879–887.
16. Nakamura Y, Ohya Y, Abe I, Fujishima M. Sodium-potassium pump current in smooth muscle cells from mesenteric resistance arteries of the guinea-pig. J Physiol 1999; 519:203–212.
17. Archer SL, Huang JMC, Reeve HL, Hampl V, Tolarova S, Michelakis E, Weir EK. Differential distribution of electrophysiologically distinct myocytes in conduit and resistance arteries determines their response to nitric oxide and hypoxia. Circ Res 1996; 78:431–442.
18. Clapp LH, Gurney AM. ATP-sensitive K^+ channels regulate resting potential of pulmonary arterial smooth muscle cells. Am J Physiol 1992; 262: H916–H920.
19. Evans AM, Osipenko ON, Gurney AM. Properties of a novel K^+ current that is active at resting potential in rabbit pulmonary artery smooth muscle cells. J Physiol 1996; 496:407–420.
20. Smirnov SV, Robertson TP, Ward JPT, Aaronson PI. Chronic hypoxia is associated with reduced delayed rectifier K^+ current in rat pulmonary artery muscle cells. Am J Physiol 1994; 266:H365-H370.
21. Peng W, Karwande SV, Hoidal JR, Farrukh IS. Potassium currents in cultured human pulmonary arterial smooth muscle cells. J Appl Physiol 1996; 80: 1187–1196.
22. Nakao M, Gadsby DC. [Na] and [K] dependence of the Na/K pump current-voltage relationship in guinea pig ventricular myocytes. J Gen Physiol 1989; 94:539–565.
23. Nelson MT, Quayle JM. Physiological roles and properties of potassium channels in arterial smooth muscle. Am J Physiol 1995; 268:C799–C822.
24. Casteels R, Kitamura K, Kuriyama H, Suzuki H. Excitation-contraction coupling in the smooth muscle cells of the rabbit main pulmonary artery. J Physiol 1977; 271:63–79.
25. Clapp LH, Gurney AM. Outward currents in rabbit pulmonary artery cells dissociated with a new technique. Exp Physiol 1991; 76:677–693.
26. Yuan X-J. Voltage-gated K^+ currents regulate resting membrane potential and $[Ca^{2+}]_i$ in pulmonary arterial myocytes. Circ Res 1995; 77:370–378.
27. Clapp LH, Gurney AM, Standen NB, Langton PD. Properties of the ATP-sensitive K^+ current activated by levcromakalim in isolated pulmonary arterial myocytes. J. Membr Biol 1994; 140:205–213.

28. Wiener CM, Dunn A, Sylvester JT. ATP-dependent K^+ channels modulate vasoconstrictor responses to severe hypoxia in isolated ferret lungs. J Clin Invest 1991; 88:500–504.
29. Pinheiro JM, Malik AB. K^+ ATP-channel activation causes marked vasodilation in the hypertensive neonatal pig lung. Am J Physiol 1992; 263: H1532–H1536.
30. Weir EK, Reeve HL, Huang JMC, Michelakis E, Nelson DP, Hampl V, Archer SL. Anorexic agents aminorex, fenfluramine, and dexfenfluramine inhibit potassium current in rat pulmonary vascular smooth muscle and cause pulmonary vasoconstriction. Circulation 1996; 94:2216–2220.
31. Shimoda L, Sylvester JT, Sham JSK. Inhibition of voltage-gated K^+ current in rat intrapulmonary arterial myocytes by endothelin-1. Am J Physiol 1998; 18:L842–L853.
32. Jaggar JH, Porter VA, Lederer WJ, Nelson MT. Calcium sparks in smooth muscle. Am J Physiol 2000; 278:C235–C256.
33. Remillard CV, Zhang WM, Shimoda LA, Sham, JSK. Physiological properties and functions of Ca^{2+} sparks in rat intrapulmonary arterial smooth muscle cells. Am J Physiol 2002; 283:L433–L444.
34. Salter KJ, Turner JL, Albarwani S, Clapp LH, Kozlowski RZ. Ca^{2+}-activated Cl^- and K^+ channels and their modulation by endothelin-1 in rat pulmonary arterial smooth muscle cells. Exp Physiol 1995; 80:815–824.
35. Archer SL, Huang JMC, Hampl V, Nelson DP, Shultz PJ, Weir EK. Nitric oxide and cGMP cause vasorelaxation by activation of a charybdotoxin-sensitive K channel by cGMP-dependent protein kinase. Proc Natl Acad Sci USA 1994; 91:7583–7587.
36. Bolotina VM, Najibi S, Palcino JJ, Pagano PJ, Cohen RA. Nitric oxide directly activates calcium-dependent potassium channels in vascular smooth muscle. Nature 1994; 368:850–853.
37. Okabe K, Kitamura K, Kuriyama H. Features of 4-aminopyridine sensitive outward current observed in single smooth muscle cells from the rabbit pulmonary artery. Pflügers Arch 1987; 409:561–568.
38. Post JM, Gelband CH, Hume JR. $[Ca^{2+}]_i$ inhibition of K^+ channels in canine. Circ Res 1995; 77:131–139.
39. Osipenko ON, Alexander D, MacLean MR, Gurney AM. Influence of chronic hypoxia on the contributions of non-inactivating and delayed rectifier K currents to the resting potential and tone of rat pulmonary artery smooth muscle. Br J Pharmacol 1998; 124:1335–1337.
40. Patel AJ, Lazdunski M, Honore E. $K_v2.1/K_v9.3$, a novel ATP-dependent delayed-rectifier K^+ channel in oxygen-sensitive pulmonary artery myocytes. EMBO J 1997; 16:6615–6625.
41. Yuan JX-J, Aldinger AM, Juhaszova M, Wang J, Conte JV, Gaine SP, Orens JB, Rubin LJ. Dysfunctional voltage-gated K^+ channels in pulmonary artery smooth muscle cells of patients with primary pulmonary hypertension. Circulation 1998; 98:1400–1406.
42. Yuan X-J, Wang J, Juhaszova M, Gaine SP, Rubin LJ. Attenuated K^+ channel gene transcription in primary pulmonary hypertension. Lancet 1998; 351: 726–727.

43. Reeve HL, Weir EK, Archer SL, Cornfield DN. A maturational shift in pulmonary K^+ channels, from Ca^{2+} sensitive to voltage dependent. Am J Physiol 1998; 19:L1019–L1025.
44. Overturf KE, Russell SN, Carl A, Vogalis F, Hart PJ, Hume JR, Sanders KM, Horowitz B. Cloning and characterization of a $K_V1.5$ delayed rectifier K^+ channel from vascular and visceral smooth muscles. Am J Physiol 1994; 267:C1231–C1238.
45. Archer SL, Souil E, DinhXuan AT, Schremmer B, Mercier JC, El Yaagoubi A, Nguyen-Huu L, Reeve HL, Hampl V. Molecular identification of the role of voltage-gated K^+ channels, Kv1.5 and Kv2.1, in hypoxic pulmonary vasoconstriction and control of resting membrane potential in rat pulmonary artery myocytes. J Clin Invest 1998; 101:2319–2330.
46. Yuan X-J, Wang J, Juhaszova M, Golovina VA, Rubin LJ. Molecular basis and function of voltage-gated K^+ channels in pulmonary arterial smooth muscle cells. Am J Physiol 1998; 274:L621–L635.
47. Hulme JT, Coppock EA, Felipe A, Martens JR, Tamkun MM. Oxygen sensitivity of cloned voltage-gated K^+ channels expressed in the pulmonary vasculature. Circ Res 1999; 85:489–497.
48. Wang J, Juhaszova M, Rubin LJ, Yuan X-J. Hypoxia inhibits gene expression of voltage-gated K^+ channel α subunits in pulmonary artery smooth muscle cells. J Clin Invest 1997; 100:2347–2353.
49. Pozeg ZI, Michelakis ED, McMurtry MS, Thebaud B, Wu X-C, Dyck JRB, Hashimoto K, Wang SH, Harry G, Sultanian R, Koshal A, Archer SL. In vivo gene transfer of the O_2-sensitive potassium channel Kv1.5 reduces pulmonary hypertension and restores hypoxic pulmonary vasoconstriction in chronically hypoxic rats. Circulation 2003; 107:2037–2044.
50. Osipenko ON, Evans AM, Gurney AM. Regulation of the resting potential of rabbit pulmonary artery myocytes by a low threshold, O_2-sensing potassium current. Br J Pharmacol 1997; 120:1461–1470.
51. Evans AM, Osipenko ON, Haworth SG, Gurney AM. Resting potentials and potassium currents during development of pulmonary artery smooth muscle cells. Am J Physiol 1998; 44:H887–H899.
52. Gurney AM, Osipenko ON, MacMillan D, McFarlane KM, Tate RJ, Kempsill FE. Two-pore domain K channel, TASK-1, in pulmonary artery smooth muscle cells. Circ Res 2003; 93:957–964.
53. Okabe K, Kitamura K, Kuriyama H. The existence of a highly tetrodotoxin sensitive Na channel in freshly dispersed smooth muscle cells of the rabbit main pulmonary artery. Pflügers Arch 1988; 411:423–428.
54. Choby C, Mangoni ME, Boccara G, Nargeot J, Richard S. Evidence for tetrodotoxin-sensitive sodium currents in primary cultured myocytes from human, pig and rabbit arteries. Pflügers Arch 2000; 440:149–152.
55. Yuan XJ. Role of calcium-activated chloride current in regulating pulmonary vasomotor tone. Am J Physiol 1997; 272:L959–L968.
56. Clapp LH, Turner JL, Kozlowski, RZ. Ca^{2+}-activated Cl^- currents in pulmonary arterial myocytes. Am J Physiol 1996; 39:H1577–H1584.
57. Greenwood I, Ledoux J, Leblanc N. Differential regulation of Ca^{2+}-activated Cl^- currents in rabbit arterial and portal vein smooth muscle cells by Ca^{2+}-calmodulin-dependent kinase. J Physiol 2001; 534:395–408.

58. Yamazaki J, Duan D, Janiak R, Kuenzli K, Horowitz B, Hume JR. Functional and molecular expression of volume-regulated chloride channels in canine vascular smooth muscle cells. J Physiol 1998; 507:729–736.
59. Greenwood IA, Large WA. Properties of a Cl^- current activated by cell swelling in rabbit portal vein vascular smooth muscle cells. Am J Physiol 1998; 275:H1524–H1532.
60. Large WA, Wang Q. Characteristics and physiological role of the Ca^{2+}-activated Cl^- conductance in smooth muscle. Am J Physiol 1996; 271:C435–C454.
61. Yuan XJ, Goldman WF, Tod ML, Rubin LJ, Blaustein MP. Hypoxia reduces potassium currents in cultured rat pulmonary but not mesenteric arterial myocytes. Am J Physiol 1993; 264:L116–L123.
62. ObejeroPaz CA, Auslender M, Scarpa A. PKC activity modulates availability and long openings of L-type Ca^{2+} channels in A7r5 cells. Am J Physiol 1998; 275:C535–C543.
63. Salvaterra CG, Goldman WF. Acute hypoxia increases cytosolic calcium in cultured pulmonary arterial myocytes. Am J Physiol 1993; 264:L323-L328.
64. McDaniel SS, Platoshyn O, Wang J, Yu Y, Sweeney M, Krick S, Rubin LJ, Yuan JX-J. Capacitative Ca^{2+} entry in agonist-induced pulmonary vasoconstriction. Am J Physiol 2001; 280:L870–L880.
65. Ng LC, Gurney AM. Store-operated channels mediate Ca^{2+} influx and contraction in rat pulmonary artery. Circ Res 2001; 89:923–929.
66. Robertson TP, Hague D, Aaronson PI, Ward JPT. Voltage-independent calcium entry in hypoxic pulmonary vasoconstriction of intrapulmonary arteries of the rat. J Physiol 2000; 525:669–680.
67. Aickin CC, Brading AF, Walmsley D. An investigation of sodium-calcium exchange in the smooth muscle of guinea-pig ureter. J Physiol 1987; 391: 325–346.
68. Lamont C, Burdyga TV, Wray S. Intracellular Na^+ measurements in smooth muscle using SBFI—changes in $[Na^+]$, Ca^{2+} and force in normal and Na^+-loaded ureter. Pflügers Arch 1998; 435:523–527.
69. Hagemeijer F, Rorive G, Schoffeniels E. Cationic composition of different rat tissues during experimental arterial hypertension. Arch Int Physiol Biochim 1966; 74:807–811.
70. Borin ML, Tribe RM, Blaustein MP. Increased intracellular Na^+ augments mobilization of Ca^{2+} from SR in vascular smooth muscle cells. Am J Physiol 1994; 266:C311–C317.
71. Mulvany MJ, Aalkjaer C, Petersen TT. Intracellular sodium, membrane potential, and contractility of rat mesenteric small arteries. Circ Res 1984; 54: 740–749.
72. Siegel G, Roedel H, Nolte J, Hofer HW, Bertsche O. Ionic composition and ion exchange in vascular smooth muscle. In: Bülbring E, Shuba MF, eds. Physiology of Smooth Muscle. New York: Raven Press, 1976:19–39.
73. Jones AW, Feigl EO, Peterson LH. Water and electrolyte content of normal and hypertensive arteries in dogs. Circ Res 1964; 15:386–392.

2

Excitation–Contraction Coupling in the Pulmonary Vasculature

Luke J. Janssen
Firestone Institute for Respiratory Health, St. Joseph's Hospital and McMaster University, Hamilton, Ontario, Canada

I. INTRODUCTION

In addition to their role in producing changes in mechanical tone, smooth muscle cells can perform other important functions such as cytokine production, migration, proliferation, and even antigen presentation. However, most of the clinically important pulmonary vascular pathologies involve defects pertaining to the contractile state of the smooth muscle; examples of this include hypoxic pulmonary vasoconstriction and ventilation–perfusion mismatching as well as pulmonary hypertension. Ionic mechanisms play key roles in many aspects of pulmonary vascular biology; this is particularly true of contraction and relaxation. Other authors in this volume will expound on each of the different ion channels and ionic mechanisms in the pulmonary vasculature. The purpose of the current chapter is to put these channels and mechanisms into the general perspective of excitation–contraction coupling.

Vascular smooth muscle function is regulated by mediators secreted by many different cell types in the vicinity of the smooth muscle (the endothelium, innervation, and inflammatory cells) as well as by bloodborne products derived from more distally located tissues. These autacoids act through diverse signaling pathways (receptors, enzymes, ion channels and pumps, etc.) that eventually terminate at the contractile apparatus and produce a change in tone. We will refer to those sequences of events that link receptor activation to a mechanical response as "excitation–contraction coupling" (applying this term as well to vasodilators even though, precisely speaking, vasodilators evoke the opposite of excitation and contraction).

II. EXCITATION–CONTRACTION COUPLING IN MUSCLE—GENERAL CONCEPTS

The walls of the pulmonary vasculature are encircled by a layer of smooth muscle, the shortening or lengthening of which regulates vessel diameter and thus resistance to blood flow. According to Poiseuille's law, resistance (R) is inversely related to the fourth power of vessel diameter ($R = 8\mu L/\pi r^4$, where μ is the blood viscosity and L is the length of the vessel). The smooth muscle cells within this layer are interconnected via proteins (collagens, elastin, fibronectin), proteoglycans, and glycoproteins, which in turn adhere to external cell–cell contacts referred to as adherens junctions, intermediate contacts, and desmosome-like structures (1,2) (Fig. 1). The latter are elaborate macromolecular complexes compring proteins such as α-actinin,

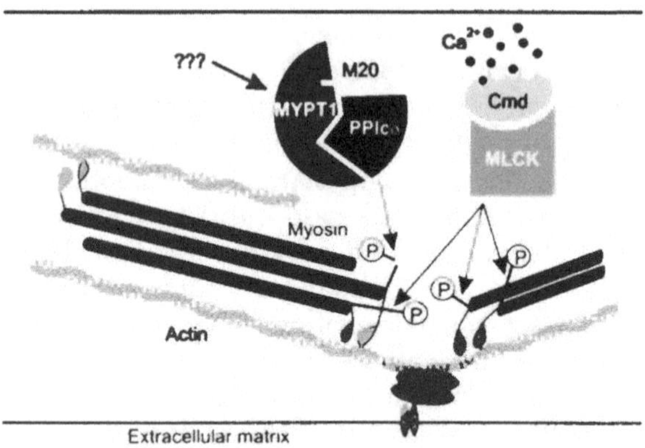

Figure 1 Sliding filament theory of contraction Actin fibers attach to the extracellular matrix via macromolecular complexes. Myosin molecules associate with the actin fibers via high affinity binding sites on their globular heads and associate with other myosin molecules via their long filamentous tails. Phosphorylation of myosin by MLCK (activated by Ca^{2+}-calmodulin) causes the globular head to detach, undergo swiveling conformational change, and reattach at another actin binding site. MLCP [made up of a catalytic subunit (PP1cδ), a targeting subunit (MYPT1), and a subunit of unknown function (M20)], dephosphorylates myosin, thereby inactivating it. The signaling mechanisms by which MLCK and MLCP are controlled are summarized in Figs. 4 and 5.

vinculin, laminin, vimentin, desmin, talin, and tensin (1) (Fig. 1), the function of which we are only beginning to understand. Projecting internally from the dense bodies are long fibers of smooth muscle α-actin.

Prior to the development of the "sliding filament" theory of excitation–contraction coupling by H. E. Huxley, it would have been surprising to learn that shortening does not occur within the connective tissue proteins external to the plasmalemma or within the actin fibers inside the cell. Instead, according to that theory, shortening occurs when the actin fibers attached to the plasmalemma are pulled inward through the catalytic activity of another muscle protein—myosin—the inward pulling force in turn being transmitted to the external contacts on the membrane and then to the connective tissue between the cells.

Actin accounts for almost half of the total protein content of smooth muscle cells, existing as a globular monomer (G-actin) with molecular weight of 42 kDa, or as a filamentous polymer (F-actin). There are six different isoforms of actin, each encoded by a distinct gene, that can be separated into three types by isoelectric focusing. The three most acidic isoforms are grouped together as α-actin (α-skeletal, α-cardiac, and α-vascular actins), and the two least acidic isoforms as γ-actin (γ-cytoplasmic and γ-enteric); the sixth isoform is referred to as β-actin or β-cytoplasmic actin. It appears that these different isoforms play somewhat unique roles, because their relative expression varies considerably between tissues and even during different stages of the life cycle of the cells within a given tissue. For example, γ-actin predominates in esophageal smooth muscle (one of the so-called phasic smooth muscles), whereas α-actin predominates in vascular smooth muscle (a "tonic" smooth muscle); also, β-actin is present to some extent in all smooth muscle tissues, but its expression decreases (and the relative amounts of α- or γ-actins increases) during cell development and maturation.

Myosin was the first molecular motor to be identified [preceding the discoveries of kinesin and dynein by decades (3)] largely on the basis of circumstantial evidence: its sheer abundance in skeletal muscle and its ATPase catalytic activity. More recently, biophysical experiments using laser tweezers, video microscopy, and in vitro motility assays confirmed and characterized its motor properties directly. Myosin is a polymer composed of two identical heavy chains (200–220 kDa each) and two pairs of light chains (17 kDa and 20 kDa, respectively) (Fig. 1). The N-terminal ends of the heavy chains intertwine and form an extended rodlike structure (≈150 nm long), which condenses with other such myosin structures to form a long brush or thick filament, out of which protrude the globular C-terminal myosin heads. The latter contain high-affinity binding sites for filamentous actin and ATP as well as an enzyme catalytic site: an Mg^{2+}-dependent ATPase. The regulatory light chains bind to a flexible linker region that bridges the globular heads and rodlike N-termini of myosin. As such, they are strategically positioned and equipped for their role in muscle contraction: their activation triggers a major conformational change in the globular head and linker region of the myosin heavy chain, causing the head to swivel while it remains attached to actin (3). As it does so, the thick and thin filaments translocate past one another. Myosin then releases actin, swivels back to its original conformation, and binds to another actin monomer in the actin filament.

The fundamental unit of muscle contraction, then, is the "step" taken by the myosin head from one actin monomer to another, with the actin and myosin filaments sliding past each other by 10 nm (the distance between actin monomers in the actin filament) and generating a force of 3–7 pN, accompanied by hydrolysis of ATP (3). These forces, acting in parallel and in series, add together to give the millinewton forces that can be detected at the tissue level.

The popular view is that the translocation of actin is driven directly by ATP hydrolysis, analogous to an artificial motor that uses chemical or electrical energy to exert a dynamic force on some lever or armature. However, a newer interpretation is that of a molecular ratchet in which the actin and myosin fibers are constantly moving randomly owing to their internal molecular thermal energy, with the myosin head constantly swiveling back and forth, but that ATP hydrolysis at the right moment in the kinetic cycle makes the backward motion thermodynamically unfavorable, thereby rectifying the random motion into a smooth forward motion. In this case, the myosin effectively acts like a "filter," selecting out certain thermodynamic states and resisting others. Two fundamental differences between these models can be highlighted. First, the force that actually moves the actin fiber derives from ATP hydrolysis in the traditional model but from the thermal energy of the fibers themselves in the other model (hence, the latter is referred to as the "thermal capture" model). Second, the traditional model requires that a great deal of torque be exerted within the myosin neck region (and transmitted through the globular head) to physically translocate the actin and thus pull on the cell membrane, whereas the thermal capture model requires the myosin head to merely form a stiff "backstop" in order to prevent backward motion of actin.

Relaxation, on the other hand, is a passive event; that is, there is no motor protein that runs "in reverse," forcing the actin fibers and connective tissue proteins outward. Instead, tension developed by the contractile apparatus is released, and unknown elastic/compressive forces restore the cells to their original length. These expansionary forces appear to be resident within the smooth muscle cells per se, at least in part, because relaxation or elongation is seen even in single enzymatically isolated cells that lack any external connections (4,5). The exact details underlying this elongation—whether they involve some form of fluid volume regulation or compression of an internal spring, for example—are entirely unclear.

III. EXCITATION–CONTRACTION COUPLING IN SMOOTH MUSCLE—ROLES OF MYOSIN LIGHT CHAIN KINASE AND PHOSPHATASE

How, then, is the interaction between actin and myosin triggered within the smooth muscle cell? Even as early as the 19th century, it had been recognized through the work of Sydney Ringer that, ultimately, contraction is a Ca^{2+}-dependent event. However, the role played by Ca^{2+} in this process differs markedly between smooth and skeletal muscles.

When myosin extracted from skeletal muscle is mixed with an extract of actin filaments, these two proteins interact spontaneously, leading to hydrolysis of ATP and sliding of the two filaments past each other. In skeletal and cardiac muscles, this actomyosin ATPase activity is regulated by troponin, which binds to high-affinity sites on actin and thereby occludes the myosin binding site: troponin is in turn displaced from actin by Ca^{2+} (more specifically, calmodulin with four bound Ca^{2+} ions).

When a similar experiment is performed using myosin derived from smooth muscle, however, the outcome is quite different. Using actomyosin ATPase activity as an index of the interaction between actin and myosin (and, thus, of contraction), Sobieszek and Small (6) first showed that actin does not stimulate smooth muscle–derived myosin directly, but myosin was stimulated in a dose-dependent fashion when they also included increasing amounts of a tropomyosin extract. Moreover, they found that this smooth muscle myosin was phosphorylated and, more important, that there was a linear relationship between actomyosin ATPase activity and myosin phosphorylation, suggesting a causal relationship between the two. Later experiments revealed central roles for myosin light chain kinase and calmodulin in all of these, thus accounting for the Ca^{2+} dependence of contraction.

Phosphorylation that results in contraction occurs at serine-19 of the 20 kDa myosin light chain (MLC_{20}). Addition of this single negative charge to the regulatory subunit of myosin appears to disrupt ionic interactions within the molecule, causing unfolding and the other conformational changes underlying contraction.

Dephosphorylation of myosin (e.g., during relaxation) is catalyzed by myosin light chain phosphatase (MLCP). This enzyme is a type I Ser/Thr protein phosphatase made up of three subunits: a 37 kDa catalytic subunit (PP1cδ), a 110–130 kDa targeting subunit (MYPT1), and a 20 kDa subunit (M20) whose function is not entirely clear (Fig. 1). The targeting subunit binds to phosphorylated myosin, bringing the catalytic subunit of MLCP into proximity for dephosphorylation of myosin.

IV. HETEROGENEITY IN THE PULMONARY VASCULATURE

Much of what we currently know about lung vascular physiology at the cellular and molecular levels has been gained using main branch segments of pulmonary artery, primarily from the rat. This is unfortunate, however, because the pulmonary vascular bed is a very heterogeneous preparation, with many species-, age-, and size-specific differences, as follows.

A. Artery Versus Vein

Many groups have reported fundamental differences in the structure or function of pulmonary veins as compared to the pulmonary arteries taken from the same animals. For example, thromboxane-, leukotriene-, hypoxia-, and isoprostane-evoked contractions are large in the vein but relatively smaller in the artery, whereas the opposite is true of noradrenaline- and tachykinin-evoked relaxations (7–11) (see Fig. 2). Conversely, relaxations evoked by prostaglandins E_2 and I_2 are considerably larger in

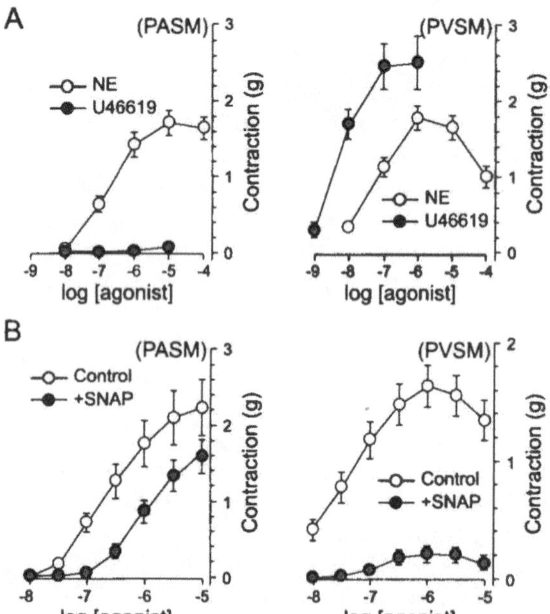

Figure 2 Differential responsiveness of pulmonary artery and vein (A) Norepinephrine (NE) shows comparable efficacy in pulmonary artery (PASM; left panel) and pulmonary vein (PVSM; right panel), although potency is slightly higher in the latter (almost a full log unit difference). The thromboxane A2 agonist U46619, on the other hand, evokes powerful and potent contractions in PV but none in the PA. (B) In another study, the nitric oxide donor SNAP markedly suppressed PASM responses to submaximal adrenergic stimulation and partially reduced those to maximal adrenergic stimulation but essentially abolished all adrenergic responses in PVSM. (Data reproduced with permission from Refs. 84 and 73.)

the newborn lamb pulmonary vein than in the pulmonary artery (12); nitric oxide also seems to play a greater role in the vein than in the artery (13) (Fig. 2). Angiotensin II constricts the artery but relaxes the vein (14), and the opposite is true of acetylcholine (15). The artery and vein even differ with respect to metabolism (11), which might account for the larger hypoxic response in the latter. In addition to such functional and metabolic differences, there are many examples of structural differences. The wall of the pulmonary vein includes cardiomyocytes and inward rectifier K^+ channels, whereas that of the pulmonary artery does not (16). The artery expresses ET_A receptors for endothelin and LT-1 receptors for the cysteinyl leukotrienes, whereas the vein expresses ET_B and LT-2 receptors (13,17,18). These receptor-related differences become important if it is proposed that selective antagonists be used to reverse pulmonary vasoconstriction.

B. Conduit Versus Resistance Vessels

Within a given vascular bed, there can be marked differences between conduit and resistance vessels. The responses to many agonists (noradrenaline, histamine, serotonin, leukotrienes, acetylcholine, nitric oxide) and to hypoxia are much greater in small vessels than in main branch vessels (10,19–23). These functional differences may be due in part to differences in the expression of ion channels and pumps across the vascular bed. For example, resistance arteries have a higher density of voltage-dependent Ca^{2+} current (22), Ca^{2+}-dependent K^+ current (19), and a voltage-, Ca^{2+}-, and ATP-insensitive K^+ current (24). Ca^{2+}-dependent Cl^- channels, on the other hand, are more abundant in the main trunk artery than in smaller vessels (e.g., 3rd to 4th division) (25,26). In the smaller vessels, hypoxia increases the magnitude of voltage-dependent Ca^{2+} currents and shifts the conductance–voltage relationship to more negative voltages, whereas the opposite changes are produced in the larger vessels (22). Related to this, hypoxia reduces intracellular calcium ion concentration, ($[Ca^{2+}]_i$), and abolishes spontaneous Ca^{2+} spikes in conduit arteries but elevates $[Ca^{2+}]_i$, and modulates Ca^{2+}-spike amplitude in resistance vessels (27). Finally, removal of external Na^+ evokes a brief hyperpolarization in the rat main trunk artery but a sustained depolarization in the small artery (28), which may reflect differences in Na^+/K^+-ATPase or Na^+/Ca^{2+} exchange activities between these two regions of the vascular bed.

C. Cell–Cell Variabilities

There can be important differences even within a given "slice" of a vascular preparation. Two distinct types of cells are obtained upon dissociation of the pulmonary artery. Some are large and elongated with a relatively low density of nitric oxide–sensitive Ca^{2+}-dependent K^+ channels, whereas others are smaller, with a perinuclear bulge and high density of nitric oxide–insensitive delayed rectifier K^+ current (19,26,29). There is evidence that such morphologically different cells are found in distinct layers in a given segment of artery and may differ with respect to expression of various contractile and cytoskeletal proteins (29).

D. Species- and Age-Related Differences

The magnitude of the vasoconstrictor response to hypoxia varies markedly between species. PGI_2 is a potent vasodilator in the human, is somewhat less so in the dog, and is ineffective in the rabbit, whereas the converse seems to be true of contractions to norepinephrine (30,31). Leukotrienes are potent vasoconstrictors in the human pulmonary vein but not in the human pulmonary artery, whereas the opposite is true in the pig (8,9). The responses to adenosine in the human and rat [dilation via A_2 receptors (32,33)] are opposite to that seen in the cat [vasoconstriction via A_1 receptors (34)]. Also, several authors have described maturational changes in the structure of the PASM cell [including expression of various contractile and cytoskeletal proteins (29)], responses to various agonists [including prostanoids and nitric oxide (15,23)], and the expression of different K^+ channels (29,35). The latter point could explain the finding that membrane potential in PASM is determined primarily by Ca^{2+}-dependent K^+ channels early in life, after which voltage-gated K^+ channels (K_V) predominate (36).

E. Conclusion

The extensive list of comparisons provided above is not a mere academic exercise but is given to highlight the need for studies using resistance vessels of both human arteries and veins. It has been unfortunate that most studies examining ion channels and/or signaling pathways have used main branch pulmonary arterial preparations, usually those of the rat. The pulmonary artery and pulmonary vein are roughly equally important in determining overall pulmonary resistance to blood flow, and the pulmonary vein is capable of generating as large a contractile response to many agonists as that of the pulmonary artery (Figs. 2 and 5). Redistribution of blood during ventilation–perfusion matching, therefore, can be effected just as well by constriction of the vein as by arterial constriction. It could be said that the vein is better positioned to sense inadequate ventilation (because it is "downstream" of the gas-exchange event) than the pulmonary artery.

V. EXCITATION–CONTRACTION COUPLING IN VASCULAR SMOOTH MUSCLE

In general, spasmogens evoke contraction by elevating $[Ca^{2+}]_i$ to stimulate MLCK, whereas relaxants cause the opposite changes (more recently discovered mechanisms will also be considered later). One major pathway by which this is accomplished involves regulation of Ca^{2+} influx through changes in membrane potential: this is appropriately referred to as electromechanical coupling. Several decades ago, smooth muscle physiologists began to appreciate that contraction can also involve pathways that are voltage-independent. These were initially referred to collectively as "pharmacomechanical" coupling mechanisms; however, this term has since fallen out of use, because we now know that it brings together so many disparate and unrelated mechanisms. For example, one of these pathways involves changes in $[Ca^{2+}]_i$ mediated by an internal Ca^{2+} pool (the sarcoplasmic reticulum), another does not require changes in $[Ca^{2+}]_i$ (altered Ca^{2+} sensitivity of the contractile apparatus), and yet others are essentially Ca^{2+}-independent (certain thin-filament-mediated mechanisms). Being voltage-independent, these pathways are intractable to the classical Ca^{2+} channel blockers and K^+ channel agonists that are widely used in the treatment of systemic hypertension. The various excitation–contraction coupling pathways are described in more detail in the following pages.

A. Electromechanical Coupling

Voltage-Dependent Ca^{2+} Influx

Many groups have examined the Ca^{2+} currents present in pulmonary arterial preparations (5,22,37,38) (see Chapter 4). Unfortunately, however, there are no published reports pertaining to Ca^{2+} currents in the pulmonary vein; it is possible that they are different than those in the artery, given the long and growing list of reported differences between these two tissues (summarized in Sec. IV). A detailed description of these channels is given elsewhere within this volume (Chapter 3). However, in order to consider their roles in excitation–contraction coupling, it will be necessary for us to summarize briefly certain of their properties.

One important characteristic of calcium ion channels is their ability to transition stochastically between an open state and a closed state with a rate constant that is dependent upon the voltage gradient across the membrane in which they are situated. Although the probability of finding them in the open state is low (but nonzero) at very negative membrane potentials, it increases dramatically as V_m rises above $-60\,mV$ and is maximal (unity) at positive potentials (Fig. 3) (38,39). Activation of these currents is rapid compared to cellular events such as contraction, occurring on a time scale of less than a few hundred milliseconds.

In addition to these open/closed state transitions, these channels can undergo another conformational change and thereby enter into a third state—the inactivated state (not to be confused with the deactivated or closed state)—in a voltage- and time-dependent fashion. At the whole-cell level, Ca^{2+} current inactivation can begin to develop at potentials that are subthreshold for activation, is typically half-maximal at potentials in the

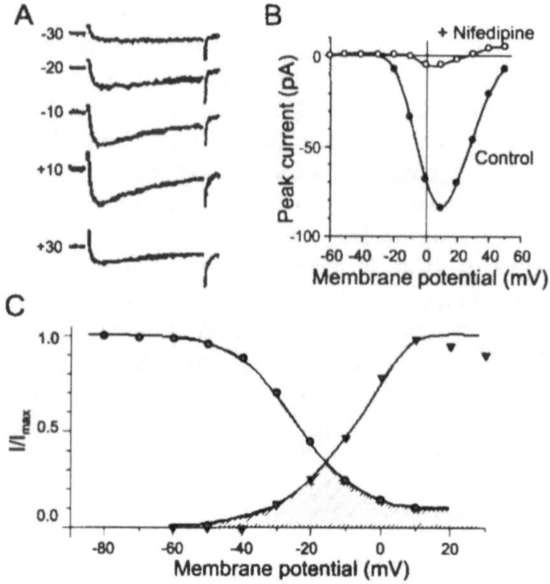

Figure 3 Voltage-dependent Ca^{2+} currents in pulmonary arterial smooth muscle. (A) Actual tracings of Ca^{2+} currents evoked by depolarizing pulses [100 ms duration; to potentials stated in figure; holding potential of −80 mV], illustrating the voltage and time dependence of activation and inactivation. (B) Mean currentvoltage relationship in the presence and absence of the dihydropyridine nifedipine (2 μM). (C) Voltage dependence of activation and inactivation are superimposed to illustrate the "window current" (shaded region) in these cells. (Data used with permission from Ref. 38.)

vicinity of the resting membrane potential, and is maximal (though not complete) at positive potentials (Fig. 3). Inactivation occurs much more slowly than activation, requiring several seconds to reach a stable equilibrium.

These activation/inactivation properties give rise to a physiologically important phenomenon referred to as "window current", alluding to a range ("window") of voltages at which the Ca^{2+} current is activated (more positive than −70 mV) but not completely inactivated (more negative than ≈0 mV) (Fig. 3). As such, any stimulus that triggers depolarization above the resting membrane potential (typically ≈ −60 mV) increases Ca^{2+} influx across the membrane (and thus increases vasomotor tone), whereas those that hyperpolarize the membrane decrease Ca^{2+} influx and tone.

Thus, many vasoconstrictors act by depolarizing the membrane [one group has estimated a doubling of Ca^{2+} influx with a depolarization as small as 3 mV (40)] whereas vasodilators typically act in part through membrane hyperpolarization (19,41), as outlined below.

Resting Membrane Potential

At rest, V_m as determined by using intracellular microelectrodes ranges from −50 to −60 mV (21,28,42). When V_m was determined using the patch clamp technique, some also found that it fell somewhere in the upper end of that range (4,43–45), but many others found that it ranged from −45 to −20 mV (19,36,39,41,46–53). Whereas the intracellular microelectrode technique is presumed to leave the intracellular ionic environment relatively intact, the patch clamp technique inevitably involves marked changes in ionic gradients, $[Ca^{2+}]_i$, cytosolic [ATP], pH, osmolarity, etc. In particular, the chloride equilibrium potential is almost always set artificially high at 0 mV, several tens of millivolts more positive than what is believed to be the physiological level (54). This would distort estimates of the membrane potential depending on the extent to which chloride channels are active at rest (see below); also, this insult could disrupt volume regulation, leading to changes in the activation state of volume-sensitive chloride channels, which have been shown to be present in these tissues (55). Others have described marked changes in V_m as cytosolic [ATP] was altered (45), suggesting an important role for ATP-dependent K^+ channels.

Having said all this, V_m at rest is generally within the voltage "window" described above (Fig. 3), allowing for exquisite regulation of Ca^{2+} influx by depolarizing and hyperpolarizing stimuli. K^+ channels play a prominent role in setting V_m at this level. However, the relative contributions of Ca^{2+}-dependent and voltage-dependent K^+ channels seem to differ in pulmonary myocytes from those of systemic myocytes.

In many systemic vascular smooth muscle cells, large conductance Ca^{2+}-dependent K^+ channels are primarily important in this respect. These channels are activated by bursts of Ca^{2+}—referred to as "Ca^{2+} sparks"—from ryanodine receptors on the sarcoplasmic reticulum immediately underneath the plasmalemma. The sparks produce a marked elevation of $[Ca^{2+}]_i$ (10–100 μM) in a very localized region of the cell (≈1% of total cell volume) while increasing overall global $[Ca^{2+}]_i$ by less than 2 nM (56). An individual Ca^{2+} spark spreads immediately under the plasmalemma (rise time of ≈20 ms) and quickly dissipates (decay rate of 50–60 ms) as $[Ca^{2+}]_i$ is restored to resting levels via diffusion, reuptake of Ca^{2+} into the sarcoplasmic reticulum, extrusion by the plasmalemmal Ca^{2+} pump, and/or Ca^{2+}-buffering proteins. In the process, Ca^{2+}-dependent K^+ channels in the vicinity of the spark are briefly activated, giving rise to a "spontaneous transient outward current" (STOC). The physiological importance of these STOCs in providing an ongoing hyperpolarizing influence in the systemic vascular preparation is indicated by the membrane depolarization and contraction that are evoked upon depletion of the sarcoplasmic reticulum (e.g., using cyclopiazonic acid) or by inhibition of Ca^{2+} sparks (using ryanodine) or of Ca^{2+}-dependent K^+ channels.

Although Ca^{2+} sparks (57) and STOCs (51) have both been observed in PASM, they do not appear to be involved in setting resting V_m in the pulmonary vasculature, because charybdotoxin, iberiotoxin, and TEA generally do not cause membrane depolarization, elevate $[Ca^{2+}]_i$, or evoke contraction in these tissues (19,39,44,46,49,58). Instead, voltage-dependent K^+ channels appear to be responsible in the rat (19,39,43,46,48,52,58–60), dog (49), rabbit (4,44,50) and human, as indicated by the marked sensitivity of the outward currents in these tissues to 4-aminopyridine. These channels are available for activation at membrane potentials as negative as −60 mV (39,43,61) and are half-inactivated at potentials ranging from −45 to −30 mV (4,43,44,50). Resting membrane potential in rabbit pulmonary arterial smooth muscle cells appears to also derive from a novel noninactivating K^+ current (44,48,62) as well as ATP-sensitive K^+ channels (4,45,62).

Other ionic mechanisms may also contribute to the setting of V_m at rest. Ca^{2+} dependent Cl^- currents have been identified in certain pulmonary vascular preparations (25,63–66). The same mechanism which gives rise to STOCs at positive membrane potentials (i.e., Ca^{2+} sparks and Ca^{2+}-dependent K^+ currents) may cause these chloride currents to be activated at rest, manifesting as spontaneous transient inward currents (STICs), these have, in fact, been observed in rabbit PASM (64). Paradoxically, another group examined STICs in rabbit PASM, finding them to comprise nonselective cation currents (51). Whether or not these spontaneous currents represent Cl^- or nonselective cation currents, the net result is the displacement of V_m in the positive direction. Others have described volume-regulated chloride currents in PASM (55); these might also contribute to resting V_m.

How do agonists change membrane potential and thereby regulate voltage-dependent Ca^{2+} influx? According to Ohm's law, a change in voltage is directly related to a change in the product of current and resistance. At rest, there is no net change in current across the membrane, inward currents being balanced by outward currents. Depolarization, then, occurs when net inward current exceeds net outward current (e.g., an increase in inward current and/or decrease in outward current), whereas the reverse holds for hyperpolarization. With this in mind, several ionic mechanisms can be proposed for agonist-evoked membrane potential changes in pulmonary vasculature, some of which now have supporting experimental evidence. Given that vascular smooth muscle cells typically exhibit an input resistance on the order of 2–20 GΩ (4,50), only a small change in outward or inward currents can lead to substantial changes in membrane potential. For example, opening of a single large conductance Ca^{2+}-dependent K^+ channel or of a few smaller conductance channels can produce a membrane current of at least 1 pA (depending on the membrane potential at the time); in a pure resistor with input resistance of 10 GΩ, this would produce an instantaneous change in potential of 10 mV. However, in reality, this voltage change is filtered by the capacitance of the cell membrane, which is in series with the resistor (the ion channel per se). As such, the voltage change follows a trajectory determined by the time constant of the membrane (generally on the order of several seconds). In this way, the instantaneous changes in membrane current produced by flickering activity of hundreds or thousands of channels are smoothed out.

Hypoxia-Induced Membrane Depolarization

Hypoxia suppresses K^+ currents in pulmonary vascular smooth muscle cells (19,43,46,59,67,68). A great number of studies have been directed at elucidating the mechanism underlying K^+ current suppression during hypoxic pulmonary vasoconstriction. Its existence in single cells and in deendothelialized tissues (69) suggest that it is in part a direct effect on the muscle. Moreover, many of these studies indicate that the K^+ channel that is suppressed by hypoxia appears to be a member of the K_V family of K^+ channels (43,44,46,58,61), the same channels that are key in setting the resting membrane potential (above): their blockade pharmacologically is sufficient to evoke repetitive action potentials, elevate $[Ca^{2+}]_i$, and cause contraction (39,49).

There is still debate as to what exactly serves as the oxygen sensor. NADPH oxidase, an important oxygen sensor in other cell types, seems to have been ruled out in the pulmonary artery. Several lines of evidence indicate that the channels themselves might be the oxygen sensors. Other possibilities include P450, the mitochondrial electron transport chain, and/or the free radicals produced by them; K_V channels are apparently quite sensitive to the cellular redox potential (50,53,58). Others have shown that hypoxia triggers a release of internally sequestered Ca^{2+} that precedes the K^+ current suppression and depolarization (61,70) which suggests that the oxygen sensor is "upstream" of the K^+ channel and might be associated somehow with the sarcoplasmic reticulum. In addition to this relatively immediate effect on K^+ channel function, prolonged exposure to hypoxic conditions also leads to downregulation of the expression of K_V channels (67).

Hypoxia has other effects on ionic mechanisms. It suppresses voltage-dependent Ca^{2+} (22,37) and Ca^{2+}-dependent K^+ (68) currents. Although the latter effect may be due in part to the effect on voltage-dependent Ca^{2+} current, it was also shown that hypoxia causes a 30–50 mV shift in the voltage–activation relationship for the K^+ currents and reduced their sensitivity to nitric oxide and cyclic GMP (68). Finally, hypoxia also impairs Na^+/Ca^{2+} exchange (71) and Na^+/K^+-ATPase activities (69,72).

Agonist-Induced Membrane Depolarization

Voltage-dependent K^+ current is also suppressed by autacoids such as norepinephrine (73), endothelin (46,60,74), and angiotensin (46). This suppression is sensitive to inhibitors of protein kinase C (60); however, the specific role of PKC is yet unclear (i.e, whether it phosphorylates the channel or some other target).

Vasoconstrictors may also act through chloride channels (Fig. 4). In intact vascular smooth muscle cells, the chloride equilibrium potential (E_{Cl}) is somewhat more positive than the resting membrane potential (≈ -30 mV) (54), indicating an active pumping of chloride ion out of the cell. Patch-clamp electrophysiological recordings have revealed the presence in PASM of small conductance Cl^- channels that are gated by Ca^{2+}. These channels are activated by voltage-dependent Ca^{2+} influx, caffeine (which releases internally sequestered Ca^{2+}) (25,64–66,75), photolytically released Ca^{2+} (25,66), or spontaneous bursts of Ca^{2+} from the sarcoplasmic reticulum (64). As such, vasoconstrictors that trigger the classical phosphoinositide cascade and IP_3-induced Ca^{2+} release (see next section) can depolarize the membrane through activation of Ca^{2+}-dependent Cl^- current: these include norepinephrine (63,64,75), ATP (75), endothelin

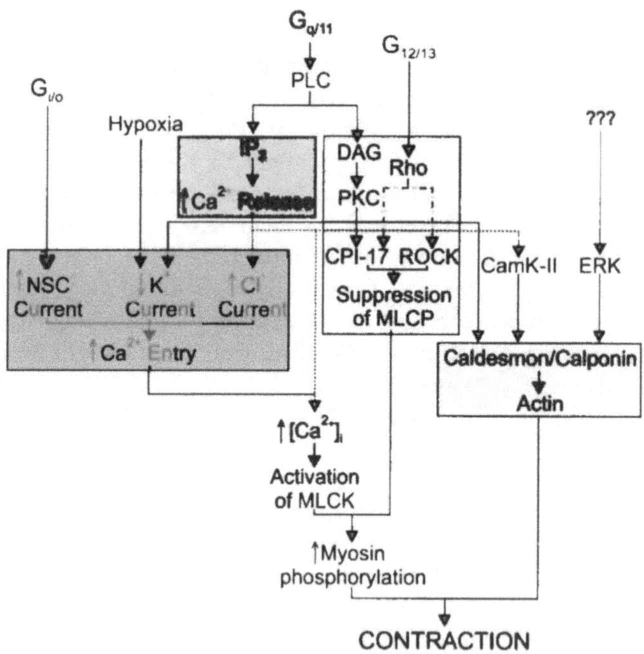

Figure 4 Excitatory signaling pathways. Overview of excitatory signaling events involving membrane depolarization, Ca^{2+} release, changes in Ca^{2+} sensitivity, and thin filament-mediated mechanisms. Vasoconstrictors act on receptors (not shown) coupled to the G proteins $G_{q,11}$, $G_{12,13}$, or Rho, which in turn trigger one or more of these signaling pathways, concluding with a constrictor response. See text for details. Abbreviations not defined in the text: DAG, diacylglycerol; NSC, nonselective cation; PKC, protein kinase C; PLC, phospholipase C.

(60,74), and histamine (75). These channels are also activated by metabolic inhibitors such as cyanide, apparently through disruption of Ca^{2+} handling and sustained elevation of $[Ca^{2+}]_i$ (63). Volume-regulated chloride currents present in these tissues (55) might also become activated during contraction owing to stretching of the membrane.

In addition to suppressing outward K^+ currents and/or increasing inward Cl^- currents, vasoconstrictors can depolarize vascular smooth muscle cells through activation of non selective cation channels (Fig. 4). These have been detected in rabbit PASM (51) [but were absent in rat small-order PASM (74)] and found to be Ca^{2+}-dependent. Therefore, they should also become activated during agonist-triggered release of internal Ca^{2+}, although this has not yet been shown.

Voltage-dependent Na^+ currents have been found in PASM (5) (see Chapter 10). These would not contribute to depolarization from the resting level, because the threshold for their activation is −30 mV; however, they could account for the action potentials observed when the membrane is sufficiently depolarized by other mechanisms (52,53). Like voltage-dependent Na^+ currents in other excitable cells, these rapidly inactivate in a voltage-dependent fashion.

Vasodilator-Induced Membrane Hyperpolarization

Membrane hyperpolarization, on the other hand, generally involves a net increase in outward current via activation of K^+ channels, although the type of K^+ channel and signaling pathway involved depends on the agonist used (Fig. 5).

Although K_{Ca} channels may be relatively unimportant in setting resting V_m of pulmonary vascular smooth muscle cells (above), they do mediate the hyperpolarizing effect of nitric oxide (19,38) or oxygen (41), because responses to these gases are generally blocked by TEA, charybdotoxin, or iberiotoxin. The Ca^{2+} dependence of these channels might suggest that the signaling pathway involves elevation of $[Ca^{2+}]_i$, perhaps via release of internally sequestered Ca^{2+} through ryanodine receptors into the subplasmalemmal space; paradoxically, however, fluorimetric recordings in PASM in fact show that global $[Ca^{2+}]_i$ is decreased by nitric oxide (52) (although it is still possible that $[Ca^{2+}]_i$ is elevated in discrete regions immediately under the membrane via release through ryanodine receptors). Pharmacological studies indicate that activation of these channels by nitric oxide and oxygen is a result of their phosphorylation by cGMP-dependent protein kinase (41,68). It is yet unclear whether this phosphorylation opens the channels directly or perhaps increases their sensitivity to Ca^{2+} such that basal $[Ca^{2+}]$ is sufficient for their activation. Vasodilators that act through cGMP seem to also enhance a plasmalemmal cGMP-dependent Na^+/K^+ ATPase activity (72), which could hyperpolarize the membrane and contribute to relaxation.

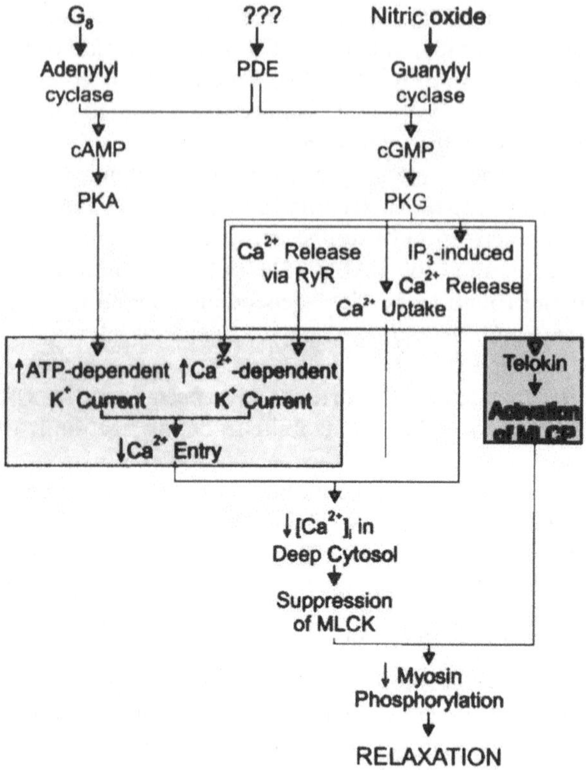

Figure 5 Inhibitory signaling pathways. Overview of inhibitory signaling events involving membrane depolarization, Ca^{2+} release, and changes in Ca^{2+} sensitivity. Vasodilators act through receptors (not shown) that couple through either adenylyl or guanylyl cyclases, which in turn activate cAMP- or cGMP-dependent protein kinases, respectively. The latter in turn exert a variety of effects on the signaling pathways, leading to relaxation. See text for details. Abbreviations not defined in the text: PKA, protein kinase A; PKG, protein kinase G.

On the other hand, vasodilators that act through receptors coupled to adenylate cyclase and cAMP production (e.g., adenosine, β-adrenergic agonists, and the prostaglandins E_2 and I_2) activate AT*P*-dependent K^+ currents (12) (Fig. 5). Endogenous phosphodiesterases (PDEs) regulate these effects via the breakdown of the key signaling molecule cAMP. Although PDE-1, -3, -4, and -5 isoforms are all present in PASM, pharmacological studies show that PDE-3, -4 and -5 are the most important in the control of pulmonary vascular tone (76).

Also, depending on the extent to which membrane potential is set by tonically active Cl^- or nonselective cation currents, suppression of these currents by vasodilators could also lead to membrane hyperpolarization. However, this has not yet been reported for pulmonary vasculature.

Suppression of Ca^{2+} Currents by Vasodilators

Some suggest that vasodilators can act by directly suppressing Ca^{2+} currents, as opposed to decreasing their activation through membrane hyperpolarization. The nitric oxide donor nitroprusside, for example, can reduce the peak magnitude of Ca^{2+} currents by nearly half in isolated rabbit pulmonary arterial smooth muscle cells (38); in addition, it accelerated inactivation of these currents. These effects required the presence of ATP in the electrode solution, suggesting that they involve a phosphorylation of some kind.

B. Release of Internally Sequestered Ca^{2+}

$[Ca^{2+}]_i$ at Rest

At rest, $[Ca^{2+}]_i$ in pulmonary arterial smooth muscle cells seems to be approximately 50–150 nM (20,52,70,77–80). This relatively low level is maintained through Ca^{2+} extrusion by pumps and Na^+/Ca^{2+} exchangers on the sarcolemma as well as through Ca^{2+} sequestration into the sarcoplasmic reticulum (by the internal Ca^{2+} pump, or SERCA) and into mitochondria [via an electrophoretic uniporter driven by the large electric potential across the inner membrane (71,78)].

The Superficial Buffer Barrier Hypothesis and Ca^{2+} Release

The sarcoplasmic reticulum not only serves to decrease $[Ca^{2+}]_i$ via Ca^{2+} uptake but also represents an important source of Ca^{2+} for physiological responses. In many nonpulmonary vascular, airway, and uterine smooth muscle preparations, the sarcoplasmic reticulum is arrayed in sheets around the internal periphery of the cell, thereby dividing the cytosol into two spaces: the peripheral space immediately underneath the plasmalemma, where ion channels are found (many of them being regulated by Ca^{2+}), and the deep cytosolic space where the contractile apparatus is found. In this way, the cell can dissociate the influence of $[Ca^{2+}]$ on mechanical and electrical activities; that is, plasmalemmal ion channels are sensitive to changes in $[Ca^{2+}]$ within the subsarcolemmal space, whereas the contractile apparatus is sensitive to such changes within the deep cytosol. The superficial buffer barrier hypothesis proposes that (1) the sarcoplasmic reticulum "buffers" the rise in $[Ca^{2+}]$ in the deep cytosolic space due to Ca^{2+} influx and (2) to unload the store, Ca^{2+} is preferentially directed toward the sarcolemmal Ca^{2+} pump and/or Na^+/Ca^{2+} exchangers. This arrangement has major implications for lung vascular physiology, as outlined below.

Release of sequestered Ca^{2+} involves two classes of Ca^{2+}-selective channels on the sarcoplasmic reticulum membrane. One, the IP_3 receptor, is a tetrameric complex possessing high affinity binding sites for the signaling molecule IP_3, the binding of which triggers a conformational change leading to the opening of a Ca^{2+}-selective aqueous pore down the central axis of the receptor and, thus, Ca^{2+} release from the sarcoplasmic reticulum. The second, often referred to as the ryanodine receptor (for its high affinity binding of that plant alkaloid), is regulated by a number of structurally unrelated agents including Ca^{2+}, caffeine, ryanodine, and cyclic ADP ribose.

In certain other types of smooth muscle, the IP_3 and ryanodine receptors are uniformly distributed or colocalized on the sarcoplasmic reticulum (SR) (57). In PASM, however, several studies suggest that the portions of sarcoplasmic reticulum bearing IP_3 receptors are distinct from those bearing ryanodine receptors (57). The functional significance of this spatial heterogeneity is unclear, but it may be related to the fact that constrictors act through IP_3-induced Ca^{2+} release (into the deep cytosol), whereas vasodilators act through Ca^{2+} sparks (in the subplasmalemmal space), as described in more detail below.

The ryanodine- and IP_3-gated channels are highly selective for Ca^{2+}. As such, loss of this divalent cation from the sarcoplasmic reticulum results in the accumulation of negative charge on the inner face of the SR membrane and a rising trans-SR membrane potential that impedes further Ca^{2+} release. Thus, efficient or sustained Ca^{2+} release requires the additional presence of ion channels that dissipate this trans-SR membrane potential. The channels involved in this function in pulmonary vasculature have not yet been investigated. However, in other cell types, these include various voltage-dependent K^+- and Cl^-- selective and nonselective cation channels; the voltage dependence of these channels directly couples their activation to Ca^{2+} release.

Refilling of the Sarcoplasmic Reticulum

Intuitively, the importance of Ca^{2+} release implies an equally important role for refilling of the internal Ca^{2+} pool. Of course, SERCA plays a major role in this context. However, given that a certain proportion of internal Ca^{2+} is ejected from the cell by the plasmalemmal Ca^{2+}-ATPase, Ca^{2+} store refilling also requires some Ca^{2+}-influx pathway to replace this lost fraction of Ca^{2+}, a process often referred to as "capacitative Ca^{2+} entry" (an allusion to the charging of a capacitor after it has been discharged). The entry of Ca^{2+} may be mediated by voltage-dependent Ca^{2+} channels and/or nonselective cation channels (if they are shown to be permeable to Ca^{2+}), both of which are activated upon agonist stimulation. In other cell types, refilling involves ion channels of the "transient receptor potential" or TRP family; RT-PCR studies have shown five different subtypes of these channels to be present in PASM (82). The relative contributions of voltage-dependent Ca^{2+} channels, nonselective cation channels, and TRP channels to store refilling is still unclear owing to the lack of sufficiently discriminating tools. For example, store refilling in PASM is sensitive to Ni^{2+} (82), which antagonizes all three types of channels, and to SKF96365 (80,81), which acts non-specifically on a wide variety of Ca^{2+}-related mechanisms. Many have shown that tyrosine kinase inhibition dramatically interferes with refilling of the sarcoplasmic reticulum (80,83) and markedly suppresses contractions in pulmonary arterial tissues (84,85), whereas PKC inhibition augments store refilling (83). However, little is known about the intracellular targets of these enzymes.

Agonist-Evoked Ca^{2+} Release

Many pulmonary vasoconstrictors act through classical heptahelical, G-protein-coupled receptors that enhance the activity of phospholipase C, leading to the generation of IP_3 and release of stored Ca^{2+}. These include norepinephrine (49,77,82,84), angiotensin II (20,65), endothelin (47), and ATP (65,78). The Ca^{2+} responses to these agents are typically biphasic, with a large initial spikelike elevation produced by IP_3-mediated release, followed by a smaller sustained elevation due to Ca^{2+} influx across the membrane (47).

Hypoxia (20,77,81) and inhibition of glycolysis (53) also cause release of internal Ca^{2+} through ryanodine receptors (77,81). This effect apparently precedes the K^+ current suppression and depolarization described above (61,70), which suggests that the sarcoplasmic reticulum or some related entity (e.g., the ryanodine receptor itself) might be the oxygen sensor. The mechanism by which hypoxia triggers this release is as yet unclear.

Vasodilators, on the other hand, cause a global decrease in $[Ca^{2+}]_i$ (52), driven largely by SERCA-mediated uptake of Ca^{2+} into the sarcoplasmic reticulum and/or extrusion from the cell by the plasmalemmal Ca^{2+} pump and Na^+/Ca^{2+} exchange. At the same time, the superficial buffer barrier hypothesis allows for the vasodilators to simultaneously trigger Ca^{2+} release from the sarcoplasmic reticulum; in this case, however, Ca^{2+} release is directed into the subplasmalemmal space and not the deep cytosol. In this way, the released Ca^{2+} (1) does not activate the contractile apparatus; (2) can activate Ca^{2+}-dependent K^+ channels, leading to membrane hyperpolarization and decreased Ca^{2+} influx; and (3) is available for extrusion from the cell by PMCA and Na^+/Ca^{2+} exchange, thereby increasing the buffering capacity of the sarcoplasmic reticulum. It is unlikely that vasodilator-induced Ca^{2+} release involves the IP_3-gated channels that mediate vasoconstriction. Instead, they may involve ryanodine receptors on regions of the sarcoplasmic reticulum that are distinct from those bearing IP_3-gated channels and may also be primarily facing the plasmalemma. According to this hypothesis, ryanodine receptors and IP_3 receptors play diametrically opposed roles in excitation–contraction coupling (vasodilation and vasoconstriction, respectively). Consistent with this, it has been shown in PASM that nitric oxide donors suppress Ca^{2+} release via IP_3 receptors but not that through ryanodine receptors (79) and that they increase STOC frequency (38) (also consistent with the Ca^{2+} spark model described above).

Calcium Ion Oscillations

One particularly interesting Ca^{2+}-related phenomenon seen in many cell types is the recurring change in $[Ca^{2+}]_i$ (referred to as "Ca^{2+}oscillations") that propagates throughout cells as "Ca^{2+} waves". These waves can convey information within their amplitudes (peak height as well as the mean or "plateau" amplitude) and in their frequency; this information may be decoded by Ca^{2+}/calmodulin-dependent kinase (Cam kinase II) (86,87), myosin light chain kinase (86), the SR Ca^{2+} pump (86), calpain, adenylyl cyclase, or mitochondria. Ca^{2+} oscillations are also seen in pulmonary vasculature, being evoked by α-adrenergic agonists (49,80), endothelin-1 (65,66,79,88), angiotensin-II (20,65), and ATP (65,78,79) in PASM of the rat (65,66,78,79,88), dog (49,80), sheep (20), and rabbit (5). Little is known about the cellular mechanisms underlying these events in the pulmonary artery—other than that they are mediated by IP_3 receptors (65,79,88) and are sensitive to cGMP but not to cGMP-dependent protein kinase (79)—and their physiological relevance in pulmonary artery/vein is completely unknown.

C. Changes in the Ca^{2+} Sensitivity of the Contractile Apparatus

As researchers continued to investigate excitation–contraction coupling in smooth muscle, evidence began to accumulate that although there was usually a tight correlation between $[Ca^{2+}]_i$, MLC_{20} phosphorylation, and contraction for a brief time after stimulation with certain spasmogens, this relationship broke down during long periods of stimulation ($[Ca^{2+}]_i$ and myosin phosphorylation both decreasing while contraction remained sustained) and/or during stimulation with certain other spasmogens. Clearly there must be some other mechanism underlying contraction. One solution to this apparent paradox involves an increased sensitivity of the contractile apparatus to Ca^{2+} such that even basal levels of $[Ca^{2+}]_i$ become sufficient to trigger contraction.

Recently, it was shown that excitatory agonists activate the monomeric G protein Rho, which goes on to activate Rho-activated kinase (ROCK); the latter is a serine/threonine kinase that phosphorylates the MLCP targeting subunit at threonine-695 and serine-854, dissociating MLCP and preventing it from binding to myosin (89). Because the phosphorylation of myosin by MLCK is a Ca^{2+}-dependent event, the suppression of MLCP activity by excitatory agonists effectively increases the Ca^{2+} sensitivity of the contractile apparatus (i.e., a greater net amount of myosin is phosphorylated for a given change in $[Ca^{2+}]_i$). Rho and ROCK have been visualized in PASM, and agonists that act in the pulmonary

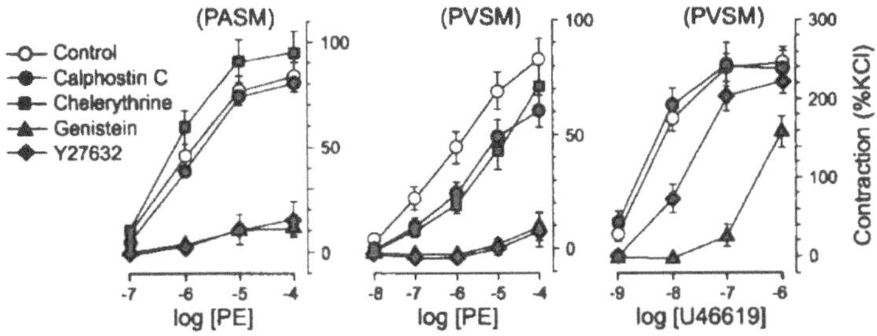

Figure 6 Pharmacological sensitivities of agonist-evoked responses Concentration–response relationships for phenylephrine (PE) or a thromboxane A2 analog (U46619) in pulmonary arterial or venous segments (PASM or PVSM, respectively) in the absence or presence of the protein kinase C inhibitors calphostin C (10^{-6}) or chelerythrine (10^{-6}), the tyrosine kinase inhibitor genistein (10^{-4}), or the Rho kinase inhibitor Y27632 (10^{-5}). (Data reproduced with permission from Ref. 84.)

vasculature through these signaling molecules include endothelin-1 and thromboxane A_2 (47,59,90) (see Fig. 6). The relative contribution of this pathway to excitatory responses appears to vary in an agonist-dependent fashion (84,89), which may have important implications for the treatment of pulmonary hypertension. Recent data suggest that the Rho/ROCK pathway may also be triggered by membrane depolarization alone (91).

In other vascular preparations, MLCP has been shown to be regulated by agonists in other ways. For example, CPI-17, an endogenous phosphoprotein, is the target of several kinases including protein kinase C, protein kinase N, and ROCK (Fig. 4); when phosphorylated by these proteins, CPI-17 inhibits MLCP activity. Nitric oxide, on the other hand, acts through PKG to phosphorylate telokin, which may then enhance MLCP activity (Fig. 4), although telokin's marked sequence homology with MLCK leads some researchers to conclude that it acts by competing with MLCK for myosin. It remains to be seen whether the same events occur in the pulmonary vasculature and whether or not agonists acting through PKA also modulate MLCP activity.

D. Thin-Filament-Mediated Excitation–Contraction Coupling Mechanisms

The excitation–contraction coupling mechanisms summarized above are all directed at the thick filament (myosin); that is, they are focused on the phosphorylation/dephosphorylation of MLC_{20}. Emerging data from smooth muscles other than pulmonary vasculature now also point to a number of thin filament- or actin-directed mechanisms underlying smooth muscle contraction. These pathways are summarized here, but it should be kept in mind that there is not yet any evidence that they are operative in the pulmonary circuit.

Calponin is a 35 kDa protein that interacts with F-actin and myosin and inhibits actomyosin ATPase activity (92). It is a substrate for PKC and Ca^{2+}/calmodulin-dependent protein kinase II (92) and the mitogen-activated protein kinase ERK (93) and is therefore subject to regulation by autacoids (Fig. 1). Upon stimulation with phenylephrine, for example, the mitogen-activated protein kinase ERK and protein kinase C (94,95) colocalize with calponin and then translocate to the cell membrane; thus, calponin might serve as an adapter protein, targeting ERK and PKC to the membrane. PKC activity increases upon association with calponin (95). ERK phosphorylation of calponin causes a conformational change in the latter, leading to removal of inhibition of actin. Finally, calponin also binds to other proteins associated with the contractile apparatus, including calmodulin and desmin, although the significance of this is unclear.

Caldesmon (90–100 kDa) is another thin-filament-associated protein that may play a role in excitation–contraction coupling. Like calponin, it binds to actin, myosin, and calmodulin and inhibits actomyosin ATPase activity. Upon PE stimulation, caldesmon becomes phosphorylated and associates with MAP kinase, whereupon both translocate to the membrane (93,96); inhibition of these events interferes with contraction, indicating a causal relationship (97). The affinity of caldesmon for actin (and thus its ability to inhibit actomyosin activity) is decreased by Ca^{2+}/calmodulin (via two high affinity binding sites on caldesmon), PKC, p21-activated kinase, or casein kinase, II, thereby providing regulatory pathways through which autacoids can act.

E. Kinases and Phosphatases in Excitation–Contraction Coupling

Most of the autacoids described above act through membrane-delimited receptors (an exception being nitric oxide, which acts on a cytosolic "receptor," guanylate cyclase) that in turn couple to a variety of enzymatic effectors and their downstream targets. Hypoxia can trigger similar enzymatic changes. At this point, then, it would be useful to collect the concepts described above into an overall scheme of excitation–contraction coupling in PASM (Figs. 4 and 5). At the same time, it is appropriate to summarize briefly a number of interesting parallels and divergences between the excitation-contraction coupling events and the biochemical events that result in cell proliferation, because the same stimuli that cause contraction upon acute exposure also cause hyperplasia and/or hypertrophy during chronic or sustained exposure.

Excitatory Stimuli

Many excitatory autacoids act on receptors coupled to $G_{q,11}$, which in turn triggers the phosphoinositide signal cascade, leading to the generation of IP_3, activation of MLCK (via IP_3-induced Ca^{2+} release), and contraction. Certain of these autacoids also act on receptors coupled to $G_{12/13}$, which activates Rho and its downstream target ROCK, leading to the suppression of MLCP.

Diacylglycerol is produced concurrently with IP_3 and goes on to enhance PKC activity. However, the specific PKC isoform that is activated seems to be stimulus-dependent; the Ca^{2+}-independent PKC-δ isozyme/CaM-dependent kinase III is enhanced by norepinephrine (98), angiotensin (98), and hypoxia (99), whereas Ca^{2+}-dependent PKC isozymes are activated only by angiotensin (98), and neither is activated by serotonin or the thromboxane analog U46619 (98). The target molecules for PKC include K^+ channels (46,60,73,74,98) and entities related to capacitative Ca^{2+} entry (83); downstream target(s) may also include enzymes of the eicosanoid pathway (e.g., cyclo-oxygenase).

Tyrosine kinases are also activated by autacoids (norepinephrine and angiotensin II) (84) and by hypoxia (85). However, little is known about the upstream effectors (unlike the receptors for many growth factors and mitogen-activated protein kinases, the receptors for spasmogens such as norepinephrine do not exhibit any tyrosine kinase activity) or the downstream targets, other than to say that tyrosine kinase inhibitors suppress capacitative Ca^{2+} entry and sarcoplasmic reticulum refilling (83) as well as K^+ channel activity (100).

Inhibitory Stimuli

Generally speaking, vasodilators produce the opposite change in MLCK activity via several pathways that culminate in decreased global $[Ca^{2+}]_i$. For example, nitric oxide acts though cGMP-dependent protein kinase to stimulate Ca^{2+}-dependent K^+ channels (19,38), while other agonists (e.g., adenosine, β-adrenergic agonists, and the prostaglandins E_2 and I_2) act through cAMP-dependent protein kinase to stimulate ATP-dependent K^+ channels (12); both actions lead indirectly to decreased voltage-dependent Ca^{2+} influx (via membrane hyperpolarization). Vasodilators can also inhibit voltage-dependent Ca^{2+} channels directly (38), enhance uptake of Ca^{2+} into the sarcoplasmic reticulum, and suppress its release by IP_3 (38,79).

Presumably, vasodilators could also act by directly stimulating MLCP activity and/or through some modulation of tyrosine kinase/phosphatase activities. However, this has not yet been reported for PASM.

Tyrosine Kinases

There is a complex relationship between tyrosine kinase activation and contraction. Whereas several of the autacoids listed above act on receptors that do not exhibit tyrosine kinase activity but nonetheless trigger tyrosine kinase–dependent contraction (84), they also stimulate tyrosine phosphorylation, which does not result in contraction. For example, endothelin-1 (101) and serotonin (102) enhance the activities of the mitogen-activated protein kinases ERK-1 and ERK-2, leading to a marked increase in threonine/tyrosine phosphorylation of p38 and JNK1, which in turn phosphorylate and activate the nuclear factor *c-jun* (101); likewise, the responses to serotonin appear to be mediated through stimulation of p21ras and p120 (GTPase-activating protein) (102). However, agonist-evoked contractions in these tissues are abolished by tyrosine kinase inhibitors but unaffected by inhibitors of p38 kinase (84).

Peroxide elicits tyrosine/threonine phosphorylation of ERK as well as a tyrosine kinase–dependent contraction, and both effects are suppressed by inhibition of PKC, of Ca^{2+} influx, and/or of Ca^{2+} release (103,104); however, PD98059 abolishes ERK activity with no effect on peroxide-evoked contraction (103). Like the response to autacoids, peroxide stimulation of ERK activity increases the expression of the early immediate gene *c-jun* (and *fra-1*) (104).

Finally, chronic hypoxia also stimulates phosphorylation and activation of JNK, followed several days later by similar changes in ERK and p38 kinase activities. Interestingly, this results in decreased gene expression of *c-jun* and *c-fos* (but up regulation of *egr-1* expression) (105), even though stimulation of JNK, ERK, and p38 by autacoids leads to up regulation of *c-jun* (101).

VI. PATHOPHYSIOLOGICAL PERSPECTIVE

To the same extent that excitation–contraction coupling is the physiologically relevant endpoint in smooth muscle, dysfunctions in this coupling can lead to devastating pathophysiological consequences. In this section we summarize some of these, highlighting in particular the excitation–contraction coupling mechanisms that contribute to them.

A. Chronic Hypoxia

The hypoxic pulmonary vasoconstrictor response in isolated subsegmental regions of the lung appears to play an important physiological role in ventilation–perfusion matching. However, chronic hypoxia or more globalized hypoxia (e.g., as in pulmonary embolism; lung diseases involving the airways and parenchyma, such as asthma chronic obstructive pulmonary disorder and acute respiratory distress syndrome; high altitude) can lead to pathological changes that mimic many of the sequellae of pulmonary hypertension. For this reason, chronic hypoxia has been used as a model of pulmonary hypertension in the hope that it might reveal the pathophysiological mechanisms underlying the latter. Resting $[Ca^{2+}]_i$ (20,47,70) and resting V_m (43,47,48,59) are markedly elevated in cells obtained from chronically hypoxic animals compared to controls, apparently as a result of altered expression of K^+ channel proteins (67), suppression of K^+ currents (summarized above), and Na^+/K^+ ATPase activity (69,72). Other relevant changes associated with hypoxia include suppression of Na^+/Ca^{2+} exchange (71), Ca^{2+} currents (37), and nitric oxide production (106).

Despite its many similarities with pulmonary hypertension, however, experimentally induced chronic hypoxia may not be an adequate model for this disease state. Although preventing Ca^{2+} influx (e.g., using channel blockers or removing external Ca^{2+}) is highly effective in reversing the hypoxic response in tissues or cells (20,53,70), it is generally ineffective in pulmonary hypertension (see Sec. VI. D). Clearly, other mechanisms are responsible for pulmonary hypertension.

B. Inflammation

Inflammation is a prominent feature in pulmonary hypertension and acute lung injury but not necessarily in chronic hypoxia. Inflammation, in turn, triggers many pathological changes in vascular function. Experimentally induced inflammation (allergen sensitization) markedly increases the sensitivity of pulmonary vascular smooth muscle to vasoconstrictors (107,108) (interestingly, this is particularly true of the venous vasculature, again emphasizing the need to include venous preparations in experimental studies). The proinflammatory cytokines interleukin-1β and tumor necrosis factor α induce a marked increase in synthesis and release of inflammatory mediators (thromboxane A_2, leukotrienes B_4, C_4, D_4, and 15-HETE) (109) and endothelin (110) from PASM. Powerful constrictor responses are evoked by cysteinyl leukotrienes (7,18), TXA_2 (10,90), and endothelin (10,47,66,74), and these responses are further augmented by hypoxia (7,59).

C. Oxidative Stress and Isoprostanes

Hypoxia and inflammation are both accompanied by the generation of a wide variety of free radicals and reactive oxygen species. These may act directly on ion channels, ion pumps, and the contractile apparatus, potentially leading to changes in excitation–contraction coupling (103). In addition, they act on membrane lipids, producing a variety of "membrane breakdown products." One of these is a class of molecules derived (nonenzymatically) from arachidonic acid and collectively referred to as isoprostanes (111); pulmonary hypertension and acute lung injury are both accompanied by marked accumulation of isoprostanes (112,113). Isoprostanes have generally been used as markers of oxidative stress, but without any apparent consideration that they might in fact be mediators in this process. Recently, several groups described powerful vasoconstrictor effects of isoprostanes on pulmonary vascular smooth muscle (90,111). This vasoconstriction appears to be exerted primarily through a thromboxane-selective prostanoid receptor (111), with an additional contribution in the pulmonary vein from a prostaglandin E_2-selective receptor (90), although the possibility that there is an isoprostane-selective receptor is still debated (111).

Acute lung injury and pulmonary hypertension are associated with increased metabolism of arachidonic acid and are sensitive to inhibitors of TP receptors (114–118). One interpretation of these data poses a central role for TXA_2, but recent data linking superoxide and peroxide to these changes, coupled with the finding that these disease states are accompanied by accumulation of isoprostanes (112,113,119), raise the possibility that isoprostanes may play one or more important causal roles in these pathological states. Isoprostanes are released by pulmonary arterial endothelial cells stimulated with H_2O_2 (120) and by deendothelialized pulmonary arterial smooth muscle cells upon stimulation with growth factors (platelet-derived growth factor, transforming growth factor β), proinflammatory cytokines (TNFα, interferon γ, and IL-1β), peroxide, or superoxide (121,122). Exposure of vascular smooth muscle cells to peroxide causes accumulation of isoprostanes, expression of preproendothelin mRNA, and production of endothelin-1 (123). Another group showed that isoprostanes stimulate production of endothelin-1 in pulmonary arterial smooth muscle cells and that hypoxia-induced pulmonary hypertension (as indicated by hypertrophy and increased levels of endothelin-1 and isoprostane) could be prevented by a thromboxane receptor blocker (L670596) but not a COX-2 inhibitor (114,124), suggesting strongly that isoprostanes play a key role in pulmonary hypertension.

D. Primary Pulmonary Hypertension

Primary pulmonary hypertension is that clinical label given to pulmonary hypertension (mean resting pulmonary arterial pressure greater than 25 mmHg) that cannot be attributed to some specific cause such as hypoxia (as outlined above). Many have investigated whether excitation–contraction coupling is altered as a result of the release of one or more autacoids from the endothelium, platelets, or various inflammatory cells. However, the possibility also exists that there is some change intrinsic to the vascular smooth muscle per se. One group has described changes in the function of voltage-dependent K^+ channels in cells taken from patients with primary pulmonary hypertension (125). There is also renewed interest in the role of α_1-adrenoceptors in this disease state (126). In addition to the functional changes described above, there is marked hypertrophy of the vessel wall; the mechanisms underlying this change are beyond the scope of the current review but are likely related to the overlap between the signaling pathways mediating excitation–contraction coupling and proliferation, as outlined above.

In light of the success experienced with vasodilator treatments for systemic hypertension, the same approach was taken for treating pulmonary hypertension, beginning with an α-adrenoceptor antagonist (tolalozine), later to be accompanied by Ca^{2+} channel blockers (e.g., verapamil, nifedipine) (127), nitric oxide donors (e.g., hydralazine) (128), and inhaled nitric oxide (106,129). Although perhaps useful in some cases, in general the results have been disappointing; these agents can often markedly drop systemic blood pressures but bring about little or no therapeutic benefit in the pulmonary circuit (127).

Prostacyclin is a powerful vasodilator, and recently prostacyclin analogs such as iloprost and epoprostanol have become the gold standard for treatment of pulmonary hypertension. However, even this approach is not effective in all patients, and "responders" are often plagued by the development of tolerance (likely via desensitization of the IP receptor), requiring repeated dose escalation. Given that prostacyclin acts through cAMP generation, phosphodiesterase inhibitors have proven useful in amplifying and/or prolonging the vasodilator actions of this drug (76).

What is needed, then, is a vasodilator that has a greater effect in the pulmonary circuit than in the systemic circuit. One approach is to selectively deliver the drug to the pulmonary vessels—e.g., via inhalation and/or providing a drug that becomes activated as it passes through the lungs—and minimize delivery to the systemic circulation. Alternatively, it might become possible to identify or design a class of drugs that capitalize on some excitation–contraction coupling mechanism that is unique to the pulmonary circulation. However, this approach has not yet met with success. Before this can happen, it is paramount that further studies be conducted to gain a better understanding of excitation–contraction coupling pathways in the lung.

VII. FUTURE DIRECTIONS

Of course, a major objective for the near future is to devise newer and better treatments for pulmonary hypertension and other pulmonary vascular disorders. To this end, the studies of pulmonary vascular physiology that have been done have been very limited—the majority having used the pulmonary artery, usually conduit rather than resistance portions, and often from the rat—which may account for the relative lack of success in solving the problem of pulmonary hypertension. As outlined earlier in Section V, there is just too much heterogeneity (species-, tissue-, and size-related) to justify this approach, especially given that the hypoxic vasoconstrictor response is relatively stronger in the pulmonary vein than in the artery (11). Likewise, the overwhelming use of rat tissues may be shortsighted, given that rat pulmonary artery relaxes poorly or may even contract (31) in response to prostacyclin, which is presently the gold standard for therapy of pulmonary hypertension in humans. The use of smaller vessels, both artery and vein (since both are equally important in determining pulmonary vascular resistance), is strongly advocated.

Also, there has been a strong emphasis on electromechanical mechanisms, particularly the role of K^+ channels in hypoxia. However, given that Ca^{2+} channel blockers are not very effective in the therapy of pulmonary hypertension, a great deal more effort should be directed toward the study of other excitation–contraction coupling mechanisms. The phenomenon of increased Ca^{2+} sensitivity of the contractile apparatus (particularly that mediated by Rho and Rho-activated kinase [ROCK]) has garnered much attention in the systemic vasculature but has received little attention in the pulmonary vascular field. Even less has been done with respect to thin-filament-mediated mechanisms of excitation–contraction coupling in pulmonary vasculature.

REFERENCES

1. Davies P, Burke G, Reid L. The structure of the wall of the rat intraacinar pulmonary artery: an electron microscopic study of microdissected preparations. Microvasc Res 1986; 32:50–63.
2. Small JV, Gimona M. The cytoskeleton of the vertebrate smooth muscle cell. Acta Physiol Scand 1998; 164:341–348.
3. Vale RD, Milligan RA. The way things move: looking under the hood of molecular motor proteins. Science 2000; 288:88–95.
4. Clapp LH, Gurney AM. Outward currents in rabbit pulmonary artery cells dissociated with a new technique. Exp Physiol 1991; 76:677–693.
5. Okabe K, Kitamura K, Kuriyama H. The existence of a highly tetrodotoxin sensitive Na channel in freshly dispersed smooth muscle cells of the rabbit main pulmonary artery. Pflügers Arch 1988; 411:423–428.
6. Sobieszek A, Small JV. Regulation of the actin-myosin interaction in vertebrate smooth muscle: activation via a myosin light-chain kinase and the effect of tropomyosin. J Mol Biol 1977; 112:559–576.
7. Paterson NA, Hamilton JT, Yaghi A, Miller DS. Effect of hypoxia on responses of respiratory smooth muscle to histamine and LTD4. J Appl Physiol 1988; 64:435–440.
8. Ohtaka H, Tsang JY, Foster A, Hogg JC, Schellenberg RR. Comparative effects of leukotrienes on porcine pulmonary circulation in vitro and in vivo. J Appl Physiol 1987; 63:582–588.
9. Schellenberg RR, Foster A. Differential activity of leukotrienes upon human pulmonary vein and artery. Prostaglandins 1984; 273:475–482.
10. Kemp BK, Smolich JJ, Cocks TM. Evidence for specific regional patterns of responses to different vasoconstrictors and vasodilators in sheep isolated pulmonary arteries and veins. Br J Pharmacol 1997; 121:441–450.
11. Zhao Y, Packer CS, Rhoades RA. The vein utilizes different sources of energy than the artery during pulmonary hypoxic vasoconstriction. Exp Lung Res 1996; 22:51–63.

12. Gao Y, Zhou H, Ibe BO, Raj JU. Prostaglandins E_2 and I_2 cause greater relaxations in pulmonary veins than in arteries of newborn lambs. J Appl Physiol 1996; 81:2534–2539.
13. Zellers TM, McCormick J, Wu Y. Interaction among ET-1, endothelium-derived nitric oxide, and prostacyclin in pulmonary arteries and veins. Am J Physiol 1994; 267:H139–H147.
14. Sai Y, Okamura T, Amakata Y, Toda N. Comparison of responses of canine pulmonary artery and vein to angiotensin II, bradykinin and vasopressin. Eur J Pharmacol 1995; 282:235–241.
15. Steinhorn RH, Morin FC, Gugino SF, Giese EC, Russell JA. Developmental differences in endothelium-dependent responses in isolated ovine pulmonary arteries and veins. Am J Physiol 1993; 264:H2162–H2167.
16. Michelakis ED, Weir EK, Wu X, Nsair A, Waite R, Hashimoto K, et al. Potassium channels regulate tone in rat pulmonary veins. Am J Physiol Lung Cell Mol Physiol 2001; 280:L1138–L1147.
17. Sudjarwo SA, Hori M, Takai M, Urade Y, Okada T, Karaki H. A novel subtype of endothelin B receptor mediating contraction in swine pulmonary vein. Life Sci 1993; 53:431–437.
18. Labat C, Ortiz JL, Norel X, Gorenne I, Verley J, Abram TS, et al. A second cysteinyl leukotriene receptor in human lung. J Pharmacol Exp Ther 1992; 263:800–805.
19. Archer SL, Huang JM, Reeve HL, Hampl V, Tolarova S, Michelakis E, et al. Differential distribution of electrophysiologically distinct myocytes in conduit and resistance arteries determines their response to nitric oxide and hypoxia. Circ Res 1996; 78:431–442.
20. Cornfield DN, Stevens T, McMurtry IF, Abman SH, Rodman DM. Acute hypoxia increases cytosolic calcium in fetal pulmonary artery smooth muscle cells. Am J Physiol 1993; 265:L53–L56.
21. Madden JA, Dawson CA, Harder DR. Hypoxia-induced activation in small isolated pulmonary arteries from the cat. J Appl Physiol 1985; 59: q113–118.
22. Franco-Obregon A, Lopez-Barneo J. Differential oxygen sensitivity of calcium channels in rabbit smooth muscle cells of conduit and resistance pulmonary arteries. J Physiol 1996; 491:511–518.
23. Domkowski PW, Cockerham JT, Kot PA, Myers JL, Wallace RB, Hopkins RA. The role of N omega-nitro-L-arginine in modulation of pulmonary vascular tone in the maturing newborn pig. J Thoracic Cardiovasc Surg 1995; 110:1486–1492.
24. Albarwani S, Heinert G, Turner JL, Kozlowski RZ. Differential K^+ channel distribution in smooth muscle cells isolated from the pulmonary arterial tree of the rat. Biochem Biophys Res Commun 1995; 208:183–189.
25. Clapp LH, Turner JL, Kozlowski RZ. Ca^{2+}-activated Cl- currents in pulmonary arterial myocytes. Am J Physiol 1996; 270:H1577–H1584.
26. Smani T, Iwabuchi S, Lopez-Barneo J, Urena J. Differential segmental activation of Ca^{2+}-dependent $Cl^-$and K^+ channels in pulmonary arterial myocytes. Cell Calcium 2001; 29:369–377.

27. Urena J, Franco-Obregon A, Lopez-Barneo J. Contrasting effects of hypoxia on cytosolic Ca^{2+} spikes in conduit and resistance myocytes of the rabbit pulmonary artery. J Physiol 1996; 496:103–109.
28. Suzuki H, Twarog BM. Membrane properties of smooth muscle cells in pulmonary arteries of the rat. Am J Physiol 1982; 242:H900–H906.
29. Frid MG, Moiseeva EP, Stenmark KR. Multiple phenotypically distinct smooth muscle cell populations exist in the adult and developing bovine pulmonary arterial media in vivo. Circ Res 1994; 754:669–681.
30. Hadhazy P, Malomvolgyi B, Magyar K, Debreczeni LA, Hutas I. Species dependent relaxation of intrapulmonary arteries (IPA) of rabbits, dogs and humans by prostacyclin. Prostaglandins 1985; 29:673–688.
31. Zhao YJ, Wang J, Tod ML, Rubin LJ, Yuan XJ. Pulmonary vasoconstrictor effects of prostacyclin in rats: potential role of thromboxane receptors. J Appl Physiol 1996; 81:2595–2603.
32. Haynes J Jr, Obiako B, Thompson WJ, Downey J. Adenosine-induced vasodilation: receptor characterization in pulmonary circulation. Am J Physiol 1995; 268:H1862–H1868.
33. McCormack DG, Clarke B, Barnes PJ. Characterization of adenosine receptors in human pulmonary arteries. Am J Physiol 1989; 256:H41–H46.
34. Neely CF, Haile DM, Cahill BE, Kadowitz PJ. Adenosine and ATP produce vasoconstriction in the feline pulmonary vascular bed by different mechanisms. J Pharmacol Exp Ther 1991; 258:753–761.
35. Evans AM, Osipenko ON, Haworth SG, Gurney AM. Resting potentials and potassium currents during development of pulmonary artery smooth muscle cells. Am J Physiol 1998; 275:H887–H899.
36. Reeve HL, Weir EK, Archer SL, Cornfield DN. A maturational shift in pulmonary K^+ channels, from Ca^{2+} sensitive to voltage dependent. Am J Physiol 1998; 275:L1019–L1025.
37. Franco-Obregon A, Lopez-Barneo J. Low PO_2 inhibits calcium channel activity in arterial smooth muscle cells. Am J Physiol 1996; 271: H2290–H2299.
38. Clapp LH, Gurney AM. Modulation of calcium movements by nitroprusside in isolated vascular smooth muscle cells. Pflügers Arch 1991; 418:462–470.
39. Yuan XJ. Voltage-gated K^+ currents regulate resting membrane potential and $[Ca^{2+}]_i$ in pulmonary arterial myocytes. Circ Res 1995; 77:370–378.
40. Nelson MT, Quayle JM. Physiological roles and properties of potassium channels in arterial smooth muscle. Am J Physiol 1995; 268:C799–C822.
41. Cornfield DN, Reeve HL, Tolarova S, Weir EK, Archer S. Oxygen causes fetal pulmonary vasodilation through activation of a calcium-dependent potassium channel. Proc Natl Acad Sci USA 1996; 93:8089–8094.
42. Fujii K, Kuriyama H. Effects of YM-12617, an alpha adrenoceptor blocking agent, on electrical and mechanical properties of the guinea-pig mesenteric and pulmonary arteries. J Pharmacol Exp Ther 1985; 235:764–770.
43. Smirnov SV, Robertson TP, Ward JP, Aaronson PI. Chronic hypoxia is associated with reduced delayed rectifier K^+ current in rat pulmonary artery muscle cells. Am J Physiol 1994; 266:H365–H370.

44. Osipenko ON, Evans AM, Gurney AM. Regulation of the resting potential of rabbit pulmonary artery myocytes by a low threshold, O_2-sensing potassium current. Br J Pharmacol 1997; 120:1461–1470.
45. Clapp LH, Gurney AM. ATP-sensitive K^+ channels regulate resting potential of pulmonary arterial smooth muscle cells. Am J Physiol 1992; 262: H916–H920.
46. Shimoda LA, Sylvester JT, Sham JSK. Chronic hypoxia alters effects of endothelin and angiotensin on K^+ currents in pulmonary arterial myocytes. Am J Physiol 1999; 277:L431–L439.
47. Shimoda LA, Sham JSK, Shimoda TH, Sylvester JT. L-type Ca^{2+} channels, resting $[Ca^{2+}]_i$, and ET-1-induced responses in chronically hypoxic pulmonary myocytes. Am J Physiol Lung Cell Mol Physiol 2000; 279:L884–L894.
48. Osipenko ON, Alexander D, MacLean MR, Gurney AM. Influence of chronic hypoxia on the contributions of non-inactivating and delayed rectifier K currents to the resting potential and tone of rat pulmonary artery smooth muscle. Br J Pharmacol 1998; 124:1335–1337.
49. Doi S, Damron DS, Ogawa K, Tanaka S, Horibe M, Murray PA. K^+ channel inhibition, calcium signaling, and vasomotor tone in canine pulmonary artery smooth muscle. Am J Physiol Lung Cell Mol Physiol 2000; 279:L242–L251.
50. Park MK, Bae YM, Lee SH, Ho WK, Earm YE. Modulation of voltage-dependent K^+ channel by redox potential in pulmonary and ear arterial smooth muscle cells of the rabbit. Pflügers Arch 1997; 434:764–771.
51. Bae YM, Park MK, Lee SH, Ho WK, Earm YE. Contribution of Ca^{2+}-activated K^+ channels and non-selective cation channels to membrane potential of pulmonary arterial smooth muscle cells of the rabbit. J Physiol 1999; 514:747–758.
52. Yuan XJ, Tod ML, Rubin LJ, Blaustein MP. NO hyperpolarizes pulmonary artery smooth muscle cells and decreases the intracellular Ca^{2+} concentration by activating voltage-gated K^+ channels. Proc Natl Acad Sci USA 1996; 93:10489–10494.
53. Yuan XJ, Tod ML, Rubin LJ, Blaustein MP. Deoxyglucose and reduced glutathione mimic effects of hypoxia on K^+ and Ca^{2+} conductances in pulmonary artery cells. Am J Physiol 1994; 267:L52–L63.
54. Chipperfield AR, Harper AA. Chloride in smooth muscle. Prog Biophys Mol Biol 2000; 74:175–221.
55. Yamazaki J, Duan D, Janiak R, Kuenzli K, Horowitz B, Hume JR. Functional and molecular expression of volume-regulated chloride channels in canine vascular smooth muscle cells. J Physiol 1998; 507:729–736.
56. Jaggar JH, Porter VA, Lederer WJ, Nelson MT. Calcium sparks in smooth muscle. Am J Physiol Cell Physiol 2000; 278:C235–C256.
57. Janiak R, Wilson SM, Montague S, Hume JR. Heterogeneity of calcium stores and elementary release events in canine pulmonary arterial smooth muscle cells. Am J Physiol Cell Physiol 2001; 280:C22–C33.
58. Yuan XJ, Tod ML, Rubin LJ, Blaustein MP. Hypoxic and metabolic regulation of voltage-gated K^+ channels in rat pulmonary artery smooth muscle cells. Exp Physiol 1995; 80:803–813.

59. Doggrell SA, Wanstall JC, Gambino A. Functional effects of 4-aminopyridine (4-AP) on pulmonary and systemic vessels from normoxic control and hypoxic pulmonary hypertensive rats. Naunyn Schmiedebergs Arch Pharmacol 1999; 360:317–323.
60. Shimoda LA, Sylvester JT, Sham JSK. Inhibition of voltagegated K^+ current in rat intrapulmonary arterial myocytes by endothelin-1. Am J Physiol 1998; 274:L842–L853.
61. Post JM, Gelband CH, Hume JR. $[Ca^{2+}]_i$ inhibition of K^+ channels in canine pulmonary artery. Novel mechanism for hypoxia-induced membrane depolarization. Circ Res 1995; 77:131–139.
62. Evans AM, Osipenko ON, Gurney AM. Properties of a novel K^+ current that is active at resting potential in rabbit pulmonary artery smooth muscle cells. J Physiol 1996; 496:407–420.
63. Wang Q, Wang YX, Yu M, Kotlikoff MI. Ca^{2+}-activated Cl^- currents are activated by metabolic inhibition in rat pulmonary artery smooth muscle cells. Am J Physiol 1997; 273:C520–C530.
64. Hogg RC, Wang Q, Helliwell RM, Large WA. Properties of spontaneous inward currents in rabbit pulmonary artery smooth muscle cells. Pflügers Arch 1993; 425:233–240.
65. Guibert C, Marthan R, Savineau JP. Oscillatory Cl^- current induced by angiotensin II in rat pulmonary arterial myocytes: Ca^{2+} dependence and physiological implication. Cell Calcium 1997; 21:421–429.
66. Salter KJ, Turner JL, Albarwani S, Clapp LH, Kozlowski RZ. Ca^{2+}-activated Cl^- and K^+ channels and their modulation by endothelin-1 in rat pulmonary arterial smooth muscle cells. Exp Physiol 1995; 80:815–824.
67. Platoshyn O, Yu Y, Golovina VA, McDaniel SS, Krick S, Li L, et al. Chronic hypoxia decreases K_V channel expression and function in pulmonary artery myocytes. Am J Physiol Lung Cell Mol Physiol 2001; 280:L801–L812.
68. Peng W, Hoidal JR, Karwande SV, Farrukh IS. Effect of chronic hypoxia on K^+ channels: regulation in human pulmonary vascular smooth muscle cells. Am J Physiol 1997; 272:C1271–C1278.
69. Hoshino Y, Morrison KJ, Vanhoutte PM. Mechanisms of hypoxic vasoconstriction in the canine isolated pulmonary artery: role of endothelium and sodium pump. Am J Physiol 1994; 267:L120–L127.
70. Salvaterra CG, Goldman WF. Acute hypoxia increases cytosolic calcium in cultured pulmonary arterial myocytes. Am J Physiol 1993; 264: L323–L328.
71. Wang YX, Dhulipala PK, Kotlikoff MI. Hypoxia inhibits the Na^+/Ca^{2+} exchanger in pulmonary artery smooth muscle cells. FASEB J 2000; 14: 1731–1740.
72. Tamaoki J, Tagaya E, Yamawaki I, Konno K. Hypoxia impairs nitrovasodilator-induced pulmonary vasodilation: role of Na-K-ATPase activity. Am J Physiol 1996; 271:L172–L177.
73. Janssen LJ, Mardi K, Netherton S, Betti PA. Nitric oxide inhibits human and canine pulmonary vascular tone via a postjunctional, nonelectromechanical, cGMP-dependent pathway. Can J Physiol Pharmacol 1999; 77:320–329.

74. Salter KJ, Kozlowski RZ. Differential electrophysiological actions of endothelin-1 on Cl^- and K^+ currents in myocytes isolated from aorta, basilar and pulmonary artery. J Pharmacol Exp Ther 1998; 284:1122–1131.
75. Helliwell RM, Wang Q, Hogg RC, Large WA. Synergistic action of histamine and adenosine triphosphate on the response to noradrenaline in rabbit pulmonary artery smooth muscle cells. Pflügers Arch 1994; 426:433–439.
76. Rabe KF, Tenor H, Dent G, Schudt C, Nakashima M, Magnussen H. Identification of PDE isozymes in human pulmonary artery and effect of selective PDE inhibitors. Am J Physiol 1994; 266:L536–L543.
77. Vadula MS, Kleinman JG, Madden JA. Effect of hypoxia and norepinephrine on cytoplasmic free Ca^{2+} in pulmonary and cerebral arterial myocytes. Am J Physiol 1993; 265:L591–L597.
78. Drummond RM, Tuft RA. Release of Ca^{2+} from the sarcoplasmic reticulum increases mitochondrial [Ca^{2+}] in rat pulmonary artery smooth muscle cells. J Physiol 1999; 516:139–147.
79. Pauvert O, Marthan R, Savineau J. NO-induced modulation of calcium-oscillations in pulmonary vascular smooth muscle. Cell Calcium 2000; 27: 329–338.
80. Doi S, Damron DS, Horibe M, Murray PA. Capacitative Ca^{2+} entry and tyrosine kinase activation in canine pulmonary arterial smooth muscle cells. Am J Physiol Lung Cell Mol Physiol 2000; 278:L118–L130.
81. Jabr RI, Toland H, Gelband CH, Wang XX, Hume JR. Prominent role of intracellular Ca^{2+} release in hypoxic vasoconstriction of canine pulmonary artery. Br J Pharmacol 1997; 122:21–30.
82. McDaniel SS, Platoshyn O, Wang J, Yu Y, Sweeney M, Krick S, et al. Capacitative Ca^{2+} entry in agonist-induced pulmonary vasoconstriction. Am J Physiol Lung Cell Mol Physiol 2001; 280:L870–L880.
83. Horibe M, Kondo I, Damron DS, Murray PA. Propofol attenuates capacitative calcium entry in pulmonary artery smooth muscle cells. Anesthesiology 2001; 95:681–688.
84. Janssen LJ, Lu-Chao H, Netherton S. Excitation–contraction coupling in pulmonary vascular smooth muscle involves tyrosine kinase and Rho kinase. Am J Physiol Lung Cell Mol Physiol 2001; 280:L666–L674.
85. Uzun O, Demiryurek AT, Kanzik I. The role of tyrosine kinase in hypoxic constriction of sheep pulmonary artery rings. Eur J Pharmacol 1998; 358:41–47.
86. Davis JP, Tikunova SB, Walsh MP, Johnson JD. Characterizing the response of calcium signal transducers to generated calcium transients. Biochemistry 1999; 38:4235–4244.
87. Dupont G, Goldbeter A. CaM kinase II as frequency decoder of Ca^{2+} oscillations. Bioessays 1998; 20:607–610.
88. Hyvelin JM, Guibert C, Marthan R, Savineau JP. Cellular mechanisms and role of endothelin-1-induced calcium oscillations in pulmonary arterial myocytes. Am J Physiol 1998; 275:L269–L282.
89. Shin HM, Je HD, Gallant C, Tao TC, Hartshorne DJ, Ito M, Morgan KE. Differential association and localization of myosin phosphatase subunits

during agonist-induced signal transduction in smooth muscle. Circ Res 2002; 90:546–553.
90. Janssen LJ, Tazzeo T. Involvement of TP and EP_3 receptors in vasoconstrictor responses to isoprostanes in pulmonary vasculature. J Pharmacol Exp Ther 2002; 301:1060–1066.
91. Mita M, Yanagihara H, Hishinuma S, Saito M, Walsh MP. Membrane depolarization-induced contraction of rat caudal arterial smooth muscle involves Rho-associated kinase. Biochem J 2002; 364:431–440.
92. Winder SJ, Allen BG, Clement-Chomienne O, Walsh MP. Regulation of smooth muscle actin-myosin interaction and force by calponin. Acta Physiol Scand 1998; 164:415–426.
93. Gerthoffer WT. Regulation of the contractile element of airway smooth muscle. Am J Physiol 1991; 261:L15–L28.
94. Menice CB, Hulvershorn J, Adam LP, Wang CA, Morgan KG. Calponin and mitogen-activated protein kinase signaling in differentiated vascular smooth muscle. J Biol Chem 1997; 272:25157–25161.
95. Leinweber B, Parissenti AM, Gallant C, Gangopadhyay SS, Kirwan-Rhude A, Leavis PC, et al. Regulation of protein kinase C by the cytoskeletal protein calponin. J Biol Chem 2000; 275:40329–40336.
96. Khalil RA, Menice CB, Wang CL, Morgan KG. Phosphotyrosine-dependent targeting of mitogen-activated protein kinase in differentiated contractile vascular cells. Circ Res 1995; 76:1101–1108.
97. Dessy C, Kim I, Sougnez CL, Laporte R, Morgan KG. A role for MAP kinase in differentiated smooth muscle contraction evoked by alpha-adrenoceptor stimulation. Am J Physiol 1998; 275:C1081–C1086.
98. De Witt BJ, Kaye AD, Ibrahim IN, Bivalacqua TJ, D'Souza FM, Banister RE, Arif AS, Dossaman BD. Effects of PKC isozyme inhibitors on constrictor responses in the feline pulmonary vascular bed. Am J Physiol Lung Cell Mol Physiol 2001; 280:L50–L57.
99. Barman SA. Effect of protein kinase C inhibition on hypoxic pulmonary vasoconstriction. Am J Physiol Lung Cell Mol Physiol 2001; 280:L888–L895.
100. Smirnov SV, Aaronson PI. Inhibition of vascular smooth muscle cell K^+ currents by tyrosine kinase inhibitors genistein and ST 638. Circ Res 1995; 76:310–316.
101. Yamboliev IA, Hruby A, Gerthoffer WT. Endothelin-1 activates MAP kinases and *c-Jun* in pulmonary artery smooth muscle. Pulm Pharmacol Ther 1998; 11:205–208.
102. Lee SL, Wang WW, Finlay GA, Fanburg BL. Serotonin stimulates mitogen-activated protein kinase activity through the formation of superoxide anion. Am J Physiol 1999; 277:L282–L291.
103. Pelaez NJ, Osterhaus SL, Mak AS, Zhao Y, Davis HW, Packer CS. MAPK and PKC activity are not required for H_2O_2-induced arterial muscle contraction. Am J Physiol Heart Circ Physiol 2000; 279:H1194–H1200.
104. Zhang J, Jin N, Liu Y, Rhoades RA. Hydrogen peroxide stimulates extracellular signal-regulated protein kinases in pulmonary arterial smooth muscle cells. Am J Respir Cell Mol Biol 1998; 19:324–332.

105. Jin N, Hatton N, Swartz DR, Xia X, Harrington MA, Larsen SH, Rhoades RA. Hypoxia activates jun-N-terminal kinase, extracellular signal-regulated protein kinase, and p38 kinase in pulmonary arteries. Am J Respir Cell Mol Biol 2000; 23:593–601.
106. Hampl V, Herget J. Role of nitric oxide in the pathogenesis of chronic pulmonary hypertension. Physiol Rev 2000; 80:1337–1372.
107. Kong SK, Stephens NL. Pharmacological studies of sensitized canine pulmonary blood vessels. J Pharmacol Exp Ther 1981; 219:551–557.
108. Kong SK, Stephens NL. Mechanical properties of pulmonary arteries from sensitized dogs. J Appl Physiol 1983; 55:1669–1673.
109. Wen FQ, Watanabe K, Yoshida M. Eicosanoid profile in cultured human pulmonary artery smooth muscle cells treated with IL-1 beta and TNF alpha. Prostaglandins Leukot Essent Fatty Acids 1998; 59:71–75.
110. Markewitz BA, Farrukh IS, Chen Y, Li Y, Michael JR. Regulation of endothelin-1 synthesis in human pulmonary arterial smooth muscle cells. Effects of transforming growth factor-β and hypoxia. Cardiovasc Res 2001; 49:200–206.
111. Janssen LJ. Isoprostanes: an overview and putative roles in pulmonary pathophysiology. Am J Physiol Lung Cell Mol Physiol 2001; 280:L1067–L1082.
112. Cracowski JL, Cracowski C, Bessard G, Pepin JL, Bessard J, Schwebel C, Stanke-Labesque F, Pison C. Increased lipid peroxidation in patients with pulmonary hypertension. Am J Respir Crit Care Med 2001; 164:1038–1042.
113. Carpenter CT, Price PV, Christman BW. Exhaled breath condensate isoprostanes are elevated in patients with acute lung injury or ARDS. Chest 1998; 114:1653–1659.
114. Jankov RP, Belcastro R, Ovcina E, Lee J, Massaeli H, Lye SJ, Tanswell AK. Thromboxane A_2 receptors mediate pulmonary hypertension in 60% oxygen-exposed newborn rats by a cyclooxygenase-independent mechanism. Am J Respir Crit Care Med 2002; 166:208–214.
115. Gonzalez PK, Zhuang J, Doctrow SR, Malfroy B, Benson PF, Menconi MJ, Fink MP. EUK-8, a synthetic superoxide dismutase and catalase mimetic, ameliorates acute lung injury in endotoxemic swine. J Pharm Exp Ther 1995; 275:798–806.
116. Orr JA, Shams H, Karla W, Peskar BA, Scheid P. Transient ventilatory responses to endotoxin infusion in the cat are mediated by thromboxane A2. Resp Physiol 1993; 93:189–201.
117. Walmrath D, Pilch J, Scharmann M, Grimminger F, Seeger W. Severe VA/Q mismatch in perfused lungs evoked by sequential challenge with endotoxin and *E. coli* hemolysin. J Appl Physiol 1994; 76:1020–1030.
118. Zamora CA, Baron DA, Heffner JE, Zhang R, Ogletree ML, Moreland S. Thromboxane contributes to pulmonary hypertension in ischemia-reperfusion lung injury. Characterization of thromboxane A2/prostaglandin endoperoxide receptors in aorta. J Appl Physiol 1993; 74:224–229.
119. Razavi HM, Werhun R, Scott JA, Weicker S, Wang IF, McCormack DG, Mehta S. Effects of inhaled nitric oxide in a mouse model of sepsis-induced acute lung injury. Crit Care Med 2002; 30:868–873.

120. Hart CM, Karman RJ, Blackburn TL, Gupta MP, Garcia JG, Mohler ER, III. Role of 8-*epi* $PGF_{2\alpha}$, 8-isoprostane, in H_2O_2-induced derangements of pulmonary artery endothelial cell barrier function. Prostaglandins Leukot Essent Fatty Acids 1998; 58:9–16.
121. Jourdan KB, Evans TW, Goldstraw P, Mitchell JA. Isoprostanes and PGE_2 production in human isolated pulmonary artery smooth muscle cells: concomitant and differential release. FASEB J 1999; 13:1025–1030.
122. Natarajan R, Lanting L, Gonzales N, Nadler J. Formation of an F_2-isoprostane in vascular smooth muscle cells by elevated glucose and growth factors. Am J Physiol 1996; 271:H159–H165.
123. Ruef J, Moser M, Kubler W, Bode C. Induction of endothelin-1 expression by oxidative stress in vascular smooth muscle cells. Cardiovasc Pathol 2001; 10:311–315.
124. Jankov RP, Luo X, Cabacungan J, Belcastro R, Frndova H, Lye SJ, et al. Endothelin-1 and O_2-mediated pulmonary hypertension in neonatal rats: a role for products of lipid peroxidation. Pediatr Res 2000; 48:289–298.
125. Weir EK, Reeve HL, Johnson G, Michelakis ED, Nelson DP, Archer SL. A role for potassium channels in smooth muscle cells and platelets in the etiology of primary pulmonary hypertension. Chest 1998; 114:200S–204S.
126. Salvi SS. α_1-adrenergic hypothesis for pulmonary hypertension. Chest 1999; 115:1708–1719.
127. Archer SL, Yankovich RD, Chesler E, Weir EK. Comparative effects of nisoldipine, nifedipine and bepridil on experimental pulmonary hypertension. J Pharmacol Exp Ther 1985; 233:12–17.
128. Fishman AP. Pulmonary hypertension—beyond vasodilator therapy. N Engl J Med 1998; 338:321–322.
129. Weinberger B, Weiss K, Heck DE, Laskin DL, Laskin JD. Pharmacologic therapy of persistent pulmonary hypertension of the newborn. Pharmacol Ther 2001; 89:67–79.

3

Ion Channel Heterogeneity in the Pulmonary Vascular Bed

A Basis for Site-Specific Responses to Vasoactive Stimuli

Stephen L. Archer
University of Alberta, Edmonton, Alberta, Canada

Nancy J. Rusch
Medical College of Wisconsin, Milwaukee, Wisconsin, U.S.A.

I. INTRODUCTION

Variety is not only the "spice of life"; it is also intrinsic to the normal functioning of all vascular beds in the body. All blood vessels have certain common features, but closer examination reveals important regional variations in structure and function. This diversity exists not only between vessels of different vascular beds but also between large and small arteries within a single organ. Indeed, cellular electrophysiology has revealed that the medial layer of the arterial wall is not homogeneous but instead is composed of a mosaic of electro physiologically diverse smooth muscle cells (SMCs). Different levels of expression and types of ion channels may contribute to this electrical heterogeneity within a single type of blood vessel. On a larger scale, the heterogeneity of ion channels between vascular beds may partly explain the site-specific responses of different arteries to vasoactive stimuli including altered oxygen tension and pH. Further diversity of ion channel expression has been noted during conditions of cardiovascular disease, in which the abnormal expression and possibly properties of ion channels may establish pathological levels of excitability in the affected SMCs. For example, in both pulmonary and systemic hypertension there is a characteristic loss of K^+ channel function and expression in the SMC membranes, causing membrane depolarization and predisposing the affected arteries to vasoconstriction and vascular remodeling.

Section II briefly reviews the heterogeneous populations of calcium ion (Ca^{2+}) and potassium ion (K^+) channels in the pulmonary vasculature and focuses on three families of ion channels that regulate pulmonary vascular tone: the voltage-gated "L-type" calcium (Ca_L) channel, the voltage-gated K^+ (Kv) channel, and the high-conductance, calcium-sensitive K^+ (BK_{Ca}) channel. Section III reviews the evidence that ion channel expression differs between single pulmonary SMCs and between the conduit and resistance arteries. Section IV discusses the role of Ca_L, Kv, and BK_{Ca} channels in the site-specific responses of the pulmonary vasculature to hypoxia and pH. For example, it has been known for decades that hypoxia and acidosis constrict the pulmonary resistancevessels, thereby minimizing ventilation–perfusion mismatch. The same stimuli dilate the large pulmonary arteries and the arteries of other vascular beds, including the coronary circulation. The concept that the pulmonary and systemic vasculatures of the same animal express unique ion channel populations and that this diversity underlies the heterogeneous responses to stimuli such as hypoxia and acidosis is important to understanding the physiological mechanisms that protect critical organs and enhance survival. *Ionic-diversity* also raises many interesting questions of how the ontogeny and local milieu of different vascular beds influences ion channel expression and function. Although there is important heterogeneity in the expression and function of other vascular ion channels (e.g., Cl^-, K_{ir}, TRP channels), details regarding the molecular components and functional roles of these and other channel proteins are discussed elsewhere in this monograph.

II. MOLECULAR IDENTIFICATION AND FUNCTION OF Ca_L, Kv, AND BK_{Ca} CHANNELS

A. Long-Lasting Calcium (Ca_L) Channels

Voltage-gated, long-lasting Ca^{2+} (Ca_L) channels represent the major pathway by which Ca^{2+} enters the pulmonary SMCs to cause vasoconstriction. Although the subunit composition of Ca_L channels in pulmonary SMCs is unknown, diverse populations of Ca_L channels have been characterized in neurons (1), and the multi-subunit structure of the Ca_L

channel implies that heterogeneity will also be observed in pulmonary SMCs. Briefly, the pore-forming α subunit ($\alpha_{1C\text{-b}}$) of Ca_L channels in vascular SMCs is distinct from the α subunit ($\alpha_{1C\text{-a}}$) expressed by cardiac myocytes and is produced by alternative splicing of the same gene (2). It consists of a single polypeptide composed of four repeat domains (I–IV), each containing six transmembrane segments (S1–S6) (Fig. 1A). The α subunit can function independently as a voltage-sensing pore and contains the primary binding sites for the classical Ca^{2+} channel blocking drugs that are therapeutically available to lower vascular tone (e.g., the dihydropyridine drug nifedipine). The expression of the α subunit and its functional and pharmacological properties are highly modulated by association with β and $\alpha_2\delta$ subunits, at least in heterologous expression systems in which these proteins are highly expressed (3–8). Notably, splice variants of the α subunit assemble with several types of β subunits to confer a complex phenotype to native Ca^{2+} currents in neurons (9), but the mechanisms that regulate subunit expression in vascular SMCs and the

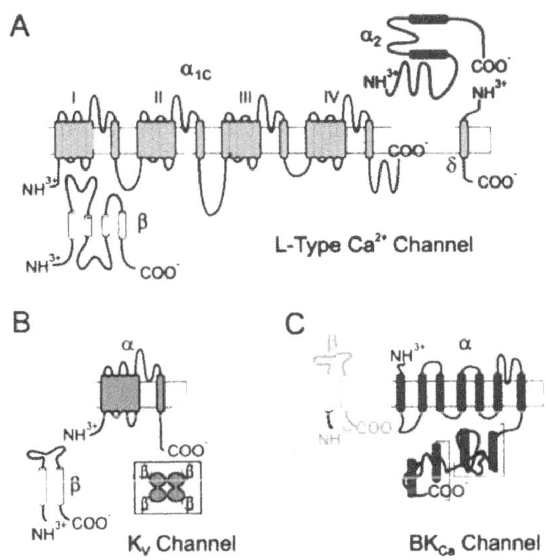

Figure 1 Proposed topology of ion channels expressed in VSMC membranes. (A) The L-type Ca^{2+} channel may consist of a single α_{1C} subunit that forms the channel pore, and ancillary β and α_2/δ subunits. (B) The α subunit of the voltage-gated K^+ (Kv) channel assembles with a β subunit. The inset indicates that four α subunits form a tetrameric channel. (C) The α subunit of the high conductance Ca^{2+}-activated K^+ (BK_{Ca}) channel is associated with a β subunit that may be membrane-delineated. BK_{Ca} channels also assemble as tetramers (not shown). See text for further details.

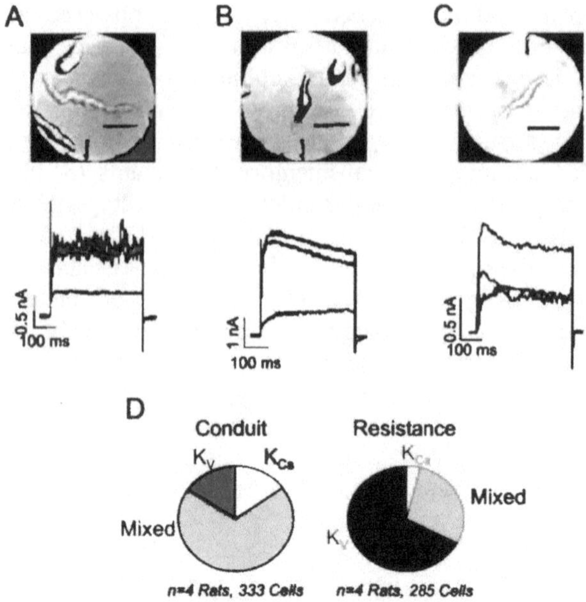

Figure 2 Light microscopy and electrophysiology identify three distinct types of SMCs in rat pulmonary arteries. (A) Large "BK_{Ca} cells" showed small, noisy currents inhibited by TEA but not by 4-AP. Currents were elicited by depolarizing pulses from −70 to +70 mV. (B) In contrast, small "Kv cells" showing a perinuclear prominence displayed large smooth currents more sensitive to 4-AP than to TEA. (C) In "mixed cells," the proportions of K^+ current inhibited by 4-AP and TEA were approximately the same. (D) The SMCs of the conduit pulmonary arteries primarily express a mix of K_{Ca} and Kv current, whereas the resistance pulmonary arteries are enriched in Kv current. (Modified from Ref. 44 with permission.)

precise identity of the ancillary β and $\alpha_2\delta$ subunits that participate in the formation of Ca_L channel complexes remain unclear.

Regardless, it has been estimated that at least several thousand Ca_L channels are expressed in a single vascular SMC, and the low unitary conductance (10–25 pS) of these channels coupled to their maintained activation during membrane depolarization finely regulates voltage-gated Ca^{2+} influx during arterial excitation (10). To judge from a single patch-clamp study, pulmonary SMCs appear to highly express Ca_L channels, with resistance arteries showing a higher density of Ca_L channel current than conduit vessels (11). Additionally, Ca^{2+} influx through Ca_L channels may enhance Ca^{2+} release events ("Ca^{2+} sparks") from thesarcoplasmic reticulum in pulmonary SMCs, resulting in graded depolarization and excitation of the SMCs (12).

B. Voltage-Gated Potassium Ion (Kv) Channels

The voltage-gated K^+ (Kv) channels are a highly diverse superfamily of K^+ channels that share the common properties of K^+ selectivity and voltage-dependent activation. Structural homology has classified Kv channels into nine gene families (Kv1–Kv9) that share a common α-subunit topology (Fig. 1B). The pore region contains a highly conserved K^+ recognition sequence, GYGD, which largely confers the channel's specificity for potassium (13), and Ca^{2+}-binding domains confer Ca^{2+} inhibition of channel gating (14,15). In contrast to the single large α_{1C} subunit that forms the Ca_L channel pore, the amino terminus of the Kv α subunit has a tetramerization (T1) domain that permits four different α subunits from the same gene family to "mix and match" to form the channel pore (16,17). The Kv1–4 α subunits form active channels when they assemble as tetramers. These tetramers may be composed of a single type of α subunit (e.g., homotetramers with all four α subunits being Kv1.5), or they may be heterotetramers (e.g., two Kv1.5 and two Kv1.2 α subunits forming a channel). Thus, Kv1.*x* family members form heterotetramers with each other but not with Kv2.*x* family members. In contrast, the Kv5–9 family members, also referred to as "γ subunits," are structurally similar to α subunits but form active channels (e.g., are electrically conductive) only when coassembled with certain Kv1–4 α subunits. The resulting heterotetramers composed of α and γ subunits may show altered voltage-dependent profiles, further broadening the potential for Kv channels to show widely diverse biophysical and pharmacological properties within or between vascular beds (18,19).

Additional mechanisms that generate heterogeneity of Kv channels include alternative splicing, post transcriptional modifications, and association of α subunits with β subunits. Local variation in promoters and silencers also may be important, particularly in light of the short half-life of Kv channel mRNA and protein (~8 for Kv1.5) (20). Of these further mechanisms for heterogeneity, the small β subunits (~30 kDa) that associate intimately with the channels are the best characterized, and four β-subunit genes (Kvβ1–4) have been identified that show several splice variants (14). The Kv β subunits createheterogeneity by modifying the gating and kinetics of the Kv channels and are members of the aldose reductase superfamily of NADPH oxidoreductases (21,22). Because they may dock to cytosolic domains of the Kv channel tetramer (22) they are positioned to transduce the cytosolic redox state of the cell to changes in channel activity. Thus, it has been suggested that the β subunits provide a mechanism for coupling the chemistry of the cell to membrane excitability via their regulation of Kv channel activity. In addition, β subunits may selectively alter the cell-surface expression of Kv channels (e.g., increasing Kv1.5 and Kv1.2 but decreasing Kv1.4 expression) to influence membrane K^+ conductance (16,23).

As is evident from the preceding discussion, the Kvchannels have a remarkable propensity for heterogeneity, and the pulmonary SMCs appear to take full advantage of this to generate diverse populations of Kv channels. Although coimmunoprecipitation studies have not defined the full complement of α and β subunits involved in channel formation, it appears that representatives from most of the Kv channel families (Kv1–Kv9) are expressed by the SMCs of the pulmonary circulation. A full complement of Kv β subunits also are available to interact with the channels (24). For example, homo- or heterotetramers composed of Kv1.2, Kv1.5, Kv2.1, Kv3.1b, and Kv2.1/Kv9.3 channels have been proposedas potential "oxygen-sensitive" channels, defined as thosechannels that are inhibited by hypoxia (25–27). The heteromultimeric channels may have kinetic, functional and pharmacological profiles that exhibit hybrid properties reflecting the subunit components. For example, heterotetramers of Kv1.2/1.5 have been suggested to be more sensitive to inhibition by hypoxia at physiological membrane potentials (E_m) than the respective homotetramers of Kv1.2/1.2 or Kv1.5/1.5 (28). Similarly, Kv2.1 may associate with Kv9.3 to form Kv2.1/9.3 channels that activate at more negativevoltages and show greater hypoxia sensitivity than homotetameric Kv2.1 channels (18,28). It has also been hypothesized that the Kv β subunits may play a role in cellular oxygen sensing, based on findings that Kvβ2.1 subunits confer oxygen sensitivity to Kv4.2 channels in HEK-293 cells that are otherwise unaffected by hypoxia (27). Thus, in addition to providing multiple pathways to regulate the resting E_m of pulmonary SMCs under normal conditions, the complex expression of Kv channels in pulmonary SMCs may provide a "safety net" to ensure that a plethora of Kv channels are available to fine-tune the critical adaptive responses of the pulmonary circulation to physiological or pathophysiological stimuli, including changes in oxygen tension and pH.

C. High-Conductance Ca^{2+}-Activated K^+ (BK_{Ca}) Channels

High-conductance Ca^{2+}-activated K^+ channels, named "BK_{Ca} channels" because of their "big" unitary conductances (150–300 pS), are ubiquitously expressed in all vascular beds. The BK_{Ca} α subunit shows partial homology with the Kv α subunit in six (S1–S6) of its seven (S0–S6) transmembrane segments, which include the intrinsic voltage sensor (S4) and the pore region (S5–S6) (29,30). An additional seventh transmembrane segment (S0) on the N-terminus interacts with one of at least four types of BK_{Ca} β subunits, an interaction that greatly increases channel sensitivity to voltage and intracellular calcium (Fig. 1C). Four additional hydrophobic segments (S7–S10) in the C-terminus contain key domains that regulate channel structure and function. A tetramerization domain between S6 and S7 permits four α subunits to assemble into the BK_{Ca} channel tetramer, whereas a "calcium bowl" residing within the S9–S10 linker and the S10 hydrophobic segment confers Ca^{2+} sensitivity to the channel (31,32). Unlike the Kv channels that originate from multiple gene families, $BK_{Ca}\alpha$ subunits appear to arise from a single gene family. However, phenotypic diversity may be generated by a high level of alternative splicing of the common primary transcript (33), and BK_{Ca} channel properties including unitary conductance and Ca^{2+} sensitivity vary greatly between vascular beds (34–36). Thus, like the Kv channels, the possibilities for diversity of BK_{Ca} channels are enormous because the impact of heterotetramer formation and splice variants on channel heterogeneity is multiplied by the ability of the resulting channels to associate with β subunits.

In the pulmonary circulation, the splice variants thatcompose the BK_{Ca} channels are unknown. It is presumed that the BK_{Ca} β1 subunit, which is highly expressed in most types of SMCs, also confers calcium and voltage sensitivity to the BK_{Ca} channel in pulmonary arteries (30,36). Perhaps the lack of knowledge regarding BK_{Ca} channel properties in the mature pulmonary circulation relates, at least in part, to findingsindicating that this channel is not the primary contributor to the resting E_m and tone of small pulmonary arteries (37,39). Neither has it been implicated in the pathogenesis of hypoxia-induced vasoconstriction or pulmonary hypertension (40–43). Rather, the BK_{Ca} channel is thought to function as a "brake" to buffer SMC excitation during these pathologies, in which depolarization and calcium loading of the SMCs may act synergistically to activate BK_{Ca} channels as a protective mechanism to limit further increases in vascular tone.

III. DIVERSITY OF Ca_L, Kv, AND BK_{Ca} CHANNELS WITHIN THE PULMONARY CIRCULATION

A. General Features of the Pulmonary Circulation

The adult pulmonary circulation is a unique low-resistance circuit designed for gas exchange and metabolism. It is perfused by a thin-walled right ventricle that is intolerant of high levels of afterload. With each heartbeat, the pulmonary circulation must accommodate the entire cardiac output at low pressure and resistance (one-fifth of that in the systemic vasculature). In fact, the pulmonary circulation of a healthy adult accommodates four-fold increases in cardiac output without any increase in pulmonary vascular resistance. The pulmonary circulation consists of extraparenchymal large arteries, which serve as conduits, and intrapulmonary arteries, which control pulmonary vascular resistance. In healthy adults, the small intrapulmonary resistance arteries are the site of hypoxic pulmonary vasoconstriction (HPV). In most forms of pulmonary hypertension, the burden of pathology also is localized to these small arteries. This proximal–distal, conduit–resistance distinction is relevant because the proximal and distal pulmonary arteries have not only different functions and electrophysiology (44) but also different embryological origins (45,46). The large proximal pulmonary arteries are derived from the 6th aortic arch, whereas the intrapulmonary arteries appear to be derived from a continuous expansion of the primary capillary plexus and originate by vasculogenesis from the mesenchymal cells of the lung bud. The pulmonary capillary bed serves a fundamental role in survival as the site of gas exchange for all air-breathing creatures and serves important roles in metabolism. Thus, it appears logical that the intrapulmonary arteries that dynamically regulate their diameter to optimize gas exchange are embryologically linked to the capillary plexus. The pulmonary venous circulation completes the "lesser" circulation of the lung, and, although it has been understudied, it is involved in the pathogenesis of HPV, pulmonary edema, pulmonary hypertension, and cardiac arrhythmias.

Some of the properties of the pulmonary circulation relate to the anatomy of the vessels, but ion channels in the vascular SMCs participate in controlling the active properties of the proximal and distal pulmonary arteries. Likewise, the pulmonary veins are not passive conduits but rather are dynamic, contractile structures that, as they approach the left atrium within the lung parenchyma, have a coaxial coating of cardiac myocytes indistinguishable from those in the left atrium. Regardless of the close proximity of the pulmonary arteries, pulmonary veins, and the heart, the pulmonary veins have their own electrical diversity, and the cardiac myocytes have a very different ionic portfolio than the contiguous pulmonary arterial SMCs. As will be discussed shortly, the differential distribution of Ca_L, Kv, and BK_{Ca} channels within the pulmonary circulation and the local milieu to which the SMCs are subjected are important regional determinants of vascular tone, although they clearly represent only the "tip of the iceberg" in terms of all aspects of pulmonary heterogeneity.

B. Regulation of Membrane Potential and Excitability in Pulmonary SMCs

Under resting conditions, the basal opening of K^+ channels mediates K^+ efflux across the plasma membrane, which results in a resting E_m value in pulmonary SMCs between ≈-60 and -40 mV. The precise families and isoforms of K^+ channels that control the level of resting E_m probably vary between animal species, between genders of the same species, between vascular beds, and during development from fetus to adult. For example, the resting E_m in the pulmonary arteries of the healthy adult is largely controlled by Kv channels(42–44,47–49), whereas BK_{Ca} channels contribute more heavily to the resting E_m of pulmonary arteries in fetal sheep (50).

Regardless of the origins of variability, similarities in the properties of ion channels permit a general paradigm to be established to explain how the E_m of the vascular SMCs is coupled to changes in arterial tone. First, depolarization of the vascular SMCs is tightly coupled to the opening of voltage-gated Ca_L channels. The Ca_L channels inactivate slowly during sustained depolarization, so that the Ca^{2+} influx mediated by a small fraction of the total number of channels may be sufficient to maintain pulmonary vascular tone. However, in the negative range of E_m found inpulmonary SMCs, the minimal Ca^{2+} influx may permit the pulmonary vascular resistance to be maintained at the low levels found in healthy individuals. Furthermore, the rise in intracellular calcium during SMC excitation will act synergistically with depolarization to activate BK_{Ca} channels. The resulting K^+ efflux will mediate hyperpolarization of the SMC membrane to help maintain the appropriately low levels of Ca^{2+} influx, intracellular calcium, and force generation. The effects of SMC excitation on the open-state probability of Kv channels are more complex, however, and may vary between tissues depending on the types of Kv channels that are present. Although Kv channels are active and contribute to the resting E_m of pulmonary SMCs, several findings suggest that rises in intracellular calcium during SMC excitation result in the closure of Kv channels in pulmonary SMCs, despite their sensitivity to voltage. Thus, diverse stimuli including endothelin, angiotensin II, and hypoxia have been shown to reduce Kv channel current in patch-clamped pulmonary SMCs, presumably through Ca^{2+}-mediated inhibition of Kv channels, resulting in SMC depolarization (42,43). In healthy individuals, the complex interactions between Ca_L, Kv, and BK_{Ca} channels apparently set the diameter of the small vessels to provide for the optimal perfusion of the pulmonary capillary bed. In vasospastic diseases such as pulmonary hypertension, these interactions may be disturbed and pathological vasoconstrictor responses may result, as discussed elsewhere in this monograph.

C. Cell- and Size-Dependent Expression of Ion Channels in the Pulmonary Circulation

Patch-clamp "surveys" have revealed a differential distribution of vascular SMCs that exhibit distinctly different expression levels of Ca_L, Kv, and BK_{Ca} channels along the length of the pulmonary arterial tree. As indicated earlier, the molecular mechanisms and signals from the environmental milieu that regulate the expression of these channels are poorly understood. Yet, it is intriguing that cell-to-cell variability exists in ion channel expression and that the ion channel profile of the intraparenchymal pulmonary resistance arteries is consistent with their role as vasoactive vessels compared to the profile of the less contractile conduit vessels.

In this regard, studies in vascular SMCs freshly dispersed from the rabbit pulmonary arterial tree indicate that Ca_L current density is enhanced more than two-fold in the SMCs of the fine tertiary arterial branches compared to those of the main pulmonary trunk (11). The increased Ca_L current in the SMCs of the distal arteries corresponds with the functional role of these vessels as contractile and dynamic regulators of local blood flow and gas exchange in the lung. Interestingly, the expression levels of Kv and BK_{Ca} channels also appear to differ between conduit and intraparenchymal resistance pulmonary arteries. For example, the vascular SMCs of the rat pulmonary arterial tree manifest phenotypically and electrophysiologically distinct cell populations coexisting side by side (Fig. 3) (44,51,52). In this circulation, for example, the SMCs of conduit pulmonary arteries are large and predominantly express BK_{Ca} current, evident as small, noisy whole-cell K^+ currents inhibited by tetraethylammonium (TEA) but insensitive to the Kv channel blocker 4-aminopyridine (4-Ap) (Fig. 3A). Inversely, the resistance arteries are enriched in smaller SMCs that show a perinuclear prominence. These SMCs show a high density of 4-AP sensitive Kv current but demonstrate sparse levels of BK_{Ca} current sensitive to blocking by TEA (Fig. 3B). A third phenotypically "mixed" cell type, found in both conduit and resistance arteries, has intermediate current density, and its whole-cell K^+ current is inhibited equally by 4-AP and TEA, suggesting the mixed presence of both Kv and BK_{Ca} channels (Fig. 3C). The characterization of large populations of SMCs from the rat pulmonary circulation indicates that SMCs characterized by predominant Kv current are more pronounced in distal than in to proximal pulmonary arteries (Fig. 3D). Consistent with this finding, small arteries vigorously contract in response to inhibition of Kv channels by 4-AP but do not respond to pharmacological blocking of BK_{Ca} channels, indicating that K^+ efflux through Kv channels is the primary contributor to the resting E_m of the SMCs (44).

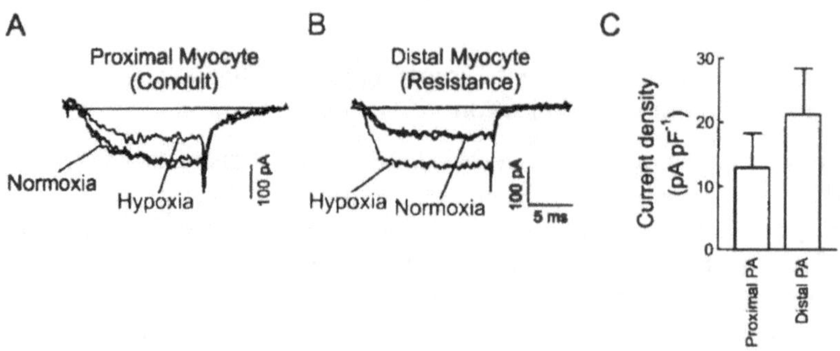

Figure 3 Opposing modulation of Ca_L channel current by hypoxia in proximal versus distal pulmonary myocytes. (A) Hypoxia inhibits Ca_L current in SMCs from proximal pulmonary arteries. Whole-cell currents were elicited by depolarizing steps from –80 to +10 mV. (B) In contrast, Ca_L current in SMCs from distal pulmonary arteries was activated by hypoxia. (C) The membrane density of Ca_L current was higher in SMCs from distal pulmonary arteries than in proximal pulmonary arteries. (Modified from Ref. 11 with permission.)

At present, the identity of the Kv channel families that are densely expressed in the SMCs of pulmonary resistance arteries is unclear. Initial attempts to identify the specific Kv channels have relied on introducing antibodies into SMCs via a patch pipette. These antibodies are directed against specific epitopes in the carboxy terminus that may inhibit channel function (53). Using this approach, the cytosolic introduction of either anti-Kv2.1 or anti-Kv1.5 has been shown to inhibit whole-cell K^+ current and depolarize the vascular SMCs isolated from rat resistance pulmonary arteries, whereasantibodies directed against other types of K^+ channels (e.g., K_{ir} channels) had no effect (53). Subsequent biophysical and pharmacological analyses also inferred that Kv1.5 homo- and heterotetramers contributed primarily to whole-cell K^+current in these cells, whereas the properties of K^+ current in SMCs of conduit arteries were consistent with a "mixed"population of SMCs expressing Kv2.1 and Kv1.5 familychannels (52). Thus, complementary approaches suggest that distal pulmonary arteries densely express Kv channels that are minimally composed of Kv1.5 and Kv2.1 α subunits and that these channels contribute to the resting E_m of the SMCs.

IV. HETEROGENEOUS POPULATIONS OF OXYGEN-SENSITIVE ION CHANNELS

Although the net response of the pulmonary circulation to acute hypoxia is to increase pulmonary vascular resistance, not all parts of the pulmonary vasculature behave the same. Proximal pulmonary arteries respond to hypoxia much like systemic arteries, with a biphasic change in tone characterized by a small initial constriction followed by a sustained relaxation below baseline (54,55). In contrast, the small distal pulmonary arteries respond to hypoxia with a sustained constriction. What mechanisms underlie the different responses of the vascular segments of the pulmonary circulation to hypoxia? Answering this question may rely, at least in part, on defining the site-specific expression of ion channels in the pulmonary circulation and defining their interaction with the unique local milieu to which pulmonary SMCs aresubjected in the lung.

A. Diversity in the Redox Environment

In this regard, there are a myriad of stimuli external to ion channels and their cofactors that dramatically regulate SMC function. Only one will be described in detail here, namely, the local variation in the redox environment, because this topic is broadly relevant to O_2 sensing, the regulation of ion channel function, and pulmonary SMC excitability. Redox chemistry may be viewed as the movement of electrons down potential gradients. The "redox hypothesis," as it relates to the resistance arteries of the lung, states that there is a tonic, basal production of active oxygen species (AOS) in the pulmonary SMCs under normoxic conditions that establishes a basal level of ion channel oxidation, thereby setting the physiological levels of channel activity (56–58). These AOS are most likely derived from the mitochondria, although contributions from other sources, such as plasmalemmal NADPH oxidase, cannot be excluded. It appears that many ion channels are regulated by changes in the redox state of the cell, including Ca_L, BK_{Ca}, and Kv channels (25–27,40,59,60). However, because Kv channels (e.g., Kv1.5) contribute heavily to the resting E_m of pulmonary SMCs and are equipped to respond to redox stimuli via their sulfhydryl-containing cysteine groups, it has been proposed that the rapid loss of AOS during hypoxia withdraws the tonic oxidant signal from the pulmonary resistance arteries (61,62). The resulting reduction of key amino acids on the Kv channels inhibits K^+ channel activity and induces SMC depolarization. Thus, the dynamic modulation of basal AOS production by the mitochondria may represent one key link between changes in Po_2, ion channel activity, and the regulation of resting E_m in pulmonary SMCs.

It is uncertain whether the diminution of AOS production directly alters ion channel gating or is a marker for altered electron transport. The resulting cytosolic accumulation of reduced forms of other redox couples, such as NADP/NADPH or GSSG/GSH, also could modulate channel function. Two major sensors have been proposed that could act asphysiological sources of AOS and fulfill the sensor role, namely, nicotinamide adenine dinucleotide phosphate (NADPHoxidase) and the mitochondrial electron transport chain. The evidence for each potential source of signaling AOS has been reviewed (25). In terms of heterogeneity, it is noteworthy that the existence of functionally different mitochondria has recently been reported in the pulmonary versus systemic arteries. Owing to different mitochondrial properties, it has been proposed that SMCs of pulmonary resistance arteries are relatively oxidized under basal conditions by the tonicproduction of a mitochondria-derived vasodilator factor, possibly H_2O_2, that establishes a high basal level of K^+ channeloxidation, channel activity, and resting E_m (56,57). Compared to the SMCs of systemic arteries, ion channel activity and the resting E_m in SMCs of pulmonary resistance arteries may be highly dependent on physiological levels of oxygen tension and, conversely, highly sensitive to inhibition by hypoxia and the resulting imposition of a different redox environment.

B. Diversity of Ion Channel Responses to Hypoxia and pH

One explanation for the diverse oxygen-sensitive responses of vascular SMCs, as discussed in the previous section, is that the SMCs of small pulmonary arteries are exposed to a highly oxidative environment that confers a high level of O_2 sensitivity to ion channel function in the SMCs. However, considered alone, this hypothesis does not seem to adequately explain the diametrically opposite responses to hypoxia of constriction of the small pulmonary arteries versus dilation of the largepulmonary arteries and the systemic resistance arteries. This phenomenon may relate more to the intrinsic differences in the oxygen sensitivity of Ca^{2+} and K^+ channels in SMCs from different arterial sites. Indeed, patch-clamp studies have shown that hypoxia reduces Ca_L current in isolated SMCs of rat proximal pulmonary arteries but enhances Ca_L current in SMCs isolated from the distal pulmonary arteries of the same animal (Figs. 3A,3B) (11). In the same proximal and distal SMCs, hypoxia induced hyperpolarizing and depolarizing shifts, respectively, in the voltage required for Ca_L channel activation. These opposing oxygen-induced shifts in the voltage sensitivity of Ca_L channels resulted in the activation of Ca_L current at more negative E_m in the distal SMCs than in the proximal SMCs and established a nearly two-fold higher Ca^{2+} current density in the SMCs of the small pulmonary arteries. Thus, longitudinal differences in Ca_L current density and O_2 sensitivity in the SMCs of the pulmonary vasculature offer one explanation for the increased reactivity to hypoxia of the distal compared to the proximal pulmonary arteries (11).

In this regard, it was observed nearly a decade ago that thiol oxidants activated Ca_L current in cardiac myocytes, a response that was reversed by thiol reductants (59). These findings suggested that there was a "redox switch" on the Ca_L channel structure that was an important determinant of channel activity. More recently, Fearon *et al.* (63) examined the oxygen sensitivity of three naturally occurring splice variants of the pore-forming α_{1C} subunit of the Ca_L channel that were expressed in HEK-293 cells. Hypoxia reversibly inhibited the Ca_L current resulting from only one of the three α_{1C} variants, whereas the remaining two variants were insensitive to Po_2 levels. In the same study, selective restriction of the spliced insert revealed that a 39-amino-acid region in the C-terminal conferred oxygen sensitivity to the channel in HEK-293 cells, in which ancillary subunits of the Ca_L channel were not expressed. This initial discovery of a unique O_2-sensitive structural region in the Ca_L channel generated by alternative splicing raised the possibility that a regional distribution of mRNAs encoding α_{1C} variants could contribute to the divergent Po_2 responses of the channel in distal versus proximal pulmonary SMCs and between the SMCs of thedistal pulmonary arteries and the systemic arteries in which hypoxia reduces Ca_L current.

Although Ca_L channels clearly appear to be "oxygen-sensitive," the unique vasoconstrictor response of the small pulmonary arteries to hypoxia could also be explained if hypoxia selectively inhibited one or more Kv channels in the distal SMCs. Indeed, several laboratories have reported that low Po_2 attenuates a Kv current in SMCs isolated from distal pulmonary arteries (44,64,65). Physiological inhibition of this Kv current by hypoxia, or pharmacological block by 4-AP, triggered membrane depolarization of the SMCs, a rise in intracellular calcium, and vasoconstriction. Thus, the experimental loss of functional Kv channels reproduces the depolarizing response of distal pulmonary SMCs to hypoxia, although the debate continues regarding which α and β subunitscompose these channels.

Based on a comparison of the pharmacology and electrophysiology of a large number of recombinant channels, several "candidates" have been identified as O_2-sensitive Kv channels. Channels composed of Kv1.2, Kv2.1, Kv3.1b, and Kv9.3 α subunits have been primarily considered. As reviewed in detail elsewhere (27), Kv1.2/1.5 and Kv2.1/9.3 heterotetrameric channels possess adequate voltage sensitivity to contribute to the resting E_m of pulmonary SMCs and are inhibited by hypoxia at negative membrane potentials. Thus, these channels may be potentially important O_2-sensing proteins under physiological conditions. Kv3.1b homotetramers also generate macroscopic and single-channel currents inhibited by low Po_2, but these channels appear to lack the voltage sensitivity required to contribute to the resting E_m of pulmonary SMCs. Thus, their role in the O_2 regulation of resting pulmonary vascular tone has been met with skepticism.

Unfortunately, pharmacological probes lack the specificity to distinguish the contribution of a single type of Kv channel to native K^+ current. Thus, gene deletion studies in mice have been designed to examine the contribution of Kv1.5 α subunits to pulmonary vascular resistance and to hypoxia-induced vasoconstriction (66). In this regard, the pulmonary SMCs of the Kv1.5 knockout mouse display reduced Kv current, and its pulmonary arteries show a blunted vasoconstrictor response to hypoxia, inferring that Kv1.5-containing channels normally contribute to the O_2-sensitive Kv current of the SMCs. However, the residual presence of O_2-sensitive Kv current in distal pulmonary SMCs from Kv1.5 knockout mice reinforces the hypothesis that at least several types of Kv channels contribute to the hybrid K^+ current regulated by oxygen. As expected, the depolarizing response to hypoxia in pulmonary SMCs appears to represent a complex series of events ultimately culminating in an intense vasoconstriction.

Interestingly, the BK_{Ca} channels show minimal sensitivity to hypoxia in the distal pulmonary SMCs and may actually be activated under conditions of reduced Po_2 (64). For example, hypoxia has little effect on BK_{Ca} current in canine pulmonary SMCs (Fig. 4A) but profoundly reduces Kv current (Fig. 4B). In isolated patches from the samepreparation that demonstrate the presence of both BK_{Ca} and Kv channels (Fig. 4C), the BK_{Ca} channels also failed to respond to hypoxia whereas Kv channel activity was markedly suppressed, consistent with the O_2-induced inhibition of these channels in whole-cell recording (Figs. 4D and 4E, respectively). Because both BK_{Ca} and Kv channels in pulmonary SMCs are reportedly activated by oxidizing conditions and inhibited by reduction, it is difficult to explain the selective oxygen sensitivity of the Kv channels based solely on the redox environment of the SMC (40,41). One alternative possibility is that only the Kv channel structure possesses the appropriate domain to "sense" changes

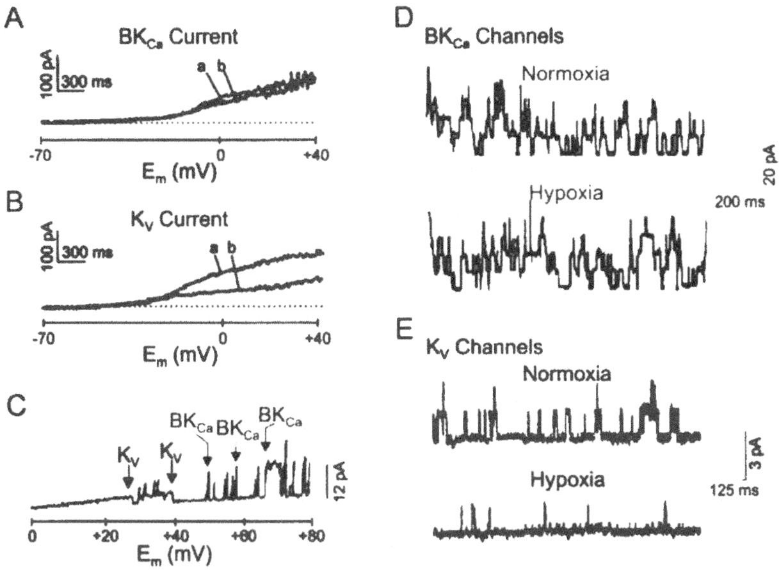

Figure 4 Hypoxia inhibits Kv current but has little effect on BK_{Ca} current in canine pulmonary resistance arteries. (A) Potassium current in an SMC pretreated with 4-AP to block Kv channels and thereby isolate BK_{Ca} current was unresponsive to hypoxia (a = normoxia, b = hypoxia). The K^+ current was elicited by a depolarizing ramp from −70 to +40 mV. (B) Potassium current in an SMC pretreated with tetraethylammonium to block BK_{Ca} channels and thereby isolate Kv current was inhibited by hypoxia (a = normoxia, b = hypoxia). (C) The Kv and BK_{Ca} channels showing low and high amplitudes, respectively, were evident in a single patch. The single-channel K^+ currents were elicited by a depolarizing ramp from 0 to +80 mV. (D) Hypoxia had no significant effect on the open-state probability of single BK_{Ca} channel currents in an inside-out patch. (E) In contrast, hypoxia inhibited single Kv channel currents in an inside-out patch. (Modified from Ref. 64 with permission.)

in Po_2 under patch-clamp conditions, whereas the lack of a similar domain in the BK_{Ca} channel results in its apparent insensitivity to changes in Po_2.

It is important to recognize that the Kv channels of the distal pulmonary SMCs are not regulated solely by hypoxia; there are other unique responses to metabolic challenge that appear to rely on Kv channel heterogeneity. For example, intracellular acidosis (pH of 6.4 compared to control pH of 7) activates whole-cell K^+ current in SMCs of rat coronary arteries (Fig. 5A) but inhibits K^+ current in pulmonary SMCs from the same animal (Fig. 5B) (67). These opposing responses to acidosis persist after BK_{Ca} channels are blocked by iberiotoxin (IBTX) but are eliminated by

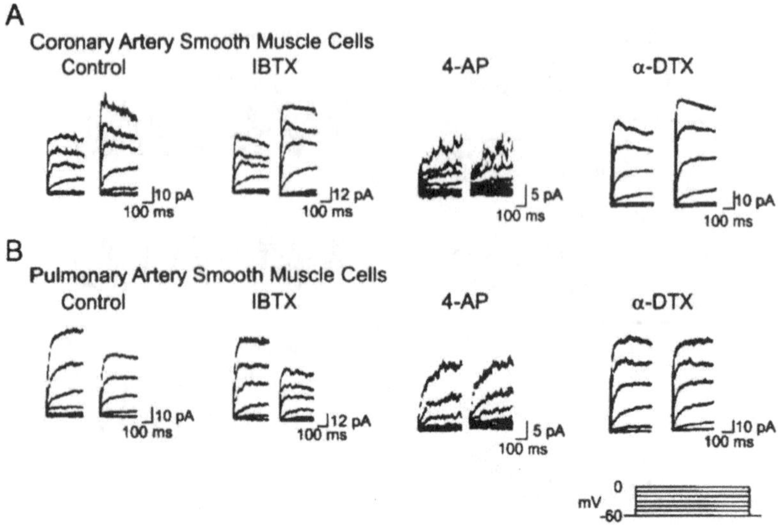

Figure 5 Changing intracellular pH from 7 to 6.4 has opposing effects on K^+ current in rat coronary and pulmonary SMCs. (A) and (B), left to right sets of tracings. Acidosis increases K^+ current in coronary SMCs but reduces K^+ current in pulmonary SMCs. In both types of SMCs, the sensitivity of K^+ current to pH persists after BK_{Ca} channels are blocked by iberiotoxin (IBTX, 100 nmol /L). However, block of Kv channels by 4-aminopyridine(4-Ap) eliminates the acidosis-induced changes in K^+ current in coronary and pulmonary SMCs, identifying Kv channels as mediators of pH sensitivity. Only the pH sensitivity of coronary SMCs remained in the presence of α-dendrotoxin (α-DTX), an inhibitor of Kv1.1, Kv1.2, and Kv1.6 channel subtypes. Thus, Kv channels composed of these α subunits uniquely respond to pH in pulmonary SMCs, whereas the identity of the pH-sensitive Kv channels in coronary SMCs appears to be different. (Modified from Ref. 67 with permission.)

pharmacological block of Kv channels by 4-AP. Thus, similar to hypoxia, the Kv channels in vascular SMCs appear to be responsible for the opposing responses to low pH of the systemic and pulmonary vascular beds. Furthermore, α-dendrotoxin(α-DTX), which blocks only Kv channels composed of Kv1.1, Kv1.2, and Kv1.6 α subunits, does not affect the acidosis-induced increase in Kv current in coronary SMCs but abolishes the corresponding decrease in pulmonary SMCs. One interpretation of these findings is that a unique population of Kv1 family members exclusively confers pH sensitivity mediated by changes in K^+ currents to pulmonary resistance arteries, whereas the systemic vascular beds express other subtypes of Kv channels that confer the opposite response to changes in intracellular protonation.

V. CONCLUSIONS

It appears that a common strategy to differentially regulate vascular tone is to enlist patterns of variability in ion channel expression or regulation within and between tissues to enable the differential regulation of vascular tone. To illustrate the functional importance of distinct patterns of ion channel expression, one need only examine the correlation between the pulmonary resistance arteries that manifest hypoxic pulmonary vasoconstriction and the distribution of O_2-sensitive Kv channels. For example, both the large and small pulmonary arteries express Ca_L, BK_{Ca}, and Kv channels. However, compared to the large arteries (Fig. 6A), the small arteries of the lung express a higher density of Ca_L and Kv channels (Fig. 6B). Hypoxia activates Ca_L channels in the SMCs of small arteries, and the resulting rise in intracellular calcium combined with the loss of the oxidative environment inactivates Kv channels. The sparse BK_{Ca} channels are unable to counteract the resulting depolarization and vasoconstriction of the resistance vessels.

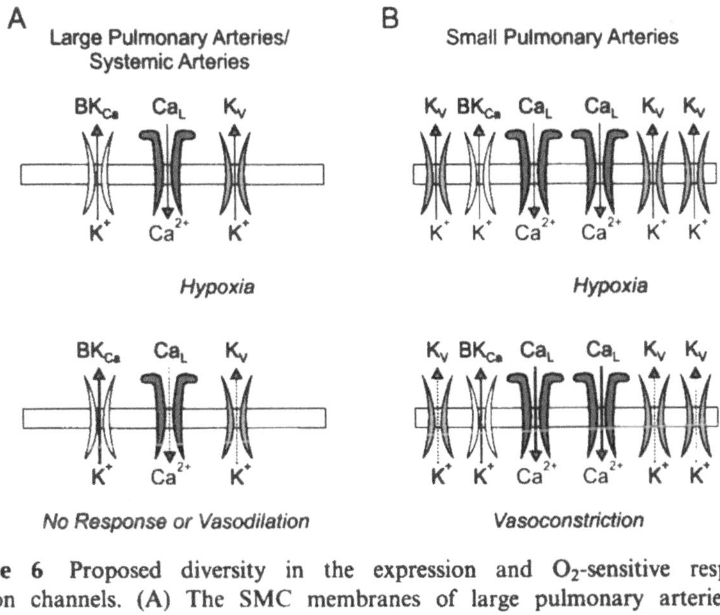

Figure 6 Proposed diversity in the expression and O_2-sensitive responses of ion channels. (A) The SMC membranes of large pulmonary arteries and systemic arteries express a medley of BK_{Ca}, Ca_L, and Kv channels. Hypoxia inhibits the Ca_L channels to reduce Ca^{2+} influx, whereas BK_{Ca} channels are slightly activated or unaffected. Although Kv channels may close, the overall vasoactive effect is little change or vasodilation. (B) The SMCs of small pulmonary arteries densely express Ca_L and Kv channels and express fewer BK_{Ca} channels. Hypoxia activates the Ca_L channels to increase Ca^{2+} influx and concurrently inhibits the Kv channels to induce depolarization and promote further Ca^{2+} entry. The resulting vasoactive effect is a strong vasoconstriction.

In contrast, the large arteries express more BK_{Ca} channels that are relatively O_2-insensitive, and, surprisingly, the Ca_L channels expressed in theconduit arteries are inhibited by hypoxia. As discussed in this chapter, the molecular mechanisms for many of these responses are poorly understood, but the impetus to understand the subunit basis of the ion channels and their interaction with the redox environment of the SMCs should lead to new insights into the regulation of pulmonary vascular tone.

REFERENCES

1. Pichler M, Cassidy TN, Reimer D, Haase H, Kraus R, Ostler D, Striessnig J. β Subunit heterogeneity in neuronal L-type Ca^{2+} channels. J Biol Chem 1997; 272:13877–13882.
2. Koch WJ, Ellinor PT, Schwartz A. cDNA cloning of a dihydropyridine-sensitive calcium channel from rat aorta. J Biol Chem 1990; 265: 17786–17791.
3. Berrow NS, Campbell V, Fitzgerald EM, Brickley K, Dolphine AC. Antisense depletion of β subunits modulates the biophysical and pharmacological properties of neuronal calcium channels. J Physiol 1995; 482:481–491.
4. Birmbaumer L, Qin N, Olcese R, Tareilus E, Platano D, Costantin J, Stefani E. Structures and functions of calcium channel β subunits. J Bioenerg Biomembr 1998; 30:357–375.
5. Cens T, Restituito S, Vallentin A, Charnet P. Promotion and inhibition of L-type Ca^{2+} channel facilitation by distinct domains of the β subunit. J Biol Chem 1998; 273:18308–18315.
6. Chien J, Zhao X, Shirokov RE, Piru TS, Chang CF, Sun D, Rios E, Hosey MM. Roles of a membrane-localized β subunit in the formation and targeting of functional L-type Ca^{2+} channels. J Biol Chem 1995; 270:30036–30044.
7. Gurnett CA, Felix R, Campbell KP. Extracellular interaction of the voltage-dependent Ca^{2+} channel α_2/δ and α_1 subunits. J Biol Chem 1997; 272:18508–18512.
8. Varadi G, Mori Y, Mikala G, Schwartz A. Molecular deteminants of Ca^{2+} channel function and drug action. Trends Pharmacol Sci 1995; 16:43–49.
9. Wei X, Pan S, Lang W, Kim H, Schneider T, Perez-Reyes E, Birnbaumaer L. Molecular determinants of cardiac Ca^{2+}channel pharmacology. J Biol Chem 1995; 270:27106–27111.
10. Nelson MT, Patlak JB, Worley JF, Standen NB. Calcium channels, potassium channels, and voltage-dependence of arterial smooth muscle tone. Am J Physiol 1990; 259:C3–C18.
11. Franco-Obregon A, Lopez-Barneo J. Differential oxygen sensitivity of calcium channels in rabbit smooth muscle cells of conduit and resistance pulmonary arteries. J Physiol 1996; 491:511–518.
12. Remillard CV, Zhang W, Shimoda LA, Sham JSK. Physiological properties and functions of Ca^{2+} sparks in rat intrapulmonary arterial smooth muscle cells. Am J Physiol 2002; 283:L433–L444.
13. Heginbotham L, Lu Z, Abramson T, MacKinnon R. Mutations in the K^+ channel signature sequence. Biophys J 1994; 66:1061–1067.

14. Post JM, Gelband CH, Hume JR. Calcium inhibition of K^+ channels in canine pulmonary artery. Novel mechanism for hypoxia-induced membrane depolarization. Circ Res 1995; 77:131–139.
15. Cox RH, Petrou S. Calcium influx inhibits voltage-dependent and augments Ca^{2+}-dependent K^+ currents in arterialmyocytes. Am J Physiol 1999; 277:C51-C63.
16. Pongs O. Molecular biology of voltage-gated K^+ channels. In: Archer SL, Rusch NJ, eds. Potassium Channel in Cardiovascular Biology. New York: Kluwer Academic Plenum, 2001:35–48.
17. Kreusch A, Pfaffinger PJ, Stevens CF, Choe S. Crystal structure of the tetramerization domain of the Shaker potassium channel. Nature 1998; 392: 945–948.
18. Patel AJ, Lazdunski M, Honore E. Kv2.1/Kv9.3, a novel ATP-dependent delayed-rectifier K^+ channel in oxygen-sensitive pulmonary artery myocytes. EMBO J 1997; 16:6615–6625.
19. Salinas M, Duprat F, Heurteaux C, Hugnot JP, Lazdunski M. New modulatory α subunits for mammalian Shab K^+ channels. J Biol Chem 1997; 272: 24371–24379.
20. Levitan ES, Gealy R, Trimmer JS, Takimoto K. Membrane depolarization inhibits Kv1.5 voltage-gated K^+ channel gene transcription and protein expression in pituitary cells. J Biol Chem 1995; 270:6036–6041.
21. Heinemann SH, Rettig J, Graack HR, Pongs O. Functional characterization of Kv channel β-subunits from rat brain. J Physiol 1996; 493: 625–633.
22. Gulbis JM, Mann S, MacKinnon R. Structure of a voltage-dependent K^+ channel β subunit. Cell 1999; 97:943-952.
23. Shi G, Nakahira K, Hammond S, Rhodes KJ, Schechter LE, Trimmer JS. Beta subunits promote K^+ channel surface expression through effects early in biosynthesis. Neuron 1996; 16:843–852.
24. Yuan XJ, Wang J, Juhaszova M, Golovina VA, Rubin LJ. Molecular basis and function of voltage-gated K^+ channels in pulmonary arterial smooth muscle cells. Am J Physiol 1998; 274:L621–L635.
25. Archer SL, Michelakis E. The mechanism of hypoxic pulmonary vasoconstriction: potassium channels, redox O_2 sensors, and controversies. News Physiol Sci 2002; 17:131 137.
26. Sweeney M, Yuan J X-J. Hypoxic pulmonary vasoconstriction: role of voltage-gated potassium channels. Respir Res 2000; 1:40–48.
27. Coppock EA, Martens JR, Tamkun MM. Molecular basis of hypoxia-induced pulmonary vasoconstriction: role of voltage-gated K^+ channels. Am J Physiol 2001; 281:L1–L12.
28. Hulme JT, Coppock EA, Felipe A, Martens JR, Tamkun MM. Oxygen sensitivity of cloned voltage-gated K^+ channels expressed in the pulmonary vasculature. Circ Res 1999; 85:489–497.
29. Meera P, Wallner M, Toro L. Molecular biology of high-conductance, Ca^{2+}-activated potassium channels. In: Archer SL, Rusch NJ, eds. Potassium Channels in Cardiovascular Biology. New York: Kluwer Academic/Plenum, 2001:49–70.

30. Orio P, Rojas P, Ferreira G, Latorre R. New disguises for an old channel: MaxiK channel subunits. News Physiol Sci 2002; 17:156–161.
31. Quirk JC, Reinhart PH. Identification of a novel tetramerization domain in large conductance K_{Ca} channels. Neuron 2001; 32:13–23.
32. Bian S, Favre I, Moczydlowski E. Ca^{2+}-binding activity of a COOH-terminal fragment of the *Drosophila* BK channel involved in Ca^{2+}-dependent activation. Proc Natl Acad Sci USA 2001; 98:4776–4781.
33. Shipston MJ. Alternative splicing of potassium channels: a dynamic switch of cellular excitability. Trends Cell Biol 2001; 11:353–357.
34. Jackson WF, Blair KL. Characterization and function of Ca^{2+}-activated K^+ channels in arteriolar muscle cells. Am J Physiol 1998; 274:H27–H34.
35. Sansom SC, Stockand JD. Differential Ca^{2+}-sensitivities of BK_{Ca} isochannels in bovine mesenteric vascular smooth muscle. Am J Physiol 1994; 266: C1182–C1189.
36. Toro L, Vaca L, Stefani E. Calcium-activated potassium channels from coronary smooth muscle reconstituted into lipid bilayers. Am J Physiol 1991; 260:H1779–H1789.
37. Bae YM, Park MK, Lee SH, Ho W-K, Earm YE. Contribution of Ca^{2+}-activated K^+ channels and non-selective cation channels to membrane potential of pulmonary arterial smooth muscle cells of the rabbit. J Physiol 1999: 747–758.
38. Farrukh IS, Peng W, Orlinska U, Hoidal JR. Effect of dehydroepiandrosterone on hypoxic pulmonary vasoconstriction: a Ca^{2+}-activated K^+ channel opener. Am J Physiol 1998; 274:L186–L198.
39. Tristani-Firouzi M, Reeve HL, Tolarova S, Weir EK, Archer SL. Oxygen-induced constriction of the rabbit ductus arteriosus occurs via inhibition of a 4-aminopyridine-sensitive potassium channel. J Clin Invest 1996; 98: 1959–1965.
40. Lee S, Park M, So I, Earm YE. NADH and NAD modulates Ca^{2+}-activated K^+ channels in small pulmonary arterial smooth muscle cells of the rabbit. Pflügers Arch 1994; 427:378–380.
41. Park MK, Lee SH, Lee SJ, Ho WK, Earm YE. Different modulation of Ca-activated K channels by the intracellular redox potential in pulmonary and ear arterial smooth muscle cells of the rabbit. Pflügers Arch 1995; 430: 308–314.
42. Karamsetty MR, Wadsworth RM, Kane KA. Effect of K^+ channel blocking drugs and nitric oxide synthase inihibition on the response to hypoxia in rat pulmonary artery rings. J Auton Pharmacol 1998; 18:49–56.
43. Shimoda LA, Sylvester JT, Sham JSK. Chronic hypoxia alters effects of endothelin and angiotensin on K^+ currents in pulmonary arterial myocytes. Am J Physiol 1999; 277:L431–L439.
44. Archer SL, Huang JMC, Reeve HL, Hampl V, Tolarova S, Michelakis E, Weir EK. Differential distribution of electrophysiologically distinct myocytes in conduit and resistance arteries determines their response to nitric oxide and hypoxia. Circ Res 1996; 78:431–442.
45. Hall SM, Hislop AA, Haworth SG. Origin, differentiation, and maturation of human pulmonary veins. Am J Respir Cell Mol Biol 2002; 26:333–340.

46. Hall SM, Hislop AA, Pierce CM, Haworth SG. Prenatal origins of human intrapulmonary arteries: formation and smooth muscle maturation. Am J Respir Cell Mol Biol 2000; 23:194–203.
47. Yuan XJ, Wang J, Juhaszova M, Golovina VA, Rubin LJ. Molecular basis and function of voltage-gated K^+ channels in pulmonary arterial smooth muscle cells. Am J Physiol 1998; 274:L621–L635.
48. Yuan XJ, Aldinger AM, Juhaszova M, Wang J, Conte JV, Gaine SP, Orens JB, Rubin LJ. Dyfunctional voltage-gated K^+ channels in pulmonary artery smooth muscle cells of patients with primary pulmonary hypertension. Circulation 1998; 98:1400–1406.
49. Platoshyn O, Yu Y, Golovina VA, McDaniel SS, Krick S, Li L, Wang J-Y, Rubin LJ, Yuan JX-J. Chronic hypoxia decreases Kv channel expression and function in pulmonary artery myocytes. Am J Physiol 2001; 280:L801–L812.
50. Cornfield D, Reeve H, Tolarova S, Weir E, Archer S. Oxygen causes fetal pulmonary vasodilation through activation of a calcium-dependent potassium channel. Proc Natl Acad Sci USA 1996; 93:8089–8094.
51. Archer SL. Diversity of phenotype and function of vascular smooth muscle cells. J Lab Clin Med 1996; 127:524–529.
52. Smirnov SV, Beck R, Tammaro P, Ishii T, Aaronson PI. Electrophysiologically distinct smooth muscle cell subtypes in rat conduit and resistance pulmonary arteries. J Physiol 2002; 538:867 878.
53. Archer SL, Souil E, Dinh-Xuan AT, Shcremmer B, Mercier J-C, El Yaagoubi A, Nguyen-Huu L, Reeve HL, Hampl V. Molecular identification of the role of voltage-gated K channels, Kv1.5 and Kv2.1, in hypoxic pulmonary vasoconstriction and control of resting membrane potential in rat pulmonary artery myocytes. J Clin Invest 1998; 101:2319–2330.
54. Bennie RE, Packer CS, Powell DR, Jin N, Rhoades RA. Biphasic contractile response of pulmonary artery to hypoxia. Am J Physiol 1991; 261:L156–L163.
55. Jin N, Packer C, Rhoades R. Pulmonary arterial hypoxic contraction: signal transduction. Am J Physiol 1992; 263:L73–L78.
56. Archer SL, Weir EK, Reeve HL, Michelakis E. Molecular identification of O_2 sensors and O_2-sensitive potassium channels in the pulmonary circulation. Adv Exp Med Biol 2000; 475:219–240.
57. Michelakis ED, Hampl V, Nsair A, Wu X, Haromy G, Harry A, Guetu R, Archer SL. Diversity in mitochondrial function explains differences in vascular oxygen sensing. Circ Res 2002; 90:1307–1315.
58. Michelakis ED, Rebeyka I, Wu X, Nsair A, Thepaud B, Hashimoto K, Dyck JR, Haromy A, Harry G, Barr A, Archer SL. O_2 sensing in the human ductus arteriosus: regulation of voltage-gated K^+ channels in smooth muscle cells by a mitochondrial redox sensor. Circ Res 2002; 91:478–486.
59. Campbell DL, Stamler JS, Strauss HC. Redox modulation of L-type calcium channels in ferret ventricular myocytes. Dual mechanism regulation by nitric oxide and S-nitrosothiols. J Gen Physiol 1996; 108:277–293.
60. Park MK, Le SH, Lee SJ, Ho WK, Earm YE. Different modulation of Ca-activated K channels by the intracellular redox potential in pulmonary and ear arterial smooth muscle cells of the rabbit. Pflugers Arch 1995; 430:308–314.

61. Ruppersberg J, Stocker M, Pongs O, Heinemann S, Frank R, Koenen M. Regulation of fast inactivation of cloned mammalian $I_K(A)$ channels by cysteine oxidation. Nature 1991; 352:711–714.
62. Archer SL, Nelson DP, Weir EK. Simultaneous measurement of oxygen radicals and pulmonary vascular reactivity in the isolated rat lung. J Appl Physiol 1989; 67:1903–1911.
63. Fearon AM, Varadi G, Koch S, Isaacsohn I, Ball SG, Peers C. Splice variants reveal the region involved in oxygen sensing by recombinant human L-type Ca^{2+} channels. Circ Res 2000; 87:537–539.
64. Post J, Hume J, Archer S, Weir E. Direct role for potassium channel inhibition in hypoxic pulmonary vasoconstriction. Am J Physiol 1992; 262:C882–C890.
65. Yuan X-J, Goldman W, Tod M, Rubin L, Blaustein M. Hypoxia reduces potassium currents in cultured rat pulmonary but not mesenteric arterial myocytes. Am J Physiol 1993; 264:L116–L123.
66. Archer SL, London B, Hampl V, Wu X, Nsair A, Puttagunta L, Hashimoto K, Waite RE, Michelakis ED. Impairment of hypoxic pulmonary vasoconstriction in mice lacking the voltage-gated potassium channel Kv1.5. FASEB J 2001; 15:1801–1803.
67. Berger MG, Vandier C, Bonnet P, Jackson WF, Rusch NJ. Intracellular acidosis differentially regulates Kv channels in coronary and pulmonary vascular muscle. Am J Physiol 1998; 275:H1351–H1359.

4

Voltage-Gated Ca^{2+} Channels in the Pulmonary Vasculature

Gregory A. Knock and Philip I. Aaronson
Centre for Cardiovascular Biology and Medicine, King's College, London, U.K.

I. INTRODUCTION

Although most vascular smooth muscles (VSMs) do not exhibit action potentials, changes in membrane potential are almost always integral to vascular responses to both constricting and dilating stimuli. Under resting conditions in vivo, the VSM membrane potential is sufficiently depolarized that Ca^{2+} influx through *voltage-gated Ca^{2+} channels* (VGCCs) makes an important contribution to basal tone. The opening of these channels is enhanced by depolarization and suppressed by hyperpolarization, leading to alterations in the intracellular calcium concentration ($[Ca^{2+}]_i$) that correspondingly potentiate or diminish force development and therefore vascular resistance.

Studies over the past two decades have provided an enormous amount of information as to the molecular classification, structures, regulation, and roles of VGCCs in the *systemic* vasculature. However, remarkably few direct studies of these channels have been carried out in the *pulmonary* vasculature, although a certain amount is known about the manner in which VGCCs contribute to the regulation of the pulmonary circulation, particularly with regard to hypoxic pulmonary vasoconstriction (HPV).

Accordingly, we have divided the remainder of this chapter into two sections. Section II describes the classification, structure, and regulation of VGCCs in the systemic vasculature, as it is likely that these properties will carry over into pulmonary vascular smooth muscle. Section III then describes the much smaller amount of information available about the properties of VGCCs in pulmonary arteries (PAs), and reviews the literature concerning the role these channels play in controlling the responses of pulmonary arteries to endogenous constrictors, changes in pressure, and, most important, hypoxia.

II. VGCCs IN SYSTEMIC VASCULAR SMOOTH MUSCLE

A. Structure of Voltage-Gated Calcium Channels; Subunit mRNA and Protein Expression; Splice Variants and Tissue Distributions

Voltage-gated calcium channels are members of a gene superfamily of transmembrane ion channel proteins that also includes voltage-gated potassium and sodium channels. Each channel is a composite protein, comprising the products of four or five genes: a central pore-forming α_1 subunit and several auxiliary subunits, including an intracellularly located β subunit and an extracellularly located α_2/δ subunit. The fifth, transmembrane subunit, γ, is present in some but not all tissues.

The α_1 Subunit

The α_1 subunit is the largest (190–250 kDa). It incorporates the conducting core, the voltage sensor, and gating apparatus, as well as most of the known sites for regulation by second messengers and drugs. The electrophysiological and pharmacological diversity of VGCCs is derived primarily, but not exclusively, from the existence of multiple forms of the α_1 unit (1–3). In mammals, there are at least 10 distinct α_1 genes, which are classified numerically into three main groups, Ca_v1, Ca_v2, and Ca_v3, according to amino acid sequence homology (4). $Ca_v1.2$, which is responsible for the high-threshold, dihydropyridine sensitive L-type current (see below) has at least three splice variants, of which $Ca_v1.2b$ (formerly known as $\alpha_{1C\text{-}b}$) is the predominant form in smooth muscle. Some smooth muscle containing tissues may also express the mainly cardioselective $Ca_v1.2a$. $Ca_v3.1$, $Ca_v3.2$, and $Ca_v3.3$ (formerly α_{1G}, α_{1H}, and α_{1I}), may also be present in some smooth muscles because they are known to mediate the high threshold T-type current (4) (also see below).

The $\alpha_{1C}/Ca_v1.2$ channel-forming proteins possess a transmembrane structure consisting of four repeat units (I, II, III, IV) that each consist of six putative transmembrane segments, the fourth of which (S_4) contains three to five positively charged amino acid residues that presumably form the voltage sensor. Both NH_2 and COOH terminals are cytoplasmic, and the longer COOH tail contains the two Ca^{2+}-sensing domains L and K, which are believed to possess multiple binding sites for Ca^{2+} ion and Ca^{2+}-calmodulin (5). There are several transmembrane segments and Ca^{2+}-sensing motifs that are encoded by up to 15 alternative exons, thus accounting for a large number of possible channel subunit splice variants with different potentially tissue- and species-specific functional properties (reviewed in Ref. 5).

The β Subunit

There are four distinct isoforms of the β subunit, coded for by four distinct genes (β_1, β_2, β_3 and β_4). Additional heterogeneity of channel function is conferred by the tissue-specific expression of one or more of these isoforms and splice variants thereof (6). β subunits are intracellularly located and are believed to bind tightly to the intracellular surface of the α1 subunit. Cotransfection studies with mouse brain Ca^{2+} channels have shown that in the presence of a β_2 subunit, currents were larger, activated faster and inactivated more rapidly, implying that β subunits facilitate gating (7). β_2 and β_3 are expressed in smooth muscle, but only β_3 participates in channel formation in rabbit aorta as determined by immunoprecipitation of (+)-[^{3}H]isradipine-prelabeled α_1 channels (6).

The α_2/δ Subunit

The α_2 and δ components of the α_2/δ protein are the products of the same gene and are linked posttranslationally by a disulfide bridge. α2 is located in the membrane, whereas δ extends into the extracellular space. At least three α_2/δ genes exist (α_2/δ-1, α_2/δ-2, and α_2/δ-3), and, like α_1 and β subunits, they may also express multiple splice variants (8). When coexpressed with α_1 and β_2 subunits in HEK-293 cells, the cardiac α_2/δ subunit speeds activation and deactivation kinetics and significantly increases channel conductance, suggesting that it too facilitates Ca^{2+} channel gating (9).

The γ Subunit

To date, eight distinct γ subunits have been cloned (10). Little is known about the regulation, if any, of the $Ca_v1.2b$ Ca^{2+} channel in smooth muscle by γ subunits, but in expression systems the γ1 protein shifts the voltage dependence of inactivation of complexes of α_{1C} ($Ca_v1.2a$) coexpressed with β and α_2/δ to more negative potentials and alters the current kinetics (11).

B. Electrophysiological and Pharmacological Characteristics of Ca^{2+} Currents in Vascular Smooth Muscle

All vascular smooth muscles possess at least one type of inward Ca^{2+} current that is activated by depolarisation: the "L-type" or "high voltage-activated" current, which is mediated by the $Ca_v1.2b$-base channel. The channel current has a conductance of ~25 pS in isotonic Ba^{2+} solution and is sensitive to dihydropyridines (e.g., nifedipine), phenylalkylamines (e.g., verapamil), and benzothiazepines (e.g., diltiazem) (12). High-affinity binding sites for all three classes of channel blockers are located on transmembrane segments of the α_1 subunit in close proximity to the pore opening (13). L-type Ca^{2+} currents are also sensitive to dihydropyridine-type agonists, such as BayR 5417, which promote arterial smooth muscle Ca^{2+} channel opening at steady-state membrane potentials (14). Also present in most types of VSMs that have been studied is the small "T-type" or "low-voltage-activated" current (15), which is insensitive to dihydropyridines, phenylalkylamines, and benzothiazepines and is mediated by a Ca_v3 channel with a conductance of ~8 pS in isotonic Ba^{2+} solution. Its physiological relevance in vascular smooth muscle remains in doubt (16), because it is likely to be substantially or completely inactivated in most VSMs except perhaps during and immediately after hyperpolarizing vasodilation in resistance arteries.

Voltage-gated calcium channels exist in at least three states, namely, the resting, open, and inactivated states. Movement from the resting to the open and from the open to the inactivated state occurs upon depolarization and is both voltage- and time-dependent (17). Single-channel and whole-cell patch-clamp studies have demonstrated that single Ca^{2+} channels in VSM cells have a low steady-state probability of opening at membrane potentials between −60 and −40 mV, and that open probability increases steeply with depolarizations from relatively hyperpolarized membrane potentials (14,18). The opposing processes of channel opening and inactivation give rise to a "window current," which reaches a peak at about −20 mV (15) and represents the sustained potential–dependent Ca^{2+} influx that underlies arterial tone (19).

C. Intracellular Pathways of Ca^{2+} Channel Regulation

The L-type Ca^{2+} channel in VSM cells is thought to be modulated by a number of cellular second messenger systems that are activated in response to vasoactive substances such as norepinephrine, endothelin, angiotensin II, 5-HT, and nitric oxide. Stimulation of protein kinase G (PKG), which occurs in response to nitric oxide, inhibits the L-type current (20,21). On the other hand, stimulation of protein kinase C (PKC), which occurs in response to the activation of most G-protein-linked vasoconstrictors, has consistently been shown to potentiate the L-type current in VSM.

Stimulation of the adenylate cyclase/cAMP/protein kinase A (PKA) system has been shown in various studies to inhibit, not affect, or increase this current (21). The bulk of the evidence favors the concept that PKA acts to enhance the current, as it does in cardiac cells. Notably, in 1993 Ishikawa et al. (22) showed in rabbit portal vein VSM that the small increase in the Ca^{2+} current induced by stimuli that activated PKA was replaced by an inhibition when high concentrations of these stimuli were used. Inhibition also occurred with 8-bromo-cGMP, which stimulates protein kinase G. Ishikawa et al. argued that PKA was acting to stimulate the current but that high levels of cAMP were inhibiting the current because PKG was also being stimulated.

In 2001, Keef et al. (21) suggested the unifying hypothesis that activation of various receptors linked to G proteins may act to stimulate PKC and therefore enhance the Ca^{2+} current through a common mechanism involving $\beta\gamma$ G-protein subunits.

There is also evidence that nonreceptor tyrosine kinases, in particular c-Src, act to enhance the L-type current (e.g., Ref. 23). This pathway is potentially of great importance in mediating the responses of arteries and arterioles to changes in flow and pressure. Recent work suggests that activation of the fibronectin receptor, one of the integrins involved in linking the vascular extracellular matrix to the VSM actin cytoskeleton, stimulates Ca^{2+} influx through the L-type channel via c-Src or a similar tyrosine kinase (24).

D. Role of Ca^{2+} Channels in Myogenic Tone

Myogenic tone develops in response to graded depolarization of the smooth muscle cell membrane caused by increases in perfusion pressure. The contribution of this response to the overall arterial tone and hence to vascular resistance may vary between vascular beds but appears to be important, at least in rat cerebral and rat mesenteric arteries (25,26), in which it is abolished by the removal of extracellular Ca^{2+} and by dihydropyridine Ca^{2+} channel antagonists. In the rat cerebral model, direct involvement of the voltage-sensitive Ca^{2+} current was confirmed by its response to stretch in isolated voltage-clamped smooth muscle cells (25).

III. VGCCs IN PULMONARY VSM

A. Ca^{2+} Channels in Lung

Of α_1 subunits, only $Ca_v1.2b$ is expressed in human lung (27,28). The rabbit lung $Ca_V1.2b$ differs from the rabbit heart $Ca_V1.2a$ with sequence homologies of between 55% and 70% at two intracellular and two transmembrane sites (27). It is worth noting that, although in studies of whole lung no distinction has been made between pulmonary vascular and airway smooth muscles, it can reasonably be assumed from electrophysiological data (see below) that $Ca_V1.2b$ is expressed in both. α_2/δ-2 mRNA is highly expressed in lung (8,29), but, interestingly, its protein is apparently absent (8). γ_4, γ_6, and γ_7 have also been detected in rat lung (10), but it is not known which of the two β-subunits found in smooth muscle, β_2 and β_3, is preferentially expressed in this tissue.

B. Resting Membrane Potentials and Ca^{2+} Channel Activity in the Pulmonary Artery

Several studies on membrane properties and Ca^{2+} currents in VSM have used the main pulmonary artery (PA) of the rabbit as an example of a large elastic artery. For example, Ito et al. (30) used it to show that diltiazem did not modify the membrane potential (-56 mV) or length constant (1.47 mm) but did suppress mechanical responses induced either by direct stimulation of the muscle or by neural activation and suppressed K^+-induced contraction without affecting K^+-induced depolarization. They also showed that under voltage-clamp conditions, diltiazem raised the critical membrane potential displacement necessary to evoke contraction from 5 mV to 12 mV (30). However, the small PA likely to be responsible for pulmonary vascular resistance may behave very differently from those in the main PA. In the rat, this issue was addressed by Suzuki and Twarog (31). Resting membrane potentials were similar in both the small and main pulmonary arteries (~52 mV), and cells displayed no spontaneous electrical activity. The maximum membrane depolarization produced by a tenfold increase in extracellular [K^+] was also similar (47–48 mV) (31).

It appears that the rat main PA possesses no basal tone in young healthy rats, because Ca^{2+}-free salt solution containing 2 mM EGTA does not relax isolated main PA rings under resting conditions. In accordance with this finding, the L-type VGCC agonist BayK8644 itself produces little or no contraction unless applied in the presence of submaximal, slightly depolarizing concentrations of K^+ (32). This suggests that the channel open probability is very low at the resting membrane potential, at least in vitro.

C. VGCC Currents in PA

Calcium ion currents have been characterized under whole-cell voltage-clamp conditions in freshly isolated smooth muscle cells derived from rabbit main PA (20,33,34). Small inward currents were observed when Cs-TEA was present in the pipette solution. These currents demonstrated L-type-like characteristics, including a voltage dependence of activation and inactivation with an apparent activation threshold at about –50 mV (33) or –40 mV (20), a maximum inward amplitude at about 0 mV, and a half-inactivation potential of –40 mV (33) or –22mV (20). There is no obvious indication from slight differences in experimental protocols to explain the rather large difference in half-inactivation potentials between these two studies. In any case, the currents were enhanced by increasing the extracellular calcium concentration or by replacing it with Ba^{2+}, were blocked by nicardipine and Mn^{2+} ions (33,34) or by nifedipine and Cd^{2+} ions, and were insensitive to tetrodotoxin (20). Similar "L-type" currents have been described in smooth muscle cells of the canine main PA (35).

It is noteworthy that none of the electrophysiological characterizations of the Ca^{2+} current in the PA of any species have revealed the existence of a T-type current.

Almost nothing is known about the regulation by agonists and cellular signal transduction pathway of VGCCs in pulmonary VSM. In the pioneering study of Clapp and Gurney (20), the NO donor sodium nitroprusside (NP), presumably acting via cGMP/PKG activation, reversibly inhibited the Ca^{2+} channel current (~45% block of peak amplitude by 1 μM) in freshly isolated smooth muscle cells of rabbit main PA. This inhibition was characterized by an enhanced current decay rate and occurred equally over all membrane potentials tested. NP also induced spontaneous outward currents in these cells. Whether the inhibition of I_{Ca} by NP contributes to the relaxant effect of the artery remains to be determined. There is also indirect evidence from a study by Shimoda et al. (36) that endothelin may act directly, rather than via depolarization, to activate VGCC in the rat intrapulmonary arteries.

D. Role of VGCCs in Regulating PA Constriction

There is little doubt that in pulmonary arterial smooth muscle, L-type Ca^{2+} channels are functionally coupled to contraction. This is readily demonstrated by their apparent involvement in myogenic tone (see below) and the contractile responses to high K^+ depolarization in isolated arteries of all sizes, from the main extralobar (32) down to the smallest manageable sizes of the intrapulmonary branches (37). Work in Fura-2 loaded arteries demonstrates that, not surprisingly, these contractions are associated with elevations in $[Ca^{2+}]_i$.

The dependence of K^+-induced contractions on Ca^{2+} influx through voltage-gated channels in rat main PA is made clear by the sensitivity of these contractions to organic L-type channel antagonists and their dependence on extracellular Ca^{2+} (32). Indeed, high K^+ contractions, at least in rat intrapulmonary arteries (37), are often greater in magnitude than the maximal contractions induced by most agonists, excluding perhaps ET-1 and U46619.

E. Myogenic Tone in Pulmonary Arteries

Human pulmonary veins apparently display spontaneous myogenic tone (38), and in the rat the main extralobar PA and small PA both depolarize in response to mechanical stretch (31). This occurs to a greater degree in the small PA (31).

There is evidence for a role for myogenic tone in the pulmonary circulation of the fetal and/or neonatal lung. For example, in the isolated guinea pig large extralobar pulmonary artery, the myogenic response appears more pronounced in the neonate than in the adult (39), and in an in vivo chronically instrumented fetal lamb model, partial occlusion of the ductus arteriosus caused pulmonary vascular resistance to gradually decrease, but when nitric oxide synthesis was inhibited, blood flow quickly decreased to a plateau whereas vascular resistance steadily rose with time (40). This has implications for fetal pulmonary hypertension where endothelial damage and impaired NO production may result in an enhanced myogenic response (41). The importance of VGCCs in the myogenic response within the pulmonary circulation was also confirmed in a neonatal sheep perfused-lung model (42), in which verapamil substantially inhibited increases in pulmonary arterial pressure induced by elevations in end-expiratory pressure.

F. Dependence on VGCCs of Vasoconstrictor-Induced Contractions in PA

The involvement of L-type VGCCs in controlling vascular force development evoked by vasoconstrictors has been extensively assessed using organic Ca^{2+} channel antagonists such as nifedipine, diltiazem, and verapamil. This method suffers from a number of drawbacks, including most notably the trade-off between incomplete channel block and drug nonselectivity. Not withstanding this problem, however, it is clear that there is enormous species-, site-, and vasoconstrictor-related variability in the contribution of these channels to contraction [see review by Godfraind et al. (43)]. In the systemic circulation, the role of L-type channels in vasoconstrictor-induced contractions appears to be larger in resistance arteries than in conduit arteries [see, e.g., Cauvin et al. (44)], a finding that is consistent with observations that agonist-induced depolarization is more prominent in the former.

Although fewer studies have been carried out in the pulmonary vasculature, it seems generally to be the case that L-type channels make a relatively minor contribution to vasoconstrictor-induced tone. Our own recent example aside (Fig. 1A), a number of groups have observed that even high-K^+-induced contractions, which are generally assumed to reflect only entry of Ca^{2+} through L-type channels, are not completely blocked by Ca^{2+} antagonists at concentrations that abolish this contraction in other arteries (43,45,46).

With respect to the contraction caused by α-adrenergic receptor activation, Haeusler (47) reported that norepinephrine caused only a small

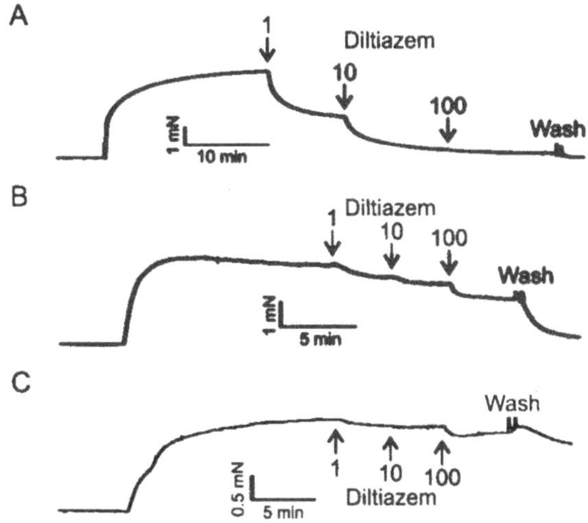

Figure 1 Examples of the effect of the VGCC blocker diltiazem (1, 10, and 100μM, indicated by arrows) added cumulatively upon contractions to 80 mM K^+ (A), 100 nM U46619 (B), and 20 nM ET-1 (C) in isolated rat small PA.

depolarization of rabbit main PA and that Ca^{2+} antagonists caused a correspondingly minor inhibition of contraction. Similarly, felodipine and diltiazem inhibited the contractile responses of the rat main PA to norepinephrine by 28% and 20%, respectively (48–50). Janssen et al. (51) saw no inhibition of norepinephrine-induced contractions by nifedipine, or indeed removal of extracellular Ca^{2+}, in third to fifth generation canine PA. In isolated smooth muscle cells of the canine main PA, phenylephrine induced oscillations in intracellular Ca^{2+} concentration (35). Despite the fact that these oscillations were dependent on the presence of extracellular Ca^{2+} and that phenylephrine also caused oscillations in membrane potential, verapamil and nifedipine were without effect, suggesting the involvement of a calcium influx pathway other than that of L-type VGCCs.

Analogous results have been obtained for $PGF_2\alpha$ and related agonists, which strongly constrict pulmonary arteries. Felodipine inhibited the $PGF_2\alpha$ contraction by only 11–30% in the rat main PA (48,49). Moreover, nifedipine had no effect on the responses to the TXA_2 analog U-46619 or to the isoprostanes 8-*iso* PGE_2 and 8-*iso* $PGF_2\alpha$ in canine PA, both of which also mainly act via TP receptors (51,52). Figure 1B shows that in our hands, however, diltiazem causes a dose-dependent but incomplete inhibition of the response to 100 nM U46619 in rat small PA, and similar results were obtained with 20 μM $PGF_2\alpha$ (not shown). Similarly, in rabbit main PA, nifedipine and verapamil both reduced the contraction to U46619 by ~25% (53).

5-Hydroxytryptamine (5-HT) also constricts the pulmonary vasculature. In sheep small PA, this response was only slightly decreased by nifedipine. On the other hand, felodipine reduced the 5-HT contraction by almost half in rat small PA (48,49), and in blood-perfused canine lung, 10 μM verapamil completely blocked the response to 5-HT (54).

The role of L-type channels in the response to endothelin is unresolved, because different laboratories have reported divergent observations, even in the same preparation. Cardell et al. (55) and Hyvelin et al. (56) have reported that nifedipine inhibited the endothelin contraction in rabbit and guinea pig small PA by 35% and 16%, respectively. On the other hand, the endothelin response in rat small PA has generally been found to be negligibly suppressed by Ca^{2+} channel blockers (37,48,49). In our hands, for example (Fig. 1C), diltiazem at concentrations up to 100 μM had almost no effect on the response to endothelin in rat small PA. On the other hand, Shimoda et al. (45) observed that 1 μM nifedipine reduced the contraction to endothelin by almost half in the same preparation. Moreover, this partial inhibition of contraction was associated with a virtually complete block by nifedipine of the sustained endothelin-induced rise in the intracellular Ca^{2+} concentration, measured using PA cells in short term culture.

G. Role of VGCCs in Hypoxic Pulmonary Vasoconstriction

As described in detail elsewhere in this book, Hypoxic Pulmonary Vasoconstriction (HPV) is generally (but not universally) held to depend upon a hypoxia-induced inhibition of voltage-gated K^+ channels. This causes membrane depolarization and the opening of L-type VGCCs. This hypothesis therefore posits an essentially passive role for Ca^{2+} channels in mediating HPV.

However, there is also evidence that a direct effect of hypoxia on VGCC may occur and could contribute to HPV. Franco-Obregón and López-Barneo (57) examined the effect of hypoxia on the L-type (as defined by its nifedipine sensitivity) VGCC current in VSM cells isolated from the main and small (third-order) PA arteries of the rabbit. They observed that hypoxia inhibited the VGCC current in the cells from the main PA while strongly enhancing the current in the cells from the small PA. Both effects were most pronounced at negative potentials close to the current threshold and were associated with shifts in the voltage dependency of current activation. The hyperpolarizing shift of 6 mV in the cells from the smaller PA might be sufficient to itself cause depolarization and Ca^{2+} influx leading to HPV and would also be expected to potentiate any Ca^{2+} influx caused by any depolarization due to K^+ channel inhibition. Subsequently the same group reported on the effect of hypoxia on basal $[Ca^{2+}]_i$ and the spontaneous Ca^{2+} spikes that they observed in VSM cells from conduit and resistance PA (58). Hypoxia abolished the Ca^{2+} spikes in cells from small PA and lowered basal $[Ca^{2+}]_i$ in cells from the conduit PA. In 40% of cells from resistance PA, hypoxia increased basal $[Ca^{2+}]_i$ and reduced spike amplitude, whereas in the rest of these cells hypoxia decreased basal $[Ca^{2+}]_i$ and enhanced spike amplitude. These results suggest that the effect of hypoxia on Ca^{2+} influx through VGCCs in the pulmonary vasculature is likely to involve a complex and site-specific interplay between changes in the activity of both voltage-gated Ca^{2+} and K^+ channels.

H. Role of Voltage-Gated Calcium Channels in Chronic Hypoxia

Chronic hypoxia is known to depolarize the resting membrane potential of small PA (45,59,60), although hyperpolarization occurs in the main PA (61). The mechanism underlying the depolarization remains unresolved, although a reduced expression of voltage-gated K^+ channels (59) has been demonstrated in the rat. This would be expected to raise basal influx through VGCCs, and in accordance with this finding Ca^{2+} removal relaxes basal tone (62) and Ca^{2+} channel antagonists are more effective in small PA from rats with pulmonary hypertension induced by chronic hypoxia in relaxing contractions to $PGF_{2}\alpha$ than in those from normoxic rats (63). On the other hand, although Shimoda et al. (45) confirmed that rat small PA cells in short term culture are depolarized and have an increased basal $[Ca^{2+}]_i$, they also found that nifedipine did not reverse the latter effect, suggesting that it is not due to VGCCs. They also demonstrated that although the force development evoked by endothelin was similar in the small PAs of normoxic and hypoxic rats, the rise in $[Ca^{2+}]_i$ was much smaller with chronic hypoxia, and the contraction became insensitive to nifedipine. The contribution of VGCCs to raised basal tone in pulmonary arteries therefore remains somewhat obscure.

REFERENCES

1. Mikami A, Imoto K, Tanabe T, Niidome T, Mori Y, Takeshima H, Narumiya S, Numa S. Primary structure and functional expression of the cardiac dihydropyridine-sensitive calcium channel. Nature 1989; 340:230–233.
2. Mori Y, Friedrich T, Kim MS, Mikami A, Nakai J, Ruth P, Bosse E, Hofmann F, Flockerzi V, Furuichi T. Primary structure and functional expression from complementary DNA of a brain calcium channel. Nature 1991; 350:398–402.
3. Tanabe T, Takeshima H, Mikami A, Flockerzi V, Takahashi H, Kangawa K, Kojima M, Matsuo H, Hirose T, Numa S. Primary structure of the receptor for calcium channel blockers from skeletal muscle. Nature 1987; 328:313–318.
4. Ertel EA, Campbell KP, Harpold MM, Hofmann F, Mori Y, Perez-Reyes E, Schwartz A, Snutch TP, Tanabe T, Birnbaumer L, Tsien RW, Catterall WA. Nomenclature of voltage-gated calcium channels. Neuron 2000; 25:533–535.
5. Abernethy DR, Soldatov NM. Structure-functional diversity of human L-type Ca^{2+} channel: perspectives for new pharmacological targets. J Pharmacol Exp Ther 2002; 300:724–728.

6. Reimer D, Huber IG, Garcia ML, Haase H, Striessnig J. Beta subunit heterogeneity of L-type Ca^{2+} channels in smooth muscle tissues. FEBS Lett 2000; 467:65–69.
7. Massa E, Kelly KM, Yule DI, MacDonald RL, Uhler MD. Comparison of fura-2 imaging and electrophysiological analysis of murine calcium channel α_1 subunits coexpressed with novel β_2 subunit isoforms. Mol Pharmacol 1995; 47:707–716.
8. Gong HC, Hang J, Kohler W, Li L, Su TZ. Tissue-specific expression and gabapentin-binding properties of calcium channel α_2/δ subunit subtypes. J Membr Biol 2001; 184:35–43.
9. Bangalore R, Mehrke G, Gingrich K, Hofmann F, Kass RS. Influence of L-type Ca^{2+} channel α_2/δ -subunit on ionic and gating current in transiently transfected HEK 293 cells. Am J Physiol 1996; 270:H1521–H1528.
10. Chu PJ, Robertson HM, Best PM. Calcium channel γ subunits provide insights into the evolution of this gene family. Gene 2001; 280:37–48.
11. Eberst R, Dai S, Klugbauer N, Hofmann F. Identification and functional characterization of a calcium channel gamma subunit. Pflügers Arch 1997; 433:633–637.
12. Ferrari R. Major differences among the three classes of calcium antagonists. Eur Heart J 1997; 18:A56–A70.
13. Hockerman GH, Peterson BZ, Johnson BD, Catterall WA. Molecular determinants of drug binding and action on L-type calcium channels. Annu Rev Pharmacol Toxicol 1997; 37:361–396.
14. Quayle JM, McCarron JG, Asbury JR, Nelson MT. Single calcium channels in resistance-sized cerebral arteries from rats. Am J Physiol 1993; 264: H470–H478.
15. Smirnov SV, Aaronson PI. Ca^{2+} currents in single myocytes from human mesenteric arteries: evidence for a physiological role of L-type channels. J Physiol 1992; 457:455–475.
16. Cribbs LL. Vascular smooth muscle calcium channels: could "T" be a target? Circ Res 2001; 89:560–562
17. Nelson MT, Patlak JB, Worley JF, Standen NB. Calcium channels, potassium channels, and voltage dependence of arterial smooth muscle tone. Am J Physiol 1990; 259:C3–C18.
18. Gollasch M, Hescheler J, Quayle JM, Patlak JB, Nelson MT. Single calcium channel currents of arterial smooth muscle at physiological calcium concentrations. Am J Physiol 1992; 263:C948–C952.
19. Gollasch M, Nelson MT. Voltage-dependent Ca^{2+} channels in arterial smooth muscle cells. Kidney Blood Press Res 1997; 20:355–371.
20. Clapp LH, Gurney AM. Modulation of calcium movements by nitroprusside in isolated vascular smooth muscle cells. Pflügers Arch 1991; 418: 462–470.
21. Keef KD, Hume JR, Zhong J. Regulation of cardiac and smooth muscle Ca^{2+} channels ($Ca_V1.2a,b$) by protein kinases. Am J Physiol Cell Physiol 2001; 281:C1743–C1756.
22. Ishikawa T, Hume JR, Keef KD. Regulation of Ca^{2+} channels by cAMP and cGMP in vascular smooth muscle cells. Circ Res 1993; 73:1128–1137.

23. Wijetunge S, Lymn JS, Hughes AD. Effects of protein tyrosine kinase inhibitors on voltage-operated calcium channel currents in vascular smooth muscle cells and pp60(c-src) kinase activity. Br J Pharmacol 2000; 129:1347–1354.
24. Waitkus-Edwards KR, Martinez-Lemus LA, Wu X, Trzeciakowski JP, Davis MJ, Davis GE, Meininger GA. $\alpha_4\beta_1$ Integrin activation of L-type calcium channels in vascular smooth muscle causes arteriole vasoconstriction. Circ Res 2002; 90:473–480.
25. McCarron JG, Crichton CA, Langton PD, MacKenzie A, Smith GL. Myogenic contraction by modulation of voltage-dependent calcium currents in isolated rat cerebral arteries. J Physiol 1997; 498:371–379.
26. VanBavel E, Wesselman JP, Spaan JA. Myogenic activation and calcium sensitivity of cannulated rat mesenteric small arteries. Circ Res 1998; 82:210–220.
27. Biel M, Ruth P, Bosse E, Hullin R, Stuhmer W, Flockerzi V, Hofmann F. Primary structure and functional expression of a high voltage activated calcium channel from rabbit lung. FEBS Lett 1990; 269:409–412.
28. Saada N, Dai B, Echetebu C, Sarna SK, Palade P. Smooth muscle uses another promoter to express primarily a form of human $Ca_V1.2$ L-type calcium channel different from the principal heart form. Biochem Biophys Res Commun 2003; 302:23–28.
29. Gao B, Sekido Y, Maximov A, Saad M, Forgacs E, Latif F, Wei MH, Lerman M, Lee JH, Perez-Reyes E, Bezprozvanny I, Minna JD. Functional properties of a new voltage-dependent calcium channel α_2/δ auxiliary subunit gene (CACNA2D2). J Biol Chem 2000; 275:12237–12242.
30. Ito Y, Kuriyama H, Suzuki H. The effects of diltiazem (CRD-401) on the membrane and mechanical properties of vascular smooth muscles of the rabbit. Br J Pharmacol 1978; 64:503–510.
31. Suzuki H, Twarog BM. Membrane properties of smooth muscle cells in pulmonary arteries of the rat. Am J Physiol 1982; 242:H900–H906.
32. Wanstall JC, O'Donnell SR. Age influences responses of rat isolated aorta and pulmonary artery to the calcium channel agonist, Bay K 8664, and to potassium and calcium. J Cardiovasc Pharmacol 1989; 13:709–714.
33. Okabe K, Terada K, Kitamura K, Kuriyama H. Selective and long-lasting inhibitory actions of the dihydropyridine derivative, CV-4093, on calcium currents in smooth muscle cells of the rabbit pulmonary artery. J Pharmacol Exp Ther 1987; 243:703–710.
34. Okabe K, Kitamura K, Kuriyama H. Features of 4-aminopyridine sensitive outward current observed in single smooth muscle cells from the rabbit pulmonary artery. Pflugers Arch 1987; 409:561–568.
35. Hamada H, Damron DS, Hong SJ, Van Wagoner DR, Murray PA. Phenylephrine-induced Ca^{2+} oscillations in canine pulmonary artery smooth muscle cells. Circ Res 1997; 81:812–823.
36. Shimoda LA, Sham JS, Shimoda TH, Sylvester JT. L-type Ca^{2+} channels, resting $[Ca^{2+}]_i$, and ET-1-induced responses in chronically hypoxic pulmonary myocytes. Am J Physiol Lung Cell Mol Physiol 2000; 279:L884–L894.
37. Leach RM, Twort CH, Cameron IR, Ward JP. A comparison of the pharmacological and mechanical properties in vitro of large and small pulmonary arteries of the rat. Clin Sci (Lond) 1992; 82:55–62.

38. Mikkelsen E, Pedersen OL. Regional differences in the response of isolated human vessels to vasoactive substances. Gen Pharmacol 1983; 14:89–90.
39. Belik J. Large pulmonary arteries and the control of pulmonary vascular resistance in the newborn. Can J Physiol Pharmacol 1994; 72:1464–1468.
40. Storme L, Rairigh RL, Parker TA, Kinsella JP, Abman SH. In vivo evidence for a myogenic response in the fetal pulmonary circulation. Pediatr Res 1999; 45:425–431.
41. Belik J. The myogenic response of arterial vessels is increased in fetal pulmonary hypertension. Pediatr Res 1995; 37:196–201.
42. Venkataraman ST, Fuhrman BP, Howland DF, DeFrancisis M. Positive end-expiratory pressure-induced, calcium-channel-mediated increases in pulmonary vascular resistance in neonatal lambs. Crit Care Med 1993; 21:1066–1076.
43. Godfraind T, Miller R, Wibo M. Calcium antagonism and calcium entry blockade. Pharmacol Rev 1986; 38:321–416.
44. Cauvin C, Lukeman S, Cameron J, Hwang O, van Breemen C. Differences in norepinephrine activation and diltiazem inhibition of calcium channels in isolated rabbit aorta and mesenteric resistance vessels. Circ Res 1985; 56:822–828.
45. Shimoda LA, Sylvester JT, Sham JS. Mobilization of intracellular Ca^{2+} by endothelin-1 in rat intrapulmonary arterial smooth muscle cells. Am J Physiol Lung Cell Mol Physiol 2000; 278:L157–L164.
46. Drummond RM, Wadsworth RM. In vitro effect of nifedipine on KCl and 5-hydroxytryptamine-induced contractions of the sheep coronary, cerebral and pulmonary arteries. Life Sci 1994; 54:1081–1090.
47. Haeusler G. Contraction of vascular muscle as related to membrane potential and calcium fluxes. J Cardiovasc Pharmacol 1985; 7:S3–S8.
48. O'Donnell SR, Wanstall JC, Kay CS, Zeng XP. Tissue selectivity and spasmogen selectivity of relaxant drugs in airway and pulmonary vascular smooth muscle contracted by $PGF_2\alpha$ or endothelin. Br J Pharmacol 1991; 102:311–316.
49. Wanstall JC, O'Donnell SR, Kay CS. Increased relaxation by felodipine on pulmonary artery from rats with monocrotaline-induced pulmonary hypertension does not reflect functional impairment of the endothelium. Pulm Pharmacol 1991; 4:60–66.
50. Wanstall JC, O'Donnell SR. Inhibition of norepinephrine contractions by diltiazem on aorta and pulmonary artery from young and aged rats: influence of alpha-adrenoceptor reserve. J Pharmacol Exp Ther 1988; 245:1016–1020.
51. Janssen LJ, Lu-Chao H, Netherton S. Excitation-contraction coupling in pulmonary vascular smooth muscle involves tyrosine kinase and Rho kinase. Am J Physiol Lung Cell Mol Physiol 2001; 280:L666–L674.
52. Janssen LJ, Premji M, Netherton S, Coruzzi J, Lu-Chao H, Cox PG. Vasoconstrictor actions of isoprostanes via tyrosine kinase and Rho kinase in human and canine pulmonary vascular smooth muscles. Br J Pharmacol 2001; 132:127–134.
53. Liu F, Wu JY, Beasley D, Orr JA. TxA_2-induced pulmonary artery contraction requires extracellular calcium. Respir Physiol 1997; 109:155–166.
54. Barman SA, Pauly JR. Mechanism of action of endothelin-1 in the canine pulmonary circulation. J Appl Physiol 1995; 79:2014–2020.

55. Cardell LO, Uddman R, Edvinsson L. Analysis of endothelin-1-induced contractions of guinea pig trachea, pulmonary veins and different types of pulmonary arteries. Acta Physiol Scand 1990; 139:103–111.
56. Hyvelin JM, Guibert C, Marthan R, Savineau JP. Cellular mechanisms and role of endothelin-1-induced calcium oscillations in pulmonary arterial myocytes. Am J Physiol 1998; 275:L269–L282.
57. Franco-Obregon A, Lopez-Barneo J. Differential oxygen sensitivity of calcium channels in rabbit smooth muscle cells of conduit and resistance pulmonary arteries. J Physiol 1996; 491:511–518.
58. Urena J, Franco-Obregon A, Lopez-Barneo J. Contrasting effects of hypoxia on cytosolic Ca^{2+} spikes in conduit and resistance myocytes of the rabbit pulmonary artery. J Physiol 1996; 496:103–109.
59. Smirnov SV, Robertson TP, Ward JP, Aaronson PI. Chronic hypoxia is associated with reduced delayed rectifier K^+ current in rat pulmonary artery muscle cells. Am J Physiol 1994; 266:H365–H370.
60. Twarog BM, Takuno H, Petrou S, Wahlqvist I, Marcus R, Campbell GL. Pathogenesis of pulmonary hypertension in the rat model. Chest 1988; 93: 100S–101S.
61. Suzuki H, Twarog BM. Membrane properties of smooth muscle cells in pulmonary hypertensive rats. Am J Physiol 1982; 242:H907–H915.
62. Wanstall JC, Hughes IE, O'Donnell SR. Evidence that nitric oxide from the endothelium attenuates inherent tone in isolated pulmonary arteries from rats with hypoxic pulmonary hypertension. Br J Pharmacol 1995; 114:109–114.
63. Priest RM, Robertson TP, Leach RM, Ward JP. Membrane potential-dependent and -independent vasodilation in small pulmonary arteries from chronically hypoxic rats. J Pharmacol Exp Ther 1998; 285:975–982.

5

Receptor-Operated Ca^{2+} Channels

Songwei Wu, Donna L. Cioffi, and Troy Stevens
University of South Alabama College of Medicine, Mobile, Alabama, U.S.A.

I. INTRODUCTION

The pulmonary vasculature mainly comprises vascular smooth muscle of the large vessel wall and endothelium of large and small vessels that arise from embryologically distinct origins. Whereas vascular smooth muscle cells generally control vascular tone, the endothelium is a metabolically active participant in the production of numerous vasoactive autacoids and participates in control of hemostasis, white blood cell trafficking, hormone metabolism, permeability, vascular growth, and the balance between blood vessel survival and apoptosis. As in other cell systems, physiological transitions in cytosolic Ca^{2+} concentration ($[Ca^{2+}]_i$) in smooth muscle and endothelium regulate a variety of critical cellular functions, ranging from contraction or shape change to secretion, endo- and exocytosis, cell growth, differentiation, modulation of enzyme function, and progression through the cell cycle. Within the same cell, Ca^{2+} influx (i.e., entry across the plasma membrane) represents an important signal that modulates each of these functions independently, under appropriate physiological conditions. To differentiate the Ca^{2+} signals required for these disparate functions, a complex network of ion channels has evolved in mammalian cells. Plasmalemmal Ca^{2+} channels can be broadly divided into voltage-gated and voltage-independent channels. The latter category includes receptor-operated and ligand-gated Ca^{2+} channels, capacitative or store-operated Ca^{2+} channels, and a variety of Ca^{2+}-permeable nonselective cation channels including mechanosensitive and cyclic nucleotide-gated channels.

The so-called receptor-operated channels were first described by Bolton (1), van Breemen et al. (2), and Somlyo and Somlyo (3) and were defined as any plasma-membrane channel that is opened as a result of agonist binding to its receptor (e.g., metabotropic receptor)—where the receptor is separate from the channel and where the channel-opening mechanism does not involve plasma-membrane depolarization. Such "metabotropic" receptors, like G-protein-coupled receptors, generate intracellular signaling cascades involving multiple second messengers that alter cell function for minutes or hours.

This chapter provides an account of the current understanding of receptor-operated channels in pulmonary vascular smooth muscle and endothelial cells. To focus the review, we do not discuss ligand-gated, mechano-gated, cyclic nucleotide gated, or store-operated Ca^{2+} entry channels.

II. GLOBAL $[Ca^{2+}]_i$, CURRENTS, AND CHANNELS

Chemical first messengers bind receptors and trigger a complex series of biochemical changes in the plasma membrane that ultimately increase $[Ca^{2+}]_i$. We have come to learn in recent times that this global $[Ca^{2+}]_i$ rise represents a conglomerate of ion channels activated by different mechanisms, likely for different functions, that each contribute to the ultimate $[Ca^{2+}]_i$ transition. A key issue is understanding which mechanism and which channel account for particular components of the global $[Ca^{2+}]_i$ rise.

One way of better understanding the rise in global $[Ca^{2+}]_i$ is to parallel cell physiology studies with electrophysiological recordings. Utilizing Ca^{2+} conductance and permeation properties as a guide to Ca^{2+} entry pathways, it is possible to learn how very specific Ca^{2+} entry pathways are activated and inhibited. By extension, identifying which Ca^{2+} current is inhibited by a precise pharmacological tool allows parallel studies to determine what component of the global $[Ca^{2+}]_i$ transition is due to the described current. As you will see, many receptor-operated channels have been described using electrophysiological approaches, yet few have successfully linked the current to an appreciable understanding of the current contribution to global $[Ca^{2+}]_i$ responses.

Even fewer studies have successfully linked a definable current with an appropriate ion channel. Indeed, until the early 1990s molecular candidates of receptor-operated Ca^{2+} channels were poorly described. We now recognize that the best candidates belong to a class of six transmembrane-spanning domain proteins with cytosolic N- and C-termini (Fig. 1). The functional ion channel comprises four subunits, but the oligomeric state of any endogenous channel is not yet known. In very few instances have endogenous currents been fully replicated by heterologous expression of individual subunits, and even in these instances studies have not confirmed that those overexpressed subunits actually form homotetramers. The result of such complications is that our present state of understanding is quite limited.

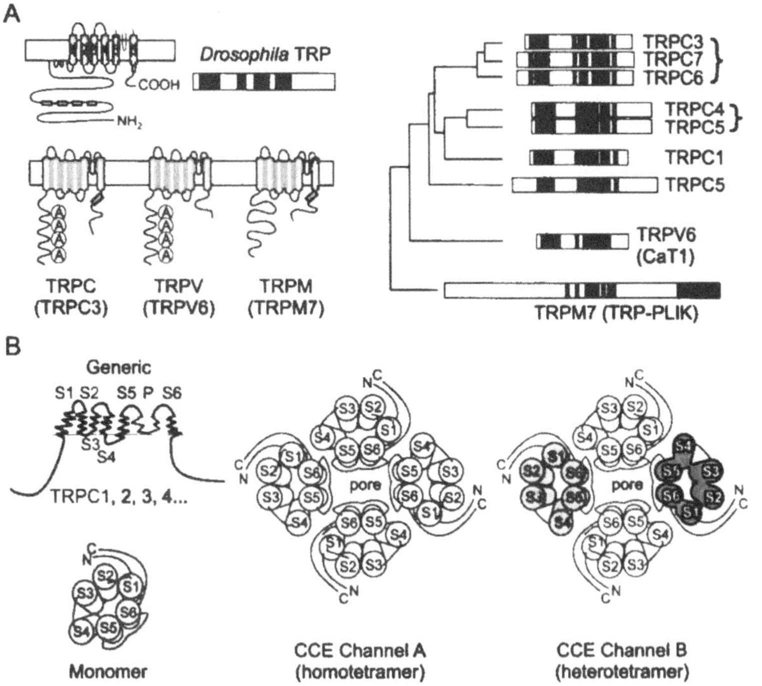

Figure 1 (A) Phylogenetic relationship between members of the TRPC protein family based on full-length amino acid sequences. Proteins are aligned around the "pore-forming" loop (green). Also shown are other transmembrane segments (gray), ankyrin-like repeats (purple), the kinase domain of TRPM7 (blue), and the "TRP box" (red). The TRP box is a small highly conserved region (amino acid sequence EWKFAR) found in *Drosophila* TRP as well as in mammalian TRPC and TRPV channels. A topological comparison of the structures of three TRP subtypes and a potassium channel are shown as well. "A" denotes ankyrin-like repeats. (B) Models of secondary and quaternary structures of capacitative Ca^{2+} entry (CCE) channels and their subunits. CCE channels are hypothesized to be made of different TRPs and/or different TRP combinations to account for CCE channels with varying ion selectivities and different forms of activation—e.g., store depletion–sensitive vs. store depletion–insensitive. It also opens the possibility that there are either diverse homomultimeric or diverse heteromultimeric CCE channels that could account for the functional heterogeneity of CCE seen in different tissues and cells. (Reproduced with permission from Refs. 109 and 113.)

The canonical subfamily of transient receptor potential proteins (TRPC) is a recently described subset of channels that may be receptor-operated. TRPC 1, 3, 6, and 7, in particular, may contribute to receptor-operated Ca^{2+} entry pathways. However, these and other TRPCs have also been suggested to be store-operated Ca^{2+} channels. The difference between receptor and store-operated channels is functional, not simply semantic. Indeed, a store-operated channel is activated by depleting Ca^{2+} in the endoplasmic reticulum—usually by using an inhibitor of the sarcoplasmic, endoplasmic reticulum Ca^{2+} ATPase. However, buffering Ca^{2+} in the endoplasmic reticulum also activates store-operated channels, as does Ca^{2+} release from the endoplasmic reticulum. On the other hand, receptor-operated Ca^{2+} channels are activated by intracellular signal transduction mechanisms that are independent of Ca^{2+} in the endoplasmic reticulum. Because receptor- and store-operated Ca^{2+} entry pathways are commonly activated by similar first messengers, it is difficult to functionally separate them. In addition, because TRPC subunits may contribute to both channel types, it is difficult to ascribe a specific role to a subunit. Thus, at the present time the molecular identity of highly characterized receptor-operated Ca^{2+} entry pathways is incompletely known.

III. SIGNAL TRANSDUCTION

The concept that receptor activation leads to Ca^{2+} entry into smooth muscle cells by mechanisms independent of membrane depolarization was introduced over two decades ago (1–4). Receptor-operated currents have been described in a variety of cell types following activation of a range of receptors. The receptor-operated currents recorded in smooth muscle and endothelial cells all exhibit nonselective cation conductances with varying degrees of Ca^{2+} selectivity (Fig. 2). In fact, there are numerous subtypes of receptor-operated currents, which can be differentiated on the basis of their selectivity for cations, mechanisms of channel opening, and physiological functions (5–7). The Ca^{2+} selectivity of receptor-operated channels varies from those that are quite Ca^{2+}-selective to those that are Ca^{2+}-nonselective (5–7). Notably, under physiological conditions, nonselective cation channels conduct Na^{+} but also admit sufficient Ca^{2+} to cause a significant $[Ca^{2+}]_i$ transition.

A variety of extracellular messengers such as hormones, neurotransmitters, neuromodulators, and growth factors act on membrane receptors to initiate cascades of intracellular second-messenger signaling with pleiotropic effects, consequently altering cellular functions including enzyme or channel activities. Second-messenger signaling cascades (Fig. 3) are activated by three major classes of receptors: guanosine triphosphate (GTP)-binding protein (G protein)-coupled receptors (GPCRs), receptor tyrosine kinases, and receptor guanylyl cyclases.

A. G-Protein-Coupled Receptors

The largest family of characterized transmembrane receptors comprises G-protein-coupled receptors. They form a gene superfamily with overall structural similarity composed of heptahelical hydrophobic transmembrane

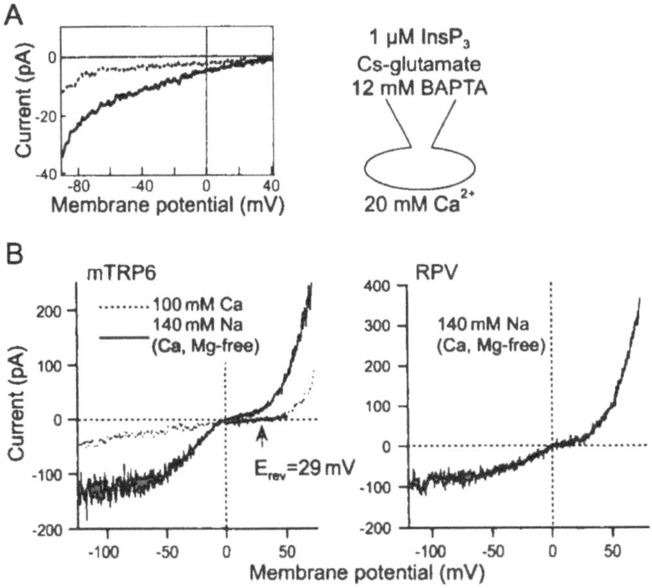

Figure 2 Calcium-selective store-operated currents can be distinguished from nonselective receptor-operated currents. (A) Current–voltage (I–V) relationships of Ca^{2+}-release-activated Ca^{2+} current (I_{CRAC}) obtained in bovine pulmonary artery endothelial cells dialyzed with standard internal solution containing 12 mM BAPTA and 1 μM inositol 1,4,5-trisphosphate ($InsP_3$), shown at the peak current (a) and after recovery from perfusion with 10 μM La^{3+} (b). (B) (I–V) relationships of mTRP6 under two biionic conditions and that of α_1-adrenoceptor-activated nonselective cation channels (α_1-AR–NSCC) from the rabbit portal vein (RPV) under conventional whole-cell clamp. Note the positive shift of the reversal potential in 100 mM [Ca^{2+}] external solution in the left panel and the similar shapes of I–V curves in both panels. (Reproduced with permission from Refs. 50 and 114.)

segments (8,9); they all have seven stretches of hydrophobic amino acids that form transmembrane α-helices and have been variously called seven-transmembrane receptors (7TMs), serpentine receptors, and heptahelical receptors. They have arisen by gene duplication and subsequent evolutionary specialization from an ancestral prototype possibly related to bacterial rhodopsin. Table 1 illustrates that there are G-protein-coupled receptors for all classical neurotransmitters except glysine, for certain peptides, and for a variety of other physiological stimuli as well.

G proteins are heterotrimeric molecules composed of Gα, Gβ, and Gγ subunits, Gαβγ. They are associated with the cytoplasmic side of the plasma membrane by hydrophobic anchors (covalently attached lipid or prenyl moieties) but do not have transmembrane segments. In the resting state,

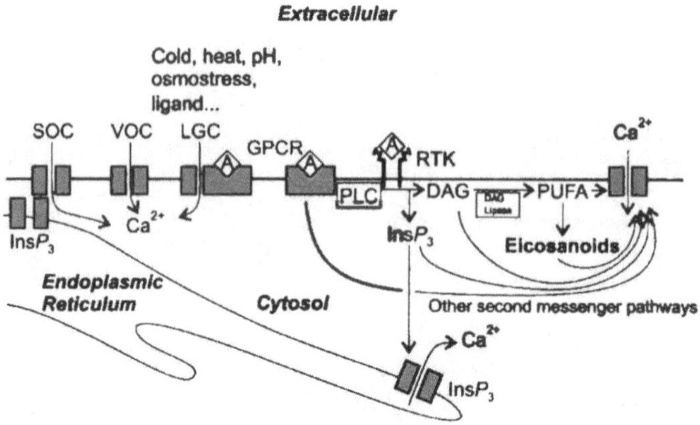

A, agonist
SOC, store-operated channel
LGC, ligand-gated channel (ionotropic receptor)
GPCR, G protein coupled receptor
RTK, receptor tyrosine kinase
ROC, receptor-operated channel (**SMOC**, second messenger–operated channel)
PLC, phospholipase C
DAG, diacylglycerol
PUFA, polyunsaturated fatty acid
ER, endoplasmic reticulum
$InsP_3R$, $InsP_3$ receptor

Figure 3 Synopsis of the main pathways proposed to activate receptor- and second-messenger-activated cation channels. Upon activation of G- protein-coupled receptor or a receptor tyrosine kinase, phospholipase C is activated. Phospatidylinositol-4,5 bisphosphate (PIP_2) is metabolized to inositol 1,4,5-trisphosphate ($InsP_3$) and diacylglycerol (DAG). $InsP_3$ depletes intracellular stores and has been proposed to activate channels directly. Store depletion per se activates store-operated channels (SOCs) through an unknown mechanism. DAG has been shown to activate channels directly or through products of its breakdown, polyunsaturated fatty acid metabolites such as arachidonic acid or linoleic acid. Other PLC-dependent but store-independent mechanisms have been proposed but are still elusive. See text for details. (Adapted with permission from Ref. 115.)

G proteins carry GDP bound in a pocket of their α subunit. If they encounter an agonist-occupied receptor, the GDP is liberated, a GTP from the cytoplasm takes its place, and the G protein heterotrimer dissociates into two membrane-associated parts, Gα-GTP and the Gβγ dimer. These are the activated forms of the G protein, capable of signaling to specific membrane-associated effectors such as ion channels.

At least 15 Gα genes and 20 different gene products have been identified. Products of these genes make up four principal G protein subfamilies: G_s, G_i, G_q, and G_{12} (10,11). Each G protein subfamily produces interesting modulation of ion channels. The first pathway is the cAMP-dependent

Table 1 G Protein-Coupled Receptors[a]

Agonist	Metabotropic G-protein-coupled receptors
Ach	Muscarinic
Glutamate	MGluR
GABA	$GABA_B$
Glycine	—
Serotonin	5-HT[b]
ATP (a purine)	P2Y
Histamine	H_1, H_2, H_3
Catecholamines	α_1, α_2, β, D_1, D_2
Anandamide	Cannabinoid R
Peptides	Opioid, tachykinin, etc.
Light	Rhodopsin
Odorants	>500 odorant receptors
Tastants	Some

[a]The nomenclature here uses the receptor classification for vertebrates. There is much direct correspondence with invertebrate families, but there are differences in detail. In invertebrates, other substances such as octopamine are neurotransmitters and some compounds (including glycine) are not known to be neurotransmitters.
[b](1,2,4–7)
Source: Ref. 116 (Adapted with permission).

pathway discovered by Sutherland (12). It uses the stimulatory G protein G_s. The second pathway inhibits adenylyl cyclase through G_i. There are separate binding sites for $G\alpha_i$ and $G\alpha_s$ on the large cytoplasmic domains of adenylyl cyclase, and agonists that activate G_i can override the cAMP-catalytic actions of agonists that stimulate G_s.

The third pathway produces two cytoplasmic second messengers and one membrane-associated second messenger. $G\alpha_q$ stimulates the membrane enzyme phospholipase Cβ. The relatively low abundance membrane phospholipid phosphatidylinositol-4,5-bisphosphate is cleaved by phospholipase C to yield two active second messengers: lipid-soluble (membrane-confined) diacylglycerol and water-soluble inositol-1,4,5-trisphosphate ($InsP_3$) (13). Diacylglycerol activates protein kinase C (14), and $InsP_3$ releases Ca^{2+} into the cytoplasm from intracellular stores that are elements of the endoplasmic reticulum (see Chapter 6). Another phospholipase, phospholipase A_2, liberates a highly unsaturated fatty acid, arachidonic acid, that is quickly metabolized to at least 20 different short-lived but extremely potent intermediates. Phospholipase A_2 is activated by Ca^{2+} and by phosphorylation. Arachidonic acid is sometimes derived from breakdown of diacylglycerol as well. A unique feature of many lipid-soluble arachidonic acid metabolites, such as prostaglandins, is that they can leave the cell and act on neighboring cells in the tissue.

B. Receptor Tyrosine Kinases and Guanylyl Cyclases

Receptor tyrosine kinases possess a single-pass transmembrane segment (1TM), dimerize on binding agonist, and activate intracellular tyrosine kinase. Growth factor–receptor binding activates the intrinsic protein tyrosine kinase activity of the receptor and consequent protein phosphorylation on tyrosine residues of numerous proteins, including the receptor itself and phospholipase Cγ (13,15–17). Activation of phospholipase Cγ induces phosphoinositide turnover and a rise in $[Ca^{2+}]_i$. Despite the structural similarities between their receptors, participation of polypeptide growth factors in phosphoinositide signaling does not appear to be universal. For example, binding of platelet-derived growth factor (PDGF), epidermal growth factor (EGF), and nerve growth factor (NGF) to their respective receptors induces phosphoinositide turnover, whereas insulin and colony-stimulating factor (CSF-1) appear to have no effect on phosphoinositide turnover. On the other hand, tyrosine phosphorylation and activation of phospholipase Cγ can also be achieved through the action of non-receptor protein tyrosine kinases in response to ligation of certain cell-surface receptors in a variety of cell types including smooth muscle (15,18). The term "non-receptor protein tyrosine kinase" was coined because of the deficiency of intrinsic protein tyrosine kinase activities on the receptor (19). Certain G-protein-coupled receptors have also been shown to induce tyrosine phosphorylation (16,20–22).

Receptor guanylyl cyclases synthesize the ubiquitous second-messenger molecule cyclic GMP (cGMP). Ligands for these receptors include α-atrial natriuretic peptide, brain natriuretic peptide, and factors from invertebrate egg jellies (23). Similar to cAMP, cGMP can activate a protein kinase. For instance, when atrial natriuretic peptide acts on kidney collecting-duct cells, cGMP rises, the resultant protein phosphorylation closes an apical cation channel, and resorption of Na^+ ions from the urine is blocked. Cyclic GMP also stimulates one type of cAMP-hydrolyzing phosphodiesterase. By activating cAMP breakdown the Ca^{2+} current, cGMP partially reverses cAMP-mediated modulation of in frog heart even while β-adrenergic agonists are continuously present (24).

IV. RECEPTOR-OPERATED Ca^{2+} CHANNELS—CONTROL BY SECOND MESSENGERS

A. Interaction Between the Channel Protein and a Trimeric G Protein

A proposed role for trimeric G proteins in the membrane-delimited activation of Ca^{2+} channels has been implicated in receptor-operated Ca^{2+} entry pathways (6,7,25–28). In some cases it seems that activated G protein subunits can interact directly with receptor-operated Ca^{2+} channels to elicit regulation, in addition to membrane-delimited G protein regulation of K^+

channels, voltage-gated Ca^{2+} channels, Na^+ channels, and Cl^- channels (29). In mast cells, intracellular nonhydrolyzable analogs of GTP such as guanosine 5′-*O*-(3-thiotriphosphate) (GTPγS), a G protein activator, increase the open probability of a Ca^{2+}-permeable cation channel of 50 pS unitary conductance in physiological solutions (Fig. 4). This channel is not activated by $InsP_3$, $InsP_4$, store depletion, or a rise in $[Ca^{2+}]_i$ (30). Currents that are presumably attributable to similar channels have been described in many other systems, including smooth muscle (26,31,32), PC-12 adrenal chromaffin tumor cell line (33), and the HL-60 neutrophil cell line (27).

Studies with A7r5 vascular smooth muscle cells (from rat embryonic thoracic aorta) (26) have shown that GTPγS activates nonselective cation channels that are most probably a receptor-operated Ca^{2+} channel subtype. The argument for direct activation of receptor-operated Ca^{2+} channels by a trimeric G protein is that in electrophysiological experiments employing the inside-out patch-clamp recording configuration, application of GTPγS to the cytoplasmic side of the membrane activates plasma membrane Ca^{2+} channels. Under these experimental conditions, any mobile intracellular messenger that might be formed as a result of the action of GTPγS would most probably be immediately diluted by rapid diffusion into the surrounding medium (27). However, although these observations provide some evidence for interaction between a direct channel protein and a trimeric G protein, they do not fully exclude the involvement of a mobile messenger (27).

Experiments with portal vein smooth muscle cells have shown that, in addition to activating SOCs, norepinephrine opens Ca^{2+}-permeable nonselective cation channels by a mechanism that does not appear to involve Ca^{2+} release from the endoplasmic reticulum (32). Studies using anti-G-protein antibodies and antisense DNA techniques have implicated $G\alpha_{11}$ in the mechanism by which norepinephrine opens nonselective cation channels (32). Thus, it is likely that G-protein-coupled α_1-adrenoreceptors use two different mechanisms to increase $[Ca^{2+}]_i$: the generation of $InsP_3$ via $G\alpha_q$ and phospholipase C, which leads to endoplasmic reticulum Ca^{2+} release and SOC entry; and the opening of Ca^{2+}-permeable nonselective cation channels via $G\alpha_{11}$ (32).

The pathway by which carbachol activation of M_3 muscarinic receptors increases $[Ca^{2+}]_i$ also provides evidence that a receptor-operated Ca^{2+} channel is activated by direct interaction with a trimeric G protein (34,35). The third cytoplasmic loop of the M_3-muscarinic receptor—which is required for Gα activation —is also required for activation of Ca^{2+} influx but not for endoplasmic reticulum Ca^{2+} release (34,35). Similarly, the *Drosophila* TRPL nonspecific cation channel (defined in Chapter 6) expressed in insect Sf9 cells is opened in response to direct interaction between $G\alpha_{11}$ and the TRPL protein (36). Although all of these studies support the idea that heterotrimeric G proteins activate Ca^{2+} entry through receptor-operated channels, the critical mechanism of coupling between a G protein and an

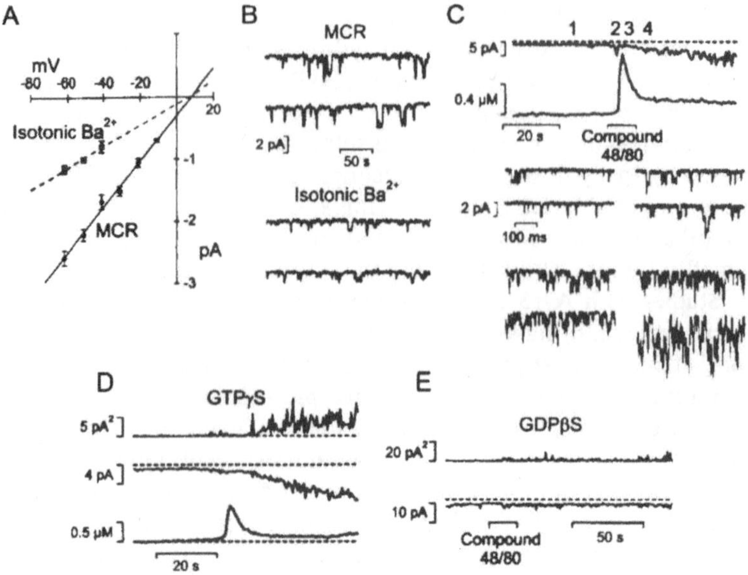

Figure 4 Properties of the 50 pS cation channel. (A,B). The 50 pS channel appears capable of carrying appreciable divalent cation current. (A) Relation of single-channel current and membrane voltage for large agonist-activated channels observed in whole-cell recordings of membrane current. (B) Examples of channel activity in mast cell Ringer solution (MCR) (upper pair of traces) and after switching the bath solution to isotonic Ba^{2} (lower pair of traces). (C) Activity of the 50 pS channel is inhibited by elevated $[Ca^{2}]_i$. Inhibition of 50 pS channel activity during Ca^{2+} transient. *Upper panel;* Traces show whole-cell membrane current and $[Ca^{2+}]_i$ in response to external application of compound 48/80 at the indicated time. *Lower panel*; Samples of single-channel activity from the times indicated by the corresponding numbers in the *upper panel*. *Pair 1*, activity in the resting state before stimulation. *Pair 2*, increased activity of 50 pS channels after applying compound 48/80 but before the Ca^{2+} transient. *Pair 3*, inhibition of activity during the Ca^{2+} transient. *Pair 4*, after the Ca^{2+} transient subsided, large activation of 50 pS channels was apparent. (D,E) The 50 pS channels are regulated by G protein. (D) Internally applied nonhydrolyzable GTP analog GTPγS (40μM) activated the 50 pS channel and induced a Ca^{2+} transient that mimics activation by external agonist [in comparison to (C)]. Top trace: Variance of the membrane current. Middle trace: Whole-cell membrane current. Bottom trace: $[Ca^{2+}]_i$. (E) Nonhydrolyzable GDP analog GDPβS reduced the activation of 50 pS channels by compound 48/80. The bottom trace of the pair is the membrane current, and the top trace is the variance of the current. (Adapted with permission from Ref. 30.)

ion channel remains unknown. Thus, demonstration of a specific physical and functional interaction between an isolated channel and a G protein remains an experimental priority (29).

B. Activation by $InsP_3$ or $InsP_4$

Inositol phosphates generated upon phospholipase activation constitute another group of second messengers, $InsP_3$ and inositol-1,3,4,5-tetrakisphosphate ($InsP_4$), which activate channel proteins. $InsP_4$ is derived from $InsP_3$ by phosphorylation. Apart from the intracellular $InsP_3$ receptor, plasma membrane channels responsive to $InsP_3$ have been reported in T-lymphocytes, mast cells, epidermal cells (30,37–40), and cultured vascular endothelial cells (41). However, the biophysical properties of $InsP_3$-responsive second-messenger-operated channels differ considerably. A cation channel directly activated by $InsP_4$ has been described in endothelial cells (42). This channel is equally permeable to Ca^{2+}, Ba^{2+}, and Mn^{2+}. To be activated, the channel requires millimolar intracellular Ca^{2+} concentrations and is unresponsive to $InsP_3$. Despite this characterization, the contribution of $InsP_3$ and $InsP_4$ responsive channels to total receptor-dependent Ca^{2+} entry has not been directly determined, and expression of similar channels in other cell types and their physiological role still remain unknown.

C. Activation by Diacylglycerol

Activation of α_1-adrenoreceptors generates diacylglycerol, which promotes a native Ca^{2+}-permeable conductance in rabbit portal vein smooth muscle (43). This conductance is activated downstream of phospholipase C, apparently not by $InsP_3$, Ca^{2+}, or Ca^{2+} store depletion. However, the conductance is activated by diacylglycerol analogs 1-oleoyl-2-acetyl-*sn*-glycerol (OAG) in a protein kinase C (PKC)-independent fashion, at concentrations as low as 10 μM, and also by inhibitors of diacylglycerol-metabolizing enzymes (e.g., diacylglycerol lipase) (43).

Electrophysiological studies determined that the diacylglycerol-activated current possessed a relative permeability favoring Ba^{2+} over Na^+ ($P_{Ba}/P_{Na} \approx 4.6$), indicating a greater Ca^{2+} permeability (44). With whole-cell and excised outside-out patches of rabbit portal vein smooth muscle cells, channel unitary conductance evoked by the selective α_1-adenoceptor agonist phenylephrine as well as the muscarinic receptor agonist acetylcholine was about 23 pS. These findings demonstrate that two different receptor types converge on the same nonselective cation channel (45). Excised outside-out patches of rabbit portal vein smooth muscle cells exhibited spontaneous single-cation currents with a unitary conductance of 23 pS. Norepinephrine and OAG evoked single-channel activity with a unitary conductance and kinetic properties that are similar to those of spontaneous channel currents, indicating that the channel appears to possess intrinsic gating and kinetic behavior once channel activity is initiated (46). In addition, norepinephrine evokes the current in Ca^{2+}-free bathing solution, suggesting that Ca^{2+} is not obligatory for current activation. Increasing external Ca^{2+} produces a marked increase (about eightfold) in the current amplitude, with an apparent equilibrium constant of about 6 μM. Increasing external Ca^{2+} above 100 μM then decreases the current amplitude with an equilibrium constant of ≈400 μM (47). This Ca^{2+} effect is seen as a bell-shaped relationship between the current amplitude and external [Ca^{2+}], with the amplitude of the norepinephrine-induced response being similar in

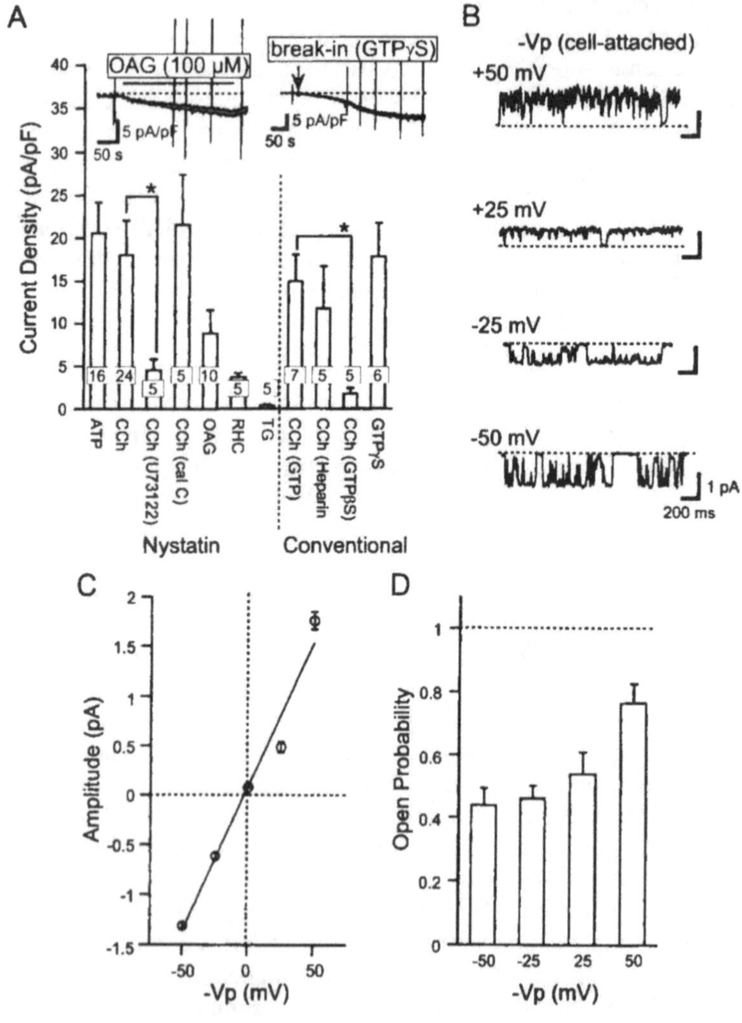

Figure 5 (*Caption on facing page*)

0 and 1.5 mM external Ca^{2+} (48). The inhibitory effect of higher external Ca^{2+} concentrations appears to be due to channel "flickery" block (49).

Recent evidence strongly suggests that the diacylglycerol-activated channels may be encoded, at least in part, by the vertebrate TRP homolog TRPC6, which accurately mimics the essential biophysical and pharmacological properties of the native current when expressed in HEK-293 cells (50) (Fig. 5). Apart from activation by diacylglycerol, these properties include an S-shaped current–voltage relationship; high divalent cation permeability; unitary conductance (30 pS); block by La^{3+}, Gd^{3+}, SKF96365, and amiloride; and a specific enhancement by flufenamate, an agent otherwise known as a cation channel blocker. Furthermore, TRPC6 immunoreactivity was detected in rabbit portal vein myocytes, and both immunoreactivity and the native current were markedly suppressed by TRPC6 antisense oligonucleotides (50). Possibly related Ca^{2+} influx pathways activated by diacylglycerol in a store- and PKC-independent manner have also been described in PC12 cells (51) and T-lymphocytes (52,53), both of which express TRPC6.

Diacylglycerol has also been reported to activate TRPC1, 3, and 7 (54–56). This effect was mimicked by various analogs of diacylglycerol and by an inhibitor of diacylglycerol metabolism. TRPC3 can also be activated by store depletion via an $InsP_3$-dependent pathway, and several studies indicate that it can interact directly with the $InsP_3$ receptor (57–59) via a domain that overlaps with a Calmodulin-binding domain on the $InsP_3$

Figure 5 (*Facing page*) Activation profile, voltage-dependent gating, and ionic selectivity of TRPC6. Characteristics of nonselective cation currents recorded in HEK-293 cells transiently expressing mouse TRPC6 proteins. (A) Amplitude of TRPC6 currents at a holding potential of −60 mV calculated as current density (pA/pF) to pharmacological receptor stimulation by 100 μM ATP or 100 μM carbachol (CCh) and to 100 μM 1-oleoyl-2-acetyl-*sn*-glycerol (OAG). The CCh-induced current was inhibited by 10 μM U73122 (PLC inhibitor) but was not affected by 10 μM calphostin C. The diacylglycerol (DAG) lipase inhibitor RHC 80267 (10 μM), which inhibits DAG metabolism in smooth muscle, also activated TRPC6 current. Thapsigargin 2 μM had no effect. With conventional whole-cell recording, GTP 100 μM, heparin 1 mg/mL, guanosine 5′-O-(2-thiotriphosphate) (GDPβS) 300 μM, and guanosine 5′-O-(3-thiotriphosphate) (GTPγS) 100 μM were added to the pipette solution to achieve intracellular application of these agents. (The insets above the histograms show experimental records of bath-applied 100 μM OAG and intracellular dialysis with 100 μM GTPγS.) (B) TRPC6 single-channel activity recorded with cell-attached recording at different patch potentials where the membrane potential was set to approximately 0 mV with high (128 mM) external K^+ solution. (C,D) Current–voltage relationship of the single-channel amplitude (C) and the effect of patch potential on channel open probability of single TRPC6 channel (D) Solid line indicates best linear fit of data points; Vp, pipette potential (Reproduced with permission from Ref. 50.)

receptor. Activation of TRPC3-dependent currents by store depletion is blocked by 2-aminoethoxydiphenyl borate (2-APB), whereas activation via diacylglycerol is unaffected (60). It is unclear whether this indicates that the same channels can be activated by diacylglycerol- and $InsP_3$-dependent pathways or whether the different biophysical properties reflect different heteromultimeric subunit compositions of endogenous TRP isoforms and/or accessory proteins. In addition, TRPC4 antisense oligonucleotides were recently reported to downregulate an endogenous diacylglycerol-sensitive conductance in HEK-293 cells (61).

D. Activation by Polyunsaturated Fatty Acids

Lipid messengers such as arachidonic acid and its metabolites activate receptor-operated Ca^{2+}-permeable channels (62–64). This raises the possibility that other signaling systems, including those of phospholipase A_2 and diacylglycerol lipase, may play a role in receptor-operated channel gating. Indeed, diacylglycerol can be metabolized by lipase to yield polyunsaturated fatty acids (PUFAs) such as arachidonic acid, which activates or modulates a range of ion channels (65).

It was first observed that EGF generates leukotriene C_4, which activates a Ca^{2+} channel with a conductance of approximately 10 pS (63). Subsequently, arachidonate was shown to activate a Ca^{2+}-selective conductance entirely distinct from capacitative or store-operated Ca^{2+} conductances (64,66,67). In addition, arachidonate is produced after agonist stimulation, not simply as a secondary consequence of Ca^{2+}-dependent phospholipase A_2 activation. Although activated by a phospholipase C-mobilizing muscarinic receptor, the pharmacology of the response indicates that arachidonate is generated by activation of a type IV cytosolic phospholipase A_2 independently of Ca^{2+} or phospholipase C (66–68). A similar observation has been made in bovine aortic endothelial cells (69).

An arachidonate-sensitive Ca^{2+} influx pathway activated via vasopressin receptors has been characterized in A7r5 vascular smooth muscle cells, but in this case the pharmacology suggests that it is activated by arachidonate generated downstream of phospholipase C and diacylglycerol lipase (62). Vasopressin, via the V_{1A} receptor, stimulates phospholipase C, leading to formation of both $InsP_3$ and diacylglycerol, each of which leads to activation of a capacitative and a noncapacitative Ca^{2+} entry pathway. The capacitative Ca^{2+} entry pathway that is activated after depletion of intracellular Ca^{2+} stores is permeable to Ca^{2+}, Ba^{2+}, and Mn^{2+}, but not to Sr^{2+}, and is blocked irreversibly by 1 μM Gd^{3+}. The noncapacitative Ca^{2+} entry pathway that is activated by arachidonate is permeable to Sr^{2+}, Ca^{2+}, and Ba^{2+}, but not to Mn^{2+}, and it is reversibly blocked by a high concentration (100 μM) of Gd^{3+}. Activation of noncapacitative Ca^{2+} entry by vasopressin is prevented by RHC-80267, a selective inhibitor of diacylglycerol lipase. Thus, in A7r5 cells both arms of the phosphoinositide pathway regulate distinct Ca^{2+} entry pathways: $InsP_3$ activates capacitative Ca^{2+} entry by emptying intracellular Ca^{2+} stores, and diacylglycerol provides the arachidonic acid that causes activation of noncapacitative Ca^{2+} entry. Other investigators using A7r5 cells indicated that a conductance activated by vasopressin was activated by diacylglycerol rather than arachidonate, similar to the diacylglycerol-activated conductance in rabbit portal vein (70).

The Ca^{2+} current underlying arachidonate-activated Ca^{2+} entry has been electrophysiologically characterized in HEK cells, the so-called arachidonate-regulated Ca^{2+} current (I_{ARC}) (71). I_{ARC} probably accounts for the arachidonate-dependent noncapacitative entry of Ca^{2+} seen in a variety of cells at low agonist concentrations. Arachidonate-regulated Ca^{2+} channels are indeed specifically activated by low agonist concentrations and provide the predominant route of Ca^{2+} entry under such conditions. Sustained elevations in $[Ca^{2+}]_i$, such as those resulting from activation of capacitative Ca^{2+} entry by high agonist concentrations, inhibit the arachidonate-regulated Ca^{2+} channels. Thus, respective activities of arachidonate-regulated Ca^{2+} and capacitative Ca^{2+} channels display a unique reciprocal regulation that is related to the specific nature of $[Ca^{2+}]_i$ signals generated at different agonist concentrations. It is clearly possible that this unique reciprocal regulation mechanism exists in many cell types. It has even been posited that, at physiologically relevant levels of stimulation, it is the noncapacitative arachidonate-regulated Ca^{2+} channels that provide the predominant route for the agonist-activated entry of Ca^{2+} (72), although this remains a controversial view (73).

Results in both A7r5 cells (74) and HEK cells (75) also suggest that capacitative and noncapacitative pathways do not operate independently. In A7r5 cells, concentrations of vasopressin that stimulate noncapacitative Ca^{2+} entry simultaneously inhibit capacitative Ca^{2+} entry. Several lines of evidence support this idea. For example, whereas exogenous arachidonic acid activates noncapacitative Ca^{2+} entry and inhibits capacitative Ca^{2+} entry, vasopressin does neither in A7r5 cells lacking diacylglycerol lipase (e.g., using selective inhibitors of phospholipase C and diacylglyercol lipase) (74). Arachidonic acid, therefore, coordinates the activities of the two vasopressin-regulated Ca^{2+} entry pathways.

This reciprocal regulation by arachidonic acid ensures that all Ca^{2+} entry via the noncapacitative pathway is followed by a brief phase of Ca^{2+} entry via the capacitative pathway when vasopressin is removed. This strictly sequential activation of two distinct Ca^{2+} entry pathways (first noncapacitative and then capacitative) after agonist addition and removal may allow Ca^{2+} to be directed first to targets that mediate a cellular response and then to targets that facilitate recovery (74,76).

Recently *Drosophila* TRP and TRPL have been shown to be activated by arachidonic acid (77), raising the possiblility that the arachidonate-activated Ca^{2+} current might be carried by a TRP homolog. However, the only indication of the molecular identity of the channels is a recent report that TRPC4 antisense oligonucleotides reduced the arachidonate-induced Ca^{2+} influx in HEK cells (61). None of the TRPs thus far cloned match the electrophysiological properties of the arachidonate-regulated Ca^{2+} current, and overexpression of TRP6 (which can be activated by lipids) in HEK cells generates a current clearly distinguishable from the arachidonate-induced Ca^{2+} current (78).

V. RECEPTOR-OPERATED Ca^{2+} CHANNELS—SMOOTH MUSCLE

Receptor-operated cation channels in vascular smooth muscle are permeable to monovalent and divalent cations. At physiological resting membrane potentials [about −45 to −75 mV in vascular smooth muscle (79)], activation of a nonselective cation conductance induces an inward current that causes membrane depolarization and activates Ca^{2+} influx through voltage-gated Ca^{2+} channels, with consequent contraction. The pertinent features of receptor-operated channels are that they have a significant Ca^{2+} permeability and that sufficient Ca^{2+} enters the cell during channel opening to activate myosin light-chain kinase and produce contraction. Therefore, this process represents a contraction mechanism in smooth muscle induced by receptor stimulation mediated at least partly by Ca^{2+} entry that is independent of voltage-gated Ca^{2+} channels (80). It also is possible that Ca^{2+} entry through receptor-operated channels is involved in other cellular processes, such as smooth muscle cell proliferation (81).

Neurotransmitters and hormones reported to activate a receptor-operated cation current in smooth muscle include ATP, noradrenaline, acetylcholine, histamine, endothelin-1, neurokinin A, substance P, and vasopressin (82). In all cases, the response is initiated following activation of G-protein-coupled receptors. The main excitatory neurotransmitters released from mammalian sympathetic nerves onto vascular smooth muscle cells are norepinephrine and ATP. ATP produces a rapid excitatory junction potential mediated by a Ca^{2+}-permeable ligand-gated channel. In addition to ATP, the response to norepinephrine on α_1-adrenoceptors involves a Ca^{2+}-permeable receptor-operated cation channel. The TRPC6 protein is an essential component of the cation channel stimulated by norepinephrine. The transduction mechanism between the α_1-adrenoceptor binding site and channel involves G protein activation and stimulation of phospholipase C. It appears that subsequent production of diacylglycerol plays a prominent role in channel opening, although it is evident that other pathways involving tyrosine kinase also can produce channel opening. Likewise, the response to vasopressin on the V_{1A} receptor involves another receptor-operated Ca^{2+} entry pathway that is activated by arachidonic acid. TRPC proteins (TRPC6) are important elements of receptor-operated channels in vascular smooth muscle, and different types of receptor-operated channels might result from other TRP proteins forming Ca^{2+}-permeable channels or other TRP protein/accessory regulatory proteins forming a heteromultimer with TRPC6.

VI. RECEPTOR-OPERATED Ca^{2+} CHANNELS—ENDOTHELIUM

Vascular endothelium modulates blood pressure and flow by producing and releasing factors that regulate the tone of underlying smooth muscle. Nitric oxide release from endothelial cells causes adjacent smooth muscle to relax (83,84). In addition, other factors including arachidonic acid and its metabolites may also contribute significantly to endothelium-mediated relaxation (85–88). Both nitric oxide and arachi donic acid production implicate a G-protein-linked enzymatic pathway, similar to the regulation of receptor-operated channels.

Various functionally different receptor-operated channels have been described in endothelial cells (89–93). Most of these channels are activated by the actions of phospholipase C, but it is not clear which second messengers are involved. Interestingly, TRPC3 and TRPC6 are present in endothelium (94,95). TRPC4 and TRPC5 may be nonselective receptor-operated channels (96), although it has been shown that TRPC4 might be at least part of a more Ca^{2+}-selective, store-operated channel (97). Endothelial receptor-operated channels have been described that are activated by an increase in $[Ca^{2+}]_i$, are permeable to Ca^{2+}, and provide a Ca^{2+} entry route that exerts a positive feedback on their own activation. Their molecular structure is not known, although members of the TRP family with Ca^{2+}-calmodulin binding sites in their primary structure are possible candidates.

Nonselective cation channels that are Ca^{2+}-permeable and are activated by vasoactive agonists in freshly isolated cells from umbilical vein (92,98–100) have recently been characterized in more detail in cultured cell lines. The channel has a conductance of approximately 25 pS and is permeable to Na^+, Cs^+, and Ca^{2+} with a permeation ratio P_{Ca}/P_{Na} that varies between 0.03 and 2 (79,90,91,101). The current slowly activates during agonist stimulation and has been observed only in the presence of physiological $[Ca^{2+}]_i$. $[Ca^{2+}]_i$ buffering with 10 mM BAPTA completely prevents current activation. On the other hand, loading cells with Ca^{2+} via the patch pipette does not activate the current. Interestingly, application of a store-depleting inhibitor of sarco plasmic, endoplasmic reticulum Ca^{2+}-ATPase pumps, such as thapsigargin, also activates this current. The influx of Ca^{2+} through this current is coupled to agonist stimulation and depends on $InsP_3$ production. Block of phospholipase C with the pyrrolidinedione derivative U73122 rapidly inhibits Ca^{2+} influx, whereas the pyrrolidinedione derivative U73343, which does not inhibit phospholipase C, is ineffective. Also

5-nitro-2-(3-phenylpropylamino)benzoic acid (NPPB), Ni^{2+}, ecanozole, and SKF-96365 inhibit the agonist-induced Ca^{2+} entry (91). This channel shares some properties with the TRPC3 channels expressed in endothelial cells that do not express this current (102). Another Ca^{2+}-permeable nonselective cation channel activated by intracellular Ca^{2+} and with a conductance of 44 pS for monovalent cations has been described (103). This channel, with a permeability ratio P_{Ca}/P_{Na} of 0.7, is half-maximally activated at 0.7 μM $[Ca^{2+}]_i$. A nonselective, agonist-induced current, which is also activated by $[Ca^{2+}]_i$ and suppressed by inhibitors of the cyclooxygenase pathway, has also been described in aortic endothelial cells (104).

Other stimuli including oxidant stress activate a 28 pS nonselective cation conductance in a calf pulmonary artery cell line. This channel is equally permeable to Na^+, K^+, and Ca^{2+}. Oxidized glutathione activates these channels, whereas reduced glutathione reverses activation (105). This channel opens in two gating modes that do not depend on intracellular Ca^{2+} stores or $[Ca^{2+}]_i$. Activation of these channels and the concomitant membrane depolarization may limit Ca^{2+} influx (106). TRPC3 has been proposed as a molecular candidate for this channel (107).

VII. RECEPTOR-OPERATED Ca^{2+} CHANNELS—RECIPROCAL REGULATION OF Ca^{2+} ENTRY

Coordinating different Ca^{2+} entry pathways is important for directing functional cues. An example of such reciprocal regulation was described above in control of capacitative and noncapacitative Ca^{2+} entry by arachidonate. Membrane potential is another means whereby the activities of different Ca^{2+} entry pathways are coordinated. Many receptor-operated channels are less Ca^{2+}-selective than store-operated Ca^{2+} entry pathways (108,109). Opening of noncapacitative channels is therefore more likely to directly depolarize the plasma membrane and influence Ca^{2+} entry via other channels by either regulating gating or reducing the electrochemical gradient for Ca^{2+} entry. Moderate stimulation of M_3 muscarinic receptors, for example, stimulates Ca^{2+} release and capacitative Ca^{2+} entry, but with more intense stimulation, a nonselective cation channel is activated [possibly by arachidonic acid, see Sect. IV. D (74)]. The resulting membrane depolarization attenuates capacitative Ca^{2+} signaling by decreasing the electrochemical gradient for Ca^{2+} entry (110). As another example, in lung endothelial cells, G_q-linked agonists cause an initial transient hyperpolarization and, subsequently, a large sustained depolarization. The $[Ca^{2+}]_i$ response to G_q-linked agonists is broadly characterized by Ca^{2+} release from intracellular stores and Ca^{2+} entry across the cell membrane following Ca^{2+} store depletion, due to activation of store-operated and receptor-operated Ca^{2+} channels that are thought to represent the principal Ca^{2+} entry pathways (111). However, recent findings resolve another mechanism of

Ca^{2+} entry in lung microvascular endothelial cells, i.e., Ca^{2+} entry through $Ca_v3.1$ (α_{1G}) T-type Ca^{2+} channels within the window current range of voltages (112). Thus, under these conditions activation of G_q signaling transitions the membrane potential into a range of voltages that activate voltage-gated Ca^{2+} channels, sufficient to contribute to the global $[Ca^{2+}]_i$ rise.

VIII. CONCLUSIONS

The past decade has seen an explosion in the number of possible molecular candidates that may contribute to receptor-operated Ca^{2+} entry pathways. However, we have not yet developed a complete understanding of how agonist first messengers may evoke a current through well-described channels. Moreover, mechanisms of channel activation and/or its ultimate biological function are still incompletely understood. This relative lack of information provides ample opportunity for significant discoveries that are yet to come.

REFERENCES

1. Bolton TB. Mechanisms of action of transmitters and other substances on smooth muscle. Physiol Rev 1979; 59:606–718.
2. Van Breemen C, Aaronson P, Loutzenhiser R. Sodium-calcium interactions in mammalian smooth muscle. Pharmacol Rev 1978; 30:167–208.
3. Somlyo AP, Somlyo AV. Electromechanical and pharmacomechanical coupling in vascular smooth muscle. J Pharmacol Exp Ther 1968; 159:129–145.
4. Bolton TB, Large WA. Are junction potentials essential? Dual mechanism of smooth muscle cell activation by transmitter released from autonomic nerves. Quar J Exp Physiol 1986; 71:1–28.
5. Berridge MJ. Capacitative calcium entry. Biochem J 1995; 312:1–11.
6. Fasolato C, Innocenti B, Pozzan T. Receptor-activated Ca^{2+}in-flux: how many mechanisms for how many channels? Trends Pharmacol Sci 1994; 15: 77–83
7. Parekh AB, Penner R. Store depletion and calcium influx. Physiol Rev 1997; 77:901–930.
8. Gudermann T, Schöneberg T, Schultz G. Functional and structural complexity of signal transduction via G-protein-coupled receptors. Annu Rev Neurosci 1997; 20:399–427.
9. Wess J. Molecular basis of receptor/G-protein-coupling selectivity. Pharmacol Ther 1998; 80:231–264.
10. Simon MI, Strathmann MP, Gautam N. Diversity of G proteins in signal transduction. Science 1991; 252:802–808.
11. Wilkie TM, Gilbert DJ, Olsen AS, Chen XN, Amatruda TT, Korenberg JR, Trask BJ, de Jong P, Reed RR, Simon MI. Evolution of the mammalian G protein alpha subunit multigene family. Nature Genet 1992; 1:85–91.
12. Sutherland EW. Studies on the mechanism of hormone action. Science 1972; 177:401–408.
13. Berridge MJ. Inositol trisphosphate and calcium signalling. Nature 1993; 361:315–325.

14. Rhee SG, Bae YS. Regulation of phosphoinositide-specific phospholipase C isozymes. J Biol Chem 1997; 272:15045–15048.
15. Rhee SG, Choi KD. Regulation of inositol phospholipid-specific phospholipase C isozymes. J Biol Chem 1992; 267:12393–12396.
16. Noh DY, Shin SH, Rhee SG. Phosphoinositide-specific phospholipase C and mitogenic signaling. Biochim Biophys Acta 1995; 1242:99–113.
17. Cockcroft S, Thomas GM. Inositol-lipid-specific phospholipase C isoenzymes and their differential regulation by receptors. Biochem J 1992; 288:1–14.
18. Tsunoda Y. Receptor-operated calcium influx mediated by protein tyrosine kinase pathways. J Recept Signal Transduct Res 1998; 18:281–310.
19. Cantley LC, Auger KR, Carpenter C, Duckworth B, Graziani A, Kapeller R, Soltoff S. Oncogenes and signal transduction. Cell 1991; 64:281–302.
20. Marrero MB, Schieffer B, Paxton WG, Schieffer E, Bernstein KE. Electroporation of $pp60^{c\text{-}src}$ antibodies inhibits the angiotensin II activation of phospholipase C-γ1 in rat aortic smooth muscle cells. J Biol Chem 1995; 270: 15734–15738.
21. Marrero MB, Venema RC, Ma H, Ling BN, Eaton DC. Erythropoietin receptor-operated Ca^{2+} channels: activation by phospholipase C-γ1. Kidney Int 1998; 53:1259–1268.
22. Rao GN, Delafontaine P, Runge MS. Thrombin stimulates phosphorylation of insulin-like growth factor-1 receptor, insulin receptor substrate-1, and phospholipase C-γ1 in rat aortic smooth muscle cells. J Biol Chem 1995; 270:27871–27875.
23. Foster DC, Wedel BJ, Robinson SW, Garbers DL. Mechanisms of regulation and functions of guanylyl cyclases. Rev Physiol Biochem Pharmacol 1999; 135:1–39.
24. Fischmeister R, Hartzell HC. Cyclic guanosine 3′,5′-monophosphate regulates the calcium current in single cells from frog ventricle. J Physiol 1987; 387: 453–472.
25. Berven LA, Hughes BP, Barritt GJ. A slowly ADP-ribosylated pertussis-toxin-sensitive GTP-binding regulatory protein is required for vasopressin-stimulated Ca^{2+} inflow in hepatocytes. Biochem J 1994; 299:399–407.
26. Iwasawa K, Nakajima T, Hazama H, Goto A, Shin WS, Toyo-oka T, Omata M. Effects of extracellular pH on receptor-mediated Ca^{2+} influx in A7r5 rat smooth muscle cells: involvement of two different types of channel. J Physiol 1997; 503:237–251.
27. Krautwurst D, Seifert R, Hescheler J, Schultz G. Formyl peptides and ATP stimulate Ca^{2+} and Na^+ inward currents through non-selective cation channels via G-proteins in dibutyryl cyclic AMP-differentiated HL-60 cells. Involvement of Ca^{2+} and Na^+ in the activation of beta-glucuronidase release and superoxide production. Biochem J 1992; 288:1025–1035.
28. von zur Mühlen F, Eckstein F, Penner R. Guanosine 5′-[β-thio] triphosphate selectively activates calcium signaling in mast cells. Proc Nat Acad Sci USA 1991; 88:926–930.
29. Wickman K, Clapham DE. Ion channel regulation by G proteins. Physiol Rev 1995; 75:865–885.

30. Matthews G, Neher E, Penner R. Second messenger-activated calcium influx in rat peritoneal mast cells. J Physiol 1989; 418:105–130.
31. Komori S, Bolton TB. Role of G-proteins in muscarinic receptor inward and outward currents in rabbit jejunal smooth muscle. J Physiol 1990; 427: 395–419.
32. Macrez-Leprêtre N, Kalkbrenner F, Schultz G, Mironneau J. Distinct functions of G_q and G_{11} proteins in coupling α_1-adrenoreceptors to Ca^{2+} release and Ca^{2+} entry in rat portal vein myocytes. J Biol Chem 1997; 272:5261–5268.
33. Reber BF, Neuhaus R, Reuter H. Activation of different pathways for calcium elevation by bradykinin and ATP in rat pheochromocytoma (PC 12) cells. Pflügers Arch 1992; 420:213–218.
34. Singer-Lahat D, Liu J, Wess J, Felder CC. The third intracellular domain of the m_3 muscarinic receptor determines coupling to calcium influx in transfected Chinese hamster ovary cells. FEBS Lett 1996; 386:51–54.
35. Singer-Lahat D, Rojas E, Felder CC. A9 fibroblasts transfected with the m_3 muscarinic receptor clone express a Ca^{2+} channel activated by carbachol, GTP and GDP. J Membrane Biol 1997; 159:21–28.
36. Obukhov AG, Harteneck C, Zobel A, Harhammer R, Kalkbrenner F, Leopoldt D, Lückhoff A, Nurnberg B, Schultz G. Direct activation of trpl cation channels by $G\alpha_{11}$ subunits. EMBO J 1996; 15:5833–5838.
37. Kiselyov KI, Mamin AG, Semyonova SB, Mozhayeva GN. Low-conductance high selective inositol (1,4,5)-trisphosphate activated Ca^{2+} channels in plasma membrane of A431 carcinoma cells. FEBS Lett 1997; 407:309–312.
38. Kiselyov KI, Semyonova SB, Mamin AG, Mozhayeva GN. Miniature Ca^{2+} channels in excised plasma-membrane patches: activation by IP_3. Pflügers Arch 1999; 437:305–314.
39. Kuno M, Gardner P. Ion channels activated by inositol 1,4,5-trisphosphate in plasma membrane of human T-lymphocytes. Nature 1987; 326:301–304.
40. Penner R, Matthews G, Neher E. Regulation of calcium influx by second messengers in rat mast cells. Nature 1988; 334:499–504.
41. Vaca L, Kunze DL. IP_3-activated Ca^{2+} channels in the plasma membrane of cultured vascular endothelial cells. Am J Physiol 1995; 269:C733–C738.
42. Lückhoff A, Clapham DE. Inositol 1,3,4,5-tetrakisphosphate activates an endothelial Ca^{2+}-permeable channel. Nature 1992; 355:356–358.
43. Helliwell RM, Large WA. α_1-Adrenoceptor activation of a non-selective cation current in rabbit portal vein by 1,2-diacyl-*sn*-glycerol. J Physiol 1997; 499:417–428.
44. Wang Q, Large WA. Noradrenaline-evoked cation conductance recorded with the nystatin whole-cell method in rabbit portal vein cells. J Physiol 1991; 435: 21–39.
45. Inoue R, Kuriyama H. Dual regulation of cation-selective channels by muscarinic and α_1-adrenergic receptors in the rabbit portal vein. J Physiol 1993; 465:427–448.
46. Albert AP, Large WA. Comparison of spontaneous and noradrenaline-evoked non-selective cation channels in rabbit portal vein myocytes. J Physiol 2001; 530:457–468.

47. Helliwell RM, Large WA. Dual effect of external Ca^{2+} on noradrenaline-activated cation current in rabbit portal vein smooth muscle cells. J Physiol 1996; 492:75–88.
48. Aromolaran AS, Large WA. Comparison of the effects of divalent cations on the noradrenaline-evoked cation current in rabbit portal vein smooth muscle cells. J Physiol 1999; 520:771–782.
49. Albert AP, Large WA. The effect of external divalent cations on spontaneous non-selective cation channel currents in rabbit portal vein myocytes. J Physiol 2001; 536:409–420.
50. Inoue R, Okada T, Onoue H, Hara Y, Shimizu S, Naitoh S, Ito Y, Mori Y. The transient receptor potential protein homologue TRP6 is the essential component of vascular α_1-adrenoceptor-activated Ca^{2+}-permeable cation channel. Circ Res 2001; 88:325–332.
51. Tesfai Y, Brereton HM, Barritt GJ. A diacylglycerol-activated Ca^{2+} channel in PC12 cells (an adrenal chromaffin cell line) correlates with expression of the TRP-6 (transient receptor potential) protein. Biochem J 2001; 358: 717–726.
52. Chakrabarti R, Kumar S. Diacylglycerol mediates the T-cell receptor-driven Ca^{2+} influx in T cells by a novel mechanism independent of protein kinase C activation. J Cell Biochem 2000; 78:222–230.
53. Gamberucci A, Giurisato E, Pizzo P, Tassi M, Giunti R, McIntosh DP, Benedetti A. Diacylglycerol activates the influx of extracellular cations in T-lymphocytes independently of intracellular calcium-store depletion and possibly involving endogenous TRP6 gene products. Biochem J 2002; 364: 245–254.
54. Hofmann T, Obukhov AG, Schaefer M, Harteneck C, Gudermann T, Schultz G. Direct activation of human TRPC6 and TRPC3 channels by diacylglycerol. Nature 1999; 397:259–263.
55. Okada T, Inoue R, Yamazaki K, Maeda A, Kurosaki T, Yamakuni T, Tanaka I, Shimizu S, Ikenaka K, Imoto K, Mori Y. Molecular and functional characterization of a novel mouse transient receptor potential protein homologue TRP7. Ca^{2+}-permeable cation channel that is constitutively activated and enhanced by stimulation of G protein-coupled receptor. J Biol Chem 1999; 274:27359–27370.
56. Lintschinger B, Balzer-Geldsetzer M, Baskaran T, Graier WF, Romanin C, Zhu MX, Groschner K. Coassembly of Trp1 and Trp3 proteins generates diacylglycerol- and Ca^{2+}-sensitive cation channels. J Biol Chem 2000; 275: 27799–27805.
57. Boulay G, Brown DM, Qin N, Jiang M, Dietrich A, Zhu X, Chen Z, Birnbaumer M, Mikoshiba K, Birnbaumer L. Modulation of Ca^{2+} entry by polypeptides of the inositol 1,4, 5-trisphosphate receptor (IP3R) that bind transient receptor potential (TRP): evidence for roles of TRP and IP3R in store depletion-activated Ca^{2+} entry. Proc Nat Acad Sci USA 1999; 96: 14955–14960.
58. Birnbaumer L, Boulay G, Brown D, Jiang M, Dietrich A, Mikoshiba K, Zhu X, Qin N. Mechanism of capacitative Ca^{2+} entry (CCE): interaction between IP_3 receptor and TRP links the internal calcium storage compartment to

plasma membrane CCE channels. Recent Prog Hormone Res 2000; 55: 127–161; discussion 161–162.
59. Kiselyov K, Xu X, Mozhayeva G, Kuo T, Pessah I, Mignery G, Zhu X, Birnbaumer L, Muallem S. Functional interaction between $InsP_3$ receptors and store-operated Htrp3 channels. Nature 1998; 396:478–482.
60. Ma HT, Patterson RL, van Rossum DB, Birnbaumer L, Mikoshiba K, Gill DL. Requirement of the inositol trisphosphate receptor for activation of store-operated Ca^{2+} channels. Science 2000; 287:1647–1651.
61. Wu X, Babnigg G, Zagranichnaya T, Villereal ML. The role of endogenous human Trp4 in regulating carbachol-induced calcium oscillations in HEK-293 cells. J Biol Chem 2002; 277:13597–13608.
62. Broad LM, Cannon TR, Taylor CW. A non-capacitative pathway activated by arachidonic acid is the major Ca^{2+} entry mechanism in rat A7r5 smooth muscle cells stimulated with low concentrations of vasopressin. J Physiol 1999; 517:121–134.
63. Peppelenbosch MP, Tertoolen LG, den Hertog J, de Laat SW. Epidermal growth factor activates calcium channels by phospholipase A2/5-lipoxygenase-mediated leukotriene C4 production. Cell 1992; 69:295–303.
64. Shuttleworth TJ, Thompson JL. Muscarinic receptor activation of arachidonate-mediated Ca^{2+} entry in HEK293 cells is independent of phospholipase C. J Biol Chem 1998; 273:32636–32643.
65. Meves H. Modulation of ion channels by arachidonic acid. Prog Neurobiol 1994; 43:175–186.
66. Shuttleworth TJ. Arachidonic acid activates the noncapacitative entry of Ca^{2+} during $[Ca^{2+}]_i$ oscillations. J Biol Chem 1996; 271:21720–21725.
67. Shuttleworth TJ, Thompson JL. Discriminating between capacitative and arachidonate-activated Ca^{2+} entry pathways in HEK293 cells. J Biol Chem 1999; 274:31174–31178.
68. Osterhout JL, Shuttleworth TJ. A Ca^{2+}-independent activation of a type IV cytosolic phospholipase A_2 underlies the receptor stimulation of arachidonic acid-dependent noncapacitative calcium entry. J Biol Chem 2000; 275: 8248–8254.
69. Fiorio Pla A, Munaron L. Calcium influx, arachidonic acid, and control of endothelial cell proliferation. Cell Calcium 2001; 30:235–244.
70. Jung S, Strotmann R, Schultz G, Plant TD. TRPC6 is a candidate channel involved in receptor-stimulated cation currents in A7r5 smooth muscle cells. Am J Physiol—Cell Physiol 2002; 282:C347–C359.
71. Mignen O, Shuttleworth TJ. I_{ARC}, a novel arachidonate-regulated noncapacitative Ca^{2+} entry channel. J Biol Chem 2000; 275:9114–9119.
72. Mignen O, Thompson JL, Shuttleworth TJ. Reciprocal regulation of capacitative and arachidonate-regulated noncapacitative Ca^{2+} entry pathways. J Biol Chem 2001; 276:35676–35683.
73. Shuttleworth TJ. What drives calcium entry during $[Ca^{2+}]_i$ oscillations?—challenging the capacitative model. Cell Calcium 1999; 25:237–246.
74. Moneer Z, Taylor CW. Reciprocal regulation of capacitative and non-capacitative Ca^{2+} entry in A7r5 vascular smooth muscle cells: only the latter operates during receptor activation. Biochem J 2002; 362:13–21.

75. Luo D, Broad LM, Bird GS, Putney JW, Jr. Mutual antagonism of calcium entry by capacitative and arachidonic acid-mediated calcium entry pathways. J Biol Chem 2001; 276:20186–20189.
76. Taylor CW. Regulation of Ca^{2+} entry pathways by both limbs of the phosphoinositide pathway. Novartis Found Symp 2002; 246:91–101; discussion 101–107.
77. Chyb S, Raghu P, Hardie RC. Polyunsaturated fatty acids activate the *Drosophila* light-sensitive channels TRP and TRPL. Nature 1999; 397:255–259.
78. Elliott AC. Recent developments in non-excitable cell calcium entry. Cell Calcium 2001; 30:73–93.
79. Nelson MT, Patlak JB, Worley JF, Standen NB. Calcium channels, potassium channels, and voltage dependence of arterial smooth muscle tone. Am J Physiol 1990; 259:C3–C18.
80. McDaniel SS, Platoshyn O, Wang J, Yu Y, Sweeney M, Krick S, Rubin LJ, Yuan JX. Capacitative Ca^{2+} entry in agonist-induced pulmonary vasoconstriction. Am J Physiol–Lung Cell Mol Physiol 2001; 280:L870–L880.
81. Yu Y, Sweeney M, Zhang S, Platoshyn O, Landsberg J, Rothman A, Yuan JX. PDGF stimulates pulmonary vas-cular smooth muscle cell proliferation by upregulating TRPC6 expression. Am J Physiol—Cell Physiol 2003; 284:C316–C330.
82. McFadzean I, Gibson A. The developing relationship between receptor-operated and store-operated calcium channels in smooth muscle. Br J Pharmacol 2002; 135:1–13.
83. Palmer RM, Ferrige AG, Moncada S. Nitric oxide release accounts for the biological activity of endothelium-derived relaxing factor. Nature 1987; 327:524–526.
84. Furchgott RF, Vanhoutte PM. Endothelium-derived relaxing and contracting factors. FASEB J 1989; 3:2007–2018.
85. Quilley J, Fulton D, McGiff JC. Hyperpolarizing factors. Biochem Pharmacol 1997; 54:1059–1070.
86. Campbell WB, Harder DR. Endothelium-derived hyperpolarizing factors and vascular cytochrome P450 metabolites of arachidonic acid in the regulation of tone. Circ Res 1999; 84:484–488.
87. Feletou M, Vanhoutte PM. The alternative: EDHF. J Mol Cell Cardiol 1999; 31:15–22.
88. Quilley J, McGiff JC. Is EDHF an epoxyeicosatrienoic acid? Trends Pharmacol Sci 2000; 21:121–124
89. Groschner K, Graier WF, Kukovetz WR. Histamine induces K^+, Ca^{2+}, and Cl^- currents in human vascular endothelial cells. Role of ionic currents in stimulation of nitric oxide biosynthesis. Circ Res 1994; 75:304–314.
90. Jow F, Numann R. Histamine increases $[Ca^{2+}]_{in}$ and activates Ca-K and nonselective cation currents in cultured human capillary endothelial cells. J Membrane Biol 2000; 173:107–116.
91. Kamouchi M, Mamin A, Droogmans G, Nilius B. Nonselective cation channels in endothelial cells derived from human umbilical vein. J Membrane Biol 1999; 169:29–38.

92. Nilius B, Schwartz G, Oike M, Droogmans G. Histamine-activated, non-selective cation currents and Ca^{2+} transients in endothelial cells from human umbilical vein. Pflügers Arch 1993; 424:285–293.
93. Nilius B, Viana F, Droogmans G. Ion channels in vascular endothelium. Ann Rev Physiol 1997; 59:145–170.
94. Freichel M, Schweig U, Stauffenberger S, Freise D, Schorb W, Flockerzi V. Store-operated cation channels in the heart and cells of the cardiovascular system. Cell Physiol Biochem 1999; 9:270–283.
95. Harteneck C, Plant TD, Schultz G. From worm to man: three subfamilies of TRP channels. Trends Neurosci 2000; 23:159–166.
96. Schaefer M, Plant TD, Obukhov AG, Hofmann T, Gudermann T, Schultz G. Receptor-mediated regulation of the nonselective cation channels TRPC4 and TRPC5. J Biol Chem 2000; 275:17517–17526.
97. Freichel M, Suh SH, Pfeifer A, Schweig U, Trost C, Weissgerber P, Biel M, Philipp S, Freise D, Droogmans G, Hofmann F, Flockerzi V, Nilius B. Lack of an endothelial store-operated Ca^{2+} current impairs agonist-dependent vasorelaxation in $TRP4^{-/-}$ mice. Nature Cell Biol 2001; 3:121–127.
98. Nilius B. Permeation properties of a non-selective cation channel in human vascular endothelial cells. Pflügers Arch 1990; 416:609–611.
99. Nilius B. Regulation of transmembrane calcium fluxes in endothelium. News Physiol Sci 1991; 6:110–114.
100. Nilius B, Riemann D. Ion channels in human endothelial cells. Gen Physiol Biophys 1990; 9:89–111.
101. Nilius B. Signal transduction in vascular endothelium: the role of intracellular calcium and ion channels. Verhandel-Koninkl Acad Geneesk Belg 1998; 60: 215–250.
102. Kamouchi M, Philipp S, Flockerzi V, Wissenbach U, Mamin A, Raeymaekers L, Eggermont J, Droogmans G, Nilius B. Properties of heterologously expressed hTRP3 channels in bovine pulmonary artery endothelial cells. J Physiol 1999; 518:345–358.
103. Baron A, Frieden M, Chabaud F, Beny JL. Ca^{2+}-dependent non-selective cation and potassium channels activated by bradykinin in pig coronary artery endothelial cells. J Physiol 1996; 493:691–706.
104. Himmel HM, Rasmusson RL, Strauss HC. Agonist-induced changes of $[Ca^{2+}]_i$ and membrane currents in single bovine aortic endothelial cells. Am J Physiol 1994; 267:C1338–C1350.
105. Koliwad SK, Elliott SJ, Kunze DL. Oxidized glutathione mediates cation channel activation in calf vascular endothelial cells during oxidant stress. J Physiol 1996; 495:37–49.
106. Koliwad SK, Kunze DL, Elliott SJ. Oxidant stress activates a non-selective cation channel responsible for membrane depolarization in calf vascular endothelial cells. J Physiol 1996; 491:1–12.
107. Balzer M, Lintschinger B, Groschner K. Evidence for a role of Trp proteins in the oxidative stress-induced membrane conductances of porcine aortic endothelial cells. Cardiovasc Res 1999; 42:543–549.
108. Clapham DE, Runnels LW, Strübing C. The TRP ion channel family. Nature Rev Neurosci 2001; 2:387–396.

109. Venkatachalam K, van Rossum DB, Patterson RL, Ma HT, Gill DL. The cellular and molecular basis of store-operated calcium entry. Nat Cell Biol 2002; 4:E263–E272.
110. Carroll RC, Peralta EG. The m3 muscarinic acetylcholine receptor differentially regulates calcium influx and release through modulation of monovalent cation channels. EMBO J 1998; 17:3036–3044.
111. Putney JW Jr. A model for receptor-regulated calcium entry. Cell Calcium 1986; 7:1–12.
112. Wu S, Haynes J Jr, Taylor JT, Obiako BO, Stubbs JR, Li M, Stevens T. $Ca_v3.1$ (α_{1G}) T-type Ca^{2+} channels mediate vasoocclusion of sickled erythrocytes in lung microcirculation. Circ Res 2003; 93:346–353.
113. Birnbaumer L, Zhu X, Jiang M, Boulay G, Peyton M, Vannier B, Brown D, Platano D, Sadeghi H, Stefani E, Birnbaumer M. On the molecular basis and regulation of cellular capacitative calcium entry: roles for Trp proteins. Proc Nat Acad USA 1996; 93:15195–15202.
114. Fasolato C, Nilius B. Store depletion triggers the calcium release-activated calcium current (I_{CRAC}) in macrovascular endothelial cells: a comparison with Jurkat and embryonic kidney cell lines. Pflügers Arch 1998; 436:69–74.
115. Bolsover S, Ashworth R, Archer F. Activator of calcium influx proves a slippery customer. J Physiol 1999; 517:2.
116. Hille B. Ion Channels of Excitable Membranes, 3rd ed. Sunderland, MA: Sinauer Associates, Inc., 2001.

6

Transient Receptor Potential Cation Channels and Store-Operated Ca^{2+} Channels

Donna L. Cioffi, Songwei Wu, and Troy Stevens

University of South Alabama College of Medicine, Mobile, Alabama, U.S.A.

I. INTRODUCTION

Cells expend energy to maintain a low cytosolic Ca^{2+} concentration ($[Ca^{2+}]_i$) relative to extracellular and organelle environments, so periodic fluctuations in cytosolic concentrations can be used to initiate intracellular signaling. Indeed, $[Ca^{2+}]_i$ is 10,000–20,000-fold lower than extracellular $[Ca^{2+}]$. Various transmembrane proteins conduct Ca^{2+}—exhibiting either high (Ca^{2+}-selective) or low (Ca^{2+} nonselective) specificity—from outside to inside the cell, in accordance with electrical and chemical ionic gradients. Protein channels open in response to distinct intracellular stimuli. Perhaps most notably, membrane depolarization opens so-called voltage-gated Ca^{2+} channels. More recently a subset of channels were identified that monitor and respond to endoplasmic reticulum Ca^{2+} concentrations; when endoplasmic reticulum Ca^{2+} concentrations decrease, membrane Ca^{2+} channels open. Transmembrane proteins have now been identified that are specifically activated following endoplasmic reticulum Ca^{2+} store depletion and thus fulfill the criterion for a "store-operatedCa^{2+} entry" (SOCE) channel.

All lung cells studied to date possess SOCE channels, although there are considerable lapses in our knowledge of cell-specific channel expression and function. It is clear from the available literature, however, that SOCE regulates the endothelial cell barrier function, production of endothelium-derived autacoids, constriction of vascular smooth muscle, and lung cell proliferation. This chapter reviews the available literature regarding SOCE, including the molecular basis of SOCE channels, mechanisms involved in channel activation, and, finally, the relevance of SOCE to physiological processes of lung cells.

II. Ca^{2+}-SELECTIVE AND NONSELECTIVE SOCE

Store-operated Ca^{2+} entry was originally proposed by Putney (1), who used the term "capacitative Ca^{2+} entry" to describe the phenomenon of coupling between endoplasmic reticulum Ca^{2+} concentration and activation of membrane Ca^{2+} entry channels. In his conception, Ca^{2+} store depletion activated Ca^{2+} entry through plasma membrane channels to refill the store, as in a capacitor. Interestingly, it is Ca^{2+} depletion of endoplasmic reticulum Ca^{2+}, and not the transient rise in $[Ca^{2+}]_i$, that triggers activation of the membrane channels. SOCE agonists induce a biphasic $[Ca^{2+}]_i$ transition, including an initial transient increase that is due to Ca^{2+} release from the endoplasmic reticulum and a sustained increase that is due to Ca^{2+} entry through channels in the plasmalemma.

Store-operated Ca^{2+} entry signaling is typically initiated by agonist binding to a G-protein-coupled receptor or receptor tyrosine kinase, resulting in the activation of phospholipase C-β or -γ, respectively (Fig. 1). Activated phospholipase C hydrolzses phosphatidylinositol 4,5-bisphosphate to the second messengers inositol 1,4,5-trisphosphate ($InsP_3$) and diacylglycerol. $InsP_3$ rapidly diffuses through the cytosol, binds to its receptor on the endoplasmic reticulum, and releases Ca^{2+} from the endoplasmic reticulum Ca^{2+} store. Many ligands relevant to pulmonary pathobiology act through SOCE-dependent mechanisms, including angiotensin II, endothelin-1, platelet-activating factor, bradykinin, thrombin, and substance P. As an example of their actions, angiotensin II and endothelin-1 stimulate SOCE in smooth muscle cells and produce pulmonary vasoconstriction. They also activate SOCE in endothelial cells, which stimulates nitric oxide and prostacyclin production, modulating the magnitude of vasoconstriction.

Because multiple parallel pathways are activated by G-protein-coupled receptors (i.e., crosstalk), it is difficult to identify the specific signaling events that mediate SOCE. However, because SOCE is activated by Ca^{2+} store depletion, and not Ca^{2+} release from the store per se, endoplasmic reticulum-specific Ca^{2+} chelators (i.e., TPEN) and inhibitors of the endoplasmic reticulum Ca^{2+}/ATPase are sufficient to stimulate plasma membrane channels. Indeed, thapsigargin, cyclopiazonic acid, and dibenzohydroquinone are endoplasmic reticulum Ca^{2+}/ATPase inhibitors that allow resolution of "true" SOCE events, i.e., Ca^{2+} entry that can be activated solely by depletion of the Ca^{2+} store (Fig. 1). Perhaps the most

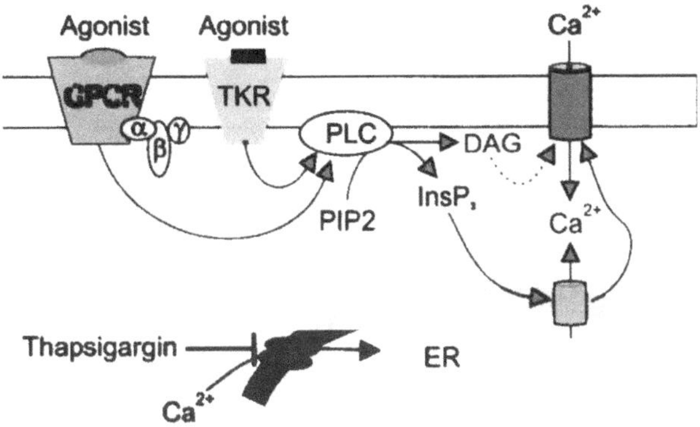

Figure 1 Activation of Gq or receptor tyrosine kinases promotes Store-operated Ca^{2+} entry (SOCE). Agonists that bind to G-protein-coupled receptors (GPCRs) or tyrosine kinase receptors (TKRs) activate phospholipase C (PLC), which cleaves phosphatidylinositol-4,5-bisphospate (PIP2) to the second messengers inositol-1,4,5-trisphosphate ($InsP_3$) and diacylglycerol (DAG). SOCE involves diffusion and binding of $InsP_3$ to its receptor on the endoplasmic reticulum (ER). Activation of the $InsP_3$ receptor results in Ca^{2+} release from the ER store. It is this Ca^{2+} store depletion that somehow triggers opening of store-operated channels on the plasma membrane. The receptor-operated pathway involves the second messenger DAG, at least, which can directly or indirectly activate channels on the plasma membrane without requiring Ca^{2+} store depletion. The plant alkaloid thapsigargin blocks Ca^{2+} reuptake into the ER and is often employed in studies of store-operated channels to avoid the confounding effects of $InsP_3$ and DAG. (Adapted from Ref. 89.)

common technique used for evaluating SOCE events is measuring thapsigargin-induced changes in global $[Ca^{2+}]_i$. Figure 2A depicts the typical global $[Ca^{2+}]_i$ response of pulmonary artery endothelial cells to thapsigargin. The initial $[Ca^{2+}]_i$ rise reflects Ca^{2+} store depletion, and the sustained $[Ca^{2+}]_i$ elevation reflects Ca^{2+} entry through channels in the plasmalemma.

The global rise in $[Ca^{2+}]_i$ depicted in Fig. 2A reflects activation of multiple SOCE channels. Electrophysiological techniques allow resolution of SOCE channel biophysical properties. In general, SOCE channels are characterized as either Ca^{2+}-selective or -nonselective. Hoth and Penner (2) originally characterized an endogenous Ca^{2+}-selective SOCE current in mast cells. This current, which they termed I_{CRAC} (Ca^{2+} release-activated current), was a small current (less than ≈50 pA at –80 mV) and exhibited selectivity for Ca^{2+} over Ba^{2+}, Mn^{2+}, and Sr^{2+} ions, with a positive reversalpotential of ≈+40 mV. Further, I_{CRAC} was not voltage-activated and possessed a strong inward rectification. I_{CRAC} was also described in Jurkat human leukemic T cells (3) and rat basophilic leukemia cells (4). A current similar to I_{CRAC} has been identified in endothelial cells by Vaca and Kunze

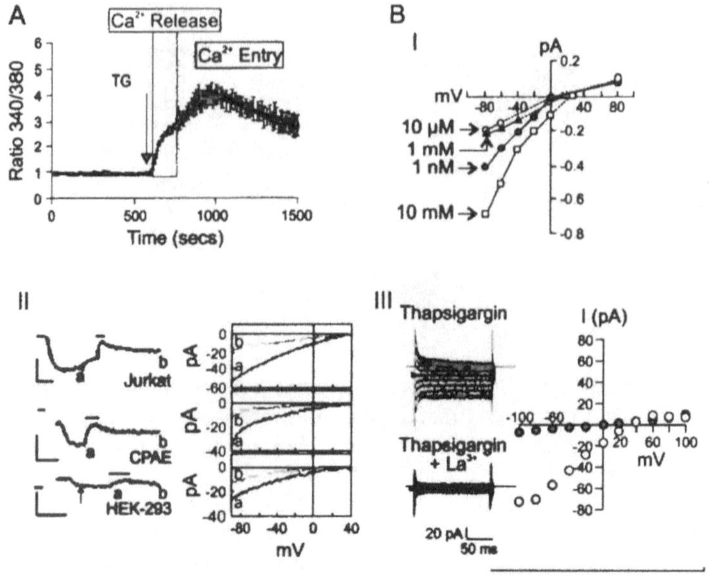

Figure 2 Calcium ion store depletion activates Ca^{2+}-selective and nonselective channels that increase global $[Ca^{2+}]_i$. (A) SOCE is activated by thapsigargin (TG). An initial rise reflects Ca^{2+} release from the endoplasmic reticulum, and the sustained elevation results from Ca^{2+} entry through SOCE channels. (Adapted from Ref. 82.) (B) Thapsigargin activates a Ca^{2+} -selective SOCE current in endothelial cells. In separate studies, Vaca and Kunze (5) (I), Fasolato and Nilius (6) (II), and Wu and coworkers (74) (III) isolated a Ca^{2+} -selective SOCE current in vascular endothelial cells. This current, generally referred to as I_{SOC}, is a small, strongly inwardly rectifying current that exhibits a positive reversal potential ($\approx +40\,mV$) and inhibition by La^{3+}. (Adapted from Ref. 90.)

(5), Fasolato and Nilius (6), and Stevens and coworkers (7). This current, generally referred to as I_{SOC} (store-operated Ca^{2+} entry), is a small inward Ca^{2+} current that reverses potential at approximately $+40\,mV$ and is strongly inwardly rectifying (Fig. 2B).

There are a far greater number of studies demonstrating activation of nonselective cation entry following Ca^{2+} store depletion. These currents are larger than the I_{CRAC} and I_{SOC} currents and usually possess a linear current–voltage relationship. Nonselective currents exhibit a $0\,mV$ reversal potential, reflecting conductance of various cationic species. Virtually every cell type studied to date possesses a nonselective current that can be activated by Ca^{2+} store depletion.

Whereas the SOCE-induced global $[Ca^{2+}]_i$ rise is well studied and the unique attributes of Ca^{2+}-selective and -nonselective currents are accepted, the molecular identities of SOCE Ca^{2+}-selective and -nonselective channels are still incompletely understood. It is not clear how the channels that makeup these respective currents are activated or, how they uniquely govern cell function. In the mid-1990s the first molecular candidates for SOCE channels were identified, initially in *Drosophila melanogaster*. More recently, mammalian homologs have been identified, several of which can be directly activated following Ca^{2+} store depletion, thus fulfilling the criteria of SOCE channels.

III. MOLECULAR BASIS FOR SOCE

The mammalian transient receptor potential (TRP) protein family is recognized as a superfamily consisting of three subfamilies (Fig. 3) (8,9). The TRPC subfamily consists of seven members (TRPC1–TRPC7) that most closely resemble the *Drosophila* TRP proteins. TRPC4 and -5 comprise a subgroup, and TRPC1, although distinct as a subgroup, is structurally most closely related to TRPC4 and -5. TRPC3, -6, and -7 also comprise a subgroup. Members of the TRPC subfamily have been identified as subunits contributing to the formation of SOCE channels (10). The TRPV subfamily, previously called OTRPC or osm TRPC, includes the vanilloid receptor 1

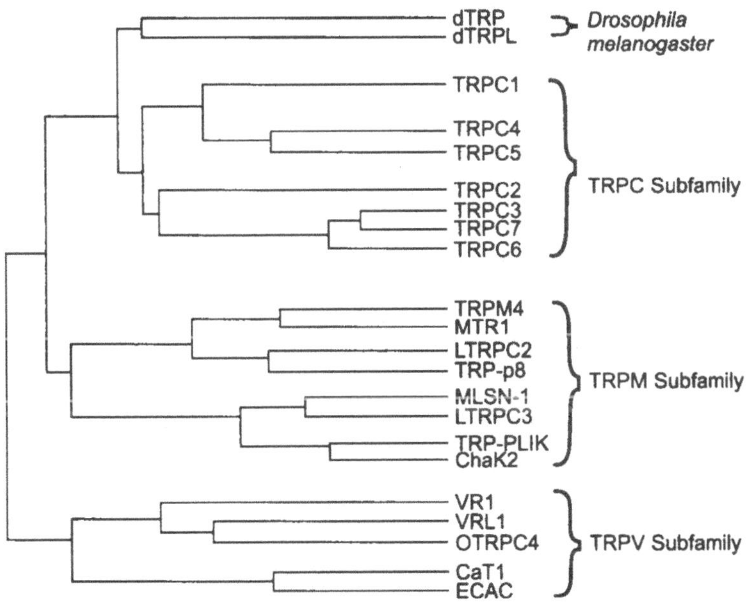

Figure 3 Phylogenetic tree of TRP proteins. The mammalian TRP protein superfamily consists of three subfamilies; TRPC, TRPM, and TRPV. The TRPC subfamily members (TRPC1–TRPC7) most closely resemble the *Drosophila melanogaster* TRP proteins, TRP and TRPL. (Adapted from Ref. 91.)

and other ion channels that are sensitive to noxious stimuli such as heat or osmotic stress. TRPV6, also referred to as CaT1, has been implicated as a SOCE channel (11). The TRPM subfamily, named for melastatin, was originally termed LTRPC and is the least understood of the subfamilies.

TRPC proteins exhibit six transmembrane domains with cytosolic N- and C-termini, ranging in size from ≈700 to 1000 amino acids. Based on analogy with voltage-gated Ca^{2+}, voltage-gated K^+, and cyclic nucleotide-gated channels, TRPC cation channels are predicted to be tetramers comprised of homo- or hetero-oligomers that coalesce to form the pore region between the fifth and sixth transmembrane domains (Fig. 4). Cytosolic

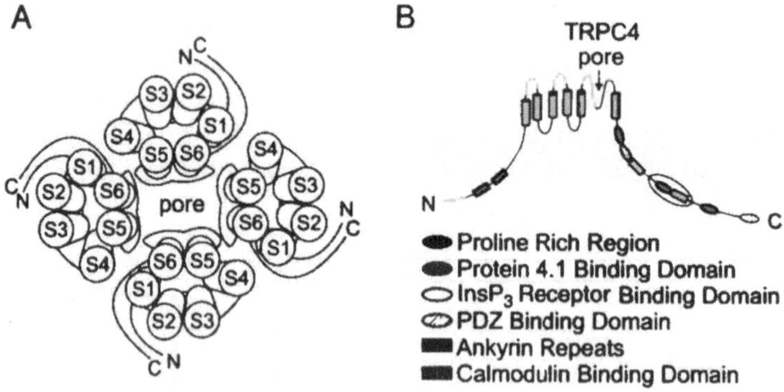

Figure 4 TRPC channel and protein structure. (A) Functional TRPC channels comprise four subunits. This tetramer can be formed from identical TRPC subunits (homotetramer) or from different TRPC subunits (heterotetramer). Although the precise oligomeric state of native channels remains to be determined, it is likely that they vary in a cell-type specific manner. Transmembrane regions 5 and 6 of each subunit coalesce to form the channel's pore region, which allows for cation entry. (Adapted from Ref. 89.) (B) TRPC protein structure. Each TRPC subfamily member exhibits six transmembrane domains with cytosolic amino (N) and carboxy (C) termini. The putative pore region resides between transmembrane regions 5 and 6. N-termini exhibit high degrees of similarity among the TRPC subfamily members. Ankyrin repeats are located in the N-terminus. Although C-termini exhibit domains common to all TRPC subfamily members, they also confer regions that are unique to a specific TRPC protein or to the TRPC subgroup. Common regions include calmodulin binding domains, proline-rich regions, and an $InsP_3$ receptor binding domain. Only TRPC4 and its closely related subgroup member, TRPC5, contain a PDZ-binding domain, which is located at the end of the C-terminus. TRPC4 contains a potential protein 4.1 binding domain, which resides in close proximity to the putative pore region. Of the other TRPC subfamily members, only TRPC3 contains a putative protein 4.1 binding domain. (Adapted from Ref. 90.)

N- and C-terminal tails possess a number of distinct domains capable of mediating specific protein–protein interactions (reviewed in Ref. 12). Some of these domains are present in all TRPC isoforms, whereas others are isoform-specific (Fig. 4). Ankyrin repeats are present in all TRPC isoforms, although the number of repeats varies. The functional relevance of these domains remains to be determined. It was originally suggested that ankyrin repeats are involved in the oligomerization of individual TRPC subunits to form the tetrameric channel. However, a recent study by Engelke et al. (13) demonstrated that it was the coiled-coil region and not ankyrin repeats that promote homodimerization of TRPC1 subunits. Although this study suggested that ankyrin repeats are not critical for homo-oligomerization of TRPC1 subunits, it is possible that ankyrin repeats are required for hetero- or homo-oligomerization of other TRPC subunits.

The C-terminus of mammalian TRPCs is the most varied of isoforms and possesses sites for protein–protein interactions that are likely critical for channel function. Most protein–protein interactions that occur at the C-terminus are presently unresolved, even though elucidating the identity and nature of these interactions is critical to resolving functional and regulatory properties of TRPC channels. Indeed, studies of *Drosophila* TRP and human TRPC1 (hTRPC1) by Schilling and coworkers (14,15) and Ambudkar and coworkers (16), respectively, demonstrated that the C-terminus is responsible for channel activation. *Drosophila* TRP is activated upon store depletion, whereas *Drosophila* TRP-like (TRPL) is constitutively active and insensitive to store depletion. C-terminal tail swaps between TRP and TRPL conferred store sensitivity to TRPL and converted TRP into a constitutively active channel. Similarly, when truncated C-terminal TRPC1 was expressed in human submandibular gland cells, Ca^{2+} entry in response to store depletion was reduced.

Several domains on the C-terminus have been identified and, in some cases, studied functionally. TRPC1 and -4 have two calmodulin-binding sites (17,18). Calmodulin binding to the more distal domain regulates Ca^{2+}-dependent feedback inhibition of SOCE in TRPC1 (18). Additionally, all seven TRPC isoforms contain a common calmodulin/$InsP_3$ receptor ($InsP_3R$) binding site (19). Coupling between $InsP_3$ receptors and TRPC1, -3, and -4 is isoform-specific. Indeed, endogenously expressed TRPC1 interacts with $InsP_3R$ type II but not type I or III in human platelets (20), dependent on endoplasmic reticulum Ca^{2+} store depletion (21,22). In contrast, heterologously expressed TRPC3 constitutively interacts with the $InsP_3R$ (23–25), whereas TRPC4α (but not TRPC4β) constitutively interacts with $InsP_3R$ types I, II, and III (26).

Proline-rich regions are present in all TRPC isoforms and in *Drosophila* TRP (and TRPL), although sequences and distribution of these regions vary widely among isoforms (12). Proline-rich regions mediate protein–protein interactions in signal transduction events (reviewed in Refs.

27–30), and the role of these regions in TRPC channel activity is only beginning to be explored. Schilling's group (31) presented evidence supporting a regulatory role of proline-rich regions in *Drosophila* TRPL, which binds to the immunophilin FKBP59 in part through an LP dipeptide contained in a proline-rich region on the C-terminus. FKBP59 binding to TRPL contributed to regulation of channel activity. Interestingly, this LP dipeptide is located near the putative pore region of the channel and, further, is conserved in all the TRPC isoforms. Additional proline- rich regions reside in various locations throughout the C-terminus, however, the functions of these regions have not been examined.

Certain TRPC isoforms directly interact with the membrane skeleton. For example, we recently identified a putative protein 4.1-binding domain near the proline-rich region of the C-terminus in TRPC4. A similar sequence is found in TRPC3. Structural and functional studies in rat pulmonary artery and pulmonary microvascular cells revealed that protein 4.1 binds to TRPC4 and, further, that the nature of this interaction is dynamic. A role for protein 4.1 in gating the TRPC4 channel was supported by experiments in which the protein 4.1-binding domain and proline rich regions were deleted from TRPC4 (unpublished results). Heterologous expression of this deletion mutant exhibited decreased SOCE compared to expression of wild-type TRPC4. Thus, direct linkage between TRPC4 and the membrane skeleton occurs through protein 4.1, an interaction necessary for channel activation.

Specific protein–protein interactions are also required for assembly of proteins into a signaling complex, the signalplex or transducisome, which enables rapid and efficient signal transduction events (32). In the *Drosophila* phototransduction system, TRP is retained in the rhabdomere-localized signalplex through its interaction with the scaffolding protein INAD (33). Further, this TRP-INAD complex is essential for correct spatial arrangement of additional proteins involved in the signaling cascade, e.g., PLC and PKC. INAD has also been implicated in regulating the preassembly of these complexes (34). Similar to *Drosophila* TRP, the mammalian TRPC4 and -5 possess C-terminal PDZ binding domains that were shown to bind to the Na^+/H^+ exchanger regulatory protein NHERF in HEK-293 cells (35). NHERF possesses two PDZ domains and interacts with PLCβ and G-protein -coupled receptors, thus implicating its function as a scaffolding protein similar to INAD (35–37). While the N-terminal PDZ domains of NHERF bind to membrane-bound signaling proteins and mediate NHERF dimerization, its C-terminus interacts with ezrin-radixin-moesin proteins (38–40). Ezrin-radixin-moesin proteins are actin-interacting proteins (reviewed in Ref. 41) that can indirectly tether TRPC4 and-5 to the cytoskeleton through interaction with NHERF. The cytoskeletal interaction is likely important for signaling complex scaffolding and anchoring. Recent work by Mery et al. (42) demonstrated expression of TRPC4 lacking the PDZ-binding domain mislocalized away from the plasma membrane.

IV. ROLE OF INDIVIDUAL TRPC PROTEINS IN SOCE

Four TRPC proteins fulfill the criterion of SOCE channels, because Ca^{2+} store depletion is sufficient for their activation; indeed, TRPC1, -2, -4, and -5 are the best-characterized SOCE channels. Although it is clear that the functional channels are tetramers, there is no description of the oligomeric state—or subunit composition—of any endogenous SOCE channel. This issue is important because subunit composition may underlie cell-specific channel properties. In addition, heterologous expression systems may form unusual subunit compositions that generate channels with properties that are not physiologically relevant. Indeed, recent compelling work by Schilling and coworkers (43) demonstrated that subunit-specific interaction occurs between TRPC isoforms, important for their proper membrane targeting. Considerable work is still required to understand how cell-specific TRPC channels form to regulate Ca^{2+} transitions.

TRPC1 contributes to SOCE. Evidence for TRPC1 as a SOCE channel in heterologous expression systems has been inconsistent, possibly because the protein is mislocalized when heterologously expressed by itself (44). In some instances TRPC1 overexpression slightly increased the global $[Ca^{2+}]_i$ response to thapsigargin, whereas in other instances TRPC1 overexpression formed a constitutively active, non-selective and Ca^{2+} store-insensitive channel (45). In contrast, several investigators have now demonstrated that antisense or iRNA inhibition of TRPC1 in endogenous systems reduces the global $[Ca^{2+}]_i$ response to thapsigargin (22,46–50). Early overexpression studies suggested that TRPC1 formed a nonselective cation channel, but there is now good evidence that the endogenous TRPC1-containing channel(s) may be either Ca^{2+}-selective or nonselective. Indeed, antisense inhibition of TRPC1 in A549 and endothelial cells decreased the Ca^{2+}-selective I_{SOC} current by 50% but did not left-shift the reversal potential, suggesting that TRPC1 contributes one or more subunits to the functional channel (7,46). Supporting evidence was subsequently reported in *Xenopus* oocytes (49), HSG cells, and CHO cells (50). In contrast, TRPC1 contributes one or more subunits to a nonselective SOCE current found in smooth muscle cells (51,52).

TRPC2 has also been implicated as a component of SOCE channels. Whereas the human homolog of TRPC2 is a pseudogene (4,53,54), mouse TRPC2 is a functional channel (55). COS-M6 cells transfected with TRPC2 revealed an enhanced thapsigargin-induced SOCE (54). Thus, TRPC2 may indeed be part of SOCE channels in some species and in some cell types; however, further studies using endogenous systems must be performed before TRPC2's role in SOCE can be clearly resolved.

TRPC4 and TRPC5 are structurally related SOCE channels. Whereas TRPC4 is expressed in vascular tissue like endothelium, TRPC5 is enriched in the brain (56). Flockerzi and coworkers (57,58) first reported the amino acid sequence of TRPC4, which they initially referred to as bovine CCE1. Expression of TRPC4 in HEK cells resulted in a thapsigargin-induced SOCE. The TRPC4-dependent current exhibited strong inward rectification and selectivity for Ca^{2+} over Na^{+} and Cs^{+} but not over Ba^{2+}. Subsequent findings from other laboratories (49,59) generally supported this initial work [with two exceptions (60,61)], providing more detailed support for the idea that TRPC4 encodes a Ca^{2+}-selective I_{SOC} channel. Indeed, Warnat et al. (59) transfected TRPC4 into CHO and rat basophilic leukemia cells, where it exhibited high selectivity for Ca^{2+}, as judged by both the >+40 mV reversal potential and anomalous mole fraction behavior. Furthermore, the aortic endothelial cell SOCE current was almost completely abrogated in the TRPC4 knockout ($TRPC4^{-/-}$) mouse (62), and the reversal potential was left-shifted from ≈50 mV to ≈0 mV, indicating loss of Ca^{2+} selectivity. These results are consistent with TRPC4 contributing to a Ca^{2+}-selective SOCE current, and suggest that TRPC4 may be the subunit that senses store depletion as well as regulating Ca^{2+} selectivity.

TRPC3, -6 and -7 are usually considered receptor-operated channels and not SOCE channels, per se, because diacylglycerol and other components of G-protein-coupled receptor signaling pathways activate the channels. However, in certain instances inhibition of endogenous protein expression decreases thapsigargin-induced Ca^{2+} entry, indicating that either in some cell types or under specified experimental conditions these proteins contribute one or more subunits to SOCE channels. As an example of this idea, Yuan and coworkers (63) demonstrated that platelet-derived growth factor upregulated TRPC6 expression with concomitant enhancement of cyclopiazonic acid–induced SOCE in rat pulmonary artery smooth muscle cells. Further, TRPC6 antisense oligonucleotides significantly attenuated SOCE in these cells. The cyclopiazonic acid–induced current was large (≈450 pA at −80 mV), nonselective (reversal potential near 0 mV), and inhibited by Ni^{2+} and SK&F-96365, nonspecific blockers of SOCE. Thus, this TRPC6-mediated SOCE in pulmonary artery smooth muscle cells appears to be a nonselective cation entry path.

TRPV6, also known as CaT1, is a member of the TRPV subfamily of mammalian TRP proteins. Several studies suggested that this protein is the molecular basis for I_{CRAC}, whereas other studies have concluded that CaT1 does not generate I_{CRAC}. Clapham and coworkers (11) originally reported that expression of CaT1 in CHO cells resulted in a Ca^{2+}-selective current that possessed many of the same features as I_{CRAC}, e.g., Ca^{2+} selectivity, anomalous mole fraction effect, activation by store depletion, and block by La^{3+}. These findings were challenged by Nilius and coworkers (64), who determined that the electrophysiological properties of CaT1 channels expressed in HEK cells were not similar to those of endogenous I_{CRAC} in RBL cells. This conclusion was further supported by Schindl et al. (65), who, compared heterologously expressed CaT1 in HEK cells to endogenous

I_{CRAC} in RBL cells, and also expressed CaT1 in RBL cells. The principal observations in this study were that endogenous I_{CRAC} in RBL cells could be discriminated from expressed CaT1 in RBL cells and that expressed CaT1 properties depend upon the cell type used as well as the level of expression attained. Even greater controversy was introduced when Flockerzi and coworkers (66) determined that CaT1 channels were not activated by store depletion. Thus, the role of CaT1 in SOCE is presently unclear.

V. ACTIVATING SOCE CHANNELS

Store-operated Ca^{2+} entry channels are activated following Ca^{2+} store depletion, and TRPC proteins TRPC1, -2, -4, and -5 comprise channel subunits (54,67). Critical questions remain as to how Ca^{2+} store depletion activates Ca^{2+} entry through SOCE channels. Indeed, mechanisms communicating the Ca^{2+} store-filling state with channel activation are unknown, although several models have been advanced (Fig. 5); experimental support for each proposed model has been reported (reviewed in Refs. 68–71). The soluble messenger model proposes that Ca^{2+} store depletion releases a soluble molecular species from the endoplasmic reticulum that diffuses through the cytosol and activates SOCE channels. The conformational coupling model suggests that the SOCE channel and $InsP_3R$ directly interact. An extension of the conformational coupling model indicates that the

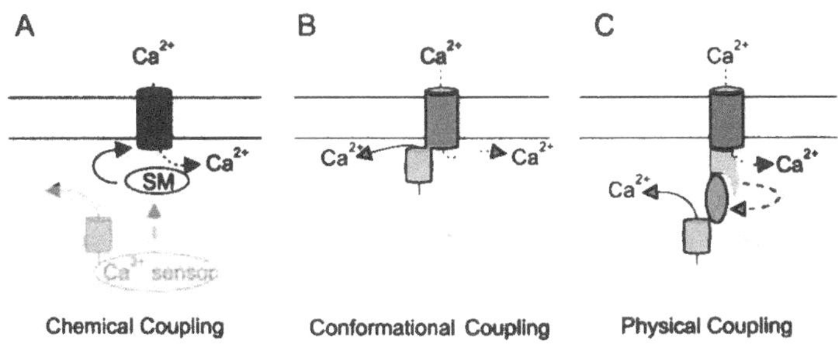

Figure 5 Proposed mechanisms coupling store release to SOCE channel activation. (A) The chemical coupling model proposes that depletion of endoplasmic reticulum Ca^{2+} triggers the release of a soluble mediator (SM) from the endoplasmic reticulum. SM diffuses through the cytosol to bind to and activate the SOCE channel on the plasma membrane. (B) Conformational coupling purports a direct physical interaction between $InsP_3$ receptors and SOCE channels. (C) In the physical coupling model, the endoplasmic reticulum is physically, yet indirectly, tethered to the SOCE channel. This interaction is mediated by one or more scaffolding proteins, likely involving the cytoskeleton. Depletion of endoplasmic reticulum Ca^{2+} initiates a conformational change (dashed arrow) that results in channel activation. (Adapted from Ref. 92.)

endoplasmic reticulum Ca^{2+}-filling state may be communicated to SOCE channels through the cytoskeleton, and the secretion-like coupling model purports that Ca^{2+} store depletion initiates endoplasmic reticulum translocation and presentation to the SOCE channel necessary for activation. Considering the diversity of cell-specific SOCE channels, it is not surprising that considerable diversity in activation properties has been reported.

The architecture of f-actin is a critical determinant of SOCE activation. Holda and Blatter (72) revealed that disruption of actin microfilaments prevented agonist-induced SOCE without altering either basal $[Ca^{2+}]_i$ or Ca^{2+} release. Several other laboratories have confirmed this finding using various cell types. The general idea advanced by these studies is that disruption of f-actin acutely activates nonselective cation entry, whereas over time, as the endoplasmic reticulum condenses around the nucleus away from the plasmalemma, the link between Ca^{2+}-filling state and channel activation becomes uncoupled. This concept was extended by Patterson et al. (73), who proposed that the cortical actin rim prevents coupling between endoplasmic reticulum and SOCE channels in the inactivated state. Reorganization of f-actin was required to traffic endoplasmic reticulum to the plasmalemma and activate SOCE channels.

Although many studies implicate a dynamic role for f-actin in activation of SOCE, these findings are based upon pharmacological approaches that potentially exert nonspecific effects. Moreover, f-actin does not interact directly with transmembrane proteins, indicating that its regulation of SOCE must be away from the channel itself. Spectrin is a principal component of the membrane skeleton that cross-links f-actin and binds protein 4.1 and ankyrin, which interact directly with transmembrane proteins. Our group (74) therefore explored the role for specific spectrin–actin interactions in regulation of SOCE and I_{SOC} channel activity. Somewhat surprisingly, disruption of the spectrin–actin interaction did not decrease thapsigargin-induced SOCE or I_{SOC}. However, disruption of the spectrin–protein 4.1 interaction decreased thapsigargin-induced SOCE by ≈50% and abolished I_{SOC}. The protein 4.1 binding site on β-spectrin is only 21 amino acids downstream from the actin-binding site. Thus, this study represents the first demonstration that endothelial I_{SOC} channel activation is regulated by a very specific protein–protein interaction within the actin cytoskeleton, the spectrin–protein 4.1 interaction. These findings also indicate that not all SOCE channels are activated or regulated by the same mechanism. Indeed, only TRPC3 and TRPC4 possess a protein 4.1 binding domain. Thus, it is important that disruption of the spectrin–protein 4.1 interaction only abolished I_{SOC} and did not influence activation of nonselective cation channels. Subsequent intensive studies will be required to more rigorously address the mechanisms through which the Ca^{2+}-filling state of the endoplasmic reticulum is selectively coupled to proteins that underlie Ca^{2+}-selective and nonselective SOCE channels.

VI. TRPC EXPRESSION AND FUNCTION IN THE LUNG

Endogenous TRPC expression has been demonstrated in various tissues and cells (75–77). TRPC1, -3, -4, -5, and -6 have been detected in lung tissue as well as pulmonary artery smooth muscle cells and pulmonary artery endothelial cells (Table 1). Although there is still some discrepancy regarding the particular TRPCs present in these cells, the overall ubiquitous expression suggests the presence of both store-dependent and store-independent channels in lung. In particular, TRPC1, -4, and -6 contribute to endogenous SOCE channels in the pulmonary vasculature.

A. Endothelial Cell Barrier Function

Store-operated Ca^{2+} entry represents the principal mode of Ca^{2+} entry in nonexcitable cells such as the endothelium (78,79). Physiological transitions in $[Ca^{2+}]_i$ trigger interendothelial cell gap formation and increased permeability. Multiple receptor-G_q-linked inflammatory agonists (e.g., thrombin, histamine, bradykinin) elevate $[Ca^{2+}]_i$ as a requisite signal that increases permeability. Through a series of studies, Stevens and coworkers (7,80–82) evaluated the independent effects of SOCE on endothelial cell permeability. In pulmonary artery endothelial cells, thapsigargin dose-dependently increased $[Ca^{2+}]_i$ with an $EC_{50} \approx 30\,nM$, identical to its IC_{50} for the sarcoplasmic/endoplasmic reticulum Ca^{2+} ATPase (83). Thapsigargin similarly increased permeability in cultured PAECs, suggesting that activation of SOCE is sufficient to trigger intercellular gap formation and increase

Table 1 TRPC Proteins in the Lung

	TRPC isoform detected	TRPC isoform not detected	Ref
Lung tissue			
Human fetal	1	—	53
Human adult	1, 3, 4, 5, 6	7	77
Rat	1, 3, 4, 6	5	75
Rat	4	—	93
Smooth muscle cells			
Canine pulmonary artery	4, 6, 7	1, 2, 3, 5	94
Rat pulmonary artery	1, 3, 4, 5, 6	—	86
Rat pulmonary artery	1, 2, 4, 5, 6	3	52
Human pulmonary artery	1, 4, 6	3	51, 63, 88
Endothelial cells			
Murine lung vascular	1, 3, 4, 6	2, 5	85
Rat pulmonary artery	1	3, 6	81
Rat pulmonary artery	1, 2, 3, 5	4, 6	52
Human pulmonary artery	1	3, 6	81

permeability. As in cultured pulmonary artery endothelial cells, activation of SOCE produced a dose-dependent increase in lung permeability (84). One physiological response to activation of SOCE is therefore increased lung permeability.

Lung endothelial cells principally express TRPC1 and TRPC4. In rat pulmonary artery endothelial cells, TRPC1 contributes to the SOCE response and, in particular, the Ca^{2+}-selective I_{SOC} current (46). TRPC4 also contributes to I_{SOC} and is probably the subunit that senses the Ca^{2+} store depletion necessary for I_{SOC} activation (62). Recently, Malik and coworkers (85) demonstrated that thrombin-induced stress fiber and gap formation is diminished in endothelial cells obtained from $TRPC4^{-/-}$ mice and that $TRPC4^{-/-}$ lungs were ≈50% less permeable to thrombin than were wild-type lungs. Thus, activation of the TRPC1/4-dependent I_{SOC} induces intercellular gap formation and increases permeability in lung endothelium.

Not all endothelia respond similarly to activation of SOCE entry, however. Interestingly, in whole lung experiments, activation of SOCE induced interendothelial cell gaps only in intermediate and large arteries and veins. Gaps were not detected in small vessels, including capillaries. The thapsigargin-induced $[Ca^{2+}]_i$ response is significantly lower in pulmonary microvascular endothelial cells than in pulmonary artery endothelial cells (81), and activation of SOCE alone is not sufficient to increase pulmonary microvascular endothelial cell permeability (83). Further, thapsigargin alone is unable to activate the Ca^{2+}-selective I_{SOC} current in pulmonary microvascular endothelial cells. However, an I_{SOC} current was obtained in pulmonary microvascular endothelial cells when thapsigargin-induced Ca^{2+} release was combined with inhibition of phosphodiesterase type 4, using the inhibitor rolipram (unpublished results). Under these same experimental conditions, significant gap formation occurred in pulmonary microvascular endothelial cell monolayers, suggesting that I_{SOC} activation is an important trigger for endothelial barrier disruption.

B. Vasoconstriction

In smooth muscle cells, an increase in $[Ca^{2+}]_i$ promotes cell contraction through the activation of myosin light chain kinase, which phosphorylates the myosin light chain, allowing for actomyosin interaction. Activation of voltage-gated Ca^{2+} channels is generally thought to represent the principal mode of Ca^{2+} entry that regulates smooth muscle contraction, although, clearly, Gq-linked agonists produce vasoconstriction. The question of whether SOCE contributes to smooth muscle cell contraction was recently addressed in several studies. McDaniel et al. (52) treated isolated rat pulmonary arteries with phenylephrine while they were exposed to a Ca^{2+}-free solution. This treatment resulted in a transient arterial contraction due to Ca^{2+} release from the endoplasmic reticulum. Following the transient phase,

Ca^{2+} was restored to the solution along with phentolamine (to block α receptors) and verapamil (to block voltage-dependent Ca^{2+} channels). This treatment resulted in a second contraction due to SOCE initiated by the phenylephrine-induced store depletion. Contraction was inhibited in the presence of Ni^{2+} or La^{3+}, nonspecific SOCE blockers, as was the global $[Ca^{2+}]_i$ response and the cyclopiazonic acid – or phenylephrine-induced cation current. Ng and Gurney (86) similarly evaluated the role of SOCE in smooth muscle cell contraction. Endothelium-denuded rat pulmonary arteries contracted following store depletion induced by thapsigargin and cyclopiazonic acid. Calcium ion fluorescence revealed a cyclopiazonic acid–induced cation entry path sensitive to inhibition by Ni^{2+}, Cd^{2+}, and SK&F-96365, SOCE channel inhibitors. Cyclopiazonic acid–induced contraction, in the presence of nifedipine, was also sensitive to these inhibitors. The cyclopiazonic acid–induced current demonstrated linear voltage dependence at negative potentials, was slightly inwardly rectifying, and reversed potential at -1 ± 7mV, indicative of a nonselective cation current. In contrast to the results obtained in pulmonary artery smooth muscle cells, Beech and coworkers (87) found that SOCE was not a contributory factor to vasoconstriction in precapillary cerebral arterioles. They suggested that SOCE channels in cerebral arteriolar smooth muscle cells provide for Ca^{2+} influx into distinct, noncontractile cellular compartments. Collectively, these data suggest that SOCE may contribute to contraction in some smooth muscle cells, e.g., pulmonary artery smooth muscle cells, although the molecular identity of the channel(s) is unknown.

C. Nitric Oxide-Induced Vasorelaxation

Vasoconstriction in the lung is modulated by release of endothelium-derived vasodilators, including nitric oxide and prostacyclin. Physiological transitions in $[Ca^{2+}]_i$ promote synthesis of both of these substances. Interestingly the TRP4$^{-/-}$ mouse developed by Freichel et al. (62) exhibited impaired vasorelaxation. In precontracted aortic rings isolated from TRP4$^{-/-}$ mice, acetylcholine-induced vasorelaxation was less than 50% of that attained in wild-type mice. When precontracted rings from wild-type mice were treated with La^{3+}, the vasorelaxation response was reduced to a level similar to that observed with the TRPC4$^{-/-}$ mice, suggesting that vasorelaxation is a SOCE-mediated response. Thus, endothelial TRPC4-mediated SOCE plays a physiological role in regulation of blood vessel tone. Although this study was performed in systemic vessels, it is likely that a similar mechanism occurs in the pulmonary arteries.

D. Vascular Remodeling

Smooth muscle cell growth is a characteristic of normal lung development and the abnormal reorganization that occurs in response to hypertensive stimuli. Yuan and coworkers (51,63,88) evaluated the contribution of SOCE to pulmonary artery smooth muscle cell proliferation. Proliferating cells exhibited higher resting $[Ca^{2+}]_i$ levels and greater cyclopiazonic acid–induced Ca^{2+} release and Ca^{2+} entry. TRPC1 expression was increased in proliferating human pulmonary artery smooth muscle cells compared to that in growth-arrested cells. This effect appeared to be specific for TRPC1, because expression of TRPC3 and the human voltage-dependent Ca^{2+} channel β_2 subunit was not affected by cell proliferation. Moreover, antisense inhibition of TRPC1 produced a 67% decrease in mRNA and a 40% decrease in protein expression that decreased smooth muscle cell proliferation. Thus, TRPC1-dependent SOCE is involved in smooth muscle cell proliferation.

Growth responses may involve more than one SOCE subunit or channel, however. Platelet-derived growth factor upregulated TRPC6, corresponding to increased resting $[Ca^{2+}]_i$ levels and cyclopiazonic acid–induced SOCE. TRPC6 antisense oligonucleotides decreased both basal and mitogen-induced upregulation of TRPC6 protein expression and inhibited SOCE and PDGF-mediated proliferation. Thus, SOCE partly mediates cell proliferation, potentially related to pathophysiological states such as pulmonary hypertension.

VII. SUMMARY

Considerable progress has been made in our understanding of SOCE since it was first proposed in 1986 by Putney (1). Discovery in the mid-1990s that *Drosophila melanogaster* TRP and mammalian homologs were candidate SOCE channels resulted in a rapid expansion of knowledge regarding their subunit composition, activation/inactivation properties, and putative gating mechanisms. Still, we are quite limited in what we know. A functional oligomeric state of any endogenous channel has yet to be determined. Cell-specific channel formation and function are incompletely understood. Moreover, an understanding of how any specific channel uniquely regulates cell function, or any physiological function, is lacking. Thus, as the last 10 years have produced considerable advances in our understanding of proteins that underlie SOCE, so too must the next 10 years produce advances in our understanding of how these proteins are expressed and how they operate to uniquely govern cell physiology.

REFERENCES

1. Putney JW Jr. A model for receptor-regulated calcium entry. Cell Calcium 1986; 7:1–12.
2. Hoth M, Penner R. Depletion of intracellular calcium stores activates a calcium current in mast cells. Nature 1992; 355:353–356.

3. Zweifach A, Lewis RS. Mitogen-regulated Ca^{2+} current of T lymphocytes is activated by depletion of intracellular Ca^{2+} stores. Proc Nat Acad Sci USA 1993; 90:6295–6299.
4. Bakowski D, Parekh AB. Voltage-dependent conductance changes in the store-operated Ca^{2+} current I_{CRAC} in rat basophilic leukemia cells. J Physiol 2000; 529:295–306.
5. Vaca L, Kunze DL. Depletion of intracellular Ca^{2+} stores activates a Ca^{2+}-selective channel in vascular endothelium. Am J Physiol 1994; 267:C920–C925.
6. Fasolato C, Nilius B. Store depletion triggers the calcium release-activated calcium current (I_{CRAC}) in macrovascular endothelial cells: a comparison with Jurkat and embryonic kidney cell lines. Pflügers Arch 1998; 436:69–74.
7. Moore TM, Brough GH, Babal P, Kelly JJ, Li M, Stevens T. Store-operated calcium entry promotes shape change in pulmonary endothelial cells expressing Trp1. Am J Physiol 1998; 275:L574–L582.
8. Montell C, Birnbaumer L, Flockerzi V, et al. A unified nomenclature for the superfamily of TRP cation channels. Mol Cell 2002; 9:229–231.
9. Montell C, Birnbaumer L, Flockerzi V. The TRP channels, a remarkably functional family. Cell 2002; 108:595–598.
10. Vennekens R, Voets T, Bindels RJ, Droogmans G, Nilius B. Current understanding of mammalian TRP homologues. Cell Calcium 2002; 31:253–264.
11. Yue L, Peng JB, Hediger MA, Clapham DE. CaT1 manifests the pore properties of the calcium-release-activated calcium channel. Nature 2001; 410: 705–709.
12. Minke B, Cook B. TRP channel proteins and signal transduction. Physiol Rev 2002; 82:429–472.
13. Engelke M, Friedrich O, Budde P, et al. Structural domains required for channel function of the mouse transient receptor potential protein homologue TRP1β. FEBS Lett 2002; 523: 193–199.
14. Sinkins WG, Vaca L, Hu Y, Kunze DL, Schilling WP. The COOH-terminal domain of *Drosophila* TRP channels confers thapsigargin sensitivity. J Biol Chem 1996; 271:2955–2960.
15. Vaca L, Sinkins WG, Hu Y, Kunze DL, Schilling WP. Activation of recombinant TRP by thapsigargin in Sf9 insect cells. Am J Physiol 1994; 267: C1501–C1505.
16. Singh BB, Liu X, Ambudkar IS. Expression of truncated transient receptor potential protein 1α (TRP1α): evidence that the TRP1 C terminus modulates store-operated Ca^{2+} entry. J Biol Chem 2000; 275:36483–36486.
17. Trepakova ES, Csutora P, Hunton DL, Marchase RB, Cohen RA, Bolotina VM. Calcium influx factor directly activates store-operated cation channels in vascular smooth muscle cells. J Biol Chem 2000; 275:26158–26163.
18. Singh BB, Liu X, Tang J, Zhu MX, Ambudkar IS. Calmodulin regulates Ca^{2+}-dependent feedback inhibition of store-operated Ca^{2+} influx by interaction with a site in the C terminus of TRPC1. Mol Cell 2002; 9:1–20.
19. Tang J, Lin Y, Zhang Z, Tikunova S, Birnbaumer L, Zhu MX. Identification of common binding sites for calmodulin and inositol 1,4,5-trisphosphate receptors on the carboxyl termini of TRP channels. J Biol Chem 2001; 276:21303–21310.

20. Rosado JA, Sage SO. Coupling between inositol 1,4,5-trisphosphate receptors and human transient receptor potential channel 1 when intracellular Ca^{2+} stores are depleted. Biochem J 2000; 350:631–635.
21. Rosado JA, Sage SO. Activation of store-mediated calcium entry by secretion-like coupling between the inositol 1,4,5-trisphosphate receptor type II and human transient receptor potential (hTrp1) channels in human platelets. Biochem J 2001; 356:191–198.
22. Rosado JA, Brownlow SL, Sage SO. Endogenously expressed Trp1 is involved in store-mediated Ca^{2+} entry by conformational coupling in human platelets. J Biol Chem 2002; 277:42157–42163.
23. Boulay G, Brown DM, Qin N, et al. Modulation of Ca^{2+} entry by polypeptides of the inositol 1,4,5-trisphosphate receptor (IP_3R) that bind transient receptor potential (TRP):evidence for roles of TRP and IP_3R in store depletion-activated Ca^{2+} entry. Proc Nat Acad Sci USA 1999; 96:14955–14960.
24. Kiselyov K, Xu X, Mozhayeva G, et al. Functional interaction between $InsP_3$ receptors and store-operated Htrp3 channels. Nature 1998; 396:478–482.
25. Kiselyov K, Mignery GA, Zhu MX, Muallem S. The N-terminal domain of the IP_3 receptor gates store-operated hTrp3 channels. Mol Cell 1999; 4:423–429.
26. Mery L, Magnino F, Schmidt K, Krause K-H, Dufour J-F. Alternative splice variants of hTrp4 differentially interact with the C-terminal portion of the inositol 1,4,5-trisphosphate receptors. FEBS Lett 2001; 487:377–383.
27. Suzuki-Inoue K, Tulasne D, Shen Y, et al. Association of fyn and lyn with the proline-rich domain of glycoprotein VI regulates intracellular signaling. J Biol Chem 2002; 277:21561–21566.
28. Yudowski GA, Efendiev R, Pedemonte CH, Katz AI, Berggren P, Bertorello AM. Phosphoinositide-3 kinase binds to a proline-rich motif in the Na^+,K^+-ATPase α subunit and regulates its trafficking. Proc Nat Acad Sci USA 2000; 97:6556–6561.
29. Williamson MP. The structure and function of proline-rich regions in proteins. Biochem J 1994; 297:249–260.
30. Kay BK, Williamson MP, Sudol M. The importance of being proline: the interaction of proline-rich motifs in signaling proteins with their cognate domains. FASEB J 2000; 14:231–241.
31. Goel M, Garcia R, Estacion M, Schilling WP. Regulation of *Drosophila* TRPL channels by immunophilin FKBP59. J Biol Chem 2001; 276:38762–38773.
32. Tsunoda S, Sierralta J, Sun Y, et al. A multivalent PDZ-domain protein assembles signaling complexes in a G-protein-coupled cascade. Nature 1997; 388:243–249.
33. Li HS, Montell C. TRP and the PDZ protein, INAD, form the core complex required for retention of the signalplex in *Drosophila* photoreceptor cells. J Cell Biol 2000; 150:1411–1422.
34. Tsunoda S, Sun Y, Suzuki E, Zuker C. Independent anchoring and assembly mechanisms of INAD signaling complexes in six *Drosophila* photoreceptors. J Neurosci 2001; 21:150–158.
35. Tang Y, Tang J, Chen Z, et al. Association of mammalian trp4 and phospholipase C isozymes with a PDZ domain-containing protein, NHERF. J Biol Chem 2000; 275:37559–37564.

36. Hwang JI, Heo K, Shin KJ, Kim E, Yun C-HC, Rya SH, Shin H-S, Suh P-E. Regulation of phospholipase C-β_3 activity by Na /H^+ exchanger regulatory factor 2. J Biol Chem 2000; 275:16632–16637.
37. Hall RA, Premont RT, Chow CW, Blitzer JT, Pitcher JA, Claing A, Stoffei RH, Barak LS, Shenolikae S, Weinman EJ, Grinstein S, Lefi Kowite RJ. The β_2-adrenergic receptor interacts with the Na /H^+-exchanger regulatory factor to control Na^+/H exchange. Nature 1998; 392:626–630.
38. Shenolikar S, Minkoff CM, Steplock DA, Evangelista C, Liu M-Z, Weinman EJ. N-terminal PDZ domain is required for NHERF dimerization. FEBS Lett 2001; 489:233–236.
39. Reczek D, Berryman M, Bretscher A. Identification of EBP50: a PDZ-containing phosphoprotein that associates with members of the ezrin-radixin-moesin family. J Cell Biol 1997; 139:169–179.
40. Murthy A, Gonzalez-Agosti C, Cordero E, Pinney D, Candia C, Solomon F, Gusella J, Ramesh V. NHE-RF, a regulatory cofactor for Na^+-H exchange, is a common interactor for merlin and ERM (MERM) proteins. J Biol Chem 1998; 273:1273–1276.
41. Bretscher A, Reczek D, Berryman M. Ezrin: a protein requiring conformational activation to link microfilaments to the plasma membrane in the assembly of cell surface structures. J Cell Sci 1997; 110:3011–3018.
42. Mery L, Straub B, Dufour JF, Krause KH, Hoth M. The PDZ-interacting domain of TRPC4 controls its localization and surface expression in HEK293 cells. J Cell Sci 2002; 115:3497–3508.
43. Goel M, Sinkins WG, Schilling WP. Selective association of TRPC channel subunits in rat brain synaptosomes. J Biol Chem 2002; 277:48303–48310.
44. Hofmann T, Schaefer M, Schultz G, Gudermann T. Subunit composition of mammalian transient receptor potential channels in living cells. Proc Nat Acad Sci USA 2002; 99:7461 7466.
45. Sinkins WG, Estacion M, Schilling WP. Functional expression of TrpC1: a human homologue of the *Drosophila* Trp channel. Biochem J 1998; 331: 331–339.
46. Brough GH, Wu S, Cioffi D, et al. Contribution of endogenously expressed Trp1 to a Ca^{2+}-selective, store-operated Ca^{2+} entry pathway. FASEB J 2001; 15:1727–1738.
47. Chen J, Barritt GJ. Evidence that TRPC1 forms a Ca^{2+} permeable channel linked to the regulation of cell volume in liver cells obtained using siRNA targeted against TRPC1. Biochem J 2003; 373:327–36.
48. Liu X, Wang W, Singh BB, Lockwich T, Jadlowier J, O'Connevi B, Wellner R, Zhu MK, Ambuckar I. Trp1, a candidate protein for the store-operated Ca^{2+} influx mechanism in salivary gland cells. J Biol Chem 2000; 275:3403–3411.
49. Tomita Y, Kaneko S, Funayama M, Kondo H, Satoh M, Akaike A. Intracellular Ca^{2+} store-operated influx of Ca^{2+} through TRP-R, a rat homolog of TRP, expressed in *Xenopus* oocytes. Neurosci Lett 1998; 248:195–198.
50. Vaca L, Sampieri A. Calmodulin modulates the delay period between release of calcium from internal stores and activation of calcium influx via endogenous TRP1 channels. J Biol Chem 2002; 277:42178–42187.

51. Sweeney M, Yu Y, Platoshyn O, Zhang S, McDaniel SS, Yuan JX. Inhibition of endogenous TRP1 decreases capacitative Ca^{2+} entry and attenuates pulmonary artery smooth muscle cell proliferation. Am J Physiol Lung Cell Mol Physiol 2002; 283:L144–L155.
52. McDaniel SS, Platoshyn O, Wang J, et al. Capacitative Ca^{2+} entry in agonist-induced pulmonary vasoconstriction. Am J Physiol Lung Cell Mol Physiol 2001; 280:L870–L880.
53. Wes PD, Chevesich J, Jeromin A, Rosenberg C, Stetten G, Montell C. TRPC1, a human homolog of a *Drosophila* store-operated channel. Proc Nat Acad Sci USA 1995; 92:9652–9656.
54. Vannier B, Peyton M, Boulay G, Brown D, Qin N, Jiang M, Zhu X, Birabaumee L. Mouse trp2, the homologue of the human trpc2 pseudogene, encodes mTrp2, a store depletion-activated capacitative Ca^{2+} entry channel. Proc Nat Acad Sci USA 1999; 96:2060–2064.
55. Zhu X, Jiang M, Peyton M, Bozlac G, Fluust R, Stefani E, Birabaumee L. trp, a novel mammalian gene family essential for agonist-activated capacitative Ca^{2+} entry. Cell 1996; 85:661–671.
56. Philipp S, Hambrecht J, Braslavski L, Stroth G, Freichei M, Murakami M, Cavalie A, Flockerzi V. A novel capacitative calcium entry channel expressed in excitable cells. EMBO J 1998; 17:4274–4282.
57. Philipp S, Cavalié A, Freichel M, Wisserbach U, Zimmee S, Teost C, Marquart A, Murakami M, Flockerzi V. A mammalian capacitative calcium entry channel homologous to *Drosophila* TRP and TRPL. EMBO J 1996; 15:6166–6171.
58. Philipp S, Trost C, Warnat J, Fiautmann J, Himmerkus N, Schreth G, Kertz O, Nastairezyk W, Caualie A, Hoth M, Flockerzi V. TRP4 (CCE1) protein is part of native calcium release-activated Ca^{2+}-like channels in adrenal cells. J Biol Chem 2000; 275:23965–23972.
59. Warnat J, Philipp S, Zimmer S, Flockerzi V, Cavalié A. Phenotype of a recombinant store-operated channel: highly selective permeation of Ca^{2+}. J Physiol 1999; 518:631–638.
60. Schaefer M, Plant TD, Obukhov AG, Hofmann T, Gudermann T, Schultz G. Receptor-mediated regulation of the nonselective cation channels TRPC4 and TRPC5. J Biol Chem 2000; 275:17517–17526.
61. Wu X, Babnigg G, Zagranichnaya T, Villereal ML. The role of endogenous human Trp4 in regulating carbachol-induced calcium oscillations in HEK-293 cells. J Biol Chem 2002; 277:13597–13608.
62. Freichel M, Suh SH, Pfeifer A. Lack of an endothelial store-operated Ca^{2+} current impairs agonist-dependent vasorelaxation in $TRP4^{-/-}$ mice. Nature Cell Biol 2001; 3:121–127.
63. Yu Y, Sweeney M, Zhang S, Platoshyn O, Landsberg J, Rothman A, Yuan JX-J. PDGF stimulates pulmonary vascular smooth muscle cell proliferation by upregulating TRPC6 expression. Am J Physiol Cell Physiol 2003; 284:C316–C330.
64. Voets T, Prenen J, Fleig A, Vennekers R, Watanabe H, Hoendrop JE, Bindels RJ, Drougmans E, Penner R, Nilius B. CaT1 and the calcium release-activated calcium channel manifest distinct pore properties. J Biol Chem 2001; 276: 47767–47770.

65. Schindl R, Kahr H, Graz I, Groschner K, Romanin C. Store depletion-activated CaT1 currents in rat basophilic leukemia mast cells are inhibited by 2-aminoethoxydiphenyl borate. Evidence for a regulatory component that controls activation of both CaT1 and CRAC (Ca^{2+} release-activated Ca^{2+}) channel) channels. J Biol Chem 2002; 277:26950–26958.
66. Bodding M, Wissenbach U, Flockerzi V. The recombinant human TRPV6 channel functions as Ca^{2+} sensor in human embryonic kidney and rat basophilic leukemia cells. J Biol Chem 2002; 277:36656–36664.
67. Hofmann T, Schaefer M, Schultz G, Gudermann T. Transient receptor potential channels as molecular substrates of receptor-mediated cation entry. J Mol Med 2000; 78:14–25.
68. Berridge MJ. Capacitative calcium entry. Biochem J 1995; 312:1–11.
69. Lewis RS. Store-operated calcium channels. Adv Second Messenger Phosphoprotein Res 1999; 33:279–307.
70. Parekh AB, Penner R. Store depletion and calcium influx. Physiol Rev 1997; 77:901–930.
71. Putney JW Jr, Ribeiro CM. Signaling pathways between the plasma membrane and endoplasmic reticulum calcium stores. Cell Mol Life Sci 2000; 57: 1272–1286.
72. Holda JR, Blatter LA. Capacitative calcium entry is inhibited in vascular endothelial cells by disruption of cytoskeletal microfilaments. FEBS Lett 1997; 403:191–196.
73. Patterson RL, van Rossum DB, Gill DL. Store-operated Ca^{2+} entry: evidence for a secretion-like coupling model. Cell 1999; 98:487–499.
74. Wu S, Sangerman J, Li M, Brough GH, Goodman SR, Stevens T. Essential control of an endothelial cell I_{SOC} by the spectrin membrane skeleton. J Cell Biol 2001; 154:1225–1233.
75. Garcia RL, Schilling WP. Differential expression of mammalian TRP homologues across tissues and cell lines. Biochem Biophys Res Commun 1997; 239: 279–283.
76. Freichel M, Schweig U, Stauffenberger S, Freise D, Schorb W, Flockerzi V. Store-operated cation channels in the heart and cells of the cardiovascular system. Cell Physiol Biochem 1999; 9:270–283.
77. Riccio A, Medhurst AD, Mattei C, et al. mRNA distribution analysis of human TRPC family in CNS and peripheral tissues. Brain Res Mol Brain Res 2002; 109:95–104.
78. Putney JW Jr, Bird GS. The signal for capacitative calcium entry. Cell 1993; 75:199–201.
79. Berridge MJ. Elementary and global aspects of calcium signalling. J Physiol 1997; 499:291–306.
80. Moore TM, Norwood NR, Creighton JR, Babal P, Bouugh EH, Shasby DM, Stevens T. Receptor-dependent activation of store-operated calcium entry increases endothelial cell permeability. Am J Physiol Lung Cell Mol Physiol 2000; 279:L691–L698.
81. Kelly JJ, Moore TM, Babal P, Diwan AH, Stevens T, Thompson WJ. Pulmonary microvascular and macrovascular endothelial cells: differential regulation of Ca^{2+} and permeability. Am J Physiol 1998; 274:L810–L819.

82. Norwood N, Moore TM, Dean DA, Bhattacharjee R, Li M, Stevens T. Store-operated calcium entry and increased endothelial cell permeability. Am J Physiol Lung Cell Mol Physiol 2000; 279:L815–L824.
83. Stevens T, Thompson WJ. Regulation of pulmonary microvascular endothelial cell cyclic adenosine monophosphate by adenylyl cyclase: implications for endothelial barrier function. Chest 1999; 116:32S–33S.
84. Chetham PM, Babal P, Bridges JP, Moore TM, Stevens T. Segmental regulation of pulmonary vascular permeability by store-operated Ca^{2+} entry. Am J Physiol 1999; 276:L41–L50.
85. Tiruppathi C, Freichel M, Vogel SM, Paria BC, Mehta D, Flockerzi V, Malik AB. Impairment of store-operated Ca^{2+} entry in $TRPC4^{-/-}$ mice interferes with increase in lung microvascular permeability. Circ Res 2002; 91:70–76.
86. Ng LC, Gurney AM. Store-operated channels mediate Ca^{2+} influx and contraction in rat pulmonary artery. Circ Res 2001; 89:923–929.
87. Flemming R, Cheong A, Dedman AM, Beech DJ. Discrete store-operated calcium influx into an intracellular compartment in rabbit arteriolar smooth muscle. J Physiol 2002; 543:455–464.
88. Golovina VA, Platoshyn O, Bailey CL, Wang I, Linsenton A, Sweeney M, Rubin-J, Yuan JX-J. Upregulated TRP and enhanced capacitative Ca^{2+} entry in human pulmonary artery myocytes during proliferation. Am J Physiol Heart Circ Physiol 2001; 280:H746–H755.
89. Li SW, Westwick J, Poll CT. Receptor-operated Ca^{2+} influx channels in leukocytes: a therapeutic target? Trends Pharmacol Sci 2002; 23:63–70.
90. Cioffi DL, Wu S, Stevens T. On the endothelial cell I_{SOC}. Cell Calcium 2003; 33:323–336.
91. Zitt C, Halaszovich CR, Lückhoff A. The TRP family of cation channels: probing and advancing the concepts on receptor-activated calcium entry. Prog Neurobiol 2002; 66:243–264.
92. Venkatachalam K, van Rossum DB, Patterson RL, Ma HT, Gill DL. The cellular and molecular basis of store-operated calcium entry. Nat Cell Biol 2002; 4:E263–E272.
93. Satoh E, Ono K, Xu F, Iijima T. Cloning and functional expression of a novel splice variant of rat TRPC4. Circ J 2002; 66:954–958.
94. Walker RL, Hume JR, Horowitz B. Differential expression and alternative splicing of TRP channel genes in smooth muscles. Am J Physiol Cell Physiol 2001; 280:C1184–C1192.

7

Ca^{2+} Releasing Channels in Pulmonary Vascular Smooth Muscle Cells

Yuji Imaizumi and Katsuhiko Muraki
Nagoya City University, Nagoya, Japan

I. INTRODUCTION

Changes in intracellular Ca^{2+} concentration play fundamental roles in the regulation of contraction and relaxation of smooth muscle cells (SMCs). The Ca^{2+} required for the activation of contractile apparatus is supplied by the influx from extracellular space through Ca^{2+}-permeable channels in the plasma membrane and/or by the release from storage sites, mainly the sarcoplasmic reticulum (SR), through Ca^{2+} releasing channels. Two families of Ca^{2+}-releasing channels are present in Ca^{2+} storage sites in SMCs: ryanodine receptors (RyRs) and inositol trisphosphate receptors (IP_3Rs). This chapter provides a general overview of Ca^{2+}-releasing channels: their structure, regulation, and expression in SMCs and specific information about them in pulmonary vascular SMCs (PVSMCs). Furthermore, the regulation of ion channel activity in the plasma membrane by local Ca^{2+} transients following the activation of RyRs and IP_3Rs in SMCs (1,2) will be discussed. Additional reviews about local Ca^{2+} transients in the pulmonary artery are available in Chapter 25.

II. MOLECULAR BASIS OF Ca^{2+} RELEASING CHANNELS

A. Ryanodine Receptors

Three different RyR isoforms have been defined in several species (3). In mammals, the isoforms RyR1, RyR2, and RyR3 are encoded by three different genes and on distinctive chromosomes. The three isoforms each consist of approximately 5000 amino acids, which share ~65% identity with each other. Analysis of the primary amino acid sequences has demonstrated that the membrane-spanning domains of RyRs are clustered near the carboxy (C) terminus and that several consensus motifs for binding of ligands such as ATP, Ca^{2+}, caffeine, and calmodulin (CaM) and also for phosphorylation are in the large amino (N) terminal cytoplasmic domain. The sequence necessary for the direct interaction with dihydropyridine-sensitive voltage-dependent Ca^{2+} channels (VDCCs) is located at the corners of the cytoplasmic assembly of RyR1, but part of it is absent from RyR2 and RyR3. Proteins to which FK506, an immunosuppressant, binds (FKBPs) associate with RyRs, and the stoichiometry of the binding has been found to be one molecule of FKBP per RyR subunit (4). Cryoelectron microscopy and three-dimensional (3-D) reconstitution studies have confirmed that RyRs are formed by the assembly of four subunits (5).

It has been shown that mutations of amino acid residue between the M3 and M4 transmembrane domains can change channel conductance and pharmacological response to caffeine and ryanodine (6). Ryanodine locks RyRs in a subconductance opening level, explaining the ability of ryanodine to release Ca^{2+}. Recent studies with RyR2 have demonstrated that ryanodine can sensitize the channel to Ca^{2+} (7). The C-terminal region of RyRs is important for their localization and functional activity. High- and low-affinity binding sites of ryanodine have also been confirmed between amino acid 4475 and the C-terminus of RyR1 (8). The channel characteristics of RyRs, which are reconstituted in liposomes and planar lipid bilayers and heterologously expressed in *Xenopus* oocytes and mammalian cell lines, are summarized in Table 1.

B. IP_3 Receptors

Three different mammalian IP_3R isoforms have been identified that share 60–80% similarity of approximately 3000 overall amino acids. IP_3R1 and probably IP_3R2 can be alternatively spliced (9). The subtypes are expected to form similar structures, with the N-termini containing the binding site of IP_3 and apocalmodulin. Basic residues in the binding site possibly mediate the interaction with phosphate groups of IP_3 (10). Many regulatory sites in IP_3R, which potentially interact with Ca^{2+}, ATP, FKBP12 (a receptor of FK506), and calcineurin, are also demonstrated. Purified IP_3Rs have been demonstrated to function as cation channels gated by IP_3 when prepared in planar lipid bilayers (11), much as RyRs do. The C-terminus includes six transmembrane segments, the last two of which, with the intervening loop, make up the pore of the channel. The functional channel is assembled as large homo- or heterotetrameric IP_3R complexes. Although the structure of IR_3R bears a similarity to RyRs, the channel properties are different in

Table 1 Characteristics of RyR and IP_3R

Characteristic	RyR	IP_3R
Subtypes	RyR1, RyR2, RyR3	IP_3R1, IP_3R2, IP_3R3
Molecular weight	500–566 kDa	300–313 kDa
Morphology	Quatrefoil	Quatrefoil
Conductance (50–55 mM Ca^{2+})	100–150 pS	~50 pS
Mechanism of activation	Direct coupling, Ca^{2+} (cADPR, NAADP)	IP_3, CaBP/caldendrin
Regulation by Ca^{2+}	Biphasic: activation (< 10 μM Ca^{2+}), inhibition (1–10 mM Ca^{2+})	Biphasic: activation (< 0.3 μM Ca^{2+}), inhibition (> 0.3 μM Ca^{2+})
Regulation by ATP	Yes. RyR1 (highly sensitive), RyR2 (weak), RyR3 (weak)	Yes (biphasic). IP_3R1 (highly sensitive), IP_3R2 (insensitive?), IP_3R3 (weak)
Phosphorylation	PKA, PKC, CaMKII,	PKA, PKC, PKG, CaMKII, PKT
Binding and interacting protein	FKBP12, FKBP12.6, CaM, TRPC 3?	FKBP12 (IP_3R1), CaM (IP_3R1,2), TRPC 3? (IP_3R1)
Distribution in smooth muscle	RyR2, RyR3, RyR3', (RyR1)	IP_3R1, IP_3R2 (neonatal, proliferation phenotype), IP_3R3 (proliferation phenotype)

several ways (Table 1). In particular, the unitary current and mean open time of IP_3R are much less than those of RyR, suggesting that the Ca^{2+} influx through a single opening of IP_3R is ~5% of that associated with RyR.

III. RYRs: CHANNEL CHARACTERISTICS, EXPRESSION, AND PHYSIOLOGICAL FUNCTIONS IN SMCs

A. Regulation and Expression of RyRs

Although cytoplasmic Ca^{2+} (<10 μM) is a primary activator of RyRs, high Ca^{2+} concentrations (1–10 mM) inhibit the activity. The Ca^{2+} binding site has been identified on the RyR1 sequence between amino acid residues 4011 and 4765. Glutamate 3885 in the transmembrane segment in rabbit RyR3 is also a Ca^{2+} sensor of the channel (12). A low affinity Ca^{2+} binding site mediating Ca^{2+}-dependent inactivation of the channel is located between residues 3726 and 5037 at the C-terminus of RyR1 (13). RyR isoforms have at least three CaM binding sites: two sites in the center of the RyR and another in the C-terminus (14). CaM shows a biphasic effect on RyRs, depending on Ca^{2+} concentration, and the effects are subtype-specific.

Cyclic ADP-ribose (cADPR), a metabolite of nicotinic acid adenine dinucleotide phosphate NAADP, is a putative endogenous activator of RyRs (15). Ca^{2+} stores sensitive to cADPR have been reported in a variety of cell types (16). The functional significance of cADPR has been established in pancreatic β cells. A membrane-bound protein, CD38, is a bifunctional enzyme for synthesis and also degradation of cADPR, and the activation of this protein is the key step in cADPR-mediated Ca^{2+} mobilization in response to agonists. Although there is controversy over the effects of cADPR on RyRs in muscle cells, a line of evidence suggesting its contribution to Ca^{2+} release following specific receptor stimulation has been accumulated for SMCs including PVSMCs (17,18).

FKBP12 and FKBP12.6, which are included in the FKBP family, have been found to associate with RyRs (19). The association is subtype-specific: FKBP12 binds both RyR1 and RyR3, and FKBP12.6 binds both RyR2 and RyR3. Removal of FKBP12 inhibited excitation–contraction coupling (E-C coupling) in skeletal muscle, suggesting that FKBP12 may be a physiological coupler between VDCCs and RyR1 (20). In mice lacking FKBP12.6, channel gating of RyR2 was substantially altered (21). Although it has been strongly suggested that FKBP12.6 may functionally stabilize RyR2 to the closed state in cardiac myocytes, the abnormality of the heart in knockout mice is not severe and the modulation of RyR2 by FKBP12.6 is not consistent. The binding of FK506 or rapamycin to FKBP suppresses the interaction of the protein with RyR and thereby increases cardiac Ca^{2+} sparks. It has been suggested that the binding of FKBP12.6 to RyR2 is prevented by cADPR (22). The expression and similar functions of FKBP12.6 in the mechanisms for the regulation of RyR2 activity by cADPR have been shown in vascular SMCs and reconstituted preparations from SMCs (23).

RyRs have been demonstrated to form a multiprotein complex that includes calsequestrin, junctin, triadin, and junctophilins (24,25). These proteins play important roles in the localization of RyRs within the endoplasmic (ER)/sarcoplasmic reticulum (SR) and the functional coupling to plasma membrane proteins as well as the regulation of RyRs. Junctophillin 2 may be particularly important in SMCs as an essential molecule to form adequate junctional structure between the cell membrane and SR.

The expression of the different RyR isoforms is tissue-specific. In skeletal muscle, RyR1 is dominant, whereas RyR2 is abundant in cardiac muscle. In contrast, RyR3 shows ubiquitous expression among tissues including skeletal muscle, neuronal cells, and SMCs. The physiological functions of RyR3 have not yet been fully determined. The research on heteromeric channel formation of these RyRs has revealed that RyR2 is capable of forming functional heteromeric channels with both RyR1 and RyR3, whereas functional heteromerization between RyR1 and RyR3 is impossible (26). Subcellular localization of RyR1 and RyR2 has been extensively studied in striated muscles, and these RyRs were condensed in the junctional region between the SR and *t-tubules*.

In smooth muscles, RyR2 and RyR3 are the primary isoforms, although RyR1 has also been present in some smooth muscle tissues (27,28). RyR3 in skeletal muscle may amplify Ca^{2+} release originally elicited by activation of RyR1 (29,30). Although the presence of the RyR3 isoform is recognized in numerous tissues and organs, the predominant expression over RyR1 or RyR2 has been shown only in non-pregnant uterus, where RyR3 may contribute Ca^{2+} signaling only when the SR is overloaded with Ca^{2+} (31). Based on results from arterial vascular SMCs of RyR3-deficient mice (32), RyR3 may contribute to the regulation of Ca^{2+} spark frequency. A similar contribution of RyR3 to cellular Ca^{2+} signaling has been suggested in Ca^{2+}-overloaded cultured rat portal vein SMCs (31). It has been found, however, that the RyR3 splice variant predominantly expressed in smooth muscle is not a functional Ca^{2+} releasing channel, although it could function in a dominant negative fashion (33).

B. Functions of RyRs in SMC: Contribution to Ca^{2+} Sparks and CICR

A spontaneous cytosolic Ca^{2+} transient in a discrete local area through RyRs, Ca^{2+} spark, was first found in quiescent cardiac myocytes and then in skeletal and smooth muscle (34–36). All three isomers of RyR are capable of generating Ca^{2+} sparks. Spatiotemporal features of Ca^{2+} sparks in quiescent cardiac myocytes are compared with those in smooth muscle cells in Table 2. One of the most important features of Ca^{2+} sparks in smooth muscle is that a small number of discrete SR elements, called "frequently discharged sites," evoke most of the Ca^{2+} sparks in the cell. This discretely localized Ca^{2+} release by activation of RyRs located near the plasma membrane stimulates Ca^{2+} activated K^+ channels (K_{Ca} channels), causing spontaneous transient outward currents (STOCs). Similar spatiotemporal properties between Ca^{2+} sparks and STOC (37,38), and histocytochemical analysis between Ca^{2+} spark sites and location of RyR, strongly suggest that Ca^{2+} sparks caused by channel opening of RyRs activates nearby iberiotoxin-sensitive large-conductance K_{Ca} channels (BK channels) to elicit STOCs (39). The major K_{Ca} channel responsible for STOCs elicited by Ca^{2+} sparks appeared to be the BK channel in most types of smooth muscles examined, whereas the apamin-sensitive small-conductance K_{Ca} channel (SK channel) contributes to mouse colon STOC-like outward currents

Table 2 Comparison Between Ca^{2+} Sparks and Ca^{2+} Puffs

	Ca^{2+} sparks in smooth muscles	Ca^{2+} puffs in smooth muscles (mouse colon)	Ca^{2+} sparks in cardiac myocytes
Change in Ca^{2+}	50–460 nM	nd (larger than Ca^{2+} spark)	200–300 nM
Frequency	0.24–2 Hz	nd	100 sparks/cell/s
Size	0.9–2.4 μm	nd	1.5–2 μm
Rise time	20–95 ms	160 ms	10 ms
Half-decay time	27–61 ms	742 ms	24, 40 ms
Ryanodine (> 10 μM)	Inhibition	No effect	Inhibition
Caffeine (> 50 μM)	Activation	Global Ca^{2+} increase	Activation
2-APB, xestospongin C	nd	Inhibition	No effect?
Coupling to ion conductance	BK, Cl_{Ca}	BK, SK	Cl_{Ca} (atrium)

nd = not determined

caused by a local Ca^{2+} transient that is sensitive to an inhibitor of IP_3Rs [Ca^{2+} puff (40)].

The activity of STOCs recorded in SMCs was affected by application of FK506 and rapamycin and infusion of cADPR (41,42). The increase in cellular cAMP or cGMP, presumably via stimulation of protein kinase A (PKA) and protein kinase G (PKG), respectively, enhanced the frequency of STOCs and Ca^{2+} sparks, whereas the activation of protein kinase C (PKC) reduced both responses (43). It should be emphasized that spontaneous Ca^{2+} sparks in a discrete local area never contribute to activation of the contractile system but regulate the activities of Ca^{2+}-dependent ion channels on the plasma membrane.

Hyperpolarization caused by STOCs leads to closure of VDCCs and decreases global Ca^{2+} and arterial contraction as a negative feedback pathway (Fig. 1) (44). Iberiotoxin, a selective blocker of BK channels, as well as ryanodine, therefore depolarize arterial smooth muscle and increase the muscle tone (45). In mice lacking the β1 subunit of the BK channel where BK channel activity was depressed, the blood pressure was significantly increased, whereas Ca^{2+} sparks in arterial myocytes had characteristics similar to those in control mice (46), supporting the idea that the basal activity of BK channels is one of the important determinants of muscle tone.

However, in arterial SMCs isolated from RyR3 knockout mice, unexpectedly, Ca^{2+} sparks were unaffected and STOC frequency was significantly increased (32). An incomplete but possible explanation of this result was recently obtained in the analysis of RyR3 splice variants

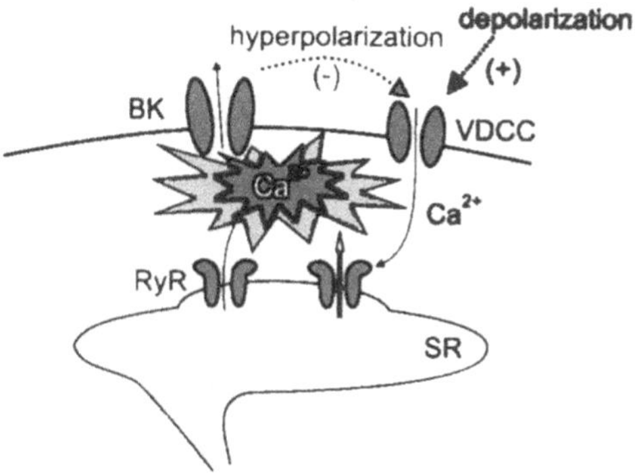

Figure 1 Schematic diagram for the mechanisms underlying BK channel activation by Ca^{2+} spark and CICR.

(26,33). Most smooth muscles express two isoforms of RyR3: RyR3 previously described and a splice variant RyR3 (RyR3′), which is abundant in smooth muscles and functions as a dominant negative channel unit for RyR2 and RyR3 to form heteromeric channels. Although the expression of RyR3' has been confirmed only at the mRNA level from some smooth muscle tissues, it is possible that the channel function of RyR2 is inhibited by RyR3' under control conditions where arterial myocytes express both RyR2 and RyR3'. Ca^{2+} sparks can be recorded from SMCs in the intact vascular wall (47), also indicating that STOCs and Ca^{2+} sparks may have significant functional roles in vascular tone control.

Ca^{2+} sparks activate Cl^- current as well as K^+ current in several types of smooth muscles (48,49). Spontaneous transient inward currents (STICs) caused by opening of Ca^{2+}-activated Cl^- channels (CKa channels) have been recorded in SMCs of the artery, vein, trachea, esophagus, and some other tissues (50). In these myocytes, STIC often occurs together with STOC, presumably activated by the same Ca^{2+} sparks (49). At a resting membrane potential of −50 to −60 mV, the activation of Cl^- current induces membrane depolarization. Therefore, Ca^{2+} sparks could contribute to the increase in muscle tone as a positive feedback pathway if Cl^- current is more prominent than K^+ current.

In cardiac myocytes, a Ca^{2+} spark can also be triggered by membrane depolarization as the unitary events of Ca^{2+}-induced Ca^{2+} release (CICR) in E-C coupling. The opening of a single VDCC increases local Ca^{2+} and thereby activates RyRs via CICR in the junction of the t-tubule and the junctional SR (jSR), where VDCCs and RyRs colocalize in counterparts of the junction at a ratio of one VDCC to several RyRs (51). Similar CICR can be a potential mechanism underlying E-C coupling in SMCs, but its functions during physiological activation are not established. Rather, initial experiments suggested that Ca^{2+} required for CICR during depolarization in smooth muscle was too high to participate in the initiation of contraction (52). Indeed, evidence for CICR was not provided in portal vein and tracheal myocytes (53,54).

However, in some smooth muscles, CICR may have essential roles in activation of ion channels and contraction during E-C coupling. In guinea pig urinary bladder and rat portal vein myocytes, CICR resulted in transient and delayed increases in Ca^{2+} following depolarization, respectively (55,56). In vas deferens and urinary bladder myocytes, 5–20 evoked Ca^{2+} sparks (Ca^{2+} hot spots) appeared within the initial 15 ms of depolarization and progressively enlarged within ~50 ms (57). These evoked Ca^{2+} sparks were sensitive to Cd^{2+} as well as ryanodine and caffeine, strongly suggesting that CICR is responsible for the Ca^{2+} sparks. In addition, Ca^{2+}-activated K^+ current (I_{KCa}) was activated in parallel with an initiation of these evoked Ca^{2+} sparks. The evoked Ca^{2+} spark sites are also identical to spontaneous Ca^{2+} spark discharge sites activating STOCs at resting conditions (Fig. 2). This number of initially evoked Ca^{2+} sparks (~5–20) may be considered to be unexpectedly small if CICR is available in every SR element in a smooth muscle cell. Assuming 10 Ca^{2+} sparks in a cell and a peak I_{KCa} amplitude of 1.5 nA at 0 mV, each Ca^{2+} spark elicits 150 pA I_{KCa}. Because the unitary current amplitude of a BK channel at 0 mV is ~1.5 pA, this may suggest a cluster of 100 BK channels in the junctional region of SR. It has been estimated that BK channels underlying STOCs are exposed to a mean Ca^{2+} concentration on the order of 10 μM during a Ca^{2+} spark within a 1 μm^2 area, and given the constraints imposed by the estimated channel density and the Ca^{2+} current during a spark, the BK channels are distributed at higher density at the spark site (58). Based on the activity of a high density of BK channels recorded in excised membrane patches with some SR apparently attached, the clustering of BK channels is also postulated (39,59). The discrete SR element, where Ca^{2+} sparks are frequently discharged, is possibly a main contributor to STOCs reducing muscle tone and I_{KCa} constructing action potential repolarization and afterhyperpolarization. Molecular mechanisms for the formation of junctions and BK channel clusters in the frequently discharged sites in SMCs remain to be determined.

In SMCs of the large pulmonary artery, E-C coupling and underlying CICR evoked by activation of VDCC are not functional under physiological conditions as has been reported in SMCs from large arteries. The low membrane excitability of large-artery SMCs is primarily due to lower expression of VDCC α1C subunits than that in excitable SMCs such as the small intestine, portal vein, urinary bladder, and vas deferens, whereas the expression of the BK channel is comparable (60). In SMCs from the large coronary artery, CICR was observed only when VDCC was activated by BayK8644 (61). It has also been shown that I_{KCa} elicited by depolarization in SMCs from the aorta can be markedly potentiated when VDCC activity is

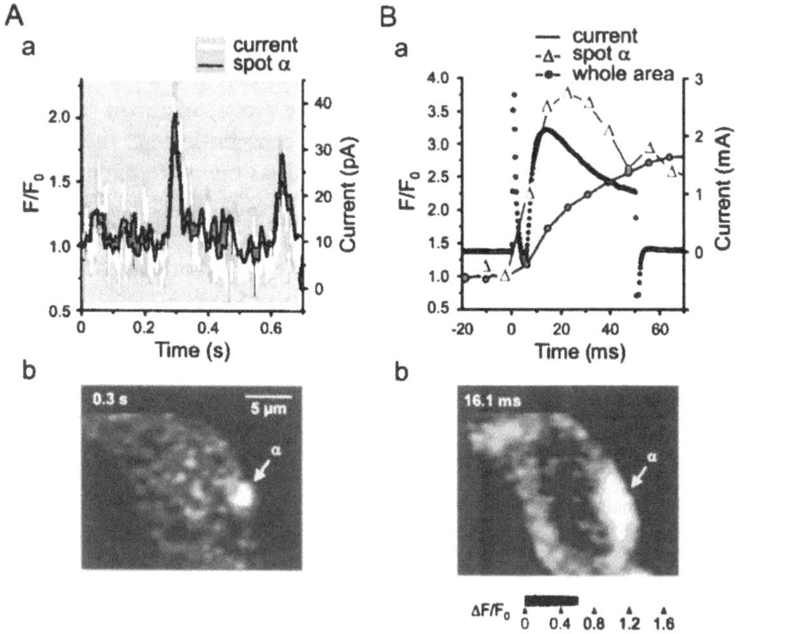

Figure 2 The relationship between spontaneously discharged Ca^{2+} sparks and Ca^{2+} transient elicited by depolarization in urinary bladder myocytes. (A) (a) The time course of membrane current at −40 mV and that of F/F_o at a spark site α, (b) The Ca^{2+} spark image in obtained at the peak F/F_o as indicated by the asterisk in (a). (B) The early Ca^{2+} transient during depolarization from −60 to 0 mV and corresponding membrane currents were measured in the same myocyte as in (A). (a) F/F_o at spot α (Δ), F/F_o in the whole-cell image (•), and membrane current (—) plotted against time. (b) The Ca^{2+} image at 16.1 ms.

increased by BayK8644 (60). This may suggest that high expression of BK channels in weakly excitable SMCs as well as in highly excitable SMCs may act as a safety margin to suppress excess Ca^{2+} influx through VDCC under some circumstances, including pathophysiological conditions. The possibility that CICR evoked by excitation can be functional in SMCs in resistant pulmonary arteries remains to be determined. Critical evidence supporting a hypothesis that small IP_3-induced Ca^{2+} release (IICR) that is induced by submaximal agonist stimulation can trigger CICR as an amplifying mechanism of Ca^{2+} release has not been obtained in SMCs.

Information about the localization of Ca^{2+} spark sites in SMCs has been limited and not consistent. In vas deferens and urinary bladder myocytes, Ca^{2+} sparks at rest and spotlike Ca^{2+} transients upon depolarization occur at the same discrete subplasmalemmal areas (39). In cerebral artery

SMCs, over 90% of spontaneous Ca^{2+} sparks occur in a superficial area $< 1.0\,\mu m$ from the cell membrane (47). On the other hand, in rat portal vein myocytes, all the sites of a cell section have similar probability of being the origin of spontaneous Ca^{2+} sparks (48). The recent work on feline esophageal cells also indicates that Ca^{2+} sparks occur both near the surface and deeper within the cell (38). Of importance is that there are particular regions of frequently discharged Ca^{2+} spark sites in SMCs (39,58,69). These regions of vas deferens and urinary bladder myocytes most likely represent functional differences within the SR and/or distinctive structures where the junctional areas of plasmalemma and SR fragments appear, and BK channels and RyR may colocalize densely in junctions to effectively translate a local Ca^{2+} event (spark) into an electrical signal (STOC). Consistently, simulations using data of esophageal cells demand that BK channels exist at higher than average density at the Ca^{2+} spark sites (58).

IV. IP_3Rs: THEIR EXPRESSION, REGULATION OF ACTIVITY, AND FUNCTIONS IN SMCs

A. Regulation and Expression of IP_3Rs

The channel open probability of IR_3R is regulated by many factors as well as cytosolic IP_3. It has been revealed that cytosolic Ca^{2+} itself, which is an activator of RyRs, also affects the channel opening of IP_3R in a biphasic manner: facilitating Ca^{2+} release by IP_3 at lower concentrations of Ca^{2+} ($< 300\,nM$) and inhibiting it at higher concentrations ($>300\,nM$). Thus the initial release of Ca^{2+} provides a positive feedback loop that ensures rapid and sufficient Ca^{2+} release, while the high level of cytosolic Ca^{2+} provides negative feedback for the release of Ca^{2+}. This biphasic regulation of IP_3-induced Ca^{2+} release by Ca^{2+} may play an obligatory role in forming Ca^{2+} waves, global propagation of the Ca^{2+} signal, and spontaneous Ca^{2+} release from IP_3Rs (Ca^{2+} puffs) when plasma membrane receptors are stimulated to liberate IP_3. Point mutation of glutamate residue at 2100 in rat IP_3R1 decreased Ca^{2+} sensitivity of IP_3R1 by one-tenth and abolished agonist-induced Ca^{2+} oscillation, suggesting that the glutamate residue is a Ca^{2+} sensor (63). However, the molecular mechanisms of this Ca^{2+}-dependent regulation of IP_3R are still complicated because several proteins sensitive to cytosolic Ca^{2+} are also involved in the regulation of IP_3R activity. CaM regulates IP_3-induced Ca^{2+} release (IICR) in a Ca^{2+}-dependent and biphasic manner (64). However, mutational studies suggest that the interaction of CaM with the binding site in the domain of IP_3R does not play an obligatory role in the biphasic regulation (65). Recently, it was reported that CaBP/caldendrin, a subfamily of the EF-hand-containing neuronal Ca^{2+} sensor family of calmodulin-related proteins (66), binds to the IP_3-binding domain of IP_3R in a Ca^{2+}-dependent manner and activates the channel even in the absence of IP_3. Taken together, several factors that are susceptible to Ca^{2+} may be involved in the Ca^{2+}-dependent regulation of IP_3R.

Protein kinases such as PKG, tyrosine kinase (PKT), and Ca^{2+}/CaM kinase II (CaMKI) phosphorylate IP_3R and increase the channel activity (67). However, the functional consequence of PKA-dependent phosphorylation is not fully determined. On the other hand, phosphorylation of IR_3P1 by PKC, which facilitates the channel activity, is modulated by calcineurin, a Ca^{2+}/CaM-dependent phosphatase and a target of FK506, rapamycin, and cyclosporine A. Because FKBP12 could serve as an adapter for calcineurin, FKBP12 modulates IP_3R as well as RyR through PKC phosphorylation.

Physiological ATP concentrations (1–2 mM) stimulate IICR. In contrast, the binding of IP_3 to IP_3R is inhibited by higher ATP concentrations with a steep concentration dependence Hill coefficient (nH: ~5.5). Decrease in cytosolic ATP concentration, which is observed under the ischemic conditions, could enhance the effect of IP_3, hence possibly in part explaining ischemic Ca^{2+} overload in several types of cells.

Most tissues including smooth muscles express all subtypes of IP_3R, although they differ in their level of expression. IP_3R1 is a predominant subtype in vascular smooth muscles. However, the expression is changed during cell development and cell differentiation (68–70). In neonatal rat portal vein and aorta, IP_3R3 is a major subtype. During the development, expression of IP_3R1 was replaced with that of IP_3R3, while the physiological significance of switching in isoforms of the IP_3R is not clear. On the other hand, proliferation of vascular myocytes increased the expression of IP_3R2 and IP_3R3, which were distributed in the nucleus and plasma membrane, and around the nucleus, respectively. Indeed, it has been shown that IP_3 mobilizes Ca^{2+} from ER/SRs but also from the nuclear envelope, Golgi apparatus, and secretory vesicles. Expression of IP_3Rs in caveolae-rich plasma membrane regions is also confirmed in some cells. Physiological functions of these IP_3Rs have not, however, been elucidated. Moreover, even distribution of IP_3Rs within the ER and possibly within the SR is not uniform. In pancreatic acinar cells, IP_3Rs are predominantly distributed in the apical secretary pole. Although direct evidence of the heterodistribution of IP_3Rs in each organelle of smooth muscles is not provided, the tight coupling of IP_3-induced Ca^{2+} events to activation of ion channels expressed in the plasma membrane indicates their heterogeneous expression in the SR.

B. Functions of IP_3R; Contribution to Ca^{2+} Puffs and IICR in SMCs

Release of Ca^{2+} from Ca^{2+} store sites via IP_3R regulates diverse cellular processes. Extensive studies of the role of IP_3R in native tissues including smooth muscles have therefore been carried out. However, the lack of a specific cell-permeable antagonist for IP_3R has prevented total understanding of the physiological role of IP_3R. Although heparin, xestospongin C, and 2-amino-ethoxydiphenyl (2-APB) are useful, their nonspecific effects are also reported (67). Nevertheless, these pharmacological tools have revealed the substantial contribution of IP_3Rs to certain biological events in smooth muscles. Localized Ca^{2+} transients in mouse colon myocytes are resistant to ryanodine, which effectively inhibits Ca^{2+} sparks (40). Because these Ca^{2+} transients were blocked by U73122 [a phospholipase C (PLC) inhibitor] as well as xestospongin C, activation of 5–10 IP_3Rs following spontaneous production of IP_3 is responsible for these events (Ca^{2+} puffs, Table 2). These Ca^{2+} puffs corresponded to STOCs that consisted of BK and SK channel activation. Moreover, augmented Ca^{2+} puffs recorded after the stimulation of a Gq-coupled receptor (GPCRs), P_{2y2}, by 2-methylthio-ATP were in part sensitive to ryanodine, suggesting that RyRs might be recruited during the receptor stimulation to amplify the Ca^{2+} release through IP_3R.

In rabbit portal vein myocytes, similar crosstalk between RyRs and IP_3Rs occurs without receptor stimulation and is a major factor in the modulation of spontaneous Ca^{2+} release (71). Not proved directly, evidence of effects of xestospongin C, 2-APB, and U73122 on Ca^{2+} transients indicates that spontaneous basal activity of PLC produces IP_3. However, Ca^{2+} transients recorded in rabbit portal vein were not Ca^{2+} puffs because a relatively high concentration of ryanodine (100 μM) abolished these events, hence suggesting the coordinated opening of IP_3Rs and RyRs in these myocytes. This may be explained by following functional basis: basal production of IP_3 and subsequent activation of IICR, which in turn may activate the neighboring RyRs via CICR.

RyRs may not be involved in IICR by muscarinic receptor agonists in tracheal myocytes (72). In contrast, carbachol-induced stimulation of muscarinic receptors in guinea pig ileal myocytes increases the frequency of Ca^{2+} sparks and develops periodically propagating Ca^{2+} waves (62). Stimulation of adrenoceptors in rabbit portal vein also increased the frequency of Ca^{2+} sparks (73). Therefore, it is likely that the coordination of RyRs and IP_3Rs and/or presumably their colocalization in the SR vary from cell to cell. IP_3-induced Ca^{2+} oscillation elicited by stimulation of GPCRs induces oscillatory activation of Ca^{2+}-activated Cl^- current (I_{ClCa}) in several smooth muscles (50), whereas it is not determined whether Ca^{2+} puffs couple to the activation of I_{ClCa}. Although characteristics of Ca^{2+} puffs have not been well defined because of the limited number of observations (Table 2), it seems that the increase in cytosolic Ca^{2+} by Ca^{2+} puffs is greater than that by Ca^{2+} sparks. Therefore, like Ca^{2+} sparks, Ca^{2+} puffs may be an effective regulator of Ca^{2+}-dependent ion conductance in SMCs. In mutant mice lacking IP_3R1, electrical slow waves in gastric myocytes almost disappear, implying that IP_3R may have an obligatory role in the generation of Ca^{2+} oscillation and the underlying electrical slow waves (74). Mechanisms involved in the generation of Ca^{2+} puffs and Ca^{2+} oscillations in SMCs are not defined in detail. Monitoring of cytosolic IP_3 changes during activation of these events will provide a clue to the mechanism (75).

V. Ca^{2+} RELEASING CHANNELS AND PULMONARY VASCULAR DISEASES

Hypoxia, which relaxes systemic arteries, specifically contracts pulmonary arteries, and the vasoconstriction results in pulmonary hypertension when the hypoxia is global (76). During hypertension, pulmonary edema and right heart failure can often appear. The hypoxia-induced contraction is triggered by Ca^{2+} release from storage sites (77) sensitive to ryanodine (78,79). ADP-ribosyl cyclase and cADPR hydrolase in PASMC may serve as redox sensors (80), and hypoxia enhances cADPR production at a much higher rate in PASMC homogenate than that from systemic arteries (17). The mechanisms underlying hypoxic coronary vasodilation however, are more complicated (76).

Moreover, it has been shown that exposure of the pulmonary artery to normoxic levels of O_2 in the perinatal stage may release Ca^{2+} through RyRs and facilitate the activity of STOCs, and subsequent hyperpolarization causes progressive and sustained pulmonary vasodilation after birth (81). It is expected that abnormalities of these subcellular responses to an acute increase in O_2 tension play an important role in developing perinatal pulmonary vascular disease.

VI. SUMMARY

In SMCs of the large pulmonary artery, VDCC is rather poorly expressed in comparison with highly excitable SMCs and CICR triggered by Ca^{2+} influx, through VDCC rarely occurs under physiological conditions. Therefore, IICR through IP_3R1 via IP_3 formation by activation of GPCRs is the fundamental signal transduction to initiate contraction in PASMCs. Spontaneous opening of RyRs, assumed to be mainly RyR2, contributes to Ca^{2+}-spark generation and subsequent activation of KCa channels and/or ClCa channels to generate STOCs/STICs. STOCs and/or STICs indirectly regulate VDCC activity via the modulation of the resting membrane potential. Ca^{2+} release through RyRs could have additional functional roles, via production of cADPR, possibly in pathophysiological conditions such as hypoxia. The exact relation between hypoxia-induced PASMC contraction and Ca^{2+} releasing channels and also the possible functional crosstalk between IP_3R and RyR in PASMCs under physiological and pathophysiological conditions remain to be elucidated.

REFERENCES

1. Imaizumi Y, Ohi Y, Yamamura H, Ohya S, Muraki K, Watanabe M. Ca^{2+} spark as a regulator of ion channel activity. Jpn J Pharmacol 1999; 80:1–8.
2. Herrera GM, Nelson MT. Sarcoplasmic reticulum and membrane currents. Novartis Found Symp 2002; 246:189–203.
3. Rossi D, Sorrentino V. Molecular genetics of ryanodine receptor Ca^{2+}-release channels. Cell Calcium 2002; 32:307–319.
4. Jayaraman T, Brillantes AM, Timerman AP, Fleischer S, Erdjument-Bromage H, Tempst P, Marks AR. FK506 binding protein associated with the calcium release channel (ryanodine receptor). J Biol Chem 1992; 267:9474–9477.
5. Radermacher M, Rao V, Grassucci R, Frank J, Timerman AP, Fleischer S, Wagenknecht T. Cryo-electron microscopy and three-dimensional reconstruction of the calcium release channel/ryanodine receptor from skeletal muscle. J Cell Biol 1994; 127:411–423.
6. Gao L, Balshaw D, Xu L, Tripathy A, Xin C, Meissner G. Evidence for a role of the lumenal M3–M4 loop in skeletal muscle Ca^{2+} release channel (ryanodine receptor) activity and conductance. Biophys J 2000; 79:828–840.
7. Masumiya H, Li P, Zhang L, Chen SR. Ryanodine sensitizes the Ca^{2+} release channel (ryanodine receptor) to Ca^{2+} activation. J Biol Chem 2001; 276: 39727–39735.
8. Callaway C, Seryshev A, Wang JP, Slavik KJ, Needleman DH, Cantu C 3rd, Wu Y, Jayaraman T, Marks AR, Hamilton SL. Localization of the high and low affinity [^{3}H]ryanodine binding sites on the skeletal muscle Ca^{2+} release channel. J Biol Chem 1994; 269:15876–15884.
9. Patel S, Joseph SK, Thomas AP. Molecular properties of inositol 1,4,5-trisphosphate receptors. Cell Calcium 1999; 25:247–264.
10. Yoshikawa F, Iwasaki H, Michikawa T, Furuichi T, Mikoshiba K. Cooperative formation of the ligand-binding site of the inositol 1,4,5-trisphosphate receptor by two separable domains. J Biol Chem 1999; 274:328–334.
11. Ramos-Franco J, Galvan D, Mignery GA, Fill M. Location of the permeation pathway in the recombinant type 1 inositol 1,4,5-trisphosphate receptor. J Gen Physiol 1999; 114:243–250.
12. Chen SR, Ebisawa K, Li X, Zhang L. Molecular identification of the ryanodine receptor Ca^{2+} sensor. J Biol Chem 1998; 273:14675–14678.
13. Nakai J, Gao L, Xu L, Xin C, Pasek DA, Meissner G. Evidence for a role of C-terminus in Ca^{2+} inactivation of skeletal muscle Ca^{2+} release channel (ryanodine receptor). FEBS Lett 1999; 459:154–158.
14. Guerrini R, Menegazzi P, Anacardio R, Marastoni M, Tomatis R, Zorzato F, Treves S. Calmodulin binding sites of the skeletal, cardiac, and brain ryanodine receptor Ca^{2+} channels: modulation by the catalytic subunit of cAMP-dependent protein kinase?Biochemistry 1995; 34:5120–5129
15. Lee HC. Mechanisms of calcium signaling by cyclic ADP-ribose and NAADP. Physiol Rev 1997; 77:1133–1164.
16. Lee HC. Physiological functions of cyclic ADP-ribose and NAADP as calcium messengers. Annu Rev Pharmacol Toxicol 2001; 41:317–345.
17. Dipp M, Evans AM. Cyclic ADP-ribose is the primary trigger for hypoxic pulmonary vasoconstriction in the rat lung in situ. Circ Res 2001; 89:77–83.

18. Boittin FX, Dipp M, Kinnear NP, Galione A, Evans AM. Vasodilation by the calcium-mobilizing messenger cyclic ADP-ribose. J Biol Chem 2003; 278: 9602–9608.
19. Timerman AP, Ogunbumni E, Freund E, Wiederrecht G, Marks AR, Fleischer S. The calcium release channel of sarcoplasmic reticulum is modulated by FK-506-binding protein. Dissociation and reconstitution of FKBP-12 to the calcium release channel of skeletal muscle sarcoplasmic reticulum. J Biol Chem 1993; 268:22992–22999.
20. Lamb GD, Stephenson DG. Effects of FK506 and rapamycin on excitation-contraction coupling in skeletal muscle fibres of the rat. J Physiol 1996; 494:569–576.
21. Xin HB, Senbonmatsu T, Cheng DS, Wang YX, Copello JA, Ji GJ, Collier ML, Deng KY, Jeyakumar LH, Magnuson MA, Inagami T, Kotlikoff MI, Fleischer S. Oestrogen protects FKBP12.6 null mice from cardiac hypertrophy. Nature 2002; 416:334–338.
22. Noguchi N, Takasawa S, Nata K, Tohgo A, Kato I, Ikehata F, Yonekura H, Okamoto H. Cyclic ADP-ribose binds to FK506-binding protein 12.6 to release Ca^{2+} from islet microsomes. J Biol Chem 1997; 272:3133–3136.
23. Tang WX, Chen YF, Zou AP, Campbell WB, Li PL. Role of FKBP12.6 in cADPR-induced activation of reconstituted ryanodine receptors from arterial smooth muscle. Am J Physiol Heart Circ Physiol 2002; 282:H1304-H1310.
24. Zhang L, Kelley J, Schmeisser G, Kobayashi YM, Jones LR. Complex formation between junctin, triadin, calsequestrin, and the ryanodine receptor. Proteins of the cardiac junctional sarcoplasmic reticulum membrane. J Biol Chem 1997; 272:23389–23397.
25. Takeshima H, Komazaki S, Nishi M, Iino M, Kangawa K. Junctophilins: a novel family of junctional membrane complex proteins. Mol Cell 2000; 6:11–22.
26. Xiao B, Masumiya H, Jiang D, Wang R, Sei Y, Zhang L, Murayama T, Ogawa Y, Lai FA, Wagenknecht T, Chen SR. Isoform-dependent formation of heteromeric Ca^{2+} release channels (ryanodine receptors). J Biol Chem 2002; 277:41778–41785.
27. Giannini G, Conti A, Mammarella S, Scrobogna M, Sorrentino V. The ryanodine receptor/calcium channel genes are widely and differentially expressed in murine brain and peripheral tissues. J Cell Biol 1995; 128:893–904.
28. Neylon CB, Richards SM, Larsen MA, Agrotis A, Bobik A. Multiple types of ryanodine receptor/Ca^{2+} release channels are expressed in vascular smooth muscle. Biochem Biophys Res Commun 1995; 215:814–821.
29. Ogawa Y, Kurebayashi N, Murayama T. Ryanodine receptor isoforms in excitation-contraction coupling. Adv Biophys 1999; 36:27–64.
30. Yang D, Pan Z, Takeshima H, Wu C, Nagaraj RY, Ma J, Cheng H. RyR3 amplifies RyR1-mediated Ca^{2+}-induced Ca^{2+} release in neonatal mammalian skeletal muscle. J Biol Chem 2001; 276:40210–40214.
31. Mironneau J, Coussin F, Jeyakumar LH, Fleischer S, Mironneau C, Macrez N. Contribution of ryanodine receptor subtype 3 to Ca^{2+} responses in Ca^{2+}-overloaded cultured rat portal vein myocytes. J Biol Chem 2001; 276:11257–11264.
32. Lohn M, Jessner W, Furstenau M, Wellner M, Sorrentino V, Haller H, Luft FC, Gollasch M. Regulation of calcium sparks and spontaneous transient

outward currents by RyR3 in arterial vascular smooth muscle cells. Circ Res 2001; 89:1051–1057.

33. Jiang D, Xiao B, Li X, Chen SR. Smooth muscle tissues express a major dominant negative splice variant of the type 3 Ca^{2+} release channel (ryanodine receptor). J Biol Chem 2003; 278:4763–4769.
34. Cheng H, Lederer WJ, Cannell MB. Calcium sparks: elementary events underlying excitation-contraction coupling in heart muscle. Science 1993; 262: 740–744.
35. Tsugorka A, Rios E, Blatter LA. Imaging elementary events of calcium release in skeletal muscle cells. Science 1995; 269:1723–1726.
36. Nelson MT, Cheng H, Rubart M, Santana LF, Bonev AD, Knot HJ, Lederer WJ. Relaxation of arterial smooth muscle by calcium sparks. Science 1995; 270:633–637.
37. Perez GJ, Bonev AD, Patlak JB, Nelson MT. Functional coupling of ryanodine receptors to K_{Ca} channels in smooth muscle cells from rat cerebral arteries. J Gen Physiol 1999; 113:229–238.
38. Kirber MT, Etter EF, Bellve KA, Lifshitz LM, Tuft RA, Fay FS, Walsh JV, Fogarty KE. Relationship of Ca^{2+} sparks to STOCs studied with 2D and 3D imaging in feline oesophageal smooth muscle cells. J Physiol 2001; 531:315–327.
39. Ohi Y, Yamamura H, Nagano N, Ohya S, Muraki K, Watanabe M, Imaizumi Y. Local Ca^{2+} transients and distribution of BK channels and ryanodine receptors in smooth muscle cells of guinea-pig vas deferens and urinary bladder. J Physiol 2001; 534:313–326.
40. Bayguinov O, Hagen B, Bonev AD, Nelson MT, Sanders KM. Intracellular calcium events activated by ATP in murine colonic myocytes. Am J Physiol Cell Physiol 2000; 279:C126–C135.
41. Weidelt T, Isenberg G. Augmentation of SR Ca^{2+} release by rapamycin and FK506 causes K^+-channel activation and membrane hyperpolarization in bladder smooth muscle. Br J Pharmacol 2000; 129:1293–1300.
42. Cheung DW. Modulation of spontaneous transient Ca^{2+}-activated K^+ channel currents by cADP-ribose in vascular smooth muscle cells. Eur J Pharmacol 2003; 458:57–59.
43. Porter VA, Bonev AD, Knot HJ, Heppner TJ, Stevenson AS, Kleppisch T, Lederer WJ, Nelson MT. Frequency modulation of Ca^{2+} sparks is involved in regulation of arterial diameter by cyclic nucleotides. Am J Physiol 1998; 274:C1346-C1355.
44. Nelson MT, Cheng H, Rubart M, Santana LF, Bonev AD, Knot HJ, Lederer WJ. Relaxation of arterial smooth muscle by calcium sparks. Science 1995; 270:633–637.
45. Knot HJ, Standen NB, Nelson MT. Ryanodine receptors regulate arterial diameter and wall $[Ca^{2+}]$ in cerebral arteries of rat via Ca^{2+}-dependent K^+ channels. J Physiol 1998; 508:211–221.
46. Pluger S, Faulhaber J, Furstenau M, Lohn M, Waldschutz R, Gollasch M, Haller H, Luft FC, Ehmke H, Pongs O. Mice with disrupted BK channel beta1 subunit gene feature abnormal Ca^{2+} spark/STOC coupling and elevated blood pressure. Circ Res 2000; 87:E53–E60.

47. Jaggar JH, Stevenson AS, Nelson MT. Voltage dependence of Ca^{2+} sparks in intact cerebral arteries. Am J Physiol 1998; 274:C1755–C1761.
48. Mironneau J, Arnaudeau S, Macrez-Lepretre N, Boittin FX. Ca^{2+} sparks and Ca^{2+} waves activate different Ca^{2+}-dependent ion channels in single myocytes from rat portal vein. Cell Calcium 1996; 20:153–160.
49. ZhuGe R, Sims SM, Tuft RA, Fogarty KE, Walsh JV Jr. Ca^{2+} sparks activate K^+ and Cl^- channels, resulting in spontaneous transient currents in guinea-pig tracheal myocytes. J Physiol 1998; 513:711–718.
50. Large WA, Wang Q. Characteristics and physiological role of the Ca^{2+}-activated Cl^- conductance in smooth muscle. Am J Physiol 1996; 271:C435–C454.
51. Guatimosim S, Dilly K, Santana LF, Saleet Jafri M, Sobie EA, Lederer WJ. Local Ca^{2+} signaling and EC coupling in heart: Ca^{2+} sparks and the regulation of the $[Ca^{2+}]_i$ transient. J Mol Cell Cardiol 2002; 34:941–950.
52. Iino M. Calcium-induced calcium release mechanism in guinea pig taenia caeci. J Gen Physiol 1989; 94:363–383.
53. Kamishima T, McCarron JG. Depolarization-evoked increases in cytosolic calcium concentration in isolated smooth muscle cells of rat portal vein. J Physiol 1996; 492:61–74.
54. Fleischmann BK, Murray RK, Kotlikoff MI. Voltage window for sustained elevation of cytosolic calcium in smooth muscle cells. Proc Natl Acad Sci USA 1994; 91:11914–11918.
55. Loirand G, Faiderbe S, Baron A, Geffard M, Mironneau J. Autoanti-phosphatidylinositide antibodies specifically inhibit noradrenaline effects on Ca^{2+} and Cl^- channels in rat portal vein myocytes. J Biol Chem 1992; 267:4312–4316.
56. Ganitkevich VY, Isenberg G. Contribution of Ca^{2+}-induced Ca^{2+} release to the $[Ca^{2+}]_i$ transients in myocytes from guinea-pig urinary bladder. J Physiol 1992; 458:119–137.
57. Imaizumi Y, Torii Y, Ohi Y, Nagano N, Atsuki K, Yamamura H, Muraki K, Watanabe M, Bolton TB. Ca^{2+} images and K^+ current during depolarization in smooth muscle cells of the guinea-pig vas deferens and urinary bladder. J Physiol 1998; 510:705–719.
58. Zhuge R, Fogarty KE, Tuft RA, Walsh JV Jr. Spontaneous transient outward currents arise from microdomains where BK channels are exposed to a mean Ca^{2+} concentration on the order of 10 μM during a Ca^{2+} spark. J Gen Physiol 2002; 120:15–27.
59. Xiong ZL, Kitamura K, Kuriyama H. Evidence for contribution of Ca^{2+} storage sites on unitary K^+ channel currents in inside-out membrane of rabbit portal vein. Pflügers Arch 1992; 420:112–114.
60. Ohya S, Yamamura H, Muraki K, Watanabe M, Imaizumi Y. Comparative study of the molecular and functional expression of L-type Ca^{2+} channels and large-conductance, Ca^{2+}-activated K^+ channels in rabbit aorta and vas deferens smooth muscle. Pflügers Arch 2001; 441:611–620.
61. Ganitkevich V, Isenberg G. Efficacy of peak Ca^{2+} currents (I_{Ca}) as trigger of sarcoplasmic reticulum Ca^{2+} release in myocytes from the guinea-pig coronary artery. J Physiol. 1995; 484:287–306.
62. Bolton TB, Gordienko DV. Confocal imaging of calcium release events in single smooth muscle cells. Acta Physiol Scand 1998; 164:567–575.

63. Miyakawa T, Mizushima A, Hirose K, Yamazawa T, Bezprozvanny I, Kurosaki T, Iino M. Ca^{2+}-sensor region of IP_3 receptor controls intracellular Ca^{2+} signaling. EMBO J 2001; 20:1674–1680.
64. Taylor CW, Laude AJ. IP_3 receptors and their regulation by calmodulin and cytosolic Ca^{2+} Cell Calcium 2002; 32:321–334
65. Nosyreva E, Miyakawa T, Wang Z, Glouchankova L, Mizushima A, Iino M, Bezprozvanny I. The high-affinity calcium—calmodulin-binding site does not play a role in the modulation of type 1 inositol 1,4,5-trisphosphate receptor function by calcium and calmodulin. Biochem J 2002; 365:659–667.
66. Yang J, McBride S, Mak DO, Vardi N, Palczewski K, Haeseleer F, Foskett JK. Identification of a family of calcium sensors as protein ligands of inositol trisphosphate receptor Ca^{2+} release channels. Proc Natl Acad Sci USA 2002; 99:7711–7716.
67. Bultynck G, Sienaert I, Parys B, Callewaert G, De Smedt H, Boens N, Dehaen W, Missiaen L. Pharmacology of inositol trisphosphate receptors. Pflugers Arch 2003; 445:629–642.
68. Tasker PN, Michelangeli F, Nixon GF. Expression and distribution of the type 1 and type 3 inositol 1,4,5-trisphosphate receptor in developing vascular smooth muscle. Circ Res 1999; 84:536–542.
69. Tasker PN, Taylor CW, Nixon GF. Expression and distribution of $InsP_3$ receptor subtypes in proliferating vascular smooth muscle cells. Biochem Biophys Res Commun 2000; 273:907–912.
70. Taylor CW, Genazzani AA, Morris SA. Expression of inositol trisphosphate receptors. Cell Calcium 1999; 26:237–251.
71. Gordienko DV, Bolton TB. Crosstalk between ryanodine receptors and IP_3 receptors as a factor shaping spontaneous Ca^{2+}-release events in rabbit portal vein myocytes. J Physiol 2002; 542:743–762.
72. Wang YX, Kotlikoff MI. Muscarinic signaling pathway for calcium release and calcium-activated chloride current in smooth muscle. Am J Physiol. 1997; 273:C509-C519.
73. Bolton TB, Gordienko DV, Pucovsky V, Parsons S, Povstyan O. Calcium release events in excitation-contraction coupling in smooth muscle. Novartis Found Symp 2002; 246:154–168.
74. Suzuki H, Takano H, Yamamoto Y, Komuro T, Saito M, Kato K, Mikoshiba K. Properties of gastric smooth muscles obtained from mice which lack inositol trisphosphate receptor. J Physiol 2000; 525:105–111.
75. Hirose K, Kadowaki S, Tanabe M, Takeshima H, Iino M. Spatiotemporal dynamics of inositol 1,4,5-trisphosphate that underlies complex Ca^{2+} mobilization patterns. Science. 1999; 284:1527–1530.
76. Weissmann N, Grimminger F, Olschewski A, Seeger W. Hypoxic pulmonary vasoconstriction: a multifactorial response? Am J Physiol Lung Cell Mol Physiol 2001; 281:L314–L317.
77. Gelband CH, Gelband H. Ca^{2+} release from intracellular stores is an initial step in hypoxic pulmonary vasoconstriction of rat pulmonary artery resistance vessels. Circulation 1997; 96:3647–3654.

78. Dipp M, Nye PC, Evans AM. Hypoxic release of calcium from the sarcoplasmic reticulum of pulmonary artery smooth muscle. Am J Physiol Lung Cell Mol Physiol 2001; 281:L318–L325.
79. Morio Y, McMurtry IF. Ca^{2+} release from ryanodine-sensitive store contributes to mechanism of hypoxic vasoconstriction in rat lungs. J Appl Physiol 2002; 92:527–534.
80. Wilson HL, Dipp M, Thomas JM, Lad C, Galione A, Evans AM. ADP-ribosyl cyclase and cyclic ADP-ribose hydrolase act as a redox sensor, a primary role for cyclic ADP-ribose in hypoxic pulmonary vasoconstriction. J Biol Chem 2001; 276:11180–11188.
81. Porter VA, Reeve HL, Cornfield DN. Fetal rabbit pulmonary artery smooth muscle cell response to ryanodine is developmentally regulated. Am J Physiol Lung Cell Mol Physiol. 2000; 279:L751–L757.

8

Agonist-Mediated Regulation of Ca^{2+} Transients in PASMCs

Jean-Pierre Savineau, Christelle Guibert, and Roger Marthan
Institut National de la Santé et de la Recherche Médicale, and Université Victor Ségalen Bordeaux2, Bordeaux, France

I. INTRODUCTION

Pulmonary artery tone is controlled by both the membrane potential of pulmonary artery smooth muscle cells (PASMCs) and a variety of circulating and locally released mediators (1–3). Vascular tone is mainly dependent on the value of the cytoplasmic calcium concentration ($[Ca^{2+}]_i$), which is generally considered the main factor controlling the activation process of smooth muscle contraction (4,5). Agonists can thus positively or negatively modulate pulmonary tone by acting on the calcium signaling pathway. An increase in $[Ca^{2+}]_i$ can result from an influx of extracellular calcium, a release of intracellular stored calcium, or a decrease of calcium efflux and reuptake (6). Extracellular calcium ions enter the smooth muscle cells mainly following the activation of voltage-gated calcium channels (L-type calcium channels), receptor-operated channels, or store-operated channels, whereas intracellular calcium originates mainly from the sarcoplasmic reticulum (SR) via the activation of two types of receptors or channels: the inositol 1,4,5 trisphosphate receptor/channel (RIP_3) and the ryanodine receptor/channel (RyR) (7,8). However, the kinetics, the pattern of $[Ca^{2+}]_i$ increase, and its temporal correlation with the contractile response are not yet clearly understood. Techniques such as enzymatic isolation of smooth muscle cells, microspectrofluorimetry (using fluorescent indicators such as indo1, fura 2, fluo 3), allowing measurement of the $[Ca^{2+}]_i$ in single cells, sometimes combined with electrophysiological (patch-clamp) experiments, are now widely used and have brought about new and important information in the field of cellular calcium signaling and the control of the $[Ca^{2+}]_i$ by agonists.

II. CHARACTERISTICS OF AGONIST-INDUCED Ca TRANSIENT IN ISOLATED PASMCs

Studies from our laboratory and others have revealed that agonists controlling smooth muscle tone via activation of membrane receptors, such as angiotensin II (ANG II), endothelin-1 (ET-1), extracellular ATP and UTP, noradrenaline, and serotonin (5HT) induce a complex temporal $[Ca^{2+}]_i$ response in PASMCs. The pattern of the response depends on several factors, including the type of arteries (proximal vs. distal), the species, the phenotype of the cells (e.g., fresh vs. cultured cells), and the agonist considered. As a general feature, two main patterns of the agonist-induced $[Ca^{2+}]_i$ response are present in PASMCs: a peak plus plateau type of response and an oscillatory type of response (Figs. 1 and 2).

In freshly isolated myocytes from proximal arteries (extrapulmonary and intralobar arteries), the agonist-induced $[Ca^{2+}]_i$ response is composed

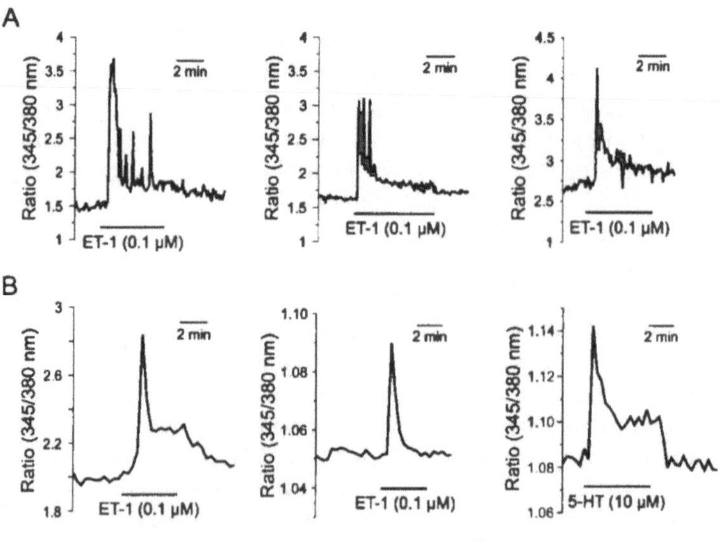

Figure 1 Various patterns of agonist-induced $[Ca^{2+}]_i$ responses in (A) freshly isolated or (B) primary cultured (48–72 h) smooth muscle cells from rat small intrapulmonary arteries (OD 200 μm). Horizontal bars indicate bath application of endothelin-1 (ET-1 0.1 μM) and serotonin [5-HT 10 μM]. $[Ca^{2+}]_i$ is indicated as the ratio of 345/380 nm signals from cells loaded with the calcium-sensitive dye fura-PE3.

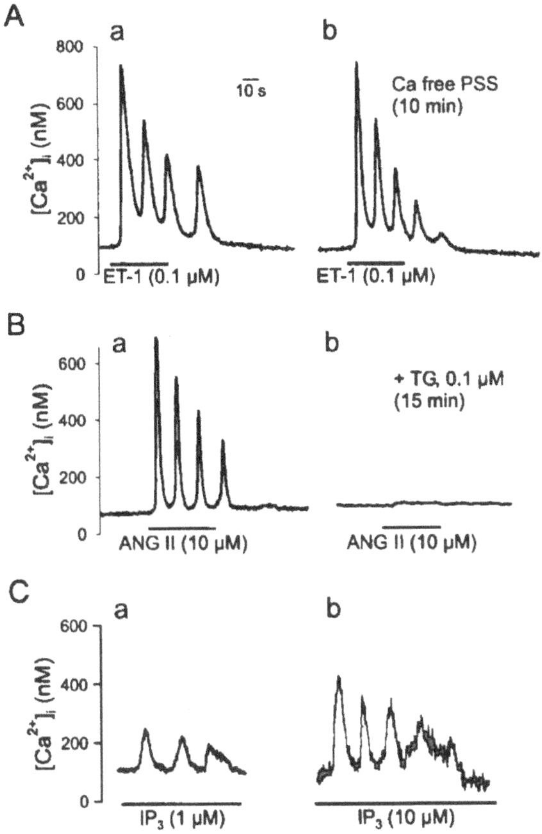

Figure 2 Agonist-induced calcium oscillations in freshly isolated smooth muscle cells from the rat main pulmonary artery. Short (30 s) afflication of endothelin-1 (Aa) (ET-1, 0.1 μM) or angiotensin II (Ba) (ANG II, 10 μM) near the cell induced oscillations in $[Ca^{2+}]_i$.These Ca oscillations were not altered when PASMCs were superfused with a Ca^{2+}-free physiological salt solution (PSS) (Ab) but disappeared when PASMCs were superfused for 15 min with 0.1 μM thapsigargin (TG) (Bb). Application of exogenous inositol 1,4,5-trisphosphate (IP_3) on permeabilized PASMCs directly induces concentration-dependent oscillations in $[Ca^{2+}]_i$ (C). These results suggest that agonist-induced calcium oscillations are mainly due to a release of intracellular calcium via the IP_3 signaling pathway. Each trace was recorded from a different cell and is typical of 8–10 cells.

of a series of cyclical increases in the $[Ca^{2+}]_i$, so-called Ca^{2+} oscillations. The $[Ca^{2+}]_i$ rises, after a delay of 5–10 s, from a resting value of 60–70 nM to a peak value of 400–800 nM (10–12). This first increase is transient and is followed by successive peaks of constant duration (Fig. 2). In some cases the

$[Ca^{2+}]_i$ returns to its resting value before each increase (10,13,14), whereas in others $[Ca^{2+}]_i$ remains above its resting value between increases (12) (Figs. 2A, 2B). These two patterns correspond to *baseline spiking* and *sinusoidal* types of oscillations, respectively. The frequency varies from 4–6 to 25–30/min^{-1}, according to the cell type and/or the agonist concentration. The average percentage of oscillating cells is 50–80% under identical experimental conditions. The concentration of agonist is the main factor that modulates the pattern of Ca^{2+} oscillations. However, this modulation depends on both the type of tissue and the agonist considered. In some cases (canine cultured PASMCs), both amplitude and frequency of the Ca^{2+} oscillations increase with the agonist concentration (13). In some other cases (freshly isolated rat PASMCs), the overall pattern of oscillations appears to be mainly independent of the mediator concentration, but the percentage of cells exhibiting Ca^{2+} oscillations in response to mediator stimulation does depend on the mediator concentration (10,12). In this latter case, the combination of the number of responding cells with the amplitude of the first $[Ca^{2+}]_i$ peak also reveals a relationship between the concentration of the mediator and the $[Ca^{2+}]_i$ response (11,12).

Although functional and phenotypical differences have been observed in proximal vs. distal (OD 2 mm vs. 300 µm) pulmonary arteries, calcium responses to agonist (ET-1) (12) show similar oscillating profiles with the involvement of the same calcium sources. However, the calcium response to ET-1 is ET_A receptor-mediated for main PASMCs and both ET_A,and ET_B receptor-mediated for small intrapulmonary smooth muscle cells (12). Moreover, in our laboratory various calcium responses to ET-1 in PASMCs from small intrapulmonary arteries (OD 200 µm) have been observed: a peak-plus-plateau type or an oscillatory type of response (Fig. 1).

In PASMCs from the main pulmonary artery, culture conditions modify the profiles of the calcium signals induced by various agonists (ET-1, ANG II, ATP). Progressively (from zero to four passages), the oscillatory response is replaced by a peak-plus-plateau response (Figs. 3 and 4). In primary cultured cells from small intrapulmonary arteries, the calcium response to ET-1 becomes transient, either followed by a small plateau (OD 300–500 µm) (9) or not (OD 200 µm), and oscillations disappear (Fig. 1B). The amplitude of the peak is dependent on the ET-1 concentration from 0.1 to 10 nM (9). Serotonin elicits a similar response in primary cultured myocytes from small (resistance) arteries (OD 200 µm) (Fig. 1B).

In contrast to agonists acting at cell-surface membrane receptors, caffeine and ryanodine, known to act directly on the SR and to potentiate the so-called mechanism of calcium-induced calcium release, always induce a transient or monotonic increase of $[Ca^{2+}]_i$ that is never followed by oscillations in PASMCs (10,12,15). The amplitude of this transient $[Ca^{2+}]_i$ response is dependent on the concentration of caffeine used from 0.1 to 10 mM.

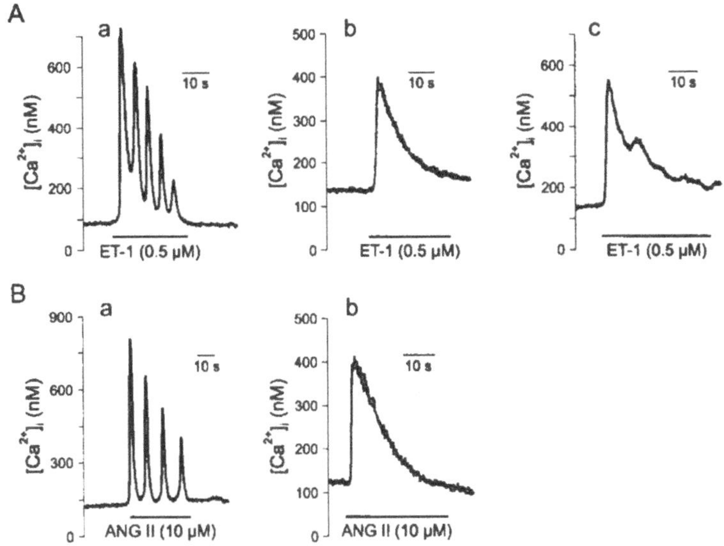

Figure 3 Evolution of the agonist-induced $[Ca^{2+}]_i$ response to ET-1 0.5 μM (A) and ANG II 10 μM (B) according to culture stage. Typical calcium responses in smooth muscle cells isolated from the rat main pulmonary artery and loaded with the calcium-sensitive dye indo-1 are shown in control conditions (Aa, Ba), primary culture (48–72 h) (Ab), and secondary culture (two to four passages) (Ac, Bb). Horizontal bars indicate bath application of the respective agonists.

III. CELLULAR MECHANISMS OF AGONIST-INDUCED $[Ca^{2+}]_i$ RESPONSES IN PASMCs

The first step in the cascade of events linking an extracellular agonist to variation in $[Ca^{2+}]_i$ is the interaction of the agonist with its membrane receptors. Agonists bind to specific subtypes of the seven-transmembrane domain, G-coupled surface membrane receptors. Using selective membrane receptor subtype inhibitors, it was demonstrated that $[Ca^{2+}]_i$ responses of PASMCs to ANG II, ET-1, ATP, serotonin, and phenylephrine are mainly due to activation of AT_1, ET_A and ET_B in small arteries, P2Y and P2X, $5HT_{2A}$ and $5HT_{1B/D}$ according to species, and α receptors, respectively (3,10–13).

A. Peak-Plus-Plateau Type of Response

The agonist-induced $[Ca^{2+}]_i$ responses observed in cultured PASMCs are generally significantly altered in the absence of extracellular calcium with the disappearance of the plateau and relatively good preservation of the peak. In contrast, the peak is fully abolished when PASMCs are pretreated

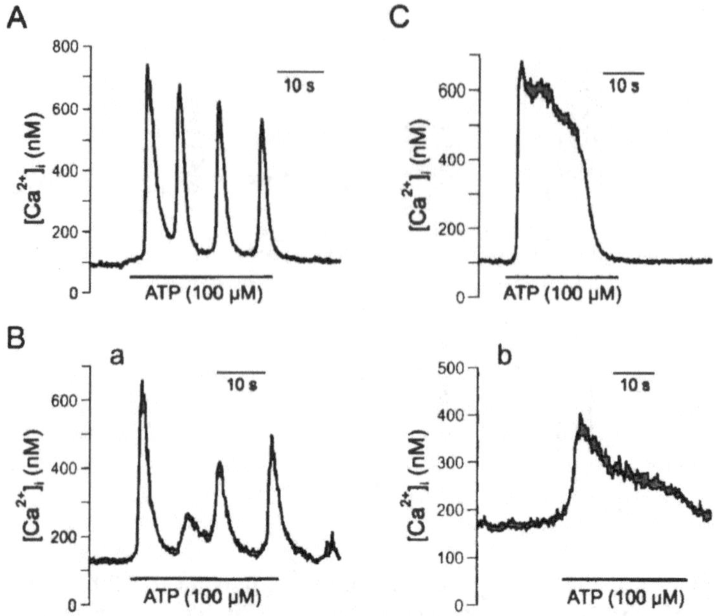

Figure 4 Evolution of the ATP-induced $[Ca^{2+}]_i$ response according to culture stage. Typical calcium responses in smooth muscle cells isolated from the rat main pulmonary and loaded with the calcium-sensitive dye indo-1 are shown in control conditions (A), primary culture (48–72 h) (Ba, Bb), and secondary culture (two to four passages) (C). Horizontal bars indicate bath application of ATP (100 µM).

with thapsigargin (TG), a specific blocker of the sarcoplasmic reticulum (SR) Ca^{2+}-ATPase pump (9). These results suggest that the peak-plus-plateau type of response is due to both a release of calcium from an intracellular store (mainly the SR) responsible for the transient peak and an influx of calcium through the plasma membrane responsible for the plateau. However, the exact sequence of events underlying this response and the nature of the Ca entry pathway are not yet fully elucidated. Both voltage-dependent calcium channels and store-operated calcium channels responsible for the so-called capacitative calcium influx (19) are involved in the maintained agonist-induced $[Ca^{2+}]_i$ increase. In the case of voltage-dependent channels, ET-1 and ANG II induce a PKC-mediated inhibition of potassium channels producing membrane depolarization and opening of the channels (9,16–18). In the case of store-operated channels, they are activated by calcium store depletion induced by agonists. For a variety of tissues, there is more and more evidence suggesting that the molecular basis for store-operated channels would be a protein encoded by a novel gene family, transient receptor potential (TRP) (20). TRP genes have been recently identified in PASMCs from both rat and human (19,21,22).

B. Ca^{2+} Oscillations

In rat PASMCs, Ca^{2+} oscillations are modified neither by the presence of organic Ca^{2+} channel blockers (verapamil or nifedipine) nor by La^{3+} or removal of extracellular Ca^{2+} (Fig. 2A) (10,12), whereas in canine PASMCs, Ca^{2+} oscillations progressively disappear when external Ca^{2+} is removed but are maintained in the presence of Ca^{2+} blockers (13). In all fresh or cultured PASMCs, agonists fail to induce Ca^{2+} oscillations when they are pretreated with specific blockers of the SR Ca^{2+}-ATPase pump, TG, or cyclopiazonic acid (CPA) (Fig. 2B) (23). This result suggests that the main Ca^{2+} compartment involved in Ca^{2+} oscillations, or at least in the triggering of Ca^{2+} oscillations, is an intracellular store (mainly the SR). Hence, agonist-induced Ca^{2+} oscillations appear to be underlain by a *cytosolic Ca^{2+} oscillator*. Agonist-induced Ca^{2+} oscillations are (1) inhibited by neomycin or U73122, potent inhibitors of the phosphoinositide phospholipase C (10–13), 2-aminoethyldiphenylborate (2 APB), and heparin, potent inhibitors of the RIP_3, and (2) mimicked by exogenous applied IP_3 on permeabilized PASMCs (Fig. 2C). These results indicate that the IP_3 pathway is implicated in the mechanism of Ca^{2+} oscillations. The cyclical character of $[Ca^{2+}]_i$ variation could be due to either a cyclical discontinuous production of IP_3 (*receptor-controlled oscillator*) or a cyclical opening and closing of the RIP_3 (*second-messenger-controlled oscillator*). So far, no direct evidence for cyclical agonist-mediated production of IP_3 has been reported in smooth muscle cells. In contrast, regulation of RIP_3 is complex and involves positive and negative feedback controls by cytosolic and/or luminal Ca^{2+} (24,25). Ca^{2+} acts as a cofactor at the site of RIP_3. At low $[Ca^{2+}]_i$ (<300 nM), Ca^{2+} potentiates the IP_3 effect whereas at high $[Ca^{2+}]_i$ (>300 nM), it antagonizes the IP_3 effect (24). In smooth muscle, as in nonmuscle cells, RIP_3s are encoded by three different genes, resulting in three isoforms: type 1, type 2, and type 3 RIP_3 (8,26). Recent studies performed on RIP_3 reconstituted in the lipid bilayer revealed important functional differences between the three isoforms. Interestingly, one type of RIP_3, type 1, is biphasically regulated by cytosolic Ca^{2+} (27–29). Preliminary results from our laboratory show that type 1 RIP_3 is predominantly expressed in PASMCs from rats.

The biphasic regulation of the RIP_3 together with the activity of the sarcoplasmic and plasmalemmal Ca^{2+} pumps can explain the cyclical nature of the agonist-induced $[Ca^{2+}]_i$ increase. The amplitude of each $[Ca^{2+}]$ spike may represent the balance between Ca^{2+} release, the loss of Ca^{2+} from the cell, and the sequestration of Ca^{2+} into intracellular stores. The termination of the spike would occur when the release process is inactivated, allowing extrusion of Ca^{2+} from the cell and the sequestration of Ca^{2+} into intracellular stores (Fig. 5). However, the SR of PASMCs has a limited capacity for Ca^{2+} storage. Therefore, prolonged stimulation by agonists depletes the internal Ca^{2+} store, which has to be replenished by entry of Ca^{2+} from extracellular space. Depletion of the internal Ca^{2+} store by agonist-induced Ca^{2+} release triggers a Ca^{2+} influx, the so-called capacitative Ca^{2+} influx, which has been clearly identified in PASMCs (19,21,23,30). Capacitative Ca^{2+} influx is implicated in the maintenance of phenylephrine-induced Ca^{2+} oscillations in canine PASMCs (30).

Although the caffeine-induced $[Ca^{2+}]_i$ response disappears in PASMCs pretreated with TG, it is not altered by modulators of the IP_3 pathway but,

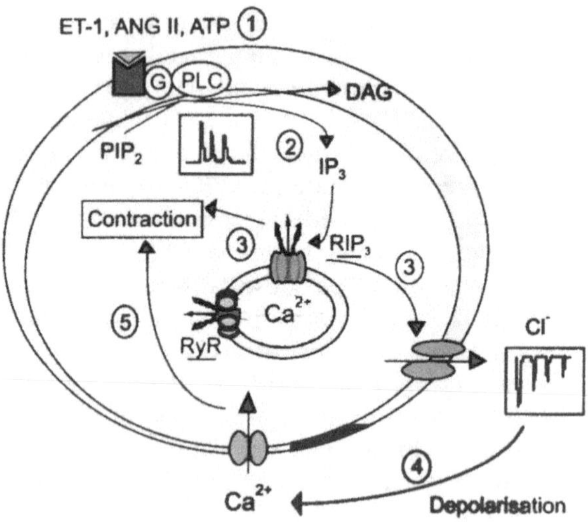

Figure 5 Proposed mechanism of agonist-induced Ca^{2+} oscillations in rat PASMCs. Agonists bind to specific G-protein-coupled membrane receptors and activate the phospholipase C (PLC), which hydrolyzes phosphatidylinositol 4,5-bisphosphate (PIP_2) in diacyglycerol (DAG) and inositol 1,4,5-trisphosphate (IP_3) (1). IP_3 diffuses in the cytosol and binds to specific receptor/channel (RIP_3) at the site of the sarcoplasmic reticulum (SR) membrane (2). The cyclical opening of this channel due to its biphasic regulation by cytosolic Ca^{2+} ions induces oscillations both in the $[Ca^{2+}]_i$ and in transmembrane chloride current (I_{Cl}) (3). Activation of I_{Cl} leads to membrane depolarization and opening of voltage-operated calcium channels (4). The resulting Ca^{2+} influx and Ca oscillations participate in the contractile response (5). Calcium ion oscillations and Ca influx through voltage-operated calcium channels contribute to a maintained contraction. The SR membrane contains another Ca release receptor/channel: the ryanodine receptor/channel (RyR), the activation of which by the pharmacological compound caffeine induces a transient $[Ca^{2+}]_i$ response. In some species and/or pulmonary vessels, RyR could also be involved in Ca oscillations and contraction.

conversely, is fully antagonized by tetracaine, a potent inhibitor of the CICR mechanism (11). It thus clearly appears that PASMCs exhibit two Ca^{2+} release systems located at the site of the SR membrane. One is the RIP_3 underlying Ca^{2+} oscillations through the IP_3-induced Ca^{2+} release (IICR) mechanism, and the other is the ryanodine receptor/channel protein (RyR) responsible for the CICR mechanism (Fig. 5). Like RIP_3, RyRs are encoded by three genes resulting in three isoforms, RyR1, RyR2, and RyR3 (8). Preliminary results from our laboratory show that PASMCs express preferentially RyR2 and RyR3. The contribution of these RyRs in agonist-induced Ca^{2+} oscillations remains a subject of controversy and deserves a more detailed investigation.

IV. FUNCTIONAL ROLE OF Ca^{2+} OSCILLATIONS

In smooth muscle, as in nonexcitable cells, the role of Ca^{2+} oscillations has not yet been clearly elucidated. As discussed in Section I, in many cell types the oscillation frequency is sensitive to the agonist concentration. It is thus suggested that oscillations may represent a digitalization of the Ca^{2+} signal, allowing frequency-dependent control of the cellular response. Calcium ion oscillations are also implicated in the control of the membrane potential through the activation of Ca^{2+}-activated ionic currents (chloride, potassium, or nonspecific cationic currents) (31,32). In rat PASMCs, clamped at a value near the resting potential, agonists (ANG II, ET-1, and ATP) induce an oscillatory inward current, the pattern of which is similar to that of Ca^{2+} oscillations (Fig. 6A). This current is mainly independent of extracellular Ca^{2+} but disappear after treatment of cells with TG (12,31,32). Electrophysiological and pharmacological characteristics indicate that this oscillatory current is carried by Cl^- ions (Fig. 6C) (12,32). Moreover, simultaneous measurement of membrane current (by means of the patch-clamp technique) and $[Ca^{2+}]_i$ in the same single smooth muscle cell has revealed that (1) each peak of inward current corresponds to a peak of $[Ca^{2+}]_i$; (2) there is a relationship between the amplitude of each $[Ca^{2+}]_i$ peak and that of the corresponding membrane current (Fig. 6A); (3) heparin (added to the pipette solution) inhibits both the current and Ca oscillations; and (4) niflumic acid, which inhibits the current, has no effect on Ca oscillations (12,32). These data clearly demonstrate that oscillations in the membrane current are induced by oscillations in $[Ca^{2+}]_i$. Depending on the electrophysiological conditions, the resulting calcium-activated chloride current could participate in the membrane depolarization that secondarily opens voltage-gated calcium channels leading to implication of the extracellular calcium source in the agonist-induced contractile response (Figs. 5 and 6B) (12,32).

Finally, oscillations may allow calcium to function as a messenger while limiting the toxic effects of a sustained elevation of $[Ca^{2+}]_i$. Sustained

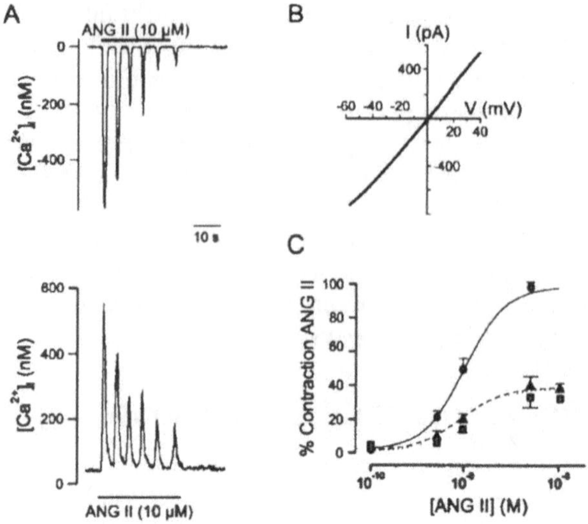

Figure 6 Role of agonist-induced Ca^{2+} oscillations in rat PASMCs. Calcium ion oscillations control the membrane potential value and contribute to the contractile response. (A) ANG II induces oscillations in both $[Ca^{2+}]_i$ and membrane current. (B) The I–V relation obtained for a ramp pulse (from −60 to +40 mV) delivered at the peak of the first current oscillation induced by ANG II shows a reversal potential (0 mV) that is close to the theoretical equilibrium potential for chloride ions in these experimental conditions. Cells were voltage-clamped at −60 mV and dialyzed with cesium solution. (C) Effect of ANG II on isometric contraction of rings isolated from the rat main pulmonary artery. Concentration–response curves for the action of ANG II alone (•) or in the additional presence of niflumic acid, a selective blocker of calcium-activated chloride currents (▲), or niflumic acid plus nifedipine, a selective blocker of votlage-activated calcium currents (■). Ordinate: Contraction expressed as a percentage of the KCl (80 mM)-induced response obtained at the beginning of the experiments. Data points are means ± SE, $n = 6$.

elevation may desensitize calcium-sensitive cellular response elements (contractile apparatus through the activation of the Ca^{2+}-calmodulin kinase II). Moreover, sustained elevation in cytosolic calcium may increase energy loss due to stimulation of calcium-activated ATP-dependent enzymes (Ca^{2+} pumps).

V. MODULATION OF AGONIST-INDUCED Ca^{2+} OSCILLATIONS BY PHYSICAL, CHEMICAL, OR PHARMACOLOGICAL AGENTS: IMPLICATION IN THE PATHOPHYSIOLOGY OF THE PULMONARY CIRCULATION

Agonist-induced Ca^{2+} oscillations are modulated by a variety of both endogenous and exogenous factors.

A. Nitric Oxide and Nitric Oxide Donors

The endothelium-derived factor nitric oxide (NO) is known to relax vascular smooth muscles including pulmonary arteries via both Ca^{2+}-dependent and Ca^{2+}-independent pathways. The generally admitted cellular mechanism of action of NO is related to its activation of the cytosolic guanylyl cyclase and the subsequent increase of the cGMP level. In rat PASMCs, NO donors (SNP, SIN1, or SNAP) inhibit ET-1- and ATP-induced Ca^{2+} oscillations (Fig. 7A). This effect is mimicked by 8Br-cGMP (33). In cultured PASMCs,

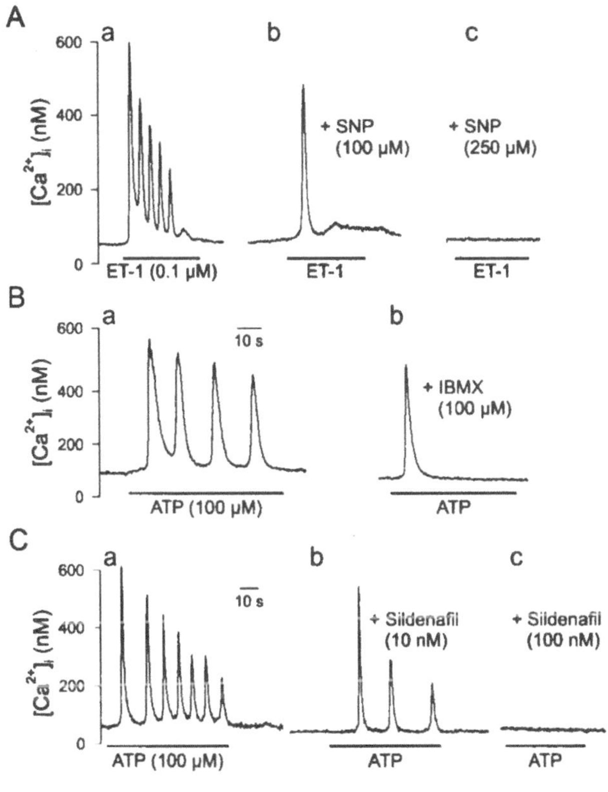

Figure 7 Modulation of agonist-induced calcium oscillations by an NO donor and different cyclic nucleotide-dependent phosphodiesterase (PDE) inhibitors. (A) Sodium nitroprusside (SNP), an NO donor, concentration-dependently inhibits endothelin-1 (ET-1)-induced $[Ca^{2+}]_i$ oscillations in rat PASMCs. (B) Isobutyl methylxanthine (IBMX), and (C) sildenafil, non-specific and specific PDE5 inhibitors, respectively, also concentration-dependently inhibit ATP-induced induced $[Ca^{2+}]_i$ oscillations. In each panel, the first record (left trace) is the control response. Each trace was recorded from a different cell and is typical of 8–10 cells.

NO also inhibits serotonin-induced Ca^{2+} oscillations (34). However, these compounds do not alter the caffeine-induced $[Ca^{2+}]_i$ response, showing that NO and NO donors alter specifically the IP_3 pathway of Ca^{2+} release (33).

B. Cyclic Nucleotide–Dependent Phosphodiesterase Inhibitors

Cyclic nucleotides (cAMP, cGMP) are involved in the control of vascular tone. The family of cyclic nucleotide phosphodiesterases (PDEs) that hydrolyzes, cAMP and cGMP represents the unique degradation pathway for these intracellular compounds. As a consequence, PDE activity is implicated in the control of vascular tone, and the pharmacological modulation of this activity (e.g., using PDE inhibitors) can also control vascular tone. In rat pulmonary artery, nonspecific (e.g., IBMX) as well as specific PDE inhibitors induce a concentration-dependent inhibition of Ca^{2+} oscillations (Fig. 7B). Among the variety of PDE inhibitors, sildenafil (Viagra), a potent PDE5 inhibitor, concentration-dependently relaxes the pulmonary artery ($IC_{50} = 10\,nM$) (35) and decreases both the amplitude and frequency of agonist-induced Ca^{2+} oscillations (Fig. 7C). The effect of sildenafil is clearly related to its action on the PDE5, which is abundantly expressed in the pulmonary artery (35). Thus, the combined treatment with an NO donor and a PDE5 inhibitor could be relevant for the treatment of pulmonary vascular diseases such as pulmonary artery hypertension (PAHT).

C. Hypoxia

Acute hypoxia specifically induces a vasoconstriction in the pulmonary circulation, whereas chronic hypoxia (CH) induces PAHT. However, the effect of hypoxia along the pulmonary vascular tree reveals some heterogeneity in the mechanical response: a vasoconstriction in small (resistant) arteries and a vasodilatation in large (conduit) arteries. The effect of acute hypoxia on Ca^{2+} signaling also depends on the origin of the PASMCs. In rabbit PASMCs originating from conduit arteries, acute hypoxia reduces basal $[Ca^{2+}]_i$ and inhibits spontaneous Ca^{2+} oscillations. However, the amplitude of such spontaneous oscillations (about 140 nM) is less than that of agonist-induced Ca^{2+} oscillations (36). In PASMCs originating from resistance arteries, acute hypoxia exhibits differential effects on basal $[Ca^{2+}]_i$ although in the majority of PASMCs it increases the amplitude of Ca^{2+} oscillations (36). Very little information is available about the interaction between acute hypoxia and the agonist-induced Ca^{2+} response. In distal pulmonary artery myocytes from fetal lamb, angiotensin II induces small Ca^{2+} oscillations (amplitude 30 nM), which were attenuated under acute hypoxic conditions (37).

Most of the studies investigating the effect of CH on $[Ca^{2+}]_i$ responses were performed on pulmonary arteries obtained from a commonly used animal model, i.e., the chronically hypoxic rat. As a general feature, CH increases the resting $[Ca^{2+}]_i$ value by approximately 60%, i.e., from 70–75 nM to 115–120 nM (38). This increase disappears in the absence of extracellular calcium but is resistant to organic inhibitors of L-type calcium channels (nifedipine, verapamil) (39), suggesting that it is due to a different Ca^{2+} entry pathway that could be upregulated by CH. The exact nature of this Ca^{2+} influx has not yet been identified. In freshly isolated arterial myocytes from CH rats, agonist-induced $[Ca^{2+}]_i$ responses are drastically altered. The main change is a decrease in the percentage of responding cells (15–30%) and the disappearance of the oscillatory profile. This change is not due to a CH-induced change in the calcium sources implicated in the $[Ca^{2+}]_i$ responses (40). As under control conditions, ANG II- or ET-1-induced $[Ca^{2+}]_i$ responses in PASMCs from CH rats were altered neither in Ca^{2+}-free solution nor in the presence of the voltage-dependent calcium channel blocker D600 but vanished after pretreatment of the cells with thapaigargin, indicating that they also involved the mobilization of an intracellular Ca^{2+} source, presumably the SR (40). In contrast, CH did not modify the percentage of cells responding to caffeine or the amplitude of the Ca^{2+} transient induced by caffeine (39,40). Collectively these data demonstrate that CH alters Ca^{2+} oscillations via an action at the site of the IP_3-signaling pathway and not the CICR mechanism.

D. Intravenous Anesthetics and Benzodiazepines

General anesthetics may modify pulmonary vasomotor tone (41). Intravenous anesthetics alter in a concentration-dependent manner agonist-induced Ca^{2+} oscillations in PASMCs. In canine PASMCs, ketamine and propofol reduce the amplitude but not the frequency of phenylephrine-induced Ca^{2+} oscillations, whereas thiopental decreases both the amplitude and the frequency of such oscillations (42). The action of propofol on Ca^{2+} oscillations involves inhibition of the capacitative Ca^{2+} influx that is necessary to replenish the internal Ca^{2+} store and therefore to maintain agonist-induced Ca^{2+} oscillations (43). The effects of ketamine and thiopental but not that of propofol are observed at clinically relevant concentrations.

Benzodiazepines are widely used in anesthetic practice as a premedication sedative-amnesiac and/or induction agent. Hemodynamic alteration induced by benzodiazepines is mediated in part through effects on the sympathetic nervous system, but direct effects on smooth muscle have also been reported (44,45). Benzodiazepines differentially alter Ca^{2+} oscillations in canine PASMCs (46). Lorazepam (1 μM) inhibits the amplitude but not the frequency of phenylephrine-induced Ca^{2+} oscillations in PASMCs, whereas diazepam (1 μM) decreases the frequency but not the amplitude of these oscillations. In contrast, midazolam (1–30 μM) has no effect on either the amplitude or the frequency of Ca^{2+} oscillations. These effects of lorazepam and diazepam are observed at clinically relevant concentrations (46).

VI. SUMMARY AND CONCLUSIONS

In PASMCs, agonists acting on G-protein-coupled membrane receptors induce Ca^{2+} transients that trigger contraction. The amplitude and the general pattern of these Ca^{2+} transients are dependent on the type of pulmonary arteries, the nature of the agonist, and the experimental conditions. However, two general patterns are generally expressed in PASMCs: a peak-plus-plateau type of response and a Ca^{2+} oscillation response. In both patterns, the release of Ca^{2+} ions from intracellular stores (mainly the SR) is a key step of the agonist-induced $[Ca^{2+}]_i$ response. Calcium ion oscillations are mainly due to a cyclical release of Ca^{2+} from the SR through the RIP_3 as a consequence of the dual effect of cytosolic Ca^{2+} itself on the control of the channel.

Although the analysis of the precise role of these oscillations requires further investigations, as a general rule they may allow calcium to function as a messenger while obviating the deleterious effect of sustained elevation of $[Ca^{2+}]_i$. Moreover, the oscillations can contribute to frequency-dependent control of smooth muscle cell response and control of the value of membrane potential via the activation of calcium-dependent membrane ion channels.

The fact that agonist-induced Ca^{2+} oscillations are modulated by physical, chemical, and pharmacological agents suggests that they require further investigations for a better understanding of the pathophysiology and treatment of pulmonary smooth muscle diseases such as pulmonary hypertension and remodeling of the pulmonary vascular wall.

ACKNOWLEDGMENTS

Work from our laboratory was funded by Conseil Régional d'Aquitaine (Grant 20020301301) and ADEME Primequal (Grant 0262019). We are grateful to our coworkers O. Pauvert and S. Bonnet.

REFERENCES

1. Osipenko ON, Alexander D, MacLean MR, Gurney AM. Influence of chronic hypoxia on the contribution of non-inactivating and delayed rectifier K currents to the resting potential and tone of rat pulmonary artery smooth muscle. Br J Pharmacol 1998; 124:1335–1337.
2. Yuan XJ. Voltage-gated K^+ currents regulate resting membrane potential and $[Ca^{2+}]_i$ in pulmonary arterial myocytes. Circ Res 1995; 77:370–378.
3. Barnes PJ, Liu SF. Regulation of pulmonary vascular tone. Pharmacol Rev 1995; 47:87–131.
4. Somlyo AP, Somlyo AV. Signal transduction and regulation in smooth muscle. Nature 1994; 372:231–234.

5. Savineau JP, Marthan R. Modulation of the calcium sensitivity of the smooth muscle contractile apparatus: molecular mechanisms, pharmacological and pathophysiological implications. Fund Clin Pharmacol 1997; 11:289–299.
6. Karaki H, Ozaki H, Hori M, Mitsui-Saito M, Amano Ki, Harada KI, Miyamoto S, Nakazawa H, Won KJ, Sato K. Calcium movements, distribution, and functions in smooth muscle. Pharmacol Rev 1997; 49:127–130.
7. Berridge MJ. Elementary and global aspects of calcium signalling. J Physiol 1997; 499:291–306.
8. Berridge MJ, Lipp P, Bootman MD. The versatility and universality of calcium signaling. Nature Rev Mol Cell Biol 2000; 1:11–21.
9. Shimoda LA, Sylvester JT, Sham JS. Mobilization of intracellular Ca^{2+} by endothelin-1 in rat intrapulmonary arterial smooth muscle cells. Am J Physiol Lung Cell Mol Physiol 2000; 278:L157–L164.
10. Guibert C, Marthan R, Savineau JP. Angiotensin II-induced Ca^{2+}-oscillations in vascular myocytes from the rat pulmonary artery. Am J Physiol Lung Cell Mol Physiol 1996; 270:L637–L642.
11. Guibert C, Pacaud P, Loirand G, Marthan R, Savineau JP. Effect of extracellular ATP on cytosolic Ca^{2+} concentration in rat pulmonary artery myocytes. Am J Physiol Lung Cell Mol Physiol 1996; 271:L450–L458.
12. Hyvelin JM, Guibert C, Marthan R, Savineau JP. Cellular mechanisms and role of endothelin-1-induced calcium oscillations in pulmonary arterial myocytes. Am J Physiol Lung Cell Mol Physiol 1998; 275:L269–L282.
13. Hamada H, Damron DS, Hong SJ, Van Wagoner DR, Murray PA. Phenylephrine-induced Ca^{2+}oscillations in canine pulmonary artery smooth muscle cells. Circ Res 1997; 81:812–823.
14. Nicholls JA, Greenwell JR, Gillespie JL. Agonist concentration influences the pattern and time course of intracellular Ca^{2+} oscillations in human arterial smooth muscle cells. Pflügers Arch 1995; 429:477–484.
15. Kang TM, Park MK, Uhm DY. Characterization of hypoxia-induced $[Ca^{2+}]_i$ rise in rabbit pulmonary arterial smooth muscle cells. Life Sci 2002; 70: 2321–2333.
16. Peng W, Michael JR, Hoidal JR, Karwande SV, Farukh IS. ET-1 modulates K_{Ca} channel activity and arterial tension in normoxic and hypoxic human pulmonary vasculature. Am J Physiol Lung Cell Mol Physiol 1998; 275: L729–L739.
17. Shimoda LA, Sylvester JT, Sham JSK. Inhibition of voltage-gated K^+ current in rat intrapulmonary arterial smooth myocytes by endothelin-1. Am J Physiol Lung Cell Mol Physiol 1998; 274:L842–L853.
18. Shimoda LA, Sylvester JT, Sham JSK. Chronic hypoxia alters effects of endothelin and angiotensin on K^+ current in pulmonary arterial myocytes by endothelin-1. Am J Physiol Lung Cell Mol Physiol 1999; 277:L431–L439.
19. McDaniel SS, Platoshyn O, Wang J, Yu Y, Sweeney M, Krick S, Rubin LJ, Yuan JX-J. Capacitative Ca^{2+} entry in agonist-induced pulmonary vasoconstriction. Am J Physiol Lung Cell Mol Physiol 2001; 280:L1870–L1880.
20. Minke B, Cook B. TRP channel proteins and signal transduction. Physiol Rev 2002; 82:429–472.

21. Ng LC, Gurney AM. Store-operated channels mediates Ca^{2+} influx and contraction in rat pulmonary artery. Circ Res 2001; 89:923–929.
22. Golovina VA, Platoshyn O, Bailey CL, Wang J, Limsuwan A, Sweeney M, Rubin LJ, Yuan JX-J. Upregulated TRP and enhanced capacitative Ca^{2+} entry in human pulmonary artery myocytes during proliferation. Am J Physiol Heart Circ Physiol 2001; 280:H746–H755.
23. Gonzalez De La Fuente P, Savineau JP, Marthan R. Control of pulmonary vascular smooth muscle tone by sarcoplasmic reticulum Ca^{2+} pump blockers: thapsigargin and cyclopiazonic acid. Pflügers Arch 1995; 429:617–624.
24. Iino M. Biphasic Ca^{2+} dependence of inositol 1,4,5-trisphosphate-induced Ca release in smooth muscle cells of the guinea pig taenia caeci. J Gen Physiol 1990; 95:1103–1122.
25. Missiaen L, Parys JB, Weidema AF, Sipma H, Vanlingen S, De Smet P, Callewaert G, De Smedt H. The bell-shaped Ca^{2+} dependence of the inositol 1,4,5-trisphosphate-induced Ca^{2+} release is modulated by Ca^{2+}/calmodulin. J Biol Chem 1999; 274:13748–13751.
26. Patel S, Joseph SK, Thomas AP. Molecular properties of inositol 1,4, 5-trisphosphate receptors. Cell Calcium 1999; 25:247–264.
27. Hagar RE, Burgstahler AD, Nathanson MH, Ehrlich BE. Type III $InsP_3$ receptor channel stays open in the presence of increased calcium. Nature 1998; 396: 81–84.
28. Ramos-Franco J, Fill M, Mignery GA. Isoform-specific function of single inositol 1,4,5-trisphosphate receptor channels. Biophys J 1998; 75:834–839.
29. Trower EC, Hagar RE, Ehrlich BE. Regulation of $Ins(1,4,5)P_3$ receptor isoforms by endogenous modulators. Trends Pharm Sci 2001; 11:580–586.
30. Doi S, Damron DS, Horibe M, Murray PA. Capacitative Ca^{2+}entry and tyrosine kinase activation in canine pulmonary arterial smooth muscle cells. Am J Physiol Lung Cell Mol Physiol 2000; 278:L118–L130.
31. Salter KJ, Kozlowski RZ. Endothelin receptor coupling to potassium and chloride channels in isolated rat pulmonary arterial myocytes. J Pharmacol Exp Ther 1996; 279:1053–1062.
32. Guibert C, Marthan R, Savineau JP. Oscillatory Cl^- current induced by angiotensin II in rat pulmonary arterial myocytes: Ca^{2+} dependence and physiological implication. Cell Calcium 1997; 21:421–429.
33. Pauvert O, Marthan R, Savineau JP. NO-induced modulation of calcium-oscillations in pulmonary vascular smooth muscle. Cell Calcium 2000; 27: 329–338.
34. Yuan XJ, Bright RT, Aldinger AM, Rubin LJ. Nitric oxide inhibits serotonin-induced calcium release in pulmonary artery smooth muscle cells. Am J Physiol Lung Cell Mol Physiol 1997; 272:L44–L50.
35. Pauvert O, Lugnier C, Keravis T, Marthan R, Rousseau E, Savineau JP. Effect of sildenafil on cyclic nucleotide phosphodiesterase activity, vascular tone and calcium signaling in rat pulmonary artery. Br J Pharmacol 2003, 139:513–522.
36. Urena J, Franco-Obregon A, Lopez-Barneo J. Contrasting effects of hypoxia on cytosolic Ca^{2+} spikes in conduit and resistance myocytes of the rabbit pulmonary artery. J Physiol 1996; 496:103–109.

37. Cornfield DM, Stevens T, McMurtry IF, Abman SH, Rodman DM. Acute hypoxia increases cytosolic calcium in fetal pulmonary artery smooth muscle cells. Am J Physiol Lung Cell Mol Physiol 1993; 265:L53–L56.
38. Bonnet S, Hyvelin JM, Bonnet P, Marthan R, Savineau JP. Chronic hypoxia-induced spontaneous and rhythmical contractions in the rat main pulmonary artery. Am J Physiol 2001; 281:L183–L192.
39. Shimoda LA, Sham JSK, Shimoda TH, Sylvester JT. L-type Ca^{2+} channels, resting $[Ca^{2+}]_i$ and ET-1-induced responses in chronically hypoxic pulmonary myocytes. Am J Physiol Lung Cell Mol Physiol 2000; 279:L884–L894.
40. Bonnet S, Belus A, Hyvelin JM, Roux E, Marthan R, Savineau JP. Effect of chronic hypoxia on agonist-induced tone and calcium signaling in rat pulmonary artery. Am J Physiol 2001; 281:L193–L201.
41. Park WK, Lynch C III, Johns RA. Effects of propofol and thiopental in isolated rat aorta and pulmonary artery. Anesthesiology 1992; 77:956–963.
42. Hamada H, Damron DS, Murray PA. Intravenous anesthetics attenuate phenylephrine-induced calcium oscillations in individual pulmonary artery smooth muscle cells. Anesthesiology 1997; 87:900–907.
43. Horibe M, Kondo I, Damron DS, Murrau PA. Propofol attenuates capacitative calcium entry in pulmonary artery smooth muscle cells. Anesthesiology 2001; 95:681–688.
44. Marty J, Gauzit R, Lefevre P, Couderc E, Farinotti R, Henzel C, Desmonts JM. Effects of diazepam and midazolam on baroreflex control of heart rate and on sympathetic activity in humans. Anesth Analg 1986; 65:113–119.
45. Koga Y, Sato S, Sodeyama N, Takahasi M, Kato M, Iwatsuki N, Hashimoto Y. Comparison of the relaxant effects of diazepam, flunitrazepam and midazolam on airway smooth muscle. Br J Anaesth 1992; 69:65–69.
46. Hong SJ, Damron DS, Murray PA. Benzodiazepines differentially inhibit phenylephrine-induced calcium oscillations in pulmonary artery smooth muscle cells. Anesthesiology 1998; 88:792–799.

9

Epithelial Sodium Channel Function in Health and Disease in the Adult Lung

Ian C. Davis, Lawrence S. Prince, and Sadis Matalon
University of Alabama at Birmingham, Birmingham, Alabama, U.S.A.

I. INTRODUCTION: THE ROLE OF SODIUM CHANNELS IN LUNG PHYSIOLOGY

For gas exchange to occur, the epithelium of the lung must maintain a humidified atmosphere with only a thin layer of fluid lining the airway surface. Absorption of fluid out of the airway and alveolar lumen requires active transport of sodium ions (Na^+) from the apical surface of the pulmonary epithelium, across the apical and basolateral membranes of epithelial cells, and into the interstitial space and/or bloodstream. Pharmacological inhibitors and genetic manipulations that disrupt Na^+ transport result in fluid accumulation within the lung and failure of gas exchange. The importance of Na^+ transport in the lung is also demonstrated in several human disease processes, where abnormal absorption of Na^+ contributes to the pathophysiology of pulmonary disease.

Whereas type I alveolar pneumocytes line >95% of the distal lung surface, alveolar type II pneumocytes (ATII cells) may mediate most of the ion and fluid transport (1). ATII cells, which make up 67% of the total number of alveolar epithelial cells, can be isolated with high purity and grown as confluent monolayers (2,3). Electrophysiological studies of cultured ATII cells have identified apical plasma membrane cation channels, referred to as epithelial Na^+ channels (ENaC) (reviewed in Ref. 4). These channels have a higher permeability to Na^+ than other cations and can be blocked by the diuretic drug amiloride (5). Na^+ ions diffuse passively into ATII cells (and possibly ATI cells, which have been shown to express ENaC subunit proteins and to transport Na^+ ions in vitro (6,7) through these apical cation channels (8,9) and are extruded across the basolateral membranes by the ouabain-sensitive Na^+,K^+-ATPase (10). Although the driving force for Na^+ transport is produced by the basolateral Na^+,K^+-ATPase, it is the apical entry of Na^+ ions through ENaC that is the rate-limiting step for Na^+ flux. Indeed, the apical plasma membrane ENaC channels offer more than 90% of the overall resistance to transepithelial Na^+ transport.

The expression and function of ENaC are highly regulated. Multiple hormones and signaling pathways influence not only expression of the channels but also posttranslational modifications that regulate channel function. By understanding Na^+ transport at the molecular level, we can better understand the molecular pathogenesis of lung disease and design more appropriate therapies and interventions.

II. BIOLOGY OF ENaC IN THE LUNG

An epithelial Na^+ channel is a composed of three transmembrane subunits (α, β, and γ), which are expressed in unequal proportions in respiratory epithelia (11), although the exact stoichiometry remains controversial. Some studies have indicated that ENaC forms a tetrameric complex (2α, β, γ) (12), and others have provided data indicating that the ENaC channel is a much larger complex (3α, 3β, 3γ) (13). Messenger RNA for all three subunits of ENaC is present in the lungs of both humans and mice (14), but the Na^+ channels identified to date in airway epithelia display variable biophysical characteristics [single-channel conductance, P_{Na}/P_k, and affinity for amiloride and its ethylisopropyl analog (4)]. For example, expression of α, β, and γ ENaC in *Xenopus* oocytes is associated with formation of highly selective cation (HSC) channels (4–6 pS; $P_{Na}/P_k > 80$) (11), but the predominant channel found in ATII cells is a nonselective cation (NSC) channel (21 pS; $P_{Na}/P_k = 1$) (15,16). It appears that αENaC is sufficient to form functional amiloride-sensitive NSC channels, but the presence of β and γ subunits significantly enhances channel activity and substantively changes gating characteristics of the channel to the HSC form (8,11,17).

Epithelial Na^+ channels are constitutively open at the plasma membrane and do not appear to require additional activation (11). However, factors that influence both ENaC mRNA and protein levels can potentially modulate amiloride-sensitive Na^+ transport in the lung. Second messengers and signaling molecules may be able to alter the open probability of ENaC either by direct modification (phosphorylation/dephosphorylation) or by altering protein–protein interactions. Although ENaC expression and function are known to be influenced by diverse factors such as oxygen tension, glucocorticoids (18), cytoskeletal proteins (19–21), and β-adrenergic/cAMP agonists, this review will concentrate on two systems that we have found to be involved in the pathogenesis of ENaC dysfunction in adult lung disease: the purinergic nucleotide system and reactive species.

III. ENaCs IN ADULT LUNG DISEASE

Sodium ion transport appears to be essential for maintenance of a normal gas diffusion distance in the adult lung. In adults with acute respiratory distress syndrome (ARDS), Matthay and Wiener-Kronish (22) found a positive correlation between the ability of the alveolar epithelium to transport Na^+ actively and the rate of resolution of noncardiogenic pulmonary edema. Similarly, instillation of the epithelial Na^+ channel blocker phenamil into the lungs of rats exposed to hyperoxia resulted in higher levels of extravascular lung fluid volumes 24 h later (23). Interestingly, the venom of a South American scorpion (*Tityus serrulatus*), which causes fatal respiratory failure and pulmonary edema, also decreases lung liquid clearance, probably by downregulating Na^+,K^+-ATPase in the alveolar epithelium (24). Finally, patients with systemic pseudohypoaldosteronism (PHA), caused by loss of function mutations in the genes encoding ENaC subunits, completely lack electrogenic Na^+ transport in the upper and lower airways. In some cases, PHA results in a doubling of ALF volume, persistent rhinorrhea, and recurrent respiratory illness (25).

IV. EFFECT OF PULMONARY PATHOGENS ON Na^+ TRANSPORT

Despite the fact that fluid and mucus accumulation in airways and lung tissue is a major component of most respiratory infections (26), the effect of pathogens on respiratory epithelial Na^+ transport has not been studied in detail. Several lung pathogens have been shown to inhibit Na^+ transport by respiratory epithelia in vitro. *Mycoplasma pulmonis* inhibits amiloride-sensitive Na^+ absorption and cholinergic-stimulated Cl^- secretion by C57BL/6 mouse tracheal epithelial cells (27). Similarly, *Pseudomonas aeruginosa* rhamnolipids inhibit amiloride-sensitive Na^+ transport by ovine tracheal epithelium (28), and the hemolysin blocks active Na^+ uptake and Cl^- secretion by canine bronchial epithelium (29). *Mycobacterium tuberculosis* (30) and pneumotropic, but not neurotropic, influenza A virus (31) have also been shown to inhibit ENaC activity in vitro. Although the mechanism of this effect was not defined for *M. tuberculosis*, influenza A virus rapidly (within 60 min of infection) inhibits amiloride-sensitive Na^+ transport by MTE cells. This inhibition is mediated by binding of viral hemagglutinin to cell-surface sialic acid moieties and subsequent activation of phospholipase C and PKC.

Interestingly, the inhibitory effects of pathogens on ENaC found in vitro have not always been found in vivo. For example, in rats with *P. aeruginosa* pneumonia, alveolar fluid clearance (AFC), which is a functional index of ENaC function, increased 24 h after infection, and this increase, which was inhibited by amiloride, was at least partially mediated by TNF-α Z (32). Similarly, instillation of *Escherichia coli* endotoxin into the lungs of rats resulted in a significant increase in AFC at 24 and 40 h (33). Whether such increases in AFC have detrimental pathophysiological consequences or whether they are the result of sublethal injury to the alveolar epithelium resulting in its repopulation with increased numbers of ATII cells remain to be determined. Nevertheless, some pulmonary pathogens may, in contrast, induce hypoxemia as a result of inhibition of AFC. For example, we recently reported that replicating respiratory syncytial virus (RSV) reduces the AFC capacity of the bronchoalveolar epithelium in vivo (Fig. 1), without inducing detectable epithelial cell death or an increase in alveolar permeability to albumin (34). Interestingly, we found that RSV-mediated inhibition of AFC was not due to reduced ENaC subunit gene transcription (Fig. 2) but was mediated by uridine triphosphate (UTP) acting in autocrine fashion on P2YR on bronchoalveolar epithelial cells (Fig. 3). Moreover, reduced AFC was associated with increased lung water content and peripheral hypoxemia (Ian Davis, unpublished observations). Reduced AFC may result in formation of an increased volume of fluid mucus, airway congestion, and rhinorrhea, all features of severe RSV disease.

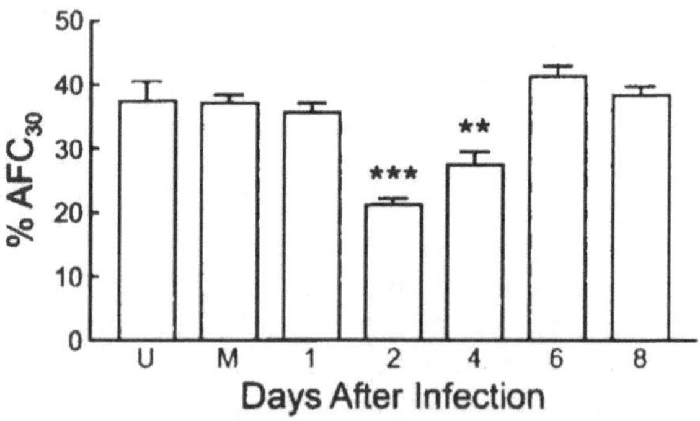

Figure 1 Intranasal infection of BALB/c mice with RSV results in significant inhibition of alveolar fluid clearance (AFC) at days 2 and 4 after infection. Mock infection (M) had no effect on AFC. AFC was inhibited by 43% at day 2 and by 26% at day 4. AFC was evaluated in live mice with normal oxygenation and acid–base balance. $n = 6$–23 per group. Values are means ± SE. (**) $p < 0.005$, (**) $p < 0.0005$, compared with uninfected mice (U).

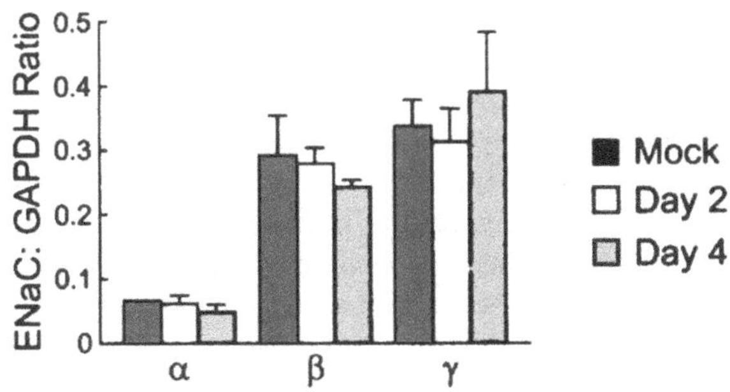

Figure 2 Infection with RSV does not alter whole–lung ENaC subunit gene expression at days 2 and 4 after infection. αEnaC/GAPDH, βENaC/GAPDH, and γEnaC/GADPH mRNA ratios in lung homogenates from mock-infected mice ($n = 2$–6) and mice infected with RSV for 2 ($n = 4$) or 4 ($n = 3$) days were measured by real-time PCR following reverse transcription to cDNA. Three separate PCR reactions were performed per animal for each gene product. In each reaction, five cDNA replicates were subjected to PCR. Values are means ± SE. Reprinted from Ref. 34. with permission.

V. ENaC MODULATION BY PURINERGIC NUCLEOTIDES

Purinergic 5′-nucleotides are known modulators of ENaC activity in respiratory epithelial cells. Relatively large amounts of adenosine triphosphate (ATP) and UTP are released by human respiratory epithelial cells in vitro, although the underlying pathway for nucleotide release remains undefined (35,36). Released ATP is rapidly metabolized to a mixture of ADP, AMP,

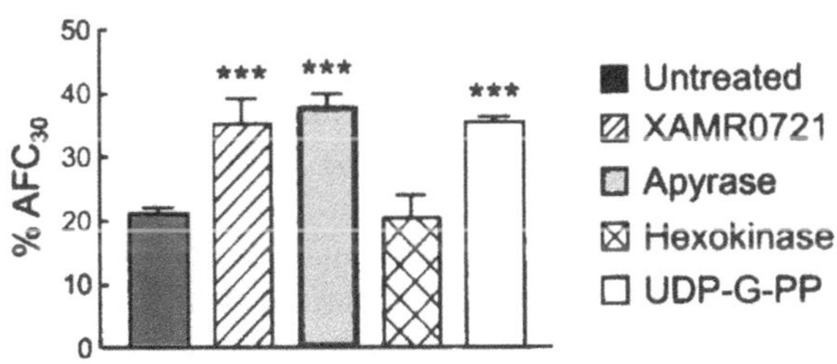

Figure 3 Effects of purinergic receptor antagonists and purinolytic enzymes on RSV-mediated inhibition of AFC at day 2 after infection. XAMR0721 200 μM, apyrase 2 U/mL, hexokinase 2 U/mL (in the presence of 10 mM glucose), and UDP-glucose pyrophosphorylase (UDP-G-PP) 2 U/mL in the presence of 10 mM glucose-1-phosphate and 2 U/mL inorganic pyrophosphatase), respectively, were added to the AFC instillate for >each group. $n = 7$–10 per treatment group. Values are means ± SE. (***)$p < 0.0005$, compared with untreated, RSV-infected group ($n = 23$).

and adenosine (ADO). ATP, its metabolites, and UTP each have inhibitory effects on ENaCs, mediated via interaction with purinergic receptors expressed on respiratory epithelial cells (37,38). Both ATP and UTP are known to inhibit respiratory epithelial Na^+ absorption in vitro (39–42), via interaction with P2Y purinoceptors (P2YR). In vivo, UTP administered at pharmacological doses (100 μM) to human subjects has also been shown to induce Cl^- secretion by nasal epithelium (43) and, when given by aerosol, to promote mucociliary clearance, although, interestingly, in the presence of amiloride it also induced mild hypoxemia (44).

VI. PROTEIN KINASE C AS A CENTRAL REGULATOR OF ENaC FUNCTION?

Until recently, the mechanism by which nucleotide binding to P2YR might induce reduced ENaC activity remained unclear. Although downstream signaling events mediating ENaC downregulation have not yet been fully defined, it is known that P2YR are G-protein-coupled and act via the inositol phosphate pathway to stimulate calcium release from intracellular stores but can also act via multiple secondary signal transduction pathways including protein kinase C (PKC) (37). Activation of PKC has been shown to reduce ENaC activity and modify its subunit composition, although the isoforms of PKC involved have not been defined. Inhibition of PKC rapidly increased P_o and caused the appearance of new channels in patches of A6 cells (45). In contrast, stimulation of PKC inhibited whole-cell currents in *Xenopus* oocytes (46). Likewise, PKC activation decreased expression of both β and γ, but not α ENaC subunit proteins in A6 cells by 3 h and 14 h, respectively, and also resulted in a decrease in transepithelial Na^+ reabsorption (47).

Recent data indicate that P2YR-mediated ENaC downregulation may also involve activation of the ubiquitin–proteosome pathway, which is an important regulator of ENaC function. The half-life of ENaC in mammalian cell membranes is short (less than 1 h). ENaC is ubiquitinated in vivo on the α and γ, but not β, subunits (48). Inhibition of ubiquitination or the proteosome results in increased channel activity, owing to an increase in the number of channels present at the plasma membrane (49). Ubiquitination (ATP-dependent serial addition of ubiquitin monomers to lysine residues on proteins), which targets proteins for rapid degradation by the proteosome, is catalyzed by the sequential action of ubiquitin-activating, ubiquitin-conjugating, and ubiquitin protein ligase enzymes (50). Neural precursor cell–expressed developmentally downregulated protein 4 (Nedd4) is the ubiquitin protein ligase required for ubiquitination of EnaC (51). Nedd4 directly regulates basal ENaC activity by modulating channel stability at the cell surface. In the lung, Nedd4 is mainly expressed in the epithelia lining the airways and in the distal respiratory epithelium, a pattern of

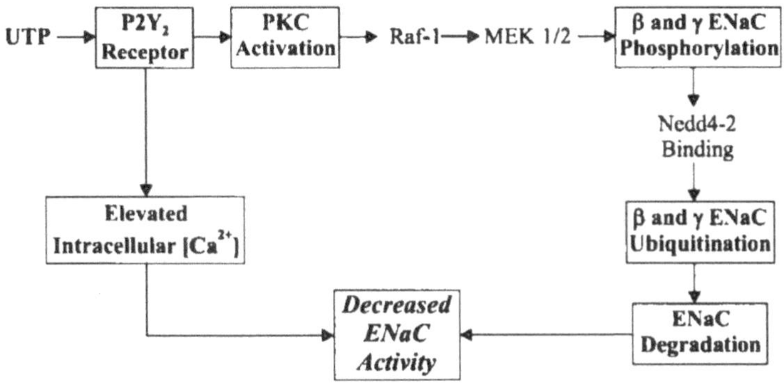

Figure 4 Proposed mechanism by which UTP binding to P2Y purinergic receptors results in reduced ENaC activity in respiratory epithelial cells.

expression similar to that of EnaC (52). Interestingly, the interaction between ENaC and Nedd4 is disrupted in Liddle syndrome, a hereditable form of salt-sensitive hypertension (53). Liddle syndrome mutations in the βENaC cytoplasmic domain disrupt the association of Nedd4 with the C-terminus of βENaC. As a result, ENaC has a longer half-life in the plasma membrane and is less efficiently internalized and degraded. This leads to increased amiloride-sensitive current at the apical membrane and increased salt absorption.

The link between PKC and the ubiquitin–proteosome pathway has just recently been made clear. In A6 cells, PKC has been shown to activate the mitogen-activated protein (MAP) kinase kinase Raf-1, and the MAP kinase kinases MAPK/ERK (MEK) 1 and 2. Activation of MEK 1 and 2 was shown to enhance phosphorylation of β and γ, but not α EnaC (54). This phosphorylation event facilitates binding of Nedd4-2 to ENaC, which may then promote ENaC internalization and its removal from the cell surface (51). Therefore, purinergic stimulation and PKC activation may decrease ENaC function through both altered ENaC phosphorylation and altered ENaC degradation. This pathway is summarized in Fig. 4.

VII. INFLAMMATORY MEDIATORS OF ENaC DYSFUNCTION IN PULMONARY DISEASE

Reactive oxygen/nitrogen species (RONS), such as the free radicals nitric oxide (•NO) and/or peroxynitrite ($ONOO^-$), are known to inhibit the activity of both EnaC (15,55–58) and the ATII cell Na^+/K^+ ATPase (59) in vitro (60), via both cGMP-dependent and cGMP-independent mechanisms. In pulmonary inflammatory disease, increased levels of RONS may directly modify ion transporters, disrupt their association with chaperone or structural proteins (such as actin), or alter signal transduction pathways, all of which may result in impaired Na^+ absorption across the alveolar epithelium. Nitrotyrosine [the stable by-product of $ONOO^-$ reaction with tyrosine residues in proteins (61)] has been detected in the lungs of patients with ARDS (62) and those with Hantavirus cardiopulmonary syndrome (HCPS) (63) and severe acute respiratory syndrome (Ian Davis, unpublished observations). Likewise, both nitrotyrosine and large amounts of nitrate have been found in the lavage fluids of patients with ARDS (Sadis Matalon, unpublished observations) and the plasma of HCPS patients (63). These findings indicate that $ONOO^-$ is produced in the lungs of patients with inflammatory disease and may contribute to the pathogenesis of the disease. In a recent study, Modelska et al. (64) showed that absorption of isotonic fluid, secondary to Na^+ absorption across the alveolar space, was inhibited following prolonged hemorrhagic shock. Moreover, instillation of aminoguanidine, a nitric oxide synthase inhibitor, restored fluid absorption to normal levels. Thus, increased production of •NO by lung epithelial or inflammatory cells may modify molecules required for Na^+ transport across the alveolar epithelium.

It should also be noted that certain proinflammatory cytokines have been shown to alter Na^+ transport by respiratory epithelial cells in vitro. Na^+ transport is inhibited by IFN-γ (65), and IL-4 (66), and TNF-α has been shown to both increase (32,67) and reduce (68) Na^+ transport.

VIII. SUMMARY AND CONCLUSIONS

Sodium ion transport in the distal lung is required for normal lung function. Defective Na^+ absorption may contribute to the pathogenesis of acute and chronic lung disease. As the molecular mechanisms of lung injury and disease are better characterized, we may better understand the contribution of ENaC function to pulmonary disease. The demonstration that RONS released by activated alveolar macrophages downregulate the activity of FDLE and ATII cells Na^+ channels (56,69,70) provides an example of how mediators of lung injury could influence Na^+ absorption during the progression of pneumonia or ARDS. Manipulating ENaC function may provide new treatments for both ARDS and pulmonary infectious diseases. For example, strategies that inhibit UTP-P2YR interaction can now be evaluated as therapeutics for RSV pneumonitis, a condition for which specific antiviral drugs are sadly lacking. Identification of additional targets for regulating ENaC expression and function in the lung may provide further opportunities for clinicians to target Na^+ absorption in the lung. Moreover, by studying Na^+ channel physiology in the context of human lung disease, we may learn more about the basic physiology of distal lung transport.

REFERENCES

1. Matalon S, Davis IC. Vectorial sodium transport across the mammalian alveolar epithelium: it occurs but through which cells? Circ Res 2003; 92: 348–349.
2. Dobbs LG. Isolation and culture of alveolar type II cells. Am J Physiol 1990; 258:L134–L147.
3. Matalon S, Benos DJ, Jackson RM. Biophysical and molecular properties of amiloride-inhibitable Na^+ channels in alveolar epithelial cells. Am J Physiol 1996; 271:L1–L22.
4. Matalon S, O'Brodovich H. Sodium channels in alveolar epithelial cells: molecular characterization, biophysical properties, and physiological significance. Annu Rev Physiol 1999; 61:627–661.
5. Benos DJ. Amiloride: a molecular probe of sodium transport in tissues and cells. Am J Physiol 1982; 242:C131–C145.
6. Borok Z, Liebler JM, Lubman RL, Foster MJ, Zhou B, Li X, Zabski SM, Kim KJ, Crandall ED. Na^+ transport proteins are expressed by rat alveolar epithelial type I cells. Am J Physiol Lung Cell Mol Physiol 2002; 282: L599–L608.
7. Johnson MD, Widdicombe JH, Allen L, Barbry P, Dobbs LG. Alveolar epithelial type I cells contain transport proteins and transport sodium, supporting an active role for type I cells in regulation of lung liquid homeostasis. Proc Natl Acad Sci USA 2002; 99:1966–1971.
8. Jain L, Chen XJ, Ramosevac S, Brown LA, Eaton DC. Expression of highly selective sodium channels in alveolar type II cells is determined by culture conditions. Am J Physiol Lung Cell Mol Physiol 2001; 280:L646–L658.
9. Yue G, Shoemaker RL, Matalon S. Regulation of low-amiloride-affinity sodium channels in alveolar type II cells. Am J Physiol 1994; 267:L94–L100.
10. Factor P, Senne C, Dumasius V, Ridge K, Jaffe HA, Uhal B, Gao Z, Sznajder JI. Overexpression of the Na^+,K^+-ATPase α_1 subunit increases Na^+,K^+-ATPase function in A549 cells. Am J Respir Cell Mol Biol 1998; 18:741–749.
11. Canessa CM, Schild L, Buell G, Thorens B, Gautschi I, Horisberger JD, Rossier BC. Amiloride-sensitive epithelial Na^+ channel is made of three homologous subunits. Nature 1994; 367:463–467.
12. Firsov D, Gautschi I, Merillat AM, Rossier BC, Schild L. The heterotetrameric architecture of the epithelial sodium channel (ENaC). EMBO J 1998; 17: 344–352.
13. Snyder PM, Cheng C, Prince LS, Rogers JC, Welsh MJ. Electrophysiological and biochemical evidence that DEG/ENaC cation channels are composed of nine subunits. J Biol Chem 1998; 273:681–684.
14. Burch LH, Talbot CR, Knowles MR, Canessa CM, Rossier BC, Boucher RC. Relative expression of the human epithelial Na^+ channel subunits in normal and cystic fibrosis airways. Am J Physiol 1995; 269:C511–C518.
15. Jain L, Chen XJ, Brown LA, Eaton DC. Nitric oxide inhibits lung sodium transport through a cGMP-mediated inhibition of epithelial cation channels. Am J Physiol 1998; 274:L475–L484.

16. Yue G, Hu P, Oh Y, Jilling T, Shoemaker RL, Benos DJ, Cragoe EJ Jr, Matalon S. Culture-induced alterations in alveolar type II cell Na^+ conductance. Am J Physiol 1993; 265:C630–C640.
17. Ismailov II, Awayda MS, Jovov B, Berdiev BK, Fuller CM, Dedman JR, Kaetzel M, Benos DJ. Regulation of epithelial sodium channels by the cystic fibrosis transmembrane conductance regulator. J Biol Chem 1996; 271: 4725–4732.
18. Venkatesh VC, Katzberg HD. Glucocorticoid regulation of epithelial sodium channel genes in human fetal lung. Am J Physiol 1997; 273:L227–L233.
19. Berdiev BK, Prat AG, Cantiello HF, Ausiello DA, Fuller CM, Jovov B, Benos DJ, Ismailov II. Regulation of epithelial sodium channels by short actin filaments. J Biol Chem 1996; 271:17704–17710.
20. Ismailov II, Berdiev BK, Shlyonsky VG, Fuller CM, Prat AG, Jovov B, Cantiello HF, Ausiello DA, Benos DJ. Role of actin in regulation of epithelial sodium channels by CFTR. Am J Physiol 1997; 272:C1077–C1086.
21. Rotin D, Bar-Sagi D, O'Brodovich H, Merilainen J, Lehto VP, Canessa CM, Rossier BC, Downey GP. An SH3 binding region in the epithelial Na^+ channel (alpha rENaC) mediates its localization at the apical membrane. EMBO J 1994; 13:4440–4450.
22. Matthay MA, Wiener-Kronish JP. Intact epithelial barrier function is critical for the resolution of alveolar edema in humans. Am Rev Respir Dis 1990; 142:1250–1257.
23. Yue G, Matalon S. Mechanisms and sequelae of increased alveolar fluid clearance in hyperoxic rats. Am J Physiol 1997; 272:L407–L412.
24. Comellas AP, Pesce LM, Azzam Z, Saldias FJ, Sznajder JI. Scorpion venom decreases lung liquid clearance in rats. Am J Respir Crit Care Med 2003; 167:1064–1067.
25. Kerem E, Bistritzer T, Hanukoglu A, Hofmann T, Zhou Z, Bennett W, MacLaughlin E, Barker P, Nash M, Quittell L, Boucher R, Knowles MR. Pulmonary epithelial sodium-channel dysfunction and excess airway liquid in pseudohypoaldosteronism. N Engl J Med 1999; 341:156–162.
26. Malhotra A, Krilov LR. Influenza and respiratory syncytial virus. Update on infection, management, and prevention. Pediatr Clin North Am 2000; 47: 353–72, vi–vii.
27. Lambert LC, Trummell HQ, Singh A, Cassell GH, Bridges RJ. *Mycoplasma pulmonis* inhibits electrogenic ion transport across murine tracheal epithelial cell monolayers. Infect Immun 1998; 66:272–279.
28. Graham A, Steel DM, Wilson R, Cole PJ, Alton EW, Geddes DM. Effects of purified *Pseudomonas* rhamnolipids on bioelectric properties of sheep tracheal epithelium. Exp Lung Res 1993; 19:77–89.
29. Stutts MJ, Schwab JH, Chen MG, Knowles MR, Boucher RC. Effects of *Pseudomonas aeruginosa* on bronchial epithelial ion transport. Am Rev Respir Dis 1986; 134:17–21.
30. Zhang M, Kim KJ, Iyer D, Lin Y, Belisle J, McEnery K, Crandall ED, Barnes PF. Effects of *Mycobacterium tuberculosis* on the bioelectric properties of the alveolar epithelium. Infect Immunol 1997; 65:692–698.

31. Kunzelmann K, Beesley AH, King NJ, Karupiah G, Young JA, Cook DI. Influenza virus inhibits amiloride-sensitive Na^+ channels in respiratory epithelia. Proc Natl Acad Sci USA 2000; 97:10282–10287.
32. Rezaiguia S, Garat C, Delclaux C, Meignan M, Fleury J, Legrand P, Matthay MA, Jayr C. Acute bacterial pneumonia in rats increases alveolar epithelial fluid clearance by a tumor necrosis factor-alpha-dependent mechanism. J Clin Invest 1997; 99:325–335.
33. Garat C, Rezaiguia S, Meignan M, D'Ortho MP, Harf A, Matthay MA, Jayr C. Alveolar endotoxin increases alveolar clearance in rats. J Appl Physiol 1995; 79:2021–2028.
34. Davis IC, Sullender WM, Hickman-Davis JM, Lindsey JR, Matalon S. Nucleotide-mediated inhibition of alveolar fluid clearance in BALB/c mice following respiratory syncytial virus infection. Am J Physiol Lung Cell Mol Physiol 2004; 286:L112–L120.
35. Homolya L, Steinberg TH, Boucher RC. Cell to cell communication in response to mechanical stress via bilateral release of ATP and UTP in polarized epithelia. J Cell Biol 2000; 150:1349–1360.
36. Lazarowski ER, Boucher RC. UTP as an extracellular signaling molecule. News Physiol Sci 2001; 16:1–5.
37. Burnstock G, Williams M. P2 purinergic receptors: modulation of cell function and therapeutic potential. J Pharmacol Exp Ther 2000; 295:862–869.
38. Kishore BK, Ginns SM, Krane CM, Nielsen S, Knepper MA. Cellular localization of $P2Y_2$ purinoceptor in rat renal inner medulla and lung. Am J Physiol Renal Physiol 2000; 278:F43–F51.
39. Inglis SK, Collett A, McAlroy HL, Wilson SM, Olver RE. Effect of luminal nucleotides on Cl^- secretion and Na^+ absorption in distal bronchi. Pflügers Arch 1999; 438:621–627.
40. Inglis SK, Olver RE, Wilson SM. Differential effects of UTP and ATP on ion transport in porcine tracheal epithelium. Br J Pharmacol 2000; 130:367–374.
41. Iwase N, Sasaki T, Shimura S, Yamamoto M, Suzuki S, Shirato K. ATP-induced Cl secretion with suppressed Na^+ absorption in rabbit tracheal epithelium. Respir Physiol 1997; 107:173–180.
42. Mall M, Wissner A, Gonska T, Calenborn D, Kuehr J, Brandis M, Kunzelmann K. Inhibition of amiloride-sensitive epithelial Na^+ absorption by extracellular nucleotides in human normal and cystic fibrosis airways. Am J Respir Cell Mol Biol 2000; 23:755–761.
43. Knowles MR, Clarke LL, Boucher RC. Activation by extracellular nucleotides of chloride secretion in the airway epithelia of patients with cystic fibrosis. N Engl J Med 1991; 325:533–538.
44. Olivier KN, Bennett WD, Hohneker KW, Zeman KL, Edwards LJ, Boucher RC, Knowles MR. Acute safety and effects on mucociliary clearance of aerosolized uridine 5′-triphosphate +/− amiloride in normal human adults. Am J Respir Crit Care Med 1996; 154:217–223.
45. Ling BN, Eaton DC. Effects of luminal Na^+ on single Na^+ channels in A6 cells, a regulatory role for protein kinase C. Am J Physiol 1989; 256: F1094–F1103.

46. Awayda MS, Ismailov II, Berdiev BK, Fuller CM, Benos DJ. Protein kinase regulation of a cloned epithelial Na^+ channel. J Gen Physiol 1996; 108:49–65.
47. Stockand JD, Bao HF, Schenck J, Malik B, Middleton P, Schlanger LE, Eaton DC. Differential effects of protein kinase C on the levels of epithelial Na^+ channel subunit proteins. J Biol Chem 2000; 275:25760–25765.
48. Staub O, Gautschi I, Ishikawa T, Breitschopf K, Ciechanover A, Schild L, Rotin D. Regulation of stability and function of the epithelial Na^+ channel (ENaC) by ubiquitination. EMBO J 1997; 16:6325–6336.
49. Malik B, Schlanger L, Al Khalili O, Bao HF, Yue G, Price SR, Mitch WE, Eaton DC. ENaC degradation in A6 cells by the ubiquitin-proteosome proteolytic pathway. J Biol Chem 2001; 276:12903–12910.
50. Hochstrasser M. Ubiquitin, proteasomes, and the regulation of intracellular protein degradation. Curr Opin Cell Biol 1995; 7:215–223.
51. Staub O, Abriel H, Plant P, Ishikawa T, Kanelis V, Saleki R, Horisberger JD, Schild L, Rotin D. Regulation of the epithelial Na^+ channel by Nedd4 and ubiquitination. Kidney Int 2000; 57:809–815.
52. Brochard L, Lemaire F. Tidal volume, positive end-expiratory pressure, and mortality in acute respiratory distress syndrome. Crit Care Med 1999; 27: 1661–1663.
53. Abriel H, Loffing J, Rebhun JF, Pratt JH, Schild L, Horisberger JD, Rotin D, Staub O. Defective regulation of the epithelial Na^+ channel by Nedd4 in Liddle's syndrome. J Clin Invest 1999; 103:667–673.
54. Shimkets RA, Lifton R, Canessa CM. In vivo phosphorylation of the epithelial sodium channel. Proc Natl Acad Sci USA 1998; 95:3301–3305.
55. Duvall MD, Zhu S, Fuller CM, Matalon S. Peroxynitrite inhibits amiloride-sensitive Na^+ currents in *Xenopus* oocytes expressing α, β, γ-rENaC. Am J Physiol 1998; 274:C1417–C1423.
56. Guo Y, Duvall MD, Crow JP, Matalon S. Nitric oxide inhibits Na^+ absorption across cultured alveolar type II monolayers. Am J Physiol 1998; 274: L369–L377.
57. Hu P, Ischiropoulos H, Beckman JS, Matalon S. Peroxynitrite inhibition of oxygen consumption and sodium transport in alveolar type II cells. Am J Physiol 1994; 266:L628–L634.
58. Nielsen VG, Baird MS, Chen L, Matalon S. DETANONOate, a nitric oxide donor, decreases amiloride-sensitive alveolar fluid clearance in rabbits. Am J Respir Crit Care Med 2000; 161:1154–1160.
59. Sznajder JI, Olivera W, Ridge KM, Rutschman DH, Olivera WG, Ridge KM. Mechanisms of lung liquid clearance during hyperoxia in isolated rat lungs. Am J Respir Crit Care Med 1995; 151:1519–1525.
60. Youssef JA, Thibeault DW, Rezaiekhaligh MH, Mabry SM, Norberg MI, Truog WE. Influence of inhaled nitric oxide and hyperoxia on Na,K-ATPase expression and lung edema in newborn piglets. Biol Neonate 1999; 75:199–209.
61. Beckman JS, Koppenol WH. Nitric oxide, superoxide, and peroxynitrite: the good, the bad, and the ugly. Am J Physiol 1996; 271:C1424–C1437.
62. Haddad IY, Pataki G, Hu P, Galliani C, Beckman JS, Matalon S. Quantitation of nitrotyrosine levels in lung sections of patients and animals with acute lung injury. J Clin Invest 1994; 94:2407–2413.

63. Davis IC, Zajac AJ, Nolte KB, Botten J, Hjelle B, Matalon S. Elevated generation of reactive oxygen/nitrogen species in hantavirus cardiopulmonary syndrome. J Virol 2002; 76:8347–8359.
64. Modelska K, Matthay MA, Pittet JF. Inhibition of inducible NO synthase activity (iNOS) after prolonged hemorrhagic shock attenuates oxidant-mediated decrease in alveolar epithelial fluid transport in rats. FASEB J 1998; 12:A39.
65. Galietta LJ, Folli C, Marchetti C, Romano L, Carpani D, Conese M, Zegarra-Moran O. Modification of transepithelial ion transport in human cultured bronchial epithelial cells by interferon-gamma. Am J Physiol Lung Cell Mol Physiol 2000; 278:L1186–L1194.
66. Galietta LJ, Pagesy P, Folli C, Caci E, Romio L, Costes B, Nicolis E, Cabrini G, Goossens M, Ravazzolo R, Zegarra-Moran O. IL-4 is a potent modulator of ion transport in the human bronchial epithelium in vitro. J Immunol 2002; 168:839–845.
67. Fukuda N, Jayr C, Lazrak A, Wang Y, Lucas R, Matalon S, Matthay MA. Mechanisms of TNF-α stimulation of amiloride-sensitive sodium transport across alveolar epithelium. Am J Physiol Lung Cell Mol Physiol 2001; 280: L1258–L1265.
68. Dagenais A, Frechette R, Yamagata Y, Yamagata T, Carmel JF, Clermont ME, Brochiero E, Masse C, Berthiaume Y. Downregulation of ENaC activity and expression by TNFα in alveolar epithelial cells. Am J Physiol Lung Cell Mol Physiol, in press, 2004.
69. Compeau CG, Rotstein OD, Tohda H, Marunaka Y, Rafii B, Slutsky AS, O'Brodovich H. Endotoxin-stimulated alveolar macrophages impair lung epithelial Na^+ transport by an L-Arg-dependent mechanism. Am J Physiol 1994; 266:C1330–C1341.
70. Ding JW, Dickie J, O'Brodovich H, Shintani Y, Rafii B, Hackam D, Marunaka Y, Rotstein OD. Inhibition of amiloride-sensitive sodium-channel activity in distal lung epithelial cells by nitric oxide. Am J Physiol 1998; 274:L378–L387.

Dave MH, [illegible] Geiser T, [illegible] Matthay [illegible] [illegible] J [illegible] 2002; [illegible]

[illegible] activity [illegible] channel [illegible] Am J Physiol [illegible]

30. [illegible] transport [illegible] Am J Physiol [illegible]

[illegible]

[illegible]

[illegible]

10

Voltage-Dependent Na^+ Channels in Pulmonary Vascular Smooth Muscle Cells

Kenji Kitamura and Hirosi Kuriyama
Fukuoka Dental College, Seinan Jogakuin University, Fukuoka, Japan

I. INTRODUCTION

The voltage-dependent Na channel is one of the principal protein molecules controlling excitability in a variety of excitable cells (including neurons and skeletal and cardiac muscle cells). In these cells, the voltage-dependent Na current, which is fast-activated and -inactivated, triggers action potentials. As a result of its electrophysiological properties, the membrane potential in these excitable cells can be kept at a low level (i.e., more negative) while still allowing voltage-dependent channel activation. It was long believed that fast Na channels did not exist in smooth muscle cells (SMCs), because action potentials were not blocked by tetrodotoxin (TTX), the puffer-fish toxin, but were inhibited by Ca channel blockers or by removal of extracellular Ca ions (1). However, application of the single-cell voltage-clamp method to dispersed cells, as in electrophysiological research carried out on SMCs in the early 1980s, revealed voltage-dependent Na channels to be present after all, and these channels have been commonly observed in neurons and cardiac muscle cells. The first to report the presence of a voltage-dependent Na current were Amédée et al. (2) (in the pregnant rat myometrium on the basis of a binding assay) and Sturek and Hermsmeyer (3) (who directly demonstrated the presence of a fast Na current in rat cultured SMCs from the azygos vein). Soon afterward, we detected a highly

TTX-sensitive Na current in freshly dispersed pulmonary arterial SMCs from mature rabbits (4). Since then, the presence of fast Na channels has been reported in various SMCs, in addition to the above tissues [human colon (5), human aorta and coronary artery (6), human esophageal cells (7), rat portal vein (8), rat vena cava (9), rat colon (5), guinea pig ureter (10), pig aorta and coronary artery (6), rabbit aorta and coronary artery (6)]. Now, although the presence of fast Na channels in various SMCs is beyond doubt, the role played by these channels remains uncertain, largely because many SMCs have a high membrane potential (i.e., more positive), at which Na channels are readily inactivated.

II. ELECTROPHYSIOLOGICAL EVIDENCE FOR VOLTAGE-DEPENDENT Na CHANNELS IN SMOOTH MUSCLE CELLS

A wide range of TTX sensitivities have been reported for fast Na currents in various SMCs (see Table 1). The voltage-dependent Na currents found in rat azygos vein and then in rabbit pulmonary artery are, respectively, the Na currents least and most sensitive to TTX reported so far (3,4). The TTX-sensitive Na current recorded in rabbit pulmonary arterial SMCs shows rapid inactivation and disappears within 10 ms. Application of a nanomolar concentration of TTX reduces the current amplitude without changing the current decay. In this arterial cell, the Na current may be inactivated at the resting membrane potential level, and it may be masked by the large Ca influx through voltage-dependent Ca channels because the TTX-sensitive Na current can be detected only in Ca-free solution (4) (Fig. 1). In the rat azygos vein, the Na current is prominent (4–5 times larger than the Ca current) but is completely inactivated at the resting membrane potential (−45 mV) (3). Although the IC_{50} value for the effect of TTX was not obtained accurately for all of the SMCs listed in Table 1, the IC_{50} values estimated from the dose–response relationship were less than 100 nM in several SMCs [similar to the values for the neuronal type of Na channels (TTX-sensitive Na channels)]. Comparative studies have shown that a larger amplitude fast Na current is observed in fewer pulmonary artery SMCs than coronary arterial SMCs (6). The same authors also demonstrated species differences in both current amplitude and the probability of Na channels existing in a cell (Fig. 2).

Recent advances in molecular biology as applied to voltage-dependent Na channels have revealed the presence of more than 10 voltage-dependent Na channel genes, and some of them are expressed in SMCs (Table 2). For example, both TTX-sensitive and -resistant Na channels have been found to be expressed in human esophageal SMCs ($Na_V1.4$ and $Na_V1.5$), as has a novel TTX-resistant Na channel (Na_X) (7). In pulmonary artery SMCs, the mRNA for a TTX-resistant Na channel ($Na_V1.5$) has been found to physiological Properties of Fast Na Current Recorded in Smooth Muscle Cells.

	V-half		
	Inactivation	Activation	IC_{50} (TTX)
	≈–60 mV	≈–20 mV	30 µM
artery	–65 mV	≈–25 mV	8.7 nM
y artery	—	–25 mV	<1 µM
y	—	–33.5 mV	<100 nM
artery	–44 mV	–25 mV	<1 µM
	—	–25 mV	<1 µM
	—	–22 mV	<100 nM
	–74.5 mV	–36.1 mV	130 nM
	–69.5 mV	–21.8 mV	14 nM
DDT_1 MF-2)	–40 mV	≈ –10 mV	150–200 nM
rcoma cell	–68.5 mV (S cell)	–15.1 mV (S cell)	47.1 nM (S cell)
	–73.4 mV (SF cell)	–18.0 mV (SF cell)	67.5 nM (SF cell)
	—	—	900 nM
ant)	–64 mV	≈–25 mV	27 nM <1 µM
	–59 mV	–21.1 mV	
l cells	–67 mV	–16 mV	20 nM

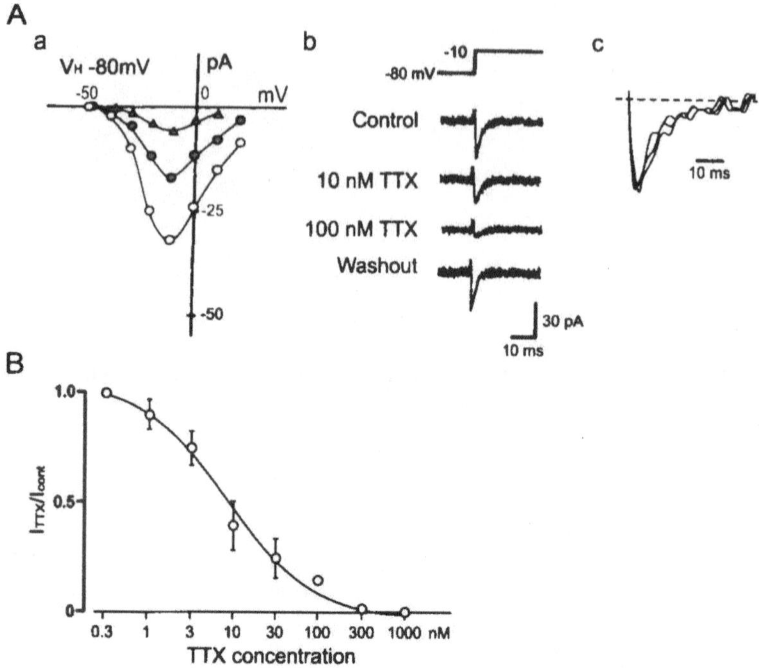

Figure 1 Effects of TTX on the Na current in rabbit main pulmonary artery in Ca-free solution. (A): I–V curves obtained in the presence [(Δ), 100 nM; (•) 10 nM] or absence (o) of TTX. (Ab) Traces of the Na current itself. (B) Relationship between TTX concentration and relative amplitude of Na current. The current was evoked by a depolarizing pulse to −10 mV from a holding potential of −80 mV. (Reproduced from Ref. 4, with permission.)

be expressed (11), although expression of the mRNA may not directly correspond to a functional expression of Na channel proteins. Be that as it may, the above results reinforce the existence of TTX-sensitive Na channels in smooth muscle cells. Molecular identification of any TTX-sensitive Na channels present in pulmonary artery SMCs should be a subject for future research, because no expression of TTX-sensitive Na channels has yet been identified in this tissue (11).

III. STRUCTURE AND FUNCTION OF VOLTAGE-DEPENDENT Na CHANNELS

Voltage-dependent Na channels are transmembrane proteins composed of α and β subunits. The former consists of approximately 1700–2000 amino acids and the latter of approximately 200 amino acids. Although more than 30 subtypes of α subunits have been identified in various species, all Na

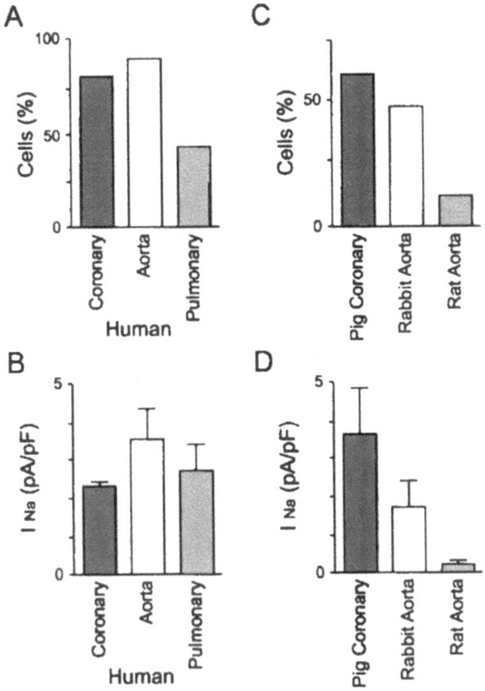

Figure 2 Probability of existence and average densities of Na current in human pulmonary and coronary arterial cells and aortic smooth muscle cells in various species. The Na current was evoked by a depolarizing pulse to −10 mV from a holding potential of −100 mV. (Reproduced from Ref. 6, with permission.)

channels (except for a few channel proteins) have been classified into a single family, called Na_V1 in the latest nomenclature published for Na channel α subunits (12). At present, Na_V1 is divided into nine subtypes; $Na_V1.1$ to $Na_V1.9$. The phylogenetic tree proposed by Goldin (12) shows that $Na_V1.1$, $Na_V1.2$, and $Na_V1.3$ are genetically close, where the members of the Na_V1 family are divided into two main groups: TTX-sensitive ($Na_V1.1$–$Na_V1.4$, $Na_V1.6$, $Na_V1.7$) and TTX-resistant ($Na_V1.5$, $Na_V1.8$, $Na_V1.9$) channels (Fig. 3). All channels have four homologous domains (domains I–IV), each with six hydrophobic transmembrane regions (S1–S6); (Fig. 4). The TTX sensitivity of voltage-dependent Na channels is thought to be determined by the amino acid sequences in the S5–S6 linker region of each domain (13–16). In Particularly, in the SS2 region of domain I, a mutation of a negatively charged glutamate (E at position 387 in the rat brain type II Na channel) to an uncharged glutamine (Q), serine (S), or tyrosine (Y) leads to a complete loss of TTX sensitivity (Fig. 5) (13,14).

nclature Used for Na Channels and their Distribution in Smooth Muscle Tissues

ne type	TTX sensitivity	Distribution in smooth muscle tissues	Distribution in othe tissues
N1A	Sensitive		CNS, heart, skeletal
N2A	Sensitive		Brain, CNS, heart, s
N3A	Sensitive	Intestine	CNS, skeletal musc
N4A	Sensitive	Esophagus	Skeletal muscle, hea
N5A	Resistant	Esophagus, pulmonary artery	Heart, denervated sk
N8A	Sensitive		Neurons, glia
N9A	Sensitive		Peripheral neurons
N10A	Resistant		DRG, trigeminal ga
N11A	Resistant		DRG, trigeminal ga
N6A, SCN7A	Resistant	Esophagus(distal), pulmonary artery	Heart
N7A	Resistant	Lung, intestine	Astrocyte, DRG, sp medulla pons, mi
N6A	Resistant	Uterus	Cardiac atria and ve
N6A	Resistant		
N7A	Resistant	Uterus	
N7A	Resistant	Lung, intestine, bladder, vas deferens	Sciatic nerve, pituita

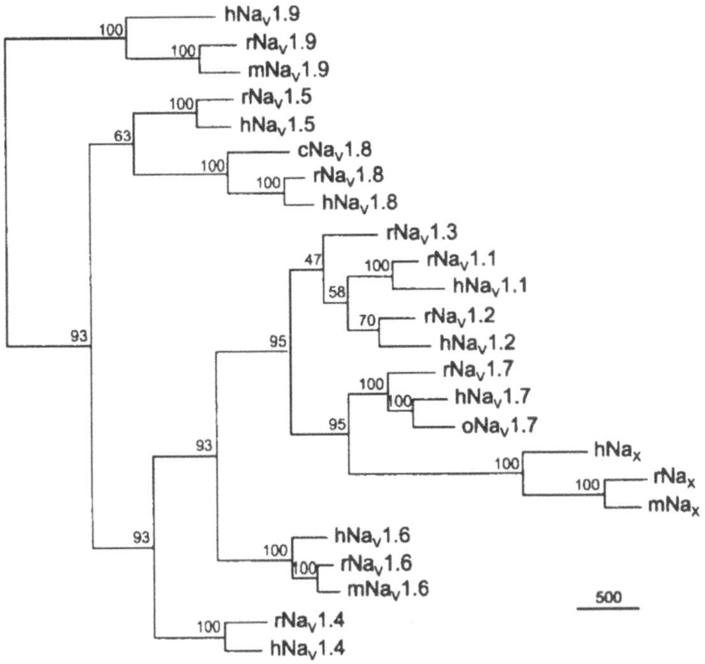

Figure 3 Proposed phylogenetic tree for mammalian fast Na channel α subunits. The scale bar represents 500 substitutions, and the numbers at the nodes indicate the bootstrap values for 100 replications. Single-letter prefixes indicate species of origin: h, *Homo sapiens* (human); r, *Rattus norvegicus* (rat); m, *Mus musculus* (mouse); c, *Canis familialis* (dog); o, *Orictolagus cuniculus* (rabbit). (Reproduced from Ref. 2, with permission.)

This negative charge may be essential for interaction with a positively charged amino radical in the TTX molecule. It has been reported that the Na channels obtained from cardiac muscle are more than 100 times as resistant to TTX as those in the brain (17). The amino acid sequences in the SS2 region showed a difference of only two amino acids between brain- and cardiac-type Na channels [phenylalanine (F) at 385 and asparagine (N) at 388 in the brain type being replaced by cysteine (C) and arginine (R), respectively, in the cardiac type] (see amino acid sequences for $Na_v1.1$–1.3 and $Na_V1.5$ in Fig. 5). A functional expression of a point mutation of the phenylalanine (F) at 385 or the asparagine (N) at 388 showed that a mutation of the former site to cysteine (C) was essential to produce a reduction in TTX sensitivity, whereas replacement of asparagine (N) at 388 by arginine (R) did not change the TTX sensitivity (18). Indeed, Ca channels, typical TTX-insensitive channels, possess an uncharged polar amino acid, threonine (T), in the SS2 region instead of glutamate (E). These pieces of evidence

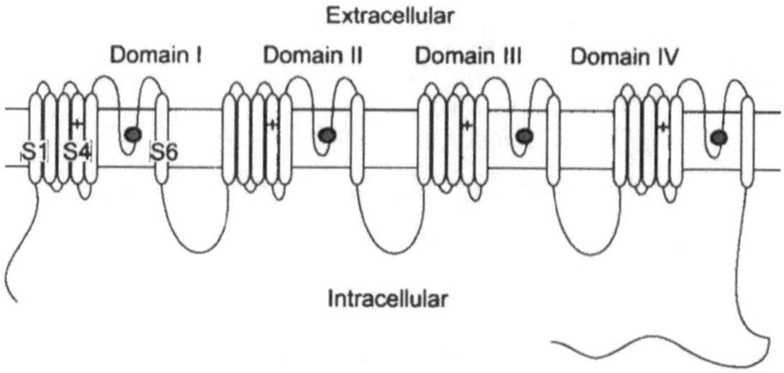

Figure 4 Schematic model of voltage-dependent Na channel α subunit. Both N and C terminals are located on the cytosolic side, and 24 transmembrane-spanning regions are present. Transmembrane-spanning regions are clustered in groups of six, and each cluster is called a domain. The six transmembrane regions in each domain are named S1–S6 segments (starting from the N-terminal side), and the amino acid chains between domains and between segments are called the linkers. The extracellular linkers S5–S6 are relatively long and contain SS-1 and SS-2 regions, which form the P-region (pore region). In the S4 segment in each domain, positively charged amino acids, arginine (R) and lysine (K), are regularly arranged; these segments are indicated by (+) in this figure. Circles indicate presumed TTX-binding sites.

indicate that a negatively charged amino acid (E) at this position [next to tryptophan (W)] is essential for TTX binding, and replacement of aromatic amino acids [phenylalanine (F) and tyrosine (Y)] with smaller ones [cysteine (C) and serine (S)] probably modifies the alignment in this region and so weakens the TTX binding.

Voltage sensing for channel opening and closing is a property of the S4 transmembrane segment in all domains (19). In this region, positively

				-											+								-				
$Na_V1.1$	T	S	F	D	T	F	S	W	A	F	L	S	L	F	R	L	M	T	Q	D	F	W	E	N	L	Y	Q
$Na_V1.2$	T	S	F	D	T	F	S	W	A	F	L	S	L	F	R	L	M	T	Q	D	F	W	E	N	L	Y	Q
$Na_V1.3$	T	S	F	D	T	F	S	W	A	F	L	S	L	F	R	L	M	T	Q	D	Y	W	E	N	L	Y	Q
$Na_V1.4$	T	S	Y	D	T	F	S	W	A	F	L	A	L	F	R	L	M	T	Q	D	Y	W	E	N	L	F	Q
$Na_V1.5$	T	S	F	D	S	F	A	W	A	F	L	A	L	F	R	L	M	T	Q	D	C	W	E	R	L	Y	Q
$Na_V1.6$	T	S	F	D	T	F	S	W	A	F	L	A	L	F	R	L	M	T	Q	D	Y	W	E	N	L	Y	Q
$Na_V1.7$	T	S	F	D	T	F	S	W	A	F	L	A	L	F	R	L	M	T	Q	D	Y	W	E	N	L	Y	Q
$Na_V1.8$	T	S	F	D	S	F	A	W	A	F	L	S	L	F	R	L	M	T	Q	D	S	W	E	R	L	Y	Q
$Na_V1.9$	T	N	F	D	N	F	G	W	S	F	L	A	M	F	R	L	M	T	Q	D	S	W	E	K	L	Y	Q
Na_X	T	N	F	D	S	F	G	W	A	L	F	A	L	F	R	L	M	A	Q	D	Y	P	E	V	L	Y	H

← SS1 → ← SS2 →

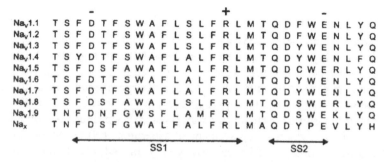

Figure 5 Amino acid sequences of S5–S6 linker region of domain I in mammalian Na channels. Each amino acid is represented by a single letter.

charged amino acids [arginine (R) or lysine (K)] are regularly aligned, but no negatively charged residue is present (Fig. 6), and the number of positively charged residues is much larger than in other transmembrane segments. Membrane depolarization reduces the electrical force between the positive charge on the inner basic residues of S4 and the negative charge on circumferential structures, and the S4 segment then rotates through 60°, which produces a 0.5 nm extrusion in the extracellular direction (20). Although neutralization of arginine (R) at the most extracellular projection of the S4 segment of domain I does not shift the *V* half-value for activation, neutralization of deeper positions in domains I and II causes a shift in the *V* half-value for activation in the positive direction, suggesting that these positively charged amino acids are important for the voltage sensing necessary for channel opening (19). However, the mechanisms involved in channel activation (and also inactivation) are quite complicated phenomena, because replacement of leucine (L), a nonpolar amino acid, by phenylalanine (F), another nonpolar amino acid with an aromatic ring, can modify the channel kinetics (21). Because replacement of the tyrosine (T) near the inner linker between domains III and IV by glutamine (Q) increases the rate of channel activation, an interaction among the S4 voltage ensor, the channel pore, and the III–IV linker would seem to be essential for channel activation (22).

The isoleucine–phenylalanine–methionine (IFM) motif in the domain III–IV linker is thought to be essential for fast channel inactivation of both TTX-sensitive and -resistant Na channels (15,23). In this region, all Na channels, except for Na_X, have almost identical sequences, and this is characterized by the presence of clustering basic, acidic, and nonpolar amino acids (Fig. 7). Replacement of phenylalanine (F) by glutamine (Q) in the III–IV inner linker produces sustained channel opening, where as replacement of the neighboring isoleucine (I) and methionine (M) by glutamine (Q) and phenylalanine (F) completely abolishes the current inactivation (23). These pieces of evidence indicated that the cluster of hydrophobic amino acids forms an inactivation particle, and a shift of the S4 segment by voltage depolarization or hyperpolarization either changed the hydrophobic properties near the channel pore or interfered with clusters of charged amino acids near the particle, or both. Replacement of hydrophobic amino acids (IFM) by uncharged hydrophilic ones may cause failure to form an inactivation particle. A pair of glycines (G) and a cluster of proline (P) residues, which form molecular hinges, are present within the linker near domains IIIS6 and IVS1 (24). A pair of tyrosine (Y) residues near the IFM motif is thought to be important for channel inactivation (22) because substitution of the two tyrosine residues by glutamine (Q) eliminates inactivation and also reduces the steady-state inactivation. Because phenylalanine (F) could replace tyrosine in this case, the hydrophobic properties or the molecular size of the amino acids near the inactivation particle would seem to be very important for channel inactivation.

Domain I

$Na_V1.1$	A	L	R	T	F	R	V	L	R	A	L	K	T	I	S	V	I	P	G	L
$Na_V1.2$	A	L	R	T	F	R	V	L	R	A	L	K	T	I	S	V	I	P	G	L
$Na_V1.3$	A	L	R	T	F	R	V	L	R	A	L	K	T	I	S	V	I	P	G	L
$Na_V1.4$	A	L	R	T	F	R	V	L	R	A	L	K	T	I	T	V	I	P	G	L
$Na_V1.5$	A	L	R	T	F	R	V	L	R	A	L	K	T	I	S	V	I	S	G	L
$Na_V1.6$	A	L	R	T	F	R	V	L	R	A	L	K	T	I	S	V	I	P	G	L
$Na_V1.7$	A	L	R	T	F	R	V	L	R	A	L	K	T	I	S	V	I	P	G	L
$Na_V1.8$	G	L	R	T	F	R	V	L	R	A	L	K	T	V	S	V	I	P	G	L
$Na_V1.9$	T	L	R	T	F	R	V	L	R	A	L	K	A	I	S	V	I	S	G	L
Na_x	T	L	Q	T	A	R	T	L	R	I	L	K	I	I	P	L	N	Q	G	L
-			+			+			+			+								

Domain II

$Na_V1.1$	V	L	R	S	F	R	L	L	R	V	F	K	L	A	K	S	W	P	T	L
$Na_V1.2$	V	L	R	S	F	R	L	L	R	V	F	K	L	A	K	S	W	P	T	L
$Na_V1.3$	V	L	R	S	F	R	L	L	R	V	F	K	L	A	K	S	W	P	T	L
$Na_V1.4$	V	L	R	S	F	R	L	L	R	V	F	K	L	A	K	S	W	P	T	L
$Na_V1.5$	V	L	R	S	F	R	L	L	R	V	F	K	L	A	K	S	W	P	T	L
$Na_V1.6$	V	L	R	S	F	R	L	L	R	V	F	K	L	A	K	S	W	P	T	L
$Na_V1.7$	V	L	R	S	F	R	L	L	R	V	F	K	L	A	K	S	W	P	T	L
$Na_V1.8$	V	L	R	T	L	R	L	L	R	V	F	K	L	A	K	S	W	P	T	L
$Na_V1.9$	F	L	A	S	L	R	V	L	R	V	F	K	L	A	K	S	W	P	T	L
Na_x	L	L	R	L	F	R	M	L	R	I	F	K	L	G	K	Y	W	P	T	F
			+			+			+			+			+					

Domain III

$Na_V1.1$	L	G	A	I	K	S	L	R	T	L	R	A	L	R	P	L	R	A	L	S	R	F
$Na_V1.2$	L	G	A	I	K	S	L	R	T	L	R	A	L	R	P	L	R	A	L	S	R	F
$Na_V1.3$	L	G	A	I	K	S	L	R	T	L	R	A	L	R	P	L	R	A	L	S	R	F
$Na_V1.4$	L	G	P	I	K	S	L	R	T	L	R	A	L	R	P	L	R	A	L	S	R	F
$Na_V1.5$	M	G	P	I	K	S	L	R	T	L	R	A	L	R	P	L	R	A	L	S	R	F
$Na_V1.6$	L	G	A	I	K	S	L	R	T	L	R	A	L	R	P	L	R	A	L	S	R	F
$Na_V1.7$	L	G	P	I	K	S	L	R	T	L	R	A	L	R	P	L	R	A	L	S	R	F
$Na_V1.8$	V	A	S	I	K	A	L	R	T	L	R	A	L	R	P	L	R	A	L	S	R	F
$Na_V1.9$	L	P	N	L	K	S	F	R	N	L	R	A	L	R	P	L	R	A	L	S	G	F
Na_x	L	-	-	-	K	P	L	I	S	M	K	F	L	R	P	L	R	V	L	S	Q	F
					+			+			+			+			+				+	

Domain IV

$Na_V1.1$	R	V	I	R	L	A	R	I	G	R	I	L	R	L	I	K	G	A	K	G	I	R
$Na_V1.2$	R	V	I	R	L	A	R	I	G	R	I	L	R	L	I	K	G	A	K	G	I	R
$Na_V1.3$	R	V	I	R	L	A	R	I	G	R	V	L	R	L	I	K	G	A	K	G	I	R
$Na_V1.4$	R	V	I	R	L	A	R	I	G	R	I	L	R	L	I	R	G	A	K	G	I	R
$Na_V1.5$	R	V	I	R	L	A	R	I	G	R	I	L	R	L	I	R	G	A	K	G	I	R
$Na_V1.6$	R	V	I	R	L	A	R	I	G	R	I	L	R	L	I	K	G	A	K	G	I	R
$Na_V1.7$	R	V	I	R	L	A	R	I	G	R	I	L	R	L	I	K	G	A	K	G	I	R
$Na_V1.8$	R	V	I	R	L	A	R	I	G	R	I	L	R	L	I	R	A	A	K	G	I	R
$Na_V1.9$	R	I	V	R	L	A	R	I	G	R	I	L	R	L	V	R	A	A	R	G	I	R
Na_x	Q	L	I	L	L	S	R	I	I	H	M	L	R	L	G	K	G	P	K	V	F	H
	+			+			+			+			+			+			+			+

Figure 6 Amino acid sequences of S4 transmembrane regions in each domain.

$Na_V1.1$	D	N	F	N	Q	Q	K	K	K	F	G	G	R	D	I	F	M	T	E	E	Q	K	K	Y	Y	N	A	M	K
$Na_V1.2$	D	N	F	N	Q	Q	K	K	K	F	G	G	Q	D	I	F	M	T	E	E	Q	K	K	Y	Y	N	A	M	K
$Na_V1.3$	D	N	F	R	Q	Q	K	K	K	F	G	G	Q	D	I	F	M	T	E	E	Q	K	K	Y	Y	N	A	M	K
$Na_V1.4$	D	N	F	N	Q	Q	K	K	K	F	G	G	K	D	I	F	M	T	E	E	Q	K	K	Y	Y	N	A	M	K
$Na_V1.5$	D	N	F	N	Q	Q	K	K	K	L	G	G	Q	D	I	F	M	T	E	E	Q	K	K	Y	Y	N	A	M	K
$Na_V1.6$	D	N	F	N	Q	Q	K	K	K	F	G	G	Q	D	I	F	M	T	E	E	Q	K	K	Y	Y	N	A	M	K
$Na_V1.7$	D	N	F	N	Q	Q	K	K	K	L	G	G	Q	D	I	F	M	T	E	E	Q	K	K	Y	Y	N	A	M	K
$Na_V1.8$	D	N	F	N	Q	A	K	K	K	L	G	G	Q	D	I	F	M	T	E	E	Q	K	K	Y	Y	N	A	M	K
$Na_V1.9$	D	N	F	N	Q	Q	Q	K	K	L	G	G	Q	D	V	F	M	T	E	E	Q	K	K	Y	Y	N	A	M	K
Na_X	D	N	F	N	K	H	K	K	I	L	G	G	X	N	I	F	I	T	V	K	Q	R	K	Q	Y	R	R	L	K
	-						+	+	+						↔				-	-		+	+						+

Figure 7 Amino acid sequences of the domain III–IV linker region in Na channels.

Was found first in human heart and uterus ($Na_V2.1$) (25) and in rat astrocytes (Na-G) (26), Na_X channel-like proteins have a unique sequence profile. In terms of sequence homology, Na_X is about 50% identical to Na_V1, and there are significant differences even in the most conserved regions, such as the transmembrane regions. One of the important differences that distinguish Na_X from ordinal Na_V1 channels is the presence of fewer positively charged residues in the S4 segments in Na_X. Arginine (R), positioned at the most extracellular projection of the S4 segment of domain I in Na_V1, is replaced by glutamine (Q) in Na_X. As mentioned above, neutralization of this position in $Na_V1.2$ by site-directed mutagenesis did not change the voltage dependence of channel activation (19), suggesting that a change in this position to glutamine (Q) might not alter the voltage dependence. The S4 segment of domain IV in Na_V1 has eight positively charged residues, whereas in Na_X two of these have mutated to neutral residues [glutamine (Q) and leucine (L)] and the rest are replaced by histidine (H), a basic amino acid that is not charged at a neutral pH (p*Ka* value of 6.5). Furthermore, in Na_X the phenylalanine (F) in the IMF motif, which is important for channel inactivation, is also mutated to isoleucine (I), and the neighboring acidic residues [aspartate (D) and glutamate (E)] are missing, suggesting that voltage-dependent channel inactivation may also be modified.

An expression of the mRNA for the Na_X channel has been found in neural tissues (such as sciatic nerve, pituitary, spinal cord, dorsal root ganglia, midbrain, medulla pons), in cardiac muscle, and in smooth muscle tissues and epithelial tissues (such as lung, intestine, bladder, vas deferens, and uterus). Unfortunately, no functional expression has been demonstrated, but a recent in vivo experiment showed that the water-intake behavior of Na_X-knockout mice differed from that of normal mice (27). In that study, the preference for hypertonic salt solution intake seen in mice with a knockout of the Na_X gene did not change after 24 h of water deprivation, although normal mice reduced their intake of such hypertonic salt solution and so avoided developing a hypernatremic condition. Because both hypovolemic and hypernatremic conditions are essential for this abnormal behavior, the authors speculated that the Na_X channel protein may act as a Na concentration sensor in and/or Na-absorbing machinery from the extracellular space and thus contribute to the control of salt water balance (27).

Three types of β subunits (β1, β2, and β3) have been identified, and of these the β1 subunit is the most abundant. Makita et al. (28) showed that current inactivation and recovery were accelerated by coexpression of the β1 subunit with $Na_V1.4$ (striated muscle) but not with $Na_V1.5$ (cardiac muscle). Coexpression of the β1 subunit with $Na_V1.3$ also moderately hastened the current decay (29). Early studies suggested that the β1 subunit did not functionally modify the Na channels, because coexpression of this subunit (1) did not significantly modify the amplitude of the peak current and (2) only slightly reduced the probability of channel opening by membrane depolarization (28,29). On the other hand, coexpression of either the β1 or β3 subunit with $Na_V1.5$ (cardiac muscle) has been demonstrated to increase the efficiency of α-subunit transport to the plasma membrane (a chaperone-like property) (30). Fahmi et al.(30) reported that the β1 subunit hastened the recovery from inactivation more than the β3 subunit, whereas the β3, but not β1, subunit shifted the steady-state inactivation curve in the depolarization direction. Because the Na channel β subunits have sequences homologous to these of cell-adhesion molecules, roles for these subunits in cell–cell interaction or high-density clustering of Na channels in special regions, such as the node of Ranvier, have also been postulated (16,31,32). Although evidence of functional roles for the β subunits is accumulating, the molecular mechanisms have not been identified.

IV. PHYSIOLOGICAL IMPORTANCE OF VOLTAGE-DEPENDENT Na CHANNELS IN PULMONARY ARTERY AND OTHER SMOOTH MUSCLE CELLS

It is well known that the fast Na current is activated and inactivated at low membrane potentials. The resting membrane potential of SMCs, including pulmonary arterial SMCs, differs both among tissues and among species, but most have resting membrane potentials of around −60 to −50 mV, a level at which most Na channels are probably inactivated. However, a few exceptions have been reported. For example, the SMCs in mesenteric arteries (guinea pig and rabbit), renal artery (guinea pig), tail artery (rat), mesenteric vein (dog), and saphenous vein (rabbit) all possess lower resting membrane potentials than other SMCs (−70 mV) (1). In these tissues, more than half of the fast Na channel population is capable of activation by a small membrane depolarization, such as the excitatory junction potentials elicited by perivascular sympathetic nerve stimulation. However, there is no evidence indicating the presence of a TTX-sensitive component in action potentials or in local responses [guinea pig mesenteric artery (33)]. Thus, the physiological relevance of fast Na channels in vascular SMCs is somewhat doubtful. On the other hand, in dog and human stomachs an Na-sensitive component of action potentials has been demonstrated (34,35). Recently, Deshpande et al. (7) demonstrated that the action potential evoked by a depolarization pulse in human esophageal muscle cells was TTX-sensitive. This may be the first report to directly reveal Na-dependent action potentials in SMCs. Although this action potential in single esophageal SMCs was generated at low membrane potentials (−80 mV) and possibly communicated with the striated muscle cells in the middle of the esophagus, a substantial number of the fast Na channels may be in the resting state. Possibly, propagation of action potentials from the proximal region of the esophagus (striated muscle cells) depolarizes the membrane to trigger opening of the fast Na channels in the distal region (SMCs). Fast Na channels might also play such a role during the rebound excitation after certain large hyperpolarizations (caused, for example, by strong activation of inhibitory neurons). Actually, there is no clear evidence for a contribution of fast Na channels to rebound excitation in smooth muscle tissues, but in an early work in smooth muscle research, Kitamura (36) showed that TTX inhibited the rebound contraction that followed the sustained relaxation induced by stimulation of the inhibitory nerves serving rabbit jejunal smooth muscle tissues. Although we could not eliminate a possible contribution by delayed excitatory responses through the neural network in this case, reactivation of TTX-sensitive Na channels during the sustained relaxation is another and simpler explanation.

Pulmonary arterial cells have been reported to show relatively high resting membrane potentials in both main and intralobar pulmonary arteries (−52 to −57 mV) (37–39). Although a blockade of K conductance by TEA, 4-AP, or procaine evoked either an action potential or a local response on depolarizing-current stimulation, no action potential could be recorded under physiological ionic conditions (37,40), suggesting that the contribution of fast Na channels to membrane excitability may be insignificant in this tissue.

Although current inactivation of voltage-dependent Na channels is very fast, a small current flows continuously during the depolarization. There is a narrow membrane potential range within which weak channel activity is shown by a small number of Na channels, called the "window current", and this survives voltage-dependent channel inactivation. The relatively high membrane potentials shown by various smooth muscle cells owe much to their possession of higher values of Na and Cl conductance than those seen in striated and cardiac muscle cells. In the case of the rabbit main pulmonary artery, the ratio of Na permeability to K permeability in the resting state is 0.22 (40). Therefore, it is plausible that continuous opening of a small number of "surviving" Na channels at the resting membrane potential could contribute to the Na-dependent component of the membrane conductance. However, this is not particularly convincing, because (1) TTX does not change the resting membrane potential and (2) low Na solution does not hyperpolarize the membrane, even though such a hyperpolarization is theoretically predicted by the Hodgkin–Huxley–Goldman equation (40).

It is well known that different types of Na channels can be alternatively expressed during an individual's development (41–43). For example, muscle denervation has been shown to enhance the expression of a TTX-resistant ($Na_V1.5$) Na channel but reduce that of a TTX-sensitive Na channel ($Na_V1.4$) (42). Further, $Na_V1.3$ is known to be an embryonic Na channel, and its expression ceases in adult neurons except under such pathological conditions as nerve injury and axotomy (44). From these results, we can postulate that expression of fast Na channels in smooth muscle tissues occurs in some specific situations, such as pathological or developmental conditions. Indeed, most reports that have demonstrated fast Na channels in smooth muscle cells have used cultured cells, myometrial cells obtained in pregnancy, or cells stored in a "power soup" containing various amino acids. The fast TTX-sensitive Na channels observed in rabbit pulmonary arterial and rat or human colonic SMCs are the only exception, having been recorded in freshly isolated cells without cultivation (4,5). Interestingly, the fast Na currents recorded from these mature specimens are of very small amplitude compared to the other Na currents recorded from cultured SMCs. Because Na currents are more frequently recorded in immature cells than in mature cells, we speculate that fast Na channels may be important at early development stages rather than in the mature condition. In this context, a difference in Na channel downregulation between immature and adult neurons was reported some years ago (45).

It is of interest that Na_X channel genes are present in the smooth muscle cells of the pulmonary artery, myometrium, vas deferens, and esophagus (7,11,25,46–48). Although no attempts to detect a functional expression of Na_X channels in oocytes or cell lines have succeeded, recent findings in in vivo experiments have suggested that Na_X channels may act as a body fluid Na concentration sensor in ependymal cells, possibly in the periventricular area of the brain, and play a key role in salt-intake behavior (27). If Na_X channels do indeed act as a Na sensor or Na absorbance machinery, as they have been postulated to do (27), this mysterious Na channel that is expressed in vascular SMCs may have important roles to play in the regulation of cell volume and/or extracellular Na concentration.

Felipe et al. (46) showed that the expression of $Na_V2.3$ changed during an individual's development, a high mRNA expression for this channel appearing only at 3 weeks after birth in skeletal muscle, whereas in cardiac and myometrial cells it peaked at birth. It is of interest that this period of high expression of $Na_V2.3$ mRNA is also the period in which myometrial cells hypertrophy, when the volume of the cells increases drastically. If we assume that the Na_X channel in the myometrium also acts as Na absorbance machinery, expression of this channel would accelerate Na uptake by the cells, and this would cause an increase in cell volume due to cotransport of water (to maintain the intracellular Na concentration). On the other hand, it has been reported that the expression of the RNA for Na-G-channel protein is highest in adult cardiac muscle and intestinal SMCs (26). These findings may indicate different roles among Na_X subtypes during cell development.

V. CONCLUSIONS

In this chapter, we have discussed some possible roles for the voltage-dependent fast Na channels in SMCs, including those of the pulmonary artery. After the initial findings of a fast Na channel current in azygos vein and of TTX binding sites in rat uterus, similar Na channel currents have been shown to be present in a variety of SMCs. Recent molecular biological investigations have further revealed the presence of a novel type of Na channel (Na_X), but its channel function has not yet been investigated. When the electrical environment surrounding SMCs is unsuitable for voltage-dependent fast Na channels to fulfill a role in cell excitation, other roles need to be considered, such as maintenance of the intracellular Na concentration, osmotic regulation for volume control, or regulation of the intracellular Ca concentration. Present evidence suggests that the roles actually played by these channels may differ at different times in an individual's development.

ACKNOWLEDGMENT

We thank Dr. Robert Timms for editing this paper.

REFERENCES

1. Kuriyama H, Kitamura K, Nabata H. Pharmacological and physiological significance of ion channels and factors that modulate them in vascular tissues. Pharmacol Rev 1995; 47:387–573.
2. Amédée T, Renaud JF, Jmari K, Lombet A, Mironneau J, Mironneau M. The presence of Na^+ channels in myometrial smooth muscle cells is revealed by specific neurotoxins. Biochem Biophys Res Commun 1986; 137:675–681.
3. Sturek M, Hermsmeyer K. Calcium and sodium channels in spontaneously contracting vascular muscle cells. Science 1986; 233:475–478.
4. Okabe K, Kitamura K, Kuriyama H. The existence of a highly tetrodotoxin sensitive Na channel in freshly dispersed smooth muscle cells of the rabbit main pulmonary artery. Pflügers Arch 1988; 411:423–428.

5. Xiong Z, Sperelakis N, Noffsinger A, Fenoglio-Preiser C. Fast Na^+ current in circular smooth muscle cells of the large intestine. Pflügers Arch 1993; 423: 485–491.
6. Choby C, Mangoni ME, Boccara G, Nargeot J, Richard S. Evidence for tetrodotoxin-sensitive sodium currents in primary cultured myocytes from human, pig and rabbit arteries. Pflügers Arch 2000; 440:149–152.
7. Deshpande MA, Wang J, Preiksaites HG, Laurier LG, Sims SM. Characterization of a voltage-dependent Na^+ current in human esophageal smooth muscle. Am J Physiol Cell Physiol 2002; 283:C1045–C1055.
8. Okabe K, Kajioka S, Nakao K, Kitamura K, Kuriyama H, Weston AH. Actions of chromakalim on ionic currents recorded from single smooth muscle cells of the rat portal vein. J Pharmacol Exp Ther 1990; 250:832–839.
9. Mironneau J, Yamamoto T, Sayet I, Arnaudeau S, Rakotoarisoa L, Mironneau C. Effect of dihydropyridines on calcium channels in isolated smooth muscle cells from rat vena cava. Br J Pharmacol 1992; 105:321–328.
10. Muraki K, Imaizumi Y, Watanabe M. Sodium currents in smooth muscle cells freshly isolated from stomach fundus of the rat and ureter of the guinea pig. J Physiol 1991; 442:351–375.
11. Mandegar M, Remillard CV, Yuan JXJ. Ion channels in pulmonary arterial hypertension. Prog Cardiovasc Dis 2002; 45:81–114.
12. Goldin AL. Resurgence of sodium channel research. Annu Rev Physiol 2002; 63:871–894.
13. Terlau H, Heinemann SH, Stühmer W, Pusch M, Conti F, Imoto K, Numa S. Mapping the site of block by tetrodotoxin and saxitoxin of sodium channel II. FEBS Lett 1991; 293:93–96.
14. Stephen MM, Potts JF, Agnew WS. The μI skeletal muscle sodium channel: mutation E403Q eliminates sensitivity to tetrodotoxin but not to μ-conotoxin GIIIA and GIIIB. J Membr Biol 1994; 137:1–8.
15. Fozzard HA, Hanck DA. Structure and function of voltage-dependent sodium channels: comparison of brain II and cardiac isoforms. Physiol Rev 1996; 76:887–926.
16. Denac H, Mevissen M, Scholtysik G. Structure, function and pharmacology of voltage-dependent sodium channels. Naunyn-Scmiedeberg's Arch Pharmacol 2000; 362:453–479.
17. Frelin C, Cognard C, Vigne P, Lazdunski M. Tetrodotoxin-sensitive and tetrodotoxin-resistant Na^+ channels differ in their sensitivity to Cd^{2+} and Zn^{2+}. Eur J Pharmacol 1986; 122:245–250.
18. Heinemann SH, Terlau H, Imoto K. Molecular basis for pharmacological differences between brain and cardiac sodium channels. Pflügers Arch 1992; 422:90–92.
19. Stühmer W, Conti F, Suzuki H, Wang X, Noda M, Yahagi N, Kubo H, Numa S. Structural parts involved in activation and inactivation of the sodium channel. Nature 1989; 339:597–603.
20. Catterall WA, Schmidt JW, Messner DJ, Feller DJ. Structure and biosynthesis of neuronal sodium channel. In: Kao CY, Levinson SR, eds. Tetrodotoxin, Saxitoxin, and the Molecular Biology of the Sodium Channel. New York: New York Acad Sci, 1986:186–203.

21. Fleig A, Fitch JM, Goldin AL, Rayner MD, Starkus JG, Ruben PC. Point mutations in IIS4 alters activation and inactivation of rat brain IIA Na channels in *Xenopus* oocyte macropatches. Pflügers Arch 1994; 427:406–413.
22. O'Leary ME, Chen LQ, Kallen RG, Horn R. A molecular link between activation and inactivation of sodium channels. J Gen Physiol 1995; 106: 641–658.
23. Hartmann HA, Tiedeman AA, Chen SF, Brown AM, Kirsch GE. Effects of III–IV linker mutations on human heart Na^+ channel inactivation gating. Circ Res 1994; 75:114–122.
24. Kellenberger S, West JW, Catterall WA, Scheuer T. Molecular analysis of potential hinge residues in the inactivation gate of brain type IIA Na^+ channels. J Gen Physiol 1997; 109:607–617.
25. George AL Jr, Knittle TJ, Tamkun MM. Molecular cloning of an atypical voltage-gated sodium channel expressed in human heart and uterus; evidence for a distinct gene family. Proc Natl Acad Sci USA 1992; 89:4893–4897.
26. Gautron S, Dos Santos G, Pinto-Henrique D, Koulakoff A, Gros F, Berwald-Netter Y. The glial voltage-gated sodium channel: cell- and tissue-specific mRNA expression. Proc Natl Acad Sci USA 1992; 89:7272–7276.
27. Watanabe E, Fujikawa A, Matsunaga H, Yasoshima Y, Sako N, Yamamoto T, Saegusa C, Noda M. Na_V2/NaG channel is involved in control of salt-intake behavior in the CNS. J Neurosci 2000; 20:7743–7751.
28. Makita N, Bennett PB Jr , George AL Jr. Voltage-gated Na^+ channel β_1 subunit mRNA expressed in adult human skeletal muscle, heart, and brain is encoded by single gene. J Biol Chem 1994; 269:7571–7578.
29. Patton DE, Isom LL, Catterall WA, Goldin AL. The adult rat brain β1 subunit modifies activation and inactivation gating of multiple sodium channel α subunits. J Biol Chem 1994; 269:17649–17655.
30. Fahmi AI, Patel M, Stevens EB, Fowden AL, John JE III, Lee K, Pinnock R, Morgan K, Jackson AP, Vandenberg JI. The sodium channel β-subunit SCN3b modulates the kinetics of SCN5a and is expressed heterogeneously in sheep heart. J Physiol 2001; 537:693–700.
31. Srinvasan J, Schmachner M, Catterall WA. Interaction of voltage-gated sodium channels with the extracellular matrix molecules tenascin-C and tenascin-R. Proc Natl Acad Sci USA 1998; 95:15753–15757.
32. Catterall WA. From ionic currents to molecular mechanisms: the structure and function of voltage-gated sodium channels. Neuron 2000; 26:13–25.
33. Itoh T, Kuriyama H, Suzuki H. Excitation-contraction coupling in smooth muscle cells of the guineapig mesenteric artery. J Physiol 1981:513–535.
34. Elsharkawy TY, Morgan KE, Szursewski JH. Intracellular electrical activity of canine and human gastric smooth muscle. J Physiol 1978; 279:291–307.
35. Fujii K, Inoue R, Yamanaka K, Yoshitomi T. Effects of calcium antagonists on smooth muscle membranes of the canine stomach. Gen Pharmacol 1985; 16:217–221.
36. Kitamura K. Comparative aspects of membrane properties and innervation of longitudinal and circular muscle layers of rabbit jejunum. Jpn J Physiol 1978; 28:583–601.

37. Hara Y, Kitamura K, Kuriyama H. Actions of 4-aminopyridine on vascular smooth muscle tissues of the guinea-pig. Br J Pharmacol 1980; 68:99–106.
38. Suzuki H, Twarog BM. Membrane properties of smooth muscle cells in pulmonary hypertensive rats. Am J Physiol 1982; 242:H907–H915.
39. Casteels R, Kitamura K, Kuriyama H, Suzuki H. Excitation-contraction coupling in the smooth muscle cells of the rabbit main pulmonary artery. J Physiol 1977; 271:63–79.
40. Casteels R, Kitamura K, Kuriyama H, Suzuki H. The membrane properties of the smooth muscle cells of the rabbit main pulmonary artery. J Physiol 1977; 271:41–61.
41. Kallen RG, Cohen SA, Barchi RL. Structure, function and expression of voltage-dependent sodium channels. Mol Neurobiol 1993; 7:383–428.
42. Yang JR, Bennett PB, Makita N, George AF, Barchi RL. Expression of the sodium channel β1 subunit in rat skeletal muscle is selectively associated with the tetrodotoxin-sensitive α subunit isoforms. Neuron 1993; 11:915–922.
43. Yang JR, Sladky J, Kallen R, Barchi RL. mRNA transcripts encoding the TTX sensitive and insensitive forms of the skeletal muscle sodium channel are independently regulated after denervation. Neuron 1991; 7:421–427.
44. Waxman SG, Kocsis JD, Black JA. Type III sodium channel mRNA is expressed in embryonic but not adult spinal sensory neurons, and is reexpressed following axotomy. J Neurophysiol 1994; 72:466–470.
45. Dargent B, Paillart C, Carlier E, Alcaraz G, Martin-Eauclair MF, Couraud F. Sodium channel internalization in developing neurons. Neuron 1994; 13: 683–690.
46. Felipe A, Knittle TJ, Doyle KL, Tamkun MM. Primary structure and differential expression during development and pregnancy of a novel voltage-dependent sodium channel in the mouse. J Biol Chem 1994; 269:30125–30131.
47. Knittle TJ, Doyle KL, Tamkun MM. Immunolocalization of the $mNa_V2.3$ Na^+ channel in mouse heart: upregulation in myometrium during pregnancy. Am J Physiol 1996; 270:C688–C696.
48. Akopian AN, Souslova V, Sivilotti L, Wood JN. Structure and distribution of broadly expressed atypical sodium channel. FEBS Lett 1997; 400:183–187.
49. Molleman A, Nelemans A, Van den Akker J, Duin M, Den Hertog A. Voltage-dependent sodium and potassium, but no calcium conductances in DDT_1 MF-2 smooth muscle cells. Pflügers Arch 1991; 417:479–484.
50. Kusaka M, Sperelakis N. Fast sodium currents induced by serum in human uterine leiomyosarcoma cells. Am J Physiol 1994; 267:C1288–C1294.
51. Yamamoto Y, Fukuta H, Suzuki H. Blockade of sodium channels by divalent cations in rat gastric smooth muscle. Jpn J Physiol 1993; 43:785–796.
52. Ohya Y, Sperelakis N. Fast Na^+ and slow Ca^{2+} channels in single uterine muscle cells from pregnant rats. Am J Physiol 1989; 257:C408–C412.
53. Yoshino M, Wang SY, Kao CY. Sodium and calcium inward currents in freshly dissociated smooth myocytes of rat uterus. J Gen Physiol 1997; 110:565–577.

11

Voltage-Gated Potassium Channels in Pulmonary Artery Smooth Muscle Cells

Kristen O'Connell, Aaron Norris, Elizabeth A. Coppock, and Michael M. Tamkun

Colorado State University, Fort Collins, Colorado, U.S.A.

I. INTRODUCTION

A. Role of K^+ Channels in Vascular Smooth Muscle Cells

In most electrically excitable cells, voltage-gated potassium (Kv) channels play an important role in determining the magnitude and duration of the action potential. Differences in the type(s) and/or levels of K^+ channel expression contribute to the heterogeneity of action potential regulation. However, in pulmonary artery vascular smooth muscle cells (VSMCs), Kv channels play a central role in establishing the resting membrane potential as opposed to regulating the action potential. Closure of VSMC K^+ channels, open at the resting membrane potential, causes membrane depolarization. This change in membrane potential activates voltage-gated Ca^{2+} channels, leading to an increase in intracellular calcium concentration and vasoconstriction (1). Activation of VSMC K^+ channels leads to hyperpolarization, inhibition of voltage-gated Ca^{2+} channels, and vasodilation (1). Vascular smooth muscle cells have a high input resistance; therefore, even a small change in K^+ channel activity can have a significant effect on membrane potential and consequently on vascular tone (2,3). Indeed, many factors that modulate vessel tone do so by activating or inhibiting VSMC K^+ channels (1).

Four main classes of potassium channels have been described in vascular smooth muscle based on their biophysical and pharmacological properties: ATP-sensitive (K_{ATP}), inward rectifier (K_{IR}), and tandem pore channels, large-conductance Ca^{2+}-activated K^+ (BK_{Ca}), and voltage-gated (Kv) (1). Of these, the Kv channels are most likely to control the pulmonary arterial VSMC membrane potential and thus regulate vessel tone (4). For example, BK_{Ca} is inhibited by low concentrations of TEA (1 mM), and K_{ATP} can be blocked by glibenclamide (1). Application of either TEA or glibenclamide to pulmonary arterial VSMCs did not result in an elevation of intracellular Ca^{2+}, whereas the application of 4-aminopyridine (4-AP) (a Kv channel blocker) resulted in reversible depolarization and an increase in intracellular Ca^{2+} (1). Thus, Kv channels blocked by 4-aminopyridine are likely the source of I_K responsible for setting the resting potential. The Kv channels are reviewed in this chapter; the BK_{Ca}, K_{ATP}, and KIR/tandem channels are reviewed in Chapters 12, 13, and 14, respectively.

B. Hypoxia-Induced Vasoconstriction Directly Involves K⁺ Channels

Hypoxic inhibition of Kv channels was first demonstrated in 1988 by Lopez-Barneo et al. in carotid body type I cells (5). Hume and coworkers (1) later showed that hypoxia causes both an inhibition of whole cell K^+ current and membrane depolarization in isolated pulmonary arterial VSMCs. Kv channel blocking agents such as 4-AP and TEA depolarized the membrane, increased pulmonary arterial ring tension, and increased pulmonary artery pressure in isolated perfused lungs (1). That hypoxia-induced VSMC membrane depolarization and arterial constriction can be mimicked by Kv channel blockers was one of the earlier findings that suggested that the depolarization induced by hypoxia is due to inhibition of Kv channels open at the resting membrane potential.

Two types of pulmonary artery VSMC K^+ channels have been suggested to be modulated by hypoxia and in turn to cause vasoconstriction. BK_{Ca} and Kv channels both exhibit modulation by hypoxia, but the majority of electrophysiological and pharmacological evidence suggests that Kv channels play the primary role in triggering vasoconstriction during hypoxia (1). The hypoxia-sensitive current described in most pulmonary artery VSMC preparations is a delayed rectifier that is sensitive to 4-AP and insensitive to charybdotoxin (CTX) block (1). In addition, the presence of BK_{Ca} channel blockers, in both single channel and whole -cell experiments (6,7), does not affect the hypoxia-sensitive component of delayed rectifier current. And last, pretreatment of isolated dog pulmonary arterial VSMCs with 1 mM 4-AP prevented the hypoxic inhibition of outward current (1). Taken together, these data suggest that Kv channels that exhibit delayed rectifier properties and are sensitive to 4-AP but insensitive to CTX are responsible for the O_2-sensitive K^+ current in pulmonary arterial VSMCs. For a review of hypoxia sensitivity of cloned Kv channels, see Chapter 17.

II. DIVERSITY OF VOLTAGE-GATED K^+ CURRENTS IN PULMONARY ARTERY VSMCs

A. Diversity of Current Phenotypes

All vascular smooth muscle cells examined to date have at least one component of voltage-sensitive K^+ current, and many studies report more than one type of current (1). These currents include "delayed rectifier" (IK_{DR}) and "transient-outward" (IK_{TO}) types (1), although many investigators downplay the role of I_{TO}-type currents. Recently, a third noninactivating Kv current (IK_N), which is activated at the resting membrane potential, has also been described in rabbit, rat, and pig pulmonary artery VSMCs (1). These channels provide an important K^+ channel conductance in the physiological membrane potential range of pulmonary arteries (3). Furthermore, several groups of investigators have shown that the membrane potential in pulmonary artery VSMCs is controlled by one or more subtypes of K_{DR} (8–12). Pharmacologically, most Kv currents can be isolated by selective inhibition to 4-aminopyridine (4-AP). Outward K^+ current in PASMCs is inhibited by low doses of 4-AP (8,11), but not by TEA (11) or CTX (11). In addition, 4-AP (10–13), but not TEA (10,11), CTX (10,11,13), iberiotoxin (10), or glibenclamide (13), depolarizes PASMCs. Furthermore, exposure to 4-AP, but not to glibenclamide or CTX, leads to an increase in $[Ca^{2+}]_i$ (1). Taken together, these studies clearly emphasize the importance of Kv channels in the regulation of PASMC membrane potential and pulmonary arterial tone.

B. Cell Specificity of Kv Current Expression

Due to the difficulties associated with obtaining pulmonary artery VSMCs from distinct regions of the pulmonary circulation, especially in the rat, there have been only a few studies addressing whether Kv currents vary as a function of location within the pulmonary vascular tree. Smirnov et al. (14) reported that 67% of the VSMCs isolated from rat conduit pulmonary artery vessels (which do not show hypoxia-induced vasoconstriction) express a rapidly activating, 4-AP sensitive but TEA-insensitive, Kv current, whereas 33% express a slowly activating, 4-AP sensitive, TEA-sensitive Kv. These currents also inactivated over different membrane potentials. In contrast, cells from resistance arteries showed a TEA-insensitive current resembling the one in conduit vessels but with altered 4-AP sensitivity. Thus, it appears that in conduit vessels there are two types of cells expressing two distinct channels, and in resistance vessels a single cell type expresses a third Kv channel type. In addition to this work, an earlier study by Archer et al.

(11) concluded that there are three different VSMC morphologies in the rat pulmonary artery along with variations in the expression of K_{Ca} and Kv channels. Cells expressing primarily BK_{Ca} were found in conduit vessels whereas cells with primarily Kv current were isolated from the resistance vessels.

III. OVERVIEW OF MOLECULAR APPROACHES TO VOLTAGE-GATED K^+ CHANNELS

Voltage-gated K^+ channels exist as tetramers formed by four six-transmembrane-spanning subunits combining to form a functional channel (15). Not only can identical subunits combine to form a functional channel, but distinct subunits can also combine to form functional heteromeric channels both in vitro and in vivo (15). These heteromeric channels have unique properties that often represent a blend of the observed properties of the corresponding homomeric channels. Furthermore, several Kv subunits are nonfunctional when expressed alone. For example, the Kv9.3 subunit does not form a functional homomeric channel itself but rather functions only in heteromeric complexes, where it confers altered voltage sensitivity and activation kinetics (16). The following section outlines the basic approaches that have contributed to our present understanding of Kv channel molecular physiology. At this point in time the Kv channel family is composed of 36 members grouped into 12 subfamilies (Kv1-Kv12), with the Kv1 family being the largest with eight members (for a recent updated of Kv channel classification, see Ref. 17.

A. The *Drosophila* Genetic Approach, Cloning-Based Chromosomal Location

The first cloned Kv channel was obtained using *Drosophila* genetics and chromosomal walking. Flies displaying the *Shaker* phenotype, which involved abnormal leg shaking in response to ether exposure, were found to be missing an I_{to} -like K^+ current from their leg and flight muscles (18). Thus, it was postulated that the defective gene responsible for the *Shaker* phenotype was a K^+ channel and that the locus of the *Shaker* mutation in the *Drosophila* genome marked the location of this channel. Isolation of this genetic locus involved extensive isolation and reisolation of genomic fragments, allowing investigators to "walk" down the *Drosophila* chromosome toward the *Shaker* defect. Using this approach, two independent groups cloned the first Kv channel (18). The original *Shaker* clone is one of the most studied proteins in terms of its structure–function relationship. Site-directed mutagenesis followed by functional expression and voltage-clamp analysis has identified sequence regions that are involved in ion permeation, gating, voltage sensing, and subunit assembly. The most impressive progress is the coupling of this mutagenesis work with the structural efforts by the MacKinnon, Perozo, and Pfaffinger laboratories, for now we have a realistic picture of both ion permeation and gating. For a recent review of Kv channel structure and function, see Ref. 19.

B. Homology Screening

Using the *Shaker* gene as a homology probe, three related *Drosophila* K^+ channel genes were isolated (18). These are referred to as the *Shaw, Shab*, and *Shal* channels, being named in part for the initials of the investigators who cloned them. Homology screening, either by probe cross-hybridization or the use of degenerate PCR primers (15), also identified numerous mammalian homologs for all the above mentioned *Drosophila* K^+ channel genes with more than eight channels being most similar to *Shaker* (17). In addition, new mammalian channels only distantly related to the *Drosophila* channels were uncovered by these techniques. Under the accepted classification scheme, mammalian Kv1 family members are most similar to *Shaker*, and the Kv2, Kv3, and Kv4 families are most similar to *Shab, Shaw*, and *Shal*, respectively (17). To account for the increasing diversity among mammals, the Kv5–Kv12 subfamilies have been added. For a current summary of Kv channel classification, see the scheme recently published by the International Union of Pharmacology (17).

C. Expression Cloning

The expression cloning strategy uses heterologous expression to screen library clones for channel activity. In this approach, cRNA is produced from pools of cDNA clones and expressed in *Xenopus* oocytes. If current is detected in the cRNA-injected oocytes, the clone pool containing the channel cDNA is subdivided and the process is repeated until cRNA derived from a single clone generates the desired current. This cloning approach was used to isolate cDNAs encoding rat *minK* and rat Kv2.1 (18).

D. Cloning Based on K^+ Channel Protein Purification

The mammalian β subunits were discovered because they copurified with Kv channel α subunits. Early purification studies of K^+ channel proteins, using the knowledge that multiple K^+ channel isoforms bind the naturally occurring toxin dendrotoxin (DTX) (18), identified a 39 kDa protein that consistently copurified with a 78 kDa DTX-binding channel of the *Shaker*-related Kv1 family (18,20). The Kv2 subfamily also is associated with β subunits, because smaller proteins also copurify from rat brain, with the Kv2.1 protein using antibodies specific for this α subunit (18). The Kv4 subfamily associates with function-altering KChIP accessory proteins (described below) as well as the aminopeptidase-related proteins that modify Kv4.2 trafficking and function (21).

E. Cloning Based on K^+ Channel Protein Interaction

Protein interaction assays have been used not only to identify proteins interacting with Kv channels [such as actinin (22)] but also to discover new channel subunits. An et al. (23) used the Kv4 channel N-terminus as bait in yeast two-hybrid screens during a search for interacting proteins or subunits that might explain the variation in inactivating currents observed between cell types natively expressing Kv4 α subunits. This approach isolated a family of clones referred to as the KChIPs (K^+-channel interacting proteins). KChIPs are members of a superfamily of 4 EF-hand-containing Ca^{2+} binding proteins that include NCS-1. These cytoplasmic accessory proteins modulate Kv4 channel function, trafficking, and regulation by intracellular Ca^{2+}(24).

Clearly, the discovery of functional K^+ channel β subunits and other accessory proteins further complicates attempts to correlate cloned vascular K^+ channels and endogenous VSMC currents. The same K^+ channel protein may be expressed in different cell types, but by virtue of being associated with various β-subunit isoforms, it may yield different electrophysiological characteristics.

F. Cloning via Database Mining

The "in silico" approach of cloning via database mining is a variant on the homology screening approach described above. Motifs common to many or all K^+ channels, such as the GYG selectivity filter motif, have been used to search databases in the hope of discovering known proteins whose role as K^+ channels were not appreciated. The two-pore TWIK channels were discovered is this fashion by simple Genbank database searching with ion conducting pore sequences (25). Additional silent α subunits were found in the human genome by searching with Kv channel-like exons (26).

G. Heterologous Expression of Cloned Kv Channels

Xenopus oocytes have been by far the expression system of choice owing to the ease of cRNA injection and the two-electrode voltage-clamp technique. For the most part, this system has been reliable in terms of producing physiologically meaningful results. However, there are at least three notable exceptions. The first is that several channels have appeared insensitive to pore-blocking drugs in the oocyte system while being readily blocked when expressed in mammalian cells. For example, quinidine blocks the Kv1.5 delayed rectifier with a dissociation constant (K_D) of 6 μM in mouse L cells, but this concentration has little effect following channel expression in oocytes. In this case, the hydrophobic yolk within the oocyte probably represents a major sink for any membrane-permeant compound. The second exception deals with the expression of the cloned *minK* protein.

Investigators were puzzled for years by the finding that the *minK* channel could be expressed reproducibly only in *Xenopus* oocytes and not in mammalian cells. This result was explained by the finding that *minK* is not a true channel but rather an accessory or β subunit that is required for the proper expression of *KvLQT1* and that oocytes express an endogenous *KvLQT1* α subunit that is silent until *minK* cRNA is injected (27). Additional, more recent, complications include the likelihood that the oocytes also express MiRP subunits (28). And last, because *Xenopus* oocytes are maintained at 18°C, there is the concern that the protein-processing machinery is not operating at a physiological temperature when dealing with mammalian membrane proteins.

Although fibroblast-like tissue culture cells are perhaps the best expression system to use in terms of their pharmacology and fast voltage clamp, they too can suffer from endogenous subunit problems. For example, human embryonic kidney (HEK 293) cells occasionally express endogenous delayed rectifier currents that resemble a number of cloned Kv channels. In addition, cell lines such as mouse L cells and Chinese hamster ovary (CHO) cells express Kv β subunits that can alter the function of heterologously expressed channels (29). And, of course, there is the constant worry that mammalian cells may express a variety of electrically silent α and/or accessory subunit proteins.

In summary, no heterologous expression system is perfect. Primary VSMC cultures derived from transgenic mice lacking the channel of interest will avoid many of these issues, but such systems are only now becoming available for a small number of channels.

IV. CLONING AND FUNCTIONAL ANALYSIS OF Kv CHANNEL EXPRESSION IN THE PULMONARY ARTERY VASCULAR SMOOTH MUSCLE CELL

Only one Kv channel protein (Kv9.3) has been actually cloned from VSMCs. In all other cases the Kv channels were cloned from other sources and then found to be expressed in the pulmonary vasculature. To date, at least 36 Kv channel α subunits have been cloned from a variety of tissue sources, most notably brain and heart, and characterized using heterologous expression systems. Of these, five are confirmed to be expressed in pulmonary artery tissue via Western blot, immunohistochemistry, and mRNA expression (1,31). Some of the subunits show differential expression as one moves down the pulmonary artery tree from the hypoxia-insensitive conduit vessel to the hypoxia-sensitive resistance arteries (see Fig. 1). In addition, extensive study of VSMCs in culture indicates that many additional isoforms may be present in native tissue. Yuan et al. (4), using RT-PCR of primary cultures of rat pulmonary artery VSMCs, confirmed expression of Kv1.1, Kv1.2, Kv1.4, Kv1.5, Kv1.6, Kv2.1, and Kv9.3

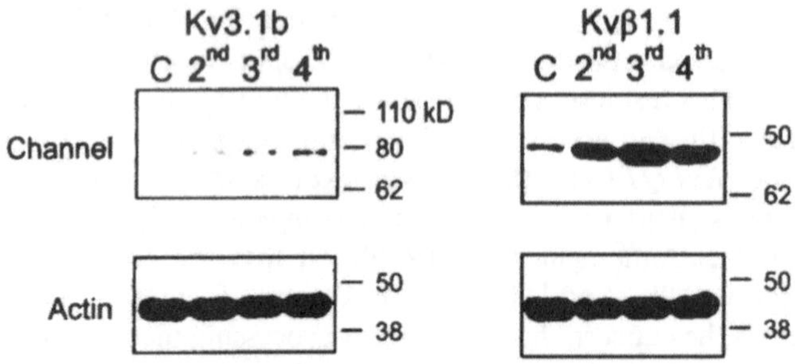

Figure 1 Western blot analysis of Kv channel expression along the pulmonary artery vascular tree. The expression of Kv3.1b and Kvβ1.1 and proteins are compared between conduit vessels and 2nd, 3rd, and 4th branch vessels. Actin expression was assayed to confirm equal sample loading. For additional data see Ref. 31.

mRNA. Using immunoblotting, they detected Kv1.2, Kv1.4, Kv1.5, but not Kv1.3 (4).

In the following sections we will summarize our current understanding of which cDNA clones represent the best molecular correlates of native Kv currents in the pulmonary circulation. Table 1 contains a summary of the literature with respect to the Kv channels that have been postulated to exist within the pulmonary circulation.

A. The Kv1.2 Channel

Kv1.2 was cloned from the rat heart and brain by homology screening (18). Northern blot, RT-PCR, and immunostaining analysis indicates that this channel isoform is expressed in the pulmonary vasculature or primary cultures of pulmonary VSMCs (1,4,30,31). Heterologous expression of Kv1.2 in mouse L cells produces K^+ currents that exhibit several notable differences compared to Kv1.2 currents recorded from *Xenopus* oocytes (15,18). For example, the activation kinetics of Kv1.2 current expressed in mouse L cells are tenfold slower than when the current is expressed in *Xenopus* oocytes. Additionally, expression of Kv1.2 in mouse L cells shifts the voltage sensitivity of activation by ≈25 mV in the depolarizing direction (Tamkun, unpublished data). Differences in protein processing between these two expression systems (15), including possible phosphorylation pathways and the presence of endogenous α and β subunits (28,29) capable of assembling with transfected α subunits, may help to explain such discrepancies.

Kv1.2 is sensitive to nanomolar concentrations of DTX, whereas 4-AP blocks only at millimolar concentrations (17). Because 200 nM DTX does not block the outward currents in VSMCs, if this channel contributes to a native current it must be as part of a heteromeric complex that is DTX-insensitive. The potential for heteromeric assembly of Kv α subunits in

Table 1 Expressions of Kv Channel Subunits in the Pulmonary Vasculature as Noted in the Literature

	mRNA		Protein	
Channel subunits	Observed	Not observed	Observed	Not observed
α1.1	4, 53–55		7	
α1.2	4, 16		1, 7, 31	
α1.3	16, 54	4	7	4
α1.4	4, 54	16	4	7
α1.5	4, 53, 54	16	4, 7, 30, 31	
α1.6	4, 54	16	7	
α1.7	54			
α2.1	4, 16, 53, 54		4, 31	
α2.2	54			
α3.1	6	54	6, 31	
α3.3		54		
α3.4	54			
α4.1	54			
α4.2	54			
α4.3	54, 56			
α5.1	54			
α6.1	54			
α8.1		54		
α9.1	54			
α9.2	54			
α9.3	4, 54			
β1.1	54, 56		31	
β1.2			31	
β1.3			31	
β2	54, 56			
β3	54, 56			

the cardiovascular system has complicated the correlation of cloned Kv channels with native currents. For example, Kv1.2 and Kv1.5 α subunits can assemble to form a functional heteromeric channel in vitro, and the presence of the Kv1.5 DTX-insensitive channel dominates the pharmacology of the heteromeric channel (30). Hulme et al. (30) postulated that Kv1.2/1.5 heteromeric channels constitute a major hypoxia-sensing current in the pulmonary circulation. Although Kv1.2 expressed alone in heterologous systems is hypoxia-sensitive, this isoform activates at potentials too depolarized to significantly influence the resting membrane potential of the pulmonary artery VSMC. However, the Kv1.2/1.5 heteromeric channel is not only hypoxia-sensitive but also activates at potentials close to the VSMC resting membrane potential. Thus, the potential for heteromeric formation may provide one explanation for the pharmacological and electrophysiological discrepancies between cloned and native K^+ currents.

B. The Kv1.5 Channel

Kv1.5 was cloned originally from rat heart and rat brain by homology screening (15,18). Of all the *Shaker*-like K^+ channels cloned to date, Kv1.5 represents the most cardiovascular-specific Kv channel based on mRNA expression (15,18). Kv1.5 mRNA is either undetectable or very low in brain tissues whereas Kv1.5 mRNA and protein are detected in rat and bovine pulmonary artery vascular smooth muscle and in cultured pulmonary artery VSMCs (4,31).

Voltage-clamp analysis of heterologously expressed Kv1.5 currents indicates that this channel is a slowly inactivating delayed rectifier sensitive to block by low concentrations of 4-aminopyridine (4-AP) and quinidine (15,18) but insensitive to block by tetraethylammonium (TEA). Based on this pharmacology, the channel's activation kinetics, and its voltage dependence, Kv1.5 was an early candidate for the O_2-sensitive current in pulmonary artery VSMCs. When Kv1.5 is expressed in heterologous systems it is not hypoxia-sensitive, but heteromeric assembly with Kv1.2 renders the complex hypoxia-sensitive, again arguing for the importance of this subunit combination in VSMCs.

C. The Kv2.1 Channel

Channel Kv2.1 was originally expression cloned by Joho and coworkers from rat brain (15,18). The mRNA for Kv2.1 is readily detected in adult rat ventricular myocytes and pulmonary artery VSMCs (4,16). A major frustration involves the attempts to immunolocalize Kv2.1 expression in the cardiovascular system in order to answer the simple question of localization. Western blot analysis indicates that Kv2.1 protein is readily detectable in rat heart (18) and bovine pulmonary artery (31), but these same antibodies do not stain any cardiac or vascular cell type (31) although they readily detect the Kv2.1 protein in transfected cells (32) and brain tissue (33). The best explanation for this negative result is that the antibody epitopes are masked in the native VSMCs.

Heterologous expression of Kv2.1 reveals slowly activating, TEA-sensitive currents (17). Heterologously expressed homomeric Kv2.1 is sensitive to hypoxia but begins to activate only at −10 mV, too depolarized a potential for the Kv2.1 subunit alone to play a role in hypoxia-sensitive currents in the VSMC (16,30). However, when coexpressed with Kv9.3, the resulting heteromeric complex is hypoxia-sensitive and activates at potentials near that of native pulmonary artery VSMCs (16,30). Thus, here again the data suggest that hypoxia-sensing currents are heteromeric α-subunit complexes.

D. Kv9.3

Kv9.3 was cloned by Patel et al. (16) from the pulmonary artery using degenerate PCR primers targeting conserved protein domains. The mRNA for this channel is most abundant in lung and is also expressed in brain, testes, intestine, and stomach (16) and in isolated VSMCs (4). Kv9.3 is a silent α subunit in that it does not generate ionic current when expressed alone. Instead, its function appears to be to form heterotetramers with other Kv-channel-forming α subunits and alter their functional properties. For example, Kv9.3 assembles with the Kv2.1 channel described above and shifts the voltage dependence of the Kv2.1/9.3 heteromer activation so that the complex begins to activate at the resting membrane potential of VSMCs.

E. Kv3.1b

Kv3.1 was originally cloned from a mouse brain cDNA library. This isoform plays a central role in the auditory system and has a pharmacology similar to that of the outward currents found in pulmonary artery VSMCs. It is for this reason that its hypoxia sensitivity and expression in the pulmonary circulation have been studied. Most recently, Osipenko et al. (6) reported expression of Kv3.1b protein in freshly dissociated pulmonary artery VSMCs from rats and rabbits using immunocytochemistry. Additionally, the Tamkun group (31) reported expression of Kv3.1b subunits in bovine resistance pulmonary artery VSMCs as shown in Fig. 1.

The effect of hypoxia on Kv3.1b was examined by Osipenko et al. (6). Hypoxia significantly and consistently reduced the whole-cell current amplitude in L929 cells expressing Kv3.1b channels by ~24% at 40 mV (6). Furthermore, an inhibitory effect of hypoxia was demonstrated at the single-channel level and in membrane patches excised from the cell. However, this inhibition was apparent only at positive potentials. These results clearly demonstrate that Kv3.1b is O_2-sensitive; however, when expressed alone as a homotetramer it is not likely to be a component of the pulmonary artery VSMC O_2-sensitive K^+ current. As with Kv2.1 and Kv1.2, it is possible that Kv3.1b functions within a heteromeric complex in native VSMCs.

F. Accessory Kv Channel Subunits

Voltage-gated K^+ β subunits were first decribed by the Dolly group (18) as accessory proteins that copurified with dendrotoxin-binding proteins from bovine brain. Cloning of the first bovine β subunit was followed by the cloning of two β subunits from rat brain that were eventually classified as Kvβ 1.1 and Kvβ 2.1 (20). Simultaneous work by three independent groups indicates that cardiovascular K^+ channel diversity is also complicated by the presence of β subunits. Two groups cloned a Kvβ 1.2 subunit from human atrium (18) and ventricle (18), and a third group cloned the equivalent protein from ferret heart (18). Another β subunit, Kvβ1.3, was cloned from human heart (18). Kvβ1.1, 1.2, and 1.3 represent splice variants derived from the same gene (18). These three proteins share a conserved COOH-terminal sequence but possess unique NH_2-termini contributed by an isoform-defining exon. It is the variable NH_2-terminal region of the three Kvβ1 family isoforms that confers fast inactivation to delayed rectifiers such as Kv1.5 (34). In the pulmonary circulation, Western blot analysis indicates that all three Kvβ1 subfamily members are present but Kvβ2.1 appears to be absent (31). Interestingly, the expression of Kvβ1.1 and 1.2 dramatically increases as one moves from the hypoxia-insensitive conduit vessel into the resistance arteries (Fig. 1) (31), suggesting that these β subunits may indeed have a role in sensing hypoxia. In fact, Kvβ subunits do bind NADPH, and it has been hypothesized that they act as redox sensors coupling the PO_2 levels to membrane potential (35). Although this is an intriguing idea, the literature is somewhat contradictory on the physiological role of the NADPH-binding domain (36–38). Because most hypoxia-sensitive outward currents in VSMCs exhibit only slow inactivation, it is also difficult to understand how these β subunits confer O_2 sensing without increasing inactivation.

Although three Kvβ subunits are expressed in the pulmonary circulation, there are no reports of either KChIP or MiRP accessory proteins in this vasculature probably because they have not been searched for as opposed to simply being absent. The possible role of these Kv channel accessory subunits in the pulmonary circulation needs to be studied.

V. SUBCELLULAR LOCALIZATION OF Kv CHANNELS IN THE PULMONARY VASCULATURE

The subcellular localization of ion channels is necessary for proper electrical signaling. One physiological consequence of such specific localization is that it places various signal transduction molecules near their ion channel substrates. Several families of intracellular proteins, such as PDZs and AKAPs, have been shown to cluster both ion channels and modulatory signaling enzymes (39). Indeed, great emphasis has been placed on the role of PDZ proteins such as PSD 95 in the targeting and localization of ion channels, and the Kv1.2 and 1.5 α subunits discussed above contain PDZ-binding domains on the C-terminus. Beta subunits also are likely to interact with the cytoskeleton and thus immobilize channels on the cell surface (40). However, not all localization or complex formation is likely to involve protein–protein interactions.

Recent advances in the study of cell membrane structure modified the original Singer–Nicholson model of the plasma membrane, with the emerging idea being that lipid microdomains exist within the fluid bilayer (41). These dynamic structures, termed lipid rafts, are rich in tightly packed sphingolipids and cholesterol. These rafts, which are present in both excitable and nonexcitable cells, localize a number of membrane proteins, including multiple signal transduction molecules, while excluding others. It is likely that the rafts serve as scaffolding regions where signal transduction pathways interface. The presence of specific marker proteins and ultrastructural data indicate the likelihood that different types of rafts exist (41).

Caveolae represent one form of lipid raft that forms an invagination at the cell surface. These structures are associated with proteins referred to as caveolins that serve as convenient markers for caveolae in cell fractionation procedures (41). The number of known proteins proposed to be associated with caveolae has increased dramatically over the past several years. Nitric oxide synthase, various tyrosine kinases, protein kinase C, and G proteins have been detected in caveolar structures (41), as have cascades involved in insulin action (42). Localization of ion channels to caveolae and rapid regulation of caveolar neck opening could mediate a channel's electrical access to the cell surface. Such a mechanism would allow rapid regulation of the number of surface channels without having to rely on the usual mechanisms of membrane protein insertion or internalization. Alternatively, because many ion channels are regulated directly by protein kinases and G proteins, it makes sense to localize them to regions that are enriched in signaling molecules.

It is clear that rafts play a major role in the cardiovascular system. Caveolae, enriched with cell-signaling enzymes such as eNOS, are abundant in muscle and endothelial cells (43,44). In cardiac myocytes, specific β-adrenergic receptor subtypes and adenylate cyclase are localized to caveolae (45), and various PKC isoforms translocate to caveolae following activation (46). In contrast, activated adenosine receptors translocate out of caveolae (47). When caveolar structure is altered by deleting the caveolin-1 protein in the mouse, these animals develop pulmonary hypertension in addition to a cardiomyopathy (48). Interestingly, Kv channels often show a highly localized pattern of surface expression in transfected fibroblasts (Fig. 2) and in native neurons (33). Martens et al. (49), showed that Kv1.5 targets to caveolar domains and that Kv2.1 targets to a noncaveolar lipid raft (32). As shown in Fig. 3, Kv2.1 is raft-associated in both conduit and resistance vessels, so it is unlikely that differential raft association is involved in the hypoxia insensitivity of the conduit vessel. Although the relationship between raft localization of Kv channels and pulmonary physiology is currently unknown, it is obvious that this type of Kv channel localization in the pulmonary vasculature must be taken into account when examining the mechanisms underlying the link between hypoxia and VSMC membrane potential.

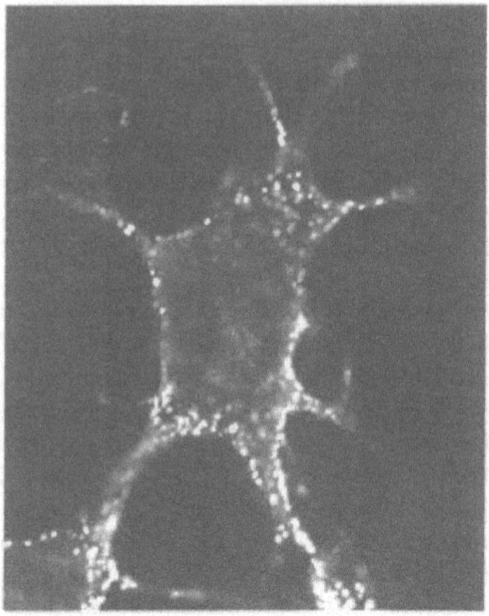

Figure 2 Localized expression of Kv2.1 in transfected HEK cells. Immunolocalization of surface Kv2.1 protein using an inserted, extracellular HA epitope. Note the restricted and highly localized expression pattern.

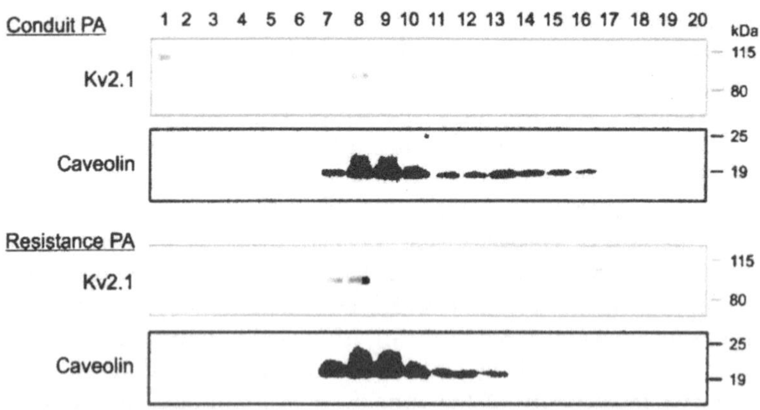

Figure 3 Raft association of Kv2.1 in bovine pulmonary artery. The detergent-free raft isolation protocol (32) was applied to both conduit and resistance vessel tissue after endothelial cell removal. Kv2.1 protein within the density gradient was then detected via Western blot analysis. In both vessel types, Kv2.1 was found in the low-density lipid raft fractions, as was the caveolar protein caveolin.

VI. RELATION OF CLONED CHANNELS WITH NATIVE CURRENTS

Although kinetic and pharmacological properties can be used to relate cloned channels to endogenous pulmonary artery VSMC currents, this approach is limited by the functional and pharmacological similarities between cloned channels. In addition, differences between native and cloned currents may reflect differences in channel subunit composition and/or post-translational modifications. Therefore, the field has emphasized the use of antibodies and transgenic knockout technologies to relate cloned cardiac channels to native VSMC currents.

A. Antibody Inhibition Studies

Antibodies against Kv channels have been added to the intracellular patch pipette solution in an attempt to dissect the O_2-sensitive K^+ current in PASMCs during whole-cell recordings in normoxic and hypoxic conditions. When Archer et al. (7) added anti-Kv2.1 to the patch pipette, they found inhibition of outward K^+ current and membrane depolarization in rat resistance pulmonary artery VSMCs, suggesting that Kv2.1 plays a role in setting the resting membrane potential . When anti-Kv1.5 was added to the patch pipette, whole-cell K^+ current was significantly decreased, and both the hypoxia- and 4-AP-induced increase in intracellular Ca^{2+} concentration of isolated pulmonary artery VSMCs were attenuated (7). However, anti-Kv1.5 antibody did not consistently depolarize the membrane in isolated pulmonary artery VSMCs. On the basis of their findings, the Archer group hypothesized that hypoxic inhibition of Kv2.1 leads to membrane depolarization, which shifts the resting membrane potential into a range where Kv1.5 is active and can thus be inhibited by hypoxia, leading to further inhibition of whole-cell K^+ current. Additionally, subsequent hypoxic challenge resulted in a further increase in intracellular Ca^{2+} with no effect on membrane potential. In related studies, Conforti et al. (50) used an antibody against Kv1.2 in the patch pipette to specifically inhibit Kv1.2 current from the whole-cell current in rat pheochromocytoma (PC12) cells (a model for oxygen sensing in the carotid body). When the cells were exposed to hypoxia, these researchers found no additional K^+ current inhibition, suggesting that the Kv1.2 current was responsible for the hypoxic effect in PC12 cells (50).

B. Transgenic Studies

The classic transgenic knockout experiment offers, in theory, a more direct approach to connect Kv clones with endogenous outward currents. It also allows examination of whole animal physiology in the absence of the channel of interest. To our knowledge, this approach has been taken only by the Archer group as of this writing (51). These investigators used a mouse generated by the London laboratory that had the Kv1.5 coding sequence exchanged with that of the Kv1.1 gene. Thus, this "SWAP" mouse expresses Kv1.1 under the control of the Kv1.5 promoter, although there was no difference in Kv1.1 mRNA expression between the SWAP mice and wild-type mice even though Kv1.5 mRNA was clearly deleted from the lung and heart. Pulmonary arterial VSMCs isolated from the SWAP mice had reduced delayed rectified current compared to those from wild-type mice (approximately 40% of normal) and showed impaired hypoxia-induced vasoconstriction (HPV). In agreement with these findings, the outward currents from the SWAP mice were less sensitive to hypoxia than those from wild-type animals. Together, these data suggest that Kv1.5 does contribute to a hypoxia-sensitive delayed rectifier current in the pulmonary circulation that plays a central role in HPV. The Kv3.1b channel has also be deleted from the mouse (52), but the effects of this deletion on pulmonary arterial VSMC currents and HPV have not yet been examined. Future studies with this mouse should also prove informative.

VII. SUMMARY AND CONCLUSIONS

During the last decade, tremendous progress has been made with respect to Kv channel molecular physiology within the nervous and cardiovascular systems. Significant data have been collected that are directly relevant to Kv channel function in the pulmonary circulation, but much remains to be done. We need a better understanding of the Kv channels expressed in the pulmonary vasculature, their subunit and macromolecular complex composition, their subcellular localization, and the mechanisms that regulate channel function and current density. Such information is especially important given the central role that Kv channels play in controlling vascular tone, especially in the lung, where hypoxia resulting from either altitude or obstructive lung diseases results in pulmonary hypertension and its associated vascular remodeling.

ACKNOWLEDGEMENT

This work was supported in part by NIH grant HL4933

REFERENCES

1. Coppock EA, Martens JR, Tamkun MM. Molecular basis of hypoxia-induced pulmonary vasoconstriction: role of voltage-gated K^+ channels. Am J Physiol Lung Cell Mol Physiol 2001; 281:L1–L12.
2. Standen NB, Quayle JM. K^+ channel modulation in arterial smooth muscle. Acta Physiol Scand 1998; 164:549–557.

3. Nelson MT, Quayle JM. Physiological roles and properties of potassium channels in arterial smooth muscle. Am J Physiol Cell Physiol 1995; 37: C799–C822.
4. Yuan XJ, Wang J, Juhaszova M, Golovina VA, Rubin LJ. Molecular basis and function of voltage-gated K^+ channels in pulmonary arterial smooth muscle cells. Am J Physiol 1998; 274:L621–L635.
5. Lopez-Barneo J, Lopez-Lopez JR, Urena J, Gonzalez C. Chemotransduction in the carotid body: K^+ current modulated by PO_2 in type I chemoreceptor cells. Science 1988; 241:580–582.
6. Osipenko ON, Tate RJ, Gurney AM. Potential role for Kv3.1b channels as oxygen sensors. Circ Res 2000; 86:534–540.
7. Archer SL, Souil E, Dinh-Xuan AT, Schremmer B, Mercier JC, El Yaagoubi A, et al. Molecular identification of the role of voltage-gated K^+ channels, Kv1.5 and Kv2.1, in hypoxic pulmonary vasoconstriction and control of resting membrane potential in rat pulmonary artery myocytes. J Clin Invest 1998; 101:2319–2330.
8. Okabe K, Kitamura K, Kuriyama H. Features of 4-aminopyridine sensitive outward current observed in single smooth muscle cells from the rabbit pulmonary artery. Pflügers Arch 1987; 409:561–568.
9. Smirnov SV, Robertson TP, Ward JP, Aaronson PI. Chronic hypoxia is associated with reduced delayed rectifier K^+ current in rat pulmonary artery muscle cells. Am J Physiol 1994; 266:H365–H370.
10. Osipenko ON, Evans AM, Gurney AM. Regulation of the resting potential of rabbit pulmonary artery myocytes by a low threshold, O_2-sensing potassium current. Br J Pharmacol 1997; 120:1461–1470.
11. Archer SL, Huang JM, Reeve HL, Hampl V, Tolarova S, Michelakis E, Weir EK. Differential distribution of electrophysiologically distinct myocytes in conduit and resistance arteries determines their response to nitric oxide and hypoxia. Circ Res 1996; 78:431–442.
12. Yuan XJ, Tod ML, Rubin LJ, Blaustein MP. Hypoxic and metabolic regulation of voltage-gated K^+ channels in rat pulmonary artery smooth muscle cells. Exp Physiol 1995; 80:803–813.
13. Yuan XJ. Voltage-gated K^+ currents regulate resting membrane potential and $[Ca^{2+}]_i$ in pulmonary arterial myocytes. Circ Res 1995; 77:370–378.
14. Smirnov SV, Beck R, Tammaro P, Ishii T, Aaronson PI. Electrophysiologically distinct smooth muscle cell subtypes in rat conduit and resistance pulmonary arteries. J Physiol 2002; 538:867–878.
15. Deal KK, England SK, Tamkun MM. Molecular physiology of cardiac potassium channels. Physiol Rev 1996; 76:49–67.
16. Patel AJ, Lazdunski M, Honore E. Kv2.1/Kv9.3, a novel ATP-dependent delayed-rectifier K^+ channel in oxygen-sensitive pulmonary artery myocytes. EMBO J 1997; 16:6615–6625.
17. Catterall WA, Chandy KG, Gutman GA. The IUPHAR Compendium of Voltage-Gated Ion Channels. 2002, Leeds: IUPHAR Media, 2002.
18. Hulme JT, Martens JR, Navarro-Polanco RA, Nishiyama A, Tamkun MM. Voltage-gated potassium channels in the myocardium. In: Archer SL, Rusch

NJ, eds. Potassium Channels in Cardiovascular Biology. New York: Kluwer Academic, 2001:337–362.
19. Choe S. Potassium channel structures. Nat Rev Neurosci 2002; 3:115–121.
20. Rettig J, Heinemann SH, Wunder F, Lorra C, Parcej DN, Dolly JO, Pongs O. Inactivation properties of voltage-gated K^+ channels altered by presence of β-subunit. Nature 1994; 369:289–294.
21. Nadal MS, Ozaita A, Amarillo Y, de Miera EV, Ma Y, Mo W, Goldberg EM, Misumi Y, Ikehara Y, Neubert TA, Rudy B. The CD26-related dipeptidyl aminopeptidase-like protein DPPX is a critical component of neuronal A-type K^+ channels. Neuron 2003; 37:449–461.
22. Maruoka ND, Steele DF, Au BP, Dan P, Zhang X, Moore EDW, Fedida D. Alpha-actinin-2 couples to cardiac Kv1.5 channels, regulating current density and channel localization in HEK cells. FEBS Lett 2000; 473(2):188–194.
23. An WF, Bowlby MR, Betty M, Cao J, Ling HP, Mendoza G, Hinson JW, Matteson KI, Strassle BW, Trimmer JS, Rhodes KJ. Modulation of A-type potassium channels by a family of calcium sensors. Nature 2000; 403:553–556.
24. Takimoto K, Ren X. KChIPs (Kv channel-interacting proteins)–a few surprises and another. J Physiol 2002; 545:3.
25. Lesage F, Guillemare E, Fink M, Duprat F, Lazdunski M, Romey G, Barhanin J. TWIK-1, a ubiquitous human weakly inward rectifying K^+ channel with a novel structure. EMBO J 1996; 15:1004–1011.
26. Ottschytsch N, Raes A, Van Hoorick D, Snyders DJ. Obligatory heterotetramerization of three previously uncharacterized Kv channel α-subunits identified in the human genome. Proc Natl Acad Sci USA 2002; 99:7986–7991.
27. Sanguinetti MC, Curran ME, Zou A, Shen J, Spector PS, Atkinson DL, Keating MT. Coassembly of K(v)LQT1 and minK (IsK) proteins to form cardiac I-Ks potassium channel. Nature 1996; 384:80–83.
28. Anantharam A, Lewis A, Panaghie G, Gordon E, McCrossan ZA, Lerner DJ, Abbott GW. RNA interference reveals that endogenous *Xenopus* MinK-related peptides govern mammalian K^+ channel function in oocyte expression studies. J Biol Chem 2003; 278:11739–11745.
29. Uebele VN, England SK, Chaudhary A, Tamkun MM, Snyders DJ. Functional differences in Kv1.5 currents expressed in mammalian cell lines are due to the presence of endogenous Kvβ2.1 subunits. J Biol Chem 1996; 271:2406–2412.
30. Hulme JT, Coppock EA, Felipe A, Martens JR, Tamkun MM. Oxygen sensitivity of cloned voltage-gated K^+ channels expressed in the pulmonary vasculature. Circ Res 1999; 85:489–497.
31. Coppock EA, Tamkun MM. Differential expression of K_V channel α- and β-subunits in the bovine pulmonary arterial circulation. Am J Physiol Lung Cell Mol Physiol 2001; 281:L1350–L1360.
32. Martens JR, Navarro-Polanco R, Coppock EA, Nishiyama A, Parshley L, Grobaski TD, Tamkun MM. Differential targeting of Shaker-like potassium channels to lipid rafts. J Biol Chem 2000; 275:7443–7446.
33. Maletic-Savatic M, Lenn NJ, Trimmer JS. Differential spatiotemporal expression of K^+ channel polypeptides in rat hippocampal neurons developing in situ and in vitro. J Neurosci 1995; 15:3840–3851.

34. Uebele VN, England SK, Gallagher DJ, Snyders DJ, Bennett PB, Tamkun MM. Distinct domains of the voltage-gated K^+ channel Kvβ1.3 β-subunit affect voltage-dependent gating. Am J Physiol Cell Physiol 1998; 274: C1485–C1495.
35. Gulbis JM, Mann S, MacKinnon R. Structure of a voltage-dependent K^+ channel β subunit. Cell 1999; 97:943–952.
36. Bahring R, Milligan CJ, Vardanyan V, Engeland B, Young BA, Dannenberg J, Waldshütz R, Edwards JP, Wray D, Pongs O. Coupling of voltage-dependent potassium channel inactivation and oxidoreductase active site of Kvβ subunits. J Biol Chem 2001; 276:22923–22929.
37. Campomanes CR, Carroll KI, Manganas LN, Hershberger ME, Gong B, Antonucci DE, Rhodes KJ, Trimmer JS. Kvβ subunit oxidoreductase activity and Kv1 potassium channel trafficking. J Biol Chem 2002; 277:8298–8305.
38. Peri R, Wible BA, Brown AM. Mutations in the Kvβ2 binding site for NADPH and their effects on Kv1.4. J Biol Chem 2001; 276:738–741.
39. Johnson BD. The company they keep: ion channels and their intracellular regulatory partners. Adv Second Messenger Phosphoprotein Res 1999: 33203–33228.
40. Nakahira K, Matos MF, Trimmer JS. Differential interaction of voltage-gated K^+ channel β-subunits with cytoskeleton is mediated by unique amino terminal domains. J Mol Neurosci 1999; 11:199–208.
41. Anderson RG, Jacobson K. A role for lipid shells in targeting proteins to caveolae, rafts, and other lipid domains. Science 2002; 296:1821–1825.
42. Baumann CA, Ribon V, Kanzaki M, Thurmond DC, Mora S, Shigematsu S, Bickel PE, Pessin JE, Saltiel AR. CAP defines a second signalling pathway required for insulin-stimulated glucose transport. Nature 2000; 407:202–207.
43. Goligorsky MS, Li H, Brodsky S, Chen J. Relationships between caveolae and eNOS: everything in proximity and the proximity of everything. Am J Physiol Renal Physiol 2002; 283:F1–F10.
44. Feron O, Zhao YY, Kelly RA. The ins and outs of caveolar signaling. m2 muscarinic cholinergic receptors and eNOS activation versus neuregulin and ErbB4 signaling in cardiac myocytes. Ann NY Acad Sci 1999; 87411–87419.
45. Rybin VO, Xu X, Lisanti MP, and Steinberg SF. Differential targeting of β-adrenergic receptor subtypes and adenylyl cyclase to cardiomyocyte caveolae: a mechanism to functionally regulate the cAMP signaling pathway. J Biol Chem 2000; 275:41447–41457.
46. Rybin VO, Xu X, Steinberg SF. Activated protein kinase C isoforms target to cardiomyocyte caveolae: stimulation of local protein phosphorylation. Circ Res 1999; 84:980–988.
47. Lasley RD, Narayan P, Uittenbogaard A, Smart EJ. Activated cardiac adenosine A_1 receptors translocate out of caveolae. J Biol Chem 2000; 275: 4417–4421.
48. Zhao YY, Liu Y, Stan RV, Fan L, Gu Y, Dalton N, Chu PH, Peterson K, Ross J Jr, Chien KR. Defects in caveolin-1 cause dilated cardiomyopathy and pulmonary hypertension in knockout mice. Proc Natl Acad Sci USA 2002; 99:11375–11380.

49. Martens JR, Sakamoto N, Sullivan SA, Grobaski TD, Tamkun MM. Isoform-specific localization of voltage-gated K^+ channels to distinct lipid raft populations. Targeting of Kv1.5 to caveolae. J Biol Chem 2001; 276:8409–8414.
50. Conforti L, Bodi I, Nisbet JW, Millhorn DE. O_2-sensitive K^+ channels: role of the Kv1.2α-subunit in mediating the hypoxic response. J Physiol 2000; 524:783–793.
51. Archer SL, London B, Hampl V, Wu X, Nsair A, Puttagunta L, Hashimoto K, Wite RE, Michelakis E. Impairment of hypoxic pulmonary vasoconstriction in mice lacking the voltage-gated potassium channel Kv1.5. FASEB J 2001; 15:1801–1803.
52. Ho CS, Grange RW, Joho RH. Pleiotropic effects of a disrupted K^+ channel gene: reduced body weight, impaired motor skill and muscle contraction, but no seizures. Proc Natl Acad Sci USA 1997; 94:1533–1538.
53. Ekhterae D, Platoshyn O, Krick S, Yu Y, McDaniel SS, Yuan JX-J. Bcl-2 decreases voltage-gated K^+ channel activity and enhances survival in vascular smooth muscle cells. Am J Physiol Cell Physiol 2001; 281:C157–C165.
54. Davies AR, Kozlowski RZ. Kv channel subunit expression in rat pulmonary arteries. Lung 2001; 179:147–161.
55. Yuan XJ, Wang J, Juhaszova M, Gaine SP, Rubin LJ. Attenuated K^+ channel gene transcription in primary pulmonary hypertension. Lancet 1998; 351: 726–727.
56. Platoshyn O, Yu Y, Golovina VA, McDaniel SS, Krick S, Li L, Wang JY, Rubin LJ Yuan JX-J. Chronic hypoxia decreases K_V channel expression and function in pulmonary artery myocytes. Am J Physiol Lung Cell Mol Physiol 2001; 280:L801–L812.

12

Ca^{2+}-Activated, Voltage-Dependent K^+ Channels

Ligia Toro, Abderrahmane Alioua, Rong Lu, Jesus Garcia-Valdes, Kazuhide Nishimaru*, Mansoureh Eghbali, and Enrico Stefani

David Geffen School of Medicine at University of California Los Angeles, Los Angeles, California, U.S.A.

Masoud M. Zarei

Center for Biomedical Studies, UTB/TSC, Brownsville, Texas, U.S.A.

I. INTRODUCTION

Calcium-activated, voltage-dependent K^+ channels, also called MaxiK or BK_{Ca} because of their large conductance (~120 pS in physiological solutions), are abundant proteins in all smooth muscles including the vasculature. MaxiK channels are key regulators of vascular tone, acting as a rheostat that fine-tunes the membrane potential and intracellular Ca^{2+} concentration according to the cell needs. Accordingly, MaxiK channels are targets of vasoactive substances including vasorelaxants (e.g., nitric oxide and arachidonic acid pathways) and vasoconstrictors (e.g., angiotensin II, 5-hydroxytryptamine, phenylephrine, thromboxane A_2). A newly discovered pathway for vasoconstriction links constricting agonist stimulation to c-Src tyrosine kinase activation followed by phosphorylation and inhibition of MaxiK channel activity, which would result in membrane depolarization, Ca^{2+} entry, and contraction. At the molecular level, MaxiK channels from vascular smooth muscle are formed by the coas-

* Current affiliation: Department of Pharmacology, Yamagata University School of Medicine, Yamagata, Japan.

sembly of four α subunits that form the channel pore with four regulatory β1 subunits. β1 subunits profoundly modify how the channel responds to Ca^{2+}, voltage, intracellular signaling, and pharmacological agents. The α subunit is the product of a single gene but with plenty of potential splice variants. The β1 subunit belongs to a family of genes that are largely tissue-specific, with β1 being the smooth muscle archetype. Because the functional properties of smooth muscle vary along the vascular tree, to understand the role of MaxiK channels in health and disease it is of the outmost importance to dissect their molecular composition, macromolecular assembly, cell targeting and traffic, and function and regulation in different vessels.

II. GENE STRUCTURE AND MOLECULAR PROPERTIES

A. Gene Structure

MaxiK channels from vascular smooth muscle are multimeric complexes formed by four α subunits (Slo) that form the K^+ channel pore and four modulatory β1 subunits (Fig. 1). The human α subunit (hSlo) is encoded by a single gene that expands ~940 kb of human chromosome 10. Alignment of hSlo cDNA including known splice inserts (Table 1) to the draft sequence of the human genome (http://www.ncbi.nlm.nih.gov/LocusLink/) predicts that the *hSlo* gene consists of at least 39 exons, of which 27 are considered constitutive exons encoding for the protein backbone (Fig. 1). Figure 1A illustrates the proposed topology of the translated constitutive exons, where arrowheads mark the beginning of each exon (except exon 1 that also contains untranslated sequences), numbers indicate exon number (missing numbers correspond to predicted alternate exons of known or experimentally undetermined protein sequence, Table 1), asterisks (*) indicate sites where alternate exons have been detected experimentally, and double asterisks (**) indicate alternate exons found experimentally but not predicted in the draft human genome. It is notable that the hSlo protein seems to be assembled by functional cassettes encoded by exons that must have been strictly selected through evolution. Examples are (1) the S4 region known to be critical for voltage sensing, (2) the pore region necessary for conduction and K^+ selectivity (linker between S5 and S6), and (3) the unique S0 domain that is necessary for β1 subunit regulation. The carboxyl terminus, on the other hand, is constituted by a large number of exons representing a big potential for functional variation underlain by modulation of alternative splicing.

The β1-subunit gene structure has been deciphered experimentally and is much simpler than the predicted α subunit gene. It is formed by four exons spanning ~29 kb of human chromosome 5. The translated constitutive protein is encoded by part of exon 2, exon 3, and part of exon 4 (1). To date, no functional splice variants have been detected for this β1 subunit; however, a truncated

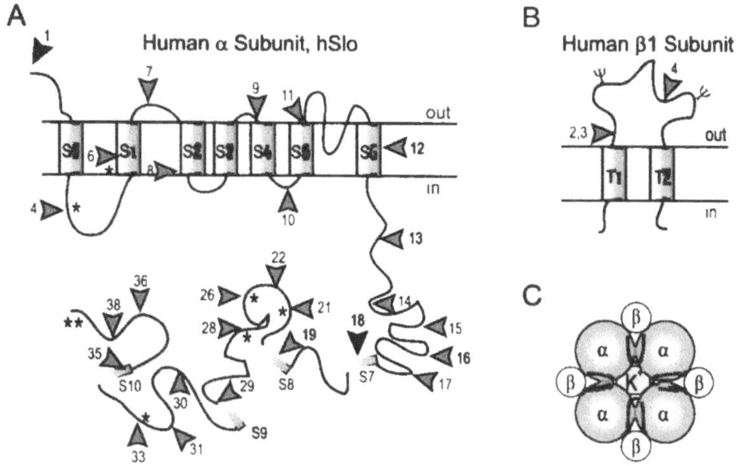

Figure 1 Topology of human MaxiK channel pore forming α (hSlo) and β1 subunits. (A) Membrane topology of hSlo. Arrows and numbers mark the constitutive exons encoding the corresponding protein domain. Missing numbers correspond to known or predicted alternate exons. ( ) Sites where sequences encoded by alternate exons have been reported. ( ) Alternate exon found experimentally but not predicted in the draft of the human genome. S0–S6, transmembrane regions. S0, necessary for β1 modulation; S4, voltage sensor; S5–S6 linker, pore region. S7–S10, hydrophobic intracellular segments. (B) Beta subunit. T1, T2, transmembrane domains. Arrows and numbers mark exon/intron boundaries. (C) MaxiK channel assembly. Four α subunits form the K pore. α : β1 stoichiometry is 1:1. Extracellular loops of β1 subunit lie near the pore.

β1-like subunit with unknown function and a predicted single, transmembrane domain has been recently reported (Accession #BC025707). Figure 1B shows the topology of the β1 subunit and the exon/intron boundaries (arrows).

B. Molecular Properties

Structure–function studies have indicated that the MaxiK channel pore-forming α subunit Slo is formed by functional cassettes. The Slo channel differs from other voltage-dependent channels in that it contains seven transmembrane domains (S0–S6). S0 is unique for the Slo channel, is necessary for β1 modulation, and leads to an extracellular N-terminus (for a review see Ref. 2). In addition, it has a very long carboxyl terminus containing another four hydrophobic segments (S7–S10). A simple scheme of the current view is depicted in Fig. 2. Methionine (M)1–M3 are three possible translation starts. Most of the studies performed to date have used clones beginning from M3. Initial studies directed to find the Ca^{2+}-sensing domain divided the protein into two parts, the "core" and the "tail." The core

Variants in Mammalian MaxiK Channel α Subunit, Slo

rotein egion[b]	Sequence[c]	Function[d]
-S1	GRKPRLQGGVIGCMFHLQPREAQ KSSSALEVHKKYGDSTGTTLE (44)	⇓ Ca^{2+}/V; $\Delta V_{1/2}$ (+) 50 m
S1	AFERSSLLARISIQKDGCQCVLF SSHFMPRLLM (33) (named SV1 exon)	Endoplasmic reticulum retention
-S9	SRKR (4)*	⇓ Ca^{2+}/V; $\Delta V_{1/2}$ (+) 10 m
	SRKRYALFVNFSSNLHPLSSLLTTGL TICQEFKKREIIYI (40)*	Unknown
-S9	IYF (3)*	Unknown
	KVAARSRYSKDPFEFKKETPNSRLVTEPV (29)*	Unknown
	IYFKVAARSRYSKDPFEFKKETPNSRLVTEPV (32)*	Unknown
	RPKMSIYKRMRRACCFDCGRSERDCSCM SGRVRGNVDTLERAFPLSSVSVNDCSTSFRAF (60)* (named the STREX exon)	⇑ Ca^{2+}/V, $\Delta V_{1/2}$ (-) 20–40 channels inhibited by PK and oxidation
-S9	RFSCPFLP (8)*	Unknown
-S10	QGMHLGVTQHQIYAVX (rabbit)	fs/sc, protein 796 amino ac
-S10	AKPAKLPLVSVNQEKNSGTHILMITEL (27)*	Unknown
OOH	NRKEMVY (7)*	Unknown
	NSTRMNRMGQEKKWFTDEPDNAYPRNIQI KPMSTHMANQINQYKSTSSLIPPIREVEDEC (60) (mouse)	Unknown

:. 1. ?, unknown.

S1, between transmembrane segments S0 and S1; S8–S9, between hydrophobic segments S8 and S9; S9–S10, between hydropho
arboxyl terminus.

ses are the numbers of amino acids inserted. Asterisks (*) indicate inserts found in the human MaxiK α subunit, hSlo (see F
ge sensitivity of the variant. $\Delta V_{1/2}$, shift in the half-activation potential induced by the insert. ⇓, decrease. ⇑, increase. (−) lef
:, frame shift found in rabbit Slo induced by 104 bp deletion leads to 15 different amino acids, a premature stop codon, and

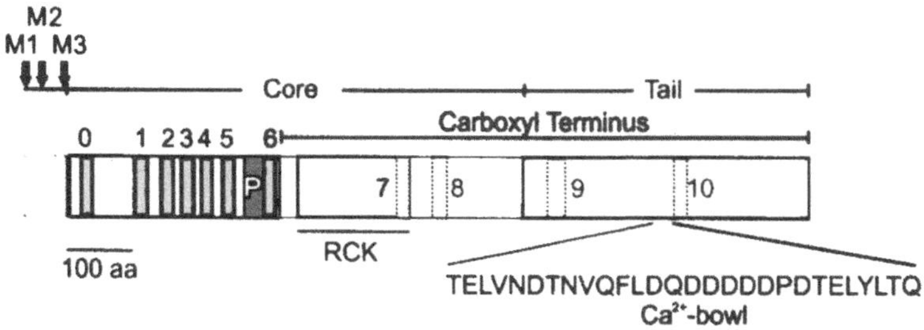

Figure 2 Linear structure of hSlo protein and functional cassettes. hSlo protein (drawn to scale) according to GenBank U11058 with 1113 amino acids (M3 start). Dotted box at the NH_2-terminus marks possible methionine starts (M1 and M2). Gray boxes (0–6) mark transmembrane domains. P, pore region. Dashed gray boxes (7–10) hydrophobic regions in intracellular carboxyl terminus. Also indicated are the positions of the "core," "tail," intracellular carboxyl terminus, regulator of conductance for K^+ domain (RCK), and "Ca bowl."

contains transmembrane segments S0–S6 and hydrophobic regions S7 and S8; the "tail" contains S9 and S10 and the "Ca^{2+}-bowl" just before S10.

Voltage Sensor

The Slo channel belongs to the S6 superfamily of K^+ channels with the S4 transmembrane region as its main voltage-sensing domain. It is now accepted that the Slo channel can be activated solely by voltage at physiological Ca^{2+} concentrations ($\leq$100 nM) and that micromolar Ca^{2+} serves as a modulator of channel activity. The first evidence for this concept was the lack of channel stimulation by Ca^{2+} concentrations $\leq$100 nM, although the channel could still be activated by depolarization (2). Further support was given by modeling the channel behavior as an allosteric protein and by directly measuring the movement of the voltage sensor (gating currents) independently of $Ca^{2+} < 100$ nM (3,4). The voltage sensor rearrangements in response to depolarization and associated pore opening are triggered by voltage and facilitated by micromolar Ca^{2+} (3). Conversely, under conditions such that the voltage sensors are not activated (voltage less than −80 mV), micromolar Ca^{2+} can increase the open probability, indicating that Ca^{2+} binding to its sensor(s) and voltage sensor activation are likely independent mechanisms (4).

Ca^{2+} Sensors

The definition of Ca^{2+} sensor(s) in Slo channels has been much more difficult than the definition of the main voltage sensor, because changes throughout the protein including the transmembrane domains can dramatically affect Ca^{2+} sensitivity. For example, the mutation R207Q in the S4 region increases Ca^{2+} sensitivity by ~1000-fold. Because Ca^{2+} sensing occurs intracellularly, most investigations have addressed the role of the intracellular carboxyl terminus as a Ca^{2+} sensor. The motif that has received much attention is the so-called Ca^{2+} bowl, which contains a string of aspartate residues that when mutated or transplanted can diminish or confer Ca^{2+} sensitivity (5) (Fig. 2). Biochemical experiments with purified protein also show that mutation of these negatively charged residues leads to a decrease in direct Ca^{2+} binding (6). However, additional sites for Ca^{2+} sensing have been proposed, including negative residues within the regulator of conductance for the K^+ domain, RCK (7), located in the first fifth of the Slo carboxyl end and a methionine at the end of hydrophobic segment S7 that lies within the RCK domain (8) (Fig. 2). These residues, when mutated, together with mutation of the Ca^{2+} bowl, practically abolish Slo physiological regulation by Ca^{2+}. In support of the RCK–Ca^{2+} bowl hypothesis for Ca^{2+} binding, the crystal structure of the *Methanobacterium thermoautotrophicum* K^+ channel (MthK) shows that eight RCK domains bind Ca^{2+} to open the K^+ pore (9). In contrast to the Ca^{2+} bowl–RCK domain hypothesis as Ca^{2+} binding domains, recent evidence suggests that neither the Ca^{2+} bowl nor the RCK domain is necessary for Ca^{2+} activation of MaxiK channels because a mutant channel lacking the whole carboxyl C-terminus is still activated by micromolar Ca^{2+} (10). It is obvious from these studies that the Ca^{2+} regulatory domain(s) are complex and not simple linear structures. Thus, at this point, we can only state that MaxiK channels probably have several Ca^{2+}-binding sites with complex 3D structures that regulate channel activity.

Mg^{2+} Sensor

Besides Ca^{2+}, MaxiK channels can also be modulated by Mg^{2+} in the millimolar range. Recent evidence indicates that Mg^{2+} binding to the Slo channel occurs at independent sites of its Ca^{2+} modulation and also within the RCK domain (11).

Splice Variant Functions

The functional diversity of the MaxiK channel arises not from different genes but from splice variation and association with β subunits. At least seven splicing sites have been found in the smooth muscle and other organs in humans (asterisks in Fig. 1A), and about 10 splice inserts (Table 1). The function of most of them remains unknown. However, there are two alternate exons that are particularly interesting: (1) a 33 amino acid insert in the S1 transmembrane region that does not modify the topology of hSlo and serves as a dominant negative regulator of surface expression (12) (Fig. 3) and (2) a 60 amino acid insert called the STREX exon that is upregulated by adrenocorticotropic hormone (13) and causes the Slo channel to be

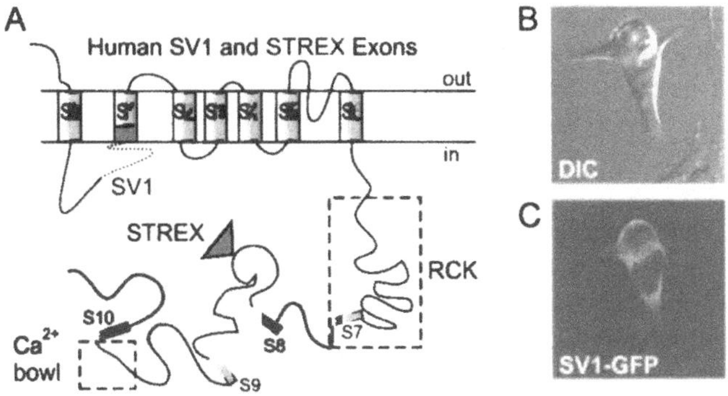

Figure 3 SV1 splice variant serves as dominant negative regulator of hSlo expression. (A) Diagram showing the positions of two functionally important splice exons, SV1 and STREX. Also shown are the relative positions of RCK domains and the "Ca^{2+} bowl." (B) DIC images of HEK 293T cells transfected with hSlo-SV1 with GFP at the carboxyl terminus. (C) hSlo-SV1-GFP fluoresecence showing that SV1 induces retention of hSlo in perinuclear organelles. (Adapted from Ref. 12.)

inhibited by oxidation (14) and to respond differentially to protein kinase A phosphorylation (15). Channels containing the STREX exon are inhibited by PKA, whereas channels without this exon are activated by PKA (15). The site in the STREX exon responsible for its dominant inhibitory PKA effect is its first serine (KMS) (Table 1). In addition, the STREX exon is slightly upregulated by β-estradiol (16) and imparts a higher degree to Ca^{2+} sensitivity to Slo channels (17). All these findings are consistent with the view that an important mechanism contributing to the functional diversity and plasticity of MaxiK channels is the expression of distinct Slo splice variants. Given the fact that MaxiK channels are important regulators of vascular tone (see below), mechanisms that regulate the expression of distinct splice variants are expected to produce important functional consequences. Much more research needs to be done to decipher which splice variants are present in each vascular bed, what are the mechanisms that regulate their temporal or constitutive expression, and their physiological impact in basic cell functions.

The β1 Subunit

The MaxiK channel β subunits form a family of four genes (β1–β4) that seem to be tissue-specific; in particular, smooth muscle is rich in the β1 subunit. The β1 subunit is formed by two transmembrane domains and a highly glycosylated extracellular loop (ψ) (Fig. 1B) with conserved cysteines that may form cross-bridges (1). When associated with the α subunit, the loop of each β1 subunit (Fig. 1C) may localize close to the K^+ conduction pathway. Evidence for this structural view comes from biochemical and pharmacological data showing that the presence of a β1 subunit alters the on-rate of blockade by toxins to the channel pore (18).

The β1 subunit extensively modifies the MaxiK channel α-subunit phenotype. Ca^{2+} sensitivity is dramatically increased by ~300-fold accompanied by a profound increase (~90 mV) in its voltage sensitivity (measured as the voltage needed to reach 50% of maximum open probability, $V_{1/2}$). This extraordinary β1 upregulation of Slo channels is switched on by micromolar Ca^{2+} (2). The functional coupling of β1 subunits with the channel pore achieved at micromolar Ca^{2+} allows arterial MaxiK channels to be tonically active and to serve as a vasodilatory force maintaining vascular tone. In resistance vessels, the Ca^{2+} necessary to couple α and β subunits comes from local Ca^{2+} sparks through ryanodine receptors in the endoplasmic reticulum, which are probably in close proximity to MaxiK channels at the plasma membrane. The role of MaxiK channels as key regulators of arterial tone was recently confirmed by silencing the β1 subunit gene. The β1 knockout (KO) mouse has decreased basal MaxiK channel activity with increased vascular reactivity and tone leading to hypertension (19).

III. REGULATION OF CHANNEL ACTIVITY AND EXPRESSION

As stated before, MaxiK channel activity is highly regulated by its molecular composition including α-subunit splice variants and association with β1 subunit. The presence or absence of both may affect how channels are regulated not only by Ca^{2+} and voltage but also by phosphorylation and hormones.

A. Phosphorylation

Serine-Threonine Kinases

MaxiK channels from the vasculature are inhibited by PKC and activated by PKG and PKA in response to exogenous stimuli such as nitric oxide and β-adrenergic stimulation (for a recent review see Ref. 20). The upregulation induced by PKA in vascular smooth muscle is consistent with a MaxiK molecular composition consisting of α subunits lacking the STREX exon, which would otherwise impart a PKA-dependent inhibitory phenotype to the channel (15). The site of PKA phosphorylation causing activation of the MaxiK α subunit has been mapped to its carboxyl terminus at the weak consensus motif $RQPS^{869}$ (15). Moreover, work performed with the *Drosophila* Slo (dSlo) channel indicates that its carboxyl residues 821–893 can directly bind to the catalytic subunit of PKA although channel phosphorylation by PKA is not required for this protein–protein interaction (21).

On the other hand, direct PKG-dependent phosphorylation of Slo has also been demonstrated, but several sites have been proposed as responsible for PKG-mediated activation of the α subunit, namely, serine 1072 and serines 855 and 869 (20). The molecular correlate for PKC-induced inhibition, however, has received no attention and needs to be explored.

Tyrosine Kinases

Tyrosine kinases are key signaling components of intracellular cascades involved in the regulation of multiple cell functions such as cell motility, proliferation, and survival and cell adhesion. In vascular smooth muscle, study of the functional role of tyrosine kinases is an emerging field and has been mostly in relation to the angiotensin II pathway and Src tyrosine kinase family. In the angiotensin II pathway, c-Src tyrosine phosphorylation is one of the earliest events of the cascade, which leads to contraction of smooth muscle (22). In support of this view, a c-Src KO mice has reduced Ca^{2+} responses to angiotensin II, and inhibition of Src by PP2 markedly reduces angiotensin II-induced contraction (22,23). We recently demonstrated that MaxiK channels form part of this signaling cascade, leading to coronary and aortic contraction (23). Moreover, it seems that the c-Src–MaxiK contractile pathway is common to other contractant agonists such as 5-hydroxytryptamine (5-HT) (23) (Figs. 4 and 5).

In isolated vascular myocytes, where c-Src is very abundant, inhibition of Src by lavendustin A produces an increase in MaxiK currents of the rat tail artery (24) and coronary arteries (23), supporting the view that MaxiK channels are inhibited by Src. Consistent with the pharmacological data, direct phosphorylation (Fig. 4) and inhibition of hSlo by c-Src tyrosine kinase has been demonstrated in heterologous systems, where hSlo and c-Src show a striking colocalization (23) and can also be coimmunoprecipitated (25). The site where c-Src phosphorylation produces inhibition in hSlo remains to be elucidated.

Interestingly, heterologous expression of active c-Src produces activation of mouse Slo (mSlo) (26) instead of the hSlo inhibition observed with native c-Src (23). It is possible that constitutively active c-Src triggers oncogenic cellular mechanisms that lead to activation of MaxiK channels. Alternatively, differences in the carboxyl end of mSlo with respect to hSlo may explain this opposite regulation. In the case of mSlo, Tyr^{766} ($GSIEY^{766}LKRE$) is an important site for phosphorylation of the active c-Src (26).

Another tyrosine kinase that interacts with hSlo is the spleen tyrosine kinase, Syk that binds to the immunoreceptor tyrosine-based activation motif (ITAM) of hSlo. However, in this case, MaxiK channel activity of the Syk-transfected human CAL-72 osteosarcoma cell line was unaffected by Syk activity (25).

In summary, experiments to understand the mechanism of MaxiK channel regulation by phosphorylation have opened a new view on the functional role of the Slo channel carboxyl terminus. We envision that it acts

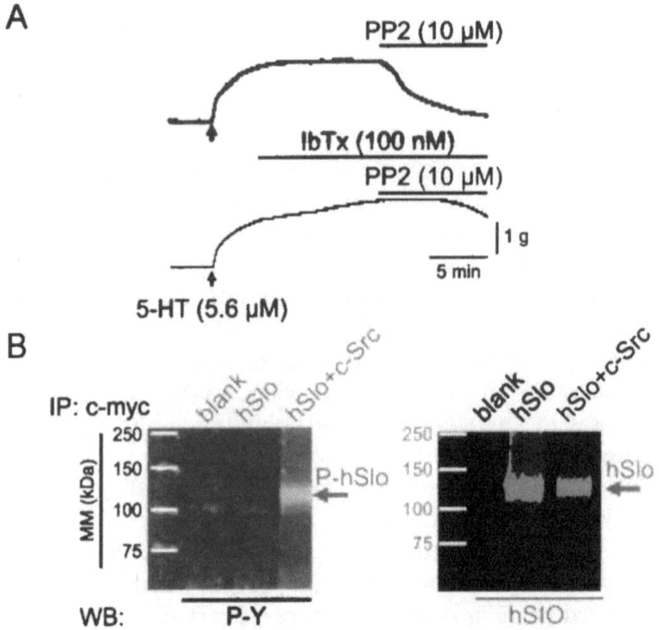

Figure 4 Phosphorylation of hSlo by c-Src mediates 5-HT-induced vasoconstriction. (A) Upper panel: 5-HT-induced contraction of aortic rings is reversed by application of Src tyrosine kinase inhibitor PP2, indicating that 5-HT-induced contraction involves Src stimulation. Lower panel: IbTx treatment after 5-HT stimulation (arrow) prevents PP2- induced relaxation, suggesting that MaxiK channels are inhibited by Src upon 5-HT stimulation. (B) MaxiK channel protein is substrate of tyrosine phosphorylation. Lysates of untransfected cells (blank) or cells transfected with hSlo or hSlo + c-Src were immunoprecipitated (IP) with anti-c-myc Ab (hSlo is c-myc tagged), resolved in SDS gels, and immunoblotted with antiphosphotyrosine (P-Y) [left Western blot (WB)] and with anti-hSlo (right WB). Images correspond to the same blot using infrared fluorescence. Tyrosine-phosphorylated band has the molecular mass of hSlo (P-hSlo) and is colabeled with anti-hSlo Ab (right blot, arrow). hSlo is also detected in hSlo-transfected cells. (Adapted from Ref. 23.)

as a scaffolding domain to bring together proteins at their correct positions to exert their modulatory and signal propagation functions.

B. Redox Regulation

In smooth muscle, redox regulation of MaxiK channels has been demonstrated in tracheal myocytes where sulfhydryl-reducing agents such as dithiothreitol (DTT) and reduced glutathione increase the channel open probability without changing the number of channels (27). The α subunit of MaxiK channels, hSlo, seems to account for these effects in native

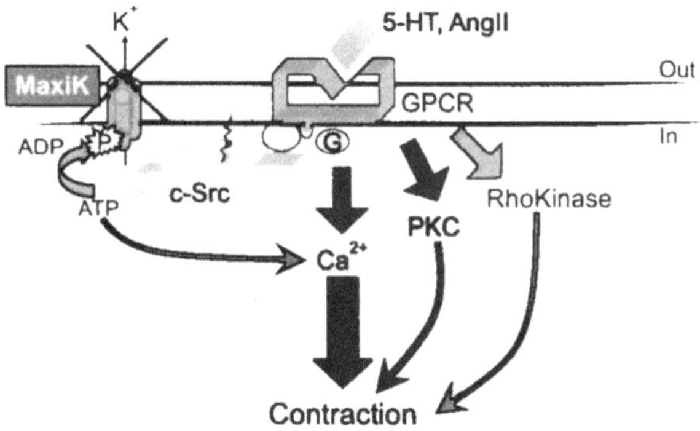

Figure 5 New G-protein coupled receptor (GPCR)–c-Src–MaxiK pathway. Stimulation of GPCRs by corresponding agonists leads to contraction via Ca^{2+}-dependent (via Ca^{2+}-induced Ca^{2+} release from intracellular stores) and Ca^{2+}-independent (via Rho Kinase or PKC) pathways. The new GPCR–c-Src–MaxiK pathway begins with 5-HT or angiotensin II stimulation of GPCRs and corresponding G proteins followed by activation of c-Src that phosphorylates and inhibits MaxiK channels. Inhibition of MaxiK channels would reduce K^+ efflux from the cell, causing depolarization, Ca^{2+} entry, and activation of the contractile machinery.

smooth muscle, because hSlo is also a target of hydrogen peroxide (H_2O_2) and DTT opposing actions (28). Oxidation of hSlo leads to lower channel open probability, but in this case, it does cause a diminution in the number of active channels. It would be interesting to determine whether coexpression with the β1 subunit reconstitutes the lack of channel number reduction seen in native smooth muscle. Reduction of hSlo with DTT leads to increased channel activity. The sites for DTT action are located in the intracellular domain of hSlo. Interestingly, the oxidative action of H_2O_2 on hSlo is Ca^{2+}-dependent and is observed at 500 nM Ca^{2+} (or 5 μM Ca^{2+} in skeletal muscle MaxiK) but not at 100 μM Ca^{2+} (28). Experiments in skeletal muscle MaxiK channels suggest that the H_2O_2 effect on hSlo activity is mediated by the free radical OH, likely involving the reduction of disulfide bonds to thiol groups in the intracellular domain of hSlo.

In addition to sulfhydryl oxidation, hSlo can also undergo methionine oxidation. Studies with chloramine-T, which preferentially oxidizes methionine, induces an increase in hSlo activity, which was partially reversed by methionine sulfoxide reductase. Because the pore blocker tetraethylammonium interferes with the chloramine-T effect, it has been proposed that the oxidizable methionine lies within the pore of hSlo (29).

C. Hormonal Regulation

Hormonal regulation of MaxiK channels has been observed at two levels, genomic and nongenomic. The main characteristic of a nongenomic effect is its rapid action through a receptor on the plasma membrane or in the cytosol, whereas a genomic effect needs hours to be established as gene activation and protein synthesis take place.

Nongenomic Regulation of MaxiK Channel Activity

Direct action of hormones on MaxiK channel activity has been shown for β-estradiol. MaxiK channels assembled by α and β1 subunits are rapidly activated by β-estradiol only at nanomolar Ca^{2+}, using the β1 subunit as binding domain (30). This view has been extended by experiments using tamoxifen and β1 subunit KO mice, where tamoxifen activation of colonic smooth muscle MaxiK channel activity is dependent on the expression of the β1 subunit (31).

Genomic Regulation of MaxiK Protein Expression

The mechanisms regulating MaxiK channel protein expression in vascular smooth muscle have received little attention. However, evidence that MaxiK channel expression is regulated at the genomic level comes from uterine smooth muscle. In this tissue, MaxiK channel expression at the plasma membrane is greatly reduced at the end of pregnancy, with a concomitant decrease in Slo mRNA levels (32) strongly indicating that the MaxiK channel gene is directly or indirectly regulated by sex hormones. This reduced protein surface expression agrees with the diminished MaxiK currents observed in late pregnant myometrium from rats and mice (33,34). However, in mice an alternative mechanism to reduced channel activity must prevail, because total protein and transcript levels augment rather than diminish at the end of pregnancy (34) and tend to be slightly higher in estradiol-treated animals (16). Beta 1 subunit mRNA from mouse myometrium also increases with β-estradiol treatment (35). It would be interesting to determine whether MaxiK channel expression changes with estrogen or progesterone treatments in the vasculature given the recent results of the Women's Health Initiative (WHI) trial of estrogen plus progestin, which had to be stopped early because of an increased risk of stroke induced by hormone therapy of postmenopausal women, and the Women's Angiographic Vitamin and Estrogen (WAVE) Trial, where estrogen (plus medroxyprogesterone acetate for women without hysterectomy) and vitamin E/C therapies increased risk for death, nonfatal myocardial infarction, or stroke of postmenopausal women with coronary disease.

D. Expression of MaxiK Regulated by Splice Variation and Cell Traffic

The cell biology of ion channels, including MaxiK, is an emerging field, and many questions need to be answered to understand how hSlo channels are assembled and traffic to reach their specific localization at the cell membrane. In this regard, we recently showed that hSlo channels possess an intrinsic signal in their carboxyl terminus for apical expression in Madin–Darby canine kidney cells. hSlo requires its carboxyl terminus for cell-surface expression and displays properties for lipid raft apical targeting that is independent of glycosylation of the channel itself or an associated protein (36). The requirement of the hSlo carboxyl terminus for surface expression was later confirmed in HEK cells and medullary thick ascending limb (mTAL) cells using the splice carboxyl-end-truncated version of rabbit Slo, which ends after S9 and has 15 unique amino acids (Table 1) (37).

One of the mechanisms to regulate surface expression of hSlo is the expression of a recently discovered splice variant, SV1 (12). This splice variant was discovered in human myometrium and is localized in the splice site at transmembrane segment S1 (Fig. 1); it replaces part of S1 and makes the S0–S1 linker longer (Fig. 3A). When expressed in HEK cells, SV1 is localized in the endoplasmic reticulum. As an example, Fig. 3B shows the perinuclear localization of SV1 tagged with green fluorescent protein (SV1-GFP). Moreover, the SV1 variant has the ability to retain insertless hSlo and β1 in the ER. These findings indicate that surface expression of the MaxiK channel can be exquisitely regulated by triggering expression of splice variants. The nature of the trigger remains unknown, but it is tempting to suggest hormones as possible regulators of splice variants.

IV. FUNCTIONAL ROLES OF THE CHANNEL

The main role of MaxiK channels in the vasculature is to control vascular tone by regulating both vasoconstriction and vasorelaxation. In addition, recent evidence indicates that they may also be tightly linked to signaling molecules and thus serve as signal transducers to modify cell functions such as growth and proliferation.

A. MaxiK Channels as Rheostats

MaxiK channels control vascular tone by responding to both contractant and relaxant stimuli. How this occurs can be simplified by viewing MaxiK channels as rheostats whereby vasorelaxants that increase channel activity and thus augment K^+ efflux (e.g., β-agonists, arachidonic acid, nitric oxide, angiotensin II via AT_2 receptors) promote hyperpolarization of the plasma membrane leading to decreased Ca^{2+} entry through voltage-dependent Ca^{2+} channels turning down Ca^{2+}-dependent contraction. Conversely, vasoconstrictors that diminish channel activity and thus reduce K^+ efflux (e.g., angiotensin II via AT_1 receptors, thromboxane A_2) would promote depolarization, increased Ca^{2+} entry and contraction.

Vasorelaxants use distinct intracellular pathways to increase MaxiK channel activity. For example, NO uses the guanylate cyclase–c-GMP-dependent pathway to directly phosphorylate the channel and increase channel activity; whereas β-adrenergic stimulation uses the adenylyl cyclase–c-AMP-dependent pathway to directly phosphorylate the channel.

The pathways used by vasoconstrictors to inhibit MaxiK channels in vascular smooth muscle are beginning to be understood. Because vasoconstrictors such as thromboxane A_2 and angiotensin II trigger PKC cascades and PKC inhibits MaxiK channels (20), PKC-dependent phosphorylation is one possible mechanism linking agonist stimulation to PKC-mediated MaxiK inhibition and contraction. However, this pathway has not been demonstrated at the cellular level.

Pharmacological evidence had indicated that agonist induced contraction involves as a primary step tyrosine kinase activation. However, most of those studies were performed using drugs of broad action, such as genistein, making it difficult to assess with accuracy the role of tyrosine kinases in agonist-induced vasoconstriction. Recently, using selective drugs for Src kinase (e.g. PP2 or PP1) and c-Src KO mice, it was demonstrated that, at least for angiotensin II, c-Src tyrosine kinase activation is one of the first steps in the contractile signaling cascade (22). Given the fact that c-Src is abundant in vascular smooth muscle as well as MaxiK channels, we put forward the hypothesis that agonist stimulation, by activating c-Src, could result in c-Src dependent phosphorylation and inhibition of MaxiK activity leading to contraction (Fig. 5). If this were the case, one could predict that (1) c-Src inhibition would reverse smooth muscle contraction and (2) blocking MaxiK channels would prevent the relaxation induced by c-Src inhibition. We recently reported that this is indeed the case (23). Figure 4A shows an example where 5-HT induced contraction in an aortic ring is reversed by application of PP2, an inhibitor of Src tyrosine kinase. Consistent with our hypothesis, treatment with a MaxiK channel blocker prevented the relaxant effect of PP2. Moreover, the Western blots of Fig. 4B show that hSlo can be directly tyrosine phosphorylated (P-Y) by coexpression with c-Src. In these experiments, we used cells that were or were not cotransfected with hSlo tagged with a c-myc epitope with or without c-Src. Immunoprecipitation (IP) was performed using anti-c-myc Ab, and Western blot (WB) was performed using the same membrane with anti-P-Y and anti-hSlo antibodies. These experiments together with electrophysiological data on native cells showing that inhibition of c-Src leads to activation of MaxiK channels and data on cotransfected cells (hSlo + c-Src) showing that tyrosine dephosphorylation leads to channel activation made us conclude that MaxiK forms part of a new signaling cascade that traduces extracellular agonist input via c-Src to intracellular pathways leading to contraction (23).

B. MaxiK Channel Macromolecular Complexes

The first evidence showing that MaxiK channels formed tight complexes with other signaling molecules came from experiments in lipid bilayers in the early 1990s when reconstituted coronary muscle channels were activated by vasorelaxant stimuli such as β-adrenergic agents (38) and inhibited by vasoconstrictors such as thromboxane A2 (39) and angiotensin II (40). Under these experimental conditions, it was expected that channels would be dissociated from other proteins in the infinite lipid environment of the bilayer; however, we could readily demonstrate that MaxiK channels were functionally coupled to receptors and G proteins, which proved that MaxiK channels formed part of tight macromolecular signaling complexes. Supporting this view and using molecular tools collected in the last decade, dSlo channels were shown to directly interact with the catalytic subunit of PKA and Src tyrosine kinase (21). Recent studies also demonstrate that hSlo and c-Src can be coimmunoprecipitated and show strong colocalization when cotransfected in heterologous systems (23,25).

Given the above evidence, it is safe to suggest that MaxiK channels are localized strategically together with G-protein-coupled receptors (GPCRs), G proteins and kinases forming macromolecular complexes via direct interactions or via scaffolding proteins (perhaps MaxiK's own carboxyl terminus acting as scaffold) to exert their functions.

V. RELATIONSHIP TO VASCULAR DISEASE AND AGING

Because MaxiK channels play such an important role in maintaining vascular tone, it is expected that their expression and/or function is altered in pathogenic states or, conversely, that alterations in their expression and/or function contribute to the pathology of disease or aging.

A. Aging

One of the main risk factors for cardiovascular disease is aging. In aging coronary smooth muscle, the functional expression of MaxiK channels is greatly diminished. This downregulation occurs in both humans and rats when protein diminishes >50% in 30-month old rats or in >60-yr-old patients (41). The decreased MaxiK expression explains the increased coronary reactivity in the elderly that makes coronaries more prone to spasm. The reduction in MaxiK channels during aging seems to be tissue specific, because a decrease in total protein was not observed in the pulmonary artery of aging rats (41). Because endothelial function, as a provider of relaxant NO, also decreases with aging, it is possible that diminution of both endothelial function and MaxiK channel expression contribute to the development of hypertension as age increases.

B. Hypertension

MaxiK channel expression is increased in the aorta and cerebral microcirculation of genetically hypertensive rats (42,43). This increase in channel expression may be a compensatory mechanism to oppose enduring hypertension in this animal model.

Pulmonary hypertension often results in profound hypoxemia and right heart failure. Two main models are available, hypoxia-induced and monocrotaline-induced pulmonary hypertension.

Chronic hypoxia causes pulmonary hypertension, resulting in inhibition of O_2-sensitive, voltage-gated potassium channels (Kv) in rat pulmonary arterial myocytes. In this rat model, recent gene transfer therapy with Kv1.5 channel improved pulmonary hypertension (44) indicating that this class of K channels plays an important role in the development of this disease. However, in early cultured human main pulmonary arterial myocytes, chronic hypoxia caused a decrease in MaxiK current without altering Kv currents (45). It is interesting to note here that chronic carbon monoxide is able to enhance MaxiK currents in rat resistance pulmonary arterial myocytes (46), providing a possible alternative treatment for pulmonary hypertension.

Similar to the in vitro human model, in monocrotaline-induced pulmonary hypertension, the Kv channel current is not reduced but MaxiK channel current is significantly diminished (47). It is possible that a reduction in MaxiK channels would make the pulmonary myocytes respond less effectively to vasorelaxant agents, promoting an increase in tension in this model.

Pulmonary hypertension has also been studied in the newborn lamb, where the activity of MaxiK channels is also decreased (48). This hypertension-induced decline in MaxiK channel currents is likely due to a diminished expression of MaxiK α-subunit protein, because its mRNA is also reduced. The decrease in MaxiK channel activity attenuates the hyperpolarization associated with an acute increase in oxygen tension; therefore, the fetus suffering from pulmonary hypertension will not be prepared to respond appropriately to an acute increase in oxygen tension at birth.

VI. CONCLUSIONS

In the last decade, we have learned much about the function and molecular properties of MaxiK channels in the vasculature. In general, MaxiK channels work as rheostats regulating membrane potential and maintaining optimum tone aided by metabolites, neurotransmitters, and hormones. Relaxants increase their activity, and vasoconstrictors inhibit their activity. MaxiK channels contribute to maintain resting membrane potential, serve as negative feedback mechanisms to restore tone after a contraction cycle, and participate in the development of stimulated contraction. Given their key role in vascular function, their activity and expression are altered in pathogenic states and aging, making them excellent candidates for molecular medicine. The recent discovery of MaxiK linkage with mitogenic pathways in the cascade comitogen agonist (e.g., angiotensin II, 5-HT)–c-Src–

MaxiK–vasoconstriction and their physical interaction with protooncogene tyrosine kinases leads to the tantalizing hypothesis that MaxiK channels may also serve as signaling (scaffolding?) molecules involved in the regulation of vascular remodeling in health and disease. We envision that in the near future it will be possible to visualize the MaxiK functional proteome in single cells and watch MaxiK channels at work.

ACKNOWLEDGMENTS

This work was supported by NIH grants HL47382, HL54970 (LT) and HL71824, HD38983 (ES).

REFERENCES

1. Jiang Z, Wallner M, Meera P, Toro L. Cloning and characterization of human and rodent MaxiK channel β subunit genes: cloning and characterization. Genomics 1999; 55:57–67.
2. Toro L, Meera P, Wallner M, Tanaka Y. $MaxiK_{Ca}$, a unique member of the voltage-gated K channel superfamily. News Physiol Sci. 1998; 13:112–117.
3. Stefani E Ottolia M, Noceti F, Olcese R, Wallner M, Latorre R, Toro L. Voltage-controlled gating in a large conductance Ca^{2+}-sensitive K^+ channel (hSlo). Proc Natl Acad Sci USA 1997; 94:5427–5431.
4. Horrigan FT, Aldrich RW. Coupling between voltage sensor activation, Ca^{2+} binding and channel opening in large conductance (BK) potassium channels. J Gen Physiol 2002; 120:267–305.
5. Schreiber M, Yuan A, Salkoff L. Transplantable sites confer calcium sensitivity to BK channels. Nat Neurosci 1999; 2:416–421.
6. Bian S, Favre I, Moczydlowski E. Ca^{2+}-binding activity of a COOH-terminal fragment of the *Drosophila* BK channel involved in Ca^{2+}-dependent activation. Proc Natl Acad Sci USA 2001; 98:4776–4781.
7. Xia XM, Zeng X, Lingle CJ. Multiple regulatory sites in large-conductance calcium-activated potassium channels. Nature 2002; 418:880–884.
8. Bao L, Rapin AM, Holmstrand EC, Cox DH. Elimination of the BK_{Ca} channel's high-affinity Ca^{2+} sensitivity. J Gen Physiol 2002; 120:173–189.
9. Jiang Y, Lee A, Chen J, Cadene M, Chait BT, MacKinnon R. Crystal structure and mechanism of a calcium-gated potassium channel. Nature 2002; 417: 515–522.
10. Piskorowski R, Aldrich RW. Calcium activation of BK_{Ca} potassium channels lacking the calcium bowl and RCK domains. Nature 2002; 420: 499–502.
11. Shi J, Krishnamoorthy G, Yang Y, Hu L, Chaturvedi N, Harilal D, Qin J, Cui J. Mechanism of magnesium activation of calcium-activated potassium channels. Nature 2002; 418:876–880.
12. Zarei MM, Zhu N, Alioua A, Eghbali M Stefani E Toro L. A novel MaxiK splice variant exhibits dominant-negative properties for surface expression. J Biol Chem 2001; 276:16232–16239.

13. Xie J, McCobb DP. Control of alternative splicing of potassium channels by stress hormones. Science 1998; 280:443–446.
14. Erxleben C, Everhart AL, Romeo C, Florance H, Bauer MB, Alcorta DA, Rossie S, Shipston MJ, Armstrong DL. Interacting effects of N-terminal variation and STREX exon splicing on Slo potassium channel regulation by calcium, phosphorylation, and oxidation. J Biol Chem 2002; 277:27045–27052.
15. Tian L, Duncan RR, Hammond MS, Coghill LS, Wen H, Rusinova R, Clark AG, Levitan IB, Shipston MJ. Alternative splicing switches potassium channel sensitivity to protein phosphorylation. J Biol Chem 2001; 276:7717–7720.
16. Holdiman AJ, Fergus DJ, England SK. 17β-estradiol upregulates distinct maxiK channel transcripts in mouse uterus. Mol Cell Endocrinol 2002; 192:1–6.
17. Saito M, Nelson C, Salkoff L, Lingle CJ. A cysteine-rich domain defined by a novel exon in a Slo variant in rat adrenal chromaffin cells and PC12 cells. J Biol Chem 1997; 272:11710–11717.
18. Meera P, Wallner M, Toro L. A neuronal beta subunit (KCNMB4) makes the large conductance, voltage- and Ca^{2+}-activated K^+ channel resistant to charybdotoxin and iberiotoxin. Proc Natl Acad Sci USA 2000; 97:5562–5567.
19. Brenner R, Perez GJ, Bonev AD, Eckman DM, Kosek JC, Wiler SW, Patterson AJ, Nelson MT, Aldrich RW. Vasoregulation by the beta1 subunit of the calcium-activated potassium channel. Nature 2000; 407:870–876.
20. Schubert R, Nelson MT. Protein kinases: tuners of the BK_{Ca} channel in smooth muscle. Trends Pharmacol Sci 2001; 22:505–512.
21. Wang J, Zhou Y, Wen H, Levitan IB. Simultaneous binding of two protein kinases to a calcium-dependent potassium channel. J Neurosci 1999; 19:RC4.
22. Touyz RM, Wu XH, He G, Park JB, Chen X, Vacher J, Rajapurohitam V, Schiffrin EL. Role of c-Src in the regulation of vascular contraction and Ca^{2+} signaling by angiotensin II in human vascular smooth muscle cells. J Hypertens 2001; 19:441–449.
23. Alioua A, Mahajan A, Nishimaru K, Zarei MM, Stefani E, Toro L. Coupling of c-Src to large conductance voltage- and Ca^{2+}-activated K^+ channels as a new mechanism of agonist-induced vasoconstriction. Proc Natl Acad Sci USA 2002; 99:14560–14565.
24. Xiong Z, Burnette E, Cheung DW. Modulation of Ca^{2+}-activated K^+ channel activity by tyrosine kinase inhibitors in vascular smooth muscle cell. Eur J Pharmacol 1995; 290:117–123.
25. Rezzonico R, Schmid-Alliana A, Romey G, Bourget-Ponzio I, Breuil V, Breittmayer V, Tartare-Deckert S, Rossi B, Schmid-Antomarchi H. Prostaglandin E2 induces interaction between hSlo potassium channel and Syk tyrosine kinase in osteosarcoma cells. J Bone Miner Res 2002; 17:869–878.
26. Ling S, Woronuk G, Sy L, Lev S, Braun AP. Enhanced activity of a large conductance, calcium-sensitive K^+ channel in the presence of Src tyrosine kinase. J Biol Chem 2000; 275:30683–30689.
27. Wang ZW, Nara M, Wang YX, Kotlikoff MI. Redox regulation of large conductance Ca^{2+}-activated K^+ channels in smooth muscle cells. J Gen Physiol 1997; 110:35–44.

28. Soto MA, Gonzalez C, Lissi E, Vergara C, Latorre R. Ca^{2+}-activated K^+ channel inhibition by reactive oxygen species. Am J Physiol Cell Physiol 2002; 282:C461–C471.
29. Tang XD, Daggett H, Hanner M, Garcia ML, McManus OB, Brot N, Weissbach H, Heinemann SH, Hoshi T. Oxidative regulation of large conductance calcium-activated potassium channels. J Gen Physiol 2001; 117:253–274.
30. Valverde MA, Rojas P, Amigo J, Cosmelli D, Orio P, Bahamonde MI, Mann GE, Vergara C, Latorre R. Acute activation of maxi-K channels (hSlo) by estradiol binding to the β subunit. Science 1999; 285:1929–1931.
31. Dick GM, Sanders KM. (Xeno)estrogen sensitivity of smooth muscle BK channels conferred by the regulatory β_1 subunit: a study of β_1 knockout mice. J Biol Chem 2001; 276:44835–44840.
32. Song M, Zhu N, Olcese R, Barila B, Toro L, Stefani E. Hormonal control of protein expression and mRNA levels of the MaxiK channel α subunit in myometrium. FEBS Lett 1999; 460:427–432.
33. Wang SY, Yoshino M, Sui JL, Wakui M, Kao PN, Kao CY. Potassium currents in freshly dissociated uterine myocytes from nonpregnant and late-pregnant rats. J Gen Physiol 1998; 112:737–756.
34. Benkusky NA, Fergus DJ, Zucchero TM, England SK. Regulation of the Ca^{2+}-sensitive domains of the maxi-K channel in the mouse myometrium during gestation. J Biol Chem 2000; 275:27712–27719.
35. Benkusky NA, Korovkina VP, Brainard AM, England SK. Myometrial maxi-K channel β_1 subunit modulation during pregnancy and after 17 β-estradiol stimulation. FEBS Lett 2002; 524:97–102.
36. Bravo-Zehnder M, Orio P, Norambuena A, Wallner M, Meera P, Toro L, Latorre R, Gonzalez A. Apical sorting of a voltage- and Ca^{2+}-activated K^+ channel α-subunit in Madin-Darby canine kidney cells is independent of N-glycosylation. Proc Natl Acad Sci USA 2000; 97:13114–13119.
37. Wang SX, Ikeda M, Guggino WB. The cytoplasmic tail of large conductance, voltage- and Ca^{2+}-activated K^+ (MaxiK) channel is necessary for its cell surface expression. J Biol Chem 2003; 278:2713–2722.
38. Scornik FS, Codina J, Birnbaumer L, Toro L. Modulation of coronary smooth muscle K_{Ca} channels by $G_s\alpha$ independent of phosphorylation by protein kinase A. Am J Physiol 1993; 265:H1460–H1465.
39. Scornik FS, Toro L. U46619, a thromboxane A2 agonist, inhibits K_{Ca} channel activity from pig coronary artery. Am J Physiol 1992; 262:C708–C713.
40. Toro L, Amador M, Stefani E. ANG II inhibits calcium-activated potassium channels from coronary smooth muscle in lipid bilayers. Am J Physiol 1990; 258:H912–H915.
41. Marijic J, Li Q-X, Song M, Nishimaru K, Stefani E Toro L. Decreased expression of voltage- and Ca^{2+}-activated K^+ channels in coronary smooth muscle during aging. Circ Res 2001; 88:210–215.
42. Liu Y, Pleyte K, Knaus HG, Rusch NJ. Increased expression of Ca^{2+}-sensitive K^+ channels in aorta of hypertensive rats. Hypertension 1997; 30:1403–1409.
43. Liu Y, Hudetz AG, Knaus HG, Rusch NJ. Increased expression of Ca^{2+}-sensitive K^+ channels in the cerebral microcirculation of genetically hyperten-

sive rats: evidence for their protection against cerebral vasospasm. Circ Res 1998; 82:729–737.

44. Pozeg ZI, Michelakis ED, McMurtry MS, Thebaud B, Wu XC, Dyck JR, Hashimoto K, Wang S, Moudgil R, Harry G, Sultanian R, Koshal A, Archer SL. In vivo gene transfer of the O_2-sensitive potassium channel Kv1.5 reduces pulmonary hypertension and restores hypoxic pulmonary vasoconstric-tion in chronically hypoxic rats. Circulation 2003; 107:2037–2044.
45. Peng W, Hoidal JR, Karwande SV, Farrukh IS. Effect of chronic hypoxia on K^+ channels: regulation in human pulmonary vascular smooth muscle cells. Am J Physiol 1997; 272:C1271–C1278.
46. Dubuis E, Gautier M, Melin A, Rebocho M, Girardin C, Bonnet P, Vandier C. Chronic carbon monoxide enhanced IbTx-sensitive currents in rat resistance pulmonary artery smooth muscle cells. Am J Physiol Lung Cell Mol Physiol 2002; 283:L120–L129.
47. Muraki S, Tohse N, Seki S, Nagashima M, Yamada Y, Abe T, Yabu H. Decrease in the Ca^{2+}-activated K^+ current of pulmonary arterial smooth muscle in pulmonary hypertension rats. Naunyn Schmiedebergs Arch Pharmacol 2001; 364:183–192.
48. Olschewski A, Hong Z, Linden BC, Porter VA, Weir EK, Cornfield DN. Contribution of the K_{Ca} channel to membrane potential and O_2 sensitivity is decreased in an ovine PPHN model. Am J Physiol Lung Cell Mol Physiol 2002; 283:L1103–L1109.
49. Korovkina VP, Fergus DJ, Holdiman AJ, England SK. Characterization of a novel 132-bp exon of the human maxi-K channel. Am J Physiol Cell Physiol 2001; 281:C361–C367.
50. Meera P, Wallner M, Toro L. Molecular biology of Ca^{2+}-activated K^+ channels. In: Archer SL, Rusch NJ, eds. Potassium Channels in Cardiovascular Biology. New York, NY: Kluwer Academic/Plenum, 2001:49–70.

13

ATP-Sensitive and Inward Rectifier K^+ Channels

Lucie H. Clapp and Brian P. Tennant
University College London, London, U.K.

I. INTRODUCTION

Inwardly rectifying K^+ channels passing current more readily in the inward rather than outward direction, have been identified in a wide range of tissues including the central nervous system, the heart, immune cells, skeletal muscle, and various types of smooth muscle (1–3). Both strong (IRK) and weakly rectifying (ATP-sensitive; K_{ATP}) K^+ channels belonging to the same superfamily (Kir) have been identified in vascular tissue. The mechanism underlying this unique rectification has been attributed to voltage-dependent block by intracellular Mg^{2+} and polyamines (2,3). These channels are important physiologically because they play a crucial role in setting the resting potential (E_m) and controlling membrane excitability. This in turn regulates Ca^{2+} entry into smooth muscle and endothelial cells and influences the level of vascular tone. Channel activity is also intrinsically linked to cell metabolism, responding to changes in ATP, K^+, pH, and O_2 (1). Whether such mechanisms contribute to the adaptive response in the pulmonary circulation of diverting blood supply away from poorly to well ventilated areas of the lung remains unclear but will be discussed in detail in this chapter. Opposing regulation by vasodilator and vasoconstrictor agents activating protein kinase A (PKA) or protein kinase C (PKC) appears to be a consistent feature of K_{ATP} channels (1), although hormone regulation has not been clearly demonstrated for IRK channels, except in endothelial cells (4). However, increasing evidence suggests that these channels may be important targets for growth factors and for the postnatal maturation of the lung. Significant strides have been made toward the molecular identification of Kir channels, although experiments involving gene "knockout" of putative subunits are extremely limited in vascular muscle, and none look at the expression pattern of these subunits during lung development or in response to hypoxia.

Seven Kir subfamilies (Kir1–Kir7) have been identified based on a subunit topology of two highly conserved transmembrane domains (M1 and M2), with intracellular N- and C-terminal tails, separated by a pore-forming loop (H5) containing a T/S-X-X-T/S-X-G-Y/F-G motif critical for K^+ ion selectivity (2,3,5). Functional Kir channels are formed by the assembly of four subunits oriented around H5 (see Fig. 1 inset), with complexes composed of either identical (homomeric) or related (heteromeric) subunits. The architecture of the pore is thought to be stabilized during channel assembly by the formation of a salt bridge between Glu and Arg residues immediately flanking the pore-forming region and also a disulfide bridge between two more distant Cys residues (Fig. 1). These residues are conserved throughout the Kir superfamily. Kir1.1 encodes the ATP-dependent K^+ channel (ROMK1) found in kidney epithelial cells, and other members of this subfamily, along with Kir4.0 and Kir7.1, appear to form K^+ transport channels in a variety of cells (2). Members of the Kir2.0 subfamily almost certainly encode the classical inward rectifiers found in the brain, heart, skeletal, and vascular muscle (1,3), and members of the Kir3.0 family exist as heteromers and constitute the G-protein-gated, inwardly rectifying K^+ (GIRK) channels found in the brain (Kir3.1 and Kir3.2) and heart (Kir3.1 and Kir3.4). Kir6.0 subunits encode the pore-forming subunit of the K_{ATP} channel, but coassembly with the sulfonylurea receptor (SUR), a member of the ATP binding cassette family of proteins, is required for functional channel expression (2,5) (Fig. 2). Kir5.1 has also been cloned but, like Kir6.0, does not form functional channels on its own but can associate with other Kir subunits to form heteromultimeric channels or interact to alter their expression at the plasma membrane (2).

II. K_{ATP} CHANNELS

A. Basic Properties of K_{ATP} Channels

Potassium channels that are ATP-sensitive (K_{ATP} channels) are widely distributed throughout the cardiovascular system and are characteristically activated by declining cytosolic ATP or elevated nucleotide diphosphate (NDP) levels, thus providing a link between metabolism and membrane excitability (1,2,5). These channels are inhibited by sulfonylurea agents such as glibenclamide and activated by K^+ channel openers (KCOs) such as

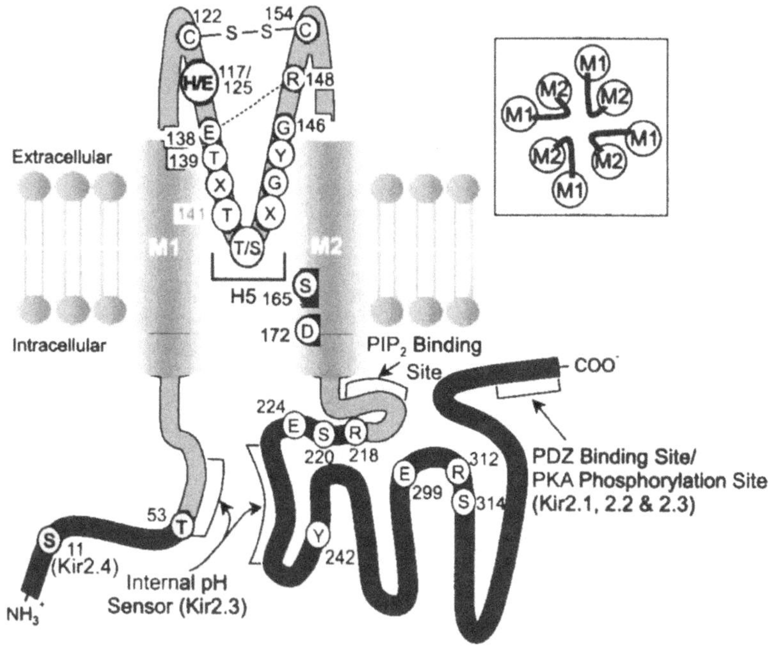

Figure 1 Proposed membrane topology of a single Kir2.0 subunit with an extracellular view of the tetrameric channel arrangement (inset). Regions of interest are indicated. Residues of interest found in all Kir2.0 subunits (white, numbered for Kir2.1) and isoform specific residues (gray) are the K^+ selectivity filter (T139–G146), located within the H5 loop; cation block at R148, E125 (Kir2.1 only), T141, S165, and D172; a salt bridge (E138 ··· R148) and a disulfide bridge (C122–S–S–C154) that form during channel assembly; external pH sensor of Kir2.3 and 2.4 involving H117 (Kir2.3) and C122 and/or C154; phosphorylation sites S11 (PKA, Kir2.4), T35 (PKC, Kir2.3), S220 and S314 (PKA, close to PIP_2-binding sites R218 and R312), and Y242 (tyrosine kinase); polyamines/Mg^{2+} bind at D172, E224, and E299. (Compiled from information found in Refs. 3, 32, and 51.)

levcromakalim and pinacidil, which in smooth muscle results in membrane hyperpolarization (Fig. 3A), closure of voltage-gated Ca^{2+} channels, and ultimately vasorelaxation. Since their initial identification in rabbit mesenteric artery, multiple types of K_{ATP} channels have been described in smooth muscle, suggesting that channels do not correspond to a single molecular entity. Broadly speaking, channels fall into two types, those that are inhibited by ATP (classical) and those that are activated by nucleotide diphosphate (K_{NDP}), with single-channel conductances reported to range from 20 to >100 pS (1,6). In general, whole-cell currents carried by these channels are time-independent, displaying little voltage dependence (See Fig. 3B), and

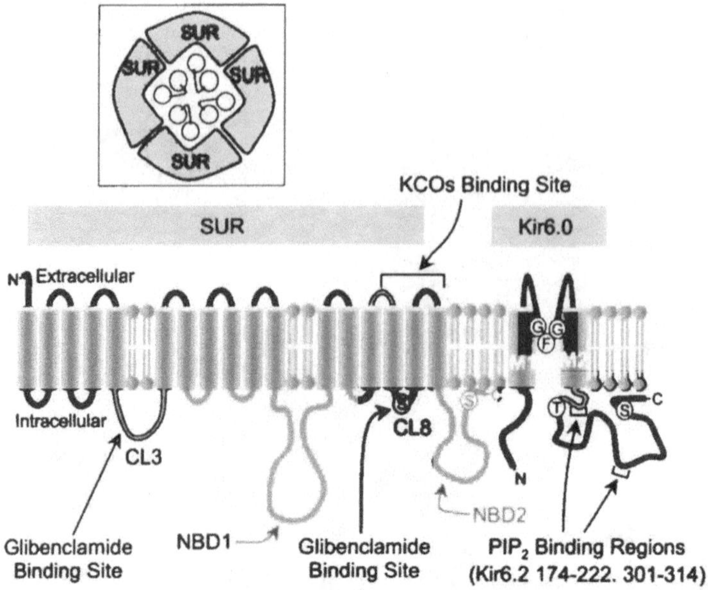

Figure 2 Proposed membrane topology of a single sulfonylurea and Kir6.0 subunit, and arrangement of an octameric channel (inset). Regions of interest indicated are cytoplasmic loops (CL) 3 and 8, thought to form the glibenclamide binding site, with S1287 of CL8 being critical; nucleotide-binding domains (NBD) 1 and 2 of SUR; the selectivity filter motif (GFG) of the Kir6.0 H5 loop; K^+channel opener (KCOs)-binding site on SUR; PIP_2-binding sites and putative phosphorylation sites Ser1571 of SUR and Thr180, Thr224, and Ser372 of Kir6.0. (Compiled from information contained in Ref. 5).

in most tissues lowering pipette ATP can significantly increase currents and enhance responses to KCOs (1). Similarly, in pulmonary arterial myocytes, dialysis of cells with low intracellular ATP causes the appearance of a time-independent background current with properties indistinguishable from those of the current activated by levcromakalim (7–9). This background current could be inhibited by photorelease of ATP or glibenclamide, confirming that ATP depletion does indeed activate K_{ATP} channels (7). Responses to levcromakalim were shown to be highly dependent on ATP in both rabbit and human pulmonary arterial smooth muscle (HPASM) cells, with the magnitude of currents being two- to threefold greater in 0.1 mM ATP than in 1 mM ATP (9,10). Reciprocal effects on membrane potential occurred, presumably because the resting membrane potential, which becomes quite hyperpolarized in low ATP (~−70 mV), cannot be driven beyond the K^+ equilibrium potential (~−82 mV) by levcromakalim (7). The single-channel conductance underlying K_{ATP} currents in pulmonary artery is small, estimated to be 20 pS from noise analysis of the

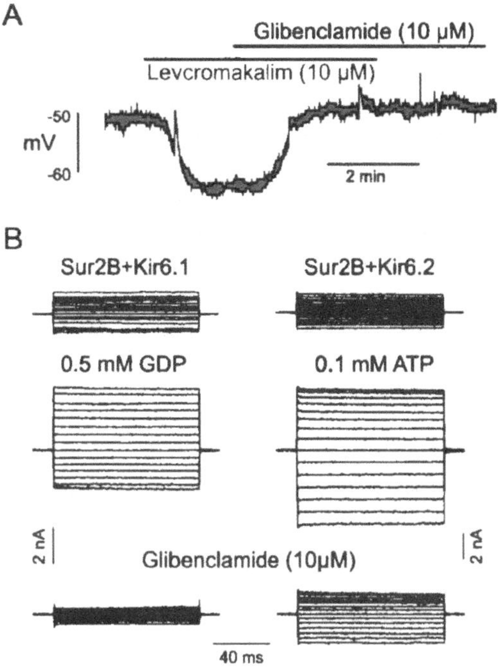

Figure 3 Basic properties of native and cloned smooth muscle K_{ATP} channels. (A) Membrane potential recording from a growth- arrested human pulmonary arterial smooth muscle cell bathed in a physiological K^+ gradient ($6_{(in)}/140_{(out)}$ mM K^+) with the pipette solution containing 1 mM ATP. Application of levcromakalim hyperpolarized the cell from −50 mV to ~−65 mV, an effect that was reversed by coapplication of glibenclamide. (B) Whole-cell currents recorded from HEK-293 cells stably tranfected with SUR2B/Kir6.1 and SUR2B/Kir6.2. Currents were activated in symmetrical 140 mM K^+ by stepping the voltage in 10 mV steps from −60 to +80 mV from a holding potential of 0 mV. Currents shown are recorded at $t = 0$ (top panels) and 5–7 min after "break-in" in the absence (middle panels) and presence (bottom panels) of 10 μM glibenclamide. With the SUR2B/Kir6.1 clone, significant run-up of the current was not observed with 0.1 mM ATP in the pipette (not shown) but was observed if GDP was present. In contrast, with SUR2B/Kir6.2, substantial increases in current were observed with time in the low ATP solution (Cui, Tinker, and Clapp, unpublished data.)

levcromakalim-activated current in rabbit myocytes (11) or 28 pS from cell-attached recordings in cultured HPASM cells (10). In the absence of ATP, intracellular GDP or UDP can activate glibenclamide-sensitive whole-cell current and single channels, in pulmonary myocytes, suggesting that NDPs are important regulators of channel function (9,10). K_{ATP} channels are inhibited by a range of chemically unrelated compounds, including PNU-99963

(IC_{50}, 10–40 nM), U-37883 (IC_{50}, 1 μM), phencyclidine (IC_{50}, > 1 μM), Ba^{2+} (IC_{50}, 100 μM), and 4-aminopyridine (IC_{50}, 0.2 mM) (1,6,12). In general, the vasorelaxant responses to KCOs in pulmonary (8,11,13) and other vascular tissues (1) can be inhibited with a pharmacological profile similar to that of channel inhibition, suggesting that activation of K_{ATP} channels is largely responsible for relaxation. The actions of KCOs are not considered to be endothelium-dependent although the endothelium plays a role in modulating responses in porcine intrapulmonary and resistance vessels (14,15). This has led some investigators to presume the existence of K_{ATP} channels in the endothelium, though so far no electrophysiological data exist to support such a claim in pulmonary endothelial cells, and their existence in this cell type remains controversial (4).

B. Molecular Identification of K_{ATP} Channels

Studies in heterologous expression systems have unequivocally demonstrated that K_{ATP} channels are octameric complexes formed by the coassembly of Kir6.0 and SUR subunits in a 4:4 stoichiometry (2,5). Only fully assembled channel complexes can express at the plasma membrane due to the masking of endoplasmic reticulum retention signals, which are exposed in partially assembled complexes (5). Structure–function studies have determined that the pore governs the single-channel conductance and contains binding sites responsible for ATP inhibition, while the SUR mediates the stimulatory effects of MgNDPs, enhances ATP sensitivity, and is the primary target for pharmacological agents such as sulfonylureas and KCOs (2) (Fig. 2). So far, two Kir6.0 genes have been isolated, Kir6.1 and Kir6.2 (2). The amino acid sequence shows that these subunits share 70% sequence homology and have the same K^+ channel signature sequence, a Gly-Phe-Gly (GFG) motif. In terms of the SUR, two genes have been identified, SUR1, which encodes a high-affinity sulfonylurea receptor, and SUR2, which encodes two low-affinity receptors, SUR2A and SUR2B (5). These splice variants differ by only 42 amino acid residues in the C-terminal end. Examination of messenger RNA expression using Northern blot and RT-PCR analysis shows ubiquitous expression of Kir6.1 and SUR2B, giving credence to the notion that these two subunits are important in smooth muscle (2). Expression of the other subunits is more restricted. Kir6.2 and SUR2A are both found in the heart, skeletal muscle, and brain, although Kir6.2 is also heavily expressed in the pancreas (2). SUR1 is found almost exclusively in the pancreas and the brain. The various Kir6.0 and SUR subunits combine to form channels with distinct conductances, nucleotide sensitivities, and pharmacology (2,16,17). Comparison of the properties of native and cloned K_{ATP} channels provides good evidence that SUR1 and Kir6.2 constitute the K_{ATP} channel in the pancreatic β cell and some neuronal cells, whereas SUR2A and Kir6.2 form the cardiac and skeletal muscle channel (2,5).

In relation to smooth muscle, two clones have been proposed, SUR2B/Kir6.2 and SUR2B/Kir6.1 (Fig. 3B). The reconstituted SUR2B/Kir6.2 channel has a conductance of ~60–80 pS in symmetrical 145 mM K^+ and is inhibited by ATP, whereas the SUR2B/Kir6.1 channel has a lower conductance of ~30 pS and is activated by NDPs and ATP (2,16) (see also Fig. 3B). It is possible that these channels underlie the classical K_{ATP} and the K_{NDP} channel, respectively, that have been reported in a number of preparations including rat and rabbit portal vein myocytes (1). However, these clones do not fully describe the properties of channels found in other tissues, particularly visceral muscle, so other pore-forming subunits may exist (6). Our own data provide strong biochemical and electrophysiological evidence that Kir6.2 and Kir6.1 can form mixed heteromultimers (16). This might explain the intermediate conductances and variable sensitivities to ATP and NDPs that have consistently been described in native smooth muscle (1). Although heteromultimerization has not been demonstrated in vivo, mRNA for Kir6.2 and Kir6.1 has nonetheless been found in the same tissue, including rat aorta, mesenteric artery, and tail artery (18). It is also interesting to note that K_{NDP} channels having conductances of ~42–44 pS in symmetrical 140 mM K^+ have consistently been reported in smooth muscle, and this corresponds closely to the conductance of cloned channels made up of two Kir6.1 and two Kir6.2 subunits (16). However, the complexity of K_{ATP} channels is not likely to be extended by mixed populations of SUR subunits, because we found no evidence for protein interaction of different subunits or observed K_{ATP} channels with altered pharmacology (17).

Studies in pulmonary artery, although limited, suggest that the molecular identity of K_{ATP} channels in this tissue is likely to be made up of SUR2B/Kir6.1. In cultured HPASM cells, the presence of SUR2B and Kir6.1 was demonstrated but not that of SUR2A, SUR1, or Kir6.2 (10). Moreover, in these cells, levcromakalim activated a glibenclamide-sensitive K^+ channel that had biophysical properties indistinguishable from those of SUR2B/Kir6.1 stably expressed in HEK-293 cells; in both cell types, levcromakalim activated a 28–29 pS channel requiring the presence of UDP for significant openings to occur in excised patches. These data are also consistent with Northern blot analysis showing expression of Kir6.1 but not Kir6.2 in whole rat lung tissue (2) and RT-PCR data in rat pulmonary artery showing clear transcripts for Kir6.1 and SUR2B but not Kir6.2 or SUR2A (18). However, we found that certain aspects of native whole-cell regulation in pulmonary cells could not be fully reconstituted by SUR2B/Kir6.1 expressed in HEK-293 cells. For one, intracellular ATP had little effect on whole-cell responses to levcromakalim, except at high concentrations (10 mM) and lowering intracellular ATP decreased rather than increased K_{ATP} current (10). The reasons for these differences are unknown, but they suggest that other cytosolic factors may be important for channel regulation in native cells.

We and others have also detected SUR1 in rat pulmonary arterial tissue (10,18). At this stage it is not clear if SUR1 is actually expressed in the medial or adventical layer of blood vessels, but SUR1 can be expressed in some neurones (2). Therefore, in future experiments, it will be important to clarify subunit distribution in vascular preparations containing a homogeneous population of cells. Systematic studies using gene "knockout" technology are decidedly lacking in smooth muscle, so conclusions about the molecular identity of K_{ATP} channels await further confirmation. However, studies in Kir6.1$^{-/-}$ and SUR2$^{-/-}$ mice suggest that Kir6.1/SUR2B is responsible for pinacidil-induced activation of K_{ATP} currents in aorta (5).

C. Regulation of K_{ATP} Channels by Intracellular Factors

There have been numerous studies indicating that K_{ATP} channels are regulated by protein kinases. In smooth muscle, activation of whole-cell current or single channels has been shown by forskolin, an activator of adenylate cyclase, by membrane-permeable analogs of cyclic AMP, or by the activated catalytic subunit of PKA (reviewed in Ref. 1). The pore is likely to be a major site for PKA phosphorylation (Ser372 or Thr224 on Kir6.2), although the SUR (Ser1571) may also be a target (5). The phosphorylation sites for smooth muscle clones are unknown, though Kir6.1, but not Kir6.2, is likely to be the target for PKA phosphorylation stimulated by Gs-coupled receptors or by forskolin (19). Direct activation of PKC by diacylglycerol, phorbol 12,13-dibutyrate, or purified PKC inhibits currents through K_{ATP} channels in native smooth muscle or in HEK-293 cells expressing SUR2B/Kir6.1 (1,20). Thus, SUR2B/Kir6.1 appears to be the major subtype for kinase regulation in smooth muscle. Recently, it was shown that the anionic membrane phospholipids phosphatidylinositol 4,5-bisphosphate (PIP_2) and phosphatidylinositol 3,4,5-trisphosphate (PIP_3) decrease the ATP sensitivity of Kir6.2 clones, thus allowing greater channel activity at higher ATP levels (2,5). Breakdown of PIP_2 by G proteins coupled to phospholipase C (Gq) may represent a physiologically relevant mechanism for K_{ATP} channel regulation, though PIP_2 regulation of native or cloned smooth muscle channels has not been studied. Little is known about the role of phosphatases, but the Ca^{2+}-dependent phosphatase calcineurin appears to be an important regulator of channel activity at physiological Ca^{2+} concentrations in rat aorta (21).

III. STRONG INWARD RECTIFIER K^+ CHANNELS

A. General Properties of Inwardly Rectifying K^+ Channels in the Lung

Strong inwardly rectifying K^+ (IRK) channels have been described in many vascular tissues from different species (1,4). These channels pass most

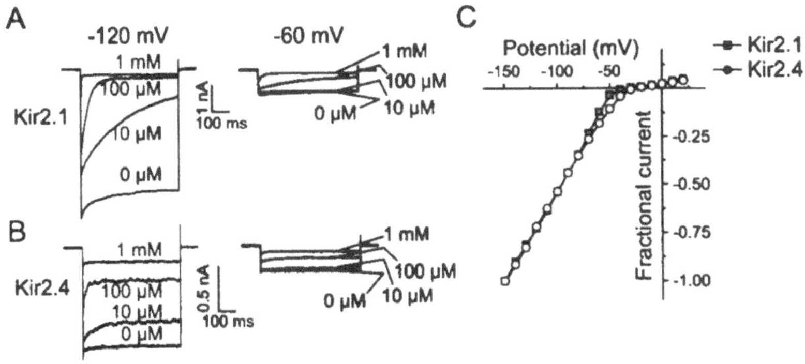

Figure 4 The effect of Ba^{2+} on whole-cell currents recorded from HEK-239 cells stably expressing mouse Kir2.1 (A) or human Kir2.4 (B). Currents were recorded in ak$^+$ gradient of $60_{(in)}$–$140_{(out)}$ mM K^+ and activated by voltage steps to −120mV and to −60 mV from a holding potential of −20 mV in the absence and presence of increasing concentrations of Ba^{2+}. Note that block by Ba^{2+} was voltage- and time-dependent for Kir2.1, but Kir2.4 showed little of these features and was much less sensitive to Ba^{2+}. (C) The current–voltage relationship for currents activated by the two Kir subunits, with current normalized to current amplitude at −150 mV. Relationships show characteristic rectification around the K^+ reversal potential, with little outward current being passed positive to this potential. (From Tennant, Tinker, and Clapp, unpublished data.)

current at potentials hyperpolarized to the K^+ equilibrium potential (Fig. 4), though the small amount of outward current carried at voltages depolarized to this potential is enough to regulate the E_m and cause vasodilatation in response to raised extracellular (10–15 mM) K^+ (1). Expression of IRK channels predominates in smaller blood vessels, making them good candidates for controlling peripheral vascular resistance. Within the respiratory system, patch-clamp studies have reported inward currents with rectification strongly dependent on membrane potential and the K^+ gradient in isolated pulmonary artery and vein endothelial cells from rat and bovine tissue (22–26), in human bronchial smooth muscle (27,28), and in human lung cancer cells (29). Such currents are potently blocked by external Ba^{2+} ions with an IC_{50} ranging from 1–2 μM at −130 mV (22,26,28) to ~50 μM at similar potentials (27,29). Where studied, block by barium is steeply voltage-dependent, increasing exponentially with hyperpolarization and taking many milliseconds to develop (27–29). External Cs^+ ions at high micromolar to millimolar concentrations (IC_{50} 57 μM at −100 mV) also block IRK currents in lung cells in a highly voltage-dependent manner, although, unlike Ba^{2+}, Cs^+ block is almost instantaneous and shows no time dependence (27,29). Other divalent cations, including Ca^{2+} and Mg^{2+}, can also inhibit native IRK currents from the outside at physiological concentrations (1), but this has not been investigated in lung cells.

Compounds known to block other K^+ channels, such as inhibitors of K_{ATP}, Ca^{2+}-activated K^+ (K_{Ca}), and voltage-dependent K^+ (Kv) channels, are largely ineffective at inhibiting IRK currents in coronary and cerebral smooth muscle (1). Likewise, neither glibenclamide (10 μM), the Kv blocker 4-aminopyridine (1–4 mM), the nonselective K^+ channel inhibitor tetraethylammonium ions (10–20 mM), nor the K_{Ca} inhibitor charybdotoxin (100 nM) blocks IRK current by more than 10% in pulmonary endothelial, bronchial smooth muscle, or lung cancer cells (24,26, 28,29). Thus, the biophysical and pharmacological features of IRK currents so far described in the lung closely resemble those of classical inward rectifiers described in other smooth muscle and skeletal muscle cell types (1,3).

B. Molecular Identity and Properties of Cloned Kir2.0 Channels

Structural Features

The Kir2.0 subfamily show the most prominent inward rectification and almost certainly encode the pore-forming subunits of strong inward rectifiers found in the brain, heart, skeletal, and vascular muscle (1,3). The pore consists of three structural features that, from the extracellular side inward, sequentially increase the pore width. First here is the outer pore-forming loop (H5), which in the Kir2.0 family contains a Gly-Tyr-Gly (GYG) motif (Fig. 1). Beyond this lies the inner pore, which is lined only by amino acid side chains from the M2 domain (3). This region binds the Mg^{2+} ions and polyamine molecules that are responsible for channel block and inward rectification, with an Asp located seven residues from the intracellular end of M2 (equivalent to D172 in Kir2.1) having been identified as critical for this. Finally, a wider cytoplasmic inner vestibule is formed from regions of the amino- and carboxy-terminal tails closest to the transmembrane domains (C54–V86, R213–S234 in Kir2.1). Hydrophobicity mapping and scanning cysteine mutagenesis suggest that hydrophobic residues within these ~30 amino acid stretches associate with the membrane, allowing loops of hydrophilic residues to protrude into the cytoplasm and construct the inner vestibule (3,30). Glu residues (E224, E299 in Kir2.1) bind polyamines, and possibly Mg^{2+}, facilitating not only the fast transfer of polyamines to block the inner pore but also the screening of local negative surface charges, resulting in reduced K^+ permeation (31).

Biophysical Properties of Kir2.0 Subunits

Four isoforms of the Kir2.0 family have been identified, Kir2.1, 2.2, 2.3, and 2.4 (3). The properties of the first three have been extensively characterized, while that of Kir2.4 has been much less studied. Nonetheless, all subunits, when expressed, produce constitutively active inwardly rectifying K^+ currents that exhibit characteristic block by external cations (see Fig. 4). Apart from Kir2.4 (32), all subunits show the blueprint of voltage- and time-dependent block with Ba^{2+} (33–35). These differences in the nature of the Ba^{2+} block in Kir2.4 (Fig. 4) along with other distinctions (see below) could prove useful in defining characteristics for determining the presence of this subunit in native tissues. There are also differences in sensitivities to Ba^{2+} among the Kir2.0 family. Ba^{2+} block is most sensitive in Kir2.2, followed by Kir2.1, 2.3, and 2.4, with the IC_{50} being ~0.5 μM, 3.2 μM, 10.3 μM, and 116 μM, respectively (32,34). This pattern of sensitivity toward cation block is, however, altered with Cs^+. Kir2.2 and 2.3 are particularly sensitive to Cs^+, being fully blocked by 50 μM at a membrane potential of −50 mV, whereas Kir2.1 and 2.4 have a much lower sensitivity with less than 10% of current being inhibited under similar conditions (32,33,36). Of the other external cations known to block, Mg^{2+} and Ca^{2+} produce a 50% inhibition of current at 10 mM in rat Kir2.1 (33), but no such information exists for the other subunits.

Several residues throughout the pore are thought to be responsible for aspects of the cation block. First, in the extra cellular regions joining M1 and M2 to the H5 loop, Arg148 (of Kir2.1) and Glu125 (in Kir2.1 only) affect the rate of blocking without affecting affinity. Residues Thr141 (in the H5 loop), Ser165, and Asp172 (of the M2 domain) are involved in the affinity of block, indicating that foreign cations can traverse the selectivity filter and block the channel deep in the pore (3). This is consistent with the high measured fractional distance of the binding site in the electrical field sensed by Cs^+ ions ($\delta = 1.6$) (32,33). A value >1 is generally accepted as evidence for multi-ion occupancy in a deep pore (3). In Kir2.4, the molecular basis for differences in Ba^{2+} and Cs^+ block is not known. However, the relative residue to Ser165 (Kir2.1) in Kir2.4 is a nonpolar Cys, which may account, in part,for the reduced sensitivity to cation block.

Molecular Distribution of Channel Isoforms in Native Tissues

Analysis of mRNA and protein levels in various tissues shows widespread distribution of Kir2.1 and Kir2.2, whereas that of Kir2.3 and Kir2.4 appears more discrete (36–38). So far most IRK currents described in smooth muscle appear to have the molecular characteristics of Kir2.1. Consistent with this, RT-PCR analysis of mRNA showed transcripts for Kir2.1, but not Kir2.2 or Kir2.3, in rat cerebral, mesenteric, and coronary arteries (33), and IRK currents were absent from cerebral arteries from neonatal Kir2.1$^{-/-}$ mice but not wild-type or Kir2.2$^{-/-}$ mice (39). In lung tissues, both RT-PCR and immunostaining experiments have supported the presence of Kir2.0 family members. Immunostaining of rat lung sections identified a high level of Kir2.1 expression in arterial and venous endothelial cells but little to none in the smooth muscle layer (24,25), whereas in cultured human bronchial smooth muscle cells, Kir2.1, but not Kir2.2 or Kir2.3, was identified by RT-PCR (28). Indeed, IRK currents were suppressed by ~75 % with antisense oligonucleotides targeted to Kir2.1 mRNA in bronchial cells. In other studies, Kamouchi et al. (23) reverse-transcribed total RNA from bovine pulmonary artery endothelial cells and designed PCR primers against conserved regions of the Kir2.0 family. Using this approach, they isolated seven clones with identical nucleotide sequences and showed 95% amino acid homology to the human Kir2.1 sequence, whereas homology with Kir2.2 and 2.3 was only 75–79%. However, subsequent identification of the Kir2.4 sequence showed amino acid substitutions in the regions used for primer generation in this study, therefore the possibility remains that Kir2.4 mRNA transcripts were present but not replicated. Kir2.1 was also identified in the small-cell lung cancer line RERF-LC-MA by both RT-PCR and Western blotting (29). Thus, strong evidence exists to suggest that Kir2.1 is a major contributor to whole-cell current in lung tissues.

In our laboratory, we have been investigating the properties of IRK currents in cultured HPASM cells. In a physiological K^+ gradient, inwardly rectifying currents could be observed, the magnitude and reversal potential of which were sensitive to changes in extracellular K^+ (40). Inward currents were significantly inhibited by 100 μM Ba^{2+}, whereas those activated in the outward direction were unaffected. RT-PCR identified transcripts encoding Kir2.1, 2.2, and 2.4 but not Kir2.3 (40), suggesting that IRK current in these cells could be made up of one or more subunits. Such a conclusion is supported by a recent report showing that real-time PCR data in rat aorta where Kir2.2 was the prominent species expressed, followed by 2.4 (41). Kir2.3 and 2.1 were also present but were far less abundant by 40- and >140-fold, respectively. In pulmonary smooth muscle we favor a major contribution from Kir2.4, because the characteristics of Ba^{2+} block showed little time or voltage dependence, and millimolar Ba^{2+} was often required for complete block (Cui and Clapp, personal communication, 2002). Nonetheless, we cannot rule out the possibility that inward current is contaminated with other Ba^{2+}- sensitive K^+ channels that may exist in pulmonary tissue, including GIRK and ROMK-1 channels (24). In this respect molecular tools are going to be important to tease out the contribution of different Kir subunits to whole-cell current.

Comparison of Single-Channel Properties

Single-channel conductances in the region of 20, 35, 10, and 15 pS in symmetrical 140 mM K^+ have been reported for Kir2.1, 2.2, 2.3, and 2.4, respectively (36,42). However, values vary somewhat depending on the expression system and the species of the clone, making direct comparisons with native tissue difficult. In general, the conductance of IRK channels in endothelial cells ranges from 23 to 30 pS (4), suggesting that Kir2.1 and/or 2.2 is the major subunit expressed. In cultured bovine pulmonary artery endothelial cells, a single-channel conductance of 31 pS was reported in symmetrical 150 mM K^+ (23). It was suggested that Kir 2.1 underlies this channel, because molecular data provided no evidence for the existence of Kir2.2. The higher conductance recorded may just reflect the higher K^+ concentration used in this study. The only single-channel data in smooth muscle report a conductance of 17 pS in cells from human small bronchioles (27), which could correspond to either Kir2.1 or 2.4. The presence of both of these subunits might explain the hybrid properties of the IRK current recorded in human bronchioles, i.e., voltage-dependent block of the whole-cell current with a low Ba^{2+} sensitivity. The situation may be even more complicated than this, because members of the Kir2.0 subfamily can coassemble in heterologous systems to form channels with altered properties (34,35), although so far there is no evidence that this happens in vivo.

C. Regulation of Kir2.0 Channels

Although very little work has been carried out on the regulation of Kir2.0 channels in the lung, the underlying principles being determined for cloned channels in heterologous expression systems could help us to understand how the native channels may be regulated.

Intra- and Extracellular pH

Some Kir2.0 isoforms show exquisite pH sensitivity over the physiological range (Kir2.3 and Kir2.4), although others (Kir2.1) show sensitivity only at extreme values. Both Kir2.3 and Kir2.4 currents are inhibited when extracellular pH becomes acidic, the effect occurring with an apparent pK_a of 6.8 and 7.1, respectively (32,43). The molecular basis for H^+ ion sensing is believed to be a residue (His117) in the M1–H5 linker region influencing one of two titratable cysteine residues (C114 and C146 of Kir2.3 and the corresponding residues in Kir2.4) located in the M1–H5 and H5–M2 linkers (43). Kir2.3 is the only isoform with any significant sensitivity to intracellular pH in the physiological range. The sensor is thought to be situated within the inner vestibule, close to the transmembrane domains. Residues Thr53, Tyr57, and Met60 in the N-terminal domain and Pro226, Try227, Met228, Thr229, and Gln230 in the C-terminal domain form a gate that under acidic conditions binds, closing the inner vestibule and therefore making it impermeable to K^+ ions (reviewed in Ref. 3). IRK currents in cultured bovine pulmonary artery endothelial cells were reported to be insensitive to intra- and extracellular pH over the range 6.4–8.4, suggesting that Kir2.3 or 2.4 subunits do not underlie native currents, but is consistent with the presence of Kir2.1.

Regulation by Protein Kinases

Strong inward rectifiers possess several putative serine/threonine phosphorylation sites, suggesting that channel regulation might occur through protein kinases. However, there have been contrasting reports regarding the regulation of Kir2.0 channels by kinases, which may indicate the subtlety of such regulation or that effects are mediated via accessory proteins not present in all cell types or the expression systems used. Thus, PKA has been described to have no effect (29), to be necessary for (44), to activate (45) or to inhibit (46) Kir2.1 channel activity. For example, transient expression of Kir2.1 channels in COS-7 cells was susceptible to a marked and rapid decrease in current by dialysis of the catalytic subunit of PKA. This was abolished when the putative phosphorylation site S425 was mutated to an Asn, suggesting that direct phosphorylation of the channel inhibits currents (46). In contrast, Dart and Leyland (45) showed that Kir2.1 channels expressed in COS-7 cells were stable in the presence of cyclic AMP but were enhanced if Kir2.1 was coexpressed with the A kinase anchoring protein, AKAP79. This regulation however, required the presence of phosphatase inhibitors. Whether AKAPs are critical for IRK regulation in native tissues remains to be examined, but colocalization of AKAP79 and Kir2.1, as demonstrated in the above study, suggests that binding of AKAP79 to Kir2.1 allows PKA to be held in close proximity to the channel, aiding site-specific phosphorylation. Regulation of Kir2.4 by PKA has not been studied but may differ from that of other Kir2.1 subunits because Kir2.4 contains a unique consensus site for PKA phosphorylation, which is located at the N-terminus (36).

Inhibition of Kir2.3 by PKC has consistently been observed in a number of studies (3). Currents in oocytes expressing Kir2.3 channels were attenuated by the phorbol ester PMA, whereas oocytes expressing Kir2.1 showed no effect (47). Mutation of the N-terminal PKC phosphorylation site in Kir2.3 (Thr53) to the equivalent residue found in Kir2.1 abolished this inhibition. Furthermore, the reciprocal mutation in Kir2.1 (I79T) rendered the channel susceptible to inhibition by PMA. However, others have observed down regulation by PKC in wild-type Kir2.1 channels. Currents in *Xenopus* oocytes expressing Kir2.1 subunits were decreased upon application of a specific PKC stimulator, SC-10 (44). Likewise, in lung cancer cells, IRK currents, presumed to be carried by Kir2.1, were decreased by around 40% with the phorbol ester PDB (29). In contrast, bovine pulmonary artery endothelial cells showed no evidence for regulation by PKA or PKC when examined using forskolin or PMA, respectively. However, in the same study, GTPγS caused inhibition of IRK currents, an effect postulated to be via G-protein-dependent activation of the phosphatase PP2A (23). Cyclic GMP has also been reported to inhibit IRK currents in pulmonary artery and microvascular endothelial cells, though this appears to be mediated by direct interaction of cyclic GMP with the channel rather than by phosphorylation via cyclic GMP-dependent protein kinase (26). Kir2.1 is also the target for tyrosine kinases, being inhibited by tyrosine phosphatase inhibitors and stabilized by the tyrosine kinase inhibitor genistein (48). Mutation of a putative tyrosine kinase phosphorylation site Y242 in the C-terminus, a site conserved throughout the Kir2.0 subfamily, produced normal currents but abolished phosphatase regulation. Other tyrosine kinase sites, such as Tyr336, may be important for channel function, because mutations at this site (Y366F) appear inhibitory in the endothelial Kir2.1 channel (49).

Regulation of Expression by Membrane Trafficking

The C-terminus of Kir2.1, 2.2, and 2.3 contains a RRESXI motif, which includes both a PKA phosphorylation site and a binding domain for the PDZ or MAGUK (membrane associated guanylate kinase) family of proteins (3) that allow for membrane clustering and cytoskeletal attachment. This motif is lacking in Kir2.4, possibly suggesting a different pattern of membrane localization to the other Kir2.0 family members (32). Both Kir2.1 and Kir2.3 have been shown to associate with the PDZ protein PSD-95. In native hippocampal cells, phosphorylation of the C-terminal PKA site detached Kir2.3 from PSD-95, whereas, coexpression of Kir2.3 with PSD-95 resulted in membrane channel clustering in COS-7 cells or a reduction in single-channel conductance in HEK-293 cells (reviewed in Ref. 3). Similarly, the MAGUK protein SAP97 binds to the C-terminus of Kir2.1, 2.2, and 2.3, the binding of which is also inhibited by PKA phosphorylation (38). Thus, the cyclic AMP/PKA-dependent pathway, through altering the binding of scaffolding proteins, may be an important pathway to regulate channel expression.

Regulation by Phosphoinositides

Kir2.0 channels are constitutively active compared to other inward rectifier channels, which require auxiliary subunits in order to carry currents (i.e., Kir6.0, SUR; Kir3.0, $G\beta\gamma$). This activity has been suggested to persist due to the high-affinity binding of phosphoinositides to Kir2.0 channels. Compared to other Kir subfamilies, Kir2.0 show considerable specificity for binding and activation by PIP_2, Kir2.1 and 2.4 being the most specific, with Kir2.2 and 2.3 also being partially activated upon PIP_3 binding (50). Numerous residues with positively charged side chains have been proposed to interact with the negatively charged phosphate groups of the PIP_2 headgroup, forming one or more binding sites for PIP_2. The most consistently recognized of these is a run of basic amino acids in the cytoplasmic C-terminal tail, close to the M2 domain, Lys/Arg-Pro/Ser-Lys-Lys-Arg (residues 185–189 in Kir2.1) (3). Two other residues potentially involved in PIP_2 binding (Arg218 and Arg312 of Kir2.1) are located adjacent to putative PKA (Ser220 and Ser314) phosphorylation sites (51). Mutation of residues within the PKA motif that preserve polar residues maintains PIP_2 interactions, whereas those that destroy this motif weaken PIP_2 binding (51). Thus, it seems plausible that PKA may modulate channel activity by altering PIP_2 binding. Interestingly, mutations of Arg218 in Kir2.1 have been identified in patients suffering with Anderson's syndrome, a disease characterized by periodic paralysis, cardiac arrhythmias, and dysmorphic features, symptoms probably caused by loss of IRK channel function.

IV. FUNCTIONAL ROLE OF K_{ATP} AND IRK CHANNELS

A. Resting Membrane Potential and the Control of Basal Tone

The resting membrane potential in most cell types is governed by background K^+ conductances that serve to modulate membrane excitability and control calcium influx. In view of the ubiquitous expression of K_{ATP} channels, this may lead one to suppose that these channels contribute to the E_m. Indeed there is strong evidence that this is the case in coronary and mesenteric vascular beds and that these channels also modulate basal tone and blood flow in these organs (reviewed in Ref. 1). In isolated myocytes from rabbit pulmonary artery, both the E_m and magnitude of the glibenclamide-induced depolarization were dependent on the intracellular ATP concentration, with the inference that a small but significant contribution from K_{ATP} channels to the E_m (~5 mV) would occur at physiological ATP concentrations (7). Similar findings were observed in HPASM cells (Fig. 3A). In rat aorta, K_{ATP} channels could be activated at high ATP levels by lowering intracellular Ca^{2+} concentration ($[Ca^{2+}]_i$) or inhibiting calcineurin activity (21). Whether Ca^{2+} regulates these channels in pulmonary artery remains to be determined, although a more hyperpolarized E_m (15 mV) was observed in HPASM cells dialyzed with high (10 mM) compared to low (1 mM) amounts of the Ca^{2+} chelator EGTA (10). In contrast, studies from a number of laboratories do not support a role for K_{ATP} channels in regulating basal tone in isolated rat perfused lung or pulmonary arterial rings (see Refs. 52–55). It should be noted that the above studies were performed under conditions where vascular tone was artificially elevated with vasoconstrictor agents and/or with cyclooxygenase inhibitors, the latter inhibiting the production of vasodilatory prostaglandins. Both interventions are likely to bring about closure of K_{ATP} channels. However, glibenclamide does elicit an increase in pulmonary artery pressure in rat and dog blood-perfused lung (56,57) and in neonatal pigs in vivo (58), providing evidence for a role in regulating basal tone in blood-perfused vessels.

Although the role of IRK channels has been far less studied than that of K_{ATP} channels, evidence to date would suggest that these channels contribute to the E_m in various pulmonary cell types. In cultured HPASM, Ba^{2+} (100 μM) causes depolarization (~10 mV) in growth-arrested cells, and overexpression of Kir2.1 produces substantial membrane hyperpolarization (40). Moreover, contractions to Ba^{2+} were observed in rat pulmonary arteries precontracted with noradrenaline (59) or in pulmonary venous resistance vessels (24), regardless of whether the endothelial layer was present or not. Although tenfold higher concentrations of Ba^{2+} were required to elicit contractions (0.1–3 mM) in the former study, this is probably accounted for by the reduced blocking capabilities of Ba^{2+} ions in more depolarized vessels (1). Ba^{2+} contractions were likely to result from inhibition of K^+ channels, because they were absent under conditions where the driving force on K^+ was negligible (60 mM extracellular K^+) or after exposure to voltage-gated Ca^{2+} channel inhibitors (59).

Strong inwardly rectifying K^+ channels are also considered to be the main contributor to E_m in those endothelial cells that are quite hyperpolarized (−70 to −60 mV) (4). In cultured adult pulmonary arterial cells, E_m averaged −62 mV, and 10 μM Ba^{2+} depolarized them to −25 mV (26). The physiological consequence of altering E_m is to regulate the driving force on Ca^{2+} entry through nonselective cation channels, such that hyperpolarization increases while depolarization decreases $[Ca^{2+}]_i$. To what extent endothelial IRK channels influence pulmonary tone through regulating the release of vasoactive factors has not been studied specifically, but an increase in endothelial $[Ca^{2+}]_i$ will promote the release of nitric oxide (NO), prostacyclin (PGI_2), and endothelium-derived hyperpolarizing factor (EDHF) (4), factors that will themselves activate a combination of smooth muscle K^+ channels (6). In addition, membrane potential changes in the endothelium may be transduced to the smooth muscle via gap junctions (4).

B. Regulation by Vasoactive Agents

K_{ATP} Channels

Patch-clamp and pharmacological studies in vascular smooth muscle provide convincing evidence that K_{ATP} channels can be activated by vasodilators such as calcitonin gene-related peptide, which stimulate PKA, and inhibited by vasoconstrictors such as angiotensin II and ET-1, which activate PKC (1,6). So far there have been no comparable electrophysiological studies in isolated pulmonary smooth muscle cells. Functional studies, however, have supported a role for K_{ATP} channels in mediating pulmonary vasorelaxation to agonists known to stimulate adenylate cyclase (Gs)-coupled receptors, including isoproterenol, adenosine, and the stable PGI_2 analog iloprost (53,60). The mechanism of channel activation may involve cyclic AMP, but its role is not unequivocal, because glibenclamide failed to have any significant effect on relaxation to forskolin in isolated pulmonary rings (60). Endothelium-dependent relaxation to bradykinin also appears to involve activation of K_{ATP} channels in canine pulmonary artery, possibly through a synergistic action of NO, PGI_2, and EDHF on these channels. Whether inhibition of K_{ATP} channels underlies the effects of vasoconstrictor agents in normal lungs remains to be clearly demonstrated, although such a mechanism may be responsible in part for the contractile effects of hypoxia associated with the release of ET-1 (see Sect V.A).

IRK channels

To date no humoral modulator of classical IRK channels has been clearly identified in smooth muscle, although in some tissues these channels may be the target for EDHF, the identity of which remains controversial and has not been studied in the pulmonary circulation. Acetylcholine does, however, activate an inward current in pulmonary vein cardiomyocytes, the origin of which may be a GIRK channel (24). In endothelial cells, ET-1, vasopressin, angiotensin II, and histamine have all been reported to inhibit IRK currents in capillary and macrovascular endothelial cells through a G-protein-dependent pathway (4). It remains to be determined if such modulation occurs in pulmonary endothelial cells.

C. Maturation of the Lung

The pulmonary circulation undergoes abrupt structural and functional changes at birth, going from a high-resistance, low-flow system to a low-resistance, high-flow vascular bed. The mechanisms underlying such changes are not well understood but probably involve increased NO production (15,58) and changes in K^+ channel expression (reviewed in Chapter 27 of this volume). Recently it was shown that porcine smooth muscle cells were depolarized at birth and hyperpolarized to the adult level of −40 mV within 3 days, suggesting that K^+ channel activation could contribute to the fall in pulmonary vascular resistance at birth (61). Mechanostimulation of endothelial cells by fluid sheer stress, which is known to activate IRK currents and release NO (4), may also contribute to vasodilation. The Kir2.1 channel is a good candidate for mechanotransduction, because laminar shear stress induces K^+ currents in cells expressing the bovine endothelial Kir2.1 channel (49). In the ovine fetus, other K^+ channels may be involved in shear stress–induced pulmonary vasodilation, but probably not K_{ATP} channels (62). Developmental changes in Kir2.1 channel expression could also underlie the increased responsiveness to flow observed in pulmonary vessels soon after birth. Indeed, bovine pulmonary endothelial cells isolated from calves express much less IRK current and have more depolarized resting potentials (−26 mV) than cells isolated from adult animals (22,26). Kir2.1 channels may also play a role in the structural maturation of the lung. Valvular pulmonary stenosis has been noted in some patients with Anderson's syndrome, the underlying cause of which is associated with dominant negative-like mutations in the gene encoding Kir2.1 (63). Moreover, Kir2.1 knockout mice develop severe respiratory problems soon after birth, becoming cyanotic and gasping for breath (39). It is assumed that perinatal lethality results from the cleft palate in these animals, but respiratory function could be compromised by the inability of the lung circulation to dilate in response to increases in oxygen tension and flow because of channel loss per se.

Potassium channels sensitive to ATP do not appear to be under significant postnatal developmental, insofar as openers of these channels relax pig pulmonary resistance arteries in the newborn and adult to similar extents (14). However, maximal relaxation and sensitivity to levcromakalim is higher in these arteries than in conduit vessels, suggesting that K_{ATP} channels could help to maintain a low pulmonary vascular resistance at birth. This would at least be consistent with the observation that glibenclamide does produce small, but consistent, increases in pulmonary arterial pressure under conditions of low resting tone in neonatal pigs (58). Furthermore, this agent reverses endothelium-dependent relaxation to acetylcholine in 3-day-old (15) but not adult pigs (64). Whether, such effects are mediated by smooth muscle and/or endothelial K_{ATP} channels is unclear. The relaxant effects of levcromakalim are partially dependent on NO release from the endothelium in resistance arteries from newborn pigs (14), possibly supporting some role for endothelial K_{ATP} channels in modulating tone at birth.

V. INWARDLY RECTIFYING K^+ CHANNELS AND PULMONARY VASCULAR DISEASE

A. Hypoxic Pulmonary Vasoconstriction

Alveolar hypoxia causes acute constriction of pulmonary blood vessels, a response known as hypoxic pulmonary vasoconstriction (HPV). Such a response is unique to the pulmonary circulation, and the purpose is to divert blood away from poorly ventilated to well ventilated areas of the lung (65). Chronic hypoxia, whether due to high altitude or obstructive airways disease, eventually leads to pulmonary hypertension and vascular remodeling. The precise mechanism of HPV is controversial but is likely to involve inhibition of one or more K^+ channel types, the release of contracting factors from the endothelium, and Ca^{2+} release from the sarcoplasmic reticulum (reviewed in detail in Chapter 24 of this book). Both acute and chronic hypoxia appear to be associated with membrane depolarization and increased ET-1 production (see Ref. 55 for references; also see Chapter 24). KCOs have consistently been shown to be potent inhibitors of HPV, both in vivo and in isolated lung preparations in the adult and the newborn, suggesting that K_{ATP} channels can be opened and can oppose the effects of hypoxia (14,57,65,66). Moreover, increased sensitivity of these agents is often observed and probably accounts for their selectivity toward pulmonary versus systemic vessels seen in pulmonary hypertensive but not normotensive rats (65).

There are conflicting reports about the actual role of the K_{ATP} channel in HPV, which appears to depend on the model, species, and severity of hypoxia. In some studies, glibenclamide has been reported to have no effect on vasoconstrictor responses to hypoxia in rat isolated perfused lung or pulmonary arterial rings (53,66). In contrast, it potentiates pressor responses to hypoxia in blood-perfused dog and rat lung (54,57) (but see Ref. 56). Although the reasons for these discrepancies remain unresolved, interpretation of data may be hampered by the sole use of glibenclamide, an agent that has significant antagonistic actions at the thromboxane receptor (13), which in turn may become significantly activated during hypoxia. In contrast, the putative vascular K_{ATP} channel inhibitor U-37883A, which inhibits these channels through an interaction with the pore-forming Kir6.0 subunit (12), actually potentiates the effects of this and other constricting prostaglandins in perfused lung (13). Thus, it will be of interest to investigate the effect of this and the newer, more potent pinacidil-derived K_{ATP} channel inhibitor PNU-99963 (12) in the setting of HPV. In other studies, glibenclamide prolongs first-phase hypoxia-induced contraction by virtue of inhibiting a secondary transient relaxation phase, the latter being particularly prominent in severe hypoxia (52,66). This relaxation could be suppressed by perfusion with a hyperglycemic (15 mM) buffer, suggesting that K_{ATP} channel opening under these circumstances resulted from decreased ATP and/or increased NDP levels. ET-1 antagonists can also markedly attenuate HPV both in vivo and in isolated lung preparations via a mechanism that appears to involve reversal of ET_A receptor-mediated inhibition of K_{ATP}-channels (54,55). Such a result may not be surprising given that ET-1 and other agonists activating Gq-coupled receptors potently inhibit vascular K_{ATP} channels through a PKC-dependent mechanism (1). This would certainly fit with data showing that PKC is responsible, at least in part, for the Ca-dependent component of HPV, though K_{ATP} channel inhibition may not overlap with PKC-mediated effects on tone (55). Moreover, a rise in intracellular Ca^{2+}, which undoubtedly occurs in HPV, could promote K_{ATP} channel closure through activation of calcineurin (21). In summary, there is evidence that K_{ATP} channels could function to provide a depolarizing stimulus for subsequent pulmonary contraction by hypoxia. Equally, various mechanisms appear to operate in the lung to prevent these channels from opening during hypoxia except under extreme conditions of metabolic stress.

One can only speculate about the role of Kir channels in HPV. Whether, as the prevailing view might predict, these channels are inhibited by hypoxia has yet to be demonstrated. However, the activity of Kir channels appears to be tightly controlled by cell metabolism. In pulmonary endothelial cells, such channels are inhibited when intracellular ATP falls or when they are exposed to metabolic inhibitors (23). Likewise, several groups have found that Kir2.0 channels "run down" in whole-cell or excised patches, a process that can be reversed by exposure to ATP (3). Acidosis, which causes pulmonary constriction, is likely to occur after prolonged hypoxia. The extent to which this might influence different K^+ channel types is unclear, but K_{ATP} channels would be activated by a fall in pH (1). Cloned or native Kir2.1 channels are largely insensitive to modulation by pH (4), although Kir2.4, which we have found expressed in HPASM cells (40), is inhibited by a fall in extracellular pH within the physiological range (32). Thus, pH-dependent inhibition of IRK channels may be a viable mechanism of contraction under certain circumstances. Regulation of IRK channels by vasoconstrictors has not been described in smooth muscle, although inhibition by such agents, including ET-1, has been reported in endothelial cells, but so far not in pulmonary cells. Although closure of Kir2.0 channels could contribute to HPV, the overall effect this would have on the release of contracting and relaxing factors from the pulmonary endothelium under normoxic and hypoxic conditions is not immediately obvious and requires some detailed examination. One might suppose that synthesis of NO and EDHF would be reduced by a downregulation of Kir2.0 channels, although hypoxia itself may paradoxically indeed increase NO production.

B. Vascular Remodelling

Medial hypertrophy and hyperplasia are among the earliest and most consistent pathological features of PPH, although as the disease progresses intimal thickening becomes increasingly more apparent (67). What triggers the vascular remodeling process remains unknown, but a rise in the $[Ca^{2+}]_i$ is an essential stimulus for promoting both vasoconstriction and cell growth (this volume, Chapter 26). Moreover, patients with PPH have enhanced levels of the potent vasoconstrictor and growth-promoting agents ET-1 and thromboxane and impaired synthesis of the vasodilatory and antiproliferative agents PGI_2 and NO (67). Thus an imbalance in the production of these factors is likely to contribute to the pathogenesis of PPH, the net effect of which would lead to inhibition of K^+ channel activity (6). Increasing evidence suggests that one of the defects leading to inappropriate vasoconstriction and vascular remodeling in PPH is mediated by a reduction in the activity of K^+ channels (reviewed in Chapter 26 of this volume). Consistent with this notion, we and others have found that proliferation of cultured HPASM cells is associated with membrane depolarization and a downregulation of delayed and transient types of Kv currents (10,68). Because cell growth could be inhibited by chelating extracellular Ca^{2+} or by application of a K^+ ionophore, this suggests that Ca^{2+} influx is an important stimulus for pulmonary cell growth, whereas K^+ efflux, through preventing cell depolarization, may inhibit growth (68).

K_{ATP} channels may play a role in modulating pulmonary cell growth, because the magnitude of K_{ATP} current activated by levcromakalim in HPASM cells was twofold less in proliferating cells than in serum-starved cells (10). Because K_{ATP} channels can contribute to the E_m in pulmonary artery (7), closure or loss of this channel could explain in part the more depolarized resting potentials in proliferating cells. However, whether membrane potential per se can regulate smooth muscle cell growth remains to be rigorously tested. To this end, we have been unable to demonstrate inhibition of HPASM cell proliferation with the K_{ATP} channel opener levcromakalim (Clapp, personal communication, 2000) despite the fact that this agent causes substantial membrane hyperpolarization (~30 mV) in proliferating cells (10). Similarly, no effects on proliferation could be observed with the extremely potent pinacidil derivative P1075 (Clapp, personal communication, 2000). The simplest interpretation of such data is that the membrane potential in these experiments was not driven to a sufficiently hyperpolarized potential to switch off voltage-dependent Ca^{2+} channel entry, which in proliferating cells may also involve entry through T-type Ca^{2+} channels, channels activated at quite hyperpolarized potentials. Alternatively, lack of effect of KCOs could indicate that either membrane depolarization alone is insufficient to drive cell growth and requires additional mechanisms to be activated in concert or that voltage-insensitive Ca^{2+} entry pathways predominates to sustain cell proliferation. We have evidence for the former (but do not discount the latter), because partial reversal (~40%) of the antiproliferative response to UT-15, a stable PGI_2 analog used in the treatment of PPH, was observed with glibenclamide, which by itself had little effect on growth in HPASM cells (Fig. 5). The idea that PGI_2 analogs oppose pulmonary growth by increasing channel K^+ activity may be expected given these agents induce vasorelaxation that is almost entirely dependent on activation of K^+ channels (1,6,69). The mechanism of K_{ATP} channel activation is unknown but probably involves cyclic AMP–dependent activation of

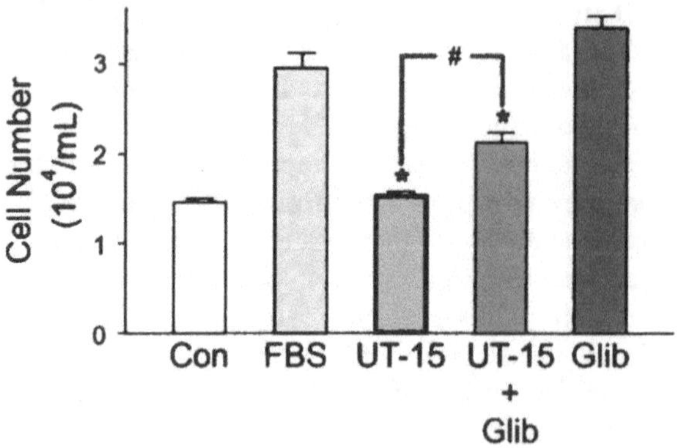

Figure 5 Glibenclamide inhibits the antiproliferative effects of the stable prostacyclin analog UT-15 in cultured human pulmonary smooth muscle cells. Cell counting was assessed in growth-arrested cells stimulated with 10% fetal bovine serum (FBS) for 48 h. UT-15 (30 nM) with or without glibenclamide (10 μM) was added at the same time as the FBS. Data are mean ± SEM ($n = 6$). (*)Significant decrease relative to FBS; (#)significant inhibition of UT-15 response ($P < 0.01$). (L. Clapp, unpublished data.)

PKA, because the antiproliferative effects of PGI_2analoges are critically dependent on cyclic AMP (70). An increase in channel activity could be direct via channel phosphorylation or indirect through increases in surface channel expression. Certainly, membrane-bound A-kinase-anchoring proteins (AKAPs), which serve to target and amplify cyclic AMP-PKA signaling, are known to inhibit smooth muscle growth (71) and increase the trafficking of certain ion channels to the membrane (72).

Studies on the relationship between cell proliferation and IRK channel activity are distinctly lacking in smooth muscle and in endothelial cells. In nonexcitable cells, expression of IRK channels appears critical for promoting cell proliferation where it is presumed that K^+ channels provide the driving force for Ca^{2+} entry through nonselective cation channels (73). Thus, it is tempting to speculate that K^+ channels may have opposing effects on smooth muscle and endothelial cell proliferation. Clearly these will be important issues to consider in future studies. Regardless of this, Kir2.1 channels appear to be regulated by a plethora of growth factors that activate receptors with inherent tyrosine kinase activity. For example, Kir2.1 channels are suppressed by epidermal, nerve, and insulin-like growth factors (48), the latter being a potent pulmonary mitogen. Interestingly, the residue (tyrosine 242) responsible for this regulation is conserved among Kir2.0 subunits but not present in other Kir subfamilies (32,36). In astrocytes, transforming growth factor β downregulates Kir2.3 via a PKC-dependent mechanism (42).

VI. CONCLUDING REMARKS

Considerable advances have been made in our knowledge concerning the properties and function of K_{ATP} and IRK channels within the cardiovascular system. Comparative studies in the lung are progressing much more slowly, particularly in relation to IRK channel function, on which only a handful of papers have been published so far. There is reasonable evidence from electrophysiological experiments that both channels function to modulate resting membrane potential; the case is particularly strong for IRK channels in endothelial cells. However, confirmation at the functional level in terms of contribution to basal or activated pulmonary vascular tone is either controversial or distinctly lacking. The role of K_{ATP} channels may be overlooked if studied under conditions where tone is artificially elevated or if glibenclamide is used under conditions where thromboxane receptors are significantly activated. So far, the function of IRK channels in the pulmonary circulation has hardly been investigated with Ba^{2+}, which still remains the only pharmacological inhibitor of these channels. Given our initial results suggesting that the molecular nature of IRK channels in pulmonary smooth muscle may differ from that of other vessels, agents with greater selectively and potency are eagerly awaited. It will be important in the future to be able to discriminate not only between different members of the Kir2.0 family, but also between members of other Kir subfamilies that have overlapping sensitivities to Ba^{2+}. Clearly, molecular techniques will be instrumental in defining channel "makeup," although with the increasing number of accessory proteins required to form K^+ channel complexes, native regulation by various signaling pathways may be difficult to reproduce in expression systems. In this respect, studies that concentrate on making comparisons of native channel properties with putative channel subunits expressed in the same system in parallel with gene targeting studies are likely to yield more conclusive results.

Clear evidence for regulation by cell metabolism makes K_{ATP} and IRK channels particularly good candidates for either initiating or, more likely, modulating the response to hypoxia in the lung. Closure of these channels could contribute to vasoconstriction or ensuing vascular remodeling of the pulmonary circulation, although the latter studies are clearly in the early stages. An intriguing question remains why K_{ATP} channels do not readily open in the lung when these channels are so readily activated by hypoxia in the systemic circulation. Lack of, or low expression of, Kir6.2 in the lung may account for some of this, because K_{ATP} channels containing Kir6.2 are particularly responsive to changes in cell metabolism, whereas Kir6.1 would theoretically close when ATP levels fall. Release of contracting factors by hypoxia in the pulmonary circulation is likely to contribute to channel inhibition of K_{ATP} and possibly IRK channels. A consistent finding is that K_{ATP} channel openers can overcome the effects of hypoxia, at least in the short term. Thus, pharmacological manipulation of these channels could have potential therapeutic value in the treatment of pulmonary hypertension.

From a disease point of view, one potential advantage of using KCOs is that physiological responses do not depend on an intact endothelium or on receptor-coupled intracellular signaling pathways. Moreover, K_{ATP} channels can function in a remodeled smooth muscle cell. Nicorandil, a K_{ATP} channel opener with NO-releasing properties, is already licensed for use in coronary artery disease, so this agent clearly warrants closer inspection in the context of vasoconstrictor disease in the lung. NO may also be beneficial because it is a potent inhibitor of platelet function and smooth muscle cell proliferation. Although it is not yet known whether KCOs might influence the remodeling process, K_{ATP} channels appear to be modulated by this process and may be the target for antiproliferative agents such as PGI_2 analogs. The potential role of Kir2.0 channels in the vascular remodeling process will be the focus of some intriguing future studies. Some evidence suggests that increased expression, coupled to activation of these channels by shear stress in the endothelium, may contribute to the structural and functional changes seen in the lung at birth. However, it will be important to clarify early on whether the role of K^+ channels in the proliferation of endothelial and smooth muscle cell types is fundamentally different.

ACKNOWLEDGMENTS

This work was supported by grants from the Medical Research Council, UK (G117/440 and G117/182) and the British Heart Foundation (PG/99176). LHC is an MRC Senior Fellow in Basic Science.

ABBREVIATIONS

EDHF	Endothelium-derived hyperpolarizing factor
E_m	Resting membrane potential
ET-1	Endothelin
GIRK	G-protein-gated inwardly rectifying K^+ channel
HEK-293	Human embryonic kidney cell
HPASM	Human pulmonary arterial smooth muscle
HPV	Hypoxic pulmonary vasoconstriction
IRK	Strong inward rectifier K^+ channel
K_{ATP}	ATP-sensitive K^+ channel
K_{Ca}	Ca^{2+}-activated K^+ channel
KCO	Potassium channel opener
Kir	Inwardly rectifying K^+ channel
Kv	Voltage-gated K^+ channel
NO	Nitric oxide
PGI_2	prostacyclin
PIP_2	Phosphatidylinositol 4,5-bisphosphate
PIP_3	Phosphatidylinositol 3,4,5-trisphosphate
PKA	Protein kinase C
PKC	Protein kinase A
PPH	Primary pulmonary hypertension
SUR	Sulfonylurea receptor

REFERENCES

1. Quayle JM, Nelson MT, Standen NB. ATP-sensitive and inwardly rectifying potassium channels in smooth muscle. Physiol Rev 1997; 77:1166–1232.
2. Fujita A, Kurachi Y. Molecular aspects of ATP-sensitive K^+ channels in the cardiovascular system and K^+ channel openers. Pharmacol Ther 2000; 85: 39–53.
3. Stanfield PR, Nakajima S, Nakajima Y. Constitutively active and G-protein coupled inward rectifier K^+ channels: Kir2.0 and Kir3.0. Rev Physiol Biochem Pharmacol 2002; 145:47–179.
4. Nilius B, Droogmans G. Ion channels in the vascular endothelium. Physiol Rev 2001; 81:1415–1459.
5. Seino S, Miki T. Physiological and pathophysiological roles of ATP-sensitive K^+ channels. Prog Biophys Mol Biol 2003; 81:133–176.

6. Clapp LH, Tinker A. Potassium channels in the vasculature. Curr Opin Nephrol Hyperten 1998; 7:91–98.
7. Clapp LH, Gurney AM. ATP-sensitive K^+ channels regulate resting potential of pulmonary arterial smooth muscle cells. Am J Physiol 1992; 262: H916–H920.
8. Clapp LH, Davey R, Gurney AM. ATP-sensitive K^+ channels mediate vasodilation produced by lemakalim in rabbit pulmonary artery. Am J Physiol 1993; 264:H1907–H1915.
9. Clapp LH. Regulation of glibenclamide-sensitive K^+ current by nucleotide phosphates in isolated rabbit pulmonary myocytes. Cardiovasc Res 1995; 30:460–468.
10. Cui Y, Tran S, Tinker A, Clapp LH. The molecular composition of K_{ATP} channels in human pulmonary artery smooth muscle cells and their modulation by growth. Am J Respir Cell Mol Biol 2002; 26:135–143.
11. Clapp LH, Gurney AM, Standen NB, Langton PD. Properties of the ATP-sensitive K^+ current activated by levcromakalim in isolated pulmonary arterial myocytes. J Membr Biol 1994; 140:205–213.
12. Cui Y, Tinker A, Clapp LH. Different molecular sites of action for the K_{ATP} channel inhibitors, PNU-99963 and PNU-37883A. Br J Pharmacol 2003; 139:122–128.
13. DeWitt BJ, Cheng DY, Mcmahon TJ, Marrone JR, Champion HC, Kandowitz PJ. Effects of U-37883A, a vascular selective $K^+{}_{ATP}$ channel antagonist, in the pulmonary and hindlimb circulation. Am J Physiol 1996; 271:L924–L931.
14. Boels PJ, Gao BR, Deutsch J, Haworth SG. ATP-dependent K^+ channel activation in isolated normal and hypertensive newborn and adult porcine pulmonary vessels. Pediatr Res 1997; 42:317–326.
15. Levy M, Souil E, Sabry S, Favatier F, Vaugelade P, Mercier JC, Dall'Ava-Santucci J, Dinh-Xuan AT. Maturational changes of endothelial vasoactive factors and pulmonary vascular tone at birth. Eur Respir J 2000; 15:158–165.
16. Cui Y, Giblin JP, Clapp LH, Tinker A. A mechanism for ATP-sensitive potassium channel diversity: functional coassembly of two pore forming subunits. Proc Natl Acad Sci USA 2001; 98:729–734.
17. Giblin JP, Cui Y, Clapp LH, Tinker A. Assembly limits the pharmacological complexity of ATP-sensitive potassium channels. J Biol Chem 2002; 277: 13717–13723.
18. Cao K, Tang G, Hu D, Wang R. Molecular basis of ATP- sensitive K^+ channels in rat vascular smooth muscles. Biochem Biophys Res Commun 2002; 296:463–469.
19. Quinn K, Tinker A. Protein kinase C and protein kinase A regulate Kir6.1/SUR2B but not Kir6.2/SUR2B in stably transfected HEK293 cells. Biophys J 2002; 82:589C.
20. Thorneloe KS, Maruyama Y, Malcolm AT, Light PE, Walsh MP, Cole WC. Protein kinase C modulation of recombinant ATP-sensitive K^+ channels composed of Kir6.1 and/or Kir6.2 expressed with SUR2B. J Physiol 2002; 541:65–80.
21. Wilson AJ, Jabr RI, Clapp LH. Calcium modulation of vascular smooth muscle ATP-sensitive K^+ channels: role of protein phosphatase-2B. Circ Res 2000; 87:1019–1025.

22. Voets T, Droogmans G, Nilius B. Membrane currents and the resting membrane potential in cultured bovine pulmonary artery endothelial cells. J Physiol 1996; 497:95–107.
23. Kamouchi M, Van Den Bremt K, Eggermont J, Droogmans G, Nilius B. Modulation of inwardly rectifying potassium channels in cultured bovine pulmonary artery endothelial cells. J Physiol 1997; 504:545–556.
24. Michelakis ED, Weir EK, Wu X, Nsair A, Waite R, Hashimoto K, Puttagunta L, Knaus HG, Archer SL. Potassium channels regulate tone in rat pulmonary veins. Am J Physiol Lung Cell Mol Physiol 2001; 280:L1138–L1147.
25. Hogg DS, McMurray G, Kozlowski RZ. Endothelial cells freshly isolated from small pulmonary arteries of the rat possess multiple distinct K^+ current profiles. Lung 2002; 180:203–214.
26. Shimoda LA, Welsh LE, Pearse DB. Inhibition of inwardly rectifying K^+ channels by cGMP in pulmonary vascular endothelial cells. Am J Physiol Lung Cell Mol Physiol 2002; 283:L297–L304.
27. Snetkov VA, Ward JPT. Ion currents in smooth muscle cells from human small bronchioles: presence of an inward rectifier K^+ current and three types of large conductance K^+ channels. Exp Physiol 1999; 84:835–846.
28. Oonuma H, Iwasawa K, Iida H, Nagata T, Imuta H, Morita Y, Yamamoto K, Nagai R, Omata M, Nakajima T. Inward rectifier K^+ current in human bronchial smooth muscle cells: inhibition with antisense oligonucleotides targeted to Kir2.1 mRNA. Am J Respir Cell Mol Biol 2002; 26:371–379.
29. Sakai H, Shimizu T, Hori K, Ikari A, Asano S, Takeguchi N. Molecular and pharmacological properties of inwardly rectifying K^+ channels of human lung cancer cells. Eur J Pharmacol 2002; 435:125–133.
30. Lu T, Nguyen B, Zhang X, Yang J. Architecture of a K^+ channel inner pore revealed by stoichiometric covalent modification. Neuron 1999; 22:571–580.
31. Xie LH, John SA, Weiss JN. Spermine block of the strong inward rectifier potassium channel Kir2.1: dual roles of surface charge screening and pore block. J Gen Physiol 2002; 120:53–66.
32. Hughes BA, Kumar G, Yuan Y, Swaminathan A, Yan D, Sharma A, Plumley L, Yang-Feng TL, Swaroop A. Cloning and functional expression of human retinal Kir2.4, a pH-sensitive inwardly rectifying K^+ channel. Am J Physiol Cell Physiol 2000; 279:C771–C784.
33. Bradley KK, Jaggar JH, Bonev AD, Heppner TJ, Flynn ERM, Nelson MT, Horowitz B. $K_{ir}2.1$ encodes the inward rectifier potassium channel in rat arterial smooth muscle. J Physiol 1999; 515:639–651.
34. Preisig-Muller R, Schlichthorl G, Goerge T, Heinen S, Bruggemann A, Rajan S, Derst C, Veh RW, Daut J. Heteromerization of Kir2.x potassium channels contributes to the phenotype of the Andersen's syndrome. Proc Natl Acad Sci USA 2002; 99:7774–7779.
35. Schram G, Melnyk P, Pourrier M, Wang Z, Nattel S. Kir2.4 and Kir2.1 K^+ channel subunits co-assemble: a potential new contributor to inward rectifier current heterogeneity. J Physiol 2002; 544:337–349.
36. Topert C, Doring F, Wischmeyer E, Karschin C, Brockhaus J, Ballanyi K, Derst C, Karschin A. Kir2.4: a novel K^+ inward rectifier channel associated with motoneurons of cranial nerve nuclei. J Neurosci 1998; 18:4096–4105.

37. Stonehouse AH, Pringle JH, Norman RI, Stanfield PR, Conley EC, Brammar WJ. Characterisation of Kir2.0 proteins in the rat cerebellum and hippocampus by polyclonal antibodies. Histochem Cell Biol 1999; 112:457–465.
38. Leonoudakis D, Mailliard W, Wingerd K, Clegg D, Vandenberg C. Inward rectifier potassium channel Kir2.2 is associated with synapse-associated protein SAP97. J Cell Sci 2001; 114:987–998.
39. Zaritsky JJ, Eckman DM, Wellman GC, Nelson MT, Schwarz TL. Targeted disruption of Kir2.1 and Kir2.2 genes reveals the essential role of the inwardly rectifying K^+ current in K^+-mediated vasodilation. Circ Res 2000; 87:160–166.
40. Cui Y, Tinker A, Clapp LH. Characterisation of inward rectifier K^+ channels in cultured human pulmonary artery smooth muscle cells. Biophys J 2002; 82:589c.
41. Alioua A, Conti L, Eghbali M, Mahajan A, Tanaka Y, Stefani E, Vandenberg C, Toro L. Inward rectifier K^+ channels (Kir) control muscle tone of a rat conduit vessel: role of Kir2.x. (abstr). Biophys J 2003; 84.
42. Perillan PR, Chen M, Potts EP, Simard JM. Transforming growth factor-β_1 regulates Kir2.3 inward rectifier K^+ channels via phospholipase C-δ in reactive astrocytes from adult rat brain. J Biol Chem 2002; 277:1974–1980.
43. Coulter KL, Perier F, Radeke CM, Vandenberg CA. Identification and molecular localization of a pH-sensing domain for the inward rectifier potassium channel HIR. Neuron 1995; 15:1157–1168.
44. Fakler B, Brandle U, Zenner HP, Ruppersberg JP. Kir2.1 inward rectifier K^+ channels are regulated independently by protein kinases and ATP hydrolysis. Neuron 1994; 13:1413–1420.
45. Dart C, Leyland ML. Targeting of an A kinase-anchoring protein, AKAP79 to an inwardly rectifying potassium channel, Kir2.1. J Biol Chem 2001; 276:20499–20505.
46. Wischmeyer E, Karschin A. Receptor stimulation causes slow inhibition of IRK1 inwardly rectifying K^+ channels by direct protein kinase A-mediated phosphorylation. Proc Natl Acad Sci USA 1996; 93:5819–5823.
47. Zhu G, Qu Z, Cui N, Jiang C. Suppression of Kir2.3 activity by protein kinase C phosphorylation of the channel protein at threonine 53. J Biol Chem 1999; 274:11643–11646.
48. Wischmeyer E, Doring F, Karschin A. Acute suppression of inwardly rectifying 2.1 channels by direct tyrosine kinase phosphorylation. J Biol Chem 1998; 273:34063–34068.
49. Hoger JH, Ilyin VI, Forsyth S, Hoger A. Shear stress regulates the endothelial Kir2.1 ion channel. Proc Natl Acad Sci USA 2002; 99:7780–7785.
50. Rohacs T, Lopes CM, Jin T, Ramdya PP, Molnar Z, Logothetis DE. Specificity of activation by phosphoinositides determines lipid regulation of Kir channels. Proc Natl Acad Sci USA 2003; 100:745–750.
51. Lopes CM, Zhang H, Rohacs T, Jin T, Yang J, Logothetis DE. Alterations in conserved Kir channel-PIP_2 interactions underlie channelopathies. Neuron 2002; 34:933–944.
52. Shigemori K, Ishizaki T, Matsukawa S, Sakai A, Nakai T, Miyabo S. Adenine nucleotides via activation of ATP-sensitive K^+ channels modulate hypoxic response in rat pulmonary artery. Am J Physiol 1996; 14:L803–L809.

53. Dumas M, Dumas JP, Rochette L, Advenier C, Giudicelli JF. Role of potassium channels and nitric oxide in the effects of iloprost and prostaglandin E_1 on hypoxic vasoconstriction in the isolated perfused lung of the rat. Br J Pharmacol 1997; 120:405–410.
54. Sato K, Morio Y, Morris KG, Rodman DM, McMurtry IF. Mechanism of hypoxic pulmonary vasoconstriction involves ET_A receptor-mediated inhibition of K_{ATP} channel. Am J Physiol Lung Cell Mol Physiol 2000; 278: L434–L442.
55. Goirand F, Bardou M, Guerard P, Dumas JP, Rochette L, Dumas M. ET_A, Mixed ET_A/ET_B receptor antagonists and protein kinase C inhibitor prevent acute hypoxic pulmonary vasoconstriction: influence of potassium channels. J Cardiovasc Pharmacol 2003; 41:117–125.
56. Feng CJ, Cheng DY, Kaye AD, Kadowitz PJ, Nossaman BD. Influence of N-omega-nitro-L-arginine methyl ester, LY83583, glybenclamide and L158809 on pulmonary circulation. Eur J Pharmacol 1994; 263:133–140.
57. Barman SA. Potassium channels modulate hypoxic pulmonary vasoconstriction. Am J Physiol 1998; 275:L64–L70.
58. Pinheiro JMB, Malik AB. K^+_{ATP}-channel activation causes marked vasodilation in the hypertensive neonatal pig lung. Am J Physiol 1992; 263: H1532–H1536.
59. Uchida K, Saito K, Kitajima T, Kamikawa Y. Effects of Ba^{2+} on F&F 96365-sensitive sustained contraction of rat pulmonary artery. J Pharm Pharmacol 2000; 52:1513–1518.
60. Sheridan BC, McIntyre RC, Meldrum DR, Fullerton DA. K_{ATP} channels contribute to β- and adenosine receptor-mediated pulmonary vasorelaxation. Am J Physiol 1997; 17:L950–L956.
61. Evans AM, Osipenko ON, Haworth SG, Gurney AM. Resting potentials and potassium currents during development of pulmonary artery smooth muscle cells. Am J Physiol 1998; 275:H887–H899.
62. Storme L, Rairigh RL, Parker TA, Cornfield DN, Kinsella JP, Abman SH. K^+-channel blockade inhibits shear stress-induced pulmonary vasodilation in the ovine fetus. Am J Physiol 1999; 20:L220–L228.
63. Andelfinger G, Tapper AR, Welch RC, Vanoye CG, George AL Jr, Benson DW. KCNJ2 mutation results in Andersen syndrome with sex-specific cardiac and skeletal muscle phenotypes. Am J Hum Genet 2002; 71:663–668.
64. Gambone LM, Murray PA, Flavahan NA. Synergistic interaction between endothelium-derived NO and prostacyclin in pulmonary artery: potential role for K^+_{ATP} channels. Br J Pharmacol 1997; 121:271–279.
65. Wanstall JC. The pulmonary vasodilator: Properties of potassium channel opening drugs. Gen Pharmacol 1996; 27:599–605.
66. Wiener CM, Dunn A, Sylvester JT. ATP-dependent K^+ channels modulate vasoconstrictor responses to severe hypoxia in isolated ferret lungs. J Clin Invest 1991; 88:500–504.
67. Gaine SP, Rubin LJ. Primary pulmonary hypertension. Lancet 1998; 352: 719–725.
68. Platoshyn O, Golovina VA, Bailey CL, Limsuwan A, Krick S, Juhaszova M, Seiden JE, Rubin LJ, Yuan JX. Sustained membrane depolarization and

pulmonary artery smooth muscle cell proliferation. Am J Physiol Cell Physiol 2000; 279:C1540–C1549.

69. Clapp LH, Turcato S, Hall SJ, Baloch M. Evidence that Ca^{2+}-activated K^+ channels play a major role in mediating the vascular effects of iloprost and cicaprost. Eur J Pharmacol 1998; 356:215–224.
70. Clapp LH, Finney PA, Turcato S, Tran S, Rubin LJ, Tinker A. Differential effects of stable prostacyclin analogues on smooth muscle proliferation and cyclic AMP generation in human pulmonary artery. Am J Respir Cell Mol Biol 2002; 26:194–201.
71. Indolfi C, Stabile E, Coppola C, Gallo A, Perrino C, Allevato G, Cavuto L, Torella D, Di Lorenzo E, Troncone G, Feliciello A, Avvedimento E, Chiariello M. Membrane-bound protein kinase A inhibits smooth muscle cell proliferation in vitro and in vivo by amplifying cAMP-protein kinase A signals. Circ Res 2001; 88:319–324.
72. Altier C, Dubel SJ, Barrere C, Jarvis SE, Stotz SC, Spaetgens RL, Scott JD, Cornet V, De Waard M, Zamponi GW, Nargeot J, Bourinet E. Trafficking of L-type calcium channels mediated by the postsynaptic scaffolding protein AKAP79. J Biol Chem 2002; 277:33598–33603.
73. Wonderlin WF, Strobl JS. Potassium channels, proliferation and G1 progression. J Membr Biol 1996; 154:91–107.

14

2P Domain K^+ Channels and Their Role in Chemoreception

Amanda J. Patel and Eric Honoré
Institut de Pharmacologie Moléculaire et Cellulaire,
Sophia Antipolis, France

I. INTRODUCTION

Environmental hypoxia evokes a rapid reflex increase in the respiration rate. This reflex is initiated in the carotid bodies located at the bifurcation of the carotid arteries (for review, see Refs. 1–4). Upon a decrease in arterial PO_2, the chemoreceptor type I carotid body cells release neurotransmitters that activate afferent sensory fibers of the sinus nerve, stimulating the brainstem respiratory centers and provoking a reflex increase in ventilation. Similarly, neuroepithelial body cells, which are innervated clusters of amine- and peptide-containing cells located within the airway mucosa, are transducers of hypoxic stimuli and function as airway chemoreceptors (for review see Refs. 3 and 4). Besides the release of neurotransmitters and the stimulation of respiration, hypoxia also has a profound adaptive effect on the pulmonary circulation (for review see Refs. 5 and 6). Hypoxia-induced vasoconstriction of resistance pulmonary artery smooth muscle (PASM) leads to a redistribution of the nonoxygenated blood toward better ventilated regions of the lung.

These specialized cells share in common a mechanism that transduces hypoxic stimuli into a rapid cellular response: the closing of O_2-sensitive K^+ channels (1,2,5,6). Hypoxia depolarizes the O_2-sensitive cells, increases excitability, provokes the opening of voltage-gated Ca^{2+} channels, increases intracellular Ca^{2+}, and triggers cellular responses including neurotransmitter release as well as myocyte contraction. Recently, it was proposed that members of the novel family of 2P domain K^+ channels play a central role in chemoreception.

Mammalian K^+ channel subunits (about 80 genes) are divided into four main structural classes comprising two, four, six, or seven transmembrane segments (TMSs) (7). The common feature of all K^+ channels is the presence of a conserved motif called the P domain that is part of the K^+ conduction pathway (8). The two TMS channels make up a single P domain and encode the inward rectifiers (IRKs), the G-protein-regulated K^+ channels (GIRKs) and the ATP-dependent K^+ channels (K_{ATP}). These K^+ channels, which operate mostly at negative membrane potentials, contribute to the setting of the resting membrane potential and to the terminal phase of the action potential repolarization. The six TMS channels, including the voltage-gated (Kv) and the small-conductance Ca^{2+}-activated K^+ channels (SKs), similarly make up a single P domain. The seven TMS channels with a single P domain encode the large-conductance Ca^{2+}-dependent K^+ channels (BKs). The six and seven TMS K^+ channels that are activated at depolarized membrane potentials and/or when intracellular Ca^{2+} or Na^+ concentrations rise, participate in the repolarization of the action potential. The recently discovered class of four TMS subunits is characterized, unlike the other K^+ channels, by the presence of two P domains in tandem (7,9–12) (Fig. 1). The 2P domain K^+ channels are open at rest and are qualified as leak or background K^+ channels. The typical baseline activity suggests that 2P domain K^+ channels will influence both the resting membrane potential and the action potential duration (7,9–12). Functional K^+ channels are tetramers of pore-forming subunits for the two, six, and seven TMS classes and dimers in the case of the four TMS class.

Although the 2P domain K^+ channel subunits display the same structural motif with four TMSs, an extended M1P1 extracellular loop, both amino- and carboxy-termini intracellular, they share moderate sequence homology outside their P regions (7,9–12). The 14 human 2P domain K^+ channels identified so far are classified into five structural subgroups: (1) TWIK-1 (KCNK1), TWIK-2 (KCNK6), and KCNK7 ; (2) TASK-1 (KCNK3), TASK-3 (KCNK9), and TASK-5 (KCNK15); (3) TREK-1 (KCNK2), TREK-2 (KCNK10), and TRAAK (KCNK4); (4) TASK-2 (KCNK5), TALK-1 (KCNK16), and TALK-2 (KCNK17); and (5) THIK-1 (KCNK13) and THIK-2 (KCNK12) (Fig. 1).

In this chapter, we will review the functional properties of the mammalian 2P domain K^+ channels. Additionally, we will discuss the recent findings concerning the role of the 2P domain K^+ channels in O_2 and pH sensing, with particular emphasis on pulmonary physiology.

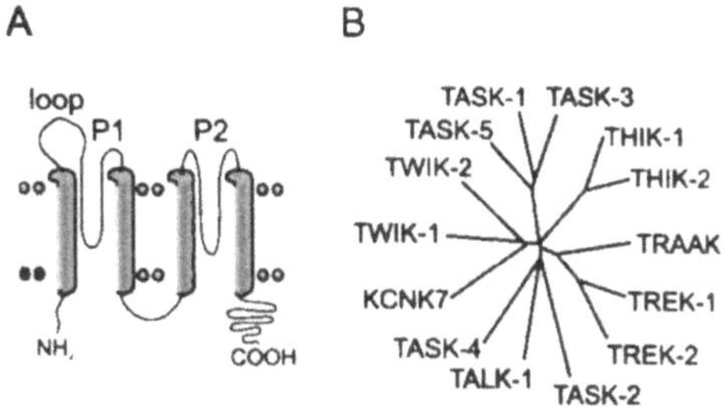

C

		Human Lung
KCNK1	TWIK-1	○
KCNK6	TWIK-2	●
KCNK7	KCNK7	●
KCNK3	TASK-1	●
KCNK9	TASK-3	○
KCNK15	TASK-5	●
KCNK2	TREK-1	○
KCNK10	TREK-2	○
KCNK4	TRAAK	○
KCNK5	TASK-2	●
KCNK16	TALK-1	○
KCNK17	TALK-2	●
KCNK13	THIK-1	ND
KCNK12	THIK-2	●

Figure 1 (A) Cartoon illustrating the transmembrane topology of a 2P domain K^+ channel subunit. A functional channel is a dimer of subunits. (B) The phylogenetic tree indicates the existence of five structural subfamilies of human 2P domain K^+ channel subunits. (C) The Hugo nomenclature and the original name of the 2P domain K^+ channel subunits are indicated in the table. 2P domain K^+ channels are expressed in the human lung. An empty circle indicates absence or very weak expression, a filled circle indicates significant expression, and ND indicates not determined (rat THIK-1 is found in the lung). (Data adapted from Refs. 15, 84, and 108.)

II. TWIK-1, TWIK-2, AND KCNK7

TWIK-1 is the first mammalian 2P domain K^+ channel that has been identified (13). TWIK-1 mRNA is widely distributed in human tissues and is particularly abundant in the brain with strong expression in the cerebellum (13–15). TWIK-1 is also found in the kidney, where it is expressed in distinct tubular segments and cells (16,17). In the human heart, TWIK-1 is more

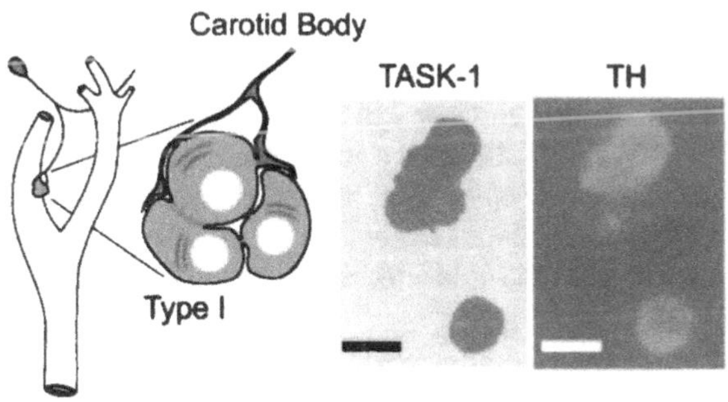

Figure 2 In situ hybridization demonstrating that TASK-1 is expressed in type I carotid body cells, which are also tyrosine hydroxylase positive. (Data adapted from Ref. 28.)

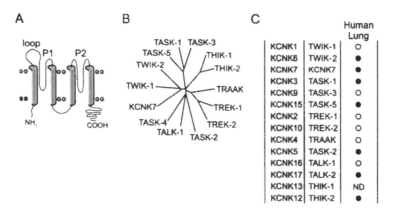

abundant in the ventricle than in the atrium (18). hTWIK-1 is barely detectable in the lung (13,15) (Fig. 1).

TWIK-1 subunits self-associate and form dimers containing an interchain disulfide bridge (19). This assembly involves a 34 amino acid domain that is localized in the extracellular M1P1 linker loop. Cysteine 69, which is part of this interacting domain, is implicated in the formation of the disulfide bond (19). Replacing this cysteine with a serine residue results in the loss of dimerization and functional expression (19). TWIK-1 currents expressed in *Xenopus* oocytes are time-independent and present a nearly linear *I–V* relationship in a symmetrical K^+ gradient that saturates for depolarizations positive to 0 mV (13). This inward rectification is abolished in the absence of internal Mg^{2+} (13). The unitary conductance of TWIK-1 is 35 pS (KCl), and the kinetic behavior is modulated by the membrane potential (13). TWIK-1 channel activity is upregulated by protein kinase C activation and downregulated by intracellular acidosis (13). Both types of regulation are, however, indirect, because they are lost in excised inside-out patches. TWIK-1 channel activity is reversibly blocked by Ba^{2+}, quinine, and quinidine (13). It should be pointed out that the amplitudes of the TWIK-1 currents recorded in *Xenopus* oocytes are very modest and that some investigators have failed to detect a significant functional expression (20). These negative results suggest that either TWIK-1 is targeted to locations other than the plasma membrane or it requires a molecular partner for efficient functional expression (10,20).

hTWIK-2 is highly expressed in the gastrointestinal tract, the vasculature including the pulmonary artery, the pancreas, and the spleen, but, in contrast to TWIK-1, is almost absent from the brain (20–22). Interestingly, hTWIK-2 is found in the thymus, the spleen, the bone marrow, and in peripheral blood leukocytes (21). Finally, hTWIK-2 is detected at a modest level in the lung (15,21) (Fig. 1).

When expressed in transfected COS cells, rat TWIK-2 currents are about 15 times larger than those of human TWIK-2 (21). Both currents exhibit outward rectification in a physiological K^+ gradient and mild inward rectification in a symmetrical K^+ condition. TWIK-2 currents are transient at depolarized potentials, and the kinetics of decay is highly temperature-sensitive (21). rTWIK-2 shows an extremely low conductance, which prevents the visualization of discrete single-channel events (21). Similarly to TWIK-1, TWIK-2 is blocked by Ba^{2+}, quinine and quinidine (21). Moreover, hTWIK-2 is also inhibited by intracellular, but not by extracellular, acidosis (22).

KCNK7, the other member belonging to this structural subfamily, has been cloned in both human and mouse (23,24). In the human, KCNK7 is mainly found in the brain with a peak expression in the cerebellum and the spinal cord (15,24). Similarly to TWIK-2, KCNK7 is found at a modest level in the lung (15,24) (Fig. 1).

Interestingly, this channel comprises a Ca^{2+}-binding EF-hand motif in the carboxy-terminal domain (24). Although KCNK7 is able to dimerize when expressed in COS cells, it remains in the endoplasmic reticulum and is unable to generate ionic channel activity (24). These results suggest that additional channel subunits, modulator substances, or cellular chaperones are required for channel function (24).

III. TASK-1, TASK-3, AND TASK-5

In humans, TASK-1 is found in the brain, with particularly strong expression in the cerebellum (15,25). Additionally, hTASK-1 is expressed in the lung, the pancreas, and the placenta (15,25–27) (Fig. 1). In situ hybridization and RT-PCR analysis (A. Patel, unpublished data) have shown that TASK-1 mRNA is abundant in rat type I carotid body cells (28) (Fig. 2). Although the specificity of the TASK-1 antibody used is questionable (see above), several studies have demonstrated the expression of TASK-1 at the protein level in type I carotid body cells (29). TASK-1 is also expressed in the O_2-sensitive pulmonary artery myocytes and H146 NEB-like cells (30,31) (Fig. 3).

TASK-1 currents show an outward rectification in a physiological K^+ gradient (25–27) (Fig. 4). The *I–V* curve of TASK-1 becomes linear in a symmetrical K^+ gradient (25–27). The rectification of TASK-1 is approximated by the Goldman–Hodgkin–Katz current equation, which predicts a curvature of the *I–V* curve in a physiological K^+ gradient (Fig. 4). In other words, TASK-1 behaves as a pure K^+-selective leak channel. However, with

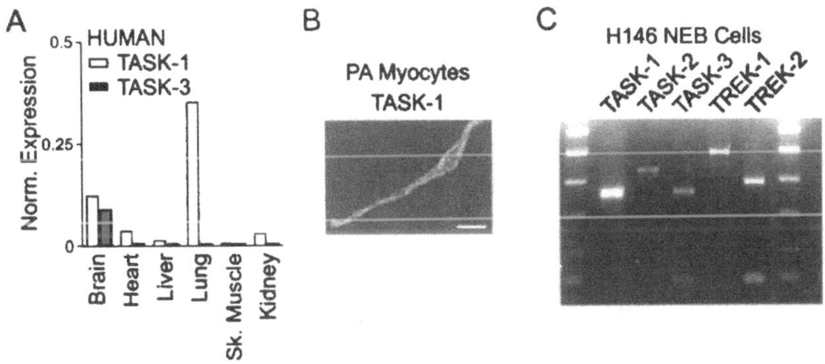

Figure 3 Expression of TASK K^+ channels in the lung chemosensitive cells. (A) TASK-1 and TASK-3 expression has been determined by real-time PCR in human tissues. (B) TASK-1 expression in pulmonary artery myocytes is visualized with a polyclonal antibody anti-TASK-1 (Alomone). (C) The expression of various 2P domain K^+ channel subunits in H146 cells, a model of neuroepithelial body cells, is shown by PCR. (Data adapted from Refs. 15, 30, and 31.)

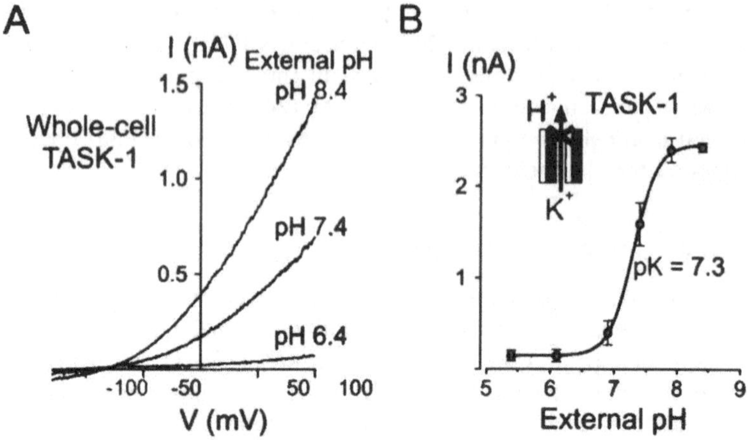

Figure 4 TASK-1 is reversibly inhibited by extracellular acidosis in the physiological range (p*K* 7.3). In these experiments TASK-1 was expressed in transfected COS cells, and currents were recorded in the whole-cell patch-clamp configuration. (Data adapted from Ref. 25.)

voltage steps, TASK-1 opens and closes in two phases; one appears to be immediate, and one is time-dependent (32). TASK-1 is very sensitive to variations in extracellular pH in a narrow physiological range (25) (Fig. 4). The p*K* of TASK-1 is about 7.3 in a physiological K^+ gradient (Fig. 4). Consistent with a pore-blocking mechanism, acidic inhibition is dependent on voltage and potassium concentration (32). Acidic block is prevented in a K^+-rich external solution. Protonation of His98 in the P1 domain is responsible for TASK-1 inhibition (33,34). H98N mutation in tandem channels was used to demonstrate that TASK-1 is indeed dimeric and that both P1 and P2 participate in the ionic pore (33). TASK-1 has a single-channel conductance of 14 pS (KCl) with a flickery behavior (25,35). At the pharmacological level, TASK-1 is blocked by Ba^{2+}, Zn^{2+}, and the local anesthetic bupivacaine (25–27,36). Additionally, TASK-1 is directly blocked by the endocannabinoid anandamide (37). Interestingly, TASK-1 is opened by halothane > isoflurane, whereas it is insensitive to chloroform and partially inhibited by diethyl ether (38–40). A halothane-responsive sequence VLRFMT has been identifed in the proximal cytosolic carboxy-terminal domain of TASK-1 (38,39). TASK-1 is downmodulated by stimulation of Gq-coupled receptors including the metabotropic glutamergic receptors mGluR1–5, the muscarinic m3 receptor, and the angiotensin II type 1a receptor (41–43). Because inibition of TASK-1 is sensitive to phosopholipase C inhibitors, it was suggested that TASK-1 downmodulation results from phospholipase C depletion of PIP2 (43,44). Alternatively, it was proposed that intracellular anandamide could be involved in this regulation

(37). More recently, it was demonstrated that volatile anesthetics and neurotransmitters share a common molecular site of action (39). The anesthetic-responsive sequence VLRFMT is indeed critical for the inhibition of TASK-1 by neurotransmitters (39).

Endogenous TASK-1-like channels have been recorded in rat heart myocytes, with the highest expression found in the right atrium (45). Block of TASK-1 was shown to contribute to the arrhythmogenic effects of platelet-activating factor and anandamide (45). In rat somatic motoneurons, locus coerulus, and cerebellar granule neurons, inhalational anaesthetics similarly activate a background TASK-1-like conductance, causing membrane hyperpolarization and suppressing action potential discharge (12,37,40,46). External acidosis to pH 6.5 completely blocks the current activated by anaesthetics (12,37,40,46). In motoneurones and cerebellar granule neurones, opening of TASK-1 likely contributes to anesthetic-induced immobilization, whereas in the locus coerulus it may support analgesic and hypnotic actions (12,37,40,46).

An oxygen- and acid-sensitive TASK-1-like background K^+ current was described in the type I chemosensitive carotid body cells (28) (Fig. 5). The primary sensory cells of the carotid body respond to hypoxia and

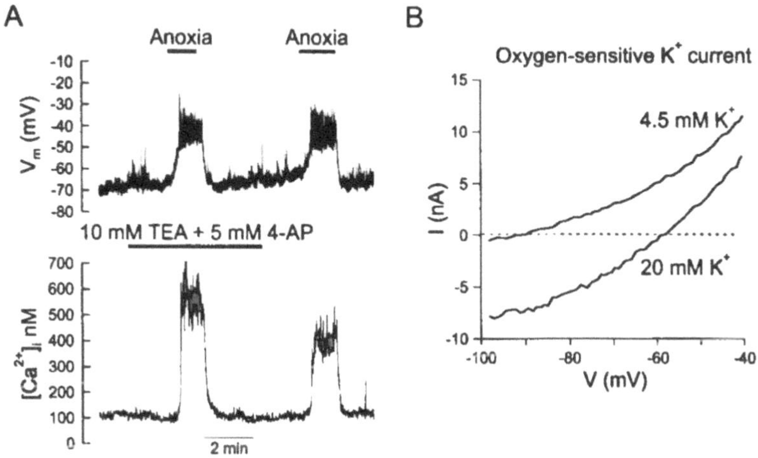

Figure 5 Inhibition of the TASK-like channel in type I carotid body cells by hypoxia, CO, and acidosis induces cell depolarization and increases intracellular calcium. (A) In these experiments the TASK-like current and the membrane potential were monitored with the perforated whole-cell patch-clamp configuration. Intracellular calcium were monitored using Indo-1 fluorescence. Hypoxic depolarization was not affected by 10 mM TEA or 5 mM 4-AP. (B) The oxygen-sensitive background K^+ current in type I carotid body cells was recorded in the presence of 4.5 mM and 20 mM K^+ in the extracellular medium. (Data adapted from Refs. 28, 47, and 113.)

acidosis with a depolarization initiating electrical activity, Ca^{2+} entry, and neurosecretion (28,47,48) (Fig. 5). A key ionic current involved in mediating these responses in rat type I cells is an O_2- and acid-sensitive background K^+ current (28,47) (Fig. 5). This current displays a baseline activity with no voltage and time dependency and shares many of the biophysical and pharmacological properties of the cloned K^+ channel TASK-1, including resistance to tetraethylammonium and 4-aminopyridine (28) (Figs. 4 and 5). Halothane, unlike chloroform, opens the endogenous background TASK-like K^+ channels in type I carotid body cells (28). This effect may be partially responsible for the suppression of hypoxic ventilatory drive under general anesthesia. In cell-attached patches of rat type I carotid body cells, hypoxia closes TASK-1-like channels, but it has no effect in the inside-out patch configuration (28). The loss of O_2 sensitivity upon excision suggests that some cytosolic messenger or cofactor may be required to confer or maintain O_2 sensitivity of TASK-1 (28). When expressed in transiently transfected COS-7 or HEK-293 cells or in mRNA-injected *Xenopus* oocytes, TASK-1 currents are not significantly altered by hypoxia (5 torr for 5 min) (Buckler and Honoré, unpublished data). However, it was recently proposed that recombinant hTASK-1 is an O_2-sensitive channel when stably expressed in HEK-293 cells (pcDNA3.1-hTASK-1 construct) (49). In this study, a mild hypoxia of 30–40 mmHg reversibly inhibits TASK-1. This current is additionally inhibited by extracellular acidosis as expected for a TASK-1 channel (49). Considering that hypoxic downmodulation of TASK-1 channels in type I carotid body cells is lost upon excision and that TASK-1 is not O_2-sensitive in COS-7, HEK-293 cells, or *Xenopus* oocytes, it is assumed that the O_2 sensor is independent of TASK-1. The fact that the stable HEK-293 cell line expressing TASK-1 displays some O_2 sensitivity suggests that the O_2 sensor may be expressed in only a subset of HEK-293 cells (49). Several inhibitors of mitochondrial respiration also mimic the effects of hypoxia and inhibit the TASK-like current in type I carotid body cells (48). The activity of background K^+ currents (i.e., the TASK channels) may therefore be related to mitochondrial respiration such that intrinsic differences between cellular metabolism in different cell types could also explain the differential sensitivity to hypoxia.

In fetal lambs with an aortopulmonary shunt showing an elevated pulmonary artery pressure and blood flow, TASK-1 mRNA is downregulated in distal lung (50). In these experimental animals, alkalosis did not affect pulmonary tone, whereas it induced vasodilation in control animals (50). These results suggest an important role for TASK-1 channels in the pulmonary circulation, particularly in alkalosis-induced dilation and possibly in hypoxic depolarization and vasoconstriction (30,50). In GABAA receptor knockout mice, TASK-1 conductance is upregulated, a form of homeostatic plasticity that allows maintainence of normal neuronal behavior (51). It is interesting to note that the anesthetic-sensitive GABAergic conductance is compensated for by TASK-1, which is also activated by volatile anesthetics. The long-term regulation of TASK-1 at the transcriptional level may therefore also be functionally important in various physiological and disease states.

Recently, the molecular mechanisms responsible for TASK-1 trafficking to the plasma membrane were identified (52–54). Both the p11 subunit of annexin II and 14-3-3 directly interact with the carboxy-terminal domain of TASK-1 (52–54). These molecular associations are essential for trafficking of TASK-1 to the plasma membrane. P11 association with TASK-1 masks an endoplasmic reticulum retention signal identified as Lys-Arg-Arg (52). The interaction of 14-3-3 with the carboxy-terminal domain of TASK-1 overcomes retention of the channel in the endoplasmic reticulum by dibasic signals binding to β-COP (53). 14-3-3 thus promotes forward transport of TASK-1 to the surface of the membrane (53,54). TASK-1 and 14-3-3 could be coimmunoprecipitated in synaptic membrane extracts and postsynaptic density membranes (53).

Human TASK-3 is found in the brain, with particularly strong expression in the cerebellum, but is absent from the lung (55–57) (Fig. 1). The TASK-3 amino acid sequence shares 54% identity with TASK-1, and the two channels exhibit similar macroscopic currents (Fig. 1). TASK-3 single-channel conductance is 27 pS (KCl) and external divalent cations block channel activity at negative membrane potentials (56,57). TASK-3 is reversibly inhibited at acidic extracellular pH with a p*K* of 6.5–6.7, more acidic by about one unit than TASK-1 (55–58). Again, protonation of His98 is involved in acidic inhibition of TASK-3 (56,57). TASK-3 is blocked by Ba^{2+}, quinidine, lidocaine and ruthenium red (39,56–61). The negatively charged residue E70 in P1, absent from TASK-1, is responsible for ruthenium red inhibition of TASK-3 (60). It has been postulated that a single polycationic ruthenium red molecule simultaneously binds to Glu 70 of both TASK-3 subunits (60). TASK-3 is blocked by Zn^{2+} but with a sensitivity of one order of magnitude less than TASK-1 (55–58,61). TASK-3 channel activity is stimulated by the volatile general anesthetic halothane but is inhibited by the local anesthetic bupivacaine (58). Similarly to TASK-1, a conserved anesthetic responsive sequence VLRFLT has been mapped in the proximal carboxy-terminal domain (39). TASK-3 is downmodulated by Gq-coupled receptors, but to a much lesser extent than TASK-1 (39,61). The anesthetic responsive sequence VLRFLT is also involved in this regulation. The interacting protein 14-3-3, unlike P11, interacts with the carboxy-terminal domain of TASK-3, similarly to TASK-1, and regulates channel trafficking (52–54). TASK-3 was shown to contribute to the high resting K^+ conductance of adrenal glomerulosa cells (43,59). Downmodulation of TASK-3 by angiotensin II, as well as depolarization by K^+, may be involved in the control of aldosterone secretion in these cells (43,59). Finally, in the H164 cells, a model of lung neuroepithelial body cells,

TASK-3 has been proposed to encode the O_2-sensitive K^+ channels (31,62) (Fig. 3).

TASK-1 and TASK-3 can form functional heterodimers when expressed in *Xenopus* oocytes (61). The heteromultimeric current shows intermediate pH sensitivity and ruthenium red insensitivity (characteristic of TASK-1) (61). The hybrid channel also responded to angiotensin II receptor stimulation with an inhibition that was weaker than the inhibition of homodimeric TASK-1 and greater than that shown by TASK-3 (61). Heteromultimeric assembly of 2P domain K^+ channels may thus contribute to enhance the functional diversity of this family of ion channels (61).

TASK-5 is structurally related to TASK-1 and TASK-3 (63–65). Human TASK-5 is expressed in the pancreas, liver, kidney, ovary, testis, heart, and lung (64) (Fig. 1). In the brain, rTASK-5 is found in olfactory bulb mitral cells and Purkinje cells predominantly associated with the central auditory pathway (63). hTASK-5 does not functionally express in *Xenopus* oocytes, whereas chimeric TASK-5/TASK-3 constructs containing the region between M1 and M3 of TASK-3 produce K^+ currents (63–65). TASK-5 may require some other, unidentified partner subunit(s) to form functional channels in the plasma membrane, or it may form a channel in an intracellular organelle.

IV. TREK-1, TREK-2, AND TRAAK

Human TREK-1, TREK-2, and TRAAK are found in the brain, with strong expression in the striatum (14,15,66–70). Immunocytochemistry with a polyclonal antibody demonstrated that TREK-1 is particularly well expressed in GABAergic interneurons (63–65). Using the same approach, TRAAK was found to be expressed in the soma and to a lesser degree in axons and/or dendrites in the brain and in the spinal cord (71). TREK-1 and TRAAK are present in rat sciatic nerve, and channels are transported in both directions in the axons, suggesting that they are associated with vesicles (72). TREK-2 is also functionally expressed in cortical astrocytes (73). A substantial expression of TREK-1 and TREK-2 is detected in the gastrointestinal tract (15,74). Two alternatively spliced TREK-2 channels (in the amino-terminal domain) were isolated from cDNA libraries of human kidney, and fetal brain (75). One splice variant is highly expressed in the kidney whereas the other is predominant in the brain (75). The functional characteristics of the two splice variants are identical. Similarly, a TRAAK splice variant was found in the human heart (76). TREK-1, TREK-2, and TRAAK are quasi-absent from the human lung (15) (Fig. 1). By RT-PCR analysis, TREK-1 and TREK-2 were found to be expressed at a very modest level in murine pulmonary artery myocytes (74).

TREK-1, TREK-2, and TRAAK channel activity is elicited by increasing mechanical pressure applied to the cell membrane and is independent of intracellular Ca^{2+} (66, 77–79). The single-channel conductances are in the range of 100 pS (KCl). TRAAK and TREK-2 present an inward rectification at positive potentials, whereas TREK-1 is characterized by an outward rectification at negative potentials (66,77–79). Outward rectification of TREK-1 is due to a mild voltage dependency and to an external Mg^{2+} block at negative potentials (80,81). In the inside-out patch configuration, positive pressure is significantly less effective than negative pressure in opening channels, suggesting that a specific membrane deformation (convex curving) preferentially opens these channels (77,79). At the whole-cell level, TREK-1 and TRAAK are modulated by cellular volume, with hyperosmolarity closing the channels (77). Both the number of active channels and the sensitivity to mechanical stretch are strongly enhanced by treating the cell-attached patches with the cytoskeleton-disrupting agents colchicine and cytochalasin D (79). These data suggest that mechanical force may be transmitted directly to the channel via the lipid bilayer and the cytoskeleton may tonically repress TREK channel activity (79,82). Both TREK-1 and TRAAK are blocked by amiloride and Gd^{3+}, blockers of stretch-sensitive ion channels (77,79). Heat gradually and reversibly opens TREK-1, with a sevenfold increase in current amplitude for a temperature jump of 10°C (Q10) (83). Activation of TREK-1 by temperature is specific; TASK-1 and THIK-1 display a Q10 of only 2 and 1.6, respectively (21,83,84). The strong expression of TREK-1 in the small- and medium-diameter dorsal root ganglion (DRG) sensory neurones as well as in the preoptic and anterior hypothalamus makes this background K^+ channel an attractive candidate for a temperature sensor (83). Thermal activation of TREK-1 requires cell integrity and suggests that a cytosolic factor might be involved in channel regulation (83). Lowering intracellular pH shifts the pressure–activation relationship of TREK-1 and TREK-2, but not TRAAK, toward positive values and ultimately leads to channel opening at atmospheric pressure (78,85). Acidosis essentially converts a TREK mechanogated channel into a constitutively active channel. Delegational and chimeric analysis demonstrates that the carboxy-terminus, but not the amino-terminus or the extracellular M1P1 loop, is critical for activation of TREK-1 by stretch, temperature, and intracellular acidosis (78,83,85). The conversion of a specific glutamate residue (E306) to an alanine in the proximal carboxy terminal domain locks TREK-1 in the open configuration (85). The E306A substitution mimics intracellular acidosis and rescues both lipid sensitivity and mechanosensitivity of a loss-of-function truncated TREK-1 mutant (85). Protonation of E306 tunes the TREK-1 mechanical setpoint and is probably the key intracellular proton sensor regulating TREK-1 channel activity (85). In contrast, TRAAK is opened by intracellular alkalosis (86). Pressure and alkali produce a strong synergistic activation. The carboxy-terminal domain of TRAAK, however, is not required for alkaline activation (86).

TREK-1, TREK-2, and TRAAK are reversibly opened by polyunsaturated fatty acids (PUFAs), including arachidonic acid (AA) (70,77,79,86,87). Activation of these channels is observed in excised patch configurations and in the presence of cyclooxygenase and lipoxygenase inhibitors, indicating that the effect is independent of AA metabolism (70). The threshold concentration of PUFA is 100 nM, and the effect does not saturate, even at concentrations as high as 100 μM (70). Activation induced by PUFAs is critically dependent on the length of the carbonyl chain (70,77). The long chain PUFAs, including AA and docosahexaenoic acid (DOHA), are the most effective (70,77). The extent of saturation is critical because long-chain saturated fatty acids are ineffective (70,77). Besides the length of the carbonyl chain and the unsaturation, the negative charge of the carboxyl is essential for channel activity (70,77). Substitution of the carboxyl of AA or DOHA with an alcohol or a methyl ester function prevents channel stimulation (70,77). Activation of TREK and TRAAK channels by PUFAs in the excised patch configuration indicates that the effect is direct either by interacting with the channel protein or by partitioning into the lipid bilayer (82). Micromolar concentrations of AA open TREK and TRAAK channels with onset and offset kinetics that are in the order of minutes (88). Considering that TREK and TRAAK channels are mechanogated and that activation of these channels by AA does not saturate at high doses, it is possible that the effects of PUFAs might be related to a membrane alteration resulting in a change in curvature (77,82). If such an effect occurs, chemically unrelated compounds known to modify membrane curvature should mimic the effect of AA. Anionic amphipaths including trinitrophenol (TNP) have been shown to cause erythrocyte crenation (they become like a ball), whereas cationic amphipaths such as chlorpromazine (CPZ) and tetracain increase the typical discoid-shape form (cup formers) and reverse the membrane effects of crenators (77). The bilayer couple hypothesis assumes that these effects derive entirely from interactions within the bilayer and are independent of the cytoskeleton (89). Anionic amphipaths preferentially insert in the outer leaflet (because of the natural asymmetrical distribution of negatively charged phosphatidylserines in the inner leaflet) and generate a convex curvature of the membrane (89). However, positively charged amphipaths are expected to preferentially insert in the inner leaflet of the bilayer and thus generate a concave curvature (89). Given that TREK and TRAAK channels are preferentially opened by negative (i.e., convex curvature) rather than positive mechanical pressure, it is expected that anionic amphipaths would open, and cationic amphipaths close, the channels (77). Indeed TNP, an anionic amphipath opens TREK channels, and CPZ and tetracain reverse TREK-1 opening by TNP or AA (77). Interestingly, the stimulatory effect of AA decreases by *e*-fold per 41 mV depolarization

(69). The decrease in membrane polarization may tend to induce the accumulation of AA in the inner leaflet of the membrane and thus minimize the crenation effect at depolarized potentials. Although the bilayer couple hypothesis fully accounts for the opening of TREK and TRAAK channels by PUFA, we still cannot entirely rule out the possible existence of a specific binding site on the channel protein itself (82). Lysophospholipids (LPs) including lysophosphatidylcholine (LPC), unlike phospholipids, open TREK and TRAAK channels (88). At low doses, AA and LPC produce additive activation. The effect of LP is critically dependent on the length of the carbonyl chain (longer than 10 carbons) and the presence of a large polar head (choline or inositol) (88). Activation is independent of the saturation status of the lipid, the charge of the polar head, or the presence of an acetyl group at position 2 (platelet-activating factor) (88). Patch excision produces a progressive loss of channel activation by LPC, whereas AA still produces maximal opening, demonstrating that cellular integrity is critically required for LP, but not AA, activation (88). LP and PUFA activation of TREK and TRAAK channels thus clearly involve different mechanisms (82). Deletional analysis indicates that the carboxy terminus, but not the amino terminus or the extracellular loop M1P1 of TREK-1, is critical for both AA and LPC activation (77,88). The same region was previously found to be important for stretch, temperature, and acidic activation, which suggests that chemical and mechanical activation might share a common molecular pathway (77). Deletion of the carboxy-terminal domain of TRAAK or substitution with the domain of TASK-3 does not impair AA activation as observed with TREK-1 and TREK-2, suggesting a different mechanism of activation by PUFA between TREK and TRAAK (86).

The neuroprotective agent riluzole activates TREK-1 and TRAAK (90). By contrast, sipatrigine, another neuroprotective agent, potently inhibits TREK-1 and TRAAK (91). Additionally, the Ca^{2+} antagonists penfluridol and mibefradil and the K_{ATP} channel blocker glibenclamide are inhibitors of TREK-1 (92). Both TREK-1 and TREK-2 are opened by chloroform, diethyl ether, halothane, and isoflurane (38,68). Interestingly, the other structurally and functionally related 2P domain K^+ channel TRAAK is insensitive to volatile anesthetics (38). Deletional and chimeric analysis demonstrate that the carboxy terminus, but not the amino terminus, of TREK-1 is again critical for anesthetic activation (77). The lack of effect of volatile anesthetics on TRAAK, another mechanogated 2P domain K^+ subunit, suggests that an indirect membrane effect (bilayer couple hypothesis) is unlikely and that again the mechanisms of activation of TREK and TRAAK are clearly different (93). When coexpressed with the 5HT4 receptor, serotonin inhibits TREK-1 and TREK-2 (68,77). This effect is mimicked by a membrane-permeant cAMP derivative. Protein kinase A-mediated phosphorylation of Ser333 in the carboxy terminus is responsible for TREK-1 closing (77). Phosphorylation of Ser333 by PKA has been proposed to produce a reversible conversion between leak- and voltage-dependent phenotypes, although these results have recently been challenged (80,81). TREK-1 and TREK-2, unlike TRAAK, are strongly inhibited by protein kinase C stimulation (67,75,88). The opening of TREK-1 by either LPC or AA is completely reversed by treatment with the phorbol ester PMA (88). Sodium nitroprusside and 8-Br-cGMP increase TREK-1 currents in perforated whole-cell and single-channel recordings (74). Mutation of the PKG consensus sequence at serine-351 blocks the stimulatory effects of sodium nitroprusside and 8-Br-cGMP on the open probability without affecting the inhibitory effect of cAMP (74).

Arachidonic-acid-sensitive mechanogated TREK-like K^+ channels have been identified in *Aplysia* sensory neurons, rat neurons, rat cardiomyocytes, frog stomach smooth muscle, bovine adrenal zona fasciculata cells, and mouse colonic smooth muscle (74,92,94–103). For instance, a TREK-1-like K^+ channel in adult rat cardiac cells is inhibited by β-adrenergic stimulation but activated by volatile anesthetics and by extracellular ATP (101,103). The activation of this current by ATP implies the activation of cytosolic phospholipase A2 and the release of AA (103). Opening of TREK channels during cardiac contraction and stretch of the membrane might act as negative feedback, terminating the excitation wave (98,101,103). In cardiac myocytes and in adrenocortical cells the TREK-1-like current is upregulated by intracellular ATP (92,102). This property is, however, absent from the cloned TREK-1 channel expressed in HEK cells (92). The activation of the endogenous TREK-1 current by intracellular ATP may indicate that this current may function as a sensor that couples the metabolic state of the cell membrane potential, perhaps through an associated ATP-binding protein (92). These findings suggest that indeed TREK-1 could behave as a metabolic sensor and may in addition to TASK-1 and -3 channels be involved in chemosensitivity. Interestingly, a recent report demonstrates that TREK-1 is an oxygen-sensitive K^+ channel when expressed in HEK cells (104). Acute hypoxia causes a rapid and reversible inhibition of whole-cell K^+ current amplitudes, with maximal inhibition achieved at 60 mmHg and below. TREK-1 stimulation by arachidonic acid or trinitrophenol is completely prevented by hypoxia (104). These data suggest that the potential neuroprotective role of TREK channels is questionable, because TREK-1 will be closed when ambient Po_2 is below 60 mmHg, a situation that normally exists in the CNS even during systemic normoxia (104).

V. TASK-2, TALK-1, AND TALK-2

Human TASK-2 is absent from the brain but is detected in the spinal cord. It is mostly expressed in the liver, lung, kidney, pancreas, and GI tract (105,106) (Fig. 1). In transfected cells, TASK-2 produces a slowly activating

(τ: 150 ms at +40 mV), noninactivating, outwardly rectifying K^+ current. The outward rectification is lost in a symmetrical K^+ gradient. The single-channel conductance of TASK-2 is 59 pS (KCl). TASK-2 is blocked by quinine and quinidine but not by the other classical K^+ channel blockers including TEA, 4-AP, Ba^{2+}, and Cs^+ [105]. TASK-2 is sensitive to external pH with a pK of 7.8. TASK-2 is strongly inhibited by the mitochondrial uncoupler DNP (106). TASK-2 channel activity is stimulated by hypotonic conditions (107). Interestingly, clofilium, a blocker of volume-activated K^+ channels in Ehrlich cells, blocks TASK-2. The presence of TASK-2 in these cells, its functional similarity with IK_{volume}, and its modulation by swelling suggest that TASK-2 may directly participate in the regulatory volume decrease phenomenon (107). In the kidney, TASK-2 is localized to cortical distal tubules and collecting ducts, suggesting that it may play an important role in both renal K^+ transport and volume regulation (105). Finally, TASK-2 is stimulated by halothane, isoflurane, desflurane, and chloroform, suggesting that it may play a role, perhaps in the spinal cord, during general anesthesia (106).

TALK-1 and TALK-2 are distantly related to TASK-2 (108,109). Human TALK-1 is expressed exclusively in the pancreas (108). Human TALK-2 is similarly expressed in the pancreas and additionally at a lower level in the liver, placenta, heart, and lung (108) (Fig. 1). These channels produce quasi-instantaneous and noninactivating currents that are activated at alkaline pH (108,109). These currents are inhibited by Ba^{2+}, quinine, quinidine, chloroform, halothane, and isoflurane but are not affected by TEA, 4-AP, Cs^+, AA, hypertonic solutions, activators of PKA and PKC, changes in intracellular Ca^{2+}, or activation of Gi and Gq proteins (108,109).

VI. THIK-1 AND THIK-2

THIK-1 and THIK-2 are 58% identical to each other (84). In rat, THIK-1 is expressed ubiquitously, and rTHIK-2 expression is found in the brain, spleen, kidney, liver, stomach, and lung (84) (Fig. 1). rTHIK-2 is expressed in most brain regions, wheras rTHIK-1 expression is more restricted (84). hTHIK-2 is expressed at a significant level in the lung (108) (Fig. 1). Heterologous expression of rTHIK-1 in *Xenopus* oocytes revealed a K^+ channel displaying weak inward rectification in symmetrical K^+ solution (84). The current is enhanced by arachidonic acid and inhibited by halothane. rTHIK-2 is not functionally expressed. Both THIK-1 and THIK-2 are targeted to the outer membrane. However, coinjection of rTHIK-2 does not affect the currents induced by rTHIK-1, indicating that the two channel subunits do not form heteromultimers (84).

VII. CONCLUSIONS

The 2P domain K^+ channels are characterized by a baseline, leak, or background channel activity (7,9,10). Because, these K^+ channels are active at rest, they will influence the resting membrane potential and will thus contribute to reduce cellular excitability. Up- and downmodulation of the opening of these channels by neurotransmitter or second messenger pathways as well as by pharmacological agents, including the inhalational anesthetics, will have a profound effect on cell electrogenesis (7,9,10).

The background K^+ channels TWIK-2, TASK-1, TASK-2, and TALK-2 and the nonfunctional 2P domain K^+ channels TASK-5, KCNK7, and THIK-2 are significantly expressed in the human lung (15) (Fig. 1). Additionally, TASK-1, TREK-1, TREK-2, and TWIK-2 have been detected the pulmonary circulation (21,30,74). Both TASK-1 and TREK-1 have been shown to be oxygen-sensitive when expressed in HEK cells and may thus be directly involved in hypoxic pulmonary depolarization and vasoconstriction (49,104). Recordings in rat lung thin slices have also revealed the existence of a TASK-1-like current in the endothelium of resistance pulmonary arteries (110). Acidic inhibition of this conductance may contribute to decrease the NO release by depolarizing endothelial cells and may thus participate in the hypercapnic pulmonary artery constriction. TASK channels may additionally play an important role in the excitation–secretion coupling of lung neuroepithelial body cells (3,31). Release of neurotransmitters including serotonin during hypoxia may be under the control of these background K^+ channels (3,31,111,112).

It will be interesting to determine whether the level of expression of these subunits is, similarly to the Kv channel subunits, decreased during chronic hypoxia and pulmonary artery hypertension. Interestingly, TASK-1 channel expression is decreased in a model of congenital heart disease (50). In this model, alkalosis-mediated pulmonary artery vasodilation is impaired, suggesting that indeed TASK-1 subunits may play an important role in the pH modulation of the pulmonary circulation (50).

Transgenic mice will soon tell us more about the physiological role of these novel K^+ channels in the lung, particularly in the pulmonary circulation.

ACKNOWLEDGMENTS

This work was funded by the Centre National de la Recherche Scientifique (CNRS). We are grateful to Pr. Michel Lazdunski for his support.

REFERENCES

1. Lopez-Barneo J. Oxygen-sensing by ion channels and the regulation of cellular functions. Trends Neurosci 1996; 19:435–440.
2. Peers C. Oxygen-sensitive ion channels. Trends Pharmacol Sci 1997; 18:405–408.
3. Kemp PJ, Searle GJ, Hartness ME, Lewis A, Miller P, Williams S, Wootton P, Adriaensen D, Peers C. Acute oxygen sensing in cellular models: relevance to the physiology of pulmonary neuroepithelial and carotid bodies. Anat Record Part A 2003; 270A:41–50.

4. Patel AJ, Honoré E. Molecular physiology of oxygen-sensitive potassium channels. Eur Respin J 2001; 118:221 227.
5. Weir EK, Archer SL. The mechanism of acute hypoxic pulmonary vasoconstriction: the tale of two channels. FASEB J 1995; 9:183–189.
6. Kozlowski RZ. Ion channels, oxygen sensation and signal transduction in pulmonary arterial smooth muscle. Cardiovasc Res 1995; 30:318–325.
7. Patel AJ, Honoré E. Properties and modulation of mammalian 2P domain K^+ channels. Trends Neurosci 2001; 24:339–346.
8. Doyle DA, Morais Cabral J, Pfuetzner RA, Kuo A, Gulbis JM, Cohen SL, Chait BT, MacKinnon R. The structure of the potassium channel: molecular basis of K^+ conduction and selectivity. Science 1998; 280:69–77.
9. Lesage F, Lazdunski M. Molecular and functional properties of two-pore-domain potassium channels. Am J Physiol Renal Physiol 2000; 279: F793–F801.
10. Goldstein SAN, Bockenhauer D, O'Kelly I, Zilberg N. Potassium leak channels and the KCNK family of two-P-domain subunits. Nature Rev/Neurosci 2001; 2:175–184.
11. O'Connell AD, Morton MJ, Hunter M. Two-pore domain K^+ channels—molecular sensors. Biochim Biophys Acta 2002; 1566:152–161.
12. Bayliss DA, Talley EM, Sirois JE, Lei Q. TASK-1 is a highly modulated pH-sensitive "leak" K^+ channel expressed in brainstem respiratory neurons. Respir Physiol 2001; 129:159–174.
13. Lesage F, Guillemare E, Fink M, Duprat F, Lazdunski M, Romey G, Barhanin J. TWIK-1, a ubiquitous human weakly inward rectifying K^+ channel with a novel structure. EMBO J 1996; 15:1004–1011.
14. Talley EM, Solorzano G, Lei Q, Kim D, Bayliss DA. CNS distribution of members of the two-pore-domain (KCNK) potassium channel family. J Neurosci 2001; 21:7491–7505.
15. Medhurst AD, Rennie G, Chapman CG, Meadows H, Duckworth MD, Kelsell RE, Gloger II, Pangalos MN. Distribution analysis of human two pore domain potassium channels in tissues of the central nervous system and periphery. Brain Res Mol Brain Res 2001; 86:101–114.
16. Orias M, Velazquez H, Tung F, Lee G, Desir GV. Cloning and localization of a double-pore K channel, KCNK1: exclusive expression in distal nephron segments. Am J Physiol 1997; 273:663–666.
17. Cluzeaud F, Reyes R, Escoubet B, Fay M, Lazdunski M, Bonvalet JP, Lesage F, Farman N. Expression of TWIK-1, a novel weakly inward rectifying potassium channel in rat kidney. Am J Cell Physiol 1998; 275: 1602–1609.
18. Wang Z, Yue L, White M, Pelletier G, Nattel S. Differential distribution of inward rectifier potassium channel transcripts in human atrium versus ventricle. Circulation 1998; 98:2422–2428.
19. Lesage F, Reyes R, Fink M, Duprat F, Guillemare E, Lazdunski M. Dimerization of TWIK-1 K^+ channel subunits via a disulfide bridge. EMBO J 1996; 15:6400–6407.
20. Pountney DJ, Gulkarov I, Vega-Saenz de Miera E, Holmes D, Saganich M, Rudy B, Artman M, Coetzee WA. Identification and cloning of

TWIK-originated similarity sequence (TOSS): a novel human 2-pore K^+ channel principal subunit. FEBS Lett 1999; 450:191–196.
21. Patel AJ, Maingret F, Magnone V, Fosset M, Lazdunski M, Honore E. TWIK-2 an inactivating 2P domain K^+ channel. J Biol Chem 2000; 275:28722–28730.
22. Chavez RA, Gray AT, Zhao BB, Kindler CH, Mazurek MJ, Mehta Y, Forsayeth JR, Yost CS. TWIK-2, a new weak inward rectifying member of the tandem pore domain potassium channel family. J Biol Chem 1999; 274:7887–7892.
23. Bockenhauer D, Nimmakayalu MA, Ward DC, Goldstein SA, Gallagher PG. Genomic organization and chromosomal localization of the murine 2P domain potassium channel gene Kcnk8: conservation of gene structure in 2P domain potassium channels. Gene 2000; 261:365–372.
24. Salinas M, Reyes R, Lesage F, Fosset M, Heurteaux C, Romey G, Lazdunski M. Cloning of a new mouse two-P domain channel subunit and a human homologue with a unique pore structure. J Biol Chem 1999; 274:11751–11760.
25. Duprat F, Lesage F, Fink M, Reyes R, Heurteaux C, Lazdunski M. TASK, a human background K^+ channel to sense external pH variations near physiological pH. EMBO J 1997; 16:5464–5471.
26. Leonoudakis D, Gray AT, Winegar BD, Kindler CH, Harada M, Taylor DM, Chavez RA, Forsayeth JR, Yost CS. An open rectifier potassium channel with two pore domains in tandem cloned from rat cerebellum. J Neurosci 1998; 18:868–877.
27. Kim D, Fujita A, Horio Y, Kurachi Y. Cloning and functional expression of a novel cardiac two-pore background K^+ channel (cTBAK-1). Circ Res 1998; 82:513–518.
28. Buckler K, Williams B, Honoré E. An oxygen-, acid- and anaesthetic-sensitive TASK-like background potassium channel in rat arterial chemoreceptor cells. J Physiol 2000; 525:135–142.
29. Yamamoto Y, Kummer W, Atoji Y, Suzuki Y. TASK-1, TASK-2, TASK-3 and TRAAK immunoreactivities in the rat carotid body. Brain Res 2002; 950:304.
30. Gurney AM, Osipenko ON, MacMillan D, Kempsill FEJ. Potassium channels underlying the resting potential of pulmonary artery smooth muscle cells. Clin Exp Pharmacol Physiol 2002; 29:330–333.
31. Hartness ME, Lewis A, Searle GJ, O'Kelly I, Peers C, Kemp PJ. Combined antisense and pharmacological approaches implicate hTASK as an airway O_2 sensing K^+ channel. J Biol Chem 2001; 276:26499–26508.
32. Lopes CM, Gallagher PG, Buck ME, Butler MH, Goldstein SA. Proton block and voltage gating are potassium-dependent in the cardiac leak channel Kcnk3. J Biol Chem 2000; 275:16969–16978.
33. Lopes CM, Zilberberg N, Goldstein SA. Block of Kcnk3 by protons. Evidence that 2-P-domain potassium channel subunits function as homodimers. J Biol Chem 2001; 276:24449–24452.
34. Morton MJ, O'Connell AD, Sivaprasadarao A, Hunter M. Determinants of pH sensing in the two-pore domain K^+ channels TASK-1 and -2. Pflügers Arch 2003; 445:577–583.

35. Han J, Truell J, Gnatenco C, Kim D. Characterization of four types of background potassium channels in rat cerebellar granule neurons. J Physiol 2002; 542:431–444.
36. Kindler CH, Yost CS, Gray AT. Local anaesthetic inhibition of baseline potassium channels with two pore domains in tandem. Anesthesiology 1999; 90:1092–1102.
37. Maingret F, Patel A, Lazdunski M, Honoré E. The endocannabinoid anandamide is a direct and selective blocker of the background K^+ channel TASK-1. EMBO J 2001; 20:47–54.
38. Patel AJ, Honoré E, Lesage F, Fink M, Romey G, Lazdunski M. Inhalational anaesthetics activate two-pore-domain background K^+ channels. Nature Neurosci 1999; 2:422–426.
39. Talley EM, Bayliss DA. Modulation of TASK-1 (Kcnk3) and TASK-3 (Kcnk9) potassium channels: volatile anesthetics and neurotransmitters share a molecular site of action. J Biol Chem 2002; 277:17733–17742.
40. Sirois JE, Lei Q, Talley EM, Lynch C 3rd, Bayliss DA. The TASK-1 two-pore domain K^+ channel is a molecular substrate for neuronal effects of inhalational anesthetics. J Neurosci 2000; 20:6347–6354.
41. Talley EM, Lei Q, Sirois JE, Bayliss DA. TASK-1, a two-pore domain K^+ channel, is modulated by multiple neurotransmitters in motoneurons. Neuron 2000; 25:399–410.
42. Millar JA, Barratt L, Southan AP, Page KM, Fyffe RE, Robertson B, Mathie A. A functional role for the two-pore domain potassium channel TASK-1 in cerebellar granule neurons. Proc Natl Acad Sci USA 2000; 97:3614–3618.
43. Czirjak G, Fischer T, Spat A, Lesage F, Enyedi P. TASK (TWIK-related acid-sensitive K^+ channel) is expressed in glomerulosa. Mol Endocrinol 2000; 14:863–874.
44. Czirjak G, Petheo GL, Spat A, Enyedi P. Inhibition of TASK-1 potassium channel by phospholipase C. Am J Physiol Cell Physiol 2001; 281:C700–C708.
45. Barbuti A, Ishii S, Shimizu T, Robinson RB, Feinmark SJ. Block of the background K^+ channel TASK-1 contributes to arrhythmogenic effects of platelet-activating factor. Am J Physiol Heart Circ Physiol 2002; 282: H2024–H2030.
46. Washburn CP, Sirois JE, Talley EM, Guyenet PG, Bayliss DA. Serotonergic raphe neurons express TASK channel transcripts and a TASK-like pH- and halothane-sensitive K^+ conductance. J Neurosci 2002; 22:1256–1265.
47. Buckler KJ. A novel oxygen-sensitive potassium current in rat carotid body type I cells. J Physiol 1997; 498:649–662.
48. Buckler KJ, Vaughan-Jones RD. Effects of mitochondrial uncouplers on intracellular calcium, pH and membrane potential in rat carotid body type I cells. J Physiol 1998; 513:819–833.
49. Lewis A, Hartness ME, Chapman CG, Fearon IM, Meadows HJ, Peers C, Kemp PJ. Recombinant hTASK1 is an O_2-sensitive K^+ channel. Biochem Biophys Res Commun 2001; 285:1290–1294.
50. Cornfield DN, Resnik ER, Herron JM, Reinhartz O, Fineman JR. Pulmonary vascular K^+ channel expression and vasoreactivity in a model of congenital heart disease. Am J Physiol Lung Cell Mol Physiol 2002; 283:L1210–L1219.

51. Brickley SG, Revilla V, Cull-Candy SG, Wisden W, Farrant M. Adaptive regulation of neuronal excitability by a voltage-independent potassium conductance. Nature 2001; 409:88–92.
52. Girard C, Tinel N, Terrenoire C, Romey G, Lazdunski M, Borsotto M. p11, an annexin II subunit, an auxilary protein associated with the background K^+ channel, TASK-1. EMBO J 2002; 21:4439–4448.
53. O'Kelly I, Butler MH, Zilberberg N, Goldstein SA. Forward transport: 14-3-3 binding overcomes retention in endoplasmic reticulum by dibasic signals. Cell 2002; 111:577–588.
54. Rajan S, Preisig-Muller R, Wischmeyer E, Nehring R, Hanley PJ, Renigunta V, Musset B, Schlichthorl G, Derst C, Karschin A, Daut J. Interaction with 14-3-3 proteins promotes functional expression of the potassium channels TASK-1 and TASK-3. J Physiol 2002; 545:13–26.
55. Chapman CG, Meadows HJ, Godden RJ, Campbell DA, Duckworth M, Kelsell RE, Murdock PR, Randall AD, Rennie GI, Gloger IS. Cloning, localisation and functional expression of a novel human cerebellum specific, two pore domain potassium channel. Brain Res Mol Brain Res 2000; 82:74–83.
56. Rajan S, Wischmeyer E, Liu GX, Preisig-Muller R, Daut J, Karschin A, Derst C. TASK-3, a novel tandem pore-domain acid-sensitive K^+ channel: an extracellular histidine as pH sensor. J Biol Chem 2000; 275:16650–16657.
57. Kim Y, Bang H, Kim D. TASK-3, a new member of the tandem pore K channel family. J Biol Chem 2000; 275:9340–9347.
58. Meadows HJ, Randall AD. Functional characterisation of human TASK-3, an acid-sensitive two-pore domain potassium channel. Neuropharmacology 2001; 40:551–559.
59. Czirjak G, Enyedi P. TASK-3 dominates the background potassium conductance in rat adrenal glomerulosa cells. Mol Endocrinol 2002; 16:621–629.
60. Czirjak G, Enyedi P. Ruthenium red inhibits TASK-3 potassium channel by interconnecting glutamate 70 of the two subunits. Mol Pharmacol 2003; 63:646–652.
61. Czirjak G, Enyedi P. Formation of functional heterodimers between the TASK-1 and TASK-3 two pore domain potassium channel subunits. J Biol Chem 2001; 277:5436–5442.
62. O'Kelly I, Stephens RH, Peers C, Kemp PJ. Potential identification of the O_2-sensitive K^+ current in a human neuroepithelial body-derived cell line. Am J Physiol 1999; 276:L96–L104.
63. Karschin C, Wischmeyer E, Preisig-Muller R, Rajan S, Derst C, Grzeschik KH, Daut J, Karschin A. Expression pattern in brain of TASK-1, TASK-3, and a tandem pore domain K channel subunit, TASK-5, associated with the central auditory nervous system. Mol Cell Neurosci 2001; 18:632–648.
64. Ashmole I, Goodwin PA, Stanfield PR. TASK-5, a novel member of the tandem pore K^+ channel family. Pflugers Arch 2001; 442:828–833.
65. Vega-Saenz de Miera E, Lau DH, Zhadina M, Pountney D, Coetzee WA, Rudy B. KT3.2 and KT3.3, two novel human two-pore K^+ channels closely related to TASK-1. J Neurophysiol 2001; 86:130–142.
66. Bang H, Kim Y, Kim D. TREK-2, a new member of the mechanosensitive tandem pore K^+ channel family. J Biol Chem 2000; 275:17412–17419.

67. Fink M, Duprat F, Lesage F, Reyes R, Romey G, Heurteaux C, Lazdunski M. Cloning, functional expression and brain localization of a novel unconventional outward rectifier K^+ channel. EMBO J 1996; 15:6854–6862.
68. Lesage F, Terrenoire C, Romey G, Lazdunski M. Human TREK2, a 2P domain mechano-sensitive K^+ channel with multiple regulations by polyunsaturated fatty acids, lysophospholipids, and Gs, Gi, and Gq protein-coupled receptors. J Biol Chem 2000; 275:28398–28405.
69. Meadows HJ, Benham CD, Cairns W, Gloger I, Jennings C, Medhurst AD, Murdock P, Chapman CG. Cloning, localisation and functional expression of the human orthologue of the TREK-1 potassium channel. Pflügers Arch 2000; 439:714–722.
70. Fink M, Lesage F, Duprat F, Heurteaux C, Reyes R, Fosset M, Lazdunski M. A neuronal two P domain K^+ channel activated by arachidonic acid and polyunsaturated fatty acid. EMBO J 1998; 17:3297–3308.
71. Reyes R, Lauritzen I, Lesage F, Ettaiche M, Fosset M, Lazdunski M. Immunolocalization of the arachidonic-acid and mechano-sensitive baseline TRAAK potassium channel in the nervous system. Neuroscience 2000; 95:893–901.
72. Bearzatto B, Lesage F, Reyes R, Lazdunski M, Laduron PM. Axonal transport of TREK and TRAAK potassium channels in rat sciatic nerves. Neuroreport 2000; 11:927–930.
73. Gnatenco C, Han J, Snyder AK, Kim D. Functional expression of TREK-2 K^+ channel in cultured rat brain astrocytes. Brain Res 2002; 931:56–67.
74. Koh SD, Monaghan KM, Sergeant GP, Ro S, Walker RL, Sanders KM, Horowitz B. TREK-1 regulation by nitric oxide and cGMP-dependent protein kinase. J Biol Chem 2001; 47:44338–44346.
75. Gu W, Schlichthorl G, Hirsch JR, Engels H, Karschin C, Karschin A, Derst C, Steinlein OK, Daut J. Expression pattern and functional characteristics of two novel splice variants of the two-pore-domain potassium channel TREK-2. J Physiol 2002; 539:657–668.
76. Ozaita A, Vega-Saenz de Miera E. Cloning of two transcripts, HKT4 1a and HKT4 1b, from the human two-pore K^+ channel gene KCNK4 Chromosomal localization, tissue distribution and functional expression. Mol Brain Res 2002; 102:18–27.
77. Patel AJ, Honoré E, Maingret F, Lesage F, Fink M, Duprat F, Lazdunski M. A mammalian two pore domain mechano-gated S-like K^+ channel. EMBO J 1998; 17:4283–4290.
78. Maingret F, Patel AJ, Lesage F, Lazdunski M, Honore E. Mechano- or acid stimulation, two interactive modes of activation of the TREK-1 potassium channel. J Biol Chem 1999; 274:26691–26696.
79. Maingret F, Fosset M, Lesage F, Lazdunski M, Honoré E. TRAAK is a mammalian neuronal mechano-gated K^+ channel. J Biol Chem 1999; 274: 1381–1387.
80. Maingret F, Honore E, Lazdunski M, Patel AJ. Molecular basis of the voltage-dependent gating of TREK-1, a mechano-sensitive K^+ channel. Biochem Biophys Res Commun 2002; 292:339–346.

81. Bockenhauer D, Zilberberg N, Goldstein SA. KCNK2: reversible conversion of a hippocampal potassium leak into a voltage-dependent channel. Nat Neurosci 2001; 4:486–491.
82. Patel AJ, Lazdunski M, Honoré E. Lipid and mechano-gated 2P domain K^+ channels. Curr Opin Cell Biol 2001; 13:422–428.
83. Maingret F, Lauritzen I, Patel A, Heurteaux C, Reyes R, Lesage F, Lazdunski M, Honoré E. TREK-1 is a heat-activated background K^+ channel. EMBO J 2000; 19:2483–2491.
84. Rajan S, Wischmeyer E, Karschin C, Preisig-Muller R, Grzeschik KH, Daut J, Karschin A, Derst C. THIK-1 and THIK-2, a novel subfamily of tandem pore domain K^+ channels. J Biol Chem 2000; 276:7302–7311.
85. Honoré E, Maingret F, Lazdunski M, Patel AJ. An intracellular proton sensor commands lipid- and mechano-gating of the K^+ channel TREK-1. EMBO J 2002; 21:2968–2976.
86. Kim Y, Bang H, Gnatenco C, Kim D. Synergistic interaction and the role of C-terminus in the activation of TRAAK K^+ channels by pressure, free fatty acids and alkali. Pflügers Arch 2001; 442:64–72.
87. Kim Y, Gnatenco C, Bang H, Kim D. Localization of TREK-2 K^+ channel domains that regulate channel kinetics and sensitivity to pressure, fatty acids and pH_i. Pflügers Arch 2001; 2001:952–960.
88. Maingret F, Patel AJ, Lesage F, Lazdunski M, Honoré E. Lysophospholipids open the two P domain mechano-gated K^+ channels TREK-1 and TRAAK. J Biol Chem 2000; 275:10128–10133.
89. Sheetz MP, Singer SJ. Biological membranes as bilayer couples. A molecular mechanism of drug-erythrocyte interactions. Proc Natl Acad Sci USA 1974; 71:4457–4461.
90. Duprat F, Lesage F, Patel AJ, Fink M, Romey G, Lazdunski M. The neuroprotective agent riluzole activates the two P domain K^+ channels TREK-1 and TRAAK. Mol Pharmacol 2000; 57:906–912.
91. Meadows H, Chapman CG, Duckworth M, Kelsell RE, Murdock PR, Nasir S, Rennie G, Randall AD. The neuroprotective agent sipatrigine (BW619C89) potently inhibits the human tandem pore-domain K^+ channels TREK-1 and TRAAK. Brain Res 2001; 892:94–101.
92. Enyeart JJ, Xu L, Danthi S, Enyeart JA. An ACTH- and ATP-regulated background K^+ channel in adrenocortical cells is TREK-1. J Biol Chem 2002; 277:49286–49199.
93. Patel AJ, Honoré E. Anesthetic-sensitive 2P domain K^+ channels. Anesthesiology 2001; 95:1013–1025.
94. Belardetti F, Siegelbaum SA. Up- and down-modulation of single K^+ channel function by distinct second messengers. Trends Neurosci 1988; 11:232–238.
95. Vandorpe DH, Morris CE. Stretch activation of the *Aplysia* S-channel. J Membr Biol 1992; 127:205–214.
96. Wallert MA, Ackerman MJ, Kim D, Clapham DE. Two novel cardiac atrial K^+ channels, IKAA and IKPC. J Gen Physiol 1991; 98:921–939.
97. Kim DH, Sladek CD, Aguadovelasco C, Mathiasen JR. Arachidonic acid activation of a new family of K^+ channels in cultured rat neuronal cells. J. Physiol. 1995; 484:643–660.

98. Kim D. A mechanosensitive K^+ channel in heart cells. Activation by arachidonic acid. J Gen Physiol 1992; 100:1021–1040.
99. Kim D, Duff RA. Regulation of K^+ channels in cardiac myocytes by free fatty acids. Circ Res 1990; 67:1040–1046.
100. Kim D, Clapham DE. Potassium channels in cardiac cells activated by arachidonic acid and phospholipids. Science 1989; 244:1174–1176.
101. Terrenoire C, Lauritzen I, Lesage F, Romey G, Lazdunski M. A TREK-1-like potassium channel in atrial cells inhibited by β-adrenergic stimulation and activated by volatile anesthetics. Circ Res 2001; 89:336–342.
102. Tan JH, Liu W, Saint DA. TREK-like potassium channels in rat cardiac ventricular myocytes are activated by intracellular ATP. J Membr Biol 2001; 185:201–207.
103. Aimond F, Rauzier JM, Bony C, Vassort G. Simultaneous activation of p38 MAPK and p42/44 MAPK by ATP stimulates the K^+ current I_{TREK} in cardiomyocytes. J Biol Chem 2000; 15:39110–39116.
104. Miller P, Kemp PJ, Lewis A, Chapman CG, Meadows H, Peers C. Acute hypoxia occludes hTREK-1 modulation: re-evaluation of the potential role of tandem P domain K^+ channels in central neuroprotection. J Physiol 2003; 548:31–37.
105. Reyes R, Duprat F, Lesage F, Fink M, Farman N, Lazdunski M. Cloning and expression of a novel pH-sensitive two pore domain potassium channel from human kidney. J Biol Chem 1998; 273:30863–30869.
106. Gray AT, Zhao BB, Kindler CH, Winegar BD, Mazurek MJ, Xu J, Chavez RA, Forsayeth JR, Yost CS. Volatile anesthetics activate the human tandem pore domain baseline K^+ channel KCNK5. Anesthesiology 2000; 92:1722–1730.
107. Niemeyer MI, Cid LP, Barros LF, Sepulveda FV. Modulation of the two-pore domain acid-sensitive K^+ channel TASK-2 (KCNK5) by changes in cell volume. J Biol Chem 2001; 276:43166–43174.
108. Girard C, Duprat F, Terrenoire C, Tinel N, Fosset M, Romey G, Lazdunski M, Lesage F. Genomic and functional characteristics of novel human pancreatic 2P domain potassium channels. Biochem Biophys Res Commun 2001; 282:249–256.
109. Decher N, Maier M, Dittrich W, Gassenhuber J, Bruggemann A, Busch AE, Steinmeyer K. Characterization of TASK-4, a novel member of the pH-sensitive, two-pore domain potassium channel family. FEBS Lett 2001; 492:84–89.
110. Olchewski A, Olchewski H, Brau ME, Hempelmann G, Vogel W, Saforonov BV. Basic electrical properties of in situ endothelial cells of small pulmonary arteries during postnatal development. Am J Respir Cell Mol Biol 2001; 25:285–290.
111. Fu XW, Nurse CA, Wang YT, Cutz E. Selective modulation of membrane currents by hypoxia in intact airway chemoreceptors from neonatal rabbit. J Physiol 1999; 514:139–150.
112. Youngson C, Nurse C, Yeger H, Cutz E. Oxygen sensing in airway chemoreceptors. Nature 1993; 365:153–155.
113. Barbe C, Al-Hashem F, Conway AF, Dubuis E, Vandier C, Kumar P. A possible dual site of action for carbon monoxide-mediated chemoexcitation in the rat carotid body. J Physiol 2002; 543:933–945.

15

Ca^{2+}-Activated Cl^- Channels and Pulmonary Vascular Tone

William A. Large and Angela S. Piper
St. George's Hospital Medical School, London, U.K.

I. INTRODUCTION

Calcium-activated chloride currents ($I_{Cl(Ca)}$) have been recorded in many smooth muscle preparations including vascular, airway, intestinal, and urogenital tissues (see Ref. 1). In unstimulated smooth muscle the resting chloride permeability is low (2) and the intracellular chloride concentration (or more accurately the activity) is higher than is expected from passive distribution. As a consequence, the chloride equilibrium potential is much more positive than the normal resting membrane potential in smooth muscle. Consequently any stimulus that increases the Cl^- conductance will produce Cl^- ion efflux and depolarization, with subsequent opening of voltage-dependent Ca^{2+} channels to produce contraction. Several Cl^- conductances have been described in smooth muscle (3), and one of the most widely expressed currents is $I_{Cl(Ca)}$.

$I_{Cl(Ca)}$ is activated by a rise in intracellular Ca^{2+} concentration ($[Ca^{2+}]_i$), which is normally derived from intracellular stores, mainly the sarcoplasmic reticulum (SR), or by influx of Ca^{2+} ions. $I_{Cl(Ca)}$ activated by Ca^{2+} release from the SR may occur in response to G-protein-coupled receptor stimulation, e.g., norepinephrine on α_1-adrenoceptors in vascular smooth muscle, which causes the formation of inositol trisphosphate (IP_3) with subsequent release of Ca^{2+} ions from the SR. Also, $I_{Cl(Ca)}$ may occur in nonstimulated cells due to the sporadic spontaneous release of Ca^{2+} ions from the SR, and these responses have been termed spontaneous transient inward currents (STICs) (1). These events may be manifested as random spontaneous transient depolarizations (STDs) recorded with microelectrodes in some whole-tissue preparations [e.g., guinea-pig mesenteric vein (4), guinea-pig urethra (5)]. Alternatively, these spontaneous $I_{Cl(Ca)}$ events may occur in an apparently more organized and larger manner in specialized pacemaker cells [rabbit urethra (6)]. In the latter situation it is likely that $I_{Cl(Ca)}$ is involved in sustained tone of this preparation. In addition it has been proposed that $I_{Cl(Ca)}$ may contribute to pacemaker mechanisms in the guinea-pig antrum (7).

With regard to the pulmonary artery, it has been shown that norepinephrine and histamine activate $I_{Cl(Ca)}$ in rabbit and rat pulmonary artery (1,8). Therefore it is likely that $I_{Cl(Ca)}$ contributes to the excitatory junction potential in the pulmonary artery in response to sympathetic nerve stimulation, which is mediated by the action of norepinephrine on α-adrenoceptors (9). An interesting observation is that some agonists (e.g., histamine) produce marked oscillatory activity of $I_{Cl(Ca)}$ in isolated pulmonary artery cells (10) and oscillating changes in the membrane potential in whole tissue (9). Finally it has been shown that STICs can be recorded in isolated rabbit pulmonary arterial myocytes (1), which are likely to underlie the STDs observed in some whole-tissue preparations of pulmonary artery (Large, unpublished).

In the last few years there have been several general reviews on $I_{Cl(Ca)}$ in smooth muscle (1,3,11), and in this chapter we discuss the properties of single Ca^{2+}-activated Cl^- channels; the regulation, pharmacology, and function of $I_{Cl(Ca)}$in the pulmonary artery; and finally the recent attempts to identify the molecular correlate of $I_{Cl(Ca)}$.

II. PROPERTIES OF UNITARY CA^{2+}-ACTIVATED CL^- CHANNELS IN PULMONARY ARTERY SMOOTH MUSCLE CELLS

Although many studies have described the properties of smooth muscle Ca^{2+}-activated Cl^- channels at the whole-cell recording level, until recently there were only a few reports on the properties of single-channel currents. In this section we will describe the properties of Ca^{2+}-activated Cl^- channel-currents in pulmonary artery myocytes.

A. Multiple Conductance States of Unitary $I_{Cl(Ca)}$ Currents

Initial studies in vascular smooth muscles showed that single Ca^{2+}-activated Cl^- channel currents had a small conductance, although estimates of the mean single-channel amplitude varied from 1.8 pS in human mesenteric artery (12) and rabbit aorta (13) to 2.8 pS in A7r5 cells (14). This variation in the amplitude of unitary Ca^{2+}-activated channels may be explained by a recent study by Piper and Large (15) that described the properties of single Ca^{2+}-activated Cl^- channels in rabbit pulmonary artery myocytes. We showed that single Ca^{2+}-activated Cl^- channels can exist in multiple conductance states depending on $[Ca^{2+}]_i$. Figure 1 shows current recorded from three inside-out patches from rabbit pulmonary artery myocytes with $[Ca^{2+}]_i$ of 50 nM, 250 nM, or 1 μM. When patches were exposed to 50 nM $[Ca^{2+}]_i$, a single conductance level of around 3.5 pS was evident (shown by a dotted line on the trace in Fig. 1A). When $[Ca^{2+}]_i$ was raised to 250 nM, openings to both the full conductance level and a subconductance level were detected, which are shown in Figs.1B and 1C by the two dotted lines on the trace. The presence of both sub- and full-conductance channel events meant that the mean overall single-channel conductance was 2.4 ± 0.2 pS ($n = 10$, Fig. 1F). When $[Ca^{2+}]_i$ was 1 μM, no full-conductance channel events were detected, and instead inside-out patches displayed a mixture of subconductance levels of around 1.8 and 1.2 pS (Figs. 1D and 1E), which meant that the mean overall single-channel conductance was only 1.5 ± 0.1 pS ($n = 7$, Fig. 1F). Because previous studies used relatively high $[Ca^{2+}]_i$ [e.g., 1–10 μM (12) or 2 mM (14)] to activate single $I_{Cl(Ca)}$, it is likely that the variation in the estimates of unitary Ca^{2+}-activated Cl^- channel amplitude in different preparations reflects a varying contribution of subconductance states to the overall mean conductance. It appears, therefore, that unitary Ca^{2+}-activated Cl^-channels can exist in multiple conductance states, with the smaller sublevels becoming more apparent at higher $[Ca^{2+}]_i$.

B. Voltage-Dependent Open Probability and Ca^{2+} Sensitivity of Single Ca^{2+}-Activated Cl^- Channels in Pulmonary Artery Myocytes

Piper and Large (15) showed that for $[Ca^{2+}]_i$ between 10 and 250 nM the total open probability (NP_o) of single Ca^{2+}-activated chloride channels in inside-out patches was voltage-dependent and was higher at positive than at negative membrane voltages. However, because $[Ca^{2+}]_i$ was increased to 500 nM, NP_o was no longer voltage-dependent. Further increasing $[Ca^{2+}]_i$ to 1 μM reversed the voltage dependence of NP_o to the extent that channel activity was higher at negative than at positive membrane voltages.

The Ca^{2+} sensitivity of single Ca^{2+}-activated Cl^- channels was estimated by plotting total single-channel open probability P_o against $[Ca^{2+}]_i$ at a range of membrane voltages. When this relationship was fitted by the Hill equation, it gave an estimate of the Ca^{2+} affinity of the single channels as well as the number of Ca^{2+} ions required for channel opening. The Ca^{2+} affinity of single Ca^{2+}-activated Cl^- channels in inside-out patches from rabbit pulmonary artery myocytes was found to be highly voltage-dependent and was increased at positive membrane potentials;

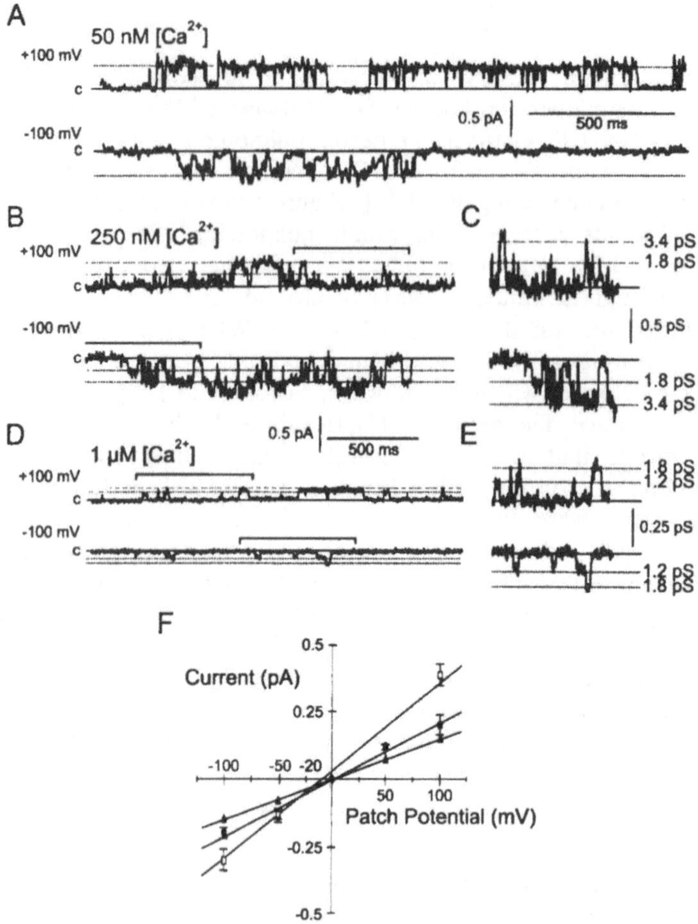

Figure 1 Single Ca^{2+}-activated Cl^- channel currents recorded in inside-out patches. (A) A trace of single-channel currents recorded at +100 mV and −100 mV from an inside-out patch with 50 nM $[Ca^{2+}]_i$. The solid line denotes the closed-channel level (c), and the dotted line represents the open-channel level. (B) Single Ca^{2+}-activated Cl channel currents recorded with 250 nM $[Ca^{2+}]_i$ at +100 mV and −100 mV. As in (A) the solid line represents the closed-channel level (c), and the dotted lines represent channel subconductance and full-conductance current levels. (C) A section of each trace indicated in (B) is shown on a greater amplification. The solid line denotes the closed-channel current level, and dotted lines through the trace show the single-channel subconductance and full-conductance current levels (1.8 pS and 3.4 pS, respectively). (D) Single-channel currents recorded at +100 mV and −100 mV from an inside-out patch with 1 μM $[Ca^{2+}]_i$. (E) Sections of the trace in (D) are shown on a greater amplification. The solid line represents the closed-channel current level, and dotted lines through the trace denote the single-channel subconductance level as well as a second smaller subconductance level (1.8 pS and 1.2 pS, respectively). (F) The overall mean single-channel *I–V* curve with 50 nM $[Ca^{2+}]_i$ (□, n=8), 250 nM $[Ca^{2+}]_i$ (•, n=10), and 1 μM $[Ca^{2+}]_i$ (▲, n=7). For each $[Ca^{2+}]_i$, the points were fitted by a straight line, the slope of which gave an estimated conductance of 3.0 pS, 2.4 pS, and 1.5 pS with 50 nM, 250 nM, and 1 μM $[Ca^{2+}]_i$, respectively. (From Ref. 15.)

for example, at $-100\,mV$ the apparent dissociation constant (K_d) was 250 nM, whereas at $+100\,mV$ it was around 10 nM. At the resting membrane potential (around -50 to $-60\,mV$ in rabbit pulmonary artery myocytes), the K_d for Ca^{2+} binding was estimated to be around 100 nM. Hirakawa et al. (13) showed that $[Ca^{2+}]_i$ greater than 200 nM is required to activate single $I_{Cl(Ca)}$ in rabbit aortic smooth muscle cells. This suggests that the Ca^{2+}-activated Cl^- channels of the rabbit pulmonary artery may be more sensitive to Ca^{2+} than those present in other vascular tissues. The Hill coefficient (n_H) gave an estimate of how many Ca^{2+} ions must bind in order to open single Ca^{2+}-activated Cl^- channels. This value was also voltage-dependent and decreased from 2.3 at $-100\,mV$ to 1.3 at $+100\,mV$, indicating that between one and three Ca^{2+} ions must bind for channel opening to occur. Although depolarization increased the Ca^{2+} affinity of single Ca^{2+}-activated Cl^- channels of pulmonary artery myocytes, Ca^{2+} binding was required to open the channels (15).

C. Model for Activation of Single Ca^{2+}-Activated Cl^- Channels

Given the single-channel characteristics determined by Piper and Large (15), a possible model for the activation of single Ca^{2+}-activated Cl^- channels has been proposed:

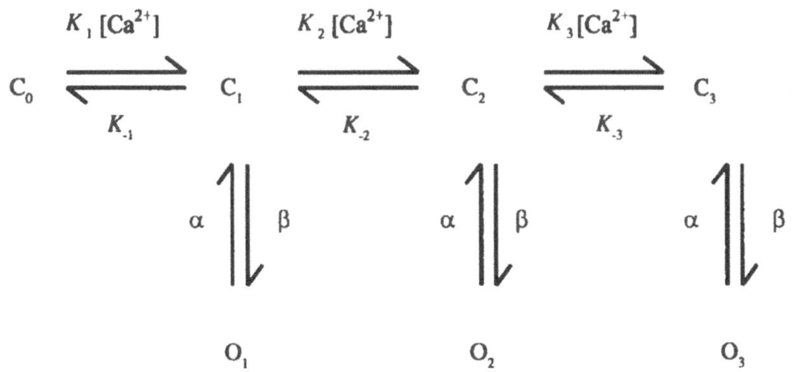

where C and O represent closed and open states, respectively. These authors identified three conductance levels and showed that the binding of Ca^{2+} opens the channel and moreover that increasing $[Ca^{2+}]_i$ reduced the unitary conductance. It was proposed that O_1, O_2, and O_3 correspond, respectively, to the 3.5, 1.8, and 1.2 pS conductance states. Piper and Large (15) suggested there are at least three Ca^{2+} binding sites on the channel protein and that the voltage dependence of K_d indicates that these sites lie within the membrane field, possibly within the channel pore itself. They proposed that the sequential binding of Ca^{2+} ions impedes current flow through the channel; i.e., as more Ca^{2+} ions are bound, the unitary conductance is reduced. Thus, a chloride channel with three Ca^{2+} ions bound has a lower conductance than a channel with a single Ca^{2+} ion, e.g., 1.2 pS vs. 3.5 pS. However, once Ca^{2+}-activated Cl^- channels are open, the probability of opening is voltage dependent with low $[Ca^{2+}]_i$. This suggests that the initial Ca^{2+}-binding/unbinding may be the point at which the voltage-dependence occurs such that depolarization reduces the dissociation of Ca^{2+} from the channel. Once a single Ca^{2+} ion has bound, transitions between O_1, O_2, and O_3 may occur in a Ca^{2+}-independent manner. Full- and sub-conductance channel events had similar distributions of open and closed times at both negative and positive membrane i.e. Ca^{2+} -independent voltages. This suggested that the channel kinetics were the same whether one or three Ca^{2+} ions cause opening at any potential. If this is the case, then the transition rate constants (α and β) between C_1, C_2, C_3 and their respective open states are similar.

III. REGULATION OF CA^{2+}-ACTIVATED CL$^-$ CHANNELS

The activity of many classes of ion channels, including Ca^{2+}-activated Cl^- channels, is modulated by various intracellular signaling pathways. In this section we will describe the regulation of $I_{Cl(Ca)}$ by both direct and indirect mechanisms.

A. Role of Phosphorylation by Ca^{2+}-Calmodulin-Dependent Protein Kinase II in the Regulation of Ca^{2+}-Activated Cl$^-$ Channels

Activation of Ca^{2+}-calmodulin-dependent protein kinase II (CaMKII) occurs in response to increases in $[Ca^{2+}]_i$ and is an important mediator of signal transduction events in smooth muscle. In addition to regulation by other protein kinases, CaMKII undergoes autophosphorylation, which prolongs enzyme activity in the absence of raised $[Ca^{2+}]_i$ (16).

Two studies investigated the role of CaMKII in the regulation of $I_{Cl(Ca)}$ in smooth muscle cells. Wang and Kotlikoff (17) showed that in equine tracheal myocytes the CaMKII inhibitor KN93 prolonged Ca^{2+}-activated Cl^- currents evoked by the addition of caffeine or ionomycin. This led these authors to speculate that CaMKII phosphorylation of Ca^{2+}-activated Cl^- channels leads to their inactivation. It is likely that CaMKII plays a similar role in pulmonary artery cells, because both KN93 and a peptide inhibitor of CaMKII increased theamplitude of $I_{Cl(Ca)}$ evoked by a pipette solution containing 500 nM $[Ca^{2+}]_i$ in rabbit pulmonary artery myocytes (18). Thus the activation of CaMKII by increases in $[Ca^{2+}]_i$ is likely to act as a negative feedback mechanism to produce inactivation of $I_{Cl(Ca)}$. When channels are activated by a brief rise in $[Ca^{2+}]_i$, it would be expected that as Ca^{2+} was removed, Ca^{2+}-activated Cl^- channels would close. However, a sustained rise in $[Ca^{2+}]_i$ could produce activation of CaMKII, which would lead to channel inactivation, effectively terminating the Cl^- current even though $[Ca^{2+}]_i$ remained elevated.

B. Regulation of Ca^{2+}-Activated Cl^- Currents by Cellular Redox State

During hypoxia, mitochondria can increase the release of reactive oxygen species such as hydrogen peroxide (H_2O_2) in the pulmonary vasculature (19), and it has been suggested that this may be a trigger for hypoxic pulmonary vasoconstriction (HPV). $I_{Cl(Ca)}$ in rabbit portal vein myocytes was enhanced by both H_2O_2 and the nonspecific oxidizing agent diamide (20). The actions of oxidizing agents appeared to be mediated partly via an increase in $[Ca^{2+}]_i$, but there was also a direct effect on Ca^{2+}-activated Cl^- channels. Although it had no effect on $I_{Cl(Ca)}$ alone, the reducing agent dithiothreitol was able to reverse the effects of diamide (20). If an increase in reactive oxygen species were to occur in response to hypoxia in pulmonary arterial smooth muscle, the resultant increase in $I_{Cl(Ca)}$ might be expected to contribute to HPV.

C. Indirect Regulation of Ca^{2+}-Activated Cl^- Currents by Nitric Oxide (NO)

It has been shown that in cat tracheal myocytes, carbachol-evoked $I_{Cl(Ca)}$ was reduced by nitric oxide (NO) donors such as *S*-nitroso-*N*-acetyl penicillamine (SNAP) via a cGMP-dependent mechanism (21). This effect of NO donors did not appear to be a direct action on Ca^{2+}-activated Cl^- channels, because both SNAP and the cGMP analog dibutyryl cGMP did not affect caffeine-evoked $I_{Cl(Ca)}$. Further evidence for the indirect modulation of Ca^{2+}-activated Cl^- channels by NO came from the study by Hirakawa et al. (13), who demonstrated that in rabbit aortic myocytes application of high concentrations of SNAP reduced the amplitude of caffeine-evoked $I_{Cl(Ca)}$. This action of NO donors did not appear to involve cGMP-dependent processes. Again SNAP did not act directly on Ca^{2+}-activated Cl^- channels, because NO applied directly to single $I_{Cl(Ca)}$ in excised inside-out membrane patches had no effect.

Although the precise mechanism by which NO regulates Ca^{2+}-activated Cl^- channels remains unclear, it is probable that there is indirect modulation of $I_{Cl(Ca)}$ by NO in pulmonary vascular myocytes via a reduction in the amount of Ca^{2+} released from intracellular stores.

IV. PHARMACOLOGY OF CA^{2+}-ACTIVATED CL^- CHANNELS

A wide variety of chemically unrelated compounds have been found to act as blockers of $I_{Cl(Ca)}$ in smooth muscle tissues. However, the potency of many of these agents varies according to the method of activation of

Ca^{2+}-activated Cl^- currents and the tissue under investigation. It is also important to consider that many compounds that inhibit $I_{Cl(Ca)}$may act as blockers of other classes of Cl^- currents as well as activators and inhibitors of other ion channels, and this will be discussed in more detail below.

A. Potency of Inhibitors of $I_{Cl(Ca)}$

The stilbene derivatives 4-acetamido-4′-isothiocyanatostilbene-2,2′-disulfonic acid (SITS) and 4,4′-diisothiocyanatostilbene-2,2′-disulfonic acid (DIDS), which are blockers of anion transporters, inhibit $I_{Cl(Ca)}$ but with low potency. The concentration that produced 50% inhibition of spontaneous Ca^{2+}-activated Cl^- currents (IC_{50}) in the rabbit portal vein for SITS was 600 μM, whereas for DIDS it was 200 μM (1). Both SITS and DIDS appear to be less effective at blocking caffeine- or agonist-evoked Ca^{2+}-activated Cl^- currents (1).

The diuretics furosemide and indanyloxyacetic acid (IAA-94) also act as blockers of $I_{Cl(Ca)}$. Like the stilbenes, furosemide and IAA-94 were not very potent inhibitors of spontaneous Ca^{2+}-activated Cl^- channels in the rabbit portal vein. The IC_{50} value for inhibition of spontaneous $I_{Cl(Ca)}$ by furosemide was 500 μM (1), whereas in the same cell type, 100 μM IAA-94 produced a 75% inhibition of spontaneous $I_{Cl(Ca)}$ current amplitude (1).

Anthracene-9-carboxylic acid (A-9-C) has been shown to block $I_{Cl(Ca)}$ in various smooth muscle tissues, includingrabbit portal vein, rabbit esophagus (see Ref. 1), sheep urethra (22), rat anococcygeus (23), and sheep lymphatic smooth muscles (24). Again, this agent is not very potent; the IC_{50} for inhibition of $I_{Cl(Ca)}$ in rat and rabbit portal vein ranged between 100 and 600 μM. The action of A-9-C is highly voltage-dependent; A-9-C was three times as potent at +50 mV as at −50 mV (25).

Another class of compounds that are known to actas Ca^{2+}-activated Cl^- channel blockers are the fenamates, including niflumic acid (NFA), flufenamic acid, mefenamic acid, dichlorodiphenylamine-2-carboxylic acid (DCDPC), and diphenylamine-2-carboxylate (DPC). Of the fenamates, NFA is the most potent and is also reasonably selective for $I_{Cl(Ca)}$. The IC_{50} for NFA-induced inhibition of spontaneous Ca^{2+}-activated Cl^- channel currents in rabbit portal vein myocytes was around 2 μM. Micromolar concentrations of NFA produce a significant inhibition of $I_{Cl(Ca)}$ in pulmonary artery smooth muscle cells; e.g., in rat pulmonary artery 10 μM NFA reduced caffeine-evoked $I_{Cl(Ca)}$ by around 60% (8) and also inhibited $I_{Cl(Ca)}$ tail currents evoked by depolarization and subsequent activation of voltage-dependent Ca^{2+} channels (26). The other fenamates are less potent than NFA, and IC_{50} values for the inhibition of spontaneous Ca^{2+}-activated Cl^- channelcurrents in rabbit portal vein ranged from 300 μM for DPC to 20 μM for flufenamic acid.

Other blockers of Ca^{2+}-activated Cl^- channels that have been used in some studies include 5-nitro-2-(3-phenylpropylamino)benzoic acid (NPPB). In rat portal vein myocytes, 10 μM NPPB produced a 60% reduction in noradrenaline-evoked $I_{Cl(Ca)}$ (27). More recently the anti-malarial compound mefloquine (Lariam) was shown to be an antagonist of $I_{Cl(Ca)}$ in a human colon carcinoma cell line with an IC_{50} of 3 μM. Also, the serotonin reuptake blocker fluoxetine inhibits Ca^{2+}-activated Cl^- channel currents in calf pulmonary artery endothelial cells (see Ref. 28). However, the actions of these compounds on $I_{Cl(Ca)}$ in smooth muscle tissues have not been determined.

B. Mechanism of Block of $I_{Cl(Ca)}$

Very few studies have investigated the mechanisms by which inhibitors block $I_{Cl(Ca)}$ in smooth muscle. It has been suggested that both the fenamates, e.g., NFA, and A-9-C act as rapidly dissociating open-channel blockers of $I_{Cl(Ca)}$ based on their effects on the kinetics of whole-cell currents (1,3).However, it appears that other agents such as the stilbene derivatives SITS and DIDS produce block of Ca^{2+}-activated Cl^- channel currents by a different mechanism that at present is unclear.

C. Selectivity of Blockers of $I_{Cl(Ca)}$

A major problem with many of the known blockers of Ca^{2+}-activated Cl^- channel currents is their poor selectivity. Most of the agents described above are known to block more than one class of Cl^- channels or even to inhibit or activate other conductances. Stilbenes such as SITS and DIDS, in addition to blocking volume-regulated Cl^- channels (29), inhibit ATP-sensitive K^+ channels in guinea pig ventricular myocytes (30). The fenamates, such as NFA and DCDPC, as well as SITS, DIDS, and A-9-C activate BK_{Ca} (31). NPPB also stimulates BK_{Ca} in rat portal vein myocytes and activates an ATP-sensitive K^+ conductance (27).

Even though most of these compounds do have actions on conductances other than $I_{Cl(Ca)}$ it is possible in functional studies to test for the nonspecific effects of Ca^{2+}-activated Cl^- channel blockers and to determine their influence on the results. For example, the activation of BK_{Ca} by the fenamates in isolated cells or in whole tissue may be prevented by the use of selective blockers of BK_{Ca} such as iberiotoxin. This means that with carefully controlled experimental conditions it is possible to investigate the role of $I_{Cl(Ca)}$ in functional studies using Ca^{2+}-activated Cl^- channel blockers.

D. Anomalous Effects of Cl^- Channel Blockers on $I_{Cl(Ca)}$

In addition to the effects described above, it has recently been shown that the Ca^{2+}-activated Cl^- channel antagonists NFA, DCDPC, and A-9-C may have unusual effects on $I_{Cl(Ca)}$ depending upon the method by which the currents are activated (32,33). In whole-cell recording studies using rabbit pulmonary artery myocytes, Ca^{2+}-activated Cl^-currents could be activated by adding 500 nM Ca^{2+} to the pipette solution and were recorded at the holding potential of −50 mV. Both NFA and DCDPC were ineffective at blocking this persistently activated $I_{Cl(Ca)}$ current. Indeed, 100 μM NFA produced an increase in Cl^- current recorded at negative membrane potentials and only a modest inhibition of $I_{Cl(Ca)}$ recorded at positive potentials (Fig. 2) (32). It was proposed that NFA and DCDPC produce a simultaneous block of outward Cl^- currents (i.e., inward Cl^- movement) and stimulation of inward Cl^- currents (i.e., outward Cl^- movement). These effects of NFA and DCDPC were revealed only when $[Ca^{2+}]_i$ was maintained at a high level (see Ref. 32 for greater details). It is likely that the reported variation in the potency of some blockers of $I_{Cl(Ca)}$ may depend on how the currents were activated (1,3,27).

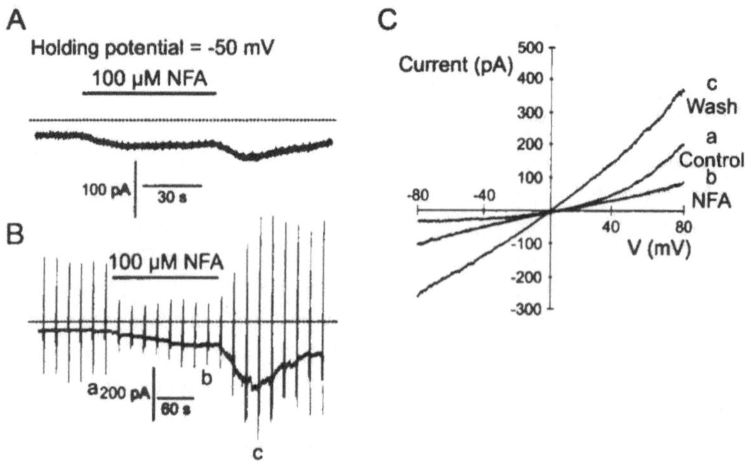

Figure 2 Effect of NFA on $I_{Cl(Ca)}$ stimulated by 500 nM $[Ca^{2+}]_i$. (A) Whole-cell current recorded from a rabbit pulmonary artery myocyte at a holding potential (V_H) of −50 mV. NFA (100 μM) was applied to the cell as indicated by the solid bar and the dotted line represents zero current. (B) Recording of current from a second pulmonary artery cell where depolarizing voltage ramps from −80 mV to +80 mV were applied at 20 s intervals from the holding potential of −50 mV. The cell was exposed to NFA (100 μM) as indicated by the solid bar; the dotted line represents zero current. (C) Plot of current recorded during the indicated voltage ramps from the cell shown in (B) against voltage (a) before (control) and (b) during the application of NFA and (c) on washout. Note that NFA increased $I_{Cl(Ca)}$ at negative potentials but decreased the current at positive potentials. (From Ref. 32.)

Anthracene-9-carboxylic acid also can have unusual effects on $I_{Cl(Ca)}$ in rabbit pulmonary artery myocytes when currents are activated by adding 500 nM Ca^{2+} to the pipette solution. However, in the case of A-9-C, although there is a modest block of outward Cl^- currents at positive potentials, the stimulation of inward Cl^- currents at negative potentials was only transient and manifested as increased "tail" currents after depolarizing steps, and there was no effect on $I_{Cl(Ca)}$ recorded at the holding potential (Fig. 3) (33).The action of A-9-C is highly voltage-dependent, so it is likely that at positive membrane potentials A-9-C binds to the channel (probably within the pore) and, like NFA and DCDPC, produces a simultaneous block of outward Cl^- currents and stimulation of inward Cl^- currents. On returning to negative membrane potentials the stimulatory effect of A-9-C is revealed. However, because the binding of A-9-C is voltage-dependent at negative potentials, it unbinds and the whole-cell currents decay in the normal manner (Fig. 3).

E. Physiological Relevance of Antagonist Selectivity

Ca^{2+}-activated Cl^- channel blockers have been used in some studies to probe the role of $I_{Cl(Ca)}$ in contraction of many smooth muscle preparations including pulmonary arteries (see Ref. 1 for more details). In the rat pulmonary artery, 10 μM NFA inhibited caffeine-evoked $I_{Cl(Ca)}$ in

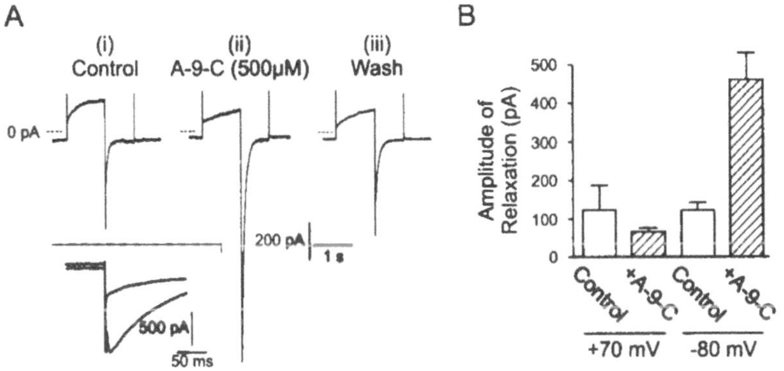

Figure 3 Effect of A-9-C on $I_{Cl(Ca)}$ stimulated by 500 nM $[Ca^{2+}]_i$. (A) A recording of current from a rabbit pulmonary artery cell (i) before and (ii) during the application of A-9-C (500 μM), and (iii) after A-9-C was removed. A section of traces (i) and (ii) is shown alongside on an expanded scale (enclosed by the box); the dotted line represents zero current. (B) Plot of amplitude of current relaxation at +70 mV or −80 mV in the absence (open; $n=12$) or presence (hatched; $n=12$) of A-9-C. Columns represent mean data ± sem; downward error bars have been omitted for clarity. (From Ref. 33.)

single cells, and both NFA and IAA-94 inhibited noradrenaline- and serotonin-evoked contractions in pulmonary artery rings (8,26). However, a lack of effect of some Cl^- channel blockers may not necessarily rule out a functional role for Ca^{2+}-activated Cl^- channels because of the anomalous effect of NFA when $[Ca^{2+}]_i$ is sustained at a high level (see above). Hirst et al. (7) showed that spontaneous potentials caused by the activation of $I_{Cl(Ca)}$ in the interstitial cells of the guinea pig gastric antrum were potentiated by NFA and further that although A-9-C did inhibit spontaneous excitatory potentials, when it was washed out the frequency of discharge of potentials was increased (7). These apparently strange effects of the Cl^- channel blockers may be a result of the potentiating effect of NFA and A-9-C described above, and it is clear, therefore, that caution must be exercised when using Cl^- channel antagonists alone in the investigation of the role of $I_{Cl(Ca)}$ in smooth muscle.

V. FUNCTION OF CA^{2+}-ACTIVATED CL^- CHANNELS IN THE PULMONARY VASCULATURE

Many studies have suggested that Ca^{2+}-activated Cl^- channels may have an important role in evoking contractile responses in many smooth muscle preparations including pulmonary artery. Moreover $I_{Cl(Ca)}$ may also be important in contributing to the resting membrane potential of pulmonary arterial myocytes. In this section we will discuss the putative functional role of Ca^{2+}-activated Cl^- channels in the pulmonary vasculature.

A. Cl^- Distribution in Vascular Smooth Muscle

Studies of the cellular distribution of Cl^- ions indicate that the intracellular Cl^- concentration ($[Cl^-]_i$) in smooth muscle myocytes is higher than would be predicted by passive distribution (2), in contrast to skeletal muscle, in which Cl^- ions is passively distributed. Cl^- ions are accumulated within vascular smooth muscle cells by three mechanisms: Cl^-/HCO_3 exchange, Na^+ K^+ Cl^- cotransport, and a third mechanism termed pump III (2). In rabbit pulmonary artery smooth muscle cells the Cl^- equilibrium potential (E_{Cl}) was estimated to be around -27 mV (26). Because the resting membrane potential (E_m) of rabbit pulmonary artery smooth muscle cells is around -50 to -60 mV (34), it is clear that the opening of Ca^{2+}-activated Cl^- channels would drive the E_m toward E_{Cl} and thus depolarize the cell. Hence $I_{Cl(Ca)}$ represents a contraction mechanism in smooth muscle, because the depolarization produced by activation of $I_{Cl(Ca)}$ will lead to the opening of voltage-gated Ca^{2+} channels (VGCCs).

B. Role of Ca^{2+}-Activated Cl^- Channels in the Regulation of E_m

It has been shown that under resting conditions the E_m of pulmonary artery myocytes is mainly controlled by K^+ permeability through 4-AP-sensitive

K_v channels (35). However, the E_m of pulmonary artery smooth muscle cells is more positive than the potassium equilibrium potential (E_K), suggesting that another membrane conductance contributes to E_m. E_{Cl} is more positive than E_K, which suggests that the E_m of pulmonary artery myocytes may be set by a balance of a resting K^+ conductance that would tend to hyperpolarize the cell and a resting Cl^- conductance that would have a depolarizing effect.

As described above, Piper and Large (15) have shown that at the E_m of rabbit pulmonary artery smooth muscle cells (~-50 mV) the K_d for Ca^{2+}-binding to single Ca^{2+}-activated Cl^- channels was close to 100 nM. The resting intracellular Ca^{2+} concentration $[Ca^{2+}]_i$ in pulmonary artery myocytes was shown to be around 100 nM (35). Together these findings suggest that in rabbit pulmonary artery myocytes a significant number of Ca^{2+}-activated Cl^- channels may be open at rest. This hypothesis is supported by the observation that replacement of external Cl^- by the more permeant anion thiocyanate (SCN^-) produced a significant outward current at -50 mV in perforated patch recordings from rabbit pulmonary artery myocytes. $I_{Cl(Ca)}$ is likely to contribute to resting conductances in other smooth muscle cell types, because niflumic acid (NFA), a blocker of $I_{Cl(Ca)}$, hyperpolarizes the resting E_m and/or reduces basal tone in guinea pig urethra (36) and opposum lower esophageal sphincter (37).

C. Role of Ca^{2+}-Activated Cl^- Channels in Agonist-Evoked Depolarization and Contraction

Various agonists, including histamine (10), norepinephrine (8,10), phenylephrine, and serotonin (26), that produce mobilization of intracellular Ca^{2+} stores have been shown to activate $I_{Cl(Ca)}$ in pulmonary artery myocytes and/or produce contraction of pulmonary artery rings. Because activation of Ca^{2+}-activated Cl^- channels leads to depolarization in pulmonary artery myocytes, it is likely that it plays animportant role in agonist-evoked depolarization and subsequent contraction.

Yuan (26) showed that NFA inhibited serotonin-evoked membrane depolarization in isolated cells from the rat pulmonary artery. In the same study NFA was shown to inhibit serotonin-mediated contraction of rat pulmonary artery rings, and both NFA and DIDS inhibited phenylephrine-evoked contraction (26). Interestingly it appears that certain agonists such as angiotensin II and ATP induce oscillations in $[Ca^{2+}]_i$ and also oscillatory Ca^{2+}-activated Cl^- currents in rat pulmonary artery myocytes (38). Both NFA and DIDS inhibited these inward Cl^- currents, and NFA also inhibited angiotensin II-induced contraction of pulmonary arterial strips (38).

Together this evidence suggests that the activation of Ca^{2+}-activated Cl^- channels is crucial to agonist-evoked membrane depolarization, which facilitates Ca^{2+} entry through VGCCs and therefore produces smooth muscle contraction.

The central tenet regarding the role of $I_{Cl(Ca)}$ in smooth muscle is that this conductance is a depolarizing mechanism that leads to the opening of VGCCs to produce contraction (1). Indeed, in many tissues the chloride channel blocker NFA reduces the contractile responses by a degree similar to that of the VGCC antagonist nifedipine. However, there is some evidence to suggest that $I_{Cl(Ca)}$ may be involved in producing contractile responses by mechanisms other than simply evoking VGCCs, although the above discussion shows that the latter mechanism is valid in some tissues. Several investigators have observed that the contraction associated with Ca^{2+}-activated chloride-current-mediated depolarization diminished greatly in conditions when the amplitude of the depolarization was reduced. For example, prolonged soaking of the rat anococcygeus muscle in low $[Cl^-]_o$ solution leads to marked reduction in the Cl^--mediated depolarization, which is associated with a reduction in the contractile response to norepinephrine (39; Large, unpublished). In this preparation there are few VGCCs, which prompted the hypothesis that $I_{Cl(Ca)}$ leads to a contractile response by mechanisms not involving VGCCs. Recently, it was pointed out that in airway smooth muscle agonists evoke large $I_{Cl(Ca)}$ responses but that the corresponding contractile responses are not inhibited greatly by VGCC antagonists (40). In this review it was postulated that the efflux of Cl^- ions from the myocyte cytosol produced by activation of $I_{Cl(Ca)}$ increased the release of Ca^{2+} ions from the SR evoked by IP_3 formation in response to agonist stimulation. Therefore the agonist-evoked contractile response is primarily caused by IP_3-induced Ca^{2+} release from the SR, and the amount of Ca^{2+} release is increased by the reduction of $[Cl^-]_i$ produced when $I_{Cl(Ca)}$ is activated (40).

A variation on this theme is that the depolarization produced by $I_{Cl(Ca)}$ increases the formation of IP_3, which leads to a greater release of Ca^{2+} from the SR. In this hypothesis it is the release of Ca^{2+} ions from the SR that is again the primary stimulus for contraction, rather than the influx of Ca^{2+} ions, and $I_{Cl(Ca)}$ increases the release of Ca^{2+} by increasing the amount of IP_3 produced in response to G-protein activation, which has been shown to be increased by depolarization in smooth muscle (41). This latter proposal was put forward from experiments in guinea pig gastric antrum (7), and therefore it seems that there may be different mechanisms by which $I_{Cl(Ca)}$ may lead to contraction. The simplest model involves opening of VGCCs to cause influx of Ca^{2+} ions, whereas the other hypotheses suggest increased release of Ca^{2+} from intracellular stores.

D. Variation in the Contribution of $I_{Cl(Ca)}$ to Agonist-Evoked Responses Within the Pulmonary Arterial Tree

Several studies have suggested that the cellular distribution of K^+ and Cl^- channels might vary in myocytes dispersed from the main branch of the pulmonary artery (conduit myocytes) compared to the smaller branches of the arterial tree (resistance myocytes) (42,43). In whole-cell patch-clamp recordings from rat pulmonary artery myocytes, conduit myocytes were more likely than resistance myocytes to exhibit a Ca^{2+}-activated Cl^- current in response to the flash photolysis of a caged Ca^{2+} compound introduced to the cytoplasm of the cells via the patch pipette (43). In contrast, Smani et al. (42) found that in cells isolated from rabbit pulmonary arteries conduit myocytes responded to an elevation of $[Ca^{2+}]_i$ (either agonist-induced or spontaneously occurring) with a hyperpolarization, suggesting a predominance of Ca^{2+}-activated K^+channels rather than $I_{Cl(Ca)}$. In contrast, in resistance vessel myocytes, agonist-evoked or spontaneous increases in $[Ca^{2+}]_i$led to depolarization, suggesting a higher proportion of Ca^{2+}-activated Cl^- channels than of K^+ channels (42). It is not clear whether these apparent differences in the relative contribution of Ca^{2+}-activated Cl^- and K^+ conductances in the rat and rabbit pulmonary arterial tree represent species differences alone. However, it is evident from these studies that the balance of $I_{Cl(Ca)}$ and K^+ conductances within the pulmonary arterial tree is not homogeneous.

Within the pulmonary vasculature the smaller resistance arteries are important regulators of vascular tone, and indeed it is within the resistance arteries that hypoxic pulmonary vasoconstriction (HPV) occurs. Hypoxia alone has been shown to produce an increase in $[Ca^{2+}]_i$ within resistance myocytes (44) and to produce contraction of small pulmonary arteries (45). It might therefore be expected that the activation of $I_{Cl(Ca)}$ by elevated $[Ca^{2+}]_i$ in response to hypoxia in resistance arteries may be important in the activation and maintenance of HPV.

VI. MOLECULAR BIOLOGY OF CA^{2+}-ACTIVATED CL^- CHANNELS

Recently a family of proteins that act as Ca^{2+}-sensitive Cl^- channels have been cloned and characterized. In this section we will describe the properties of these recombinant proteins and discuss their similarities to and differences from native Ca^{2+}-activated Cl^- channels. For a more detailed discussion, see reviews by Gruber et al. (46), Fuller et al. (47), Jentsch et al. (48), and Nilius and Droogmans (28).

A. The CLCA Family

The first member of the CLCA family to be described (bCLCA1) was isolated and purified from bovine tracheal epithelial cells (see Refs. 47 and 48). The protein formed anion-selective channels with a permeability sequence of I^- (2.1) > NO_3^- (1.7) > Br^- (1.2) > Cl^- (1.0). The single channels had a conductance of around 30 pS, and channel activity was inhibited by DIDS. The single-channel open probability was significantly increased by the elevation of $[Ca^{2+}]_i$, but only at higher than physiological levels (5–10 μM) (47). Addition of calmodulin-dependent protein kinase II (CaMKII) along with ATP and calmodulin increased the Ca^{2+} sensitivity of the channel such that maximum channel activation occurred at $[Ca^{2+}]_i$ between 600 nM and 1 μM, indicating that the channel may be regulated by CaMKII (47). When the cDNA for this putative channel was cloned and expressed in *Xenopus* oocytes, a Cl^- conductance that displayed outward rectification but none of the time dependence associated with native $I_{Cl(Ca)}$ currents (18) was recorded (47,48). Although this Cl^- conductance was blocked by DIDS, it was not affected by a second blocker of $I_{Cl(Ca)}$, niflumic acid. Expression of the cDNA clone in COS-7 cells produced a current with a linear I–V relationship (unlike native $I_{Cl(Ca)}$ currents, which display a characteristic outward rectification), and higher than physiological levels of $[Ca^{2+}]_i$ were required for activation (47).

Since these initial studies were carried out, several related proteins from different mammalian species have been identified and cloned, all with broadly similar properties. These include bCLCA2, also known as lung endothelial cell adhesion molecule 1 (Lu-ECAM-1), which was immunopurified from bovine aortic endothelial cells (46,47). bCLCA2 appears to act as both a Cl^- channel and an adhesion molecule mediating the attachment of metastatic tumor cells to endothelial cells in the lung (46).

Four human isoforms have also been described. RNA for hCLCA1 was detected by Northern blot analysis in crypt and goblet cells in the small intestine (46), and RNA encoding hCLCA2 was detected by Northern blot analysis in the trachea and mammary tissue (46). The more sensitive technique RT-PCR detected hCLCA2 RNA expression in the lung and in a human mammary epithelial cell line (46), suggesting epithelial expression in the mammary gland. Human embryonic kidney 293 (HEK-293) cells transfected with hCLCA1 cDNA displayed whole-cell Ca^{2+}-activated Cl^- currents that showed properties similar to those of bCLCA1, although both DIDS and NFA inhibited hCLCA1 currents. The single-channel slope conductance was 13 pS, but the relative permeability for anions was not determined (46). hCLCA2, like bCLCA2, is thought to play a role in cell adhesion, because the transection of hCLCA2 into a human breast carcinoma cell line reduced its tumorogenicity (46). hCLCA3 appears to be a truncated form of CLCA protein that was secreted into the culture supernatant when its cDNA was expressed in HEK-293 cells or Chinese hamster ovary (CHO) cells (46). hCLCA4 was found to be widely expressed in many tissues. RNA dot blot analysis showed hCLCA4 expression throughout the digestive tract, particularly in the colon. Expression was also detected in the trachea, bladder, mammary gland, uterus, prostate, and testis as well as in most brain regions and the spinal cord but not in the cerebellum (47).

Four murine CLCA homologs have been identified. mCLCA1 was cloned from a mouse lung cDNA library, and Northern blot analysis revealed RNA expression in the spleen, kidney, lung, liver, and brain (46). When expressed in HEK-293 cells, mCLCA1 channel currents were very similar to bCLCA1 currents. With a $[Ca^{2+}]_i$ of 2 mM, a Cl^- current was recorded that was sensitive to inhibition by DIDS and NFA (46). Again, relative anion permeability was not determined. mCLCA2 expression, as determined by Northern blot analysis, was detected in the mammary gland, and mCLCA3 RNA was found in the small intestine, colon, stomach, uterus, and trachea (46). No further electrophysiological characterization of mCLCA2 or -3 was carried out. The most recent mCLCA isoform to be described, mCLCA4, appears to be exclusively expressed in smooth-muscle-rich tissues (49) as determined by RT-PCR. When the cDNA encoding mCLCA4 was transiently expressed in HEK-293 cells, a Cl^- current activated by the Ca^{2+} ionophore ionomycin was recorded (Fig. 4A). The current had a linear *I–V* relationship and, like bCLCA1 currents, displayed none of the time dependence associated with native $I_{Cl(Ca)}$ currents (49). Antagonist selectivity and the relative anion permeability were not determined.

A single porcine CLCA (pCLCA1) with similarities to hCLCA1 was cloned (46,47), and RT-PCR analysis detected pCLCA1 RNA in ileum, salivary glands, and tracheal epithelium.

The CLCA family of proteins appears to consist of precursors around 125 kDa in size that are then cleaved to form heterodimers around 90 and 35 kDa. Although detailed glycosylation site mapping has not been carried out for many CLCA isoforms, it seems that the channel proteins consist of four or five transmembrane domains (28,46–48).

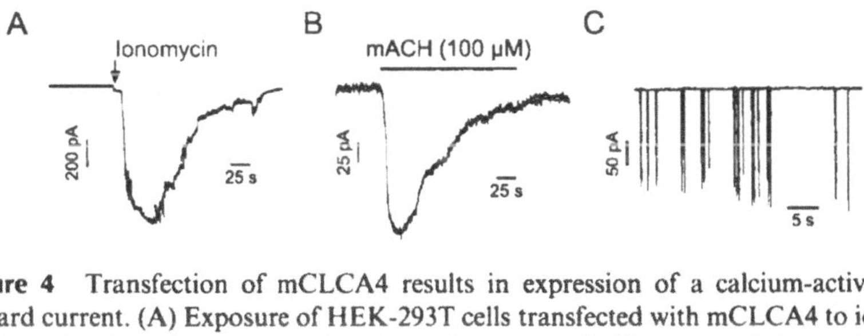

Figure 4 Transfection of mCLCA4 results in expression of a calcium-activated inward current. (A) Exposure of HEK-293T cells transfected with mCLCA4 to ionomycin (10 μM) activates a transient inward current. (B) Exposure of these cells to methacholine (mACH) evoked a similar transient current with faster activation kinetics, consistent with a release of intracellular calcium stores. (C) In some mCLCA4-transfected cells spontaneous transient inward currents were observed. These spontaneous transient inward currents were not observed in all cells but were never observed in nontransfected cells. (From Ref. 49.)

B. Relationship Between CLCA Channels and Native Ca^{2+}-Activated Cl^- Channels

It is by no means clear whether the CLCA channel proteins described above represent the channels underlying Ca^{2+}-activated Cl^- currents in pulmonary vascular smooth muscle. Although there are some similarities, there are also some major differences in the properties of CLCA proteins and $I_{Cl(Ca)}$. The unitary conductance of single Ca^{2+}-activated Cl^- channels recorded in smooth muscle tissues was estimated at between 2 and 4 pS (12–15), whereas the single-channel conductance of bCLCA1 and hCLCA1 was 30 and 13 pS, respectively (48). The Ca^{2+} sensitivity of CLCA channels and that of native Ca^{2+}-activated Cl^- channels are markedly different. We have shown that the K_D for Ca^{2+} binding to single Ca^{2+}-activated Cl^- channels in pulmonary artery myocytes was around 100 nM at −50 mV (15). In murine portal vein myocytes a $[Ca^{2+}]_i$ of 500 nM was sufficient to activate Ca^{2+}-activated Cl^- channels, although in the same study 2 mM $[Ca^{2+}]_i$ was needed to evoke Cl^- currents in HEK cells stably expressing mCLCA1 (50). The permeability sequence of anions through both CLCA channels and native Ca^{2+}-activated Cl^- channels is very similar, although the relative permeabilities are different. For example, the permeability sequence for anions permeating bCLCA 1 is I^- (2.1) > NO_3^- (1.7) > Br^- (1.2) > Cl^- (1.0) (48), whereas for $I_{Cl(Ca)}$ in the rabbit ear artery it was SCN^- (8.3) > I^- (4.7) > NO_3^- (3.1) > Br^- (2.0) > Cl^- (1.0) (1).

One mCLCA isoform (mCLCA4) is expressed exclusively in smooth-muscle-rich tissues (49), and when this CLCA was transfected into HEK-293 cells the whole-cell currents in response to the Ca^{2+} ionophore ionomycin and also the muscarinic agonist methacholine were very similar to those recorded in smooth muscle cells (Figs. 4A and 4B). In some transfected cells, spontaneous Ca^{2+}-activated Cl^- currents very similar to the spontaneous currents recorded in various smooth muscle subtypes were also recorded (49) (Fig. 4C), suggesting that mCLCA4 has a Ca^{2+} sensitivity similar to that of native Ca^{2+}-activated Cl^- channels. Britton et al. (50) showed that mCLCA1 is expressed in mouse portal vein myocytes. However, transfection of HEK-293 cells with the cDNA encoding mCLCA1 yielded currents with a lower Ca^{2+} sensitivity and different channel kinetics than native currents. These authors concluded that mCLCA alone is not responsible for the $I_{Cl(Ca)}$ recorded in mouse portal vein smooth muscle cells (50). Interestingly, the same group showed that when mCLCA1 was coexpressed with the regulatory β subunit of the BK_{Ca} potassium channel (KCNMB1) in HEK-293 cells, the Ca^{2+} sensitivity of the Cl^- channel was enhanced and time-dependent currents characteristic of native $I_{Cl(Ca)}$ were recorded (Fig. 5) (see Ref. 51).

Whether the expression of members of the CLCA family gives rise to native Ca^{2+}-activated Cl^- currents is far from clear. It is possible that there

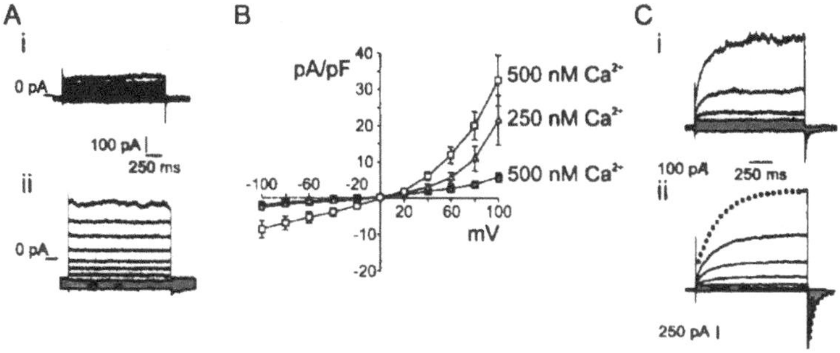

Figure 5 Ca^{2+}-activated currents in HEK cells expressing mCLCA1. (A) (i) and (ii) show an ensemble of currents evoked by 500 nM Ca^{2+} in HEK cells expressing mCLCA1 alone (i) or coexpressing KCNMB1 (ii). (B) The mean late current evoked by 500 nM Ca^{2+} in HEK cells expressed mCLCA1 alone (solid symbols, $n=12$) or mCLCA1 + KCNMB1 (open squares, $n=17$). Currents elicited by 250 nM Ca^{2+} in HEK cells expressing both genes are shown by open triangles ($n=9$). Late current was recorded at the end of the test step immediately prior to repolarization to the holding potential of −50 mV. (C) A comparison of the kinetics of $I_{Cl(Ca)}$ from one of five of the HEK cells expressing mCLCA1 and KCNMB1 that displayed time dependence to the activation and deactivation (i) with native $I_{Cl(Ca)}$ recorded from murine portal vein myocytes (ii). Currents were generated by pipette solutions containing 500 nM Ca^{2+}, and currents were recorded at test potentials between −100 and +120 mV from a holding potential of −50 mV. Currents with outward relaxations at potentials positive of +60 mV were observed in five of 17 cells expressing mCLCA1 + KCNMB1. (From Ref. 51.)

are distinct classes of Ca^{2+}-activated Cl^- channel proteins that have not yet been identified, because it has been shown that Ca^{2+}-activated Cl^- currents that have properties similar to those of native $I_{Cl(Ca)}$ can be recorded in Ehlich ascites tumor cells even though mRNA for mCLCA1–3 could not be detected in these cells (52). However, because mCLCA4 had not been identified at this time the possibility that this isoform gave rise to the Ca^{2+}-activated Cl^- currents in these cells cannot be ruled out. It appears that even if CLCA proteins are responsible for $I_{Cl(Ca)}$ recorded in smooth muscle cells there must be some additional modulation, perhaps by an accessory subunit that has not yet been identified.

VII. CONCLUSIONS

It is clear that Ca^{2+}-activated Cl^- channels have an important role to play in pulmonary arterial myocytes. They are involved, along with K^+ channels, in the regulation of cell membrane potential. Activation of Ca^{2+}-activated Cl^- channels by Ca^{2+} release from intracellular stores appears to be an important mediator of agonist-evoked depolarization and contraction. The activation of $I_{Cl(Ca)}$ by raised $[Ca^{2+}]_i$ in response to hypoxia may be significant in the development of HPV. Studies of single native Ca^{2+}-activated Cl^- channels have recently expanded our knowledge of this conductance at the level of single channels to whole tissue. However, at present there is no clear indication of the molecular identity of $I_{Cl(Ca)}$.

REFERENCES

1. Large WA, Wang Q. Characteristics and physiological role of the Ca^{2+}-activated Cl conductance in smooth muscle. Am J Physiol 1996; 271:C435–C454.
2. Chipperfield AR, Harper AA. Chloride in smooth muscle. Prog Biophys Mol Biol 2000; 74:175–221.
3. Greenwood IA, Large WA. Properties and role of chloride channels in smooth muscle. In: Kozlowski KZ, ed. Chloride Channels. Oxford: Isis Medical Media, 1999:121–135.
4. Van Helden DF. Spontaneous and noradrenaline-induced transient depolarizations in the smooth muscle of guinea-pig mesenteric vein. J Physiol 1991; 437:511–541.
5. Hashitani H, Van Helden DF, Suzuki H. Properties of spontaneous depolarizations in circular smooth muscle cells of rabbit urethra. Br J Pharmacol 1996; 118:1627–1632.
6. Sergeant GP, Hollywood MA, McCloskey KD, Thornbury KD, McHale NG. Specialised pacemaking cells in the rabbit urethra. J Physiol 2000; 526:359–366.
7. Hirst GDS, Bramich NJ, Teramoto N, Suzuki H, Edwards FR. Regenerative component of slow waves in the guinea-pig gastric antrum involves a delayed increase in $[Ca^{2+}]_i$ and Cl^- channels. J Physiol 2002; 540:907–920.
8. Wang Q, Wang Y-X, Yu M, Kotlikoff M. Ca^{2+}-activated Cl^- currents are activated by metabolic inhibition in rat pulmonary artery smooth muscle cells. Am J Physiol 1997; 273:C520–C530.
9. Suzuki H. An electrophysiological study of excitatory neuromuscular transmission in the guinea-pig main pulmonary artery. J Physiol 1983; 336:47–59.
10. Wang Q, Large WA. Action of histamine on single smooth muscle cells dispersed from the rabbit pulmonary artery. J Physiol 1993; 468:125–139.
11. Large WA, Greenwood IA, Piper AS. Recent advances on the properties and role of Ca^{2+}-activated chloride currents in smooth muscle. In: Fuller C, ed. Topics in Membranes Vol 53. New York: Elsevier Science, 2002:95–114.
12. Klöckner U. Intracellular calcium ions activate a low-conductancechloride channel in smooth-muscle cells isolated from human mesenteric artery. Pflügers Arch 1993; 424:231–237.
13. Hirakawa Y, Gericke M, Cohen RA, Bolotina VM. Ca^{2+}-dependent Cl^- channels in mouse and rabbit aortic smooth muscle cells: regulation by intracellular Ca^{2+} and NO. Am J Physiol 1999; 277:H1732–H1744.
14. Van Renterghem C, Lazdunski M. Endothelin and vasopressinactivate low conductance chloride channels in aortic smooth muscle cells. Pflügers Arch 1993; 425:156–163.

15. Piper AS, Large WA. Multiple conductance states of single Ca^{2+}-activated Cl^- channels in rabbit pulmonary artery smooth muscle cells. J Physiol 2003; 547:181–196.
16. Singer HA, Abraham ST, Schworer CM. Calcium/calmodulin-dependent protein kinase II. In: Bárány M, ed. Biochemistry of Smooth Muscle Contraction. Toronto: Academic Press, 1996:143–153.
17. Wang YX, Kotlikoff MI. Inactivation of calcium-activated chloride channels in smooth muscle by calcium/calmodulin-dependent protein kinase. Proc Natl Acad Sci USA 1997; 94:14918–14923.
18. Greenwood IA, Ledoux J, Leblanc N. Differential regulation of Ca^{2+}-activated Cl^- currents in rabbit arterial and portal vein smooth muscle cells by Ca^{2+}/calmodulin-dependent kinase. J Physiol 2001; 534:395–408.
19. Waypa GB, Chandel NS, Schumaker PT. Model for hypoxic pulmonary vasoconstriction involving mitochondrial oxygen sensing. Circ Res 2001; 88: 1259–1266.
20. Greenwood IA, Leblanc N, Gordienko DV, Large WA. Modulation of $I_{Cl(Ca)}$ in vascular smooth muscle cells by oxidising and cysteine-reactive agents. Pflügers Arch 2002; 443:473–482.
21. Waniishi Y, Inoue R, Morita H, Teramoto N, Abe K, Ito Y. Cyclic GMP-dependent but G-kinase-independent inhibition of Ca^{2+}-dependent Cl^- currents by NO donors in cat tracheal smooth muscle. J Physiol 1998; 511: 719–731.
22. Cotton KD, Hollywood MA, McHale NG, Thornbury KD. Ca^{2+} current and Ca^{2+}-activated chloride current in isolated smooth muscle cells of the sheep urethra. J Physiol 1997; 505:121–131.
23. Wayman CP, MacFadzean I, Gibson A, Tucker JF. Two distinct membrane currents activated by cyclopiazonic acid-induced store depletion in single smooth muscle cells of mouse anococcygeus. Br J Pharmacol 1996; 117:566–572.
24. Toland HM, McCloskey KD, Thornbury KD, McHale NG, Hollywood MA. Ca^{2+}-activated Cl^- current in sheep lymphatic smooth muscle. Am J Physiol Cell Physiol 2000; 279:C1327–C1335.
25. Hogg RC, Wang Q, Large WA. Effects of Cl channel blockers on Ca-activated chloride and potassium currents in smooth muscle cells from rabbit portal vein. Br J Pharmacol 1994; 111:1333–1341.
26. Yuan X-J. Role of calcium-activated chloride current in regulating pulmonary vasomotor tone. Am J Physiol 1997; 272:L959–L968.
27. Kirkup AJ, Edwards G, Weston AH. Investigation of the effects of 5-nitro-2-(3-phenylpropylamino)-benzoicacid (NPPB) on membrane currents in rat portal vein. Br J Pharmacol 1996; 117:175–183.
28. Nilius B, Droogmans G. Amazing chloride channels: an overview. Acta Physiol Scand 2003; 177:119–147.
29. Dick GM, Kong ID, Sanders KM. Effects of anion channel antagonists in canine colonic myocytes: comparative pharmacology of Cl^-, Ca^{2+} and K^+ currents. Br J Pharmacol 1999; 127:1819–1831.
30. Furukawa T, Virag L, Sawanobori T, Hiraoka M. Stilbene disulfonates block ATP-sensitive K^+ channels in guinea pig ventricular myocytes. J Membr Biol 1993; 136:289–302.

31. Ottolia M, Toro L. Potentiation of large conductance K_{Ca} channels by niflumic, flufenamic and mefenamic acids. Biophys J 1994; 67:2272–2279.
32. Piper AS, Greenwood IA, Large WA. Dual effect of blocking agents on Ca^{2+}-activated Cl^- currents in rabbit pulmonary artery smooth muscle cells. J Physiol 2002; 539:119–131.
33. Piper AS, Greenwood IA. Anomalous effect of anthracene-9-carboxylic acid on calcium-activated chloride currents in rabbit pulmonary artery smooth muscle cells. Br J Pharmacol 2003; 138:31–38.
34. Casteels R, Kitamura DV, Kuriyama H, Suzuki H. The membrane properties of the smooth muscle cells of the rabbit main pulmonary artery. J Physiol 1977; 271:41–61.
35. Yuan X-J. Voltage-gated K^+ currents regulate resting membrane potential and $[Ca^{2+}]_i$ in pulmonary arterial myocytes. Circ Res 1995; 77:370–378.
36. Hashitani H, Edwards FR. Spontaneous and neurally activated depolarizations in smooth muscle cells of the guinea-pig urethra. J Physiol 1999; 514:459–470.
37. Zhang Y, Miller DV, Paterson WG. Opposing roles of K^+ and Cl^- channels in maintenance of opossum lower esophageal sphincter tone. Am J Physiol Gastroint Liver Physiol 2000; 279:G1226–G1234.
38. Guibert C, Marthan R, Savineau JP. Oscillatory Cl^- current induced by angiotensin II in rat pulmonary arterial myocytes: Ca^{2+} dependence and physiological implication. Cell Calcium 1997; 21:421–429.
39. Bramich NJ, Hirst GD. Sympathetic neuroeffector transmission in the rat anococcygeus muscle. J Physiol 1999; 516:101–115.
40. Janssen LJ. Ionic mechanisms and Ca^{2+} regulation in airway smooth muscle contraction: do the data contradict dogma? Am J Physiol Lung Cell Mol Physiol 2002; 282:L1161–L1178.
41. Itoh T, Kajikuri K, Kuriyama H. Characteristic features of noradrenaline-induced Ca^{2+} mobilization and tension in arterial smooth muscle of the rabbit. J Physiol 1992; 457:297–314.
42. Smani T, Iwabuchi S, López-Barneo J, Ureña U. Differential segmental activation of Ca^{2+}-dependent Cl and K^+ channels in pulmonary arterial myocytes. Cell Calcium 2001; 29:369–377.
43. Clapp LH, Turner JL, Kowlowski RZ. Ca^{2+}-activated Cl^- currents in pulmonary arterial myocytes. Am J Physiol 1996; 270:H1577–H1584.
44. Ureña U, Franco-Obregon A, López-Barneo J. Contrasting effects of hypoxia on cytosolic Ca^{2+} spikes in conduit and resistance myocytes of the rabbit pulmonary artery. J Physiol 1996; 496:103–109.
45. Vadula MS, Kleinman JG, Madden JA. Effect of hypoxia and norepinephrine on cytoplasmic free Ca^{2+} in pulmonary andcerebral arterial myocytes. Am J Physiol 1993; 265:L591–L597.
46. Gruber AD, Fuller CM, Elble RC, Benos DJ, Pauli BU. The CLCA gene family: a novel family of putative chloride channels. Curr Genet 2000; 1: 201–222.
47. Fuller CM, Ji HL, Tousson A, Elble RC, Pauli BU, Benos DJ. Ca^{2+}-activated Cl^- channels: a newly emerging anion transport family. Pflügers Arch 2001; 443:S107–S110.

48. Jentsch TJ, Stein V, Weinreich F, Zdebik AA. Molecular structure and physiological function of chloride channels. Physiol Rev 2002; 82:503–568.
49. Elble RC, Ji G, Nehrke K, DeBasio J, Kingsley PD, Kotlikoff MI, Pauli BU. Molecular and functional characterization of a murine calcium-activated chloride channel expressed in smooth muscle. J Biol Chem 2002; 277:18586–18591.
50. Britton FC, Ohya S, Horowitz B, Greenwood IA. Comparison of the properties of CLCA1 generated currents and $I_{Cl(Ca)}$ in murine portal vein smooth muscle cells. J Physiol 2002; 539:107–117.
51. Greenwood IA, Miller LJ, Ohya S, Horowitz B. The large conductance potassium channel β-subunit can interact with and modulate the properties of a calcium-activated chloride channel, CLCA1. J Biol Chem 2002; 277: 22119–22122.
52. Papassotiriou J, Eggermont J, Droogmans G, Nilius B. Ca^{2+}-activated Cl^- channels in Ehrlich ascites tumor cells are distinct from mCLCA1, 2 and 3. Pflügers Arch 2001; 442:273–279.

16

Volume-Sensitive Cl^- Channels in Pulmonary Vascular Smooth Muscle and Endothelial Cells

Amy Sanguinetti and Normand Leblanc
University of Nevada School of Medicine, Reno, Nevada, U.S.A.
Iain A. Greenwood
St. George's Hospital Medical School, London, U.K.

I. INTRODUCTION

This chapter focuses on recent advancements in our understanding about the cellular and molecular properties as well as postulated function of a subset of chloride channels found in both endothelial and smooth muscle cells of the pulmonary vasculature that are sensitive to changes in osmolarity. The major aims of this review are to highlight the characteristics of these Cl^- currents and to discuss putative genes that are thought to encode the underlying channel protein. We denote this current as the swelling-activated Cl^- current or $I_{Cl(Swell)}$. However, it should be noted that various other nomenclatures are used to describe this conductance based on their ability to be activated by cell volume changes (e.g., volume-regulated anion channel, volume-regulated anion current) or their permeability to various organic anions [volume-sensitive organic osmolyte anion channel (VSOAC)]. For the sake of clarity the main focus will be on $I_{Cl(Swell)}$ in smooth muscle cells followed by a separate section on $I_{Cl(Swell)}$ in pulmonary endothelial cells.

II. CHLORIDE CURRENTS IN SMOOTH MUSCLE CELLS

Smooth muscle cells actively accumulate Cl^- ions through the Na, K, 2Cl cotransporter, Cl:HCO_3 exchanger and a mechanism termed "pump III" (1). Consequently, the opening of Cl^- channels leads to a net loss of Cl^- ions and subsequent membrane depolarization. To date, two distinct classes of Cl^- currents have been identified in smooth muscle cells. $I_{Cl(Swell)}$ is evoked as a consequence of cell swelling, whereas the other (termed I_{ClCa}; see Chapter 15) is activated by an increase in the intracellular concentration of Ca^{2+}. In comparison to the numerous studies of I_{ClCa} in smooth muscle cells (see Refs. 2 and 3 and Chapter 15 of this volume), there have been very few investigations of $I_{Cl(Swell)}$ although this conductance has been studied extensively in other cell types such as cardiac myocytes, endothelial cells, lymphocytes and carcinoma cells. To date, $I_{Cl(Swell)}$ has been recorded electrophysiologically only in smooth muscle cells isolated from guinea pig gastric antrum (4), canine pulmonary and renal arteries (5), canine colon (6), and rabbit portal vein (7). In addition, the chloride-sensitive dye 6-methoxy-*N*-ethylquinolinium revealed volume-sensitive chloride activity in human coronary artery myocytes (8). Furthermore, a stretch-sensitive Cl^- current was reported in a minority (5%) of corpus cavernosum cells (9).

III. BIOPHYSICAL CHARACTERISTICS OF $I_{Cl(Swell)}$

Both $I_{Cl(Swell)}$ and I_{ClCa} are present in freshly dispersed pulmonary artery myocytes (5,10–13). As Fig. 1 shows, both currents can be evoked contemporaneously, and therefore various criteria have to be used to isolate these separate conductances effectively. Each conductance has distinctive biophysical and pharmacological properties, and these will be highlighted in the following sections.

A. Ca^{2+} Dependence

Various methods can be used to evoke I_{ClCa} either by promoting Ca^{2+} influx, eliciting Ca^{2+} release from intracellular stores, or enriching internal recording solutions with different levels of free Ca^{2+}. Regardless of the method of activation there is an obligatory requirement for an increase in intracellular $[Ca^{2+}]$ with a whole-cell threshold of about 200 nM at –50 mV (14–16). In comparison, generation of $I_{Cl(Swell)}$ has no dependency on a rise in intracellular Ca^{2+} concentration ($[Ca^{2+}]_i$) although cell swelling evokes a transient rise in $[Ca^{2+}]_i$ in most cell types (see, e.g., Ref. 17). $I_{Cl(Swell)}$ of similar magnitude has been recorded using the perforated patch configuration, where the intracellular milieu remains relatively undisturbed and $[Ca^{2+}]_i$ is free to rise (7), and also in conventional whole-cell mode with internal solutions containing high concentrations of a Ca^{2+} chelator such as EGTA or BAPTA (e.g., Refs. 4 and 5).

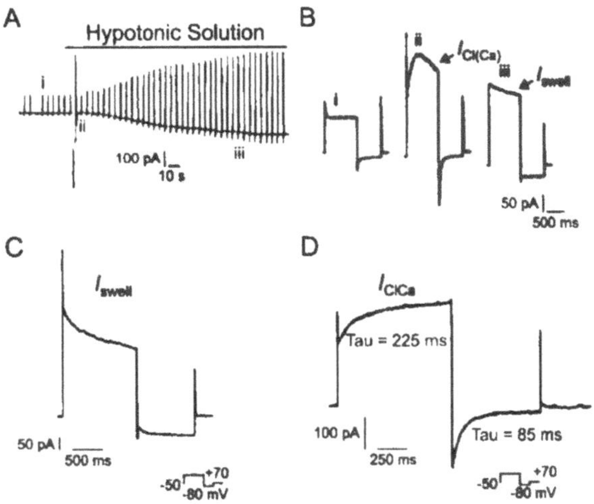

Figure 1 Comparison of swelling-activated and Ca^{2+}-activated Cl^- currents in vascular myocytes. Panel A shows the effect of replacing the isotonic extracellular solution with a hypotonic one on a smooth muscle cell held at –50 mV. Large deflections represent voltage steps from –50 mV to +90 mV followed by repolarization to –100 mV. Panel B shows currents evoked by the voltage protocol described in (A) at different time points. Numerals refer to time points in panel A. Panels C and D show the voltage-dependent kinetics of $I_{Cl(Swell)}$ and I_{ClCa} evoked by sustained stimuli in different cells. In (C) the current is recorded after the response to hypotonic extracellular solution has stabilized. In (D) the Cl current is evoked persistently by a pipette solution containing 500 nM free Ca^{2+}. The voltage protocol in each experiment is shown below the current trace.

B. Permeation and Selectivity

The ion channels underlying $I_{Cl(Swell)}$ and I_{ClCa} have a negligible permeability to cations but are affected by changes in the chloride gradient (4,5), showing that the channels are anion-selective. Although there are a number of different types of anion channel currents, each underlying channel has a distinctive anion permeability profile (18). The selectivity sequences of $I_{Cl(Swell)}$ and I_{ClCa} in smooth muscle cells conform to a lyotropic sequence of SCN > I∼ NO_3 > Br > Cl≫gluconate/isethionate (2,4,5,7,19), where ion passage is governed more by the free energy for ion hydration than by ion binding in the channel pore. However, a more illuminating and diagnostic feature of anion channels are the permeabilities of different anions relative to chloride. This gives precise information about the selectivity filter of the channel pore, and in this respect there is a marked difference in the relative permeability of more permeable anions between the two channel types. In canine pulmonary artery myocytes, SCN^- and I^- were respectively

1.36-fold and 1.18-fold more permeable than Cl^- through swelling-activated chloride channels (5). These data are similar to values for $I_{Cl(Swell)}$ determined in other cell types. In comparison, these same anions are approximately eightfold and fourfold more permeable, respectively, through chloride channels activated by a rise in Ca^{2+} regardless of the mechanism used to increase $[Ca^{2+}]_i$ (2,12,19). Consequently, observation of the magnitude of the changes in reversal potential produced by changes in the respective anions can be used to discriminate between these two types of Cl^- current recorded from the same cell type.

C. Voltage-Dependent Kinetics

Chloride ion currents evoked by cell swelling exhibit an outwardly rectifying instantaneous current–voltage relationship in symmetrical Cl^- solutions (5). Voltage steps to moderate positive potentials (0 to +40 mV) from a negative holding potential (e.g., –50 mV) produce a current that, in general, exhibits no time-dependent kinetics (4,6). However, voltage steps to more positive potentials yield an outward current that declines slowly during the test pulse (4,6) (Fig. 1). This decay can be fitted by a single exponential with a time constant of about 250 ms at +100 mV (6) and is consistent with the gradual inactivation of $I_{Cl(Swell)}$ described fully in other cell types (20). The mechanism of inactivation of $I_{Cl(Swell)}$ is not completely understood but is sensitive to external pH, divalent cations, and the nature of the permeating anion (20). Repolarization to negative potentials frequently results in the observation of an inward relaxation as the channels recover from inactivation. Such voltage-dependent kinetics are in stark contrast to those exhibited by I_{ClCa} in the same cell type (Fig. 1). Depolarizing voltage steps applied to record sustained I_{ClCa} evoked by pipette solutions containing free Ca^{2+} ions generate an outward current that develops progressively for the duration of the test pulse (see Ref. 11, Chapter 15, and Fig. 1). Repolarization to negative potentials generates an inward current that declines exponentially. The decay of this inward current, like that of transient I_{ClCa} evoked either as a consequence of Ca^{2+} influx through voltage-dependent Ca^{2+} channels or following the spontaneous release of Ca^{2+} from the sarcoplasmic reticulum, is quicker at more negative voltages (11,12,21,22). The kinetics observed at positive voltages are considered to reflect a voltage-dependent increase in the binding affinity for Ca^{2+} and a slowing of the rate of channel closure at positive potentials (23). As a consequence of the time- and voltage-dependent kinetics, I_{ClCa} is outwardly rectifying, although the current–voltage relationship of the fully activated channel is approximately linear. Although there is a marked difference in the voltage-dependent properties of $I_{Cl(Swell)}$ and I_{ClCa}, the kinetics of both currents are modified by the nature of the external anion. In canine colonic myocytes, the decay of $I_{Cl(Swell)}$ at positive potentials was slowed by replacement of the external anion by the more permeable anion I^- (6). These observations are in line with other observations in endothelial cells (20). Anions that are more permeable than Cl^- also slow the decay of I_{ClCa} in portal vein and pulmonary myocytes regardless of the mechanism used to stimulate the channel (11,12,19).

D. Single-Channel Conductance

A number of studies have investigated the single-channel properties of I_{ClCa} in smooth muscle cells (discussed in Chapter 15). Suffice it to say the unitary conductance ranges between 1 and 3 pS, and in pulmonary artery myocytes there is evidence that the channel exhibits a number of subconductance states dictated by the $[Ca^{2+}]$ in the vicinity of the channel. No studies on the single-channel properties of $I_{Cl(Swell)}$ in smooth muscle cells have been undertaken. However, the unitary properties of the channels underlying $I_{Cl(Swell)}$ have been investigated in various other cell types (18,24) and can be separated into three categories: small, intermediate, and large conductance channels. Stationary noise analysis of macroscopic currents revealed a unitary conductance of 1.1 pS in human vascular endothelial cells and some nonexcitable cells (18). A similar low-conductance channel was recorded in excised patch channel studies at hyperpolarized potentials, but in the same experiments larger conductance values (50–90 pS) were recorded at positive potentials (18,24). These observations showed that the outward rectification of the whole-cell current–voltage relationship is an intrinsic property of the swelling-activated channel pore. Cl^- channels activated by hypotonic media with a conductance in the range of ~200–400 pS have been described in neonatal rat cardiac myocytes (25) and renal collecting duct cells (26). There is clearly a wide range of unitary Cl^- conductances that might account for $I_{Cl(Swell)}$ in smooth muscle cells, and more studies need to be undertaken to confirm the unitary properties of the underlying channels.

E. Pharmacology of $I_{Cl(Swell)}$

A recent review highlighted the range of agents that block $I_{Cl(Swell)}$ in endothelial cells (18). These include conventional anion transport blockers such as DIDS and niflumic acid, antiestrogens such as tamoxifen and chlomiphen, antimalarial agents, and ATP at millimolar concentrations. To date no selective blocker of $I_{Cl(Swell)}$ exists, although the indanone DCPIB exhibits some specificity (18). $I_{Cl(Swell)}$ in smooth muscle cells is blocked by DIDS (4–7,27), external ATP (4–6), niflumic acid (4,6,7), and tamoxifen (6,7,27). Large and Piper (Chapter 15, this volume) and Large and Wang (2) showed that a number of compounds that block $I_{Cl(Swell)}$ also inhibit I_{ClCa}; however, there are marked differences in the pharmacological profiles of these conductances. DIDS blocks $I_{Cl(Swell)}$ in gastrointestinal and vascular myocytes at concentrations considerably lower than those required to block I_{ClCa}

(4–7,27), Moreover, in portal vein and colonic myocytes the inhibitory effect of DIDS against $I_{Cl(Swell)}$ was voltage-dependent (7,27), with the IC_{50} decreasing from 21 μM at +100 mV to 5 μM at −50 mV (7). In comparison, the block of I_{ClCa} in smooth muscle cells by DIDS is voltage-independent (2). Conversely, niflumic acid is a more potent blocker of I_{ClCa} (2) in smooth muscle cells than of $I_{Cl(Swell)}$ in portal vein and colonic myocytes (7,27), although its efficacy is reliant upon the method used to activate I_{ClCa} (12; see also Chapter 15). Furthermore, the effect of this agent on I_{ClCa} is more potent at positive voltages than at negative ones (2,12). Anthracene-9-carboxylic acid is also a highly voltage-dependent blocker of I_{ClCa} (2,16) that is largely ineffective against $I_{Cl(Swell)}$ (27). Consequently, although no selective blocker for either conductance in smooth muscle cells exists, there are a number of pharmacological differences that allow the two conductances to be separated.

IV. MODULATION OF $I_{Cl(Swell)}$ IN SMOOTH MUSCLE CELLS

A number of studies in cell types other than smooth muscle cells have looked at a wide range of putative modulators and pathways involved with channel activation (see Ref. 18 for a review). In comparison, the relative paucity of research on $I_{Cl(Swell)}$ in smooth muscle means that information on the regulation of this conductance in this cell type is scarce. However, there is evidence that the modulation of $I_{Cl(Swell)}$ in smooth muscle cells is very much tissue-specific, although the elicited currents have a similar appearance, pharmacological sensitivity, and pore properties. In canine colonic and pulmonary myocytes, stimulation of protein kinase C (PKC) by phorbol esters inhibits $I_{Cl(Swell)}$ (6,13) (Fig. 2). Conversely, inhibition of PKC by chelerythrine or calphostin C generated currents with properties similar to $I_{Cl(Swell)}$ under isotonic conditions. These data were similar to those from studies on rabbit and guinea pig cardiomyocytes (28) and led to the proposal of a putative scheme for activation of $I_{Cl(Swell)}$ by the cell-swelling-induced dephosphorylation of the target channel (28) (see Sec. VI). Interestingly, in pulmonary artery myocytes concentrations of bisindolylmaleimide (BIM) that are selective for conventional PKC isoforms did not evoke $I_{Cl(Swell)}$ (13), but attenuation of εPKC translocation enhanced $I_{Cl(Swell)}$ under isotonic conditions (13). These data led to the proposal that membrane-bound novel PKC isoforms regulate $I_{Cl(Swell)}$ in pulmonary artery myocytes. In comparison, stimulation of PKC in portal vein myocytes by phorbol esters or stimulation of α_1-adrenoceptors enhanced chloride currents evoked by hypoosmotic solutions (see Fig. 3) but did not affect basal currents under isotonic conditions (29). In this cell type the PKC inhibitors chelerythrine and calphostin C attenuated $I_{Cl(Swell)}$ in a concentration-dependent manner (29). Similar effects have been observed in canine atrial cells (30). These data suggest that in terms of their sensitivity

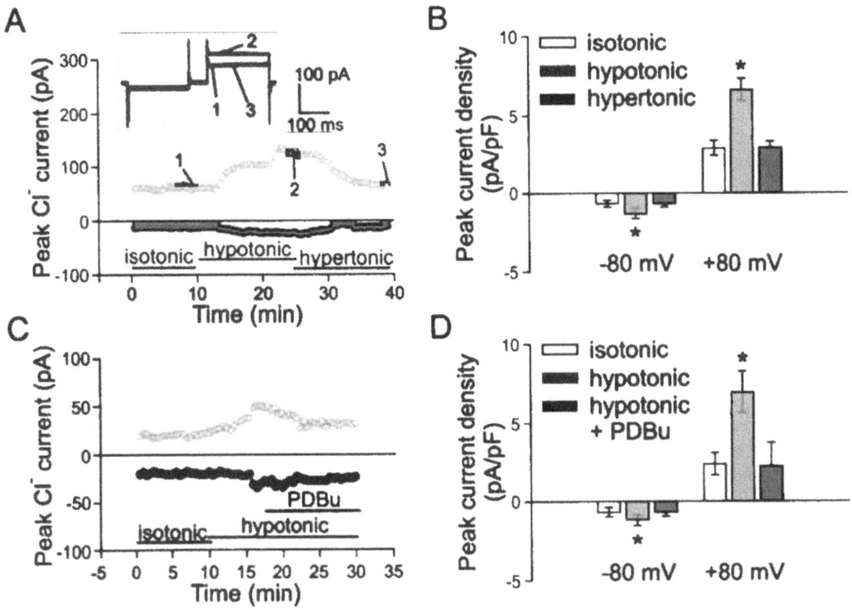

Figure 2 Effect of phorbol esters on $I_{Cl(Swell)}$ in pulmonary artery myocytes. (A) Representation of the inhibitory effect of phorbol-12, 13-dibutyrate (PDBu) on $I_{Cl(Swell)}$ in pulmonary artery myocytes. Open symbols are the current at +80 mV, and filled symbols are the current at −80 mV. (B) Mean data from five such experiments showing that the PDBu-induced inhibition of $I_{Cl(Swell)}$ was not voltage-dependent. (*) Current amplitudes significantly different from values obtained under isotonic conditions. (Reproduced from Ref. 13 with permission from the American Physiological Society.)

to PKC, two distinct populations of $I_{Cl(Swell)}$ exist in vascular smooth muscle cells. An interesting corollary to the modulation of $I_{Cl(Swell)}$ by protein kinases is that in rabbit portal vein myocytes stimulation of protein kinase A by 8-Br-cAMP or stimulation of β-adrenoceptors inhibited $I_{Cl(Swell)}$ but stimulation of protein kinase G augmented $I_{Cl(Swell)}$ (29,31). These data revealed that in portal vein myocytes the channel complex underlying $I_{Cl(Swell)}$ is regulated by a complicated interplay of kinases probably held in place by anchoring proteins and scaffold elements. Until the molecular identity of $I_{Cl(Swell)}$ is determined unequivocally, the precise role of each kinase can only be estimated.

V. $I_{Cl(Swell)}$ IN ENDOTHELIAL CELLS

Swelling-induced chloride currents have been studied in a number of endothelial cell lines, and in all cases the biophysical properties have been

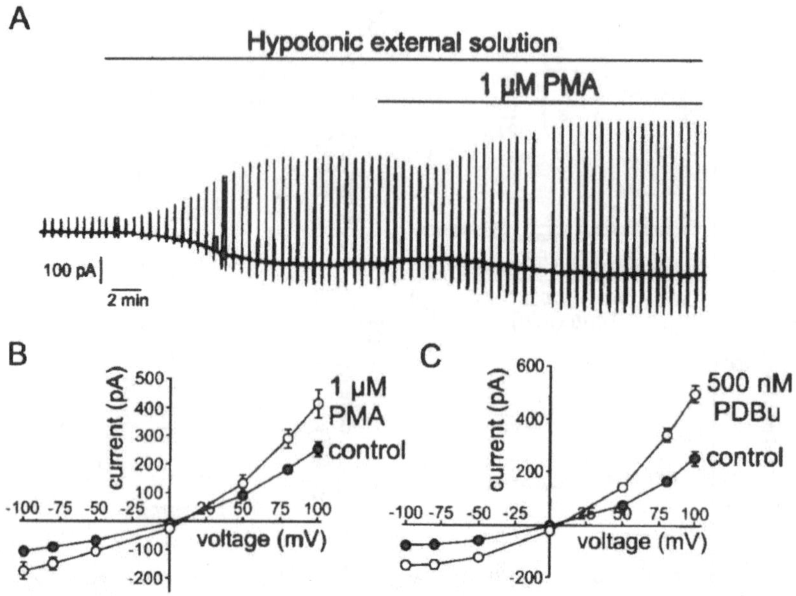

Figure 3 Effect of phorbol esters on $I_{Cl(Swell)}$ in portal vein myocytes. (A, C) Representative traces showing the stimulatory effect of phorbol-12-myrisate-13 acetate (PMA) (A) and phorbol-12, 13-dibutyrate (PDBu) (C) on $I_{Cl(Swell)}$. Cell was held at −50 mV, and deflections represent currents produced by ramp protocols (−100 mV to +100 mV at 133 mV/s). (B, D) Effect on the leak-subtracted current–voltage relationship of $I_{Cl(Swell)}$. in the absence and (o) in the presence of PMA (B) and phorbol-12, 13-dibutyrate (PDBu) (D). Each point is the mean ± S.E.M of five cells. (Reproduced from Ref. 29 with permission from Blackwell Publishing, Oxford, UK.)

similar to those described above. The presence of this conductance in these cells is particularly pertinent, because $I_{Cl(Swell)}$ in endothelial cells is activated by membrane stretch and the endothelium is continuously exposed to the shear forces associated with the turbulent flow of blood through the vessel. In contrast to work on $I_{Cl(Swell)}$ in smooth muscle cells a number of exhaustive studies have investigated the gating mechanism involved with the activation of this conductance in endothelial cells. These studies have highlighted three main regulatory pathways. A role for membrane reorganization was implicated by the observations that disruption of annexin II, a structural protein abundant in caveolae, attenuated $I_{Cl(Swell)}$ activation (18) and transfection of caveolin-1 enhanced $I_{Cl(Swell)}$ activation (18). $I_{Cl(Swell)}$ in pulmonary artery endothelial cells is inhibited by blockers of tyrosine kinases and augmented by protein tyrosine phosphatase inhibitors (32). Recent studies have shown that GTPγS activates a current similar to $I_{Cl(Swell)}$ in the absence of any cell swelling, and this appears to involve the GTPase Rho A and its downstream kinase (18). However, the gating mechanism underlying the activation of $I_{Cl(Swell)}$ remains to be defined unequivocally, and it is likely that the involvement of tyrosine phosphorylation and Rho-dependent kinase are merely permissive pathways (18).

VI. MOLECULAR CANDIDATES FOR $I_{Cl(Swell)}$

Because of the lack of a specific channel ligand and the presence of $I_{Cl(Swell)}$ in almost all cell types, the molecular identity of the channel protein remains elusive. However, various candidates have been proposed, including the ABC transporter *p*-glycoprotein and chloride conductance regulatory protein (pI_{Cln}), of which have been dismissed (18,24,33). More recently, various members of the CLC gene family were implicated to encode for $I_{Cl(Swell)}$. CLC2 encodes a Cl^- channel that is expressed ubiquitously and is activated by cell swelling, and mRNA transcripts corresponding to CLC2 have been detected in human vascular smooth muscle and endothelial cells (34). However, when expressed in mammalian cell lines, CLC2 displayed inward rectification and activated in a time-dependent fashion with membrane hyperpolarization (18,35). In contrast, $I_{Cl(Swell)}$ displays strong outward rectification and is usually time-independent, except for slow inactivation observed at very positive potentials in most cell types so far studied (see Sec. III. C and Fig. 1). In addition, the anion permeability sequence of CLC2 is opposite to native $I_{Cl(Swell)}$, with $Cl^- > Br^- > I^-$, and is relatively insensitive to DIDS. Consequently, the CLC2-encoded protein is unlikely to be responsible for generating $I_{Cl(Swell)}$ in vascular smooth muscle cells although it is possible that CLC2 might coassemble with another protein to form the endogenous channel.

A second member of the CLC gene family, CLC3, was recently proposed to underlie $I_{Cl(Swell)}$ in a number of cell types including cardiomyocytes, pulmonary and renal arteries, and colon (5,6,36). These studies showed that CLC3 is expressed at high levels in cell types shown to exhibit robust $I_{Cl(Swell)}$. Among the members of the CLC family of genes, the CLC3 transcript exhibits the highest level of expression in human blood vessels (34). Heterologous expression of CLC3 in NIH/3T3 cells generated a basally active current with biophysical and pharmacological properties similar to native $I_{Cl(Swell)}$ that was enhanced by osmotic cell swelling (36). Moreover, antibodies raised against amino acids in the C-terminus and extracellular segments of CLC3 inhibited $I_{Cl(Swell)}$ development in cardiac and pulmonary artery cells (37,38). Furthermore, CLC3 antisense oligonucleotides attenuated the development of $I_{Cl(Swell)}$ in epithelial Hela cells and *Xenopus* oocytes (39,40). The argument for CLC3 was strengthened by the observation that in CLC3-overexpressing cells, mutation of a specific serine residue (serine 51) located in a protein kinase C consensus site produced a constitutively active current that was unresponsive to cell swelling or PKC inhibitors (28). This observation and the potentiation mediated by PKC inhibitors in some cell types (see Sec. III and Fig. 2) led to the proposal that $I_{Cl(Swell)}$ was evoked by the swelling-induced removal of PKC-dependent phosphorylation of CLC3 encoded proteins (29). A necessary caveat to this proposal is that it cannot be a ubiquitous scheme, because PKC enhances $I_{Cl(Swell)}$ in some cell types, notably portal vein myocytes (30) (Fig. 3).

The credence of CLC3 as the molecular candidate for $I_{Cl(Swell)}$ has been doubted by a number of groups for various reasons. First, heterologous expression of CLC3 does not always generate $I_{Cl(Swell)}$ (see Ref. 33). Second, although native $I_{Cl(Swell)}$ is generally undetectable under isotonic conditions, cells overexpressing CLC3 exhibited robust Cl^- currents in the absence of cell swelling with biophysical properties similar to those of $I_{Cl(Swell)}$ (36). Perhaps the strongest argument against a role for CLC3 was the observation that in transgenic mice where the CLC3 gene was ablated, there was no apparent difference in native $I_{Cl(Swell)}$ compared to wild-type animals (41). This study also showed that although CLC3 was present in the plasmalemmal membrane there was significant localization in cytoplasmic organelles. These observations led to the proposal that CLC3 proteins merely regulate the endogenous swelling-activated channel protein (33). One caveat to the use of general transgenic mouse models is the possibility of compensatory mechanisms being activated, giving rise to channels displaying similar properties. More advanced molecular approaches such as the generation of inducible tissue-specific gene targeting in mice to avoid potential deleterious developmental changes (41) should be considered to assess the function of candidate genes.

There are two other CLC gene family members with a high homology to CLC3, namely CLC4 and CLC5, whose expression generates Cl^- currents. However, these conductances are not activated by changes in cell geometry and have permeability profiles different from that of native $I_{Cl(Swell)}$ (33). Regardless of the contribution of CLC proteins to the swelling-activated Cl^- channel, it is evident from the effects of different kinase modulators that even in smooth muscle cells there seem to be distinct subgroups of $I_{Cl(Swell)}$. This may reflect the contribution of different proteins to the swelling-activated Cl^- channel, and the composition of these heteromeric channels probably changes depending on the tissue under study.

VII. PHYSIOLOGICAL ROLES OF $I_{Cl(Swell)}$

Swelling-activated Cl^- currents serve a number of functions in different cell types. These include regulatory volume decrease in cells undergoing osmotic stress, development of force, cell proliferation, apoptosis, and transcellular Cl^- transport. These roles have been summarized in a number of reviews (e.g., Ref. 24). The aim of this section is to highlight roles that have relevance to the pulmonary vasculature. It is worth noting that there have been no studies that have attempted to define the role of $I_{Cl(Swell)}$ in the pulmonary circulation. Consequently, the functional role of $I_{Cl(Swell)}$ in this vascular bed can only be extrapolated from studies on other cell types.

A. Regulation of Cell Volume

Perturbations of the osmotic gradient lead to cell swelling or shrinkage. This can occur physiologically due to active solute uptake or secretion. Pathophysiologically, various disorders such as diabetes mellitus, renal failure, and congestive heart failure affect the extracellular osmolarity whereas ischemia or metabolic insufficiency increase intracellular osmolarity. In general, changes in cellular geometry are minimized by compensatory mechanisms such as the regulatory volume decrease (RVD) that is associated with most swollen mammalian cells. RVD is mediated by the efflux of K^+, Cl^-, and various organic osmolytes such as amino acids (24) through the activation of various transporters and channels. Considerable evidence has been accrued that implicates $I_{Cl(Swell)}$ in this response, and it is worth noting that this current can also be carried by anions such as taurine and proline. Most of the molecular candidates for $I_{Cl(Swell)}$ listed above have been implicated in contributing to RVD.

B. Development of Vascular Tone

In a number of blood vessels, especially in small arteries and arterioles, smooth muscle cells respond to an increase in intravascular pressure by generating tone. The smooth muscle contraction triggered by this endothelium-independent myogenic response involves membrane depolarization-induced activation of voltage-dependent L-type Ca^{2+} channels ($I_{Ca(L)}$), increased intracellular Ca^{2+} levels from a resting level of ~100 nM to ~250 nM, and enhanced sensitivity of the contractile proteins to Ca^{2+}. In spite of recent advancements in this area, the molecular mechanism by which electromechanical coupling of membrane stretch and ion channel activation occurs is not completely understood. Three main mechanisms have been proposed to underlie the membrane depolarization in vascular smooth muscle, namely, influx of monovalent cations through stretch-activated nonselective cation channels, closure of K^+ channels to prevent efflux of K^+ ions, and efflux of Cl^- through Cl^- channels. The argument in favor of a role of Cl^- currents in the development of myogenic tone extends from the observation that Cl^- channel blockers or manipulations of the Cl^- gradient altered the myogenic response in a number of beds. Thus, in rat posterior cerebral arteries, pressure-induced constriction was increased by reduction of extracellular Cl^- concentration and was blocked by the chloride channel inhibitors IAA-94 and DIDS, but not by niflumic acid (42). Similarly, 200 μM DIDS reduced myogenic tone in small endothelium-denuded pressurized rabbit mesenteric arteries (Fig. 4B) whereas 100 μM niflumic acid was without effect (Fig. 4A) (43). In this study DIDS and niflumic acid failed to inhibit KCl-induced vasoconstrictions, supporting the concept that the DIDS-induced vasodilation was not due to the direct inhibition of $I_{Ca(L)}$. The observation that $I_{Cl(Swell)}$ was present in vascular myocytes (5,7) consolidated the putative role of Cl^- currents in the myogenic response by providing a mechano sensitive conductance that could transduce the mechanical perturbation of the membrane into depolarization of the membrane potential. Further support for a Cl^- component to the myogenic response in cerebral arteries was provided by the detection of pressure-dependent Cl^- efflux by a Cl^--sensing electrode (44). The observation that $I_{Cl(Swell)}$ was active under isotonic conditions added further support to the Cl^- channel hypothesis. However, it is likely that the mechanical duress imposed on the cell by the whole-cell recording technique is sufficient to generate an artifactual resting conductance. In addition it is worth considering

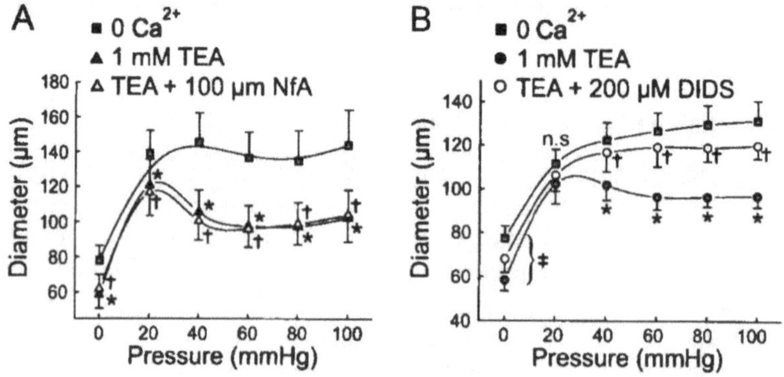

Figure 4 Effects of niflumic acid and DIDS on myogenic tone recorded from endothelium-denuded small pressurized rabbit mesenteric arteries. This figure shows the effects of (A) 100 μM niflumic acid (NfA), ($n = 6$) or (B) 200 μM DIDS ($n = 6$) on myogenic tone recorded from small pressurized rabbit mesenteric arteries. In both series of experiments, the test solution also contained 1 mM tetraethylammonium chloride (TEA) to minimize the impact of niflumic acid on large-conductance Ca^{2+}-dependent K^+ channels. The graph in each panel plots lumen diameter easured optically by edge detection as a function of transmural pressure. For each series of experiments, the passive lumen diameter relationship to pressure was obtained by exposing the preparation to a nominally Ca^{2+}-free solution containing 2 mM EGTA (0 Ca^{2+}). (*) A significant difference from the 0 Ca^{2+} level ($P < 0.05$): (†)(A) A significant difference between TEA + NfA and 0 Ca^{2+} ($P < 0.05$). (B): † significantly different from TEA alone ($P < 0.05$), (‡). All three points were significantly different from each other ($P < 0.05$). n.s., not significant. (Reproduced from Ref. 43 with permission from Elsevier Ltd., Oxford, UK.)

that because $I_{Cl(Swell)}$ is also present in endothelial cells, the role of this conductance in the generation of pressure-dependent tone is far from clear in studies carried out with an intact endothelium. Moreover, there are a number of necessary caveats to these observations. First, although Cl channel blockers such as DIDS and IAA-94 block the development of myogenic tone, these agents also inhibit the Ca^{2+}-dependent Cl^- conductance in smooth muscle cells (see Ref. 2 and Chapter 15 of this volume). More important, these agents were also shown to directly block voltage-gated calcium channels in rat cerebral arteries (45) and to block a stretch-activated cation current in cerebral arteries with a potency similar to the block of $I_{Cl(Swell)}$ (46). Unequivocal determination of the role of $I_{Cl(Swell)}$ in vascular responsiveness will rely upon the development of more selective pharmacological probes or the generation of transgenic mice in which the elusive gene responsible for the $I_{Cl(Swell)}$ has been disrupted. Furthermore it will be necessary to separate the individual contributions of $I_{Cl(Swell)}$ in smooth muscle cells from those in endothelial cells. In the latter case, activation of $I_{Cl(Swell)}$ would be predicted to maintain the cell at a relatively depolarized potential, thus reducing Ca^{2+} influx, which is crucial for the synthesis of vasoreactive mediators such as NO. Finally, the pulmonary vasculature is normally not subjected to transmural pressures greater than 20 mmHg. However, the vascular wall tension resulting from the relatively high flow rates encountered in some segments of the pulmonary circulation might be sufficient to stretch the vascular smooth muscle cells and stimulate $I_{Cl(Swell)}$.

C. Cell Proliferation

Volume-regulated chloride currents have been implicated as important regulators of the cell cycle (18). The function of the swelling-activated chloride channel is intimately related to the cell cycle in many cell types, and activation of an outwardly rectifying channel permeable to chloride and organic osmolytes coincides with cell proliferation. Cell proliferation is associated with an increase in metabolism, mitosis, and cell growth and migration compared with cells arrested in the G0/G1 stage of the cell cycle. In addition, various studies show that generation of $I_{Cl(Swell)}$ is possible only in cells undergoing proliferation and not differentiation. This would likely be associated with an increase in cell volume and intracellular solute concentration, thus making cell volume regulatory mechanisms essential during proliferation. Cells in G0 arrest exhibited a lower density of Cl^- channels than either actively proliferating cells or cells undergoing mitosis (18). Moreover, blockers of $I_{Cl(Swell)}$ impaired cell growth in a number of cell types that did not correlate with an effect on cellular metabolism (18). More specifically, inhibitors of $I_{Cl(Swell)}$ retarded vascular smooth muscle cell proliferation (47) and blocked the serum-induced proliferation of pulmonary artery endothelial cells (48). Extensive studies using a number of angiogenesis models showed that agents that blocked endothelial $I_{Cl(Swell)}$ such as mibefradil, NPPB, tamoxifen, and clomiphene inhibited microvessel formation (49). Interestingly, endothelin-induced proliferation of aortic myocytes was also attenuated by antisense oligonucleotides specific to CLC3, and the expression of this gene paralleled cell growth (50). A corollary to the above physiological role of $I_{Cl(Swell)}$ in cell growth is the observation that apoptotic cells undergo cell shrinkage that precedes the release of cellular metabolites. This volume-decrease-mediated cell death is ablated by blockers of $I_{Cl(Swell)}$. Consequently there is considerable evidence that $I_{Cl(Swell)}$ is an important component of cell proliferation, but its precise role remains to be determined. It is possible that $I_{Cl(Swell)}$, in concert with several classes of K^+ channels, plays a prime role in the remodeling of the pulmonary vasculature occurring in pulmonary hypertension.

VIII. CONCLUSIONS

Swelling-activated chloride currents are present in a wide range of excitable and nonexcitable cell types, and in the pulmonary vasculature this conductance is present in both endothelial cells and smooth muscle cells. However, the contribution of $I_{Cl(Swell)}$ from both cell types to the regulation of pulmonary artery vascular reactivity has not been determined. In that respect it is worth noting that $I_{Cl(Swell)}$ is not the only Cl^- current in the pulmonary vasculature. Endothelial cells exhibit Ca^{2+} and protein kinase A-activated Cl^- currents (18), and Ca^{2+}-activated Cl^- currents have also been recorded in pulmonary artery myocytes (e.g., 10–12). The molecular identity of the $I_{Cl(Swell)}$ channel remains a source of debate, and it seems that subpopulations of the channel exist in smooth muscle cells according to the sensitivity to various kinase modulators. Furthermore, it still remains to be determined whether the gating mechanisms described for $I_{Cl(Swell)}$ in endothelial cells occur in smooth muscle cells. Consequently, a number of questions about the molecular identity and functional roles of $I_{Cl(Swell)}$ in the pulmonary vasculature remain to be answered.

ACKNOWLEDGMENTS

This work was supported by grants from the Canadian Institutes of Health Research (NL; CIHR MOP-10863), National Institutes of Health (NL; NIH NCRR 5 P2015581), the Western Affiliate of the American Heart Association (NL; 0355060Y), and Wellcome Trust (IAG; 053794).

REFERENCES

1. Chipperfield AR, Harper AA. Chloride in smooth muscle. Biophys Mol Biol 2000; 74:175–221.

2. Large WA, Wang Q. Characteristics and physiological role of the Ca^{2+}-activated Cl^- conductance in smooth muscle. Am J Physiol 1996; 271:C435–C454.
3. Kitamura K, Yamazaki J. Chloride channels and their functional roles in smooth muscle tone in the vasculature. Jpn J Pharmacol 2001; 85:351–357.
4. Xu WX, Kim SJ, So I, Kang TM, Rhee JC, Kim KW. Volume-sensitive chloride current activated by hyposmotic swelling in antral gastric myocytes of the guinea pig. Pflügers Arch 1997; 435:9–19.
5. Yamazaki J, Duan D, Janiak R, Kuenzli K, Horowitz B, Hume JR. Functional and molecular expression of volume-regulated chloride channels in canine vascular smooth muscle cells. J Physiol 1998; 507:729–736.
6. Dick GM, Bradley KK, Horowitz B, Hume JR, Sanders KM. Functional and molecular identification of a novel chloride conductance in canine colonic smooth muscle. Am J Physiol 1998; 275:C940–C950.
7. Greenwood IA, Large WA. Properties of a Cl^- current activated by cell swelling in rabbit portal vein vascular smooth muscle cells. Am J Physiol 1998; 275:H1524–H1532.
8. Masuda T, Tomiyama Y, Kitahata H, Kuroda Y, Oshita S. Propofol inhibits volume-sensitive chloride channels in human coronary artery smooth muscle cells. Anesth Analg 2003; 97:657–662.
9. Fan SF, Christ GJ, Melman A, Brink PR. A stretch sensitive Cl^- current in human corpus cavernosal myocytes. Int J Impotence Res 1999; 11:1–7.
10. Yuan XJ. Role of calcium-activated chloride current in regulating pulmonary vasomotor tone. Am J Physiol 1997; 272:L959–L966.
11. Greenwood IA, Ledoux J, Leblanc N. Differential regulation of Ca^{2+}-activated Cl^- currents in rabbit arterial and portal vein smooth muscle cells by Ca^{2+}/calmodulin-dependent kinase. J Physiol 2001; 534:395–408.
12. Piper AS, Greenwood IA, Large WA. Dual effect of blocking agents on Ca^{2+}-activated Cl^- currents in rabbit pulmonary artery smooth muscle cells. J Physiol 2002; 539:119–131.
13. Zhong J, Wang GX, Hatton WJ, Yamboliev IA, Walsh MP, Hume JR. Regulation of volume-sensitive outwardly rectifying anion channels in pulmonary artery smooth muscle cells by PKC. Am J Physiol Cell Physiol 2002; 283:C1627–C1636.
14. Pacaud P, Loirand G, Grégoire G, Mironneau C, Mironneau J. Calcium-dependence of the calcium-activated chloride current in smooth muscle cells of rat portal vein. Pflügers Arch 1992; 421:125–130.
15. Wang YX , Kotlikoff M I. Inactivation of calcium-activated chloride channels in smooth muscle by calcium/calmodulin-dependent protein kinase. Proc Natl Acad Sci USA 1997; 94:14918–14923.
16. Piper AS, Greenwood IA. Anomalous effect of anthracene-9-carboxylic acid on calcium-activated chloride currents in rabbit pulmonary artery smooth muscle cells. Br J Pharmacol 2003; 138:31–38.
17. Taouil K, Giancola R, Morel JE, Hannaert P. Hypotonically induced calcium increase and regulatory volume decrease in newborn rat cardiomyocytes. Pflügers Arch 1998; 436:565–574.
18. Nilius B, Droogmans G. Amazing chloride channels: an overview. Acta Physiol Scand 2003; 177:119–147.

19. Greenwood IA, Large WA. Modulation of Ca^{2+}-activated Cl^- currents in rabbit portal vein smooth muscle cells by external anions. J Physiol 1999; 516: 365–376.
20. Voets T, Droogmans G, Nilius B. Modulation of voltage-dependent properties of a swelling-activated Cl^- current. J Gen Physiol 1997; 110:313–325.
21. Hogg RC, Wang Q, Large WA. Time course of spontaneous calcium-activated chloride currents in smooth muscle cells from rabbit portal vein. J Physiol 1993; 464:15–31.
22. Greenwood IA, Large WA. Analysis of the time course of calcium-activated chloride "tail" currents in rabbit portal vein smooth muscle cells. Pflügers Arch 1996; 432:970–979.
23. Arreola J, Melvin JE, Begenisich T. Activation of calcium-dependent chloride channels in rat parotid acinar cells. J Gen Physiol 1996; 108:35–47.
24. Okada Y. Volume expansion-sensing outward rectifier Cl^- channel: fresh start to the molecular identity and volume sensor. Am J Physiol 1997; 273: C755–C789.
25. Coulombe A, Corabeouf E. Large-conductance Chloride channels of new-born rat cardiac myicytes are activated by hypotonic media. Pflügers Arch 1992; 422: 143–150.
26. Schwiebert EM, Mills JW, Stanton BA. Actin-based cytoskeleton regulates a chloride channel and cell volume in a renal cortical collecting duct cell line. J Biol Chem 1994; 269:7081–7089.
27. Dick GM, Kong ID, Sanders KM. Effects of anion channel antagonists in canine colonic myocytes: comparative pharmacology of Cl^-, Ca^{2+} and K^+ currents. Br J Pharmacol 1999; 127:1819–1831.
28. Duan D, Cowley S, Horowitz B, Hume JR. A serine 3 in CLC-3 links phosphorylation-dephosphorylation to chloride channel regulation by cell volume. J Gen Physiol 1999; 113:57–70.
29. Ellershaw DC, Greenwood IA, Large WA. Modulation of swelling-activated currents by noradrenaline in rabbit portal vein myocytes. J Physical 2002; 542: 537–547.
30. Du XY, Sorota S. Protein kinase C stimulates cell swelling-induced chloride current in canine atrial cells. Pflügers Arch 1999; 437:227–234.
31. Ellershaw DC, Greenwood IA, Large WA. Dual modulation of swelling-activated chloride currents by NO and NO-donors in rabbit vascular myocytes. J Physiol 2000; 528:15–24.
32. Voets T, Manolopoulos V, Eggermont J, Ellory C, Droogmans G, Nilius B. Regulation of a swelling-activated chloride current in bovine endothelium by protein phosphorylation and G proteins. J Physiol 1998; 506:341–352.
33. Jentsch TJ, Stein V, Weinreich F, Zdebik AA. Molecular structure and physiological function of chloride channels. Physiol Rev 2002; 82:503–568.
34. Lamb FS, Clayton GH, Liu BX, Smith RL, Barna TJ, Schutte BC. Expression of CLCN voltage-gated chloride channel genes in human blood vessels. J Mol Cell Cardiol 1999; 31:657–666.
35. Gründer S, Thiemann A, Pusch M, Jentsch TJ. Regions involved in the opening of CLC-2 chloride channel by voltage and cell volume. Nature 1992; 360: 759–762.

36. Duan D, Winter C, Cowley S, Hume JR, Horowitz B. Molecular identification of a volume-regulated chloride channel. Nature 1997; 390:417–421.
37. Duan D, Zhong J, Hermoso M, Satterwhite CM, Rossow CF, Hatton WJ, Yamboliev IA, Horowitz B, Hume JR. Functional inhibition of native volume-sensitive outwardly rectifying anion channels in muscle cells and *Xenopus* oocytes by anti-CLC3 antibody. J Physiol 2001; 531:437–444.
38. Wang GX, Hatton WJ, Wang GL, Zhong J, Yamboliev I, Duan D, Hume JR. Functional effects of novel anti-CLC3 antibodies on native volume-sensitive osmolyte and anion channels in cardiac and smooth muscle cells. Am J Physiol Heart Circ Physiol 2003; 285:H1453–H1463.
39. Wang L, Chen L, Jacob TJ. The role of CLC3 in volume-activated chloride currents and volume regulation in bovine epithelial cells demonstrated by antisense inhibition. J Physiol 2000; 524:63–75.
40. Hermoso M, Satterwhite CM, Andrade YN, Hidalgo J, Wilson SM, Horowitz B, Hume JR. CLC3 is a fundamental molecular component of volume-sensitive outwardly rectifying Cl^- channels and volume regulation in HeLa and *Xenopus laevis* oocytes. J Biol Chem 2002; 277:40066–40074.
41. Stobrawa SM, Breiderhof T, Takamori S, Engel D, Schweizer M, Zdebik AA, Bösl MR, Ruether K, Jain H, Draguhn A, Jain R, Jentsch TJ. Disruption of CLC-3, a chloride channel expressed on synaptic vesicles, leads to a loss of the hippocampus. Neuron 2001; 29:185 196.
42. Nelson MT, Conway MA, Knot HJ, Brayden JE. Chloride channel blockers inhibit myogenic tone in rat cerebral arteries. J Physiol 1997; 502:259–264.
43. Remillard CV, Lupien MA, Crépeau V, Leblanc N. Role of Ca^{2+}- and swelling-activated Cl^- channels in α_1-adrenoceptor-mediated tone in pressurized rabbit mesenteric arterioles. Cardiovasc Res 2000; 46:557–568.
44. Doughty JM, Langton PD. Measurement of chloride fluxassociated with the myogenic response in rat cerebral arteries. J Physiol 2001; 534:753–761.
45. Doughty JM, Miller AL, Langton PD. Non-specificity of chloride channel blockers in rat cerebral arteries: block of the L-type calcium channel. J Physiol 1998; 507:433–439.
46. Welsh DG, Nelson MT, Eckmann DM, Brayden JE. Swelling-activated cation channels mediate depolarization of rat cerebrovascular smooth muscle by osmolarity and intravascular pressure. J Physiol 2000; 527:139–148.
47. Xiao GN, Guan YY, He H. Effects of Cl^- channel blockers on endothelin-1 induced proliferation of rat vascular smooth muscle cells. Life Sci 2002; 70: 2233–2241.
48. Voets T, Szücs G, Droogmans G, Nilius B. Blockers of volume-activated Cl currents inhibit endothelial cell proliferation. Pflügers Arch 1995; 431: 132–134.
49. Manolopoulos VG, Liekens S, Koolwijk P, Voets T, Peters E, Droogmans G, Lelkes PI, De Clercq E, Nilius B. Inhbitors of angiogenesis by blockers of volume-regulated anion channels. Gen Pharmacol 2000; 34:107–116.
50. Wang GL, Wang XR, Lin MJ, He H, Lan XJ, Guan YY. Deficiency in CLC-3 chloride channels prevents rat aortic smooth muscle cell proliferation. Circ Res 2002; 91:e28–e32.

17

Molecular Physiology of O_2-Sensitive Ion Channels

Kristen O'Connell, Elizabeth A. Coppock, Aaron Norris, and Michael M. Tamkun
Colorado State University, Fort Collins, Colorado, U.S.A.

I. INTRODUCTION

Membrane ion channels play an essential role in the maintenance of cellular excitability. In vascular smooth muscle, membrane excitability is principally controlled by voltage-gated K^+ channels, which are responsible for setting the resting membrane potential (1). Changes in K^+ channel function can profoundly affect vascular tone by regulating voltage-gated Ca^{2+} channel function; an increase in K^+ conductance hyperpolarizes the membrane, inhibiting the activation of Ca^{2+} channels, whereas a decrease in K^+ conductance results in depolarization and the subsequent activation of voltage-gated Ca^{2+} channels (1). The role of K^+ channel function in regulating PASMC contraction is summarized in Fig. 1.

Vascular tone is also affected by O_2 tension (Po_2): in the systemic circulation and larger conduit vessels of the pulmonary vasculature, low Po_2 causes arterial vasodilation, thereby increasing O_2 delivery to tissues. In contrast, the small resistance arteries of the lung constrict in response to low Po_2, shunting blood flow away from poorly ventilated areas of the lung. The response of both types of arterial smooth muscle is due in part to modulation of voltage-gated K^+ and Ca^{2+} channels by O_2 levels.

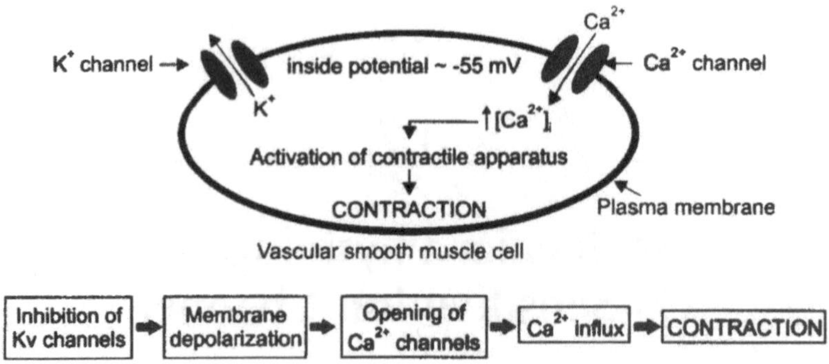

Figure 1 Role of Kv channels in controlling vascular smooth muscle contraction.

Oxygen-sensitive ion channels therefore play an important role in matching vascular tone and perfusion to ventilation and O_2 tension.

This chapter will present an overview of the oxygen-sensitive ion channels in pulmonary artery smooth muscle cells (PASMCs) and the potential mechanisms by which Po_2 alters ion channel function. For a review of the voltage-gated K^+ (Kv) channels expressed in the pulmonary vasculature, see Chapter 11.

A. Hypoxic Pulmonary Vasoconstriction

One of the most-studied examples of the physiological importance of O_2-sensitive ion channels is hypoxic pulmonary vasoconstriction (HPV) in the small resistance arteries of the pulmonary circulation. In contrast to the small arteries of the systemic circulation, which dilate in response to hypoxia, small arteries of the pulmonary circulation respond to low Po_2 by constricting (1). In the fetal circulation, HPV contributes to the high pulmonary arterial resistance, diverting blood through the ductus arteriosus (1). In the adult, HPV reduces the flow of blood through atelectatic or underventilated areas of the lung where ventilation is not adequate for oxygenation (1). In this manner, acute HPV is a mechanism that helps to match perfusion to ventilation, diverting blood flow away from poorly ventilated portions of the lung in order to maximize arterial saturation. When only a small region of the lung is hypoxic, HPV occurs without a significant effect on pulmonary arterial pressure. However, if hypoxia is generalized, as is seen with many lung diseases and with high altitude exposure, the subsequent pulmonary vasoconstriction causes an increase in pulmonary arterial pressure, which can potentially lead to pulmonary hypertension, heart failure, and death (1).

Since it was first described nearly 60 years ago (1), HPV has been extensively studied, but the exact mechanisms underlying HPV remain unknown. Although endothelium-derived vasoactive factors are clearly important and appear to be necessary for the full expression of HPV in vivo [for a review, see Ward and Aaronson (2)], it seems likely that HPV is initiated, at least partially, through a mechanism intrinsic to PASMCs. Responsiveness to acute hypoxia has been demonstrated not only in isolated lungs but also in pulmonary arterial rings denuded of endothelium and in single PASMCs (1,3,4).

It is currently hypothesized that alveolar hypoxia acts to directly depolarize the PASMC membrane, thus causing an influx of Ca^{2+} through L-type voltage-gated Ca^{2+} channels and subsequent contraction. Indeed, in isolated PASMCs, acute hypoxia has been shown to significantly depolarize the membrane potential by about 15–20 mV, leading to contraction of individual PASMCs (1,3). In the isolated perfused lung, HPV is inhibited by the voltage-gated Ca^{2+} channel antagonists verapamil and SKF 525 and potentiated by Bay K8644, an L-channel agonist (1,5,6). The hypoxia-induced constriction of small pulmonary arteries is associated with membrane depolarization that is inhibited by verapamil (1,7). Furthermore, more recent studies have demonstrated that the hypoxia-induced increase in intracellular Ca^{2+} in both adult and fetal PASMCs is inhibited by L-channel blockers (1,7). These studies clearly illustrate the importance of Ca^{2+} influx through membrane voltage-gated Ca^{2+} channels in HPV. Indeed, Franco-Obregon and Lopez-Barneo (8) showed that hypoxia causes a potentiation of the Ca^{2+} current in the majority of cells isolated from rabbit resistance pulmonary arteries (8). However, voltage-gated Ca^{2+} channels are relatively inactive at the resting membrane potential of PASMCs (8); therefore, it is likely that hypoxia acts first to depolarize the membrane by inhibiting the K^+ channels involved in setting the resting membrane potential. Hypoxic inhibition of K^+ channels was first demonstrated in 1988 by Lopez-Barneo and coworkers in carotid body type I cells (9). Later, Hume and coworkers (1) showed that hypoxia causes both an inhibition of whole-cell K^+ current and membrane depolarization in isolated PASMCs. An alternative, or perhaps additional, hypothesis is that hypoxia causes the release of Ca^{2+} from intracellular stores independent of Ca^{2+} influx and that this rise in intracellular Ca^{2+} leads to inhibition of membrane Kv channels (1). The relative importance of these mechanisms is not clear; however, the aforementioned studies suggest that hypoxia acts through multiple pathways to induce pulmonary vasoconstriction.

Vascular smooth muscle cells (VSMCs) show different responses to hypoxia according to the size and type of vessel from which they are isolated. Small resistance pulmonary arteries (3rd intrapulmonary artery or greater) constrict in response to hypoxia (1), whereas large, conduit pulmonary arteries (main pulmonary artery and right and left branches) usually do not respond, or dilate slightly (1), although hypoxic responses have been described in some preparations (1). In addition, the response of small pulmonary arteries is in marked contrast to that of small arteries isolated from the systemic circulation, which dilate in response to hypoxia (10). At the single-cell level, hypoxia causes small contractions and increased intracellular Ca^{2+} in resistance PASMCs but has little or no effect in conduit PASMCs or VSMCs isolated from small systemic arteries (11,12). Furthermore, hypoxia causes a significant depolarization of the membrane potential from approximately −51 mV to −37 mV in resistance PASMCs, whereas in conduit PASMCs the membrane potential is not significantly affected (1,11). Proposed mechanisms for the contrasting vasoactive responses to hypoxia of conduit and resistance pulmonary arteries and vessels from other vascular beds include differential expression of an O_2-sensitive K^+ channel, differential expression of O_2-sensitive L-type Ca^{2+} channels, and/or the presence of distinct O_2-sensing mechanisms (1).

B. Potassium Channels in HPV

Agents that block K^+ channels, such as 4-AP and TEA, depolarize the membrane, increase tension in pulmonary arterial rings, and increase pulmonary arterial pressure in isolated perfused lungs (1). Hypoxia acts in a similar manner to inhibit whole-cell outward K^+ current, causing membrane depolarization, constriction of small pulmonary arteries, and an increase in pulmonary artery pressure (1). The fact that PASMC membrane depolarization and pulmonary artery constriction can be mimicked by K^+ channel blockers suggests that the depolarization induced by hypoxia is due to inhibition of K^+ channels open at the resting membrane potential.

It has been suggested that two types of PASMC K^+ channels are modulated by hypoxia, leading to HPV: BK_{Ca} (13,14) and Kv (which includes IK_{DR} and IK_N). However, the majority of electrophysiological and pharmacological evidence points to members of the Kv family as the main PASMC O_2 sensors (1). The O_2-sensitive K^+ current described in most rat PASMC preparations is a delayed rectifier that is sensitive to 4-AP and insensitive to CTX. Indeed, hypoxic inhibition of PASMC K_{DR} current has been shown in whole-cell and single-channel studies in the presence of BK_{Ca} channel inhibitors. Furthermore, hypoxia and 4-AP constrict resistance arteries, whereas CTX has no effect (15,16). In addition, pretreatment of isolated dog PASMCs with 4-AP (1 mM), but not TEA (1 mM), prevents the hypoxic effect on outward K^+ current (17). Taken together, these data suggest that Kv channels that exhibit delayed-rectifier currents and are sensitive to 4-AP but insensitive to CTX are responsible for the O_2-sensitive K^+ current in native PASMCs. However, pretreatment with 4-AP does not always prevent, and in some cases may even potentiate, hypoxic constriction, as has been demonstrated in rat and dog lungs, rat resistance pulmonary arteries, and isolated pig PASMCs (1). These discrepancies may be partially explained by differential 4-AP sensitivity between Kv channel subtypes and between species homologs (18). Furthermore, in some instances, 4-AP may act as a priming agent, causing decreased background K^+ permeability and potentiation of the hypoxic response. It is likely that the pulmonary arterial O_2-sensitive K^+ current represents an ensemble of current from distinct Kv channel isoforms, some of which may be 4-AP insensitive. Thus, the variable response to hypoxia in the presence of 4-AP does not exclude a role for Kv channels in HPV.

II. O_2-SENSITIVE K^+ CHANNELS

Of the ion channels known to be expressed in the vasculature, to date four types have been identified as being O_2-sensitive: Ca^{2+}-activated K^+ channels (Maxi-K^+; BK_{Ca}), tandem pore (K_{2P}) channels, voltage-gated (Kv) channels, and voltage-gated Ca^{2+} channels. K_{ATP} channels exist in vascular smooth muscle, and although they do contribute to regulating vascular tone during hypoxia and during periods of metabolic stress, they themselves do not exhibit O_2 sensitivity and therefore will not be discussed further here (see Chapter 14 for a review of K_{ATP} channels).

A. BK_{Ca} Channels

The BK_{Ca} channel comprises four α and four β subunits (19) with a single-channel conductance of 250 pS in symmetrical K^+ and are sensitive to block by tetraethylammonium (TEA), charybdotoxin (CTX), and iberiotoxin (20). It is important that increases in intracellular Ca^{2+} shift the activation curve to more hyperpolarized potentials (19). Thus, BK_{Ca} channels play a role in the control of arterial smooth muscle membrane potential by serving as a negative feedback mechanism, regulating the degree of membrane depolarization and vasoconstriction induced by increased cytoplasmic Ca^{2+} (19,20). Although four genes encoding α subunits have been identified (*KCNMB*1–4), considerable diversity of BK_{Ca} channels is derived from extensive splice variants (19). The topologies of the S1–S6 domains of the BK_{Ca} α subunit share homology with the Kv channels, with S4 identified as the voltage sensor and the loop between S5 and S6 contributing to the ion-conducting pore. However, unlike the Kv channels, BK_{Ca} channels have a seventh transmembrane domain (S0) such that the N-terminus of these channels is extracellular. The BK_{Ca} β subunit is a two-transmembrane domain protein, with both the N- and C-termini located on the cytoplasmic side. It alters the biophysical properties of the BK_{Ca} channels, resulting in altered voltage and Ca^{2+} sensitivity (19).

PASMC BK_{Ca} channels are activated at membrane potentials positive to the resting membrane potential [which explains why CTX does not depolarize PASMCs (16,21,22)]; thus, under conditions of hypoxia, it is likely that the membrane depolarization and increased $[Ca^{2+}]_i$ activate BK_{Ca} channels, leading to membrane hyperpolarization. BK_{Ca} channels are inhibited by hypoxia, suggesting that these channels are O_2-sensitive (23). When expressed in HEK-293 cells, hypoxia induced a depolarizing shift in the voltage dependence of BK_{Ca} activation as well as decreasing single-channel conductance and NP_o. Although BK_{Ca} channels are expressed in PASMCs, it seems unlikely based on their biophysical properties that regulation of these channels by hypoxia is a triggering event in the modulation of vascular tone by low Po_2; rather, they serve as a feedback mechanism to prevent excessive vasoconstriction.

B. Tandem Pore K^+ Channels (K_{2P})

Several families of tandem pore K^+-selective channels have been recently identified (TREK, TWIK, TRAK, TASK) (24–28). The K_{2P} channels have four transmembrane domains and two pore regions and are insensitive to membrane potential. These channels are responsible for the background "leak" current in many cell types and contribute to setting the resting membrane potential. Of particular interest is the TASK family of K_{2P} channels. TASK channels have been identified as the pH-sensitive background K^+ current in carotid body cells and display inhibition by hypoxic conditions (28). The TASK channels have also been found in the oxygen-sensing cells in the neuroepithelial body in the lung, where they are also inhibited by Po_2 levels and are likely the major O_2-sensing channel in these cells (24,27). However, although these channels may be important in the oxygen-sensing cells of the carotid body and neuroepithelial body, so far they have not been identified in the pulmonary vasculature, and any contribution they may make to the O_2-sensitive current is unknown.

C. Voltage-Gated K^+ Channels

Voltage-gated K^+ (Kv) channels represent the main class of K^+ channels in pulmonary vascular smooth muscle. All vascular smooth muscle cells examined to date have at least one component of voltage-sensitive K^+ current, and many studies report more than one type of current (20). These currents include "delayed rectifier" (IK_{DR}) and "transient outward" (IK_{TO}) types (14). Recently, a third noninactivating Kv current (IK_N), which is activated at the resting membrane potential, has also been described in rabbit, rat, and pig PASMCs (21,29,30). These channels provide an important K^+ channel conductance in the physiological membrane potential range of pulmonary arteries (20), and several studies have demonstrated that PASMC membrane potentials are controlled by one or more subtypes of K_{DR} (16,21,31–33). Pharmacologically, most Kv currents can be isolated by selective inhibition to 4-AP. Outward K^+ current in PASMCs is inhibited by 4-AP (16,31), but not by TEA (16) or CTX (16). In addition, 4-AP (16,21,22,33), but not TEA (16,21), CTX (16,21), iberiotoxin, or glibenclamide (21,22), depolarizes PASMCs. Furthermore, exposure to 4-AP, but not glibenclamide or CTX, leads to an increase in $[Ca^{2+}]_i$ (34). Taken together, these studies emphasize the importance of Kv channels in the regulation of PASMC membrane potential and pulmonary arterial tone.

Voltage-dependent K^+ channels exist as tetramers of four six-transmembrane-spanning α subunits combining to form a functional channel (35). At this point in time the Kv channel α subunit family is composed of 36 members grouped into 12 subfamilies (Kv1–Kv12), with the Kv1 family being the largest, with eight members (for an update of Kv channel classification, see Ref. 36). These channels often display differences in voltage sensitivity, current kinetics, and steady-state activation and inactivation (35). Not only can identical α subunits combine to form a functional channel, but distinct α subunits can also combine to form functional heteromeric channels both in vitro and in vivo (18,35). These heteromeric channels have unique properties that often represent a blend of the observed properties of the corresponding homomeric channels. Furthermore, several Kv α subunits appear to be exclusively involved in heteromeric channel formation, because they are nonfunctional when expressed alone. For example, the Kv9.3 subunit does not form a functional homomeric channel itself but rather functions only in heteromeric complexes, where it confers altered voltage sensitivity and activation kinetics (37,38).

Accessory β subunits can combine with Kv α subunits to add even more diversity to Kv channel function (39). Four Kv β-subunit gene families have been described (40). All are cytoplasmic proteins, approximately 40 kDa in mass, with a conserved core sequence and variable N-termini. Voltage-gated K^+ channel β subunits have been shown to confer functional effects to α subunits, including both fast and slow inactivation, altered voltage sensitivity, and slowed deactivation (40). Additionally, β subunits may play a role as a cellular redox sensor; Kvβ1.2 appears to confer O_2 sensitivity to the Kv4.2 channel in heterologous expression systems (41). Thus, the roles of Kv β subunits are many, and indeed they may be important not only in the functional modulation of Kv α subunits but also in the response of PASMCs to hypoxia.

Multiple investigators, using a variety of techniques, have examined Kv channel expression in PASMCs (3,4,15,37,38,42,43) (see Ref. 1 for a more complete discussion). To summarize, these results strongly suggest the expression of the following α subunits in resistance PASMCs: Kv1.2, Kv1.5, Kv2.1, Kv3.1b, and Kv9.3 (see Table 1). Not as convincingly, the presence of Kv1.1, Kv1.4, and Kv1.6 is also suggested.

For a review of Kv channel expression and function in PASMCs, see Chapter 11.

Table 1 Hypoxia Sensitivity of Cloned Kv Channels in Heterologous Expression Systems

Kv α subunit	Protein expression confirmed in PASMCs	Hypoxia-sensitive in heterologous systems?
Kv1.2	Western (4,43)	Yes, L-cells but at positive potentials (37)
	Immunostaining (37)	Yes, in oocytes (78)
Kv1.5	Western (3,4,43)	No, in L-cells (37)
	Immunostaining (37)	No, in L929 cells (15)
Kv1.2/1.5	No assembly confirmed in PASMCs	Yes, in L-cells at negative potentials (37)
Kv2.1	Western blot (3,43)	Yes, in L-cells at positive potentials (37)
	Immunostaining (4)	Yes, in COS7 cells at positive potentials (38)
		No, in oocytes (78)
Kv9.3	No protein expression confirmed, mRNA only (3,38)	Silent subunit, no current as a homotetramer
Kv2.1/9.3	No assembly confirmed in PASMCs	Yes, in L-cells at negative potentials (37)
		Yes, in COS7 cells at negative potentials (38)
Kv3.1b	Immunostaining (15)	Yes, in L929 cells at positive potentials (15)

III. O_2 SENSITIVITY OF CLONED KV CHANNELS EXPRESSED IN HETEROLOGOUS SYSTEMS

The O_2 sensitivity of several cloned Kv channels has been studied in heterologous expression systems. Investigators have focused primarily on channels that are expressed in the pulmonary vasculature and, when expressed in heterologous expression systems, meet the profile of the PASMC O_2 sensitive current: delayed rectifier, sensitive to 4-AP, and insensitive to CTX. A noted exception here is the Kv2.1 channel, which is, in most species except rat, relatively 4-AP-insensitive (18).

A. The Kv2.1 Channel

Patel et al. examined the O_2 sensitivity of Kv2.1 expressed in COS-7 cells (38). In a subset of COS cells, Kv2.1 was reversibly inhibited by hypoxia by 34%, but this sensitivity was detected in only 21% of cells expressing Kv2.1 current (38). Hulme et al. (37) found similar results with Kv2.1 in mouse L-cells. Hypoxia significantly inhibited Kv2.1 currents by 23% at 60 mV. However, these investigators found that Kv2.1 was O_2-sensitive in nearly all of the cells studied. In both studies, only the Kv2.1 currents that were activated at more positive potentials were significantly inhibited by hypoxia. Furthermore, little Kv2.1 current was detected at potentials more negative than −20 mV. In contrast, Conforti et al. (44) found Kv2.1 currents to be O_2-in sensitive when expressed in *Xenopus* oocytes. These oocyte data indicate that the hypoxia sensitivity of Kv2.1 depends on the expression system. However, two out of three expression systems show hypoxic regulation, although this sensitivity does not occur in the voltage range of the resting membrane potential of native PASMCs.

B. The Kv2.1/Kv9.3 Heteromeric Channel

Patel et al. (38) cloned a novel subunit, Kv9.3, that does not form a functional channel itself but combines with Kv2.1, as evidenced by immunoprecipitation from metabolically labeled *Xenopus* oocytes and altered Kv2.1 biophysical and pharmacological properties. Most important, Kv9.3 causes a shift in the voltage dependence of activation into the voltage range of the resting membrane potential of PASMCs (37,38), suggesting that the Kv2.1/Kv9.3 heteromeric channel may contribute to the regulation of PASMC resting membrane potential and thus represents a PASMC O_2-sensitive K^+ current. In fact, in a subset of COS cells (56% of cells), Kv2.1/Kv9.3 current was reversibly inhibited by hypoxia by 28% (69). Hulme et al. (37) found similar results when Kv2.1/Kv9.3 was expressed in mouse L-cells. Hypoxia reversibly inhibited the Kv2.1/Kv9.3 current by 21% at 60 mV in all cells studied. In support of the role for Kv2.1/Kv9.3

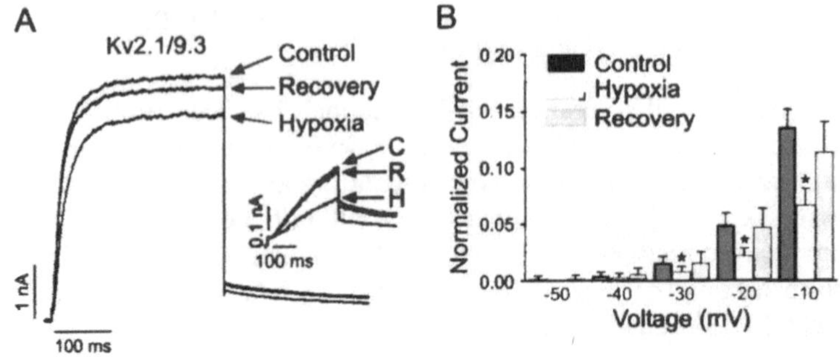

Figure 2 Hypoxia sensitivity of the Kv2.1/9.3 heteromeric channel. (A) Representative Kv2.1/Kv9.3 currents recorded from transfected L-cells at 60 mV before, during, and after 10 min of exposure to hypoxic solution. Holding potential was −80 mV. Inset shows representative Kv2.1/Kv9.3 currents recorded at −20 mV before, during, and after 10 min of exposure to hypoxic solution. (B) Bar graph highlighting effects of hypoxia on Kv2.1/Kv9.3 current at negative potentials closer to the resting potential of native vascular myocytes. (Data shown are presented in greater detail in Ref. 37.)

current in the physiological response of PASMCs to hypoxia, Kv2.1/Kv9.3 current is sensitive to hypoxia in the voltage range of the PASMC resting membrane potential (37,38). This hypoxia sensitivity is illustrated in Fig. 2.

Both Kv2.1 and Kv9.3 subunits are expressed in PASMCs (1,3,38,43), and evidence for assembly in vitro has been demonstrated (38); however, there is no direct evidence that this heteromeric channel is expressed in vivo. Furthermore, when expressed in *Xenopus* oocytes, Kv2.1/Kv9.3 current is significantly less sensitive to 4-AP than Kv2.1 current alone ($IC_{50} = 4.5$ mM mM for Kv2.1 vs. $IC_{50} = 31.6$ mM for Kv2.1/9.3) (38), making the Kv2.1/Kv9.3 heteromeric channel much less sensitive to 4-AP than the O_2-sensitive K^+ current most often described in PASMCs (1).

C. The Kv1.5 Channel

The results from studies using inhibitory anti-Kv1.5 antibodies in the patch pipette have led some investigators to hypothesize that Kv1.5 is an important component of the O_2-sensitive K^+ current in the pulmonary artery (4). Furthermore, Kv1.5 meets the profile of the O_2-sensitive K^+ current in PASMCs: delayed rectifier, sensitive to 4-AP, and insensitive to CTX (36). However, Kv1.5 is not sensitive to hypoxia when expressed as a homotetramer in L-cells (37), COS-7 cells (15), or MEL cells (15). Therefore, it is unlikely that Kv1.5 homomeric channels contribute to the O_2-sensitive current in PASMCs.

D. The Kv1.2 Channel

Although it is thought to underlie the CTX- and hypoxia-sensitive K^+ current in PC12 cells (44), Kv1.2, owing to its sensitivity to CTX, has historically been ignored as an important player in PASMC oxygen sensing (45). However, the O_2 sensitivity of this channel was examined by Hulme et al. (37), who found that, when expressed in mouse L-cells, Kv1.2 current was significantly inhibited by hypoxia (19% inhibition at 80 mV), though only at depolarized potentials of >40 mV. In agreement with this observation, Conforti et al. (44) found that Kv1.2 current was significantly inhibited by hypoxia in *Xenopus* oocytes. In contrast, when expressed in B82 cells, Kv1.2 current was not affected by hypoxia (15). Here again the importance of the expression system used to study hypoxia sensitivity is emphasized. Although these results suggest that Kv1.2 current is O_2-sensitive, at least in some preparations, because it does not activate in the voltage range of the PASMC resting membrane potential (37) and because of its sensitivity to CTX, it is unlikely that Kv1.2 homomeric channels underlie an O_2-sensitive current in PASMCs.

E. The Kv1.2/Kv1.5 Heteromeric Channel

When coexpressed, Kv1.2 and Kv1.5 assemble to form a functional heteromeric channel with kinetic and pharmacological properties distinct from those displayed by Kv1.2 and Kv1.5 homomeric channels (37). This heteromeric channel produces a delayed-rectifier current that is sensitive to 4-AP but insensitive to CTX (1). Noting that the Kv1.2/Kv1.5 current meets the characteristics of the O_2-sensitive K^+ current in PASMCs, Hulme et al. (37) examined the O_2 sensitivity of this channel. When expressed in L-cells, Kv1.2/Kv1.5 whole-cell current was reversibly inhibited by hypoxia (18% reduction at 80 mV) (37). Furthermore, in support of a role for Kv1.2/Kv1.5 current in the physiological response of PASMCs to hypoxia, this current was significantly inhibited by hypoxia in the voltage range of the PASMC resting membrane potential as shown in Fig. 3. For example, hypoxia inhibited the heteromeric current by ~65% at −40 mV (37). Although there is no direct evidence that this heteromeric channel is expressed in vivo, both individual subunits have been detected in PASMCs (3,4,37).

F. The Kv3.1b Channel

The effect of hypoxia on Kv3.1b was examined by Osipenko et al. (15). Hypoxia significantly and consistently reduced the whole-cell current amplitude in L929 cells expressing Kv3.1b channels by 24% at 40 mV (15). Furthermore, an inhibitory effect of hypoxia was demonstrated at the single-channel

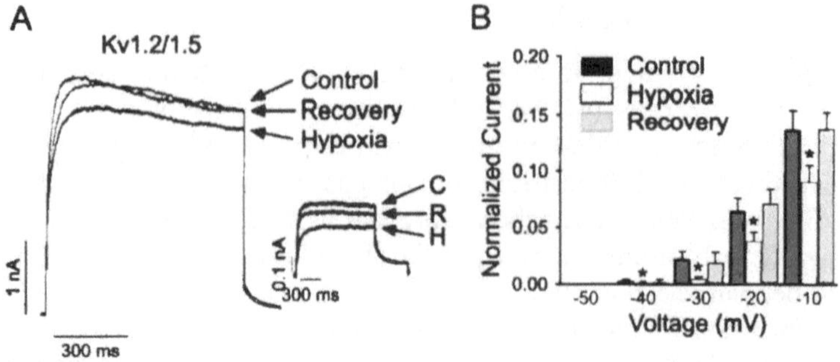

Figure 3 Hypoxia sensitivity of the Kv1.2/1.5 heteromeric channel. (A) Representative transfected L-cell currents elicited in response to step depolarization from −80 mV to 80 mV before, during, and after 10 min of exposure to hypoxic solution. Inset shows representative Kv1.2/Kv1.5 currents recorded at −20 mV before, during, and after 10 min of exposure to hypoxic solution. (B) Bar graph highlighting effect of hypoxia on Kv1.2/Kv1.5 current at more negative potentials. (Data shown are presented in greater detail in Ref. 37.)

level and in membrane patches excised from the cell. However, the inhibitory effect of hypoxia was apparent only at positive potentials. These results clearly demonstrate that Kv3.1b is O_2-sensitive; however, when expressed alone as a homotetramer it is not likely to be a component of the PASMC O_2-sensitive K^+ current. Also in support of a role for Kv3.1b in O_2 sensing in the pulmonary artery, data from our laboratory for the bovine pulmonary artery indicate that expression of Kv3.1b protein is markedly increased in the 3rd and 4th intrapulmonary resistance arteries in comparison with the main conduit pulmonary (43).

Taken together, these studies support a potential role for Kv2.1/Kv9.3 and Kv1.2/Kv1.5 heteromeric channels in the physiological response of PASMC K^+ channel to hypoxia. The Kv3.1b α subunit is also a strong candidate; although the homotetrameric Kv3.1b channel is not activated near the PASMC resting membrane potential. However, association of Kv3.1b with other α subunits to form heteromeric channels, or β-subunit assocation, may shift the activation of Kv3.1b-containing channel complexes to more hyperpolarized potentials in vivo, thereby accounting for the physiological response of PASMCs to hypoxia. It is not clear if Kv channels other than those mentioned above contribute significantly to the O_2 K^+ current. Kv1.1, Kv1.3, and Kv1.5 currents were not O_2-sensitive in all cell systems studied (15,37). The O_2 sensitivity of Kv1.4 has not been examined; however, there is some controversy as to whether it is even expressed in PASMCs, and, because it produces an A-type current, it does not meet the biophysical profile of the O_2-sensitive K^+ current in PASMCs.

IV. CALCIUM CHANNELS AND HYPOXIA

A. Calcium Channel Structure

Unlike K^+ channels, in which tetramers of α subunits form the channel, the Ca^{2+} channel α_1 subunit is a single polypeptide with four homologous repeats (I–IV), each containing six transmembrane-spanning domains (S1–S6) (46). The N- and C-termini are intracellular, as are the linkers between the repeat domains. As in Kv channels, the S4 of each repeat is the putative voltage sensor and the P-loop between S5 and S6 forms the ion-conducting pore (46). To date, 10 Ca^{2+} channel α_1-subunit genes have been cloned, and splice variants within each gene lend additional diversity to the voltage-gated Ca^{2+} channels (36). Ca^{2+} channels are functionally divided into two classes based loosely on their voltage dependence of factivation.

The high-voltage-activated (HVA) channels, as their name implies, are activated at more depolarized potentials than the LVA channels. Seven α_1 subunits have been identified so far in the HVA class. The first HVA channels identified were the L-type (long-lasting) Ca^{2+} channels in skeletal muscle. There are now at least three L-type channels identified: α_{1S} ($Ca_v1.1$), α_{1C} ($Ca_v1.2$), and α_{1D} ($Ca_v1.3$) [a fourth, α_{1F} ($Ca_v1.4$), has been cloned but not yet characterized (36)]. Four β-subunit genes, with numerous splice variants, encode cytoplasmic proteins that modulate expression of α_1 subunits and biophysical properties such as voltage dependence, kinetics of activation and inactivation, and current magnitude. Additionally, Ca^{2+} channels coassemble with α_2 and δ subunits, and some channels also have a γ subunit (46).

The L-channels are characterized by their slow activation and inactivation kinetics and by their pharmacology; they are also known as dihydropyridine receptors because of their sensitivity to modulation by dihydropyridines such as nifedipine (an antagonist) and Bay K8644 (an agonist) (46). The $Ca_v1.2$ L-channel is often referred to as the cardiac L-type Ca^{2+} channel because of its high level of expression in the heart and its key role in cardiac excitation–contraction coupling. It is widely expressed in other tissues and is expressed in pulmonary vascular smooth muscle, where it likely represents the primary Ca^{2+} influx pathway. Opening of L-channels results in Ca^{2+} influx and vasoconstriction, whereas block of Ca^{2+} channels results in vasodilation. Both in the heart and in arterial smooth muscle, the cardiac L-channel is modulated through the β-adrenergic pathway (47). Other, non-L-type, voltage-gated Ca^{2+} channels include. P/Q-type (α_{1A}; $Ca_v2.1$), N-type (α_{1B}; $Ca_v2.2$), and R-type (α_{1E}; $Ca_v2.3$) (36). Expression of P/Q-type channels has been demonstrated in rat aorta and renal arteries (48); however, none of these Ca^{2+} channels have been identified in pulmonary vascular smooth muscle. Therefore, they will not be discussed further here.

The low-voltage-activated (LVA) channels are those with an activation threshold around −40 mV, requiring only small depolarizations of the membrane. Also called T-type (for transient) channels, their activation and inactivation kinetics are faster than those of the high-voltage-activated (HVA) channels. So far, three LVA α_1 subunits have been identified: α_{1G} ($Ca_v3.1$), α_{1H} ($Ca_v3.2$), and α_{1I} (Ca_v 3.3) (36). T-channels are widely expressed in many tissues, being highly expressed in neurons and also expressed in smooth muscle, cardiac muscle, and some endocrine tissues (49).

B. O_2 Sensitivity of Voltage-Gated Calcium Channels

T-type channels are O_2-sensitive. When expressed in HEK-293 cells, α_{1H} and α_{1I} both exhibited sensitivity to changes in O_2 tension, whereas α_{1G} was relatively insensitive to hypoxic conditions (50). In this study, hypoxia did not alter the voltage dependence or kinetics of activation or inactivation, affecting only peak current levels. Although T-channel expression has been demonstrated in the lung, none of the LVA α_1 subunits have been specifically identified in the pulmonary vasculature.

There is also increasing evidence to suggest that α_{1C} is also regulated by Po_2. In systemic and coronary arteries, as well as in pulmonary conduit arteries, decreases in Po_2 (hypoxia) cause a decrease in nifedipine-sensitive Ca^{2+} current (51). This is consistent with the vasodilatory response of these artery types to hypoxia. Fearon et al. (52) identified differences in the hypoxia sensitivity of three different splice variants of the human α_{1C}ex-ressed in HEK-293 cells. The presence of a 71-amino-acid insert within the C-terminus of the hHT splice variant was necessary for the attenuation of L-current in response to hypoxia; Fearon et al. further narrowed the important region down to 39 residues that were critical for the O_2-sensing capability of the hHT L-channel, suggesting that for the cardiac L-channel O_2 sensitivity is an intrinsic property of the channel and may not require accessory subunits or other regulatory pathways.

The L-currents in resistance pulmonary arterial myocytes also exhibit O_2 sensitivity, suggesting that these channels may play a role in HPV. Under conditions of decreased Po_2, the Ca^{2+} currents in resistance myocytes are reversibly potentiated, resulting in vasoconstriction (51). These potentiated currents are blocked by nifedipine, confirming that they originate through L-channels. The nature of the differential response of conduit and resistance arterial Ca^{2+} channels to hypoxia remains unknown. Possible explanations for the difference include expression of distinct splice variants, differential expression of β subunits, or other unidentified regulatory pathways.

V. HYPOXIA-SENSITIVE KV CURRENTS IN NATIVE PASMCs

A. Antibody Dissection of the O_2-Sensitive Kv Current

Inclusion of antibodies against Kv channels in the intracellular pipette solution has been used as a method to dissect the O_2-sensitive K^+ current in PASMCs during whole-cell recordings in normoxic and hypoxic conditions.

When Archer et al. (4) added anti-Kv2.1 to the patch pipette, they found inhibition of outward K^+ current and membrane depolarization in rat resistance PASMCs, suggesting that Kv2.1 plays a role in setting the resting membrane potential. When anti-Kv1.5 was added to the patch pipette, whole-cell K^+ current was significantly decreased, and both the hypoxia and 4-AP-induced increase in intracellular Ca^{2+} concentration of isolated PASMCs were attenuated (4). However, anti-Kv1.5 did not consistently depolarize the membrane in isolated PASMCs. Based on their findings, the Archer group hypothesized that hypoxic inhibition of Kv2.1 leads to membrane depolarization, which shifts the resting membrane potential into a range where Kv1.5 is active and can thus be inhibited by hypoxia, leading to further inhibition of whole-cell K^+ current (4). Somewhat contrary to the Archer results, Hogg et al. (53) reported that in rat PASMCs the majority of the hypoxia-sensitive current is due to Kv2.1 in that anti-Kv2.1 antibodies reduce outward current under normoxic conditions and also prevent hypoxic regulation of Kv current. Thus, these data argue that Kv2.1 has a more central role than Kv1.5.

In related studies, Conforti et al. (44) used an antibody against Kv1.2 in the patch pipette to specifically inhibit Kv1.2 current in rat pheochromocytoma (PC12) cells (a model for oxygen sensing in the carotid body). They found no additional K^+ current inhibition in cells exposed to hypoxia, suggesting that the Kv1.2 current was responsible for the hypoxic effect in PC12 cells.

B. Altered Hypoxia-Sensitive Kv Current in Kv1.5-Null Mice

Further evidence to support a role for Kv1.5 in oxygen sensing in native PASMCs comes from the SWAP mouse generated in the London laboratory (54). To selectively delete Kv1.5, Kv1.5 was swapped with Kv1.1 (Kv1.1 behind the Kv1.5 promoter). Whereas expression of Kv1.5 was knocked out in the heart and lungs of these mice, the inserted transgenic rat Kv1.1 gene was expressed only in the heart, suggesting that the SWAP mouse is actually a targeted deletion of Kv1.5 in the lung (54).

If Kv1.5 is an O_2-sensitive K^+ channel that is involved in the hypoxic response in the resistance arteries of the pulmonary vasculature, then HPV should be altered in the lungs of the SWAP mouse. In accordance with this hypothesis, Archer et al. (54) found that HPV was significantly reduced but pulmonary arterial pressure was no different under normoxic conditions between the SWAP mice and wild-type mice. Additionally, PASMCs from the SWAP mice had lower I_K under normoxic conditions, consistent with the deletion of Kv1.5, and the O_2-sensitive component of these currents was smaller in the SWAP mice than in wild-type controls (54). Furthermore, both the HPV response and the hypoxia-sensitive I_K were restored following adenovirus-mediated restoration of Kv1.5 (55).

These results are consistent with Kv1.5 being an O_2-sensitive channel, although it cannot be determined from these studies whether the native O_2-sensitive current ascribed to Kv1.5 comes from homomeric Kv1.5 channels or complexes of Kv1.5 and Kv1.2. Furthermore, the hypoxia-sensitive current in the Kv1.5 knockout mice is not completely eliminated; therefore, a role of other Kv α subunits, such as Kv1.2, Kv2.1, or Kv3.1b, remains likely.

VI. MECHANISMS OF O_2 SENSING

A. Role of Kv β Subunits in O_2 Sensing

When the conserved core of Kvβ2.1 was crystallized, NADPH was detected within the solved crystal structure (39). The three-dimensional structure of the Kvβ2.1 subunit also demonstrates striking similarity to the structure of aldo-keto reductases, further suggesting that the β-subunit may couple the cellular redox state to Kv channel function (39). It has therefore been hypothesized that Kv β subunits may play a role in cellular redox sensing (39).

Multiple Kv β subunits have been detected in PASMCs. Yuan et al. (3), using RT-PCR of rat primary cultured resistance PASMCs, detected mRNA expression of Kvβ1.1, Kvβ1.2, and Kvβ2.1. Data from our laboratory indicate that Kvβ1.1, Kvβ1.2, and Kvβ1.3 proteins are expressed in bovine PASMCs (43). Furthermore, our data also suggest that protein expression of these β subunits dramatically increases as one moves from the main conduit pulmonary artery into the 3rd and 4th intrapulmonary resistance arteries. This expression gradient is interesting in light of the fact that resistance pulmonary arteries constrict in response to hypoxia whereas conduit pulmonary arteries do not (1), suggesting that Kv β-subunit expression may be partially responsible for the differential effects of hypoxia on conduit and resistance pulmonary arteries.

The Kv β subunit confers O_2 sensitivity to certain Kv α subunits. In HEK-293 cells, Kv4.2 alone was unaffected by hypoxia, but when coexpressed with Kvβ1.2 the current was significantly reduced (15.5% inhibition at 40 mV) (41). Kv β subunits do bind NADPH, and the cytoplasmic levels of NAD^+modulate Kv α/β functional interactions (56). In agreement with this finding is the fact that the mouse L-cells, used in one of the more extensive studies of the hypoxia sensitivity of cloned channels, endogenously express the Kvβ2.1 subunit (57). The NAD^+/NADPH ratio is sensitive to oxygen concentration, so the Kv β subunits may play a direct role in hypoxia sensing. Unfortunately, this idea has yet to be tested directly, i.e., no group has yet mutated the NADPH binding or catalytic sites and then determined hypoxia sensitivity, even though these mutations have been made and β effects such as trafficking and inactivation examined (58–60). Finally, there is no evidence that Kv2.1 or Kv3.1 α subunits assemble with

Kv β subunits (61), suggesting that even if Kv1 subfamily members sense hypoxia via β subunits, other Kv channels may respond via a different mechanism.

B. Membrane-Bound Heme-Linked Protein and/or NADPH Oxidase Mechanisms of O_2 Sensing

One possible explanation for the O_2 sensitivity of voltage-gated K^+ channels is the existence of a membrane-bound heme-linked protein closely associated with the channel. One possibility is that the binding of oxygen to the putative sensor directly modulates the K^+ current. Alternatively, hypoxia could decrease the production of reactive oxygen species (ROS) generated by a membrane-bound NADPH oxidase, modulating the channel through a redox mechanism (see Refs. 1 and 45). In support of a membrane-bound O_2 sensor, Kv channel inhibition has been demonstrated in excised patches from type I cells of the carotid body (1) as well as in heterologous expression systems (1,15,41). Furthermore, carbon monoxide, which in biological systems is only known to react with heme proteins, significantly reverses the hypoxic inhibition of Kv channels expressed in HEK cells (41) and in rabbit carotid body type I cells (1).

In the second hypothesis, the heme protein complex contains an NADPH oxidase that rapidly generates superoxide and H_2O_2 under normoxic conditions, creating a relatively oxidized redox state (1). During hypoxia there is less substrate for the oxidase, leading to decreased production of ROS, a more reduced state, and downregulation of redox-dependent Kv channels (1). Indeed, K^+ channel activity can be regulated by redox modulation in vitro (62,63). In support of the NADPH oxidase hypothesis, reducing agents such as dithiothreitol (DTT), reduced glutathione (GSH), and NADH mimic the effects of hypoxia on PASMCs by decreasing K^+ current (1), whereas oxidizing agents such as diamide and oxidized GSH (GSSH) increase K^+ current (1,64). NADPH oxidase is expressed in a variety of O_2-sensitive tissues, including pulmonary airway chemoreceptor cells (neuroepithelial body cells), carotid body, and PASMCs (1). Diphenyleneiodonium (DPI), an inhibitor of NADPH oxidase, has been shown to significantly inhibit HPV in isolated rat lungs, rabbit lungs, and rat pulmonary arteries (1). However, because it has been shown to inhibit both K^+ and Ca^{2+} currents, DPI has been criticized as not being a useful tool in evaluating the importance of NADPH oxidase in O_2 sensing (1). Furthermore, although DPI inhibits HPV, it does not cause sustained vasoconstriction under normoxic conditions (1).

Two independent groups of investigators used an NADPH oxidase-deficient mouse model to examine the role of NADPH oxidase in O_2 sensing. These groups studied the effects of hypoxia on K^+ current in neuroepithelial body (NEB) cells (65) and PASMCs (66) from these knockout mice and found very different results. Hypoxia had no effect on the K^+ current in NEB cells from oxidase-deficient mice, but it significantly inhibited the K^+ current in NEB cells from wild-type mice (65). Additionally, DPI significantly reduced the K^+ current by 30% in wild-type NEB cells but had no effect in oxidase-deficient NEB cells. These results clearly support a role for NADPH oxidase as an O_2 sensor in pulmonary airway chemoreceptors. In contrast are the results of Archer et al. (66) for PASMCs in the same mouse model. Although they found the production of ROS to be significantly lower in the lungs of oxidase-deficient mice than in the lungs of wild-type mice, there was no significant difference in the hypoxic inhibition of K^+ current between PASMCs from wild-type and oxidase-deficient animals. These data suggest that NADPH oxidase is not necessary for O_2 sensing in PASMCs. However, the NADPH gp91^{phox} knockout mouse experiments do not exclude a role for a "low-output" NADPH oxidase isoform (1). These seemingly contradictory results with the NADPH oxidase knockout mouse emphasize the complexity of O_2 sensing and argue for a diversity of O_2-sensing mechanisms between tissues.

C. Modulation of HPV by Protein Kinase C

There is growing evidence suggesting a role of protein kinase C (PKC) in the regulation of HPV in PASMCs, possibly by modulating K^+ channels. In one study, the PKC inhibitors staurosporine, calphostin C, and Gö-6976 blocked HPV as measured by changes in hypoxic pressor reponses (67), implicating a role of specific PKC isozymes in the initiation of HPV. A more specific approach was used by Littler et al. (68), who investigated the role of PKC in HPV using a PKC-ε knockout mouse. The lungs from the PKC-ε-null mice showed a significantly attenuated response to acute hypoxia compared to lungs from wild-type mice. Vasoconstriction in response to vasopressors such as angiotensin II was unaltered, indicating that the decrease in vasoconstriction following hypoxic challenge is specific to the absence of PKC-ε rather than an artifact of the knockout. Expression of Kv3.1b, which is O_2-sensitive in heterologous expression systems, was slightly upregulated in the PKC-ε-null mice in both whole lung and isolated PASMCs. The authors did not examine the impact of the PKC deletion on Kv3.1b function or the effects of PKC on other O_2-sensitive channels known to be expressed in the pulmonary vasculature, such as Kv2.1 or Kv1.5. Still, these results are a promising step forward in elucidating the mechanism by which low Po_2 alters Kv channel function.

D. Is Altered Channel Trafficking Involved in Hypoxia-Induced Inhibition of Kv Currents?

A growing literature suggests that PKC-mediated events regulate membrane protein surface expression by controlling the rates at which protein shuttles through the cell surface–endosome pathway. For example, PKC activation increases the delivery of NMDA receptors to the cell surface via a SNARE -dependent process (69), dopamine transporters are internalized into an endosomal compartment in response to PKC activation (70), GABA receptor internalization is enhanced by PKC activation (71), and Glut-2 glucose transporters are moved to the cell surface after PKC activation (72). Along these lines, our preliminary experiments using voltage-clamp analysis, cell surface channel labeling, and organelle fractionation suggest that PKC activation modulates the cell-surface expression of Kv2.1 protein in the L-cell system (data not shown). Interestingly, Kv2.1 targets to a noncaveolar lipid raft (73), and raft domains are implicated as an important trafficking mechanism within the cell (74). Because hypoxia-sensitive currents are downregulated with no change in kinetic properties or voltage dependence, it is plausible that this downregulation is achieved via a rapid removal of channel protein from the cell surface.

E. Is Localization to Caveolae Involved in Hypoxia-Induced Inhibition of Kv1.5 Current?

Caveolae represent one type of lipid raft that forms an invagination at the cell surface (74). Localization of ion channels to caveolae and rapid regulation of caveolar neck opening could mediate a channel's electrical access to the cell surface. Such a mechanism would allow rapid regulation of the number of surface channels without having to rely on the usual mechanisms of membrane protein insertion or internalization. In fact, such a mechanism has been suggested for cardiac Na^+ channels, which are reported to reside within cardiac myocyte caveolae (75). Alternatively, because many ion channels are regulated directly by protein kinases and G proteins, and these signaling proteins are often localized to caveolae (76), it is reasonable to localize ion channels to regions that are enriched in signaling molecules. But most relevant to the pulmonary circulation, Martens et al. (77) showed that Kv1.5 targets to caveolar domains whereas Kv2.1 targets to a noncaveolar lipid raft (77). Although the relationship between raft localization of Kv channels and pulmonary physiology is currently unknown, it is obvious that this type of compartmentalization must be taken into account when examining the mechanisms underlying the link between hypoxia and VSMC membrane potential.

VII. CONCLUSIONS

We now have a reasonable understanding of the ion channels expressed in the pulmonary vasculature that regulate the resting membrane potential, Ca^{2+} influx, and hence contraction. The cloned channels expressed in the PASMCs whose properties resemble the native outward currents have been studied in heterologous expression systems with respect to their kinetics, pharmacology, voltage dependence, and hypoxia sensitivity. This work suggests that heteromeric complexes of Kv2.1/9.3 and Kv1.2/1.5 are the leading candidates for the endogenous hypoxia-sensitive currents. Kv3.1b is probably also involved but assembled with an unknown accessory subunit that modulates its voltage dependence. However, much remains to be done. The definitive experiments with respect to the role of the Kv β subunit as a direct redox sensor for Kv1 family channels have yet to be performed. Other important areas for future study include other potential mechanisms of hypoxia sensing and how the sensor is coupled to the observed decreases in outward current. Altered trafficking and caveolar localization may be the means by which current downregulation is achieved for some Kv channels. The expanded use of knockout mice, RNA inhibition technologies, and live cell imaging approaches will be needed to further advance this sometimes confusing, but highly significant, area of pulmonary physiology.

ACKNOWLEDGMENT

This work was supported in part by NIH grant HL49330.

REFERENCES

1. Coppock EA, Martens JR, Tamkun MM. Molecular basis of hypoxia-induced pulmonary vasoconstriction: role of voltage-gated K^+ channels. Am J Physiol Lung Cell Mol Physiol 2001; 281:L1–L12.
2. Ward JP, Aaronson PI. Mechanisms of hypoxic pulmonary vasoconstriction: can anyone be right? Respir Physiol 1999; 115:261–271.
3. Yuan XJ, Wang J, Juhaszova M, Golovina VA, Rubin LJ. Molecular basis and function of voltage-gated K^+ channels in pulmonary arterial smooth muscle cells. Am J Physiol 1998; 274:L621–L635.
4. Archer SL, Souil E, Dinh-Xuan AT, Schremmer B, Mercier JC, El Yaagoubi A, Nguyen-Huu L, Reeve HL, Hampl V. Molecular identification of the role of voltage-gated K^+ channels, Kv1.5 and Kv2.1, in hypoxic pulmonary vasoconstriction and control of resting membrane potential in rat pulmonary artery myocytes. J Clin Invest 1998; 101:2319–2330.
5. McMurtry IF, Davidson AB, Reeves JT, Grover RF. Inhibition of hypoxic pulmonary vasoconstriction by calcium antagonists in isolated rat lungs. Circ Res 1976; 38:99–104.
6. McMurtry IF. BAY K 8644 potentiates and A23187 inhibits hypoxic vasoconstriction in rat lungs. Am J Physiol 1985; 249:H741–H746.
7. Cornfield DN, Stevens T, McMurtry IF, Abman SH, Rodman DM. Acute hypoxia causes membrane depolarization and calcium influx in fetal pulmonary artery smooth muscle cells. Am J Physiol 1994; 266:L469–L475.

8. Franco-Obregon A, Lopez-Barneo J. Differential oxygen sensitivity of calcium channels in rabbit smooth muscle cells of conduit and resistance pulmonary arteries. J Physiol 1996; 491:511–518.
9. Lopez-Barneo J, Lopez-Lopez JR, Urena J, Gonzalez C. Chemotransduction in the carotid body: K^+ current modulated by PO_2 in type I chemoreceptor cells. Science 1988; 241:580–582.
10. Yuan XJ, Goldman WF, Tod ML, Rubin LJ, Blaustein MP. Hypoxia reduces potassium currents in cultured rat pulmonary but not mesenteric arterial myocytes. Am J Physiol 1993; 264:L116–L123.
11. Madden JA, Dawson CA, Harder DR. Hypoxia-induced activation in small isolated pulmonary arteries from the cat. J Appl Physiol 1985; 59:113–118.
12. Sham JSK, Crenshaw BR Jr, Deng LH, Shimoda LA, Sylvester JT. Effects of hypoxia in porcine pulmonary arterial myocytes: roles of K_V channel and endothelin-1. Am J Physiol Lung Cell Mol Physiol 2000; 279:L262–L272.
13. Park MK, Lee SH, Lee SJ, Ho WK, Earm YE. Different modulation of Ca-activated K channels by the intracellular redox potential in pulmonary and ear arterial smooth muscle cells of the rabbit. Pflügers Arch 1995; 430: 308–314.
14. Post JM, Hume JR, Archer SL, Weir EK. Direct role for potassium channel inhibition in hypoxic pulmonary vasoconstriction. Am J Physiol 1992; 262: C882–890.
15. Osipenko ON, Tate RJ, Gurney AM. Potential role for Kv3.1b channels as oxygen sensors. Circ Res 2000; 86:534–540.
16. Archer SL, Huang JMC, Reeve HL, Hampl V, Tolarova S, Michelakis E, Weir EK. Differential distribution of electrophysiologically distinct myocytes in conduit and resistance arteries determines their response to nitric oxide and hypoxia. Circ Res 1996; 78(3):431–442.
17. Post JM, Gelband CH, Hume JR. $[Ca^{2+}]_i$ inhibition of K^+ channels in canine pulmonary artery—novel mechanism for hypoxia-induced membrane depolarization. Circ Res 77:131–139.
18. Deal KK, England SK, Tamkun MM. Molecular physiology of cardiac potassium channels. Physiol Rev 1996; 76:49–67.
19. Korovkina VP, England SK. Molecular diversity of vascular potassium channel isoforms. Clin Exp Pharmacol Physiol 2002; 29:317–323.
20. Nelson MT, Quayle JM. Physiological roles and properties of potassium channels in arterial smooth muscle. Am J Physiol 1995; 37:C799-C822.
21. Osipenko ON, Evans AM, Gurney AM. Regulation of the resting potential of rabbit pulmonary artery myocytes by a low threshold, O_2-sensing potassium current. Br J Pharmacol 1997; 120:1461–1470.
22. Yuan XJ. Voltage-gated K^+ currents regulate resting membrane potential and $[Ca^{2+}]i$ in pulmonary arterial myocytes. Circ Res 1995; 77:370–378.
23. Lewis A, Peers C, Ashford ML, Kemp PJ. Hypoxia inhibits human recombinant large conductance, Ca^{2+}-activated K^+ (maxi-K) channels by a mechanism which is membrane delimited and Ca^{2+} sensitive. J Physiol 2002; 540:771–780.
24. Lewis A, Hartness ME, Chapman CG, Fearon IM, Meadows HJ, Peers C, et al. Recombinant hTASK1 is an O_2-sensitive K^+ channel. Biochem Biophys Res Commun 2001; 285:1290–1294.

25. Lesage F, Guillemare E, Fink M, Duprat F, Lazdunski M, Romey G, Barhanin J. TWIK-1, a ubiquitous human weakly inward rectifying K^+ channel with a novel structure. EMBO J 1996; 15:1004–1011.
26. Gurney AM, Osipenko ON, MacMillan D, Kempsill FE. Potassium channels underlying the resting potential of pulmonary artery smooth muscle cells. Clin Exp Pharmacol Physiol 2002; 29:330–333.
27. Hartness ME, Lewis A, Searle GJ, O'Kelly I, Peers C, Kemp PJ. Combined antisense and pharmacological approaches implicate hTASK as an airway O_2 sensing K^+ channel. J Biol Chem 2001; 276:26499–26508.
28. Buckler KJ, Williams BA, Honore E. An oxygen-, acid- and anaesthetic-sensitive TASK-like background potassium channel in rat arterial chemoreceptor cells. J Physiol 2000; 525:135–142.
29. Osipenko ON, Alexander D, MacLean MR, Gurney AM. Influence of chronic hypoxia on the contributions of non-inactivating and delayed rectifier K currents to the resting potential and tone of rat pulmonary artery smooth muscle. Br J Pharmacol 1998; 124:1335–1337.
30. Evans AM, Osipenko ON, Haworth SG, Gurney AM. Resting potentials and potassium currents during development of pulmonary artery smooth muscle cells. Am J Physiol 1998; 275:H887–H899.
31. Okabe K, Kitamura K, Kuriyama H. Features of 4-aminopyridine sensitive outward current observed in single smooth muscle cells from the rabbit pulmonary artery. Pflügers Arch 1987; 409:561–568.
32. Smirnov SV, Robertson TP, Ward JP, Aaronson PI. Chronic hypoxia is associated with reduced delayed rectifier K^+ current in rat pulmonary artery muscle cells. Am J Physiol 1994; 266:H365–H370.
33. Yuan XJ, Tod ML, Rubin LJ, Blaustein MP. Hypoxic and metabolic regulation of voltage-gated K^+ channels in rat pulmonary artery smooth muscle cells. Exp Physiol 1995; 80:803–813.
34. Doi S, Damron DS, Ogawa K, Tanaka S, Horibe M, Murray PA. K^+ channel inhibition, calcium signaling, and vasomotor tone in canine pulmonary artery smooth muscle. Am J Physiol Lung Cell Mol Physiol 2000; 279: L242–L251.
35. Hulme JT, Martens JR, Navarro-Polanco RA, Nishiyama A, Tamkun MM. Voltage-gated potassium channels in the myocardium. In Archer SL, Rusch NJ, eds. Potassium channels in cardiovascular biology. New York: Kluwer Academic, 2001:337–362.
36. Catterall WA, Chandy KG, Gutman GA. The IUPHAR compendium of Voltage-Gated Ion Channels. 2002, Leeds: IUPHAR Media, 2002.
37. Hulme JT, Coppock EA, Felipe A, Martens JR, Tamkun MM. Oxygen sensitivity of cloned voltage-gated K^+ channels expressed in the pulmonary vasculature. Circ Res 1999; 85:489–497.
38. Patel AJ, Lazdunski M, Honoré E. Kv2.1/Kv2.1 Kv9.3, a novel ATP-dependent delayed-rectifier K^+ channel in oxygen-sensitive pulmonary artery myocytes. EMBO J 1997; 16:6615–6625.
39. Gulbis JM, Mann S, MacKinnon R. Structure of a voltage-dependent K^+ channel β subunit Cell 1999; 97:943–952.

40. Martens JR, Kwak YG, Tamkun MM. Modulation of Kv channel α/β subunit interactions. Trends Cardiovasc Med 1999; 9:253–258.
41. Perez-Garcia MT, Lopez-Lopez JR, Gonzalez C. Kvβ1.2 subunit coexpression in HEK293 cells confers O_2 sensitivity to Kv4.2 but not to Shaker channels. J Gen Physiol 1999; 113:897–907.
42. Wang J, Juhaszova M, Rubin LJ, Yuan XJ. Hypoxia inhibits gene expression of voltage-gated K^+ channel α subunits in pulmonary artery smooth muscle cells. J Clin Invest 1997; 100:2347–2353.
43. Coppock EA, Tamkun MM. Differential expression of K_V channel α- and β-subunits in the bovine pulmonary arterial circulation. Am J Physiol Lung Cell Mol Physiol 2001; 281:L1350–L1360.
44. Conforti L, Bodi I, Nisbet JW, Millhorn DE. O_2-sensitive K^+ channels: role of the Kv1.2-subunit in mediating the hypoxic response. J Physiol. 2000; 524: 783–793.
45. Archer SL, Weir EK, Reeve HL, Michelakis E. Molecular identification of O_2 sensors and O_2-sensitive potassium channels in the pulmonary circulation. Adv Exp Med Biol 2000:475219–475240.
46. Catterall WA. Structure and regulation of voltage-gated Ca^{2+}channels. Annu Rev Cell Dev Biol 2000:16521–16555.
47. Nelson MT, Patlak JB, Worley JF, Standen NB. Calcium channels, potassium channels, and voltage dependence of arterial smooth muscle tone. Am J Physiol 1990; 259:C3–C18.
48. Hansen PB, Jensen BL, Andreasen D, Friis UG, Skott O. Vascular smooth muscle cells express the α_{1A} subunit of a P/Q-type voltage-dependent Ca^{2+} channel, and it is functionally important in renal afferent arterioles. Circ Res 2000; 87:896–902.
49. Perez-Reyes E. Molecular physiology of low-voltage-activated T-type calcium channels. Physiol Rev 2003; 83:117–161.
50. Fearon IM, Randall AD, Perez-Reyes E, Peers C. Modulation of recombinant T-type Ca^{2+} channels by hypoxia and glutathione. Pflügers Arch 2000; 441: 181–188.
51. Lopez-Barneo J, Pardal R, Montoro RJ, Smani T, Garcia-Hirschfeld J, Urena J. K^+ and Ca^{2+} channel activity and cytosolic $[Ca^{2+}]$ in oxygen-sensing tissues. Respir Physiol 1999; 115:215–227.
52. Fearon IM, Varadi G, Koch S, Isaacsohn I, Ball SG, Peers C. Splice variants reveal the region involved in oxygen sensing by recombinant human L-type Ca^{2+} channels. Circ Res 2000; 87:537–539.
53. Hogg DS, Davies AR, McMurray G, Kozlowski RZ. K_V2.1 channels mediate hypoxic inhibition of I_{KV} in native pulmonary arterial smooth muscle cells of the rat. Cardiovasc Res 2002; 55:349–360.
54. Archer SL, London B, Hampl V, Wu X, Nsair A, Puttagunta L, Hashimoto K, Waite RE, Michelakis ED. Impairment of hypoxic pulmonary vasoconstriction in mice lacking the voltage-gated potassium channel Kv1.5. FASEB J 2001; 15:1801–1803.
55. Pozeg ZI, Michelakis ED, McMurtry MS, Thebaud B, Wu XC, Dyck JR, Hashimoto K, Wang S, Moudgil R, Harry G, Sultanian R, Koshal A, Archer SL. In vivo gene transfer of the O_2-sensitive potassium channel Kv1.5

reduces pulmonary hypertension and restores hypoxic pulmonary vasoconstriction in chronically hypoxic rats. Circulation 2003; 107:2037–2044.
56. Bhatnagar A, Kumar R, Tipparaju SM, Liu SQ. Differential pyridine nucleotide coenzyme binding to the beta-subunit of the voltage-sensitive K^+ channel: a mechanism for redox regulation of excitability? Chem Biol Intereact 2003; 143:144613–144620.
57. Uebele VN, England SK, Chaudhary A, Tamkun MM, Snyders DJ. Functional differences in Kv1.5 currents expressed in mammalian cell lines are due to the presence of endogenous Kvβ2.1 subunits. J Biol Chem 1996; 271:2406–2412.
58. Bahring R, Milligan CJ, Vardanyan V, Engeland B, Young BA, Dannenberg J, Waldshütz R, Edwards JP, Wray D, Pongs O. Coupling of voltage-dependent potassium channel inactivation and oxidoreductase active site of Kvβ subunits. J Biol Chem 2001; 276:22923–22929.
59. Campomanes CR, Carroll KI, Manganas LN, Hershberger ME, Gong B, Antonucci DE, Rhodes KJ, Trimmer JS. Kvβ subunit oxidoreductase activity and Kv1 potassium channel trafficking. J Biol Chem 2002; 277:8298–8305.
60. Peri R, Wible BA, Brown AM. Mutations in the Kvβ2 binding site for NADPH and their effects on Kv1.4. J Biol Chem 2001; 276:738–741.
61. Nakahira K, Shi GY, Rhodes KJ, Trimmer JS. Selective interaction of voltage-gated K^+ channel β-subunits with α-subunits. J Biol Chem 1996; 271:7084–7089.
62. Duprat F, Guillemare E, Romey G, Fink M, Lesage F, Lazdunski M. Honore E. Susceptibility of cloned K^+ channels to reactive oxygen species. Proc Natl Acad Sci USA 1995; 92:11796–11800.
63. Ruppersberg JP, Stocker M, Pongs O, Heinemann SH, Frank R, Koenen M. Regulation of fast inactivation of cloned mammalian $I_k(A)$ channels by custeine oxidation. Nature 1991; 352:711–714.
64. Park MK, Lee SH, Ho WK, Earm YE. Redox agents as a link between hypoxia and the responses of ionic channels in rabbit pulmonary vascular smooth muscle. Exp Physiol 1995; 80:835–842.
65. Fu XW, Wang D, Nurse CA, Dinauer MC, Cutz E. NADPH oxidase is an O_2 sensor in airway chemoreceptors: evidence from K^+ current modulation in wild-type and oxidase-deficient mice. Proc Natl Acad Sci USA 2000; 97: 4374–4379.
66. Archer SL, Reeve HL, Michelakis E, Puttagunta L, Waite R, Nelson DP, Dinauer MC, Weir EK. O_2 sensing is preserved in mice lacking the gp91 phox subunit of NADPH oxidase. Proc Natl Acad Sci USA. 1999; 96:7944–7949.
67. Barman SA. Effect of protein kinase C inhibition on hypoxic pulmonary vasoconstriction. Am J Physiol Lung Cell Mol Physiol 2001; 280:L888–L895.
68. Littler CM, Morris KG Jr, Fagan KA, McMurtry IF, Messing RO, Dempsey EC. Protein kinase C-epsilon-null mice have decreased hypoxic pulmonary vasoconstriction. Am J Physiol Heart Circ Physiol 2003; 284:H1321–H1331.
69. Lan JY, Skeberdis VA, Jover T, Grooms SY, Lin Y, Araneda RC, Zheng X, Bennett MV, Zulkin RS. Protein kinase C modulates NMDA receptor trafficking and gating. Nat Neurosci. 2001; 4:382–390.
70. Melikian HE, Buckley KM. Membrane trafficking regulates the activity of the human dopamine transporter. J Neurosci 1999; 19:7699–7710.

71. Cinar H, Barnes EM Jr. Clathrin-independent endocytosis of $GABA_A$ receptors in HEK 293 cells. Biochemistry 2001; 40:14030–14036.
72. Helliwell PA, Richardson M, Affleck J, Kellett GL. Stimulation of fructose transport across the intestinal brush-border membrane by PMA is mediated by GLUT2 and dynamically regulated by protein kinase C. Biochem J. 2000; 350:149–154.
73. Martens JR, Navarro-Polanco R, Coppock EA, Nishiyama A, Parshley L, Grobaski TD, Tamkun MM. Differential targeting of Shaker-like potassium channels to lipid rafts. J Biol Chem 2000; 275:7443–7446.
74. Anderson RG, Jacobson K. A role for lipid shells in targeting proteins to caveolae, rafts, and other lipid domains. Science 2002; 296:1821–1825.
75. Yarbrough TL, Lu T, Lee HC, Shibata EF. Localization of cardiac sodium channels in caveolin-rich membrane domains: regulation of sodium current amplitude. Circ Res 2002; 90:443–449.
76. Anderson RGW. The caveolae membrane system. Annu Rev Biochem 1998:67199–67225.
77. Martens JR, Sakamoto N, Sullivan SA, Grobaski TD, Tamkun MM. Isoform-specific localization of voltage-gated K^+ channels to distinct lipid raft populations. Targeting of Kv1.5 to caveolae. J Biol Chem 2001; 276:8409–8414.
78. Conforti L, Millhorn DE. Regulation of Shaker-type potassium channels by hypoxia. Oxygen-sensitive K^+ channels in PC12 cells. Adv Exp Med Biol 2000:475265–475274.

18

Hypoxia-Induced Modulation of O_2-Sensitive K^+ Channels in Pulmonary Vascular Smooth Muscle Cells

Carmelle V. Remillard, Oleksandr Platoshyn, Tiffany Sison, and Jason X.-J. Yuan

Department of Medicine, University of California, San Diego, California, U.S.A.

I. INTRODUCTION

The regulation of ion channel activity is key to the maintenance of cellular excitability in many cell types. In vascular smooth muscle, the activity of K^+ channels is essential to the control of membrane excitability in that K^+ channels are responsible for setting the resting membrane potential (RMP) at relatively negative membrane potentials (1). Alteration of K^+ channel activity or gene expression will therefore have a major impact on cell excitability. Indeed, dysfunctional ion channels permeable to K^+, Na^+, Ca^{2+}, and Cl^- have been involved in many forms of cardiovascular disease (2–5).

In both the systemic and pulmonary vasculature, K^+ channels play a particularly important role in controlling vascular tone. K^+ efflux through sarcolemmal K^+ channels has also been linked to apoptosis in many cell types, including pulmonary artery smooth muscle cells (PASMCs) (6,7). Previous chapters (Chapters 11–14) within this monograph have already characterized K^+ channel subtypes within the pulmonary vasculature. The preceding chapter, by O'Connell et al., explored the molecular identity and physiology of O_2-sensitive ion channels. This chapter will focus primarily on the effect of acute and chronic hypoxia on K^+ channel activity and function within the pulmonary vascular bed. We will also address the modulation of other ion channels by hypoxia in pulmonary arterial smooth muscle cells and endothelial cells.

II. K^+ CHANNELS AND THE REGULATION OF MEMBRANE POTENTIAL

Activity of K^+ channels plays a crucial role in modulating membrane potential (E_m) in both excitable and nonexcitable cells. In vascular smooth muscle cells, K^+ permeability across the plasma membrane, i.e., outward K^+ currents, determines and maintains E_m in the range of −70 to −50 mV, which is near the reversal potential for K^+ ions (E_K). The slight difference between E_m and E_K is due to the contribution of other outward currents (e.g., currents generated by Na^+ pumps and Na^+–Ca^{2+} exchangers) and inward currents (e.g., Na^+, Ca^{2+}, or Cl^- channels).

Agonist or receptor stimulation can result in membrane depolarization, i.e., a shift of E_m toward less negative and/or more positive potentials. In many situations, membrane depolarization drives E_m into a range of potentials where voltage-dependent Ca^{2+} channels (VDCCs) are activated. VDCC activation causes an influx of Ca^{2+} from the extracellular space, increasing cytoplasmic free Ca^{2+} concentration ($[Ca^{2+}]_{cyt}$) and ultimately causing contraction (8). In some cases, Ca^{2+} influx has also been linked to increased cellular proliferation (9). Voltage-dependent K^+ channels, such as the voltage-gated K^+ (Kv) channels (see Chapter 11) and Ca^{2+}-activated K^+ (K_{Ca}) channels (see Chapter 12) are also activated by membrane depolarization. Activation of K^+ channels shifts E_m toward more negative potential close to the E_K and causes membrane hyperpolarization, whereas inhibition of K^+ channels causes membrane depolarization and shifts E_m toward the threshold potentials for activating VDCCs. Therefore, "normal" activity of K^+ channels is essential for maintaining a rested state in vascular smooth muscle cells.

Five distinct K^+ channels have been identified in vascular smooth muscle (including PASMCs): Kv channels, K_{Ca} channels, inward rectifier K^+ (K_{IR}) channels, ATP-sensitive K^+ (K_{ATP}) channels, and tandem-pore two-domain K^+ (K_T) channels (1,10). In PASMCs, the activity of Kv (11–13), K_{Ca} (14), K_{ATP} (8,15), and K_T (16,17) channels appears to be important in the regulation of E_m. Indeed, many of these K^+ channels, in terms of both their subunit expression and their current characteristics, are modulated by hypoxia, as discussed further in the following sections and in Chapter 17.

III. ACUTE HYPOXIA DECREASES K^+ CHANNEL ACTIVITY

Acute alveolar hypoxia (<3 min) produces a relatively rapid cellular response that results in venous blood being diverted away from poorly

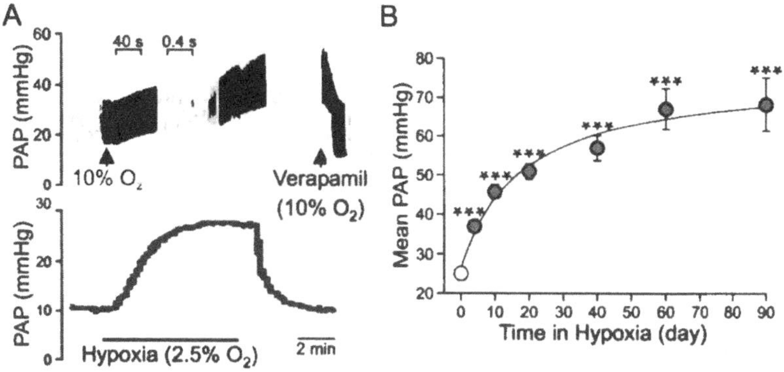

Figure 1 Acute and chronic hypoxia elevate pulmonary arterial pressure (PAP). (A) (Top panel) PAP was measured using a catheter positioned in the pulmonary artery in a rat before and during inhalation of 10% O_2 gas. Verapamil, a Ca^{2+} channel inhibitor, was injected via a femoral vein catheter during hypoxia (10% O_2). (Bottom panel) PAP was also measured in isolated, blood-perfused rat lungs in response to alveolar hypoxia (2.5% O_2). (Reproduced with permission from Ref. 126.) (B) Mean PAP was measured in rats exposed to room air (normoxic control, day 0) and in rats housed in a hypobaric hypoxia (10% O_2) chamber for 4, 10, 20, 40, 60, and 90 days. (***) $P < 0.001$ vs. day 0.

aerated regions of the lung to well-ventilated regions where adequate gas exchange can occur to maximize oxygenation of venous blood in the pulmonary artery. Because the redistribution of blood flow occurs within minutes of the onset of alveolar hypoxia, it is generally believed that the ensuing increase in pulmonary arterial pressure (PAP) (Fig. 1A) involves the modification of molecular and cellular machinery already present within the pulmonary vessels.

A. Hypoxic Pulmonary Vasoconstriction Requires Enhanced $[Ca^{2+}]_{cyt}$

The most prominent effect of acute hypoxia on the pulmonary vasculature is vasoconstriction. "Hypoxic pulmonary vasoconstriction" (HPV), as it is often called, is a phenomenon that is unique to the pulmonary vasculature (18). Many believe that HPV is intrinsic to individual PASMCs and that it is not endothelium-dependent (19–21). The mechanism(s) underlying HPV are elusive. Nonetheless, similar to the blockade of Kv channels, acute hypoxia does result in an increase in $[Ca^{2+}]_{cyt}$ (Fig. 2A). It is known that increased $[Ca^{2+}]_{cyt}$ is a major trigger for vasoconstriction, and Ca^{2+} influx through VDCCs is involved, at least in part, in acute hypoxia-mediated increase in

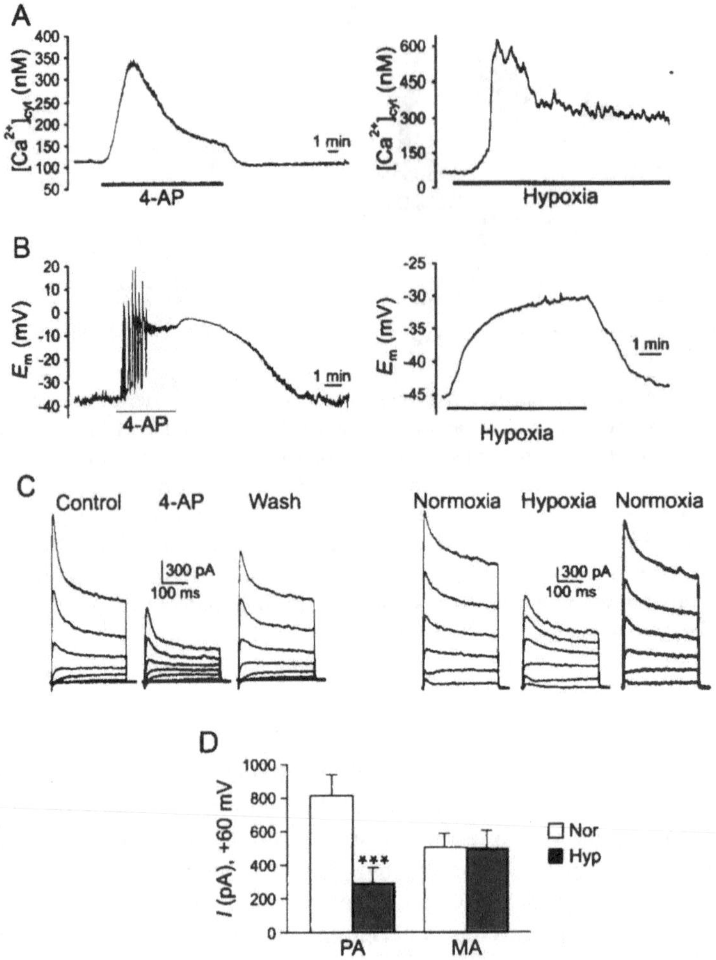

Figure 2 Modulation of $[Ca^{2+}]_{cyt}$, E_m, and K_V channels by 4-aminopyridine (4-AP) and acute hypoxia. Changes in $[Ca^{2+}]_{cyt}$ (A) and E_m (B) induced by 5 mM 4-AP and acute hypoxia (10% O_2) in PASMC. (C) Representative K^+ currents from PASMCs were elicited by test potentials ranging between −60 and +80 mV from a holding potential of −70 mV before, during, and after either application 5 mM 4-AP or a hypoxic challenge. (D) The bar graph summarizes the current amplitude measured at +60 mV in PASMCs (PA) and mesenteric artery smooth muscle cells (MA) under normoxic (Nor) and hypoxic (Hyp) conditions. (***) $P < 0.001$ vs. Nor. (Reproduced with permission from Refs. 35,38,113,124.)

$[Ca^{2+}]_{cyt}$ in PASMCs (22) (see the following section). In addition to Ca^{2+} influx through VDCCs, Ca^{2+} influx via voltage-independent Ca^{2+} channels (23) and capacitative Ca^{2+} entry (23) have been involved in increasing $[Ca^{2+}]_{cyt}$. Also, Ca^{2+} release from intracellular ryanodine-sensitive stores has been shown to be one of the initial steps contributing to HPV (24–27).

B. Membrane Depolarization and K^+ Channel Inhibition

Similar to the extracellular application of K^+ channel blocker 4-aminopyridine (4-AP), brief hypoxic episodes result in an increase in $[Ca^{2+}]_{cyt}$ (Fig. 2A) and membrane depolarization (Fig. 1B), and vasoconstriction ensues owing to activation of VDCCs. It is generally agreed upon that inhibition of Kv (and K_T) channels is the main trigger for the initial membrane depolarization induced by acute hypoxia. In PASMCs, acute hypoxia-induced depolarization has generally been associated with attenuation of Kv channel activity and a reduction in Kv current ($I_{K(V)}$) (Fig. 2C) (17,22, 28–37). The hypoxia-induced inhibitory effect on Kv channels appears to be selective to PASMCs; hypoxia has little effect on $I_{K(V)}$ in mesenteric artery smooth muscle cells (Fig. 2D) (35,38,39). Potential mechanisms by which acute hypoxia modulates Kv function are described in the following section.

Many isoforms of the voltage-independent and constitutively active K_T channels have been identified (10). In PASMCs, decreased K_T channel activity has been linked to the initial membrane depolarization and $[Ca^{2+}]_{cyt}$ rise observed during acute hypoxia (17,40). More recently, TASK-1, a pH- and oxygen-sensitive K_T channel isoform, was identified that could be responsible for the modulatory effect of pH on HPV (16).

Unlike K_T channels, K_{Ca} channels inhibition during acute hypoxia does not appear to be involved in triggering initial membrane depolarization. K_{Ca} channels are activated by membrane depolarization and a rise in $[Ca^{2+}]_{cyt}$, resulting in membrane hyperpolarization and vasodilation (1,41), a negative feedback response typical of K_{Ca} activation (1,42). However, acute hypoxia produces both membrane depolarization (e.g., due to inhibition of Kv and K_T channels) and Ca^{2+} transients in PASMCs, both of which, theoretically, should activate K_{Ca} to cause membrane repolarization and vasodilation. Nonetheless, vasoconstriction persists, implying that acute hypoxia indirectly inhibits K_{Ca} channel activity in PASMCs (30,33,43), potentially via the changes in the cell's redox state (43,44). However, there are still claims that K_{Ca} channels are activated by hypoxia (45), presumably due to the increase in intracellular Ca^{2+} levels during hypoxic challenges. There is also evidence that small-conductance K_{Ca} (SK_{Ca}) channels are inhibited by hypoxia (22). Nonetheless, acute hypoxic inhibition of K_{Ca} channels appears to be mediated by a factor that is either produced or released during hypoxia (22,44) rather than via a direct effect on channel function.

C. Mechanisms Involved in Acute-Hypoxia-Induced Inhibition of K_v Channels

A functional Kv channel is composed from four pore-forming α subunits and four regulatory β subunits. More than 20 highly homologous α subunits with different properties (pharmacology, kinetics, voltage sensitivity) have been identified in various tissues, including most types of vascular smooth muscles (46,47). Considering that the tetramers formed by these α subunits can be homomeric or heteromeric, the possible composition of native Kv channels is nearly impossible to discern. In most cells, including PASMCs, the channels are presumed to be heterotetramers of different α and β subunits (48,49).

Two hypotheses have been put forth in an attempt to characterize the mechanism by which Kv function is modulated by acute hypoxia. According to the "direct action" hypothesis, the Kv channel itself (either α or β subunit) acts as both the hypoxic sensor and effector; i.e., the Kv channel α and β subunits have amino acid residues that are sensitive to, and can be modulated by, changes in oxygen tension and redox status (50) without the need for intermediates. Studies showing that acute hypoxia reduces the current generated by recombinant Kv channels in heterologous transfection systems support this hypothesis (48,51,52) (see Chapters 11 and 17). However, studies have also shown that only currents generated by certain α subunit homotetramers (i.e., Kv1.2, Kv2.1, Kv3.2), α/α heterotetramers (i.e., Kv1.2/Kv1.5, Kv1.2/Kv9.3), or α/β heterotetramers (i.e., Kv1.2/Kvβ1.1, Kv1.5/Kvβ1.2) are altered by acute hypoxic challenges (31,51–53). Because of this, the "indirect action" hypothesis has also been put forth, proposing that acute hypoxia may cause the release or production of an intermediate or modulator (e.g., active oxygen species, endothelin-1, Ca^{2+}), which then acts upon Kv channels to modulate the currents (22,54,55). Potential elements that may modulate Kv function during acute hypoxia are discussed below.

Kv Channel β Subunits

By associating with the amino-terminal region of Kv α subunits (56,57), cytoplasmic Kv β subunits are known to modulate Kv channels in different ways (49): (1) conferring rapid inactivation onto noninactivation K_v channel α subunits (or converting noninactivating $I_{K(V)}$ into rapidly inactivating transient $I_{K(V)}$) (58) (2) modifying current kinetics (activation, deactivation) and peak amplitude by acting as an open channel blocker (56,59), and (3) participating in α subunit assembly and transport to the plasma membrane and enhancing subunit interactions with protein kinases (56,60). Its final role, the one most relevant to this discussion, is its ability to confer redox and O_2 sensitivity to Kv channels (49,61). The Kv β subunit shares homology with the NAD(P) H oxidoreductase (62), potentially allowing it to sense oxygen tension and thereby regulate channel gating properties (i.e., conductance, voltage dependence, kinetics, drug sensitivity, kinase regulation) inherent to the α subunit. In some cases, β subunits themselves have been shown to detect a decrease in oxygen tension (49,52,61), leading to direct physical interaction between the α and β subunits that results in Kv channel closure (or inactivation), membrane depolarization, Ca^{2+} influx and release from intracellular stores, and pulmonary vasoconstriction (48,51).

Redox Status and Oxygen Radicals

Reactive oxygen species (ROS) and reactive nitrogen species (RNS) produced during hypoxic challenges may also act as signaling molecules in altering Kv function. Because their production is dependent on a change in the redox status of the cell, it has been theorized that the mitochondrion (or some of its components) serves as an oxygen sensor in PASMCs. Although ROS can have a destructive effect on DNA, it has been suggested that low-level ROS generation can serve as a signaling pathway (63,64). Therefore, in a normal cell, the redox network contained within the mitochondria is constitutively active and ROS are constantly produced to maintain cellular homeostasis. When a stress such as acute hypoxia occurs, redox potential is disturbed, and the ROS may target the function or expression of ion channels or other channel modulatory proteins and disrupt cellular homeostasis.

Whether ROS levels themselves are elevated or decreased during hypoxia is controversial, and precisely how ROS mediate pulmonary vasoconstriction under hypoxic conditions is unclear. ROS and other oxidants, such as nitric oxide (NO), diamide, and hydrogen peroxide (H_2O_2) (44,65,66), have been shown to enhance K^+ channel activity, as opposed to reducing agents (e.g., dithiothreitol, reduced glutathione), which decrease K^+ currents (36,37,44,65,67) in PASMCs. Therefore, studies showing that acute hypoxia reduces ROS production and changes redox status in PASMCs (28) indicate that K^+ channels would be inhibited, leading to membrane depolarization and pulmonary vasoconstriction. However, others have demonstrated an increase in ROS (i.e., superoxide) and H_2O_2 production in acutely hypoxic microvascular PASMCs (63,64). The newly synthesized ROS and H_2O_2 then increase the release of Ca^{2+} from intracellular stores (25,64), which then inhibits Kv channels (22) and causes PASMC depolarization.

Metabolic Inhibition

The production of ATP is essential for maintaining normal cellular homeostasis. Oxidative phosphorylation and inhibition of glycolysis have been shown to induce or enhance pulmonary vasoconstriction, respectively (68,69), suggesting that alveolar hypoxia may reduce the phosphate potential ($ATP/[ADP+P_i]$), an indicator of the cells' energy status, by attenuating oxidative phosphorylation in PASMCs (68,69). Metabolic inhibitors such as 2-deoxy-D-glucose (36), carbonyl cyanide-ρ-trifluoromethoxyphenylhydrazone (FCCP) (37,41), rotenone (28,70), and antimycin A (28) decrease $I_{K(V)}$, much like acute hypoxia. On the other hand, intracellular application of ATP enhances $I_{K(V)}$ in PASMCs (71). Therefore, in addition to the global decrease in ATP production, acute hypoxia and/or metabolic inhibition may cause rapid depletion of highly localized ATP in certain regions of the cells or tissues (72). This change in energy status due to decreased ATP levels would cause membrane depolarization, Ca^{2+} influx, and pulmonary vasoconstriction subsequent to K^+ channel inhibition.

Cytochrome P450 and NAD(P) H-Dependent Oxidoreductase

The cytochrome P450 monooxygenase system (P450) is a family of heme-thiolate enzymes that catalyze oxidative reactions. P450 activity is dependent on a reducing agent, NADPH, and molecular oxygen. Its activation is oxygen-dependent, with half-saturation with oxygen occurring at oxygen pressures of 20–100 torr (73,74), at which Kv channels and vascular tone are also modulated (18,35). P450, or a related heme protein, has been proposed as an oxygen sensor in the hypoxia-mediated inhibition of Kv channels and pulmonary vasoconstriction (73,74) on the basis of two observations: (1) P450 inhibitors (37) or P450 depletion (75) cause membrane depolarization by attenuating $I_{K(V)}$ in PASMC; and (2) hypoxia inhibits P450 activity (76).

To reduce $NAD(P)^+$ to NAD(P)H, P450 must form a complex with NADPH oxidoreductase. Regulatory Kv β subunits belong to the NAD(P)H-dependent oxidoreductase superfamily of proteins (62). Therefore, it is possible that, like Kv β subunits, NADPH oxidoreductase can modulate Kv function directly or indirectly via an intermediate. Under normoxic conditions, for example, the oxygen-dependent P450–NADPH oxidoreductase complex may constantly produce an intermediate product, the oxygen-dependent channel regulator (ODCR) (e.g., oxygen radicals, epoxides, NO, cytochrome c), which acts as a link between the enzyme complex and Kv channel proteins to keep the channel open and to maintain a negative E_m. Because ODCR production is dependent on the activity of the oxygen-dependent P450–NADPH oxidoreductase complex, it is plausible that Kv channels are closed because of decreased ODCR production during hypoxic episodes. Therefore, in this scenario, the complex acts as the oxygen sensor, the ODCR is a coupler, and Kv channels are the effectors in the signaling pathway that leads to HPV. The observations supporting this contention that P450–NADPH oxidoreductase complex is an oxygen sensor in PASMC include the following:

1. P450 inhibitors decrease $I_{K(V)}$ and cause membrane depolarization (77),
2. The enzyme complex is oxygen-sensitive,

3. Diphenyleneiodonium (DPI), an NADPH oxidase inhibitor, decreases $I_{K(V)}$ (78) and blocks HPV (79), although the latter effect may be due to DPI also inhibiting Ca^{2+} channels in PASMCs (78),
4. P450-derived epoxides (e.g., epoxyeicosatrienoic acid) activate K^+ channels and lead to vasodilation (80–82).

Despite this supportive evidence, there is also evidence arguing that NADPH oxidase is *not* an oxygen sensor:

1. NADPH oxidoreductase activity (and production of ROS) is actually increased during acute hypoxic challenges (83,84),
2. DPI directly affects K^+ and VDCC channels (78),
3. Hypoxia-induced inhibition of $I_{K(V)}$ and HPV is maintained in NADPH oxidase deficient mice (lacking $gp91^{phox}$) (70),
4. The expression of hypoxia-inducible genes, such as vascular endothelial growth factor (VEGF), is normal in NADPH-deficient ($gp91^{phox}$ and $p22^{phox}$ knockout) mouse cells (85),
5. Kv channels themselves are redox-sensitive.

In native PASMCs, receptors, ion channels, enzymes, and signal transduction proteins are often compartmentalized or colocalized to form an efficient "functional" complex for certain specific processes. The hypoxia-induced local changes (either increases or decreases) in ROS production by NADPH oxidoreductase–P450 complexes that are adjacent to Kv channel proteins may play a more important role in regulating K^+ channel function and HPV (28,36,41,86) (see next section).

Finally, NO produced by nitric oxide synthase (NOS), a P450-type hemoprotein (87,88), activates Kv channels (89). Because of the dependence of NOS on oxygen tension, acute hypoxia may also exert its regulatory effect on Kv channels through changes in NOS activity and NO production. In addition, NOS can also be a source of ROS rather than NO under conditions where L-arginine is limiting (90); it is unclear whether NOS-derived ROS are involved in the development of HPV.

D. Modulation of Voltage-Gated Ca^{2+} Channels

Almost 10 years ago, López-Barneo and his associates identified Ca^{2+} channels as one of the putative targets of hypoxia. Franco-Obregón et al. showed that acute hypoxia inhibits high-voltage-gated L-type Ca^{2+} channels in systemic and main pulmonary arteries (91–93) but does not affect T-type low voltage-gated Ca^{2+} channels. Inhibition of Ca^{2+} channels by hypoxia in these vessels resulted in visible attenuation of Ca^{2+} oscillations (91) and vasodilation. On the other hand, in resistance PASMCs, acute hypoxia potentiated the Ca^{2+} current (92). Therefore, the direct modulation of voltage-gated Ca^{2+} channels by oxygen tension may be another underlying mechanism of HPV.

IV. CHRONIC HYPOXIA DOWNREGULATES K^+ CHANNEL EXPRESSION

As opposed to acute hypoxia, where vasoconstriction is the major vascular response to redirect blood flow to better-ventilated regions of the lung, chronic hypoxia (> 12 h) results not only in pulmonary vasoconstriction but also in pulmonary vascular remodeling. The latter manifests as enhanced intimal growth, thrombosis, and/or medial hypertrophy. Medial hypertrophy, which results in reduced vascular lumen and possible occlusion, results from a combination of increased PASMC proliferation and decreased PASMC apoptosis. Pathological examples of chronic hypoxia are apparent in patients diagnosed with chronic obstructive pulmonary disease (COPD) and congenital heart disease (e.g., Eisenmenger syndrome or complex) as well as in individuals living at high altitude. The ultimate outcome of the pulmonary vascular remodeling process and the increased vasoconstriction are pulmonary hypertension [i.e., increased PAP (Fig. 1B)] and, in many cases, right heart failure and death.

Over 20 years ago, McMurtry et al. (94) observed that the pressor response to acute hypoxia was impaired while that to vasoconstrictors was enhanced in lungs from chronically hypoxic rats. This early observation led to speculation that the underlying mechanisms of acute and chronic hypoxic vasoconstriction were similar. In fact, chronic hypoxia–mediated pulmonary vasoconstriction and vascular remodeling are both related to the inhibition of Kv channels in PASMCs (12,34,95–97). Changes in ROS production, cellular redox status, and cell metabolism (i.e., oxidative phosphorylation and glycolysis), as well as the increased effect of regulatory proteins (e.g., Kv β subunits, P450–NADPH oxidoreductase complex), are also common to both acute and chronic hypoxia.

Despite the apparent similarities in the regulation of vasoconstriction during acute and chronic hypoxia, the issue of the mechanisms underlying the vascular remodeling process associated with chronic hypoxia is still unresolved. Current hypotheses suggest that the cellular response to chronic hypoxia might involve altered gene expression. The common regulating factor in pulmonary vascular smooth muscle contraction and PASMC proliferation is Ca^{2+}. Therefore, it has been speculated that hypoxia-induced pulmonary vasoconstriction and PASMC proliferation use overlapping signaling processes that result in enhanced $[Ca^{2+}]_{cyt}$. As was stated earlier, attenuation of $I_{K(V)}$ is common to both acute and chronic hypoxia. The discussion that follows explores the regulation of Kv channel gene expression and regulation during chronic hypoxia.

A. Chronic Hypoxia Selectively Downregulates K_v α-Subunit Expression in PASMCs

Whole-cell $I_{K(V)}$ is determined by the number of functional channels (N), the single-channel current amplitude ($i_{K(V)}$), and the steady-state open probability (P_{open}) of individual Kv channels according to the equation $I_{K(V)} = Ni_{K(V)}P_{open}$. Based on this formula, it is apparent that the attenuation of $I_{K(V)}$ in PASMCs during hypoxia can be due not only to a decrease in Kv channel activity (i.e., decreased P_{open} and/or single-channel conductance) but also to alterations in the mRNA and/or protein expression of Kv α subunits that are essential for the proper functioning of native Kv channels and the overall regulation of E_m and $[Ca^{2+}]_{cyt}$.

Indeed, there is evidence showing that chronic hypoxia inhibits the mRNA (Fig. 3A) and protein (Fig. 3B) expression of Kv α subunits (but not β subunits) (95,97,98) and decreases whole-cell $I_{K(V)}$ (Fig. 4A) (12,34,95–97) in PASMCs. The result of decreased Kv α-subunit expression and Kv function is membrane depolarization (Fig. 4B) and enhanced $[Ca^{2+}]_{cyt}$ (Fig. 4C) in PASMCs. All of these effects of chronic hypoxia (and acute hypoxia as well) are specific to PASMCs alone; they are not observed in smooth muscle cells isolated from systemic vessels such as the

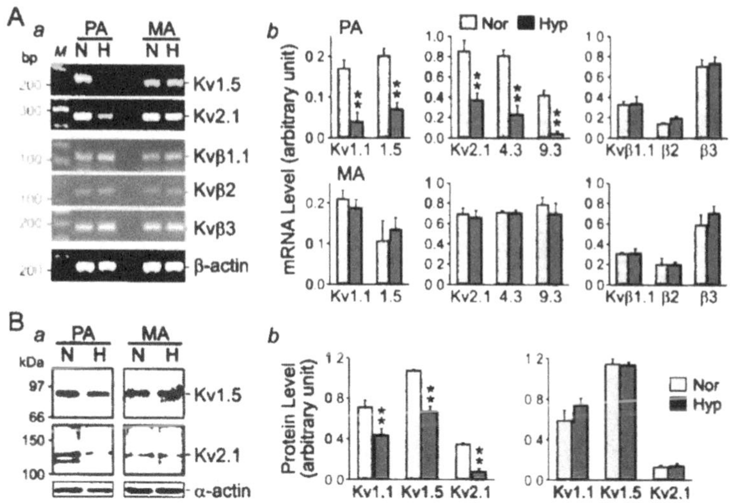

Figure 3 Chronic hypoxia alters K_V gene expression differentially in pulmonary and systemic myocytes. PCR-amplified products (A) and protein expression (B) of selected K_V α and β subunits were differentially altered by hypoxia (H) in PA and MA. Summarized mRNA and protein expression for selected Kv α and β subunits, as shown in the representative gels in (a), in normoxic (Nor) and hypoxic (Hyp) PA and MA are shown in the bar graphs (b). ( ) $P < 0.01$ vs. Nor. (Reproduced with permission from Ref. 95.)

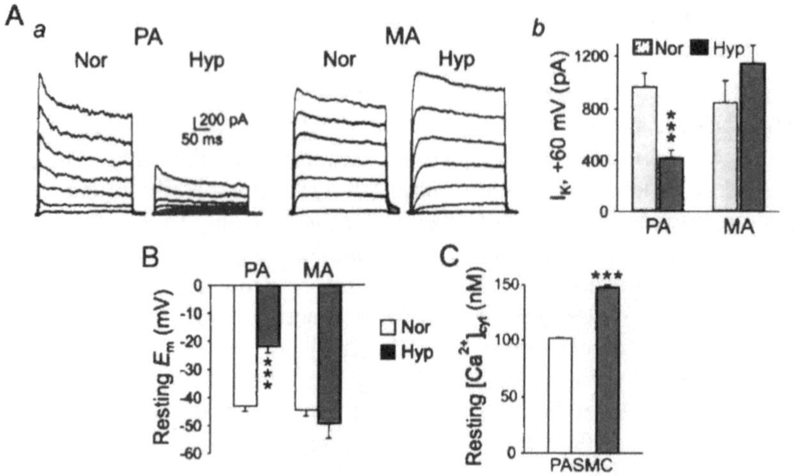

Figure 4 Chronic hypoxia alters $I_{K(V)}$, E_m, and $[Ca^{2+}]_{cyt}$ differently in PA and MA. (A)(a) $I_{K(V)}$ was recorded from normoxic and hypoxic PA and MA following step depolarizations ranging between −60 and +80 mV from a holding potential of −70 mV. (b). A bar graph summarizing the effects of normoxia (N) and hypoxia (H) on $I_{K(V)}$ at +60 mV. (B) Summarized data showing the effect of hypoxia on the resting E_m in PA and MA. (***) $P < 0.001$ vs. Nor. (C) Resting $[Ca^{2+}]_{cyt}$ is significantly [(***) $P < 0.001$ vs. Nor] increased in PASMCs. (Reproduced with permission from Ref. 95.)

mesenteric artery (Figs. 3 and 4). This suggests that pulmonary and systemic vascular smooth muscle cells are regulated by hypoxia via different cellular and/or molecular mechanisms. Therefore, the sustained pulmonary vasoconstriction caused by prolonged hypoxia, such as that seen in chronically hypoxic subjects or those suffering from hypoxic cardiopulmonary disease (e.g., COPD/emphysema and congenital heart diseases) may be due to decreased Kv channel gene expression as well as function. The identities of the Kv α subunits that make up the putative oxygen-sensitive K^+ channels in PASMCs are listed in Table 1 (34), and detailed discussions about the molecular identity of oxygen-sensitive Kv channel subunits can be found in Chapters 11 and 17.

B. Transcriptional Regulation of Kv Channel Genes

Chronic hypoxia-mediated downregulation of Kv channel expression may be due to its inhibitory effect on gene transcription and translation or an augmenting effect on mRNA and protein degradation of the channels. Transcriptional regulation of Kv channel genes involves binding transcription factors with their specific binding sequences in the promoter of the genes. In the human Kv1.5 gene, for example, there are multiple binding

Table 1 K_V α and β Subunits Expressed in the Pulmonary Vasculature Potentially Involved in O_2 Sensing

Channel subunit	mRNA expression	Protein expression	Sensitivity to hypoxia	Reference
α Subunits				
Kv1.1[a]	Yes	Yes		95,97,127–129
Kv1.2[a]	Yes	Yes	Yes	31,52,95,97,127–131
Kv1.3	Yes	Yes		52,127,128
Kv1.4	Yes	Yes		52,128,129
Kv1.5[a]	Yes	Yes	Yes	31,49,52,95,97, 127–129,132
Kv1.6	Yes	Yes		127 129
Kv1.7	Yes			128
Kv2.1[a]	Yes	Yes	Yes	31.49,52,97,127,129
Kv2.2	Yes	Yes		128
Kv3.1	Yes	Yes	Yes	49,53,131
Kv3.3	Yes			128
Kv3.4[b]	Yes			128
Kv4.1[b]	Yes			128
Kv4.2	Yes			128
Kv4.3[a]	Yes		Yes	95,128
Kv5.1	Yes			128
Kv6.1[c]	Yes			128
Kv9.1	Yes			128
Kv9.2	Yes			128
Kv9.3[c]	Yes		Yes	52,95,97,128,129
β subunits				
Kv β1.1	Yes	Yes	Yes	49,58,95,97,128,129
Kv β1.2	Yes	Yes	Yes	49,61,95,97,128,129
Kv β1.3	Yes	Yes		49
Kv β2.1	Yes			95,97,128,129
Heteromeric α/α or α/β channels				
Kv1.2/Kv1.5			Yes	31,49
Kv2.1/Kv9.3			Yes	31,49,52
Kv4.2/Kvβ1.2			Yes	61

[a]mRNA or protein expression is downregulated by chronic hypoxia (95,97).
[b]Only in small pulmonary arteries (128).
[c]Only in large pulmonary arteries (128).

sequences in the promoter region, including binding motifs for transcription factors such as activating protein-1 (AP1), hypoxia-inducible factor-1 (HIF-1), nuclear factor-κB (NF-κB), Smad, c-Myb, and Sp-1 (Fantozzi and Yuan, unpublished data).

Oxygen tension modulates gene expression via multiple pathways, such as second messenger systems (e.g., cAMP/cGMP, calmodulin, ROS), phosphorylation pathways (i.e., protein kinases), and transcription factors. Among the myriad of known transcription factors, AP-1, HIF-1, NF-κB, nuclear factor interleukin-6 (NF-IL6, also known as c/EBP_{β}), and early growth response-1 (EGR-1) are modulated by oxygen tension and play important roles in mitogenesis, cell proliferation and apoptosis, vasoreactivity, and the inflammatory response inherent to many types of pulmonary diseases (54).

HIF-1 activation during prolonged hypoxia induces pulmonary hypertension (99). Functional HIF-1 exists as a heterodimer of one α (HIF-1α) and one β (HIF-1β) subunit. Under normoxic conditions, HIF-1 is ubiquitinated and rapidly degraded, preventing the formation of functional heterodimers. During hypoxia, HIF-1α ubiquitination is inhibited and HIF-1α–HIF-1β dimers form. Under these conditions, functional HIF-1 binds with hypoxia response element (HRE; 5′-GCGTG-3′) DNA sites and targets the expression of a number of mitogenic and vasoactive genes such as those encoding for VEGF, platelet-derived growth factor (PDGF), and endothelin-1 (ET-1). Whether hypoxia-mediated HIF activation is involved directly (e.g., by binding to its binding motif in Kv1.5 gene) or indirectly (e.g., via upregulating ET-1 or other transcription repressors) in downregulating Kv channel transcription is still unclear.

Like HIF-1, AP-1 is also upregulated during sustained hypoxia, resulting in enhanced cell proliferation. AP-1 is a family of homo- (e.g., Jun/Jun) or hetero- (Jun/Fos) dimeric transcription factors such as Jun (v-Jun, c-Jun, JunB, JunD), Fos (v-Fos, c-Fos, FosB, Fra1, Fra2), and activating transcription factor (ATF2, ATF3/LRF1, B-ATF) subunits that bind to a common DNA site, the AP-1 binding site (5′-TGACTCA-3 (TRE) or 5′-TGACGTCA-3′ (CRE)) (100). c-Fos and c-Jun have been suggested as possible effectors of hypoxic gene regulation because of their ability to sense changes in redox potential and intracellular (cytoplasmic and nuclear) [Ca^{2+}] (101,102), resulting in a change in target channel function. In normoxic PASMCs, overexpression of *c-jun* results in decreased Kv channel activity by downregulating Kv channel α subunits (e.g., Kv1.5) or upregulating Kv β subunits (e.g., Kv β2.1) (103). c-Jun, a transcription activator, may indirectly regulate transcription of Kv1.5 gene by activating expression of an intermediate gene product that can subsequently downregulate Kv1.5 channel expression and decrease $I_{K(V)}$. The augmenting effect of c-Jun on Kv β2.1 transcription implies that c-Jun modulates Kv channel α- and β-subunit gene expression by different mechanisms, despite the existence of AP-1 binding sites in the promoter sequences for these two genes, as has been suggested for the human K_{Ca} gene, h*slo*, and its regulatory β subunit (104). Recently, we showed that AP-1 binding activity was enhanced during chronic hypoxia in human pulmonary artery endothelial cells (PAECs) due to upregulated transient receptor potential (TRP) cation channel expression (105). The increased AP-1 DNA binding activity would upregulate transcription and expression of genes that contain AP-1 binding sites, such as ET-1, PDGF and VEGF. The increased production of these mitogenic agonists or growth factors may indirectly downregulate Kv channels in PASMCs via a paracrine mechanism.

The AP-1 binding site (5′-TGACGTCA-2; CRE) is also the binding site for another transcription factor, the cAMP response element binding protein (CREB), which has been involved in vascular remodeling and mitogenesis. Klemm et al. (106) reported an inverse relationship between CREB content and cell proliferation in hypoxic bovine PASMCs and aortic cells, i.e., CREB content was decreased whereas proliferation was increased by hypoxia. Tokunou et al. (107,108) showed that CREB upregulation plays an important role in the vascular remodeling processes induced by thrombin during atherosclerosis, possibly via a pathway involving *c-fos* expression. Because the CRE binding site is present on some of the Kv channel genes, it is possible that CREB also modulates Kv channel expression and function, although this possibility has not been explored to date.

Finally, since we have discussed the Kv1.5 promoter and its role in regulating Kv1.5 gene expression, we would be remiss in omitting the existence of silencer binding elements. Silencers are cis-acting regulatory DNA elements that control cell-specific gene expression or prevent potentially damaging overexpression of certain proteins. Valverde and Koren (109) and Mori et al. (110) reported the existence of a Kv1.5 repressor element (KRE) located in the 5′-flanking region of the cardiac Kv1.5 gene. The KRE contains a dinucleotide repetitive element $[(GT)_{19}(GA)_1(CA)_{15}(GA)_{16}]$ that is necessary for mediating silencer activity (110). KRE selectively decreases the expression of Kv1.5 in cell lines that do not express native Kv1.5 genes, but deletion of the KRE repetitive element abolishes the KRE silencer effect altogether (110). In addition, a KRE binding factor (KBF) has also been identified that can abolish the silencer effect of KRE, regulating Kv1.5 transcription. Neither the KRE sequence nor KBF have been identified in PASMCs yet. Any effect they may (or may not) have on Kv channel expression and/or function during hypoxia is speculative. However, if they do exist in PASMCs, expression of KRE in those cells would downregulate Kv channel expression and function, causing membrane depolarization and vasoconstriction (and/or remodeling). Alternatively, if KBF expression is downregulated during hypoxia, Kv α-subunit expression can be repressed by KRE, decreasing Kv channel expression and availability.

C. K⁺ Channel Function is Modulated by Mitogens and Growth Factors

As indicated in the previous section, activation of transcription factors during chronic hypoxia can result in increased transcription and activation of genes encoding for vasoactive agonists (e.g., ET-1), mitogens (e.g., VEGF,

PDGF), and selected glycolytic enzymes (54). Some vasoactive agonists and mitogens are known to alter K^+ channel function. ET-1, which is both a vasoconstrictor and a mitogen, decreases $I_{K(V)}$ (55) and depolarizes PASMCs. However, ET-1-mediated Ca^{2+} sparks also enhance K_{Ca} channel activity in the same cells (111). During sustained hypoxia, the inhibitory effect of ET-1 on $I_{K(V)}$ is reduced in PASMCs (96), possibly due to other hypoxia-induced $I_{K(V)}$ inhibitory mechanisms. The membrane depolarization resulting from $I_{K(V)}$ inhibition by ET-1 causes a significant increase in $[Ca^{2+}]_{cyt}$, which can contribute not only to ET-1-induced vasoconstriction but also to proliferation. Activation of ET_A and ET_B receptors by ET-1 causes human PASMC proliferation (112). In the latter study, serum-stimulated PASMC proliferation was inhibited by decreasing ET-1 release or activity (112). Previously we showed that K^+ currents were also decreased in proliferating PASMCs (113). Therefore, it is possible that the inhibition of K^+ currents by ET-1 may cause the membrane depolarization and enhanced $[Ca^{2+}]_{cyt}$ necessary for proliferation to occur.

Recently we showed that PDGF could stimulate PASMC proliferation via upregulation of TRPC6 (114), which putatively encodes for receptor- or store-operated Ca^{2+} channels. In addition, ATP-induced PASMC mitogenesis may involve upregulation of TRPC4 channels (Zhang, Remillard, Fantozzi, and Yuan, unpublished observations). The latter observation is rendered more interesting by our prior discovery that TRPC4 expression and activity are also enhanced by chronic hypoxia (105) in human pulmonary artery endothelial cells. Therefore, the regulation of channel expression and function by mitogens and vasoactive agonists clearly does not limit itself to K^+ channels.

D. Modulation of K^+ Channel Expression by Auxiliary Regulatory Proteins

Potassium channel–associated proteins (KChAPs) and K^+ channel–interacting proteins (KChIPs) are auxiliary regulatory proteins that have been described in the brain and heart, where, like Kv β subunits, they interact directly with the pore-forming Kv α subunits to modulate Kv channel expression and function.

KChAPs act as chaperones for selected Kv channels (e.g., Kv1.3 and Kv4.3), resulting in their enhanced protein expression (115,116). The three KChIPs that have been identified (KChIP1–KChIP3) have the opposite effect on Kv currents in comparison to Kv β subunits, i.e., KChIPs slow channel activation and accelerate recovery from inactivation (117). These KChIPs coprecipitate with Kv4 α subunits, implying that they are an integral part of the functional K^+ channel complex. In addition, with its structure bearing a Ca^{2+}-binding site, KChIP-induced modulation of K^+ channel activity is sensitive to Ca^{2+} levels (118). Therefore, sensing of the elevated

$[Ca^{2+}]_{cyt}$ levels by KChIPs may represent yet another mechanism by which hypoxia modulates Kv channel expression and function.

Because KChAPs and KChIPs have not been characterized extensively (or even identified in the case of KChIPs) in other tissues, we can only guess at the role they might play in modulating pulmonary vascular K^+ channel function. However, we have preliminary evidence that KChAP mRNA expression is decreased in chronically hypoxic PASMCs, but not in mesenteric artery smooth muscle cells (Ying and Yuan, unpublished data), suggesting that KChAPs may indeed play a role in the hypoxic response of PASMCs.

V. COLOCALIZATION OF O_2 SENSORS AND EFFECTORS WITHIN MICRODOMAINS

Caveolae are cholesterol and caveolin- and sphingolipid-rich plasma membrane regions that form distinct invaginations (119); they have been implicated in vesicular trafficking and signal transduction. The concept that signal transduction proteins, membrane receptors, and ion channels colocalize within this type of plasmalemmal microdomain may explain how a cell can respond quickly to a given stress, such as acute hypoxia, and adapt to regulate cell function.

Caveolin proteins are required for the structural formation of caveolae. Although there are many types of caveolin proteins, caveolin-1 has been identified as a putative modulator of pulmonary hypertension. Caveolin-1-deficient (knockout) mice exhibit pulmonary hypertension, right ventricular hypertrophy, and upregulated systemic NO production (120). Because caveolae appear to be "normal" within the pulmonary vasculature, the stress response that occurs following a hypoxic challenge may involve disrupted caveolae formation and therefore altered signal transduction. Nevertheless, the revelation that caveolin-rich microdomains with Kv1.5 channels exist (121) has suggested that regulatory proteins involved in the hypoxic response may colocalize with Kv1.5 channels. In PASMCs, this microdomain may include (1) oxygen sensors (e.g., P450-NADPH oxidoreductase); (2) couplers (e.g., ODCR), auxiliary modulators (e.g., KChIPs and KChAPs), or signal transduction proteins (e.g., G proteins); and (3) effectors (e.g., Kv or Ca^{2+} channels). Figure 5 shows the idealized structural arrangement of such a microdomain.

Additional evidence is also available to support the notion that caveolae formation somehow contributes to Kv channel modulation during hypoxia. Caveolae are part of a larger family of membrane structures called lipid raft domains that are rich in arachidonic acid (122). Cytochrome P450-derived arachidonic acid derivatives such epoxyeicosatrienoic acids (EETs) and hydroxyl-eicosatetranoic acids (HETEs) can regulate vascular tone (i.e., K^+ channel-mediated vasodilation or Ca^{2+} channel-mediated vasocon-

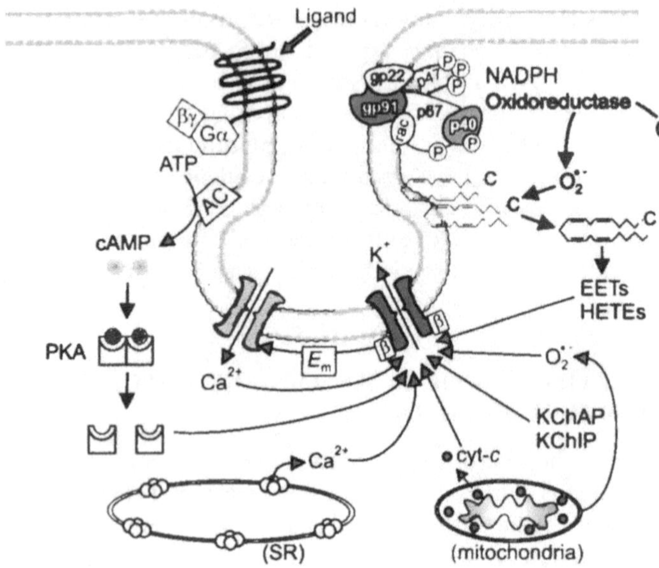

Figure 5 Schematic representation of intercaveolae organization of signaling proteins. K^+ and Ca^{2+} channels are shown as a seven-transmembrane-domain G-protein-coupled receptor associated with adenylate cyclase (AC), the NADPH oxidoreductase enzyme complex (shown here with gp91, gp22, p47, p67, rac, and p40 subunits). Ca^{2+} released from the SR, cytochrom c and ROS ($O^-{}_2$) released from the mitochondria, and protein kinase A (PKA) are indicated as K^+ channel modulators. EET/HETE produced from arachidonic acid is also depicted as a K^+ modulator.

striction) (81,82,123). In the pulmonary vasculature, cytochrome P450 4A metabolite (HETE) formation from arachidonic acid is inhibited by hypoxia (82), resulting in increased pulmonary artery pressure due to vasoconstriction. Thus, locally produced arachidonic acid derivatives within the K^+ channel-containing microdomain may also impact K^+ channel function.

Based on the evidence, it is conceivable that lipid raft domains and their localized components may contribute greatly to the development of hypoxia-mediated Kv channel inhibition, pulmonary vasoconstriction, vascular remodeling, and, ultimately, pulmonary hypertension.

VI. SUMMARY

Pulmonary vasoconstriction due to hypoxia is essential to ensure the maximal oxygenation of the venous blood in the pulmonary artery, particularly during acute hypoxic challenges. Sustained hypoxia results in persistent pulmonary vasoconstriction and causes pulmonary vascular remodeling

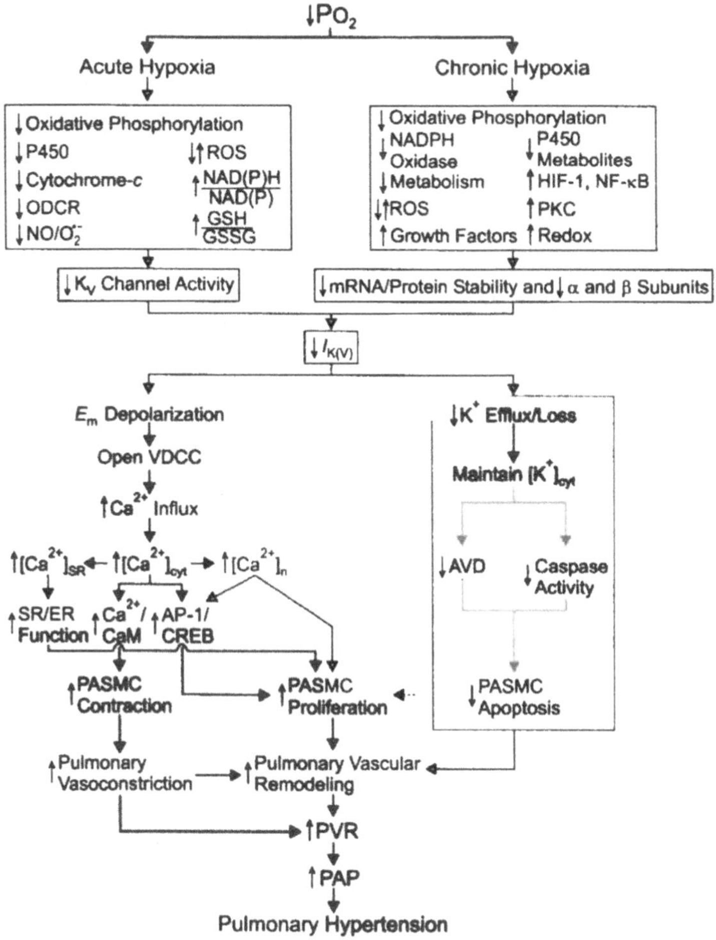

Figure 6 Flowchart showing how acute hypoxia and chronic hypoxia cause pulmonary vasoconstriction and vascular remodeling via the modulation of K_V channel function and/or expression, $[Ca^{2+}]_{cyt}$ and E_m regulation, and modulation of the apoptotic volume decrease (AVD), which leads to apoptosis (shaded box). PVR, pulmonary vascular resistance; PAP, pulmonary arterial pressure.

(e.g., excessive PASMC proliferation). K^+ channels, especially Kv channels, are intimately involved in the pulmonary responses to hypoxia. Kv channel gene expression and function are significantly altered during hypoxia. In acute hypoxia, a reduction in $I_{K(V)}$ results from (1) a change in the cellular redox state, (2) inhibited oxidative phosphorylation, (3) disrupted ROS production, (4) attenuated release or activity of Kv channel modulators such as

NO and P450-NADPH oxidoreductase metabolites, and (5) β subunit sensitivity to the decrease in oxygen tension resulting in altered $I_{K(V)}$ kinetics. In chronic hypoxia, all of these factors are also involved, but gene expression is also altered by (1) oxygen-sensitive transcription factors (e.g., AP-1, HIF-1, and NF-κB),(2) growth factors (e.g., VEGF and PDGF) and mitogens (e.g., ATP and ET-1), and (3) auxiliary proteins (e.g., KChAPs and KChIPs) (Fig. 6).

Like that between membrane depolarization and hyperpolarization, the homeostatic balance between PASMC proliferation and apoptosis is also dependent of K^+ channel activity. Although it was not directly discussed in the context of this chapter, a decrease in $I_{K(V)}$ during hypoxia can also result in maintenance of the cytosolic K^+ ($[K^+]_{cyt}$) level, which is essential in preventing apoptotic volume decrease (AVD) and apoptosis (Fig. 6, shaded box). Although part of the PASMC proliferation induced by $I_{K(V)}$ inhibition is due to the subsequent membrane depolarization and Ca^{2+} influx, inhibition of AVD and apoptosis in PASMCs further promote the progression of pulmonary medial hypertrophy during persistent hypoxia.

The progression from short-term pulmonary vasoconstriction during acute hypoxia to long-term pulmonary remodeling during chronic hypoxia is a well-coordinated cellular recovery response. Although the ultimate goal of the cell is to prevent its further injury following the hypoxic stress, the physiological results can be debilitating, not to mention life-threatening. From our overview of the mechanisms underlying PASMC responses to hypoxia-induced pulmonary vasoconstriction and vascular remodeling, it is apparent that there are many potential therapeutic targets involving ion channels in the treatment of pulmonary vascular disease.

ACKNOWLEDGMENTS

We gratefully acknowledge the contributions of Drs. I. Fantozzi, Y. Yu, and S. Zhang to unpublished work cited in this review. This work was supported by grants (HL54043, HL64945, HL66012, HL69758, and HL66941) from the National Institutes of Health.

REFERENCES

1. Nelson MT, Quayle JM. Physiological roles and properties of potassium channels in arterial smooth muscle. Am J Physiol 1995; 268:C799–C822.
2. Felix R. Channelopathies: ion channel defects linked to heritable clinical disorders. J Med Gen 2000; 37:729–740.
3. Jentsch TJ. Chloride channels. Curr Opin Neurobiol 1993; 3:316–321.
4. Mandegar M, Remillard CV, Yuan JX-J. Ion channels in pulmonary arterial hypertension. Prog Cardiovasc Dis 2002; 45:81–114.

5. Shieh C-C, Coghlan M, Sullivan JP, Gopalakrishnan M. Potassium channels: molecular defects, diseases, and therapeutic opportunities. Pharmacol Rev 2000; 52:557–293.
6. Lang F, Lepple-Wienhues A, Paulmichl M, Szabó I, Siemen D, Gulbins E. Ion channels, cell volume, and apoptotic cell death. Cell Physiol Biochem 1998; 8:285–292.
7. Remillard CV, Yuan JX-J. Activation of K^+ channels: an essential pathway in programmed cell death. Am J Physiol Lung Cell Mol Physiol 2004; 286: L49–L67.
8. Nelson MT, Patlak JB, Worley JF, Standen NB. Calcium channels, potassium channels, and voltage dependence of arterial smooth muscle tone. Am J Physiol 1990; 259:C3–C18.
9. Berridge MJ. Calcium signalling and cell proliferation. BioEssays. 1995; 17: 491–500.
10. Lesage F, Lazdunski M. Molecular and functional properties of two-pore-domain potassium channels. Am J Physiol Renal Physiol 2000; 279: F793–F801.
11. Robertson B. The real life of voltage-gated K^+ channels: more than model behaviour. Trends Physiol Sci 1997; 18:474–483.
12. Smirnov SV, Robertson TP, Ward JPT, Aaronson PI. Chronic hypoxia is associated with reduced delayed rectifier K^+ current in rat pulmonary artery muscle cells. Am J Physiol 1994; 266:H365–H370.
13. Yuan XJ. Voltage-gated K^+ currents regulate resting membrane potential and $[Ca^{2+}]_i$ in pulmonary arterial myocytes. Circ Res 1995; 77:370–378.
14. Peng W, Hoidal JR, Karwande SV, Farrukh IS. Effect of chronic hypoxia on K channels: regulation in human pulmonary vascular smooth muscle cells. Am J Physiol 1997; 272:C1271–C1278.
15. Clapp LH, Gurney AM, Standen NB, Langton PD. Properties of the ATP-sensitive K^+ current activated by levcromakalim in isolated pulmonary arterial myocytes. J Membr Biol 1994; 140:205–213.
16. Gurney AM, Osipenko ON, MacMillan D, McFarlane KM, Tate RJ, Kempsill FEJ. The two-pore domain K channel, TASK-1, in pulmonary artery smooth muscle cells. Circ Res 2003; 93:957–964.
17. Osipenko ON, Evans AM, Gurney AM. Regulation of the resting potential of rabbit pulmonary artery myocytes by a low threshold, O_2-sensing potassium current. Br J Pharmacol 1997; 120:1461–1470.
18. Yuan X-J, Tod ML, Rubin LJ, Blaustein MP. Contrasting effects of hypoxia on tension in rat pulmonary and mesenteric arteries. Am J Physiol Heart Circ Physiol 1990; 259:H281–H289.
19. Madden JA, Ray DE, Keller PA, Kleinman JG. Ion exchange activity in pulmonary artery smooth muscle cells: the response to hypoxia. Am J Physiol Lung Cell Mol Physiol 2001; 280:L264–L271.
20. Madden JA, Vadula KS, Kurup VP. Effects of hypoxia and other vasoactive agents on pulmonary and cerebral artery smooth muscle cells. Am J Physiol 1992; 263:L384–L393.

21. Murray TR, Chen L, Marshall BE, Macarak EJ. Hypoxic contraction of cultured pulmonary vascular smooth muscle cells. Am J Respir Cell Mol Biol 1990; 3:457–465.
22. Post JM, Gelband CH, Hume JR. $[Ca^{2+}]_i$ inhibition of K^+ channels in canine pulmonary artery. Novel mechanism for hypoxia-induced membrane depolarization. Circ Res 1995; 77:131–139.
23. Robertson TP, Hague D, Aaronson PI, Ward JPT. Voltage-independent calcium entry in hypoxic pulmonary vasoconstriction of intrapulmonary arteries of the rat. J Physiol 2000; 525:669–680.
24. Dipp M, Evans AM. Cyclic ADP-ribose is the primary trigger for hypoxic pulmonary vasoconstriction in the rat lung in situ. Circ Res 2001; 89:77–83.
25. Dipp M, Nye PCG, Evans AM. Hypoxic release of calcium from the sarcoplasmic reticulum of pulmonary artery smooth muscle. Am J Physiol Lung Cell Mol Physiol 2001; 281:L318–L325.
26. Gelband CH, Gelband H. Ca^{2+} release from intracellular stores is an initial step in hypoxic pulmonary vasoconstriction of rat pulmonary artery resistance vessels. Circulation 1997; 96:3647–3654.
27. Jabr RI, Toland H, Gelband CH, Wang XX, Hume JR. Prominent role of intracellular Ca^{2+} release in hypoxic vasoconstriction of canine pulmonary artery. Br J Pharmacol 1997; 122:21–30.
28. Archer SL, Huang J, Henry T, Peterson D, Weir EK. A redox-based O_2 sensor in rat pulmonary vasculature. Circ Res 1993; 73:1100–1112.
29. Archer SL, Huang JMC, Reeve HL, Hampl V, Tolarová S, Michelakis E, Weir EK. Differential distribution of electrophysiologically distinct myocytes in conduit and resistance arteries determines their response to nitric oxide and hypoxia. Circ Res 1996; 78:431–442.
30. Barman SA. Potassium channels modulate hypoxic pulmonary vasoconstriction. Am J Physiol 1998; 275:L64–L70.
31. Hulme JT, Coppock EA, Felipe A, Martens JR, Tamkun MM. Oxygen sensitivity of cloned voltage-gated K^+ channels expressed in the pulmonary vasculature. Circ Res 1999; 85:489–497.
32. Olschewski A, Hong Z, Nelson DP, Weir EK. Graded response of K^+ current, membrane potential, and $[Ca^{2+}]_i$ to hypoxia in pulmonary arterial smooth muscle. Am J Physiol Lung Cell Mol Physiol 2002; 283:L1143–L1150.
33. Post JM, Hume JR, Archer SL, Weir EK. Direct role for potassium channel inhibition in hypoxic pulmonary vasoconstriction. Am J Physiol 1992; 262:C882–C890.
34. Sweeney M, Yuan JX-J. Hypoxic pulmonary vasoconstriction: role of voltage-gated potassium channels. Respir Res 2000; 1:40–48.
35. Yuan XJ, Goldman WF, Tod ML, Rubin LJ, Blaustein MP. Hypoxia reduces potassium currents in cultured rat pulmonary but not mesenteric arterial myocytes. Am J Physiol 1993; 264:L116–L123.
36. Yuan XJ, Tod ML, Rubin LJ, Blaustein MP. Deoxyglucose and reduced glutathione mimic effects of hypoxia on K^+ and Ca^{2+} conductances in pulmonary artery cells. Am J Physiol 1994; 267:L52–L63.

37. Yuan X-J, Tod ML, Rubin LJ, Blaustein MP. Hypoxic and metabolic regulation of voltage-gated K^+ channels in rat pulmonary artery smooth muscle cells. Exp Physiol 1995; 80:803–813.
38. Yuan X-J, Salvaterra CG, Tod ML, Juhaszova M, Goldman WF, Rubin LJ, Blaustein MP. The sodium gradient, potassium channels, and regulation of calcium in pulmonary and mesenteric arterial smooth muscles: effect of hypoxia. In: Weir EK, Hume JR, Reeves JT, eds. Ion Flux in Pulmonary Vascular Control. New York: Plenum Press; 1993:205–222.
39. Yuan X-J. Mechanisms of hypoxic pulmonary vasoconstriction: The role of oxygen-sensing voltage-gated potassium channels. In: López-Barneo J, Weir EK, eds. Oxygen Regulation of Ion Channels and Gene Expression. Armonk, NY: Futura; 1998:207–233.
40. Gurney AM, Osipenko ON, MacMillan D, Kempsill FEJ. Potassium channels underlying the resting potential of pulmonary artery smooth muscle cells. Clin Exp Pharmacol Physiol 2002; 29:330–333.
41. Yuan X-J, Sugiyama T, Goldman WF, Rubin LJ, Blaustein MP. A mitochondrial uncoupler increases K_{Ca} currents but decreases Kv currents in pulmonary artery myocytes. Am J Physiol 1996; 270:C321–C331.
42. Brayden JE, Nelson MT. Regulation of arterial tone by activation of calcium-dependent potassium channels. Science 1992; 256:532–535.
43. Park MK, Lee SH, Lee SJ, Ho W-K, Earm YE. Different modulation of Ca-activated K channels by the intracellular redox potential in pulmonary and ear arterial smooth muscle cells of the rabbit. Pflügers Arch 1995; 430:308–314.
44. Lee S, Park M, So I, Earm YE. NADH and NAD modulates Ca^{2+}-activated K^+ channels in small pulmonary arterial smooth muscle cells of the rabbit. Pflügers Arch 1994; 427:378–380.
45. Bonnet P, Vandier C, Cheliakine C, Garnier D. Hypoxia activates a potassium current in isolated smooth muscle cells from large pulmonary arteries of the rabbit. Exp Physiol 1994; 79:597–300.
46. Chandy KG, Gutman GA. Voltage-gated K^+ channels. In: North RA, ed. Ligand- and Voltage-Gated Ion Channels. Boca Raton, FL: CRC; 1995:1–71.
47. Coetzee WA, Amarillo Y, Chiu J, Chow A, Lau D, McCormack T, Moreno H, Nadal MS, Ozaita A, Pountney D, Saganich M, Vega-Saenz de Miera E, Rudy B. Molecular diversity of K^+ channels. Ann NY Acad Sci 1999; 868:233–285.
48. Coppock EA, Martens JR, Tamkun MM. Molecular basis of hypoxia-induced pulmonary vasoconstriction: role of voltage-gated K^+ channels. Am J Physiol Lung Cell Mol Physiol 2001; 281:L1–L12.
49. Coppock EA, Tamkun MM. Differential expression of Kv channel α- and β-subunits in the bovine pulmonary arterial circulation. Am J Physiol Lung Cell Mol Physiol 2001; 281:L1350–L1360.
50. López-Barneo J. Oxygen-sensing by ion channel and the regulation of cellular functions. Trends Neurosci. 1996; 19:435–440.
51. Patel AJ, Honoré E. Molecular physiology of oxygen-sensitive potassium channels. Eur Respir J 2001; 18:221–227.

52. Patel AJ, Lazdunski M, Honoré E. Kv2.1/Kv9.3, a novel ATP-dependent delayed-rectifier K^+ channel in oxygen-sensitive pulmonary artery myocytes. EMBO J 1997; 16:6615–6625.
53. Osipenko ON, Tate RJ, Gurney AM. Potential role for Kv3.1b channels as oxygen sensors. Circ Res 2000; 86:534–540.
54. Semenza GL. Oxygen-regulated transcription factors and their role in pulmonary disease. Respir Res 2000; 1:159–162.
55. Shimoda LA, Sylvester JT, Booth GM, Shimoda TH, Meeker S, Undem BJ, Sham JSK. Inhibition of voltage-gated K^+ currents by endothelin-1 in human pulmonary arterial myocytes. Am J Physiol Lung Cell Mol Physiol 2001; 281:L1115–L1122.
56. Martens JR, Kwak Y-G, Tamkun MM. Modulation of Kv channel α/β subunit interactions. Trends Cardiovasc Med 1999; 9:253–258.
57. Toro L, Wallner M, Meera P, Tanaka Y. Maxi-K_{Ca}, a unique member of the voltage-gated K channel superfamily. News Physiol Sci 1998; 13:112–117.
58. Rettig J, Heinemann SH, Wunder F, Lorra C, Parcej DN, Dolly JO, Pongs O. Inactivation properties of voltage-gated K^+ channels altered by presence of β-subunit. Nature 1994; 369:289–294.
59. Rasmusson RL, Wang S, Castellino RC, Morales MJ, Strauss HC. The β subunit, Kvβ1.2, acts as a rapid open channel blocker of NH_2 terminal deleted Kv1.4 α-subunits. Adv Exp Med Biol 1997; 430:29–37.
60. Gong J, Xu J, Bezanilla M, van Huizen R, Derin R, Li M. Differential stimulation of PKC phosphorylation of potassium channels by ZIP1 and ZIP2. Science 1999; 285:1565–1569.
61. Pérez-García MT, López-López JR, González C. Kvβ1.2 subunit coexpression in HEK293 cells confers O_2 sensitivity to Kv4.2 but not to Shaker channels. J Gen Physiol 1999; 113:897–907.
62. McCormack T, McCormack K. Shaker K^+ channel β subunits belong to an NAD(P)H-dependent oxidoreductase superfamily. Cell 1994; 79:1133–1135.
63. Waypa GB, Chandel NS, Schumacker PT. Model for hypoxic pulmonary vasoconstriction involving mitochondrial oxygen sensing. Circ Res 2001; 88:1259–1266.
64. Waypa GB, Marks JD, Mack MM, Boriboun C, Mungai PT, Schumacker PT. Mitochondrial reactive oxygen species trigger calcium increases during hypoxia in pulmonary arterial myocytes. Circ Res 2002; 91:719–726.
65. Olschewski A, Hong Z, Peterson DA, Nelson DP, Porter VA, Weir EK. Opposite effects of redox status on membrane potential, cytosolic calcium, and tone in pulmonary arteries and ductus arteriosus. Am J Physiol Lung Cell Mol Physiol 2004; 286:L15–L22.
66. Wang Z-W, Nara M, Wang Y-X, Kotlikoff MI. Redox regulation of large conductance Ca^{2+}-activated K^+ channels in smooth muscle cells. J Gen Physiol 1997; 110:35–44.
67. Park MK, Bae YM, Lee SH, Ho W-K, Earm YE. Modulation of voltage-dependent K^+ channel by redox potential in pulmonary and ear arterial smooth muscle cells of the rabbit. Pflügers Arch 1997; 434:764–771.

68. Rounds S, McMurtry IF. Inhibitors of oxidative ATP production cause transient vasoconstriction and block subsequent pressor responses in rat lungs. Circ Res 1981; 48:393–400.
69. Stanbrook HS, McMurtry IF. Inhibition of glycolysis potentiates hypoxic vasoconstriction in lungs. J Appl Physiol 1983; 55:1467–1473.
70. Archer SL, Reeve HL, Michelakis E, Puttagunta L, Waite R, Nelson DP, Dinauer MC, Weir EK. O_2 sensing is preserved in mice lacking the gp91 phox subunit of NADPH oxidase. Proc Natl Acad Sci USA 1999; 96:7944–7949.
71. Evans AM, Clapp LH, Gurney AM. Augmentation by intracellular ATP of the delayed rectifier current independently of the glibenclamide-sensitive K-current in rabbit arterial myocytes. Br J Pharmacol 1994; 111:972–974.
72. Ishida Y, Paul RJ. Effects of hypoxia on high-energy phosphagen content, energy metabolism and isometric force in guinea-pig taenia caeci. J Physiol 1990; 424:41–56.
73. Miller MA, Hales CA. Role of cytochrome P-450 in alveolar hypoxic pulmonary vasoconstriction in dogs. J Clin Invest 1979; 64:666–673.
74. Sylvester JT, McGowan C. The effects of agents that bind to cytochrome P-450 on hypoxic pulmonary vasoconstriction. Circ Res 1978; 43:429–437.
75. Chen G, Cheung DW. Modulation of endothelium-dependent hyperpolarization and relaxation to acetylcholine in rat mesenteric artery by cytochrome P450 enzyme activity. Circ Res 1996; 79:827–833.
76. Harder DR, Narayanan J, Birks EK, Liard JF, Imig JD, Lombard JH, Lange AR, Roman RJ. Identification of a putative microvascular oxygen sensor. Circ Res 1996; 79:54–61.
77. Yuan X-J, Tod ML, Rubin LJ, Blaustein MP. Inhibition of cytochrome P-450 reduces voltage-gated K^+ currents in pulmonary arterial myocytes. Am J Physiol 1995; 268:C259–C270.
78. Weir EK, Wyatt CN, Reeve HL, Huang J, Archer SL, Peers C. Diphenyleneiodonium inhibits both potassium and calcium currents in isolated pulmonary artery smooth muscle cells. J Appl Physiol 1994; 76:2611–2615.
79. Thompson JS, Jones RD, Rogers TK, Hancock J, Morice AH. Inhibition of hypoxic pulmonary vasoconstriction in isolated rat pulmonary arteries by diphenyleneiodonium (DPI). Pulm Pharmacol Ther 1998; 11:71–75.
80. Campbell WB, Gebremedhin D, Pratt PF, Harder DR. Identification of epoxyeicosatrienoic acids as endothelium-derived hyperpolarizing factors. Circ Res 1996; 78:415–423.
81. Hu S, Kim HS. Activation of K^+ channel in vascular smooth muscles by cytochrome P450 metabolites of arachidonic acid. Eur J Pharmacol 1993; 230: 215–221.
82. Zhu D, Birks EK, Dawson CA, Patel M, Falck JR, Presberg K, Roman RJ, Jacobs ER. Hypoxic pulmonary vasoconstriction is modified by P-450 metabolites. Am J Physiol Heart Circ Physiol 2000; 279:H1526–H1533.
83. Fu XW, Wang DX, Nurse CA, Dinauer MC, Cutz E. NADPH oxidase is an O_2 sensor in airway chemoreceptors: evidence from K^+ current modulation in wild-type and oxidase-deficient mice. Proc Natl Acad Sci USA 2000; 97: 4374–4379.

84. Marshall C, Mamary AJ, Verhoeven AJ, Marshall BE. Pulmonary artery NADPH-oxidase is activated in hypoxic pulmonary vasoconstriction. Am J Respir Cell Mol Biol 1996; 15:633–644.
85. Wenger RH, Marti HH, Schuerer-Maly CC, Kvietikova I, Bauer C, Gassman M, Maly FE. Hypoxic induction of gene expression in chronic granulomatous disease- derived B-cell lines: oxygen sensing is independent of the cytochrome b558-containing nicotinamide adenine dinucleotide phosphate oxidase. Blood 1996; 87:756–761.
86. Yuan JX-J. Oxygen-sensitive K^+ channel(s): where and what? Am J Physiol Lung Cell Mol Physiol 2001; 281:L1345–L1349.
87. Bredt DS, Hwang PM, Glatt CE, Lowenstein C, Reed RR, Snyder SH. Cloned and expressed nitric oxide synthase structurally resembles cytochrome P-450 reductase. Nature 1991; 351:714–718.
88. White KA, Marletta MA. Nitric oxide synthase is a cytochrome P-450 type hemoprotein. Biochemistry 1992; 31:6627–6631.
89. Yuan XJ, Tod ML, Rubin LJ, Blaustein MP. NO hyperpolarizes pulmonary artery smooth muscle cells and decreases the intracellular Ca^{2+} concentration by activating voltage-gated K^+ channels. Proc Natl Acad Sci USA 1996; 93:10489–10494.
90. Pou S, Pou WS, Bredt DS, Snyder SH, Rosen GM. Generation of superoxide by purified brain nitric oxide synthase. J Biol Chem 1992; 267:24173–24176.
91. Franco-Obregón A, Ureña J, López-Barneo J. Oxygen-sensitive calcium channels in vascular smooth muscle and their possible role in hypoxic arterial relaxation. Proc Natl Acad Sci USA 1995; 92:4715–4719.
92. Franco-Obregon A, Lopez-Barneo J. Differential oxygen sensitivity of calcium channels in rabbit smooth muscle cells of conduit and resistance pulmonary arteries. J Physiol 1996; 491:511–518.
93. Franco-Obregón A, López-Barneo J. Low PO_2 inhibits calcium channel activity in arterial smooth muscle cells. Am J Physiol 1996; 271:H2290–H2299.
94. McMurtry IF, Petrun MD, Reeves JT. Lungs from chronically hypoxic rats have decreased pressor response to acute hypoxia. Am J Physiol 1978; 235:H104–H109.
95. Platoshyn O, Yu Y, Golovina VA, McDaniel SS, Krick S, Li L, Wang JY, Rubin LJ, Yuan JX-J. Chronic hypoxia decreases Kv channel expression and function in pulmonary artery myocytes. Am J Physiol Lung Cell Mol Physiol 2001; 280:L801–L812.
96. Shimoda LA, Sylvester JT, Sham JSK. Chronic hypoxia alters effects of endothelin and angiotensin on K^+ currents in pulmonary arterial myocytes. Am J Physiol 1999; 277:L431–L439.
97. Wang J, Juhaszova M, Rubin LJ, Yuan X-J. Hypoxia inhibits gene expression of voltage-gated K^+ channel α subunits in pulmonary artery smooth muscle cells. J Clin Invest 1997; 100:2347–2353.
98. Michelakis ED, McMurtry MS, Wu X-C, Dyck JRB, Moudgil R, Hopkins TA, Lopaschuk GD, Puttagunta L, Waite R, Archer SL. Dichloroacetate, a metabolic modulator, prevents and reverses chronic hypoxic pulmonary hypertension in rats: Role of increased expression and activity of voltage-gated potassium channels. Circulation 2002; 105:244–250.

99. Yu AY, Shimoda LA, Iyer NV, Huso DL, Sun X, McWilliams R, Beaty T, Sham JSK, Wiener CM, Sylvester JT, Semenza GL. Impaired physiological responses to chronic hypoxia in mice partially deficient for hypoxia-inducible factor 1α. J Clin Invest 1999; 103:691–696.
100. Michiels C, Minet, Michel G, Mottet D, Piret J-P, Raes M. HIF-1 and AP-1 cooperate to increase gene expression in hypoxia: role of MAP kinases. IUBMB Life 2001; 52:49–53.
101. Abate C, Patel L 3rd. RFJ, Curran T. Redox regulation of fos and jun DNA-binding activity in vitro. Science 1990; 24:1157–1161.
102. Bannister AJ, Cook A, Kouzarides T. In vitro DNA binding activity of Fos/Fun and BZLF1 but not C/EBP is affected by redox changes. Oncogene 1991; 6:1243–1250.
103. Yu Y, Platoshyn O, Zhang J, Krick S, Zhao Y, Rubin LJ, Rothman A, Yuan JX-J. c-Jun decreases voltage-gated K^+ channel activity in pulmonary artery smooth muscle cells. Circulation 2001; 104:1557–1563.
104. Dhulipala PDK, Kotlikoff MI. Cloning and characterization of the promoters of the maxiK channel α and β subunits. Biochim Biophys Acta 1999; 1444:254–262.
105. Fantozzi I, Zhang S, Platoshyn O, Remillard CV, Cowling RT, Yuan JX-J. Hypoxia increases AP-1 binding activity by enhancing capacitative Ca^{2+} entry in human pulmonary artery endothelial cells. Am J Physiol Lung Cell Mol Physiol 2003; e-pub; 285:L1233–L1245.
106. Klemm DJ, Watson PA, Frid MG, Dempsey EC, Schaack J, Colton LA, Nesterova A, Stenmark KR, Reusch JE-B. cAMP response element-binding protein content is a molecular determinant of smooth muscle proliferation and migration. J Biol Chem 2001; 276:46132–46141.
107. Tokunou T, Ichiki T, Takeda K, Funakoshi Y, Iino N, Takeshita A. cAMP response element-binding protein mediates thrombin-induced proliferation of vascular smooth muscle cells. Arterioscler Thromb Vasc Biol 2001; 21:1764–1769.
108. Tokunou T, Shibata R, Kai H, Ichiki T, Morisaki T, Fukuyama K, Ono H, Iino N, Masuda S, Shimokawa H, Egashira K, Imaizumi T, Takeshita A. Apoptosis induced by inhibition of cyclic AMP response element–binding protein in vascular smooth muscle cells. Circulation 2003; 108:1246–1252.
109. Valverde P, Koren G. Purification and preliminary characterization of a cardiac Kv1.5 repressor element binding factor. Circ Res 1999; 84:937–944.
110. Mori Y, Folco E, Koren G. GH3 cell-specific expression of Kv1.5 gene. Regulation by a silencer containing a dinucleotide repetitive element. J Biol Chem 1995; 270:27788–27796.
111. Zhang W-M, Yip K-P, Lin M-J, Shimoda LA, Li W-H, Sham JSK. ET-1 activates Ca^{2+} sparks in PASMC: local Ca^{2+} signaling between inositol trisphosphate and ryanodine receptors. Am J Physiol Lung Cell Mol Physiol 2003; 285:L680–L690.
112. Davie N, Haleen SJ, Upton PD, Polak JM, Yacoub MH, Morrell NW, Wharton J. ET_A and ET_B receptors modulate the proliferation of human pulmonary artery smooth muscle cells. Am J Respir Crit Care Med 2002; 165: 398–405.

113. Platoshyn O, Golovina VA, Bailey CL, Limsuwan A, Krick S, Juhaszova M, Seiden JE, Rubin LJ, Yuan JX-J. Sustained membrane depolarization and pulmonary artery smooth muscle cell proliferation. Am J Physiol Cell Physiol 2000; 279:C1540–C1549.
114. Yu Y, Sweeney M, Zhang S, Platoshyn O, Landsberg J, Rothman A, Yuan JX-J. PDGF stimulates pulmonary vascular smooth muscle cell proliferation by upregulating TRPC6 expression. Am J Physiol Cell Physiol 2003; 284:C316–C330.
115. Kuryshev YA, Gudz TI, Brown AM, Wible BA. KChAP as a chaperone for specific K^+ channels. Am J Physiol Cell Physiol 2000; 278:C931–C941.
116. Kuryshev YA, Wible BA, Gudz TI, Ramirez AN, Brown AM. KChAP/Kvβ1.2 interactions and their effects on cardiac Kv channel expression. Am J Physiol Cell Physiol 2001; 281:C290–C299.
117. An WF, Bowlby MR, Betty M, Cao J, Ling H-P, Mendoza G, Hinson JW, Mattson KI, Strassle BW, Trimmer JS, Rhodes KJ. Modulation of A-type potassium channels by a family of calcium sensors. Nature 2000; 403:553–556.
118. Patel SP, Campbell DL, Strauss HC. Elucidating KChIP effects on Kv4.3 inactivation and recovery kinetics with a minimal KChIP2 isoform. J Physiol 2002; 545:5–11.
119. Song KS, Scherer PE, Tang Z, Okamoto T, Li S, Chafel M, Chu C, Kohtz DS, Lisanti MP. Expression of caveolin-3 in skeletal, cardiac, and smooth muscle cells. Caveolin-3 is a component of the sarcolemma and co-fractionates with dystrophin and dystrophin-associated glycoproteins. J Biol Chem 1996; 271:15160–15165.
120. Zhao Y-Y, Liu Y, Stan R-V, Fan L, Gu Y, Dalton N, Chu P-H, Peterson K, Ross JJ, Chien KR. Defects in caveolin-1 cause dilated cardiomyopathy and pulmonary hypertension in knockout mice. Proc Natl Acad Sci USA 2002; 99:11375–11380.
121. Martens JR, Sakamoto N, Sullivan SA, Grobaski TD, Tamkun MM. Isoform-specific localization of voltage-gated K^+ channels to distinct lipid raft populations. Targeting of Kv1.5 to caveolae. J Biol Chem 2001; 276: 8409–8414.
122. Pike LJ, Han X, Chung K-N, Gross RW. Lipid rafts are enriched in arachidonic acid and plasmenylethanolamine and their composition is independent of caveolin-1 expression: a quantitative electrospray ionization/mass spectrometric analysis. Biochemistry 2002; 41:2075–2088.
123. Fang X, Weintraub NL, Stoll LL, Spector AA. Epoxyeicosatrienoic acids increase intracellular calcium concentration in vascular smooth muscle cells. Hypertension 1999; 34:1242–1246.
124. Krick S, Platoshyn O, McDaniel SS, Rubin LJ, Yuan JX-J. Augmented K^+ currents and mitochondrial membrane depolarization in pulmonary artery myocyte apoptosis. Am J Physiol Lung Cell Mol Physiol 2001; 281: L887–L894.
125. Mori Y, Matsubara H, Folco E, Siegel A, Koren G. The transcription of a mammalian voltage-gated potassium channel is regulated by cAMP in a cell-specific manner. J Biol Chem 1993; 268:26487–26493.

126. Archer SL, Hampl V, Nelson DP, Sidney E, Peterson DA, Weir EK. Dithionite increases radical formation and decreases vasoconstriction in the lung. Evidence that dithionite does not mimic alveolar hypoxia. Circ Res 1995; 77:174–181.
127. Archer SL, Souil E, Dinh-Xan AT, Schremmer B, Mercier JC, Yaagoubi AE, Nguyer-Huu L, Reeve HL, Hampl V. Molecular identification of the role of voltage-gated K^+ channels, Kv1.5 and Kv2.1, in hypoxic pulmonary vasoconstriction and control of resting membrane potential in rat pulmonary artery myocytes. J Clin Invest 1998; 101:2319–2330.
128. Davies ARL, Kozlowski RZ. Kv channel subunit expression in rat pulmonary arteries. Lung 2001; 179:147–161.
129. Yuan XJ, Wang J, Juhaszova M, Golovina VA, Rubin LJ. Molecular basis and function of voltage-gated K^+ channels in pulmonary arterial smooth muscle cells. Am J Physiol 1998; 274:L621–L635.
130. Conforti L, Bodi I, Nisbet JW, Milhorn DE. O_2-sensitive K^+ channels: role of the Kv1.2 α-subunit in mediating the hypoxic response. J Physiol 2000; 524:783–793.
131. Conforti L, Millhorn DE. Selective inhibition of a slow-inactivating voltage-dependent K^+ channel in rat PC12 cells by hypoxia. J Physiol 1997; 502:293–305.
132. Archer SL, London B, Hampl V, Wu X, Nsair A, Puttagunta L, Hashimoto K, Waite RE, Michelakis ED. Impairment of hypoxic pulmonary vasoconstriction in mice lacking the voltage-gated potassium channel Kv1.5. FASEB J 2001; 15:1801–1803.

19

Ion Channels and the Effects of Hypoxia in Pulmonary Artery Endothelial Cells

Andrew R. L. Davies, Dayle S. Hogg, and Roland Z. Kozlowski
University of Bristol, Bristol, U.K.

I. INTRODUCTION

The vascular endothelium forms the lumenal surface of blood vessels and exerts an essential role as a selective barrier to the vessel lumen. A host of functions are performed by the vascular endothelium, some of which are unique in relation to the vascular bed or size of the vessel in which the endothelial cells are located. The vascular endothelium is able to regulate permeability to gases, fluids, solids, cells, macromolecules, nutrients, metabolites, and autocrine and paracrine factors, not only to the endothelial cells themselves but also to the underlying smooth muscle cells. It also exerts a profound influence on vascular tone, manipulating blood pressure and flow by adjusting the caliber of the arteries and arterioles.

In addition to its roles in controlling permeability and influencing vascular tone, the endothelium is also involved in blood coagulation, transport between blood and tissues, movement of cells such as white blood cells and thrombocytes adhering to the endothelium, wound healing, angiogenesis, and immune responses. Many of these actions are facilitated by the release of a diverse range of vasoactive mediators from endothelial cells (ECs). These modulatory agents include nitric oxide (NO), endothelium-derived hyperpolarizing factor (EDHF), prostaglandins, endothelins (ET), natriuretic peptide, small signaling molecules such as substance P, ATP, growth factors, steroids, and large proteins involved in the blood-clotting cascade.

A. Regulation of Vascular Tone by the Endothelium

The ECs of pulmonary resistance arteries exert the greatest influence on blood pressure and flow. Vasoactive factors are released by these cells in response to humoral stimuli, mechanical stimuli such as shear or biaxial tensile stress, and autonomic nerves. The release of endothelium-derived relaxing factors such as NO, prostacyclin, arachidonic acid, histamine, and EDHF is balanced by the release of endothelium-derived constricting factors (EDCFs) such as ET to produce the required physiological response through their effects on the underlying smooth muscle layer of the arteries (1).

In addition to the release of vasoactive substances from the pulmonary endothelium, transmission of signals from ECs to the smooth muscle layer can also occur via the movement of ions or small molecules through myoendothelial gap junctions. Gap junction communication between ECs within the endothelium and between ECs and smooth muscle cells could therefore influence pulmonary vascular tone. Thus, the EC membrane potential (E_m) may have a direct influence on the smooth muscle cell E_m, consequently modulating the contractile state of the smooth muscle and ultimately vascular tone. Myoendothelial gap junctions have been shown to exist in pulmonary arteries (PAs) (2) and electrical coupling demonstrated between pulmonary artery endothelial cells (PAECs) in lung slice preparations (3).

B. Role of Endothelial Cell Ion Channels in Determining Release of Vasoactive Mediators

The release of many vasoactive substances from ECs is dependent upon an increase in the intracellular Ca^{2+} concentration. In turn, the E_m of ECs can regulate the driving force for Ca^{2+} influx and therefore the intracellular Ca^{2+} concentration, ultimately regulating vascular tone through the release of vasoactive factors. Because they are the determining entities of E_m, it is important to know which ion channels are present in ECs in order to facilitate an understanding of the factors that regulate them under physiological and pathological conditions. ECs from vessels of different sizes, and from different vascular beds, express a multitude of different ion channels (4), and their characterization can be hampered by the fact that the expression shows a degree of plasticity and can vary between cells. Changes in ion channel expression are known to occur under physiological conditions in a huge variety of cell types. But when evaluating a system to characterize the current profiles of expressed channels, the changes that are induced by cell isolation, culture, and growth conditions must be considered (5). These changes may begin to explain some of the highly variable and conflicting results within the published literature.

When considering the involvement of ion channels in Ca^{2+} signaling in ECs as well as the contribution to electrogenesis, ion channels can be loosely divided into two groups: (1) ion channels that provide a direct Ca^{2+} entry pathway and (2) ion channels that contribute to determining the E_m and thereby indirectly regulate the driving force for Ca^{2+} entry. The myriad of ion channels expressed in ECs have recently been extensively reviewed (4), and it is now clear that these encompass several calcium entry pathways. These include (1) nonselective cation channels, (2) store-operated or capacitative Ca^{2+} entry, and (3) members of the *trp* gene family. Critical for understanding the physiological role of PAECs is the control of E_m. K^+ channels are the most important class of ion channels involved in the control of the E_m of a cell. A number of different channels are involved in this process, including the Ca^{2+}-activated, inwardly rectifying, and, in some preparations, voltage-dependent K^+ channels. Cl^- channels, such as the volume-regulated and Ca^{2+}-activated Cl channels, in addition to calcium-impermeable nonselective cation channels, have also been shown to contribute to determining the resting E_m in various EC preparations. It is clear that the ion channel expression of endothelial cells differs depending upon the vascular bed studied and between larger conduit vessels compared to resistance vessels and capillaries, reflecting perhaps the different physiological roles of these vessels and vascular beds.

C. Role of the Endothelium in Hypoxic Pulmonary Vasoconstriction

Hypoxic pulmonary vasoconstriction (HPV) is a mechanism whereby capillary perfusion is modulated to match alveolar ventilation by diverting blood flow away from poorly ventilated regions of the lung. This is brought about by the constriction of small resistance pulmonary arteries in response to a reduction in the local oxygen tension, and detailed discussions of the mechanisms surrounding this phenomenon, unique to the pulmonary vasculature, are reviewed in Chapter 24. Vasoconstriction of isolated small PAs in response to hypoxia is now widely accepted to consist of a biphasic response (6). The initial phase consists of a rapid, transient increase in vascular tone that develops over about 5–10 min. After the initial phase begins to recede, the second phase, a slowly developing but sustained elevation of vascular constriction, ensues, reaching a plateau after about 40 min. It has been shown that the initial transient phase of HPV is intrinsic to pulmonary arterial smooth muscle, because this phase of constriction remains even after removal of the endothelium (6), although the endothelium may be able to modulate the transient phase of constriction to some extent. Similar observations of the effects of hypoxia have been recorded in conduit PAs and some systemic arteries where an initial transient constriction precedes a sustained vasodilation (7). The second phase, however, is believed to be endothelium-dependent and appears to be unique to small PAs, because the second phase of HPV is abolished after removal of the endothelium

(6). Thus it would appear that multiple oxygen-sensing mechanisms exist within PAs, all of which may be necessary for the full expression of HPV. Intuitively, however, it would seem that the physiological relevance of the second, endothelium-dependent, phase is greater than the first phase, because the second phase can be sustained (7), indicating a pivotal role for the ECs of small resistance PAs in HPV. Because it is the resistance PAs that mediate hypoxic constriction leading to a rise in PA pressure, significant differences must exist in the expression of oxygen-sensing mechanisms between the smooth muscle cells and endothelial cells of both small and large PAs. The differences in the responses to hypoxia between the smooth muscle of small and large PAs have been correlated to the phenotypic differences in pulmonary artery smooth muscle cells (PASMCs) and their K^+ current profile from these two regions (8). Clearly, understanding the effects hypoxia exerts on the pulmonary endothelium, particularly from resistance PAs, is important for our comprehension of the pulmonary response to hypoxia under physiological and pathological conditions.

Endothelial cells release an array of vasoactive agents, and many candidates have been proposed as initiators or modulators of the endothelium-dependent components of HPV. Vasoconstriction mediated in response to hypoxia could result from either the increased release of vasoconstrictors or decreased release of vasodilators (9). However, if a decrease in the release of a vasodilator were instrumental in HPV, removal of the endothelium would be expected to increase tension during hypoxia, whereas it actually reduces phase 2 to a level below the pretone (7). Furthermore, release of endothelium-derived mediators may be a prerequisite for conferring sensitivity of PASMCs to hypoxia (10).

Nitric oxide is a potent vasodilator that can be released from the pulmonary endothelium. In the majority of recent studies, hypoxia limits the production of NO (11), as might be expected because molecular O_2 is required for NO synthesis. However, studies on the contribution of NO to HPV provide little evidence of a significant involvement. Conversely, NO production may act as a physiological braking mechanism against HPV (9). Metabolites of arachidonic acid, a precursor of a number of vasoactive substances, have also been postulated to play a role in HPV. A number of reports indicate that arachidonic acid metabolites from the cyclooxygenase, lipoxygenase, and cytochrome P-450 monooxygenase pathways may potentially contribute to modulating HPV to varying extents (9).

Several reports have suggested that a vasoconstrictor released from the endothelium is central to the sustained, endothelium-dependent phase of HPV (12,13). To date, several reports have attempted to address the identity of this mediator. Endothelin 1 (ET-1), a 21-amino-acid peptide, has frequently been proposed as the identity of this mediator. ET-1 can indeed constrict PAs, raising pulmonary vascular resistance, but these observations appear to vary depending on species, level of pretone applied, and the size and/or position of vessels within the pulmonary vascular tree. These differential effects may be due in part to the existence of different subtypes of ET receptors, which modulate different PASMC membrane currents (14–16). Also, the slow reversal of ET-1-mediated vasoconstriction is in marked contrast to the effects of hypoxia, and furthermore, infusion of ET-1 does not potentiate HPV. Contradictions in studies using ET receptor antagonists have only served to increase confusion as to the role of ET receptors and ET-1 in HPV (9). A possible explanation of the results is that ET-1 may play a "priming" role in HPV rather than acting as the primary stimulus (17), which supports the evidence suggesting that PASMCs may require prior membrane depolarization by ET-1 in order to respond fully to hypoxia (10). Although the role of the vasoconstricitor ET-1 in HPV is unclear, evidence is accumulating for the role of other endothelium-derived constricting factors (12,13). A factor that is thought to be distinct from ET-1, pulmonary selective, and released in response to hypoxia seemingly sensitizes PASMCs to intracellular free Ca^{2+} and has been partially purified (13). The factor promotes a response similar to the second phase of HPV, but further work is needed to reveal its molecular identity. Although a consensus as to the identity of the EC-derived factors that contribute to HPV remains to be achieved, the mechanism whereby PAECs sense reduced Po_2 and signal the modulation of the vasoactive agent released will remain key to understanding HPV. Thus, PAEC ion channels and their effects on E_m and intracellular free Ca^{2+} are likely to be integral components of this process.

II. ION CHANNELS IN PULMONARY ARTERY ENDOTHELIAL CELLS

One of the most extensively used preparations for the study and characterization of ECs is a cell line established from ECs of proximal calf PAs (cell line CPAE; American Type Culture Collection, Rockille, MD, USA). It must be emphasized that caution must be exercised when interpreting functional data from EC preparations in relation to the membrane currents relevant to native PAECs for a number of reasons. First, as described previously, the response of PAs to hypoxia depends upon vessel size and the relative position in the PA tree. Heterogeneity in the properties of the PAECs from different-sized vessels is therefore likely to be encountered, and it is likely that the CPAE model, because it is derived from the main PAs, will not possess the oxygen-sensing mechanisms intrinsic to the ECs of small PAs. Furthermore, there is growing evidence that the expression of ion channels and receptors may be altered in many cell types following primary or long-term cell culture (5,18,19). However, the amenability of cultured ECs for electrophysiological studies has led to the membrane currents of CPAE cells being among the most characterized.

Three dominant membrane currents are displayed by CPAE cells: a prominent inwardly rectifying K^+ current, an outwardly rectifying Cl^- current, and a voltage-independent, nonselective cationic background current. Together, these three currents form the major determinants of the membrane potential (20) of these cells. A low-slope conductance in the region between −70 mV and 0 mV means that minor modulation of any one of these currents could result in a major depolarizing or hyperpolarizing change in the resting E_m. This indicates that factors influencing the conductance of these channels can have a large influence on E_m and in turn on the intracellular free Ca^{2+}, ultimately resulting in modulation of pulmonary vascular tone. This situation may provide an explanation for the observed scatter of E_m in resting CPAE cells. Cells could be observed with an E_m between –88 and +5 mV with a bimodal distribution between hyperpolarized cells and relatively depolarized cells (20). Interestingly, when short-term cultured cells (passages 4–7) from PA conduit and microvascular endothelium were compared, the bimodal distribution was present only within the population of cells from the larger vessels. Microvascular cells had a more depolarized unimodal distribution centered on –22 mV (21). When PAECs were freshly isolated from small pulmonary arteries of the rat, two populations of cells were observed, as indicated by their K^+ current profiles from voltage-clamp experiments. The minority population (~10%) of cells had an E_m distribution consistent with that shown for calf conduit PAECs. However, the majority population (~90%) had E_m values that were fitted by a single Gaussian distribution and a mean resting E_m of –36 mV (22,23), a value that is consistent with the E_m of ECs from other resistance-sized vessels (24–26). Because cell cultures may have originated from just a few ECs or even a single endothelial cell, studies performed on freshly isolated cell preparations may provide a much broader and more representative cross-sectional sample of the population of cells present in small PAs. These findings are consistent with a graded change in the properties of PAECs as vessel size decreases, which may have particular relevance to PAEC function in HPV. Furthermore, they serve to emphasize the care that must be taken in interpreting the membrane currents involved in PAEC function when taking into account the origins and suitability of the cells chosen as a model.

A. K^+ Currents in PAECs

The CPAE cell line, derived from conduit PAECs, displays a prominent inwardly rectifying potassium current (I_{KIR}) (20). I_{KIR} shows strong inward rectification and reverses close to the K^+ equilibrium potential. This current could be blocked by Ba^{2+}, had a single-channel conductance of 31 pS, and was not sensitive to changes in pH within the physiological range (27). By comparison to the properties of cloned inwardly rectifying potassium channels, it was proposed that the channel was a product of the Kir2.1 gene.

RT-PCR did indeed confirm the presence of Kir2.1 mRNA in CPAE cells (27). CPAE cells with E_m values more negative than –35 mV, out of the wide range of resting E_m in these cells, were rapidly and reversibly depolarized to around –10 mV (20) by Ba^{2+} inhibition of I_{KIR}. The importance of I_{KIR} in setting the membrane potential, coupled with the observed G-protein-dependent regulation of the channel (27), suggests a role for these channels in determining the driving force for Ca^{2+} entry during cell stimulation. The channel also appears to be sensitive to metabolic regulators, with a reduction in intracellular ATP and an induction of hypoxic conditions dramatically attenuating I_{KIR} (27). This may contribute to a mechanism for determining the release of vasoactive agents from the PAECs in response to the metabolic or redox state of the cell. Such regulation might be important during episodes of hypoxia within the PAs.

In endothelial cells freshly isolated from resistance-sized PAs, two distinct populations of cells could be distinguished from their whole-cell electrophysiological profile (Fig. 1) (23). Ten percent of the cells were characterized by a Ba^{2+}-sensitive inward rectifier K^+ conductance with properties consistent with the I_{KIR} demonstrated in CPAE cells (Figs. 1C and 1D). However, 90% of the cells were characterized by a voltage-dependent, outwardly rectifying K^+ current (I_{KV}) that activated close to the E_m (Figs. 1A and 1B). The current showed clear voltage-dependent activation with little or no time-dependent inactivation and was sensitive to inhibition by 4-aminopyridine but not tetraethylammonium chloride (22,23,28). The properties of this I_{KV} are shared by a number of cloned Kv channel subtypes, including Kv1.1, Kv1.2, Kv1.3, Kv1.5, Kv3.1, and Kv2.1, and appear to be unusual among reported K^+ currents in endothelial cells from different vascular regions, with the exception of coronary vascular endothelial cells (29). The I_{KV} in freshly isolated PAECs activates close to the resting E_m, so it may play a role in controlling this parameter. A small membrane depolarization could evoke the rapid activation of this outward current and counteract any further membrane depolarizations, because the current displays very slow inactivation. Activation of these currents could also initiate sustained hyperpolarization and alter the transmembrane flux of Ca^{2+} and therefore the release of vasoactive compounds. This might impart a particular functional relevance to this subset of cells displaying I_{KV}.

In contrast to the above studies on CPAE cells and isolated resistance-sized PAECs is a patch-clamp investigation of the electrical properties of rat pulmonary artery endothelial cells in situ, of vessels from arteries smaller than those of the previous studies (15–40 µm). This study revealed K^+ currents that were not voltage-dependent or sensitive to 4-aminopyridine, tetraethylammonium, or charybdotoxin. They were, however, pH-sensitive and thus were proposed to belong to the family of twin-pore-domain K^+ channels (3). The vessels used in this study were extremely small (15–40 µm) and so may represent another set of PAECs with different

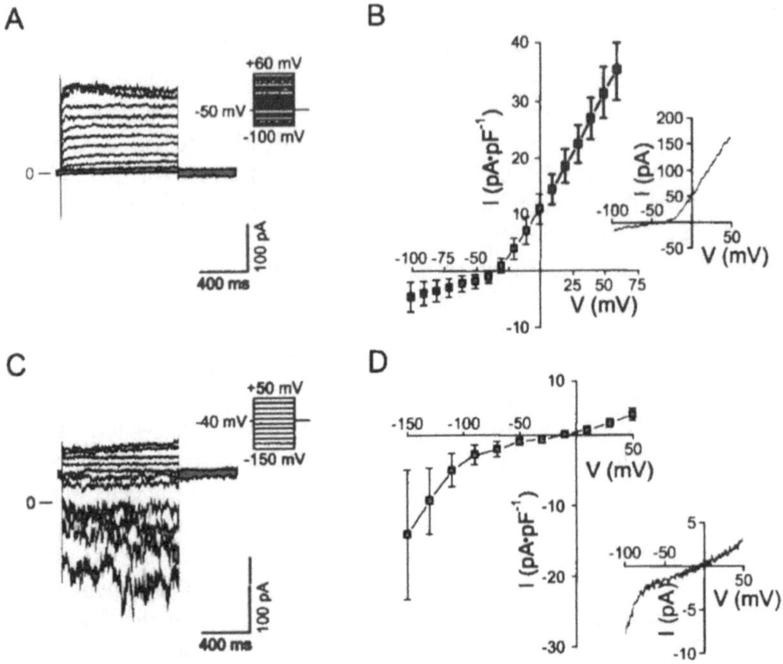

Figure 1 Membrane currents recorded under perforated-patch conditions from PAECs displaying two unique populations of cells that are characterized by either an outwardly rectifying or an inwardly rectifying electrophysiological current profile. (A) A typical family of membrane currents evoked in response to 1000 ms voltage steps from −100 mV to +60 mV in 10 mV increments from a holding potential of −50 mV (see inset), for cells that display a voltage-dependent outwardly rectifying current profile. (B) Mean steady-state *I–V* relationship for currents recorded using the voltage-step protocol described in (A) ($n = 5$). The inset illustrates typical currents recorded in response to depolarizing voltage ramps from −100 mV to +50 mV and show a profile identical to those induced using voltage steps. (C) Typical family of inward-rectifier currents recorded from PAECs in response to voltage steps from −150 mV to +50 mV in 20 mV increments (see inset). (D) Mean steady-state *I–V* relationship for currents recorded using the voltage protocol described in (C) ($n = 3$). The inset illustrates that currents evoked in response to voltage ramps from −100 mV to +50 mV show characteristics similar to those induced by voltage steps. (From Ref. 23.)

properties and functions from those of CPAE cells (from conduit vessels) or the freshly isolated PAECs (from rat vessels ranging from 200 to 400 μm). In terms of the importance of endothelial cell modulation of vascular tone, it is well established that it is the small pulmonary arteries that contribute most to pulmonary blood flow resistance (30). However, a detailed study of the anatomy of the pulmonary artery tree reveals that very small PAs, just before vessels become capillaries, possess little or no smooth muscle in the vessel walls (31). It is therefore likely to be the intermediate branches (200–400 μm in the rat) that contribute most to the modulation of PA resistance.

It is clear that the distribution of PAECs displaying different K^+ current profiles, and the molecular identity of the channels, must be understood if the functional relevance of these channels and cells is to be revealed. As stated previously, the molecular identity of channels responsible for I_{KIR} in CPAE cells has been proposed as Kir2.1 (27). Immunohistochemical localization, using anti-Kir2.1 antibody (Fig. 2), shows the presence of the channel protein in the endothelium of small PAs (23,28). The similarity of I_{KIR} in a subpopulation of PAECs from small PAs to that in CPAE cells, coupled with the identification of Kir2.1 protein, suggests that this channel may in part contribute to the I_{KIR} present in both cell preparations. However, the outwardly rectifying K^+ current expressed in the majority of freshly isolated PAECs from small PAs resembles that of a number of Kv channel subtypes, as previously stated. Both Kv1.5 (22,23,28,32) and Kv2.1 (28) have been identified in small PA endothelia by using antibody staining (Fig. 2). It is not clear from the present immunolocalization data whether Kir and Kv channels are coexpressed in the same PAECs or in different populations. However, the latter situation would provide an explanation for the two functionally distinct populations of cells from PA endothelia. More extensive studies, using a wider variety of K^+ channel antibodies and dual labeling techniques, will be required to correlate fully the electrophysiological profiles of distinct PAEC populations with particular K^+ channel expression profiles.

The electrophysiological profiles of PAECs from large and small PAs and the presence of multiple K^+ channel types are consistent with a variation in endothelial cell K^+ channel expression, dependent upon the position of the cells within the PA tree. Kir2.1 seems to be important in large PA ECs, with voltage-gated K^+ channels having greater influence in small PA ECs. More studies will be required to attribute fully the K^+ current profiles to specific K^+ channels and determine their distribution throughout the PA tree. However, it is tempting to speculate that the differences noted between large- and small-artery PAECs contribute to the different functional roles of these cells in controlling vascular tone and pulmonary arterial blood flow.

B. Cl^- Currents in PAECs

Following inhibition by Ba^{2+} of I_{KIR} in CPAE cells, the dominant current was characterized by outwardly rectifying, chloride-permeable channels (20). Superfusion of these cells with hypotonic solution results in cell swelling that activates a volume-sensitive chloride current ($I_{Cl,vol}$). Crucially,

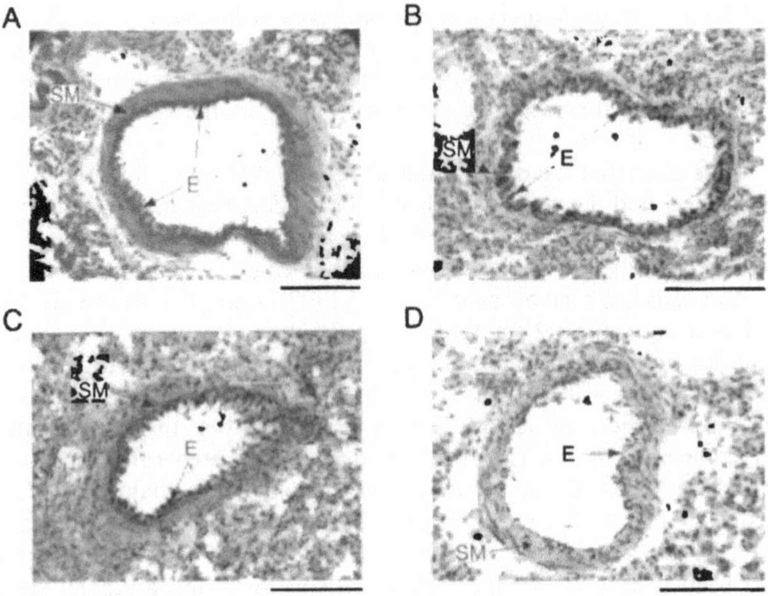

Figure 2 Immunolocalization of anti-Kv1.5, anti-Kir2.1, and anti-Kv2.1 in small pulmonary arteries (200–400 μm diameter) from sections of rat lung. (A) Immunolocalization of anti-Kv1.5 is present in the smooth muscle layer and is also very prominent in the endothelium. (B) Anti-Kir2.1 immunoreactivity is very marked in the endothelium, but very little localization is present in the smooth muscle layer. (C) Anti-Kv2.1 immunoreactivity is localized to the endothelium of pulmonary arteries and also present within the smooth muscle layer. Areas in brown represent localization of antibody immunoreactivity. (D) Representative example of a control experiment showing the absence of nonspecific staining with the secondary antibody in the absence of the primary antibodies. Note the complete absence of any immunolocalization of the channel proteins. Areas in blue represent nucleophilic staining with hematoxylin. Bar = 100 μm. E = endothelium. SM = smooth muscle. (Adapted from Ref. 23.)

shrinkage of the cells with hypertonic solutions decreases the current below the level seen in isotonic solution, indicating that the current is partially active in resting cells and may be important for the electrogenesis of the resting potential. $I_{Cl,vol}$ in CPAE cells is sensitive to 4,4′-diisothiocyanatostilbene-2,2′-disulfonic acid (DIDS), 5-nitro-2-(3-phenylpropylamino) benzoate (NPPB), quinine, quinidine, and tamoxifen (20,33). $I_{Cl,vol}$ is also activated by a reduction of intracellular ionic strength and by intracellular dialysis of GTPγS, independently of cell swelling (34,35). Clearly this current can be modulated by complex and diverse stimuli under physiological conditions, with a resulting influence on the E_m of PAECs.

In addition to $I_{Cl,vol}$, a calcium-activated chloride current, $I_{Cl,Ca}$ has also been shown to be present in CPAE cells (36). This current was strongly outwardly rectifying, was activated by increasing intracellular Ca^{2+} concentrations, and was sensitive to DIDS, niflumic acid, *N*-phenylanthracilic acid (NPA), NPPB, and tamoxifen. $I_{Cl,Ca}$ can be distinguished from $I_{Cl,vol}$ on the basis of their kinetic and rectification properties (33,36). $I_{Cl,Ca}$ displays much stronger outward rectification than $I_{Cl,vol}$. $I_{Cl,vol}$ slowly inactivates at positive potentials, whereas $I_{Cl,Ca}$ inactivates at negative potentials and shows activation at positive potentials. $I_{Cl,vol}$ also has a markedly greater current density than $I_{Cl,Ca}$. The properties of these currents are such that they will both be activated under various physiological conditions. However, cAMP-activated and voltage-dependent chloride currents are absent from CPAE cells (33).

The molecular identities of the channels responsible for $I_{Cl,vol}$ and $I_{Cl,Ca}$ are still unknown. Volume-regulated anion channels are observed, in one form or another, in the majority of mammalian cells. A number of molecular candidates for these channels have been proposed, including P-glycoprotein, ClC-2, ClC-3, and phospholemman. However, none of these appear to have the characteristics necessary to provide a convincing case for being responsible for the $I_{Cl,vol}$ observed in CPAE cells (discussed in Ref. 4 and references therein). Similarly, a number of genes have been cloned that, when expressed in HEK cells, produce currents similar to $I_{Cl,Ca}$. These include CLCA1, CLCA2, CLCA3, and the endothelial adhesion protein Lu-ECAM. However, the identity of the channel responsible for $I_{Cl,Ca}$ in CPAE cells remains to be fully elucidated (4).

A chloride conductance develops over the first 22 days of postnatal development in rat PAECs, as detected by recording from ECs, from small-diameter PAs, in situ (3). The functional relevance of the postnatal development of this current has not been determined, and the properties of the channels responsible have not yet been investigated. The presence and nature of a chloride conductance in freshly isolated PAECs from small PAs have not been studied, unlike the main cationic currents (22,23). Apart from differences in currents from CPAE cells due to the size of the donor vessels, the nature of chloride currents may vary owing to cell culture conditions. For example, the volume-regulated anion channel in mouse primary cultured aortic ECs has a lower current density and activates more slowly than the current observed in cultured cell lines (37). Although the Cl^- channels in CPAE cells have been well studied because of the common use of this cell line as a model, the lack of data from small-PA PAECs makes it difficult to determine the specific role of Cl^- channels in these cells.

In general, $I_{Cl,Ca}$ and $I_{Cl,vol}$ are each predominantly activated by their specific stimuli of vasoactive agonists and mechanical stimulation, inducing changes in cell shape and volume. They may also be coactivated under various physiological conditions. The chloride channels have a dominant effect in some stimulated endothelial cells, with the associated importance in setting the membrane potential and hence the driving force for calcium entry and direct electrical coupling through gap junctions. This will therefore be reflected in the direct and indirect endothelium-dependent modulation of the underlying smooth muscle. The mechano-sensing properties of $I_{Cl,vol}$, in response to shear stress and biaxial tensile stress, may be particularly important in EC function for determining the flow-modulated release of vasoactive mediators. In addition, anion channels may be important for the transport of amino acids, organic osmolytes, and HCO_3^-, which is important for regulation of the intracellular pH in ECs (4,38). $I_{Cl,vol}$ and $I_{Cl,Ca}$ are common to many cell types, not just ECs, and although they could influence the many functions of PAECs, it is difficult to identify how they could have a unique role in the pulmonary vasculature with the constraints of current knowledge and pharmacological tools.

C. Nonselective Cation Channels in PAECs

Both cultured CPAE cells and freshly isolated PAECs display a nonselective cation current (I_{NSC}). Inhibition of K^+ currents by ionic substitution of K^+ for Cs^+ in freshly isolated PAECs from resistance vessels revealed a whole-cell I_{NSC} with little time or voltage dependence (28,39). Ion substitution experiments and blocking of the dominant K^+ currents with 4-AP and TEA identified a permeability sequence of $K^+ > Cs^+ > Na^+ >$ *N*-methyl-D-glucamine$^+$ ($NMDG^+$). This is similar to the permeability of the I_{NSC} described in cultured CPAE cells (20) and in PASMCs (40). The reversal potential of I_{NSC} was very close to the resting E_m recorded in PAECs under K^+-free conditions, suggesting a possibly significant contribution to electrogenesis under physiological conditions (20,28,39). Under physiological conditions, the E_m of isolated PAECs was ~−35 mV (22,23), a potential at which the I_{NSC} would be active, perhaps providing a small efflux pathway for K^+ and a small influx pathway for Na^+.

Some nonselective cation channels in ECs provide an influx pathway for Ca^{2+} (4). Transmembrane Ca^{2+} influx via nonselective cation channels has been implicated in the release of a number of vasoactive substances, including NO and prostacyclin (41,42). The I_{NSC} described in freshly isolated PAECs (28,39), cultured CPAE cells (20), and PASMCs (40) was not shown to be permeable to Ca^{2+}. However, membrane currents of approximately 1 pA, as described for store depletion–activated Ca^{2+} entry into endothelial cells (43), would fall below the detection limit of the patch-clamp recording technique. The I_{NSC} of freshly isolated PAECs differs from the other two currents in that it was not inhibited by the presence of Ca^{2+}. The I_{NSC} in these cells also differs in its sensitivity to block by trivalent cations. The I_{NSC} in PAECs could be attenuated by both Gd^{3+} and La^{3+}, as could the I_{NSC} in human umbilical vein ECs (44), whereas the I_{NSC} in CPAE cells was not sensitive to Gd^{3+} (20).

The mean steady-state *I–V* relationship of I_{NSC} in freshly isolated PAECs also shows a weak inward rectification at hyperpolarized potentials, which is not observed in I_{NSC} of CPAE cells. This characteristic has been noted in ECs isolated from intrapulmonary artery (45) and in vascular endothelial cells after activation by mechanical stretch (46). It is therefore possible that a component of stretch-induced I_{NSC} present in these cells was activated during the studies on freshly isolated PAECs. Whether the differences in I_{NSC} current properties arise from altered channel expression due to either cell culture differences or the size of the PA from which the ECs originate is not clear. It would be difficult to address this question at the present time because no clear molecular candidates exist for Ca^{2+}-impermeable nonselective cation channels. They are worthy of further investigation, however, because they contribute to the resting E_m of PAECs under physiological conditions (20,39).

A number of functionally different receptor-activated cation channels have been described in ECs from various vascular beds. These are gated by agonists binding to their membrane receptor, usually via a signaling cascade involving phospholipase C, and provide a Ca^{2+} entry pathway (4). A histamine-activated cation channel has been described in rat intrapulmonary artery ECs (45). The channel shows a high permeability for Ca^{2+} but is also permeable to Na^+ and K^+, with a permeability ratio of P_K 1: P_{Na} 1: P_{Ca} 15.7. This channel is clearly distinct from the channels responsible for I_{NSC} in isolated PAECs and cultured CPAE cells, under nonstimulated conditions, as described above. However, the existence of such receptor-activated cation channels in these preparations has not been investigated and could well provide functionally important Ca^{2+} entry and signaling mechanisms.

III. EFFECTS OF HYPOXIA ON PULMONARY ARTERY ENDOTHELIAL CELL ION CHANNELS

As discussed earlier, regulation of PAEC membrane potential and cytosolic calcium concentrations are inextricably linked to the modulation of pulmonary vascular tone. The ion channels that determine these properties may therefore exert a crucial role in mediating the effects of hypoxia during HPV. The effects of hypoxia on ion channels have been implicated in the unique responses of specialized, oxygen-sensitive cells and tissues of the carotid body (47), neuroepithelial body (48), and the pulmonary vasculature (49). Indeed, much discussion about the role of oxygen-sensitive K^+ channels in the transient, smooth-muscle-dependent phase of HPV has been published (50–53) and is reviewed in Chapters 17 and 18. Most of the studies on oxygen-sensitive channels in PAs relate to channels of the PASMCs. However, there are indications that hypoxia can also modulate ionic currents in PAECs.

A. Hypoxia-Sensitive K^+ Channels in PAECs

The majority of PAECs freshly isolated from rat small pulmonary arteries express a voltage-dependent, outwardly rectifying K^+ channel (see Sec. II.A). Using the perforated-patch-clamp technique, a reduction in oxygen tension from normoxia (Po_2 ~145 mmHg) to hypoxia (Po_2 ~25 mmHg) elicited a small but significant reduction in whole-cell currents generated by depolarizing voltage ramps (28). Peak outward currents as measured at +40 mV were inhibited by ~16%. The hypoxia-sensitive current was voltage-dependent, showing strong outward rectification and a reversal potential of ~−29 mV (Fig. 3). The proximity of the reversal potential of this oxygen-sensitive component of I_{Kv} to the E_m of PAECs suggests that this current could have an important role in modulating the E_m in response to hypoxia.

A number of molecular candidates for the oxygen-sensing Kv channels in PASMCs have been proposed, including Kv1.2, Kv1.5, Kv2.1, Kv3.1b, and Kv9.3 (52,53). Immunolocalization of Kv1.5 and Kv2.1 to PAECs (see Sec. II.A) provides an indication that these subunits may be involved in mediating the hypoxia-sensitive I_{Kv}. However, from the modest effect of hypoxia on I_{Kv} in PAECs compared to that in PASMCs, a predominance of these subunits in smooth muscle would be expected. It is not possible to conclude this from the immunohistochemical studies carried out to date. Further studies, examining the distribution of a wider range of Kv channel subunits, will be required to determine which channels carry the

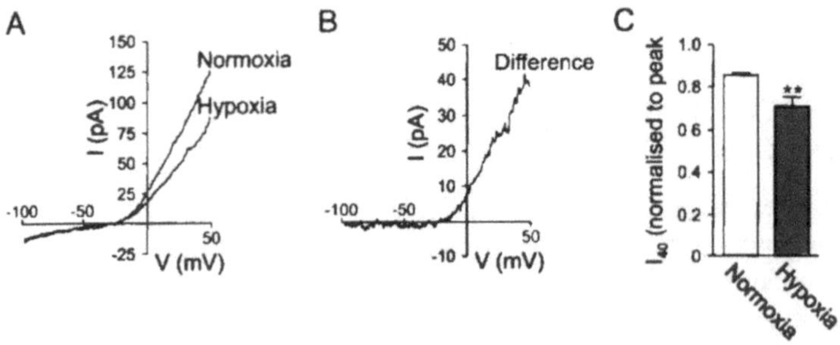

Figure 3 Effects of hypoxia on outwardly rectifying K^+ currents recorded from pulmonary arterial endothelial cells maintained in the perforated-patch configuration under physiological conditions. (A) An example of a typical I–V relationship derived from depolarizing voltage ramps from −100 mV to +50 mV under normoxic conditions. After application of hypoxia, outward currents were attenuated. (B) Representative example of the I–V relationship of the difference (hypoxia-sensitive) current. (C) Data summarizing the attenuation of the mean current recorded at +40 mV (I_{40}) during depolarization of voltage-ramp protocols under hypoxic conditions ($n = 7$). (**) $P < 0.005$ compared to control.

hypoxia-sensitive I_{Kv} in PAECs. It is also evident that expression of the proposed oxygen-sensitive Kv channel subunits is not sufficient in itself to explain the presence of an oxygen-sensitive K^+ current. For example, the presence of Kv1.5 and Kv2.1 has been shown in brain tissue and mesenteric arteries, which do not possess oxygen-sensitive K^+ currents, as well as in both small and large PAs (50). Similarly, controversy over the identity of the molecular candidates for the oxygen-sensitive Kv channels and the potential oxygen sensor in PASMCs (52,53) still remains. The facts that a correlation between the expression of Kv channels implicated as possible oxygen sensors and the magnitude of oxygen-sensitive K^+ currents between ECs and PASMCs cannot be made and that these subunits are not unique to PASMCs or PAECs would appear to support the hypothesis that a modulatory subunit or auxiliary subunit may confer oxygen sensitivity to Kv channels (51,54). It is tempting to speculate from these initial data that such hypoxia-sensitive currents will contribute to the E_m and cytosolic Ca^{2+} concentration of PAECs, as they do in PASMCs, providing a mechanism for the endothelium-dependent phase of HPV. Clearly, however, more work combining electrophysiology and functional proteomics is needed to establish such a role and identify the interacting proteins involved.

B. Hypoxia-Sensitive Nonselective Cation Channels in PAECs

As potential modulators of E_m and providers of a Ca^{2+} influx pathway, nonselective cation channels in the PA endothelium are well placed to provide a mechanism for transducing hypoxia sensitivity into changes in vascular tone. Nonselective cation currents in CPAE cell lines can be modulated in response to redox changes in the cell. Application of oxidant stress activates a current that is nonselective for monovalent cations and inwardly permeable to Ca^{2+}, depolarizing the cell and inhibiting store-dependent Ca^{2+} influx (55,56). In view of this potential for modulation of E_m and Ca^{2+} signaling, it is intriguing to consider the possibility of nonselective cation channel involvement in mediating HPV in the resistance vessels of the PA system. The examination of I_{NSC} under K^+-free conditions in PAECs freshly isolated from rat small PAs (see Sec. II.C) revealed a component of I_{NSC} that was activated following hypoxia (28,39). Hypoxia dramatically increased the inward current components at potentials more negative than -25 mV and displayed very erratic time-dependent activation. The hypoxia-activated component of I_{NSC} showed strong inward rectification and was sensitive to block by La^{3+} (Fig. 4). The kinetics of this component of I_{NSC} differ markedly from those of the basely active I_{NSC}, which was virtually time-independent and showed only mild inward rectification at very hyperpolarized membrane potentials. It is possible, therefore, that although the basal I_{NSC} was predominantly impermeable to Ca^{2+}, the hypoxia-activated I_{NSC} was mediated by a different molecular entity and could

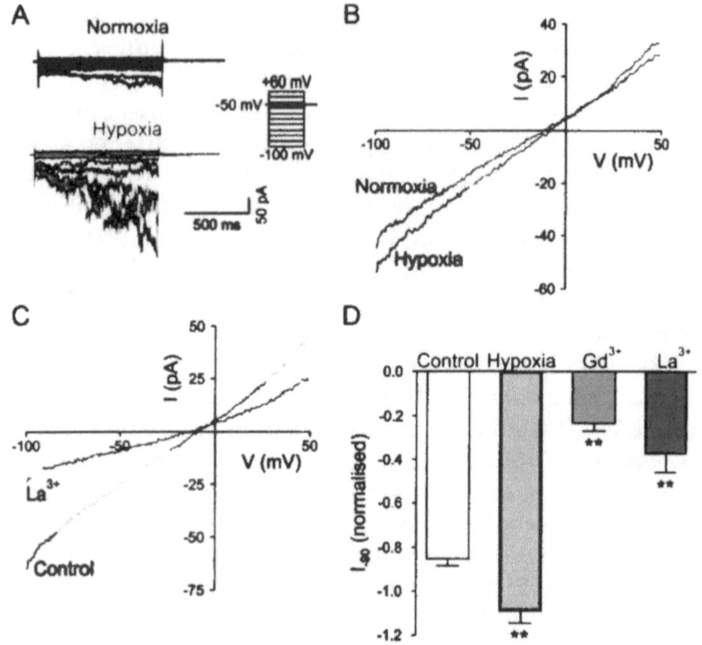

Figure 4 Effects of hypoxia and trivalent cations on the I_{NSC} recorded from PAECs under K^+-free perforated-patch conditions. (A) Voltage steps from –150 mV to +50 mV in 20 mV increments from a holding potential of 0 mV induced a typical family of membrane currents (left panel), which were significantly potentiated in the presence of hypoxia ($Po_2 \sim 25$ mmHg). Note the erratic nature and appearance of time-dependent activation of these currents at more hyperpolarized potentials. (B) Typical examples of *I–V* relationships derived from depolarizing voltage ramps from –100 mV to + 50 mV under normoxic ($Po_2 \sim 150$ mmHg) and hypoxic conditions. Note the increase in the magnitude of inward currents upon application of hypoxia. (C) Representative examples of *I–V* relationships derived from depolarizing voltage ramps from –100 mV to + 50 mV in the absence and presence of 100 μM La^{3+}. Note the inhibition of both the inward and outward components of the background currents in the presence of 100 μM La^{3+}. (D) Data summarizing the effects of hypoxia ($n = 4$), 100 μM Gd^{3+} ($n = 3$), and 100 μM La^{3+} ($n = 3$) on the mean current recorded at –90 mV (I_{-90}) in response to depolarizing voltage ramps (normalized to peak inward current) compared to control conditions ($n = 10$). (**) $P < 0.01$ compared to control. (From Ref. 39.)

provide a Ca^{2+} influx pathway. This hypothesis is supported by evidence that a rise in the intracellular free Ca^{2+} concentration is observed upon application of hypoxia in PAECs (57,58). In addition, hypoxia-induced activation of Ca^{2+} mobilization and influx in human umbilical vein endothelial cells has been recorded previously (59). Thus these hypoxia-activated Ca^{2+}

influx pathways in endothelial cells could form a common mechanism whereby the concomitant increase in intracellular Ca^{2+} is identical for many EC preparations; however, the identity of the mediator released under hypoxic conditions is a unique property of individual arteries and vascular beds.

The hypoxia-activated inward current described could be abolished by the addition of low concentrations of La^{3+} to the extracellular bath solution (28). This is a very interesting observation, because La^{3+} can also inhibit the hypoxia-induced elevation of cytosolic free calcium in PAECs (58). Furthermore, low concentrations of La^{3+} can attenuate the sustained, endothelium-dependent phase 2 of HPV (60). It would be tempting to suggest that this hypoxia-activated inward current induces an La^{3+}-sensitive Ca^{2+} influx pathway responsible for the sustained elevation of Ca^{2+} required for the second phase of HPV. This sustained rise in cytosolic free Ca^{2+} may in turn lead to the release of constricting factors in order to maintain pulmonary vasoconstriction.

IV. CONCLUSIONS

In this chapter the importance of the endothelium in the functioning of PAs has been discussed, particularly in relation to the modulation of vascular tone under hypoxic conditions. The benefits of being able to match blood perfusion to ventilation efficiency on a moment-to-moment basis in the lung are well known. However, under conditions such that ventilation impairment is widespread or prolonged, such as at high altitude or in patients with chronic obstructive pulmonary disease (COPD), widespread vasoconstriction occurs. This excessive increase in PA resistance can ultimately lead to pulmonary hypertension. The fact that the second phase of HPV is endothelium-dependent illustrates the importance of ECs in this unique vascular response of small PAs and shows that they may provide therapeutic targets for the treatment of pulmonary hypertension. The mechanisms involved when ECs sense hypoxia and transduce this signal to the modulation of the PA smooth muscle tone by the release of vasoactive agents or by direct electrical coupling are far from understood at the current time. Much work is therefore still required before specific targets for drug intervention can be identified.

The electrophysiological properties of PAECs under normal and hypoxic conditions have not received the same attention as those of PASMCs. Perhaps this is because contraction in response to hypoxia is an intrinsic property of PASMCs and preparations for studying currents in isolated PASMCs are well established. Because of the physiological importance of PAECs in HPV, it will be intriguing to follow the future progress and development relating to the understanding of ion channel regulation and the oxygen-sensing mechanisms intrinsic to PAECs.

The available research findings reveal that there is heterogeneity in the phenotypes of PAECs from different regions of the pulmonary vascular tree. The demonstration of at least two subpopulations of cells from resistance PAs, based on their electrophysiological profiles, coupled with heterogeneous staining for K^+ channel proteins, implies that the distribution of cell types is complex. In resistance vessel PAECs, most cells were characterized by the presence of I_{Kv}, whereas a small but significant number of cells were characterized by the presence of I_{KIR}. Chloride and nonselective cation currents appear to also have a role in setting E_m in PAECs. The balance of these currents is a fine one, such that modulation of any one of them can cause a dramatic change in E_m. Such changes are obviously important for the signaling role of PAECs on the underlying smooth muscle layer, but the specifics of this modulation have yet to be elucidated.

The observations that hypoxia can inhibit I_{Kv} and activate I_{NSC} in different PAECs from small PAs would suggest that these could be important components in the endothelium-dependent modulation of vasoconstriction during HPV. This modulation could be accomplished by regulating E_m or by providing a Ca^{2+} influx pathway. However, this indicates a further complexity in the response to hypoxia. Under physiological conditions, hypoxic inhibition of an outward K^+ current would tend to depolarize the cell membrane and decrease Ca^{2+} entry. In contrast, hypoxic activation of an inward current would act to hyperpolarize the cell. Because PAECs showed a marked increase of an outward current that did not show any signs of inactivation, it is possible that hypoxic inhibition of I_{Kv} acts to stabilize the E_m of endothelial cells to prevent cell damage from excessive Ca^{2+} entry subsequent to the hypoxic activation of an I_{NSC}. Ultimately this may act to prevent ischemic damage to areas of the lung during prolonged periods of oxygen deprivation. Alternatively, hypoxic inhibition of I_{Kv} in the pulmonary endothelium may act solely to modulate the E_m of the underlying smooth muscle layer during the transient phase of HPV.

In summary, recent studies have started to reveal the nature of the currents in the PAECs of the PA resistance vessels. Molecular identification of the channels responsible for these currents still remains to be elucidated. The evidence suggests, however, that there are at least two intrinsic oxygen-sensing mechanisms in these cells. These may exert an essential role in the endothelium-dependent phase of HPV as well as influencing the tone of the underlying smooth muscle layer and modulating its response to hypoxia.

REFERENCES

1. Barnes PJ, Liu SF. Regulation of pulmonary vascular tone. Pharmacol Rev 1995; 47:87–131.

2. Schneeberger EE. Segmental differentiation of endothelial intercellular junctions in intra-acinar arteries and veins of the rat lung. Circ Res 1981; 49: 1102 1111.
3. Olschewski A, Olschewski H, Bräu ME, Hempelmann G, Vogel W, Safronov BV. Basic electrical properties of in situ endothelial cells of small pulmonary arteries during postnatal development. Am J Respir Cell Mol Biol 2001; 25: 285–290.
4. Nilius B, Droogmans G. Ion channels and their functional role in vascular endothelium. Physiol Rev 2001; 81:1415–1459.
5. Hewett PW, Murray JC, Price EA, Watts ME, Woodcock M. Isolation and characterisation of microvessel endothelial cells from human mammary adipose tissue. In Vitro Cell Dev Biol 1993; 29:325–331.
6. Ward JPT, Robertson TP. The role of the endothelium in hypoxic pulmonary vasoconstriction. Exp Physiol 1995; 80:793–801.
7. Ward JPT, Aaronson PI. Mechanisms of hypoxic pulmonary vasoconstriction: can anyone be right? Respir Physiol 1999; 115:261–271.
8. Archer SL, Huang JM, Reeve HL, Hampl V, Tolarová S, Michelakis E, Weir EK. Differential distribution of electrophysiologically distinct myocytes in conduit and resistance arteries determines their response to nitric oxide and hypoxia. Circ Res 1996; 78:431–442.
9. Aaronson PI, Robertson TP, Ward JPT. Endothelium-derived mediators and hypoxic pulmonary vasoconstriction. Respir Physiol Neurobiol 2002; 132: 107–120.
10. Turner JL, Kozlowski RZ. Relationship between membrane potential, delayed rectifier K^+ currents and hypoxia in rat pulmonary arterial myocytes. Exp Physiol 1997; 82:629–645.
11. Le Cras TD, McMurtry IF. Nitric oxide production in the hypoxic lung. Am J Physiol Lung Cell Mol Physiol 2001; 280:L575–L582.
12. Gaine SP, Hales MA, Flavahan NA. Hypoxic pulmonary endothelial cells release a diffusible contractile factor distinct from endothelin. Am J Physiol 1998; 274:L657–L664.
13. Robertson TP, Ward JPT, Aaronson PI. Hypoxia induces the release of a pulmonary-selective, Ca^{2+}-sensitising, vasoconstrictor from the perfused rat lung. Cardiovasc Res 2001; 50:145–150.
14. Salter KJ, Turner JL, Albarwani S, Clapp LH, Kozlowski RZ. Ca^{2+}-activated Cl^- and K^+ channels and their modulation by endothelin-1 in rat pulmonary arterial smooth-muscle cells. Exp Physiol 1995; 80:815–824.
15. Salter KJ, Kozlowski RZ. Endothelin receptor coupling to potassium and chloride channels in isolated rat pulmonary arterial myocytes. J Pharm Exp Ther 1996; 279:1053–1062.
16. Salter KJ, Kozlowski RZ. Differential electrophysiological actions of endothelin-1 on Cl^- and K^+ currents in myocytes isolated from aorta, basilar and pulmonary artery. J Pharm Exp Ther 1998; 284:1122–1131.
17. Sato K, Morio Y, Morris KG, Rodman DM, McMurtry IF. Mechanism of hypoxic pulmonary vasoconstriction involves ET_A receptor-mediated inhibition of K_{ATP} channel. Am J Physiol Lung Cell Mol Physiol 2000; 278: L434–L442.

18. Tracey WR, Peach MJ. Differential muscarinic receptor mRNA expression by freshly isolated and cultured bovine aortic endothelial cells. Circ Res 1992; 70: 234–240.
19. Bregestovski PD, Ryan US. Voltage-gated and receptor-mediated ionic currents in the membrane of endothelial cells. J Mol Cell Cardiol 1989; 21: 103–108.
20. Voets T, Droogmans G, Nilius B. Membrane currents and the resting membrane potential in cultured bovine pulmonary artery endothelial cells. J Physiol 1996; 497:95–107.
21. Stevens T, Fouty B, Hepler L, Richardson D, Brough G, McMurtry IF, Rodman DM. Cytosolic Ca^{2+} and adenylyl cyclase responses in phenotypically distinct pulmonary endothelial cells. Am J Physiol 1997; 272:L51–L59.
22. Hogg DS, Albarwani S, Davies ARL, Kozlowski RZ. Endothelial cells freshly isolated from resistance-sized pulmonary arteries possess a unique K^+ current profile. Biochem Biophys Res Commun 1999; 263:405–409.
23. Hogg DS, McMurray G, Kozlowski RZ. Endothelial cells freshly isolated from small pulmonary arteries of the rat possess multiple distinct K^+ current profiles. Lung 2002; 180:203–214.
24. Von Beckerath N, Dittrich M, Klieber HG, Daut J. Inwardly rectifying K^+ channels in freshly dissociated coronary endothelial cells from guinea-pig heart. J Physiol 1996; 491:357–365.
25. Chen GF, Cheung DW. Characterization of acetylcholine-induced membrane hyperpolarisation in endothelial cells. Circ Res 1992; 70:257–263.
26. Rusko J, Tanzi F, Van Breemen C, Adams DJ. Calcium-activated potassium channels in native endothelial cells from rabbit aorta; conductance, Ca^{2+} sensitivity and block. J Physiol 1992; 455:601–621.
27. Kamouchi M, Van Den Bremt K, Eggermont J, Droogmans G, Nilius B. Modulation of inwardly rectifying potassium channels in cultured bovine pulmonary artery endothelial cells. J Physiol 1997; 504:545–556.
28. Hogg DS. Cationic currents in pulmonary arterial cells and their sensitivity to hypoxia. D.Phil. Thesis, University of Oxford, Oxford, UK, 2001.
29. Dittrich M, Daut J. Voltage-dependent K^+ current in capillary endothelial cells isolated from guinea pig heart. Am J Physiol 1999; 277:H119–H127.
30. Mulvany MJ, Aalkjær C. Structure and function of small arteries. Physiol Rev 1990; 70:921–961.
31. Sasaki S-I, Kobayashi N, Dambara T, Kira S, Sakai T. Structural organization of pulmonary arteries in the rat lung. Anat Embryol 1995; 191:477–489.
32. Archer SL, Souil E, Dinh-Xuan AT, Schremmer B, Mercier JC, El Yaagoubi A, Nguyen-Huu L, Reeve HL, Hampl V. Molecular identification of the role of voltage-gated K^+ channels, Kv1.5 and Kv2.1, in hypoxic pulmonary vasoconstriction and control of resting membrane potential in rat pulmonary artery myocytes. J Clin Invest 1998; 101:2319–2330.
33. Nilius B, Szücs G, Heinke S, Voets T, Droogmans G. Multiple types of chloride channels in bovine pulmonary artery endothelial cells. J Vasc Res 1997; 34: 220–228.

34. Voets T, Droogmans G, Raskin G, Eggermont J, Nilius B. Reduced intracellular ionic strength as the initial trigger for activation of endothelial volume-regulated anion channels. Proc Natl Acad Sci USA 1999; 96:5298–5303.
35. Voets T, Manolopoulos V, Eggermont J, Ellory C, Droogmans G, Nilius B. Regulation of swelling-activated Cl^- current in bovine endothelium by protein tyrosine phosphorylation and G-proteins. J Physiol 1998; 506:341–352.
36. Nilius B, Prenen J, Szücs G, Wei L, Tanzi F, Voets T, Droogmans G. Calcium-activated chloride channels in bovine pulmonary artery endothelial cells. J Physiol 1997; 498:381–396.
37. Suh SH, Vennekens R, Manolpoulos VG, Freichel M, Schweig U, Prenen J, Flockerzi V, Droogmans G, Nilius B. Characterisation of explanted endothelial cells from mouse aorta: electrophysiology and Ca^{2+} signalling. Pflügers Arch 1999; 438:612–620.
38. Strange K, Jackson PS. Swelling-activated organic osmolyte efflux: a new role for anion channels. Kidney Int 1995; 48:994–1003.
39. Hogg DS, Kozlowski RZ. Hypoxia activates a background conductance in freshly isolated pulmonary arterial endothelial cells of the rat. FEBS Lett 2002; 522:125–129.
40. Bae YM, Park MK, Lee SH, Ho W-K, Earm YE. Contribution of Ca^{2+}-activated K^+ channels and non-selective cation channels to membrane potential of pulmonary arterial smooth muscle cells of the rabbit. J Physiol 1999; 514: 747–758.
41. Iouzalen L, Lantoine F, Pernollet MG, Millanvoye-Van Brussels E, Devynck MA, David-Dufilho M. SK&F 96365 inhibits intracellular Ca^{2+} pumps and raises cytosolic Ca^{2+} concentration without production of nitric oxide and Von Willebrand factor. Cell Calcium 1996; 20:501–508.
42. Lantoine F, Iouzalen I, Devynck MA, Millanvoye-Van Brussels E, David-Dufilho M. Nitric oxide production in human endothelial cells stimulated by histamine requires Ca^{2+} influx. Biochem J 1998; 330:695–699.
43. Oike M, Gericke M, Droogmans G, Nilius B. Calcium-entry activated by store depletion in human umbilical vein endothelial-cells. Cell Calcium 1994; 16: 367–376.
44. Kamouchi M, Mamin A, Droogmans G, Nilius B. Nonselective cation channels in endothelial cells derived from human umbilical vein. J Membr Biol 1999; 169:29–38.
45. Yamamoto Y, Chen G, Miwa K, Suzuki H. Permeability and Mg^{2+} blockade of histamine-operated cation channel in endothelial cells of rat intrapulmonary artery. J Physiol 1992; 450:395–408.
46. Popp R, Hoyer J, Meyer J, Galla HJ, Gögelein H. Stretch-activated non-selective cation channels in the antiluminal membrane of porcine cerebral capillaries. J Physiol 1992; 454:435–449.
47. Prabhakar NR. Oxygen sensing by the carotid body chemoreceptors. J Appl Physiol 2000; 88:2287–2295.
48. Cutz E, Jackson A. Neuroepithelial bodies as airway oxygen sensors. Respir Physiol 1999; 15:201–214.

49. Post JM, Hume JR, Archer SL, Weir EK. Direct role for potassium channel inhibition in hypoxic pulmonary vasoconstriction. Am J Physiol 1992; 262:C882–C890.
50. Davies ARL, Kozlowski RZ. Kv channel subunit expression in rat pulmonary arteries. Lung 2001; 179:147–161.
51. Hogg DS, Davies ARL, McMurray G, Kozlowski RZ. Kv2.1 channels mediate hypoxic inhibition of I_{Kv} in native pulmonary arterial smooth muscle cells. Cardiovasc Res 2002; 55:349–360.
52. Yuan JX-J. Oxygen-sensitive K^+ channel(s): where and what? Am J Physiol Lung Cell Mol Physiol 2001; 281:L1345–L1349.
53. Coppock EA, Martens JR, Tamkun MM. Molecular basis of hypoxia-induced pulmonary vasoconstriction: role of voltage-gated K^+ channels. Am J Physiol Lung Cell Mol Physiol 2001; 281:L1–L12.
54. Patel AJ, Lazdunski M, Honoré E. Kv2.1/Kv9.3, a novel ATP-dependent delayed-rectifier K^+ channel in oxygen-sensitive pulmonary artery myocytes. EMBO J 1997; 16:6615–6625.
55. Koliwad SK, Kunze DL, Elliot SJ. Oxidant stress activates a non-selective cation channel responsible for membrane depolarisation in calf vascular endothelial cells. J Physiol 1996; 491:1–12.
56. Koliwad SK, Elliot SJ, Kunze DL. Oxidized glutathione mediates cation channel activation in calf vascular endothelial cells during oxidant stress. J Physiol 1996; 495:37–49.
57. Hampl V, Cornfield DN, Cowan NJ, Archer SL. Hypoxia potentiates nitric oxide synthesis and transiently increases cytosolic calcium levels in pulmonary artery endothelial cells. Eur Respir J 1995; 8:515–522.
58. Hu QH, Wang DX. Hypoxia increases cytosolic free calcium in porcine pulmonary arterial endothelial cells. J Tongji Med Univ 1993; 13:14–17.
59. Aono Y, Ariyoshi H, Sakon M, Ueda A, Tsuji Y, Kawasaki T, Monden M. Human umbilical vein endothelial cells (HUVECs) show Ca^{2+} mobilization as well as Ca^{2+} influx upon hypoxia. J Cell Biochem 2000; 78:458–464.
60. Robertson TP, Hague D, Aaronson PI, Ward JPT. Voltage-independent calcium entry in hypoxic pulmonary vasoconstriction of intrapulmonary arteries of the rat. J Physiol 2000; 525:669–680.

20

Aquaporins in the Vasculature

Venkataramana Sidhaye and Landon S. King
Johns Hopkins University School of Medicine, Baltimore, Maryland, U.S.A.

I. INTRODUCTION

Water constitutes 70% of the mass of most living organisms. Regulated transport of water is essential to maintaining the proper fluid balance within and between different anatomical compartments. Diffusion of water through the lipid bilayer certainly occurs; however, this low-velocity, high-resistance path is not sufficiently rapid—or regulatable—for many biological processes. Water-specific membrane channel proteins were postulated to exist for several decades, but it was not until 1992 that the first molecular water channel, now called aquaporin-1 (AQP1), was described (1). For discovery of this protein family, as well as for spearheading studies to define the unique structure–function relationships of the molecules, Peter Agre was awarded the Nobel prize in chemistry in 2003. Aquaporins have now been identified at all levels of life, including bacteria, yeast, invertebrates, plants, and animals, a conservation that strongly suggests fundamental roles in a variety of biological processes.

Several recent reviews discuss the biology of the broader aquaporin family (2,3). In this review, following a general description of the aquaporin protein family, we will discuss the regulation and function of AQP1, the primary vascular water channel.

II. THE AQUAPORIN FAMILY

Thirteen mammalian aquaporin homologs have been identified, each with distinct cellular and subcellular distribution (3). The sine qua non of these proteins is the presence of the three-amino acid sequence asparagine-proline-alanine (NPA) in both the amino- and carboxy-terminal halves of the molecule (4). This motif is generally conserved in all members of the family, with the possible exception of the two most recently identified candidates, AQP11 and AQP12. Overall, amino acid identity among the family members is ~25–40%; however, it is much higher for the sequences immediately flanking each of the NPA motifs.

The aquaporin family can be divided into two groups based on sequence analysis. The aquaporins (AQP0, 1, 2, 4, 5, 6, 8) are permeated only by water, with the exception of AQP6 and AQP8, which are also permeated by anions (AQP6) or other small molecules (AQP8). The aquaglyceroporins (AQP3, 7, 9, 10) are permeated to varying degrees by water but are highly permeable to glycerol and other small molecules. In contrast to bacteria, yeast, and plants, which have defined glycerol transporters, in mammals the aquaglyceroporins are the only known glycerol channels.

III. AQUAPORIN STRUCTURE AND FUNCTION

A. Topology

Determination of the structural aspects of the aquaporins that confer such unique permeability characteristics—permeable to water but not H_3O—has been the subject of intense investigation. Aquaporins have six transmembrane domains, with N- and C-termini that are intracellular (5). Physiologically defined inhibition of water permeability by mercury occurs at cysteine-189, adjacent to the pore-forming NPA motif (6). Mutation of residues around each of the NPA motifs reduced water permeability and led to prediction of an hourglass structure, with the NPA motifs folding into the lipid bilayer to form the pore (7). This prediction was confirmed by recent structural studies, which include cryoelectron microscopy of AQP1 to 3.8 Å resolution (8) and X-ray crystal structures of GlpF (9) and bovine AQP1 (10) to 2.2 Å and 2.1 Å resolution, respectively. Determination of the structure at an atomic level has provided insight into the mechanisms by which aquaporin mutations in select human diseases lead to changes in water permeability or protein stability (11).

A single AQP1 protein has a molecular mass of 28 kDa; however, the channel is present in the membrane as a tetramer as determined by both sedimentation (5) and membrane freeze-fracture (12). Structural studies provided insights into the apparent requirement for tetramer formation (11). The helices present on the outside of the AQP1 monomer are hydrophobic, whereas those on the internal face are hydrophilic—an asymmetrical arrangement that is stabilized by placing the hydrophilic sequences toward the center of the tetramer (13). In contrast to ion channels, in which the four subunits of the tetramer form a central pore, each of the subunits in an aquaporin tetramer contains its own channel (14).

B. Channel Selectivity and Gating

The exquisite selectivity of the channel for water has provoked keen interest from both physiologists and structural biologists. The restriction of AQP1 permeability to water arises from two principal mechanisms (13,15,16). First, the channel narrows to a diameter of 2.8 Å approximately 8 Å above the center of the bilayer, providing a physical limitation to the size of molecules that can pass through it. A bacterial aquaporin homolog, the glycerol channel GlpF, has a pore diameter approximately 1 Å wider than AQP1, sufficiently greater to allow the passage of glycerol (9). A second filter is provided by charged molecules near the NPA motifs that can interact with single water molecules passing through the pore, eliminating the possibility of H^+ transfer through the channel. This combination of size and charge restrictions provides the basis for the unique permeability characteristics of the aquaporins.

Nakhoul et al. (17) and Cooper and Boron (18) reported increased CO_2 permeability of *Xenopus* oocytes expressing AQP1; the magnitude of the increase was approximately 40%. Similarly, when AQP1 was reconstituted into *E. coli* phospholipids, CO_2-induced intracellular acidification increased four-fold (19). In each of these studies, addition of mercurial compounds blocked membrane CO_2 permeability, consistent with channel-mediated permeability through AQP1. In contrast, Yang and colleagues observed no differences in CO_2 permeability in red blood cells from wild-type and Aqp1-null mice (20), and no differences in CO_2 permeability of intact lungs or blood P_{CO_2} between wild-type, Aqp1-null, and Aqp5-null-mice (21). The discordance between these studies has not been reconciled, and the potential physiological implications for CO_2 transport in mammals—given the high partition coefficient for CO_2 into membrane lipids—remains unclear (22,23). Of note, recent investigation in plants may provide additional insight. Uehlein et al. (24) reported that an aquaporin in tobacco plants increases CO_2 permeability and facilitates both photosynthesis and leaf growth, but this was evident only in conditions where the CO_2 gradient is small.

Channel gating has been demonstrated for several members of the AQP family and may play an important role in regulation of permeability. The bovine form of AQP0 (also known as major intrinsic protein, MIP), a homolog abundant in the lens of the eye, is activated at pH 6 in *Xenopus* ooctyes (20). AQP3 permeability is reduced by low pH in oocytes (25) and by low pH and nickel in cultured lung epithelial cells (26). A reduction in AQP4 water permeability following activation by protein kinase C has been reported in oocytes (23) and LLC-PK1 renal epithelial cells (24); however, AQP4 phosphorylation by PKC in proteoliposomes reconstituted with purified protein had no effect on water permeability (Kozono and Agre, personal communication). AQP6 water and ion permeability are activated by low pH and nitrate in oocytes (6) and cultured cells (25). Channel gating provides an appealing mechanism for rapid regulation of channel permeability and is the subject of active investigation at both physiological and structural levels.

C. Aquaporins as Ion Channels

Yool et al. (27) described forskolin-stimulated ion permeability of AQP1 expressed in oocytes, however this was not reproduced in other labs (28). More recently, Yool and coworkers demonstrated cGMP-stimulated AQP1 ion conductance in oocytes (29). Reconstitution of purified AQP1 protein into lipid membranes also revealed cGMP-mediated ion conductance; however, the number of channels activated by cGMP appeared to be as low as one per million AQP1 molecules (30). The physiological implications of AQP1-mediated ion conductance remain undefined. Ion conductance has been established for AQP6, which is permeated by anions in response to low pH or nitrate (31). AQP6 colocalizes with the H^+-ATPase in acid-secreting intercalated cells of the renal collecting duct. AQP6-mediated anion conductance is believed to contribute to balancing charge as intracellular vesicles accumulate H^+.

IV. AQUAPORIN-1

At least four aquaporins have been identified in the respiratory tract. Three of these—AQP3, AQP4, and AQP5—are present in the respiratory epithelium. In the upper airways (including the nasopharynx), AQP3 is present in basal cells, AQP4 is in ciliated columnar cells, and AQP5 is in the apical membrane of the airway epithelium as well as in acinar cells of airway submucosal glands (3,32,33). In the alveolus, AQP5 is in the apical membrane of type I pneumocytes (33,34); the presence of water channels in type II cells has not been unambiguously determined. Here we will focus on AQP1, which is abundant in endothelial cells of capillaries and venules in the lung (35,36). As is true at most sites where AQP1 is expressed, the protein is present in both the apical and basolateral membranes (Fig. 1) (37). Until recently, AQP1 was the only member of the family identified in blood vessels. Amiry-Moghaddam et al. (38) identified AQP4 in the endothelium of blood vessels in the brain, a site where AQP1 is notably absent from the endothelium.

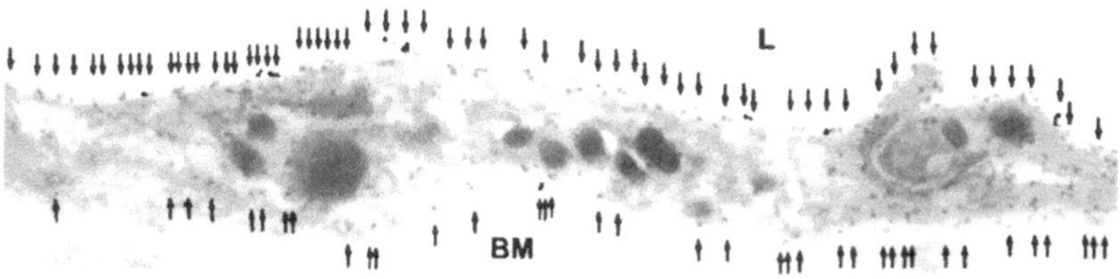

Figure 1 Electron micrograph of human capillary endothelial cell from the peribronchiolar vascular plexus reveals immunogold particle labeling (arrows) of AQP1 on both the apical and basal membranes of the cell. L, vessel lumen; BM, basement membrane. (From Ref. 37).

V. REGULATION OF AQP1

Early in the aquaporin story, AQP1 was considered to be a "constitutive" water channel (39), in no small part because its regulation clearly contrasted with that of AQP2 in the renal collecting duct, which was dynamically trafficked on or off the plasma membrane in a vasopressin-dependent fashion (40). It is increasingly evident that AQP1 is also actively regulated at multiple levels.

During development, the lung is filled with a chloride-rich, low-protein fluid until late in gestation, when the lung transitions from being secretory to being absorptive, a critical step in preparing the newborn for assumption of gas-exchange responsibilities (41). AQP1 protein is detectable in fetal rat lung late in gestation, increases severalfold in the day prior to birth, and is sustained at high levels in adult animals (35), an ontogeny that is nearly identical to that of the sodium channel αrENaC, Na^+-K^+-ATPase, and surfactant proteins, each of which is believed to play an important role in this transition (42–44). The administration of corticosteroids is known to improve pulmonary function in premature human infants. The underlying mechanisms are incompletely understood, but the benefits are believed to result at least in part from induction of surfactant proteins (45) and ENaC (43). Similarly, we observed that corticosteroids upregulate AQP1 mRNA and protein in fetal lung by fivefold (35,46) while having no effect on expression of AQP5. Corticosteroid induction of AQP1 was also observed in adult rat lung and in perinatal but not adult kidney; no induction was observed in other AQP1-expressing tissues, including the developing forepaw and red blood cells (35), indicating tissue-specific steroid induction. Additionally, other aquaporins were not induced by steroids in the rat lung. Increased AQP1 mRNA in lung resulted at least partially from transcriptional activation, and corticosteroid induction of AQP1 in mouse erythroleukemia cells could be mapped to two glucocorticoid response elements in the AQP1 promoter (47). More recently, a study of aquaporin expression in fetal sheep lung revealed that AQP1, AQP3, AQP4, and AQP5 protein could be detected during gestation, and both AQP1 and AQP5 were upregulated by administration of corticosteroids to the mother (48). While reinforcing the potential contribution of aquaporins in lung water homeostasis during development, these observations also emphasize that differences between rodents and larger mammals can complicate assignment of specific physiological roles for these proteins.

Although these observations are suggestive of a role for AQP1 in perinatal lung water clearance, direct evidence for participation in this process has not yet been demonstrated. Studies in a single strain of AQP1-null mice did not reveal an apparent difference in lung water or mortality in the perinatal period (49).

AQP1 abundance is clearly altered by a wide range of stress stimuli, as one might expect if dynamic changes in water channel expression contribute to changes in membrane permeability. Some basic insights into mechanisms underlying potential AQP1 regulation have derived from a simple model of osmotic cell stress. Cells respond to hypertonic stress by upregulating a limited number of genes, among which are those encoding transporters or enzymes that facilitate accumulation of intracellular organic osmolytes such as betaine or sodium myoinositol (50). We and others have noted that AQP1 is upregulated by hypertonicity in cultured cells, including fibroblasts (51) and renal epithelial cells (52,53). AQP1 induction requires activation of mitogen-activated protein kinases (MAPKs). Umeneshi demonstrated that hypertonic induction of AQP1 in renal IMCD cells required activation of all three MAP kinases [jun N-terminal kinase (JNK); extracellular signal-regulated kinase (ERK), and p38], and we observed that only ERK activation was required for AQP1 induction in cultured fibroblasts (L. King, unpublished observation), consistent with our findings for hypertonic induction of AQP5 in mouse lung epithelial cells (54). Umenishi and Schrier (53) demonstrated that transcriptional activation of AQP1 occurs by way of a novel osmotic response element in the AQP1 proximal promoter. The magnitude of this induction was small, perhaps reflective of the presence of osmotic response elements outside of the promoter fragment studied.

Leitch et al. (51) observed that AQP1 protein is modified by ubiquitination, the enzymatic addition of a 7–8 kDa peptide that binds to lysine residues of target proteins (55). The first (and then subsequent) ubiquitins can then be ubiquitinated on lysine residues in an iterative process that leads to generation of a polyubiquitin chain of varying lengths. In the most straightforward model for this type of processing, proteins that are polyubiquitinated are targeted to the proteasome for degradation. Consistent with this type of processing, we observed that AQP1 protein is degraded by the proteasome and has a half-life of approximately 3 hrs. (51). In cells exposed to hypertonic medium, ubiquitination of AQP1 could no longer be detected, and the half-life of the protein increased markedly. These studies provided the first example of regulation of the stability of a membrane protein as a mechanism for altering protein abundance in conditions of osmotic stress.

Inflammation is commonly associated with disruption of local water homeostasis and manifests as edema. One might anticipate that if aquaporins participate in the regulation of water homeostasis, their expression would be altered by inflammatory mediators. Indeed, evidence is mounting that this is the case. Towne et al. (56) examined the effects of adenoviral infection of the lung on lung water content and aquaporin expression. Intratracheal administration of adenovirus to mice was associated with histological evidence of inflammation. Although the lungs appeared to be morphologically intact and there was no evidence of necrosis, marked reductions in the expression of both AQP1 and AQP5 were observed. The reductions in AQP1 and AQP5 correlated temporally with increased lung water and, of some note, were observed in regions of the lung in which inflammatory infiltrates were not evident, indicating the likely contribution of humoral factors. Similarly, in a study of lung microarrays following intratracheal administration of phospholipase A_2, a model of snakebite-induced lung injury, Cher et al. (57) found that AQP1 and AQP5 mRNA and protein were reduced. In contrast, Lai et al. (58) examined the effects of macrophage migration inhibitory factor (MIF) on AQP1 expression and found that MIF and tumor necrosis factor α induced AQP1 expression in cultured endothelial cells. These investigators also reported small increases in AQP1 in lung tissue of patients with ARDS. We have observed marked increases in AQP1 expression in cultured cells exposed to both gram-positive and gram-negative bacteria as well as select bacterial products (59). In total, these observations indicate that AQP1 is regulated by a wide range of products associated with inflammation. It should be noted that the role for aquaporins in acute inflammation may not be so straightforward. It is difficult to appreciate what contribution a water-specific channel makes during the development of high protein edema, for example. Rather, aquaporins may be more important during periods of recovery and edema resolution, rather than the acute stages in which a large paracellular contribution is predicted to predominate (60).

VI. AQUAPORINS AND HUMAN PATHOPHYSIOLOGY

An increasing array of pathophysiological processes have been associated with the aquaporins, in both humans and animal models (2,3). Perhaps the most unambiguous examples of aquaporin function in humans derive from studies of the kidney. Individuals with mutations in the renal collecting duct aquaporin AQP2 have congenital nephrogenic diabetes insipidus (NDI) (61), and AQP2 has been implicated in several acquired forms of NDI (62). AQP1 is also abundant in the kidney, in the epithelium of the renal proximal tubule and descending thin limb, and in the endothelium of the descending vasa recta (62). A few humans have been identified who are AQP1-null (63). Surprisingly, these individuals have normal urinary volumes, but when deprived of water they have a limited ability to maximally concentrate their urine (64). The apparent frequency of homozygous *AQP1* mutations is extremely low (seven kindreds identified in the world), suggesting the possibility that these individuals may have as yet unidentified forms of compensation for the lack of AQP1. Additional examples of aquaporin-related pathophysiology in humans are emerging. AQP0 is a homolog abundant in the lens of the eye. Humans with mutations in AQP0 have congenital cataracts (65), and more subtle changes in AQP0 expression or function that contribute to adult onset cataracts are anticipated. Sjögren's syndrome is an immunologically mediated disease whose primary clinical manifestations are dry eyes and dry mouth. In collaboration with groups in Japan and Belgium, we recently demonstrated that AQP5 is not present in the apical membrane of secretory cells in lacrimal (66) or minor salivary glands (67) of individuals with Sjögren's syndrome, a defect that likely plays a prominent role in the clinical expression of the disease.

VII. AQUAPORIN-1 FUNCTION IN THE LUNG

As noted, rare humans with mutations in the *AQP1* gene leading to complete absence of the protein have been identified (63). In the lung, AQP1 is abundant in the vascular plexus surrounding the airways (35). In the mid-1990s, Brown et al. (68) used high-resolution computed tomography (HRCT) to examine changes in peribronchial edema in fluid-challenged dogs. We used a similar strategy to search for differences in peribronchial edema formation following fluid challenge in AQP1-null humans compared to control individuals (37). Serial HRCT scans were performed following intravenous infusion of 3 L of isotonic saline over the course of 30 min (Fig. 2). Similar to what was observed in saline-infused dogs, the bronchiolar wall thickened by approximately 40% over 30 min in control individuals following saline infusion but did not change in thickness at all in AQP1-null individuals (Fig. 3). These findings indicate that AQP1 participates in determining the membrane water permeability of the lung endothelium and are particularly notable in light of classical studies demonstrating that fluid fluxes across the vasculature of the peribronchiolar interstitial space occur early in edema formation (69) as well as during edema clearance (70).

Our findings in humans are consistent with studies in AQP1-null mice (49). In response to an osmotic gradient imposed across the lung vasculature, permeability was decreased by approximately ten-fold in AQP1-null mice, indicating that much of the osmotically driven water transport across lung microvascular endothelial cells occurs by a transcellular route through

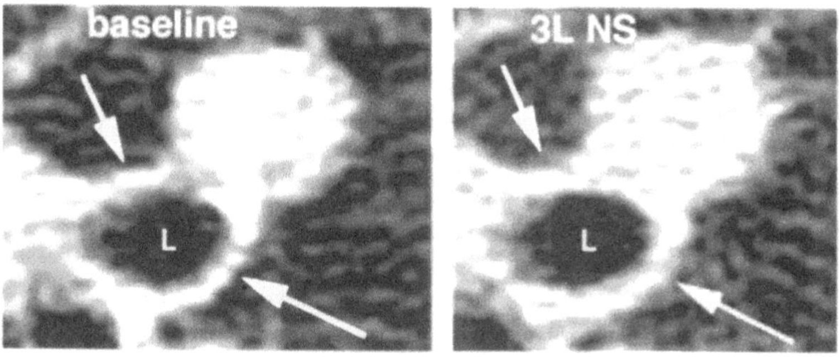

Figure 2 High-resolution computed tomographic (HRCT) scan of human lung at baseline and after 3 L of normal saline was infused intravenously over 30 min (3L NS). The airway lumen (L) is visible, and thickening of the bronchiolar wall (arrows) can be seen following saline infusion. (From Ref. 37.)

AQP1 water channels. Additionally, extravascular lung water accumulation in response to increased pulmonary artery perfusate pressure was significantly decreased in AQP1-null animals, suggesting that AQP1-mediated transport also participates in hydrostatically driven fluid movement across lung microvessels.

AQP1 has been identified as a candidate gene in a genomic analysis of nickel-induced lung injury (71), and distinct haplotypes of single-nucleotide polymorphisms in the 3′ untranslated region of the *AQP1* gene appear to confer susceptibility to or protection from sepsis and lung injury in

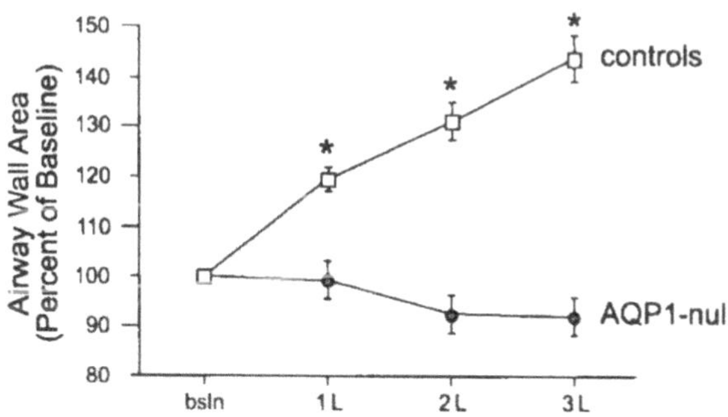

Figure 3 High-resolution computed tomographic scans were performed at baseline (bsln) and following each of 3 L of normal saline infused intravenously. Bronchiolar wall area of airways that could be identified in all four scans was measured (17–33 airways per subject) in two AQP1-null individuals and five controls, and recorded as percent of the baseline wall area. (*) $p < 0.05$ from baseline

African-Americans (72). However, direct studies of acute lung edema formation in mice have failed to demonstrate differences between AQP1-null and wild-type animals (73). Certainly strain or species differences in responses could confound definitive assignment of functional roles in these pathophysiological events. It is also possible, however, that AQP1 plays no role in the acute stages of lung injury. Indeed, it is unclear how AQP1 would participate in the formation of protein-rich edema fluid in the acute setting. Future studies examining potential roles for AQP1 during the reparative stages of lung injury, when gross barrier function has returned and fluid mobilization at the lowest energy cost is the goal, may prove informative. Similarly, results of fluid challenge studies in mice and humans suggest potential roles for AQP1 in acute and chronic heart failure models.

VIII. CONCLUSION

Discovery of the aquaporins has provoked a paradigm shift in the ways we consider regulation of membrane water transport. In particular, the presence or absence of these high-capacity, low-resistance channels can alter membrane water permeability independently of the complement of membrane solute transporters. AQP1 abundance is dynamically regulated. Both in vitro and in vivo studies indicate that AQP1 participates in modulating endothelial water permeability; however, the contexts in which AQP1 is likely to contribute to altered water homeostasis in pathophysiological conditions are incompletely defined and require further investigation.

REFERENCES

1. Preston GM, Carroll TP, Guggino WB, Agre P. Appearance of water channels in *Xenopus* oocytes expressing red cell CHIP28 protein. Science 1992; 256: 385–387.
2. Agre P, Kozono D. Aquaporin water channels: molecular mechanisms for human diseases. FEBS Lett 2003; 555:72–78.
3. King LS, Yasui M. Aquaporins and disease: lessons from mice to humans. Trends Endocrinol Metab 2002; 13:355–360.
4. Preston GM, Agre P. Isolation of the cDNA for erythrocyte integral membrane protein of 28 kilodaltons: member of an ancient channel family. Proc Natl Acad Sci USA 1991; 88:11110–11114.
5. Smith BL, Agre P. Erythrocyte Mr 28,000 transmembrane protein exists as a multisubunit oligomer similar to channel proteins. J Biol Chem 1991; 266: 6407–6415.
6. Preston GM, Jung JS, Guggino WB, Agre P. The mercury-sensitive residue at cysteine 189 in the CHIP28 water channel. J Biol Chem 1993; 268:17–20.
7. Jung JS, Bhat RV, Preston GM, Guggino WB, Baraban JM, Agre P. Molecular characterization of an aquaporin cDNA from brain: candidate osmoreceptor

and regulator of water balance. Proc Natl Acad Sci USA 1994; 91: 13052–13056.

8. Murata K, Mitsuoka K, Hirai T, Walz T, Agre P, Heymann JB, Engel A, Fujiyoshi Y. Structural determinants of water permeation through aquaporin-1. Nature 2000; 407:599–605.
9. Fu D, Libson A, Miercke LJ, Weitzman C, Nollert P, Krucinski J, Stroud RM. Structure of a glycerol-conducting channel and the basis for its selectivity. Science 2000; 290:481–486.
10. Sui H, Han BG, Lee JK, Walian P, Jap BK. Structural basis of water-specific transport through the AQP1 water channel. Nature 2001; 414:872–878.
11. Kozono D, Yasui M, King LS, Agre P. Aquaporin water channels: atomic structure molecular dynamics meet clinical medicine. J Clin Invest 2002; 109: 1395–1399.
12. Verbavatz JM, Brown D, Sabolic I, Valenti G, Ausiello DA, Van Hoek An, Ma T, Verkman AS. Tetrameric assembly of CHIP28 water channels in liposomes and cell membranes: a freeze-fracture study. J Cell Biol 1993; 123: 605–618.
13. de Groot BL, Grubmuller H. Water permeation across biological membranes: mechanism and dynamics of aquaporin-1 and GlpF. Science 2001; 294: 2353–2357.
14. Jung JS, Preston GM, Smith BL, Guggino WB, Agre P. Molecular structure of the water channel through aquaporin CHIP. The hourglass model. J Biol Chem 1994; 269:14648–14654.
15. de Groot BL, Frigato T, Helms V, Grubmuller H. The mechanism of proton exclusion in the aquaporin-1 water channel. J Mol Biol 2003; 333:279–293.
16. Tajkhorshid E, Nollert P, Jensen MO, Miercke LJ, O'Connell J, Stroud RM, Schulten K. Control of the selectivity of the aquaporin water channel family by global orientational tuning. Science 2002; 296:525–530.
17. Nakhoul NL, Davis BA, Romero MF, Boron WF. Effect of expressing the water channel aquaporin-1 on the CO_2 permeability of *Xenopus* oocytes. Am J Physiol 1998; 274:C543–C548.
18. Cooper GJ, Boron WF. Effect of PCMBS on CO_2 permeability of *Xenopus* oocytes expressing aquaporin 1 or its C189S mutant. Am J Physiol 1998; 275:C1481–C1486.
19. Prasad GV, Coury LA, Finn F, Zeidel ML. Reconstituted aquaporin 1 water channels transport CO_2 across membranes. J Biol Chem 1998; 273: 33123–33126.
20. Yang B, Fukuda N, van Hoek A, Matthay MA, Ma T, Verkman AS. Carbon dioxide permeability of aquaporin-1 measured in erythrocytes and lung of aquaporin-1 null mice and in reconstituted proteoliposomes. J Biol Chem 2000; 275:2686–2692.
21. Fang X, Yang B, Matthay MA, Verkman AS. Evidence against aquaporin-1-dependent CO_2 permeability in lung and kidney. J Physiol 2002; 542:63–69.
22. Cooper GJ, Zhou Y, Bouyer P, Grichtchenko, II, Boron WF. Transport of volatile solutes through AQP1. J Physiol 2002; 542:17–29.
23. Verkman AS. Does aquaporin-1 pass gas? An opposing view. J Physiol 2002; 542:31.

24. Uehlein N, Lovisolo C, Siefritz F, Kaldenhoff R. The tobacco aquaporin NtAQP1 is a membrane CO_2 pore with physiological functions. Nature 2003; 425:734–737.
25. Zeuthen T, Klaerke DA. Transport of water and glycerol in aquaporin 3 is gated by H^+. J Biol Chem 1999; 274:21631–21636.
26. Zelenina M, Bondar AA, Zelenin S, Aperia A. Nickel and extracellular acidification inhibit the water permeability of human aquaporin-3 in lung epithelial cells. J Biol Chem 2003; 278:30037–30043.
27. Yool AJ, Stamer WD, Regan JW. Forskolin stimulation of water and cation permeability in aquaporin 1 water channels. Science 1996; 273:1216–1218.
28. Agre P, Lee MD, Devidas S, Guggino WB. Aquaporins and ion conductance. Science 1997; 275:1490.
29. Anthony TL, Brooks HL, Boassa D, Leonov S, Yanochko GM, Regan JW, Yool AJ. Cloned human aquaporin-1 is a cyclic GMP-gated ion channel. Mol Pharmacol 2000; 57:576–588.
30. Saparov SM, Kozono D, Rothe U, Agre P, Pohl P. Water and ion permeation of aquaporin-1 in planar lipid bilayers. Major differences in structural determinants and stoichiometry. J Biol Chem 2001; 276:31515–31520.
31. Yasui M, Hazama A, Kwon TH, Nielsen S, Guggino WB, Agre P. Rapid gating and anion permeability of an intracellular aquaporin. Nature 1999; 402: 184–187.
32. Kreda SM, Gynn MC, Fenstermacher DA, Boucher RC, Gabriel SE. Expression and localization of epithelial aquaporins in the adult human lung. Am J Respir Cell Mol Biol 2001; 24:224–234.
33. Nielsen S, King LS, Christensen BM, Agre P. Aquaporins in complex tissues. II. Subcellular distribution in respiratory and glandular tissues of rat. Am J Physiol 1997; 273:C1549–C1561.
34. Borok Z, Lubman RL, Danto SI, Zhang X-L, Zabski SM, King LS, Lee DM, Agre P, Crandall ED. Keratinocyte growth factor modulates alveolar epithelial cell phenotype in vitro: expression of aquaporin 5. Am J Respir Cell Mol Biol 1998; 18:554–561.
35. King LS, Nielsen S, Agre P. Aquaporin-1 water channel protein in lung: ontogeny, steroid-induced expression, and distribution in rat. J Clin Invest 1996; 97: 2183–2191.
36. Nielsen S, Smith BL, Christensen EI, Agre P. Distribution of the aquaporin CHIP in secretory and resorptive epithelia and capillary endothelia. Proc Natl Acad Sci USA 1993; 90:7275–7279.
37. King LS, Nielsen S, Agre P, Brown RH. Decreased pulmonary vascular permeability in aquaporin-1-null humans. Proc Natl Acad Sci USA 2002; 99: 1059–1063.
38. Amiry-Moghaddam M, Xue R, Haug F-M, Neely JD, Bhardwaj A, Agre P, Adams ME, Froehner SC, Mori S, Ottersen OP. Alpha syntrophin deletion removes the perivascular but not the endothelial pool of aquaporin-4 at the blood-brain barrier and delays the development of brain edema in an experimental model of acute hyponatremia. FASEB J 2004; 18:542–544.

39. Agre P, Preston GM, Smith BL, Jung JS, Raina S, Moon C, Guggino WB, Nielsen S. Aquaporin CHIP: the archetypal molecular water channel. Am J Physiol 1993; 265:F463–F476.
40. Fushimi K, Uchida S, Hara Y, Hirata Y, Marumo F, Sasaki S. Cloning and expression of apical membrane water channel of rat kidney collecting tubule. Nature 1993; 361:549–552.
41. Bland RD, Hansen TN, Haberkern CM, Bressack MA, Hazinski TA, Raj JU, Goldberg RB. Lung fluid balance in lambs before and after birth. J Appl Physiol 1982; 53:992–1004.
42. Mendelson CR, Boggaram V. Hormonal control of the surfactant system in fetal lung. Annu Rev Physiol 1991; 53:415–440.
43. O'Brodovich H, Canessa C, Ueda J, Rafii B, Rossier BC, Edelson J. Expression of the epithelial Na^+ channel in the developing rat lung. Am J Physiol 1993; 265:C491–C496.
44. O'Brodovich H, Staub O, Rossier BC, Geering K, Kraehenbuhl JP. Ontogeny of α_1- and β_1-isoforms of Na^+-K^+-ATPase in fetal distal rat lung epithelium. Am J Physiol 1993; 264:C1137–C1143.
45. Schellhase DE, Shannon JM. Effects of maternal dexamethasone on expression of SP-A, SP-B, and SP-C in the fetal rat lung. Am J Respir Cell Mol Biol 1991; 4:304–312.
46. King LS, Nielsen S, Agre P. Aquaporins in complex tissues. I. Developmental patterns in respiratory and glandular tissues of rat. Am J Physiol 1997; 273: C1541–C1548.
47. Moon C, King LS, Agre P. Aqp1 expression in erythroleukemia cells: genetic regulation of glucocorticoid and chemical induction. Am J Physiol 1997; 273: C1562–C1570.
48. Liu H, Hooper SB, Armugam A, Dawson N, Ferraro T, Jeyaseelan K, Thiel A, Koukoulas I, Wintour EM. Aquaporin gene expression and regulation in the ovine fetal lung. J Physiol 2003; 551:503–514.
49. Bai C, Fukuda N, Song Y, Ma T, Matthay MA, Verkman AS. Lung fluid transport in aquaporin-1 and aquaporin-4 knockout mice. J Clin Invest 1999; 103:555–561.
50. Burg MB, Kwon ED, Kultz D. Osmotic regulation of gene expression. FASEB J 1996; 10:1598–1606.
51. Leitch V, Agre P, King LS. Altered ubiquitination and stability of aquaporin-1 in hypertonic stress. Proc Natl Acad Sci USA 2001; 98:2894–2898.
52. Jenq W, Mathieson IM, Ihara W, Ramirez G. Aquaporin-1: an osmoinducible water channel in cultured mIMCD-3 cells. Biochem Biophys Res Commun 1998; 245:804–809.
53. Umenishi F, Schrier RW. Identification and characterization of a novel hypertonicity-responsive element in the human aquaporin-1 gene. Biochem Biophys Res Commun 2002; 292:771–775.
54. Hoffert JD, Leitch V, Agre P, King LS. Hypertonic induction of aquaporin-5 expression through an ERK-dependent pathway. J Biol Chem 2000; 275: 9070–9077.

55. Ciechanover A. The ubiquitin-proteasome proteolytic pathway. Cell 1994; 79: 13–21.
56. Towne JE, Harrod KS, Krane CM, Menon AG. Decreased expression of aquaporin (AQP)1 and AQP5 in mouse lung after acute viral infection. Am J Respir Cell Mol Biol 2000; 22:34–44.
57. Cher CD, Armugam A, Lachumanan R, Coghlan MW, Jeyaseelan K. Pulmonary inflammation and edema induced by phospholipase A_2: global gene analysis and effects on aquaporins and Na^+/K^+-ATPase. J Biol Chem 2003; 278: 31352–31360.
58. Lai KN, Leung JC, Metz CN, Lai FM, Bucala R, Lan HY. Role for macrophage migration inhibitory factor in acute respiratory distress syndrome. J Pathol 2003; 199:496–508.
59. KVE, Li E, King LS, Landon S. Induction of aquaporin-1 by bacterial infection. Am J Respir Crit Care Med 2002; 165:A297.
60. Dudek SM, Garcia JG. Cytoskeletal regulation of pulmonary vascular permeability. J Appl Physiol 2001; 91:1487–1500.
61. Deen PM, Verdijk MA, Knoers NV, Wieringa B, Monnens LA, van Os CH, van Oost BA. Requirement of human renal water channel aquaporin-2 for vasopressin-dependent concentration of urine. Science 1994; 264:92–95.
62. Nielsen S, Frokiaer J, Marples D, Kwon TH, Agre P, Knepper MA. Aquaporins in the kidney: from molecules to medicine. Physiol Rev 2002; 82:205–244.
63. Preston GM, Smith BL, Zeidel ML, Moulds JJ, Agre P. Mutations in aquaporin-1 in phenotypically normal humans without functional CHIP water channels. Science 1994; 265:1585–1587.
64. King LS, Choi M, Fernandez PC, Cartron JP, Agre P. Defective urinary-concentrating ability due to a complete deficiency of aquaporin-1. N Engl J Med 2001; 345:175–179.
65. Berry V, Francis P, Kaushal S, Moore A, Bhattacharya S. Missense mutations in MIP underlie autosomal dominant 'polymorphic' and lamellar cataracts linked to 12q. Nat Genet 2000; 25:15–17.
66. Tsubota K, Hirai S, King LS, Agre P, Ishida N. Defective cellular trafficking of lacrimal gland aquaporin-5 in Sjogren's syndrome. Lancet 2001; 357:688–389.
67. Steinfeld S, Cogan E, King LS, Agre P, Kiss R, Delporte C. Abnormal distribution of aquaporin-5 water channel protein in salivary glands from Sjogren's syndrome patients. Lab Invest 2001; 81:143–148.
68. Brown RH, Zerhouni EA, Mitzner W. Visualization of airway obstruction in vivo during pulmonary vascular engorgement and edema. J Appl Physiol 1995; 78:1070–1078.
69. Staub NC, Nagano H, Pearce ML. Pulmonary edema in dogs, especially the sequence of fluid accumulation in lungs. J Appl Physiol 1967; 22:227–240.
70. Jayr C, Matthay MA. Alveolar and lung liquid clearance in the absence of pulmonary blood flow in sheep. J Appl Physiol 1991; 71:1679–1687.
71. Leikauf GD, McDowell SA, Wesselkamper SC, Hardie WD, Leikauf JE, Korfhagen TR, Prows DR. Acute lung injury: functional genomics and genetic susceptibility. Chest 2002; 121:70S–75S.

72. King LS, Barnes K, Ashworth R, Zambelli-Weiner A, Scott AF, Grigoryev D, Ye SQ, Garcia JGN. Aquaporin-1: a candidate gene in sepsis and lung injury. Am J Respir Crit Care Med 2003; 167:A662.
73. Song Y, Fukuda N, Bai C, Ma T, Matthay MA, Verkman AS. Role of aquaporins in alveolar fluid clearance in neonatal and adult lung, and in oedema formation following acute lung injury: studies in transgenic aquaporin null mice. J Physiol 2000; 525:771–779.

21

Functional Roles of Ion Channels in the Regulation of Membrane Potential and Pulmonary Vascular Tone

Alison M. Gurney
University of Strathclyde, Glasgow, Scotland, U.K.

I. INTRODUCTION

The smooth muscle cells (SMCs) of pulmonary arteries are electrically silent (1,2). Under normal conditions they do not fire action potentials, either spontaneously or in response to depolarizing current pulses or many depolarizing drugs. The membrane potential of pulmonary artery SMCs is nevertheless an important factor in the regulation of pulmonary vascular tone. This is illustrated by the well-known vasoconstrictor effect of raising the extracellular K^+ concentration, which depolarizes the cells by suppressing the transmembrane K^+ gradient. Contraction occurs at K^+ concentrations as low as 15 mM, which depolarizes pulmonary artery SMCs by around 15 mV, and increases with increasing K^+ concentration to a maximum above 50 mM K^+, when the membrane potential is nearly eliminated (1–3). The contractile effect of potassium requires the presence of extracellular Ca^{2+}, indicating that it depends on Ca^{2+} influx. Indeed, it is widely recognized that K^+-induced depolarization causes the opening of voltage-gated Ca^{2+} channels in the SMC plasma membrane, through which Ca^{2+} enters the cell to initiate contraction. Perhaps less widely appreciated are studies suggesting that in smooth muscle the membrane potential can influence additional pathways that regulate the intracellular Ca^{2+} concentration ($[Ca^{2+}]_i$). Thus depolarization was found to stimulate the hydrolysis of inositol phospholipids and the synthesis of inositol 1,4,5-trisphosphate (IP_3), which triggers the release of Ca^{2+} from intracellular stores (4,5). This too would raise $[Ca^{2+}]_i$ and promote contraction. Membrane potential may additionally influence the sensitivity of the contractile machinery to Ca^{2+} (6). The maintenance of a constant negative potential across the plasma membrane of pulmonary artery SMCs therefore helps to maintain $[Ca^{2+}]_i$ at a low level and inhibits cell contraction. This may be important in maintaining the low intrinsic tone that is characteristic of pulmonary arteries in vivo.

II. THE RESTING MEMBRANE POTENTIAL

The resting membrane potential of pulmonary artery SMCs, measured in intact vessels with microelectrodes, lies within the range −50 to −60 mV in several species (1,2,7–9). Resting potentials in this range have also been reported for isolated pulmonary artery SMCs, measured using patch-clamp techniques (10–13). Isolated cells often appear, however, to be more depolarized (14–16). This may reflect differences in the recording conditions, particularly in the ionic gradients across the membrane, which can be disrupted during patch-clamp recording. The ionic basis of the resting potential is determined by the concentration gradients of ions across the membrane and the selective permeability of the membrane to these ions. As in most excitable cells, the resting membrane of pulmonary artery SMCs is more permeable to K^+ than to other ions, and the concentration of K^+ in the sarcoplasm is much higher than that in the extracellular space (2,7). Thus the major determinant of the resting potential is the efflux of K^+ from the cell through K^+-selective ion channels. Although this has been long established, the nature of the K^+ channels giving rise to the resting efflux of K^+ and the resting potential in pulmonary artery SMCs is still the subject of much debate. The main focus of this chapter is on the evidence for and against the different K^+ channels that have been proposed to play this role.

If K^+ flux were the only determinant, the resting potential would be expected to have a value equal to the K^+ equilibrium potential (E_K), which is around −80 mV (7). Clearly this is not the case; the resting potential is substantially depolarized compared with E_K. Thus other ions must also contribute, most likely Cl^- or Na^+, to which the resting membrane is also permeable (2,7). The roles of these ions in regulating the resting potential and the ion channels that regulate their flux across the cell membrane are less well understood than for K^+ channels. This chapter also considers possible candidate channels that might underlie the depolarizing influence that prevents the resting potential from reaching E_K.

III. MOLECULAR IDENTIFICATION OF THE K^+ CHANNELS UNDERLYING THE RESTING MEMBRANE POTENTIAL

The pore-forming α subunits of K^+-selective channels comprise a large and diverse superfamily of proteins (17). There are four main families: the voltage-activated, Ca^{2+}-activated, inward rectifier, and two-pore-domain K^+ channels. Each of these families has many members, and in addition there are a number of auxiliary subunits that can modify the behavior of the main subunits. Members of all of these families have been identified in pulmonary artery smooth muscle. Work now is aimed at addressing the functional roles of these channels in health and disease.

A fundamental requirement for a K^+ channel to contribute to setting the resting membrane potential of pulmonary artery SMCs is that it must be open at the resting potential, between −50 and −60 mV. This is an important consideration, because many of the K^+ channels that have been identified in pulmonary artery smooth muscle cells are voltage-dependent, with an activation threshold that lies close to this voltage range or at more positive potentials. Establishing the precise threshold for K^+ channel opening can, however, be difficult, because at such negative potentials, close to E_K, the amplitude of currents flowing through K^+ channels is very small. The high input resistance of pulmonary artery myocytes (18) means that a small change in K^+ current can have a profound effect on membrane potential: at an input resistance of 10 GΩ a current of only 1 pA would change the membrane potential by 10 mV. Thus, much of the discussion over the nature of the K^+ channels giving rise to the resting potential centers on their ability to open and generate current at these negative potentials.

A. Voltage-Activated K^+ Channels

There is a general consensus that voltage-dependent K^+ channels contribute to the resting potential (12–14,16,19–21). Most studies have concluded that the important K^+ channel is a voltage-gated delayed rectifier (12,14,20). The initial evidence in favor of this was the close correlation between the inhibitory effects of 4-aminopyridine (4-AP) on membrane potential and voltage-gated K^+ currents in isolated pulmonary artery SMCs. This drug is a characteristic blocker of delayed rectifier channels, encoded by the voltage-activated K_V family of proteins. It reduces the resting potential in isolated pulmonary artery SMCs and increases resting tension in the intact vessel (8,13,21). In line with this, several members of the K_V family are expressed in the pulmonary circulation, although only a few have been seriously considered for a role in resting potential regulation. In assessing their likely contribution it is important to bear in mind that millimolar concentrations of 4-AP are required to change the resting potential or tone in pulmonary arteries, whereas most K_V channels are inhibited by 4-AP at much lower concentrations. Additional pharmacological features of the resting potential and resting tone that need to be considered include insensitivity to the K^+-channel blockers, tetraethylammonium ions (TEA) and charybdotoxin, but sensitivity to hypoxia, which inhibits the resting K^+ conductance and depolarizes pulmonary artery SMCs (12–14,21).

One of the first K_V channel subunits to be proposed as a mediator of resting potential was $K_V2.1$ (22). Studies of heterologously expressed $K_V2.1$ channels found that the concentration of 4-AP causing 50% inhibition (IC_{50}) lies in the millimolar range (17). This correlates well with the effects of 4-AP on pulmonary artery. On the other hand, the threshold for activation of homomeric $K_V2.1$ channels lies between −30 and −20 mV, so they would be closed at the resting potential of pulmonary artery SMCs. In addition, $K_V2.1$ channels are inhibited by millimolar TEA (17). The silent subunit $K_V9.3$, also found in pulmonary artery, associates with $K_V2.1$ and enables it to open at more negative potentials and also modifies its pharmacology (22). Thus, heteromeric $K_V2.1/K_V9.3$ channels were able to generate a resting potential of −50 mV when transfected into a cell line lacking a significant membrane potential, and the sensitivities to TEA and 4-AP were reduced (22). Moreover, although $K_V2.1$ channels could be inhibited by hypoxia, the sensitivities to hypoxia increased following coexpression with $K_V9.3$. Thus if $K_V2.1$ channels do contribute to the resting potential, they probably do so as part of a heteromeric channel assembly.

$K_V1.5$ channels are also expressed in pulmonary artery SMCs (see, e.g., Ref. 23) and have been considered as potential mediators of the resting K^+ conductance (15,24). The voltage threshold for activation of homomeric Kv1.5 channels is close to the resting potential of pulmonary artery SMCs (17), but other features of the channel make it an unlikely candidate. For example, 4-AP inhibits homomeric $K_V1.5$ channels with an IC_{50} below 1 mM (17), and these channels are insensitive to hypoxia (25,26). Again, if these channels do participate in setting the resting membrane potential, it is likely to be as a component of heteromeric channels, probably in association with auxiliary β subunits or $K_V1.2$ α subunits, both of which are also found in pulmonary artery and modify the properties of $K_V1.5$ (23). Strong evidence against a role for $K_V1.5$ channels in setting the resting potential is the finding that resting potential is essentially unchanged in $K_V1.5$ knockout mice (24).

It is our view that the voltage-dependent K^+ channel underlying the negative resting membrane potential of pulmonary artery SMCs is not a classical delayed rectifier or K_V channel (13,16,19). This stems from disparities between the properties of the delayed rectifier, activated by brief depolarizing voltage steps, and the K^+ current that we showed mediates the resting K^+ conductance in these cells. We found that the resting K^+ conductance has an activation threshold below −60 mV, it activates slowly (on the order of 1 s) and does not inactivate even after 30 min, and it is relatively insensitive to inhibition by the drug quinine (13,19). The noninactivating

K^+ (K_N) channels that underlie this conductance must have the same properties. The molecular correlates of these channels have not yet been identified, but they do not resemble any identified member of the K_V channel family. The kinetic properties and voltage sensitivity of K_N are similar, however, to those of the KCNQ family of voltage-activated channels (17). It is therefore of interest that two splice variants of the KCNQ1 subunit are expressed in portal vein myocytes (27). Although KCNQ channels are generally insensitive to block by 4-AP, this does not rule them out as candidates for K_N, because around 40% of the resting K^+ conductance and resting membrane potential remains unblocked in the presence of a high concentration (10 mM) of 4-AP (13,19). Thus although highly speculative at present, KCNQ channels seem like good candidates that should be considered for a role in mediating the resting K^+ conductance and setting the resting membrane potential of pulmonary artery SMCs.

B. Two-Pore-Domain K^+ Channels

In the presence of physiological concentrations of K^+, the noninactivating K^+ conductance behaves as though it were voltage-gated. Raising the extracellular K^+ concentration to 130 mM reveals that in addition to voltage-dependent current there is also a voltage-independent component (Fig. 1) (19). This is apparent as an increase in the amplitude of the inward current at negative membrane potentials (−80 to −100 mV). Because it is expected that voltage-activated K^+ channels would be closed at these potentials, changing the K^+ gradient should not alter the flow of current through such channels. The clear increase in current with increasing K^+ concentration therefore indicates that K^+ channels are open at these negative membrane potentials. This behavior is characteristic of the recently discovered two-pore-domain family of potassium channels, which have been receiving increasing interest as mediators of background K^+ conductance in a range of cell types (28). The gating of these channels lacks voltage dependence, so they have a constant probability of being open at all membrane potentials and would be open at the resting potential. Following reports that mammalian lung expresses mRNA for several members of this family (28,29), we found that mRNA and protein for the TASK-1 [TWIK (two-pore weak inward rectifier K^+)-related acid-sensitive K^+] channel are expressed in pulmonary artery SMCs (30). These channels have a characteristic pharmacological profile, which we found was also shared by the resting K^+ conductance and resting potential in pulmonary artery myocytes. Thus, in addition to the pharmacological properties described above, the resting potential and K^+ conductance are enhanced by halothane, inhibited by anandamide and low concentrations of Zn^{2+}, and exquisitely sensitive to extracellular pH, with acidosis causing inhibition (30). Thus, there is now strong evidence that the resting potential is at least partially determined by TASK-1 channels.

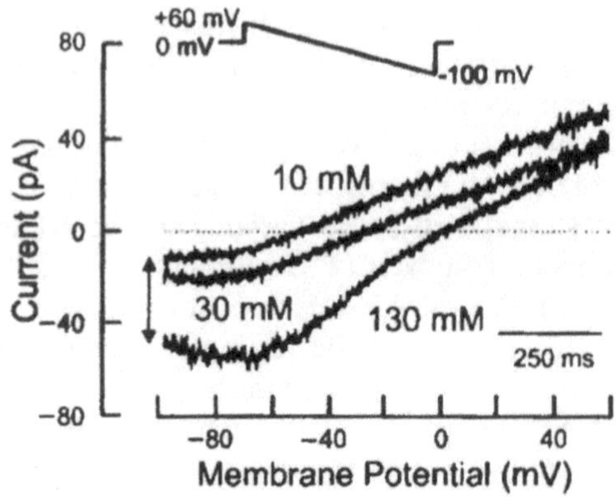

Figure 1 Effect of the extracellular K^+ concentration on the noninactivating background current (K_N). The cell was clamped at 0 mV for 10 min to inactivate K_V channels. Currents was then recorded during a 1s voltage ramp from +60 mV to −100 mV, applied in the presence of 10, 30, or 130 mM K^+. Equimolar substitution of K^+ for Na^+ maintained osmolarity. For clarity, records are shown on an inverted time base, so that the voltage axis spans from 100 mV on the left to +60 mV on the right. Raising the K^+ concentration shifted the reversal potential to more positive potentials as expected for a K^+-selective current. The arrows show the voltage-independent component apparent at −100 mV. The voltage-dependent component is indicated by rectification of the current at negative potentials at all K^+ concentrations. (Adapted from Ref. 19.)

C. Other K^+ Channels

In addition to the K^+ channels described above, pulmonary artery myocytes also express large-conductance Ca^{2+}-activated K^+ (BK_{Ca}) channels (31) and ATP-sensitive K^+ (K_{ATP}) channels (32). BK_{Ca} channels appear to be silent at the resting potential, because TEA, charybdotoxin, and iberiotoxin have essentially no effect on resting potential or resting tone (13,14,21,33). These agents do enhance the effects of a range of vasoconstrictor agents (e.g., 2,34), implying that BK_{Ca} channels open during active contraction, when $[Ca^{2+}]_i$ is elevated. Thus, it is likely that the major role of BK_{Ca} channels is to provide negative feedback regulation of Ca^{2+} influx by hyperpolarizing the membrane during active contraction. This would limit vasoconstriction and prevent vasospasm. The K_{ATP} channel is a large protein complex consisting of an inward rectifier K channel and a sulfonylurea receptor. Under normal physiological conditions, the K_{ATP} channels in resting pulmonary artery SMCs are also silent (32). They therefore contribute little to setting the resting potential, but they are well placed to modify the membrane potential when required. As discussed in Chapter 13, their main role is to hyperpolarize the SMC membrane and dilate pulmonary vessels in response to changes in the metabolic state of the cell. They also mediate hyperpolarization in response to endogenous or exogenous vasodilators acting as K^+ channel openers.

IV. ION CHANNELS MEDIATING A DEPOLARIZING INFLUENCE ON THE RESTING POTENTIAL

A role for Cl^- channels in mediating agonist-induced depolarization of pulmonary artery SMCs is well established (35,36). Their role in maintaining the resting membrane potential is less clear. The predominant channel mediating Cl^- flux in pulmonary artery SMCs is a Ca^{2+}-activated Cl^- channel (35–37). The threshold $[Ca^{2+}]_i$ at which this channel activates was found to be around 180 nM (38). Because the resting $[Ca^{2+}]_i$ in pulmonary artery myocytes may be as high as 150 nM (39), there may be sufficient Ca^{2+} present to activate a small Cl^- conductance under resting conditions. Consistent with this, a small background Cl^- current was recorded from rat pulmonary artery myocytes at physiological $[Ca^{2+}]_i$ (37). On the other hand, the resting potential of rabbit pulmonary artery SMCs was unaffected by changing the Cl^- concentration or applying Cl^- channel blockers (33). Therefore any contribution of Cl^- channels to the membrane potential in the resting state is probably small.

Although pulmonary arteries show a resting permeability to Na^+, the nature of the transport protein underlying Na^+ flux is not clear. Voltage-gated Na^+ channels are not involved, primarily because they are not evident in pulmonary artery myocytes under physiological conditions (40). A recent study on rabbit pulmonary artery myocytes identified a voltage-independent, nonselective cation conductance with an Na^+/K^+ permeability ratio of 0.6 and a reversal potential at around −10 mV (33). This conductance would provide a depolarizing current at the resting potential, mainly carried by Na^+, to counteract the K^+-selective conductance. Consistent with this, the same study found that removing the extracellular Na^+ reduced the inward current at negative potentials and caused membrane hyperpolarization. A constitutively active, nonselective cation channel with several conductance states was identified in myocytes from systemic vessels, where it was shown to be permeable to Ca^{2+} as well as Na^+ (41). The Ca^{2+} permeability of the pulmonary artery channel was not tested. It is likely to be Ca^{2+}-permeable, because pulmonary artery smooth muscle cells display substantial Ca^{2+} influx under resting conditions, as indicated by the rapidity with which Mn^{2+} quenches fura-2 fluorescence (42). Thus a constitutive channel with properties similar to those reported in systemic vessels may contribute to basal Ca^{2+} influx in pulmonary artery SMCs. If so, then constitutive Ca^{2+} influx may also contribute to the resting potential. Interestingly, extracellular Ca^{2+} also blocked the nonselective cation conductances in pulmonary and systemic artery myocytes, with an IC_{50}

in the millimolar range. This may explain the well-known depolarizing effect of Ca^{2+} removal on vascular SMCs.

V. INFLUENCE OF OTHER ION TRANSPORTERS ON RESTING POTENTIAL

The membrane potential is also influenced by the activity of electrogenic ion pumps and exchangers. For example, the ouabain-sensitive Na^+-K^+ ATPase promotes hyperpolarization (1,7). The Na^+–Ca^{2+} exchanger has been reported to generate a current of around 10 pA in rat pulmonary artery myocytes under physiological conditions (43), and, as indicated above, this could substantially depolarize the resting potential. The presence of the current was detected by switching from an Na^+-free to an Na^+-containing solution in the absence of Ca^{2+} and presence of extracellular ouabain, nisoldipine and $BaCl_2$ (1 mM) and intracellular CsCl, to inhibit the Na^+-K^+ ATPase, voltage-gated Ca^{2+} channels and K^+ channels. Although the experiments employed a standard protocol for measuring exchange current, another interpretation is possible. Because the conductance of nonselective cation channels would be largely inhibited under these conditions, the reintroduction of Na^+ could induce Na^+ current through the constitutive cation channels. Clearly, more work is needed to confidently isolate the exchange current from other components and to clarify its role in regulating the resting potential.

VI. THE RESTING POTENTIAL AND PULMONARY VASCULAR DISEASE

Changes in the resting potential have been implicated in animal models of pulmonary vascular disease. A consistent finding is that during pulmonary hypertension caused by chronic exposure to hypoxic conditions, the resting potential of pulmonary artery SMC becomes depolarized (16,44,51). This is associated with downregulation of delayed rectifier currents (16,51) and the background K^+ conductance mediated by K_N channels (16), although it is not known whether the latter effect is due to changes in the expression of voltage-dependent or voltage-independent (TASK-1) components. Pulmonary hypertension due to congenital heart disease was also found to be associated with altered K^+ channel expression (45). Interestingly, the expression of TASK-channel protein was reduced, whereas BK_{Ca} expression was increased and $K_V2.1$ unchanged. Other conductances involved in maintaining the resting potential have yet to be investigated in pulmonary disease.

A similar situation exists in the hypoxic lung of the fetus, in that fetal and newborn SMCs are significantly depolarized compared with those of older neonates and adult animals (46,47). Failure to hyperpolarize to the normal adult level may be important in pulmonary hypertension of the newborn, because exposure to hypoxia at birth prevents this developmental change from proceeding normally (46). The relationship of this developmental change in resting potential to K^+ channels is, however, unclear. Although it has been suggested that the predominant K^+ channel changes from BK_{Ca} to K_V after birth (47) and that stimulation of BK_{Ca} current underlies O_2-induced vasodilation in late gestation (48), this cannot account for the changes in resting potential recorded during the first days to weeks after birth. The depolarized fetal cells do display small voltage-activated K^+ currents relative to the adult, and the noninactivating K_N conductance is largely absent (46). However, the amplitudes of the K_V and BK_{Ca} currents actually decrease over the two weeks following birth, when the major changes in resting potential develop (46), implying that they are not responsible for normalizing the membrane potential. Perhaps BK_{Ca} channels mediate an initial hyperpolarization upon breathing, possibly caused by a rise in $[Ca^{2+}]_i$ (49) and other mechanisms are required during development to generate and stabilize the hyperpolarized potentials of adulthood. An increased contribution of K_N channels during the neonatal period may contribute (46), but changes in other conductances, perhaps nonselective cation channels, are also likely to be important.

It is not clear yet how the findings in animal models translate into human disease. Resting potentials of around −40 mV were reported for pulmonary artery SMCs from patients with secondary pulmonary hypertension (50). Although control cells from normotensive patients were not investigated, this value is within the normal range reported for other species. In contrast, the resting potentials of SMCs from patients diagnosed with primary pulmonary hypertension showed pronounced depolarization (−20 mV) associated with small K_V currents (50). Altered expression of several K_V subunits seems to be involved. However, because the molecular basis of these changes and their potential contribution to primary pulmonary hypertension are discussed in detail in Chapter 26, they are not considered further here.

VII. FUNCTIONAL IMPORTANCE OF THE RESTING POTENTIAL

As previously indicated, the main role of the resting membrane potential of pulmonary artery SMCs is to inhibit Ca^{2+} influx and release and thereby prevent vasoconstriction. Thus anything causing SMC depolarization, such as elevated K^+ or 4-AP, promotes a rise in $[Ca^{2+}]_i$ and vasoconstriction, whereas agents that cause hyperpolarization, such as K^+-channel openers (10), tend to lower $[Ca^{2+}]_i$ and promote vasodilation. It is not surprising, therefore, that the depolarized membrane potentials found in pulmonary hypertensive disease are associated with an elevated level of resting $[Ca^{2+}]_i$ (50). This is likely to play a major role in the pulmonary vasoconstriction found in pulmonary hypertensive disease. In addition, by elevating $[Ca^{2+}]_i$

sustained depolarization also stimulates the proliferation of pulmonary artery SMCs in culture (51), and this may contribute to the characteristic medial hypertrophy and vascular remodeling found in patients with pulmonary hypertension.

In addition to promoting contraction and proliferation, the depolarized membrane potentials associated with pulmonary hypertension may alter the responsiveness of pulmonary arteries to endogenous and exogenous vasoactive agents. The depolarized arteries from chronically hypoxic rats show increased responsiveness to the voltage-dependent vasodilators, verapamil and levcromakalim (52). This is hardly surprising, because these agents counteract the effect of depolarization by inhibiting Ca^{2+} influx through voltage-gated Ca^{2+} channels. A less expected effect is a pronounced increase in the sensitivity of hypertensive vessels to 4-AP (16,52). This was shown to result from a switch in the nature of the predominant K^+ channel that underlies the resting potential, from K_N with a relatively low sensitivity to block by 4-AP, to the more 4-AP-sensitive K_V (16). This change in the nature of the resting K^+ channel has important implications, because drugs or endogenous molecules that modulate K_V but do not normally affect pulmonary artery tone [e.g. quinine (13)] could become potent vasoactive agents in the hypertensive circulation. This effect may also help to explain why in vivo gene transfer of $K_V1.5$ reduced the pulmonary hypertension caused by chronic exposure of rats to hypoxia (53), despite the arguments, outlined above, against a role for this channel in regulating the resting potential of pulmonary artery SMCs. I would predict that gene transfer of most K_V channels would have the same effect.

The influence of membrane potential on the pharmacology of pulmonary arteries should be an important consideration in relation to drug therapy for pulmonary vascular disease. Pulmonary arteries from chronically hypoxic animals show altered reactivity to a range of vasoactive agents (52,54). Of particular note is the finding that membrane depolarization inhibits the vasodilator effect of nitric oxide, and as this occurs independently of the rise in SMC guanosine 3′,5′-cyclic monophosphate (cGMP), membrane potential must interfere with a step downstream of cGMP generation (55). This effect could contribute to the impaired sensitivity of hypertensive and neonatal pulmonary arteries to nitric oxide and endothelium-dependent vasodilators. Moreover, it has the potential to limit the therapeutic effectiveness of inhaled nitric oxide. On the other hand, by altering SMC responsiveness, it is possible that membrane depolarization could provide a means of selectively targeting vasodilators at the pulmonary circulation.

VIII. SUMMARY

The resting potential of pulmonary artery SMCs is an important regulator of cell $[Ca^{2+}]_i$ and therefore pulmonary vascular tone. Both acute and chronic hypoxia depolarize the membrane and elevate $[Ca^{2+}]_i$, and this is likely to contribute to pulmonary vasoconstriction as illustrated in Fig. 2. Depolarization is also likely to contribute to SMC proliferation and pulmonary vascular remodeling in disease. The resting potential is determined by the balance between K^+ efflux through K^+-selective ion channels and Na^+ influx, probably carried through nonselective cation channels. The molecular correlate of the main K^+ channel involved in setting the resting potential is not yet certain. There is strong evidence that voltage-independent TASK-1 channels are important, but a voltage-dependent channel with biophysical properties similar to those of the KCNQ family may also be involved. In addition, $K_V2.1$ channels, most likely in association with $K_V9.3$ subunits, may play a lesser role. The depolarization of SMCs in pulmonary hypertensive disease is associated with altered expression of several K^+ channels. The expression of depolarizing cation channels remains to be

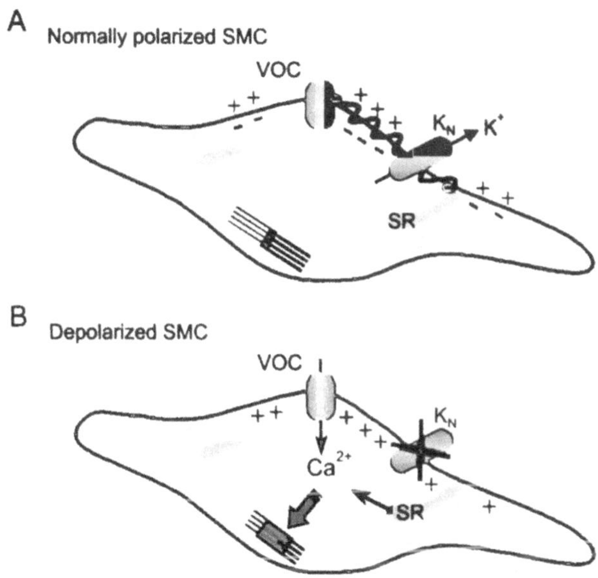

Figure 2 In normally polarized pulmonary artery SMC (A), the resting efflux of K^+ through background K^+ (mostly K_N) channels maintains a negative potential across the resting membrane. This prevents the opening of voltage-operated Ca^{2+} channels (VOC), thereby inhibiting Ca^{2+} influx, and suppresses Ca^{2+} release from the sarcoplasmic reticulum (SR). This maintains a low resting $[Ca^{2+}]_i$, which prevents contraction. The inhibition or downregulation of K_N channels blocks K^+ efflux, allowing the membrane to depolarize (B). This removes the inhibition of VOC and SR Ca^{2+} release, so that Ca^{2+} can permeate into the cytoplasm to raise $[Ca^{2+}]_i$ and promote contraction.

investigated. During pulmonary hypertension caused by chronic hypoxia, the major resting K^+ channel switches from the background channel, K_N, to a voltage-gated channel of the K_V family. Along with depolarization, this has a major impact on the pharmacology of the pulmonary vessels. This could have important implications for the design of pulmonary selective vasodilators to treat pulmonary hypertensive disease.

ACKNOWLEDGMENTS

Work in my laboratory is funded by the Biotechnology and Biological Sciences Research Council, the British Heart Foundation, the Wellcome Trust, and Tenovus Scotland.

REFERENCES

1. Suzuki H, Twarog BM. Membrane properties of smooth muscle cells in pulmonary arteries of the rat. Am J Physiol 1982; 242:H900–H906.
2. Haeusler G. Contraction, membrane potential, and calcium fluxes in rabbit pulmonary arterial muscle. Fed Proc 1983; 42:263–268.
3. Casteels R, Kitamura K, Kuriyama H, Suzuki H. Excitation-contraction coupling in the smooth muscle cells of the rabbit main pulmonary artery. J Physiol 1977; 271:63–79.
4. Ito S, Kajikuri J, Itoh T, Kuriyama H. Effects of lemakalim on changes in Ca^{2+} concentration and mechanical activity induced by noradrenaline in the rabbit mesenteric artery. Br J Pharm 1991; 104:227–233.
5. Best L, Bolton TB. Depolarisation of guinea-pig visceral smooth muscle causes hydrolysis of inositol phospholipids. Naunyn Schmiedebergs Arch Pharmacol 1986; 333:78–82.
6. Okada Y, Yanagisawa T, Taira N. BRL 38227 (levcromakalim)-induced hyperpolarization reduces the sensitivity to Ca^{2+} of contractile elements in canine coronary artery. Naunyn Schmiedebergs Arch Pharmacol 1993; 347:438–444.
7. Casteels R, Kitamura K, Kuriyama H, Suzuki H. The membrane properties of the smooth muscle cells of the rabbit main pulmonary artery. J Physiol 1977; 271:41–61.
8. Hara Y, Kitamura K, Kuriyama H. Actions of 4-aminopyridine on vascular smooth muscle tissues of the guinea-pig. Br J Pharm 1980; 68:99–106.
9. Madden JA, Dawson CA, Harder DR. Hypoxia-induced activation in small isolated pulmonary arteries from the cat. J Appl Physiol 1985; 59:113–118.
10. Clapp LH, Gurney AM. ATP-sensitive K^+ channels regulate resting potential of pulmonary arterial smooth muscle cells. Am J Physiol 1992; 262: H916–H920.
11. Smirnov SV, Robertson TP, Ward JPT, Aaronson PI. Chronic hypoxia is associated with reduced delayed rectifier K^+ current in rat pulmonary artery muscle cells. Am J Physiol 1994; 266:H365–H370.

12. Post JM, Gelband CH, Hume JR. $[Ca^{2+}]_i$ inhibition of K^+ channels in canine pulmonary artery. Novel mechanism for hypoxia-induced membrane depolarization. Circ Res 1995; 77:131–139.
13. Osipenko ON, Evans AM, Gurney AM. Regulation of the resting potential of rabbit pulmonary artery myocytes by a low threshold, O_2-sensing potassium current. Br J Pharm 1997; 120:1461–1470.
14. Yuan XJ. Voltage-gated K^+ currents regulate resting membrane potential and $[Ca^{2+}]_i$ in pulmonary arterial myocytes. Circ Res 1995; 77:370–378.
15. Archer SL, Souil E, Dinh-Xuan AT, Schremmer B, Mercier JC, El Yaagoubi A, Nguyen-Huu L, Reeve HL, Hampl V. Molecular identification of the role of voltage-gated K^+ channels, Kv1.5 and Kv2.1, in hypoxic pulmonary vasoconstriction and control of resting membrane potential in rat pulmonary artery myocytes. J Clin Invest 1998; 101:2319–2330.
16. Osipenko ON, Alexander D, MacLean MR, Gurney AM. Influence of chronic hypoxia on the contributions of non-inactivating and delayed rectifier K currents to the resting potential and tone of rat pulmonary artery smooth muscle. Br J Pharm 1998; 124:1335–1337.
17. Coetzee WA, Amarillo Y, Chiu J, Chow A, Lau D, McCormack T, Moreno H, Nadal MS, Ozaita A, Pountney D, Saganich M, Vega-Saenz de Miera E, Rudy B. Molecular diversity of K^+ channels. Ann NY Acad Sci 1999; 868:233–285.
18. Clapp LH, Gurney AM. A simple method for cell isolation: characterisation of the major outward currents in rabbit pulmonary artery. Exp Physiol 1991; 76:677–693.
19. Evans AM, Osipenko ON, Gurney AM. Properties of a novel K^+ current that is active at resting potential in rabbit pulmonary artery smooth muscle cells. J Physiol 1996; 496:407–420.
20. Archer SL, Weir EK, Reeve HL, Michelakis E. Molecular identification of O_2 sensors and O_2-sensitive potassium channels in the pulmonary circulation. Adv Exp Med Biol 2000; 475:219–240.
21. Doi S, Damron DS, Ogawa K, Tanaka S, Horibe M, Murray PA. K^+ channel inhibition, calcium signaling, and vasomotor tone in canine pulmonary artery smooth muscle. Am J Physiol Lung Cell Mol Physiol 2000; 279:L242–L251.
22. Patel AJ, Lazdunski M, Honore E. Kv2.1/Kv9.3, a novel ATP-dependent delayed-rectifier K^+ channel in oxygen-sensitive pulmonary artery myocytes. EMBO J 1997; 16:6615–6625.
23. Coppock EA, Tamkun MM. Differential expression of K_V channel α- and β-subunits in the bovine pulmonary arterial circulation. Am J Physiol Lung Cell Mol Physiol 2001; 281:L1350–L1360.
24. Archer SL, London B, Hampl V, Wu X, Nsair A, Puttagunta L, Hashimoto K. Impairment of hypoxic pulmonary vasoconstriction in mice lacking the voltage-gated potassium channel Kv1.5. FASEB J 2001; 15:1801–1803.
25. Hulme JT, Coppock EA, Felipe A, Martens JR, Tamkun MM. Oxygen sensitivity of cloned voltage-gated K^+ channels expressed in the pulmonary vasculature. Circ Res 1999; 85:489–497.
26. Osipenko ON, Tate RJ, Gurney AM. Potential role for Kv3.1b channels as oxygen sensors. Circ Res 2000; 86:534–540.

27. Ohya S, Sergeant GP, Greenwood IA, Horowitz B. Molecular variants of KCNQ channels expressed in murine portal vein myocytes: a role in delayed rectifier current. Circ Res 2003; 92:1016–1023.
28. Lesage F, Lazdunski M. Molecular and functional properties of two-pore-domain potassium channels. Am J Physiol Renal Physiol 2000; 279: F793–F801.
29. Kim Y, Bang H, Kim D. TASK-3, a new member of the tandem pore K^+ channel family. J Biol Chem 2000; 275:9340–9347.
30. Gurney AM, Osipenko ON, MacMillan D, McFarlane KM, Tate RJ, Kempsill FEJ. Two-pore domain K channel, TASK-1, in pulmonary artery smooth muscle cells. Circ Res 2003; 93:957–964.
31. Snetkov VA, Gurney AM, Ward JPT, Osipenko ON. Inward rectification of the large conductance potassium channel in smooth muscle cells from rabbit pulmonary artery. Exp Physiol 1996; 81:743–753.
32. Clapp LH, Gurney AM. ATP-sensitive K^+ channels regulate resting potential of pulmonary arterial smooth muscle cells. Am J Physiol 1992; 262: H916–H920.
33. Bae YM, Park MK, Lee SH, Ho WK, Earm YE. Contribution of Ca^{2+}-activated K^+ channels and non-selective cation channels to membrane potential of pulmonary arterial smooth muscle cells of the rabbit. J Physiol 1999; 514:747–758.
34. Peng W, Michael JR, Hoidal JR, Karwande SV, Farrukh IS. ET-1 modulates K_{Ca}-channel activity and arterial tension in normoxic and hypoxic human pulmonary vasculature. Am J Physiol 1998; 275:L729–L739.
35. Wang Q, Large WA. Action of histamine on single smooth muscle cells dispersed from the rabbit pulmonary artery. J Physiol 1993; 468:125–139.
36. Salter KJ, Turner JL, Albarwani S, Clapp LH, Kozlowski RZ. Ca^{2+}-activated Cl^- and K^+ channels and their modulation by endothelin-1 in rat pulmonary arterial smooth muscle cells. Exp Physiol 1995; 80:815–824.
37. Clapp LH, Turner JL, Kozlowski RZ. Ca^{2+}-activated Cl^- currents in pulmonary arterial myocytes. Am J Physiol 1996; 270:H1577–H1584.
38. Pacaud P, Loirand G, Gregore G, Mironneau C, Mironneau J. Calcium-dependence of the calcium-activated chloride current in smooth muscle cells of rat portal vein. Pflügers Arch 1992; 421:125–130.
39. Drummond RM, Tuft RA. Release of Ca^{2+} from the sarcoplasmic reticulum increases mitochondrial $[Ca^{2+}]_i$ in rat pulmonary artery smooth muscle cells. J Physiol 1999; 516:139–147.
40. Clapp LH, Gurney AM. Modulation of calcium movements by nitroprusside in isolated vascular smooth muscle cells. Pflügers Arch 1991; 418:462–470.
41. Albert AP, Piper AS, Large WA. Properties of a constitutively active Ca^{2+}-permeable non-selective cation channel in rabbit ear artery myocytes. J Physiol 2003; 549:143–156.
42. Ng LC, Gurney AM. Store-operated channels mediate Ca^{2+} influx and contraction in rat pulmonary artery. Circ Res 2001; 89:923–929.
43. Wang YX, Dhulipala PK, Kotlikoff MI. Hypoxia inhibits the Na^+/Ca^{2+} exchanger in pulmonary artery smooth muscle cells. FASEB J 2000; 14: 1731–1740.

44. Suzuki H, Twarog BM. Membrane properties of smooth muscle cells in pulmonary hypertensive rats. Am J Physiol 1982; 242:H907–H915.
45. Cornfield DN, Resnik ER, Herron JM, Reinhartz O, Fineman JR. Pulmonary vascular K^+ channel expression and vasoreactivity in a model of congenital heart disease. Am J Physiol Lung Cell Mol Physiol 2002; 283:L1210–L1219.
46. Evans AM, Osipenko ON, Haworth SG, Gurney AM. Resting potentials and potassium currents during development of pulmonary artery smooth muscle cells. Am J Physiol 1998; 275:H887–H899.
47. Reeve, HL, Archer SL, Weir EK, Cornfield DN. Maturational changes in K^+-channel activity and oxygen sensing in the ovine pulmonary vasculature. Am J Physiol 1998; 275:L1019–L1025.
48. Cornfield DN, Reeve HL, Tolarova S, Weir EK, Archer S. Oxygen causes fetal pulmonary vasodilation through activation of a calcium-dependent potassium channel. Proc Natl Acad Sci USA 1996; 93:8089–8094.
49. Porter VA, Rhodes MT, Reeve HL, Cornfield DN. Oxygen-induced fetal pulmonary vasodilation is mediated by intracellular calcium activation of K_{Ca}-channels. Am J Physiol Lung Cell Mol Physiol 2001; 281:L1379–L1385.
50. Yuan JX-J, Aldinger AM, Juhaszova M, Wang J, Conte JV Jr, Gaine SP, Orens JB, Rubin LJ. Dysfunctional voltage-gated K^+ channels in pulmonary artery smooth muscle cells of patients with primary pulmonary hypertension. Circulation 1998; 98:1400–1406.
51. Platoshyn O, Yu Y, Golovina VA, McDaniel SS, Krick S, Li L, Wang J-Y, Rubin LJ, Yuan JX-J. Chronic hypoxia decreases K_V channel expression and function in pulmonary artery myocytes. Am J Physiol Lung Cell Mol Physiol 2001; 280:L801–L812.
52. Priest RM, Robertson TP, Leach RM, Ward JPT. Membrane potential-dependent and -independent vasodilation in small pulmonary arteries from chronically hypoxic rats. J Pharmacol Exp Ther 1998; 285:975–982.
53. Pozeg ZI, Michelakis ED, McMurtry MS, Thebaud B, Wu XC, Dyck JR, Hashimoto K, Wang S, Moudgil R, Harry G, Sultanian R, Koshal A, Archer SL. In vivo gene transfer of the O_2-sensitive potassium channel Kv1.5 reduces pulmonary hypertension and restores hypoxic pulmonary vasoconstriction in chronically hypoxic rats. Circulation 2003; 107:2037–2044.
54. Karamsetty VS, Kane KA, Wadsworth RM. The effects of chronic hypoxia on the pharmacological responsiveness of the pulmonary artery. Pharmacol Ther 1995; 68:233–246.
55. Rapoport RM, Schwartz K, Murad F. Effect of sodium-potassium pump inhibitors and membrane-depolarizing agents on sodium nitroprusside-induced relaxation and cyclic guanosine monophosphate accumulation in rat aorta. Circ Res 1985; 57:164–170.

22

Calcium Channels, Calcium Signaling, and Lung Vascular Barrier Regulation

Bryan J. McVerry, Steven M. Dudek, and Joe G. N. Garcia
Johns Hopkins University School of Medicine, Baltimore, Maryland, U.S.A.
Dolly Mehta
University of Illinois, Chicago, Illinois, U.S.A.

I. INTRODUCTION

The endothelium is a complex, dynamic tissue that regulates multiple vascular wall processes, including smooth muscle tone, thrombogenesis, and angiogenesis, and provides a semiselective cellular barrier between the intravascular and extravascular fluid compartments. Given the vast surface area of the pulmonary microcirculation and the intimate association of the microvasculature with gas-exchanging alveolar elements, the integrity of the vascular barrier is a key consideration in lung homeostasis. Indeed, in pathological lung inflammatory states, the pulmonary endothelial barrier endures significant disruption leading to profound leakage of fluid and macromolecules into the lung interstitium, ultimately resulting in alveolar flooding when alveolar fluid clearance mechanisms are overwhelmed. The consequence of this imbalance in lung fluid homeostasis is clinically manifested as high-permeability, protein-rich pulmonary edema producing the characteristic physiological derangement of severe hypoxemia and reduced lung compliance observed in acute lung injury (ALI).

The mechanisms by which the lung vascular barrier is maintained and those by which barrier integrity is restored after inflammatory states are of immense interest and importance. The pulmonary endothelium, long considered a passive barrier, is now well appreciated as a highly metabolically active tissue regulating barrier function via highly orchestrated changes in cell shape. Cytoskeletal elements play a critical role in determining these shape changes and in the maintenance of barrier integrity, as demonstrated by multiple in vitro studies in which the interaction of actin and myosin leads to cytoskeletal rearrangement that results in endothelial cell (EC) contraction and subsequent paracellular gap formation (1). Insights into the molecular mechanisms underlying the maintenance of endothelial barrier integrity have elucidated the active participation of calcium ions (Ca^{2+}) as a vital regulatory second messenger in the signaling cascade leading to activation of the contractile apparatus, barrier disruption, and possibly barrier restoration as well. For example, Ca^{2+}-dependent signaling pathways targeting the EC cytoskeleton are important determinants of endothelial vascular leak produced by the highly edemagenic agent thrombin (2). In this chapter, we will address the role of Ca^{2+} and Ca^{2+} channels in the regulation of pulmonary endothelial barrier properties.

II. CALCIUM CHANNELS

Structural and functional aspects of Ca^{2+} channels in vascular endothelium are reviewed by Nilius and Droogmans (3), and further details regarding Ca^{2+} channels appear elsewhere in this text. Briefly, seven types of channels act in a coherent manner to regulate Ca^{2+} homeostasis and stimulus-coupling signaling in the pulmonary endothelium. Three of these channels modulate extracellular Ca^{2+} entry whereas four channel types activate Ca^{2+} release from intracellular stores (see Table 1). The nonselective cation channels (NSCs) can be activated by ligation of membrane receptors, cyclic nucleotide binding of the carboxyl terminus of the channel, or interaction of superoxide ions with the cytosolic domain of the channel (3,4). The receptor-activated nonspecific Ca^{2+} channels are members of the transient receptor potential (Trp) family of proteins originally described in *Drosophila* species, which typically function through signaling cascades involving activation of phospholipase C (PLC). Variably sensitive to endoplasmic reticulum (ER) Ca^{2+} store depletion, these channels nonspecifically allow Ca^{2+} entry into endothelial cells (ECs) along with other cations (potassium, sodium, cesium, manganese, etc.). A few of these channels, known as store-operated channels (SOCs), respond to increases in intracellular Ca^{2+} concentration ($[Ca^{2+}]_i$) coupled to inositol 1,4,5-trisphosphate production (IP_3) and subsequent ER Ca^{2+} depletion. SOCs, including Trp4 and the calcium release-activated channel (CRAC), appear to be more selective for Ca^{2+} ion than for other cations (3). These channels, also known as capacitative Ca^{2+} entry channels (CCEs), likely represent the major route of Ca^{2+} entry into ECs and open in response to depletion of ER Ca^{2+} stores either directly by compounds such as thapsigargin or by IP_3-dependent ary Endothelial Ca^{2+} Channels

	Ca^{2+} flux	Role in barrier regulation
s		
channels (NSC) ed	Minor extracellular Ca^{2+} entry pathway	Under investigation
acitative) Ca^{2+} channels	Selective extracellular Ca^{2+} influx	Trp4 expression necessary for maximal thrombin-induced barrier disruption[a]
e (NCX) responsive	Extracellular Ca^{2+} entry	Under investigation
els		
osphate receptor (IP_3R) sitive to local [Ca^{2+}]	Intracellular store release	Route for store depletion necessary f Ca^{2+} entry[b]
SERCA) modulated	Intracellular store replenishment	Maintain Ca^{2+} stores necessary for EC activation after barrier-disruption stimuli[c]
	Intracellular store depletion	Minor role in store depletion
tive		
porter	Imports Ca^{2+} into mitochondria	Links EC stretch to proinflammatory response through ROS generation[d]

ef. 5.; [d]Ref. 9.

mechanisms. The presence of extracellular Ca^{2+} is essential for SOC function, as has been reported in pulmonary artery endothelial cells (PAECs) and pulmonary microvascular endothelial cells (PMVECs) stimulated in Ca^{2+}-free media (5–7). The IP_3–receptor complex is a 310 kDa homotetramer found on the membrane of the endoplasmic reticulum. Upon activation by IP_3, the receptor forms a channel that transports Ca^{2+} across the membrane into the cytosol (4,8) regulated by local concentrations of Ca^{2+} both in the cytosol and in the ER. The IP_3 receptor (IP_3R) becomes more sensitive to IP_3 as the local cytosolic Ca^{2+} ion concentration elevates to 100–300 nM, whereas micromolar concentrations inhibit IP_3R function (4,8). In contrast, when ER luminal Ca^{2+} concentration exceeds its buffering capacity, the IP_3R complex becomes more sensitive to agonist stimulation (8). The smooth endoplasmic reticulum (ER) Ca^{2+} ATPase (SERCA), the major membrane protein of the ER, actively pumps Ca^{2+} from the cytosol back into the endoplasmic reticulum to replenish and maintain intracellular stores at millimolar concentrations (4). Thapsigargin specifically inhibits SERCA function, leading to depletion of Ca^{2+} stores via constitutively active leak channels operative on the ER membrane. Recent evidence suggests that a mitochondrial uniporter may also play an important role in regulating Ca^{2+} entry into mitochondria, which is necessary for the generation of proinflammatory reactive oxygen species after EC stretch (9,10). Finally, a reduction in the sodium (Na^+) gradient across the plasma membrane activates an Na^+–Ca^{2+} exchange (NCX) leading to increases in $[Ca^{2+}]_i$, although its role in the pulmonary vasculature is presently unknown. These channels integrate to modulate Ca^{2+} homeostasis within the endothelium and to control Ca^{2+}-dependent intracellular signal transduction. A significant body of evidence suggests that voltage-regulated Ca^{2+} channels, primary modulators of Ca^{2+} homeostasis in other cell types and present in systemic endothelial cells, are absent from cultured pulmonary endothelial cells (4).

III. CALCIUM SIGNALING

The Ca^{2+}-dependent increase in pulmonary endothelial permeability is initiated by diverse stressors including inflammatory cytokines, oxygen free radicals, transmural stress, or thrombin that stimulate hydrolysis of membrane phospholipids (1,4). Following cell stimulation, this cascade appears as an initial transient peak known as Ca^{2+} release followed by a more sustained response due to Ca^{2+} entry across the plasmalemma (7,11,12). It is well established that EC surface receptors coupled to guanosine-nucleotide binding proteins (G_q proteins) induce the activation of phospholipase C (PLC), which stimulates the production of IP_3 and diacylglycerol (DAG) from phosphatidylinositol-4,5-bisphosphate (PIP_2) by a mechanism independent of Ca^{2+}. As mentioned above, IP_3 diffuses to the ER, activating its tetrameric receptor (IP_3R) and resulting in rapid release of stored Ca^{2+} into the cytosol (4). Thrombin is a potent stimulus for Ca^{2+} release from intracellular stores in several types of endothelia including lung EC, similar to that induced by thapsigargin and independent of extracellular Ca^{2+} concentration (6). Release from the ER of IP_3R-dependent Ca^{2+} subsequently triggers the downstream release of mitochondrial Ca^{2+} stores (approximately 25% of EC stores) via a close-coupling mechanism that may contribute, albeit minimally, to the initial transient peak in $[Ca^{2+}]_i$ (4). DAG along with cytosolic Ca^{2+} activates protein kinase C (PKC), which may propagate Ca^{2+} -dependent cellular responses and may facilitate Ca^{2+}-independent signaling mechanisms. IP_3 hydrolysis and increasing local $[Ca^{2+}]_i$ combine to inhibit further activity of the IP_3R. Patch-clamp analysis demonstrates that the open probability of IP_3R decreases sharply as local $[Ca^{2+}]_i$ increases beyond 300 nM (13). Ryanodine, a plant alkaloid, promotes release of intracellular Ca^{2+} stores from a pool separate from that accessed by IP_3R via channels known as ryanodine receptor channels (14). Ryanodine stimulation typically results in a smaller transient rise in $[Ca^{2+}]_i$ than that induced by IP_3. Ryanodine receptors are variably expressed in ECs and may thus activate Ca^{2+} release; however, their role in regulating pulmonary endothelial permeability is not yet established.

The release of ER Ca^{2+} stores is essential for downstream Ca^{2+} signaling in ECs because it facilitates Ca^{2+} entry from the extracellular milieu via the activation of store-operated or capacitative plasmalemmal Ca^{2+} channels. Current concepts invoke the Trp family of proteins as the primary effectors of store-operated Ca^{2+} entry. Trp proteins comprise a family of cation channels first described in *Drosophila* that includes seven mammalian homologs (Trp1–Trp7) (discussed in detail elsewhere in this volume in Chapters 5 and 6). Multiple heterologous combinations of these Trp proteins combine to produce tetrameric channels with unique properties. Although Trp1, 2, 4, and 5 are all activated by Ca^{2+} store depletion (15), in ECs Trp1 and 4 primarily contribute to the molecular formation of the thapsigargin-activated Ca^{2+}-selective current, I_{SOC} (7,16,17), which is sensitive to the organization of the actin-based cytoskeleton (18) and therefore provides a potential direct link to the cytoskeletal rearrangements necessary for barrier modulation. Antisense depletion of Trp1 protein expression reduces I_{SOC} activity by 50% in human pulmonary artery EC (HPAEC) cultures (16), and Trp4 expression has been even more closely linked to pulmonary vascular barrier function. Lung microvascular endothelial cells, which selectively express Trp4 more abundantly than other Trp channels, were isolated from wild-type and Trp4-knockout ($Trp4^{-/-}$) mice and stimulated with the potent edemagenic agent thrombin (7). Ca^{2+} entry, actin stress fiber formation, and thrombin-induced permeability were all significantly attenuated in the $Trp4^{-/-}$ group compared to the wild-type mice (Fig. 1). Furthermore, isolated lung preparations from these animals

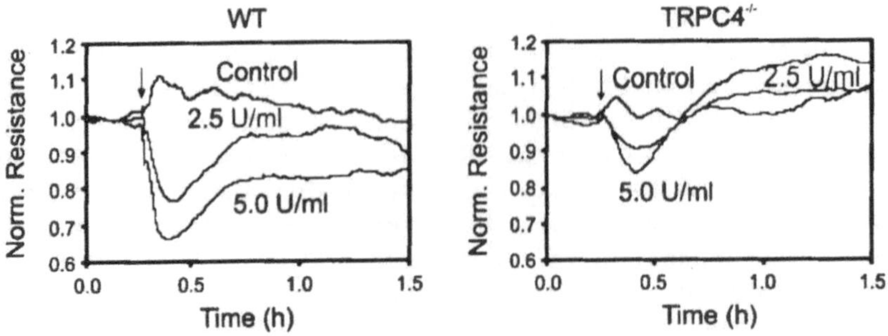

Figure 1 Effects of thrombin on wild-type and Trp4 lung MVEC transmonolayer electrical resistance (TER). The drop in TER induced by thrombin is attenuated in $Trp4^{-/-}$ cells implicating Ca^{2+} entry via the Trp4 store-operated channel in the disruption of MVEC barrier integrity. (From Ref. 7.)

demonstrated reduced thrombin-induced microvascular permeability in $Trp4^{-/-}$ vs. wild type mice (7). These results identify Trp4 as a key Ca^{2+} transport channel regulating permeability in the lung microvasculature.

IV. REGULATION OF CALCIUM ENTRY

The mechanisms directly relevant to I_{SOC} activation following depletion of ER Ca^{2+} stores are currently the focus of significant research efforts. Several coupling models have been proposed to explain the linkage between ER store depletion and I_{SOC} activation (19–21). One possibility involves the presence of an as yet unidentified diffusible second messenger, activated by Ca^{2+} release from intracellular stores, that traverses to the plasma membrane to stimulate store-operated Ca^{2+} entry. The second theory invokes the process of exocytosis with insertion of calcium channels into the plasma membrane by vesicle fusion triggered by ER store depletion. Third, it is well established that $[Ca^{2+}]_i$ inhibits nearby membrane channel function (21). Perhaps ER store depletion results in decreased $[Ca^{2+}]_i$ in the space between the ER and the plasma membrane, releasing the Ca^{2+} inhibition of membrane channels. Finally, based on the findings that Trp activation requires continued close contact with IP_3R, a widely favored conformational-coupling model has been suggested. This model presumes that depletion of ER Ca^{2+} stores leads to a conformational change in the IP_3R that is transmitted to I_{SOC} by a direct interaction between the receptor and Trp channel. However, proof favoring conformation-driven coupling between IP_3R and Trp channel is still lacking. The majority of research, however, points to that coupling between IP_3R and Trp channels potentially being mediated by kinase and phosphatase activity following Ca^{2+} store depletion, thereby altering SOC permeability to Ca^{2+} (4). An excellent candidate kinase in this paradigm is the endothelial cell myosin light-chain kinase isoform (EC MLCK), a multifunctional 210 kDa Ca^{2+}/CaM-dependent enzyme whose activation increases levels of phosphorylated MLCs, producing greater tension development, actin stress fiber formation, and barrier dysfunction in multiple models of EC permeability (1). The highly multifunctional EC MLCK isoform, first cloned by the Garcia laboratory, is essential for the operation of SOCs in response to depletion of intracellular Ca^{2+} stores in rat pulmonary artery endothelial cells (PAECs) (22). Overexpression of N-terminal MLCK deletion constructs, which lack kinase activity, attenuates store-operated calcium entry, strongly suggesting the involvement of N-terminal MLCK binding in the coupling between ER Ca^{2+} release and I_{SOC} (Stevens and Garcia, personal communication). Whether this involves a direct interaction with Trp or regulation occurs through the assembly of a spectrin protein 4.1 complex remains unclear. Mehta and colleagues recently demonstrated a role for small GTPase Rho in mediating the coupling of the Trp1 channel to IP_3R and trafficking of the complex to the plasma membrane surface, thus allowing for extracellular Ca^{2+} entry (Mehta, D, Ahmmed GJ, Paria BC, Holinstat M, Voyno-Yasenetskaya T, Tiruppathi C, Minsmall RD, Malik AB. RHOA interaction with inositol 1,4,5-triphosphate receptor and transient receptor potential channel-1 regulates Ca^{2+} entry: Role in signaling increase endothelial permeability. J. Biol Chem 2003 Vol. 278, No. 35. pp 33492–3350). This observation is particularly intriguing, becuase the activation of Rho via its intracellular target, Rho kinase, directly modulates EC permeability through its inhibitory action on MLC phosphatase (MYPT) activity (23). Thus, the coordinate regulation by EC MLCK and Rho kinase of intracellular levels of MLC phosphorylation has profound effects on EC permeability, possibly via regulation of SOCs and IP_3R.

Recent work highlighted an important role for the actin cytoskeleton in modulating I_{SOC}. Treatment of individual ECs with cytochalasin D to disrupt actin microfilaments or inhibition of MLCK resulted in significant inhibition of I_{SOC} stimulated by thapsigargin (18,22). Moreover, stabilization of actin fibers also inhibited activation of I_{SOC} by thapsigargin, suggesting an integral role for active actin rearrangement in this process (22). The multiple observations that capacitative Ca^{2+} entry (CCE) in porcine aortic ECs was differentially inhibited in proportion to the potency of MLCK pharmacological inhibitors ML-5, -7, and -9 and by MLCK antisense treatment (24–26) provide further evidence implicating MLCK in the modulation of I_{SOC}. Although these data strongly suggest a linkage between actomyosin rearrangement, permeability changes, and I_{SOC}, the mechanisms regulating this relationship are not fully defined. This linkage appears to be partially mediated through interactions of the actin binding protein spectrin with protein 4.1 at the plasma membrane, because microinjection of an antibody that specifically disrupts spectrin–protein 4.1 binding decreased the global $[Ca^{2+}]_i$ response to thapsigargin and abolished I_{SOC} (27). The small GTPase Rho may also be involved in the linkage between actomyosin arrangement and I_{SOC}, because Rho inhibition prevented actin stress fiber formation in thrombin-stimulated ECs, and the inhibition of actin

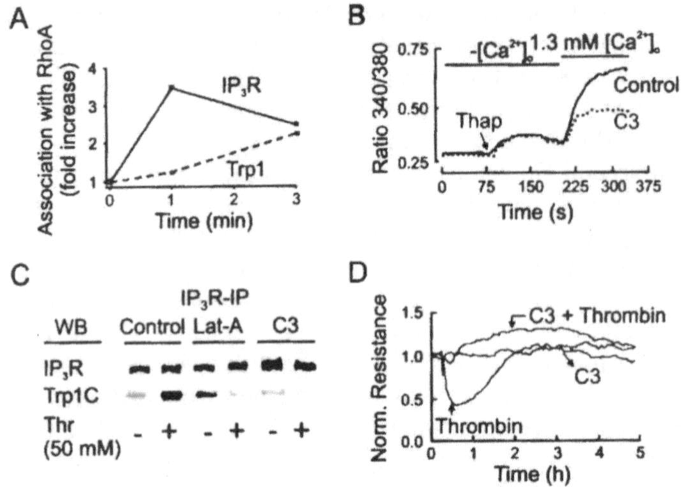

Figure 2 Role of Rho in mediating endothelial cell Ca^{2+} entry and permeability. (A) Lysates from thrombin-stimulated or unstimulated HPAEC were incubated with GST-rhotekin fusion protein to pull down activated Rho, then subjected to Western blotting with anti-IP_3R, Trpl channel, or Rho antibody. Thrombin induced a sustained association of IP_3R with activated Rho within 1 min, whereas Trpl associated with Rho 3 min after thrombin stimulation. Rho associates with IP_3R and Trpl channel in a time-dependent manner to regulate cytosolic Ca^{2+} concentration. (B) HPAEC labeled with Fura2 in a Ca^{2+}-free milieu were treated with thapsigargin (Thap) in the presence or absence of C3 transferase, which ADP-ribosylates and inhibits Rho. Inhibition of Rho had no effect on TG-induced Ca^{2+} store release but markedly attenuated store-operated Ca^{2+} entry after extracellular Ca^{2+} replenishment. These observations indicate that Rho modulates SOC directly. (C) Following thrombin administration, lysates from C3 transferase-treated, latrunculin-treated, and control HPAECs were immunoprecipitated using IP_3R antibody, then Western blotted using Trpl or IP_3R antibody. Inhibition of either Rho or actin polymerization prevented the thrombin-induced association of IP_3R with Trpl channels. Thus, Rho is required not only for trafficking of IP_3R and Trpl channel but also for IP_3R–Trpl coupling to induce Ca^{2+} entry. (D) Transmonolayer electrical resistance (TER) was measured across HPAEC monolayers treated with thrombin, C3 transferase, or C3 transferase in the presence of thrombin. C3 transferase attenuated the thrombin-induced drop in TER, implicating Rho in the mechanism of barrier dysregulation induced by thrombin. (Mehta, D, Ahmmed GJ, Paria BC, Holinstat M, Voyno-Yasenetskaya T, Tiruppathi C, Minsmall RD, Malik AB. RHOA interaction with inositol 1,4,5-triphosphate receptor and transient receptor potential channel-1 regulates Ca^{2+} entry: Role in signaling increase endothelial permeability. J. Biol Chem 2003 Vol. 278, No. 35. pp 33492–3350.)

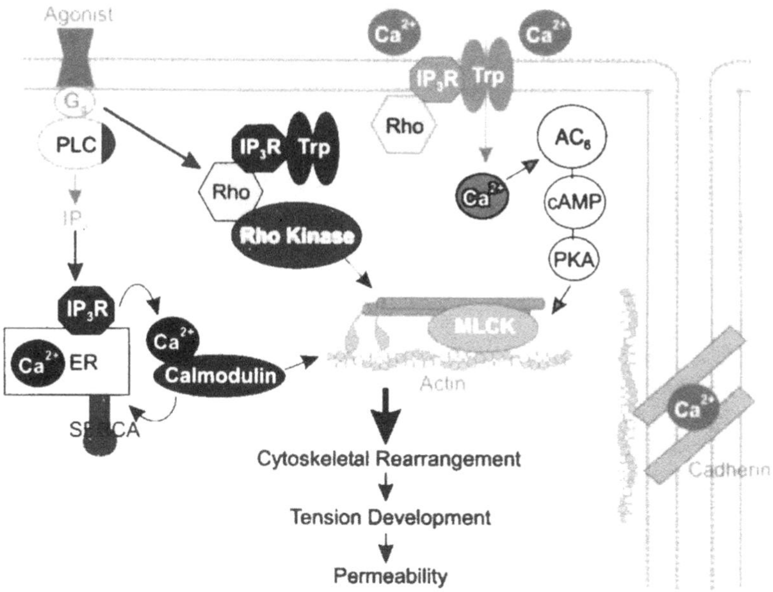

Figure 3 Summary of endothelial Ca^{2+} signaling and mechanisms linking Ca^{2+} to cytoskeletal barrier regulation. Ca^{2+} is released from intracellular stores maintained in the endoplasmic reticulum (ER) after inositol 1,4,5-trisphosphate (IP_3), generated upon cell-surface receptor stimulation, activates the transmembrane IP_3 receptor (IP_3R). Subsequently, store-operated transient receptor protein (Trp) channels traffic to the cell membrane coupled to IP_3R and activate Rho, allowing entry of extracellular Ca^{2+}. Both through binding calmodulin and activating myosin light chain kinase (MLCK) and through modulating the activity of adenylyl cyclase 6 (AC_6), intracellular Ca^{2+} induces the phosphorylation of myosin light chains, thus promoting interaction with filamentous actin, resulting in cytoskeletal rearrangement, cellular contraction, and paracellular gap formation. See text for further details. G_q = G-protein subunit q; PLC = phospholipase C, SERCA = sarco(endo) plasmic reticulum Ca^{2+} ATPase; cAMP = cyclic adenosine monophosphate; PKA = protein kinase A.

polymerization with latrunculin prevented I_{SOC}. Inhibition of Rho activation or actin polymerization also prevented the thrombin-stimulated association of IP_3R with Trp1 in HPAECs (Fig. 2) (Mehta, D, Ahmmed GJ, Paria BC, Holinstat M, Voyno-Yasenetskaya T, Tiruppathi C, Minsmall RD, Malik AB. RHOA interaction with inositol 1,4,5-triphosphate receptor and transient receptor potential channel-1 regulates Ca^{2+} entry: Role in signaling increase endothelial permeability. J. Biol Chem 2003 Vol. 278, No. 35. pp 33492–3350). Thus, intact cytoskeletal linkages and active actomyosin rearrangement are essential components of I_{SOC} regulation.

V. CALCIUM SIGNALING TO THE CYTOSKELETON AND PERMEABILITY PATHWAYS

Intracellular Ca^{2+} signaling modulates EC permeability via multiple pathways (Fig. 3) with a primary mechanism involving Ca^{2+} binding to calmodulin (CaM), a 17 kDa protein cofactor essential for activation of several Ca^{2+} sensitive enzymes. For example, the Ca^{2+}/CaM complex interacts with MLCK to induce a conformational change, exposing an MLC-binding site, increasing catalytic activity and the phosphorylation of myosin light chains, an event that increases myosin filament formation and interaction with filamentous actin, resulting in cytoskeletal rearrangement and prominent development of stress fibers (28). Thrombin, a rapid-acting and potent Ca^{2+} secretagogue, rapidly activates EC MLCK, with peak enzymatic activity at 2 min (28,29). Similar results are observed in BPAECs 5 min after stimulation with thapsigargin (6). Activation of EC MLCK by ischemia/reperfusion (30) or excessive mechanical stress (31), events that also increase Ca^{2+}, leads to increased MLC phosphorylation and vascular permeability. Thus in specific models of vascular permeability, increases in intracellular Ca^{2+} evoke a signaling cascade that culminates in contraction of neighboring endothelial cells, formation of intercellular gaps, and separation of the ECs from the underlying matrix, all of which lead to barrier disruption and increased permeability to fluid and solute.

However, several models of EC permeability exist in which $[Ca^{2+}]_i$ is directly increased but EC MLCK activity and levels of MLC phosphorylation are not enhanced (1,32). For example, the potent Ca^{2+} ionophore ionomycin produces pulmonary EC barrier dysfunction by MLCK-independent mechanisms, again suggesting the existence of additional Ca^{2+} signaling pathways involved in permeability regulation (32). Sandoval et al. (2) reported MLCK-independent barrier dysfunction in human umbilical vein ECs treated with thapsigargin. Increased Ca^{2+}/calmodulin availability may target kinases other than MLCK as well as cytoskeletal components other than actin and myosin. For example, filamin, a 280 kDa homodimer found in the cell periphery, participates in organizing a three-dimensional actin network and in the interaction of actin with plasma membrane glycoproteins. Ca^{2+}/calmodulin-dependent kinase II (CaM kinase II) phosphorylates filamin, decreasing its actin filament cross-linking activity, therefore potentially disrupting the membrane–cytoskeleton network. Borbiev et al. (33) demonstrated CaM kinase II activation following BPAEC stimulation with thrombin, and pharmacological inhibition of CaM kinase II attenuated the decline in transendothelial electrical resistance and the permeability to albumin in EC monolayers treated with thrombin (33). The Ca^{2+}/CaM complex also participates in permeability-modulating pathways through feedback inhibition of Ca^{2+} entry via store-operated Trp channels and facilitates Ca^{2+} store replenishment via activation of SERCA (Fig. 3).

Increases in the cyclic nucleotide cAMP have long been correlated with barrier enhancement (34,35), which may involve both direct and indirect Ca^{2+}-elicited signals. In addition to binding calmodulin, Ca^{2+} directly inhibits adenylyl cyclase 6 (AC_6) (12), which may be essential for microvascular barrier disruption associated with increased Ca^{2+} entry via SOCs (36). Interestingly, AC_6 appears to colocalize with store-operated channels near the plasma membrane (37,38) as well as near sites of cell–cell contact (12). Infection of PMVECs with AC_8, an isoform that reverses Ca^{2+} inhibition of cAMP production, abolished the formation of gaps in PMVECs treated with thrombin (12), suggesting that inhibition of AC_6 is essential for barrier dysregulation. One possible mechanism invoked by the declining levels of cAMP involves decreasing activity of the cAMP target, protein kinase A (PKA), which under normal homeostatic conditions exerts multiple barrier regulatory effects including tonic inhibition of EC MLCK via phosphorylation (29) (Fig. 3). Therefore, the overall effect of Ca^{2+} inhibition of AC_6 is the downstream activation of MLCK, which results in increased centripetal force generation, cytoskeletal rearrangement, intercellular gap formation, and increased permeability.

Adding complexity to the effects of intracellular Ca^{2+} signaling pathways on vascular permeability is the protective effect of elevated $[Ca^{2+}]_i$ on endothelial barrier function via activation of gelsolin, an 80 kDa actin-binding protein that alters cytoskeletal rearrangement by severing and capping actin filaments (39). Gelsolin activity is necessary for maintenance of optimal barrier function; gelsolin-deficient mice exhibit increased BAL protein concentration and osmotic reflection coefficient for albumin compared to wild-type mice, indicating elevated vascular leak in these knockout mice, findings augmented following oxidant stress exposure (40). The duration of ischemia-induced increased permeability is also prolonged in gelsolin knockout mice relative to controls (40). In addition to gelsolin's direct effects on the actin cytoskeleton, gelsolin overexpression studies reveal biphasic modulation of phospholipase C activity (41), which, by regulating phosphoinositide levels inside the cell, may provide a further link to signaling mechanisms integral to cytoskeletal rearrangements involved in permeability regulation. Given the more recently described role of EC MLCK in barrier restoration (42) it is clear that elevated $[Ca^{2+}]_i$ can stimulate a barrier-protective mechanism that may function to partially compensate for or modulate the multiple barrier-disrupting activities outlined above.

Extracellular Ca^{2+} may also play an important role in the maintenance of pulmonary endothelial barrier integrity. Cadherins of neighboring cells bind together in a Ca^{2+}-dependent, homotypical fashion. The depletion of extracellular Ca^{2+} may lead to dissociation of these bonds, resulting in paracellular gap formation as noted with disrupted EC–EC and EC–extracellular matrix interactions in frog microvascular cells in a Ca^{2+} -depleted environment (43). Therefore, sufficient extracellular Ca^{2+} is necessary for maintenance of intact cell–cell interactions integral to optimal barrier integrity.

VI. CALCIUM-INDEPENDENT PERMEABILITY MECHANISMS

Despite substantial evidence supporting an essential role for Ca^{2+} in endothelial barrier regulation, some studies point to additional Ca^{2+}-independent pathway involvement. Cioffi et al. (12) demonstrated increasing PAEC monolayer permeability related to increased intercellular gap formation with increasing doses of thrombin. However, this increase in permeability was associated with decreases in Ca^{2+} influx as thrombin doses escalated, implying involvement of a Ca^{2+}-independent mechanism. In further support of this hypothesis, increased permeability has been observed in PAEC monolayers after treatment with calyculin, a serine/threonine phosphatase inhibitor, without alterations in intracellular Ca^{2+} concentration (44,45). Furthermore, inhibitors of MLCK demonstrated no effect on these changes. He et al. (46) demonstrated increased hydraulic conductivity in the absence of increased $[Ca^{2+}]_i$ in isolated perfused rat and frog microvessels treated with cGMP analogs. Bradykinin has been demonstrated to increase microvascular permeability both in vivo and in vitro (46,47) (Dull, in press). This effect is potentiated by treatment with cGMP analogs and inhibited by treatment with guanylate cyclase inhibitors, suggesting a Ca^{2+}-independent permeability mechanism (46). Finally, Mehta and colleagues postulated a role for the small GTPase Rho, via Rho-kinase activation, in store-operated Ca^{2+} channel trafficking to the plasma membrane (Mehta, D, Ahmmed GJ, Paria BC, Holinstat M, Voyno-Yasenetskaya T, Tiruppathi C, Minsmall RD, Malik AB. RHOA interaction with inositol 1,4,5-triphosphate receptor and transient receptor potential channel-1 regulates Ca^{2+} entry: Role in signaling increase endothelial permeability. J. Biol Chem 2003 Vol. 278, No. 35. pp 33492–3350). Rho-kinase directly inhibits Myosin Light Chain (MLC) phosphatase to increase MLC phosphorylation and subsequent actomyosin interaction, cytoskeletal rearrangement, contraction, gap formation, and increased permeability. Ultimately, the maintenance and disruption of endothelial barrier integrity likely occurs through complex interplay involving both Ca^{2+}-dependent and -independent pathways.

VII. MICROVASCULAR VERSUS MACROVASCULAR ENDOTHELIAL PERMEABILITY

The majority of studies to date addressing the issue of Ca^{2+} signaling in pulmonary endothelial cells have examined conduit vessels. However, the microvasculature is the presumed site of the majority of physiologically relevant permeability changes, and in these cells the data appear to be equivocal. Clearly, phenotypic differences exist between conduit endothelial

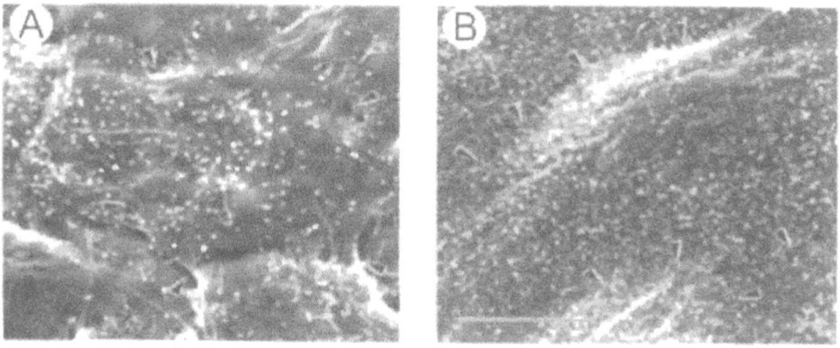

Figure 4 Scanning electron microscopic photographs of rat pulmonary artery (RPA) (A) and rat pulmonary microvascular (RPMV) (B) endothelial cells in culture on semipermeable membranes. Immediately after termination of permeability experiments, transwells with cultured ECs were washed in PBS and fixed in 3% glutaraldehyde. Cell junctions (arrowheads) of RPAECs formed visible gaps unlike the RPMVEC tight intercellular junctions. MVECs showed a greater number of dense hairy fingerlike cytoplasmic protrusions on their surface compared with RPAECs. Bar = 10 μm. (From Ref. 14.)

cells and those found in the microvasculature, with pulmonary microvascular endothelial cells (PMVECs) forming a tighter, less permeable barrier to fluid and solute than pulmonary artery endothelial cells (PAECs) (48); this differential barrier function is ascribed to a significantly greater population of focal adhesion complexes in PMVECs (48). Modulation of the focal adhesion complex by focal adhesion kinase (FAK) is essential in the pathogenesis of thrombin-induced pulmonary endothelial barrier disruption (49). Scanning electron micrographs depicting cell-surface differences between neighboring cultured PAECs and PMVECs after permeability studies (Fig. 4) (14) disclosed visible junctional gaps between conduit vessel endothelial cells, whereas microvascular cells form tight intercellular junctions without visible gaps.

Until recently, few investigations examined the signaling mechanisms within PMVECs or the roles of Ca^{2+} ions and cAMP in the signaling process. Basal intracellular Ca^{2+} concentration appears lower and the response to thapsigargin or ATP stimulation is attenuated both in amplitude and in duration of plateau response in PMVECs compared to PAECs (50). Similarly, the Ca^{2+} response to thapsigargin in rat PMVECs is attenuated compared to PAECs (14). The presence of extracellular Ca^{2+} contributed significantly to the peak increase in Ca^{2+} in MVECs, suggesting a greater role for Ca^{2+} entry relative to store release in these cells in contrast to conduit endothelial cells (14). Cioffi et al. (12) compared the responses of PAECs and PMVECs to thrombin stimulation in vitro. Each cell type demonstrated a dose-dependent response to Ca^{2+}; however, the coupling between Ca^{2+} release and Ca^{2+} entry differed between groups. Thrombin produced a bell-shaped response in PAECs, where Ca^{2+} release and entry increased initially but subsequently decreased at higher thrombin doses. In contrast, MVECs displayed a sigmoidal response to thrombin, with Ca^{2+} entry and release sustained at higher doses of thrombin (12). Release of Ca^{2+} was 40% lower in PMVECs than in PAECs in response to thrombin. This observation may be related to the fact the IP_3 is rapidly hydrolyzed in the cytosol and the ER resides at a greater distance from the plasma membrane in PMVECs than in PAECs (12).

Cyclic AMP, which is known to protect barrier integrity by promoting cell–cell and cell–matrix interactions, is found in greater concentration in MVECs than in PAECs (14,51), although the turnover from ATP to cAMP is decreased in MVECs (51). Recent evidence suggests that cAMP promotes MVEC barrier integrity via inhibition of the Rho-mediated signal pathway (52). Inhibition of phosphodiesterase 4 activity with rolipram increased the turnover of ATP to cAMP in MVECs, whereas ß-adrenergic stimulation increased cAMP levels in PAECs by stimulating adenylyl cyclase activity (51). Both cell types express Ca^{2+}-inhibited adenylyl cyclase (AC_6), a pivotal molecule involved in PAEC barrier disruption. Compared to the inhibition of AC_6 by thapsigargin-induced store depletion in PAECs, activation of store-operated Ca^{2+} channels by thapsigargin had no effect on AC_6 activity in rat PMVECs (51) and no discernible effect on intercellular gap formation. Further experimentation demonstrated that this effect is related to decreased store-operated Ca^{2+} entry into PMVECs in response to thapsigargin. Following rolipram administration, however, thapsigargin administration attenuated the production of cAMP in MVECs due to Ca^{2+}-induced inhibition of AC_6 (51,53). Subsequent testing revealed significant intercellular gap formation in MVECs after thapsigargin administration in the presence of rolipram, further supporting the role of AC_6 and cAMP in endothelial barrier regulation (Stevens, personal communication).

Bradykinin, an important nonapeptide inflammatory mediator involved in modulation of vascular tone, pain sensation, and bronchoconstriction, has been demonstrated to alter endothelial macromolecular permeability (46,47). Recent data suggest that bradykinin-induced albumin permeability is up to 2.5-fold greater in bovine PAECs than that induced in bovine PMVECs (Dull, in press). Furthermore, the alterations in albumin flux across these cell layers is effected through different receptor cascades; HOE 140, a competitive antagonist at the kinin B_2 receptor on the EC membrane, attenuated the permeability response in conduit cells but failed to do so in MVECs (Dull, in press).

Clearly, the signaling pathways in PMVECs differ from those in PAECs; however, the extent to which this alters barrier regulatory responses is unclear. Intercellular gap formation was demonstrated within 10 min of thrombin stimulation in both PAEC and PMVEC monolayers (12). Gaps in microvascular cells resolved within 30–60 min, whereas conduit cell gaps persisted for up to 120 min. However, despite the rapid resolution of gaps in PMVECs, these gaps were significantly larger than those formed in PAECs (12). Thapsigargin does not significantly alter PMVEC monolayer permeability to dextran, and furthermore, elevations in intracellular $[Ca^{2+}]$ to levels comparable to those seen in PAECs in response to thapsigargin similarly failed to increase permeability to dextran even in the presence of physiological extracellular $[Ca^{2+}]$ (14). This finding may be related to an apparent lack of Ca^{2+}-induced AC_6 inhibition in PMVECs (Stevens, personal communication). In contrast, Tiruppathi et al. (7) evaluated thrombin-induced permeability changes in cultured endothelial cells and isolated perfused lungs from wild-type and $Trp4^{-/-}$ mice. The drop in transendothelial electrical resistance induced by thrombin was attenuated in the $Trp4^{-/-}$ mice (Fig. 1), which exhibited significantly less actin stress fiber formation in response to thrombin compared to ECs derived from wild-type mice. The increased filtration coefficient, $K_{f,c}$, in response to thrombin receptor agonism was also attenuated in perfused $Trp4^{-/-}$ mouse lungs compared to wild-type mouse lungs (7). These data support a role for extracellular Ca^{2+} entry via store-operated Trp channels in the maintenance of microvascular barrier integrity. In Stevens's model of thapsigargin-induced increase in rat lung microvascular permeability, decreasing extracellular Ca^{2+} or increasing intracellular cAMP attenuated the permeability response (54). In these in vivo models, however, gaps between capillary and microvascular ECs were not observed. Inhibition of phosphodiesterase 4 activity (with rolipram) unmasked thapsigargin's ability to induce intercellular gap formation in rat MVECs by translocating the ER to the abluminal surface of the cell, increasing store-operated Ca^{2+} current and unmasking the inhibition of AC_6, which is imperative for endothelial barrier disruption (53) (Stevens, personal communication). In summary, existing data support the notion that increases in intracellular Ca^{2+} concentration alone are insufficient to alter MVEC permeability in the absence of AC_6 inhibition. Further investigation is clearly necessary to elucidate the complex signaling mechanism and interaction between Ca^{2+} influx, cAMP, and alterations in microvascular permeability.

VIII. SUMMARY AND FUTURE DIRECTIONS

Although our understanding of the cellular events that regulate pulmonary endothelial permeability is expanding, clinically useful modulation of EC barrier function remains an elusive goal in the treatment of the vascular leak syndrome associated with many inflammatory conditions. Ca^{2+} signaling plays a central role in many models of endothelial barrier regulation and therefore may provide an avenue into the development of effective therapeutic interventions for highly morbid clinical conditions such as acute lung injury. The rapid advance of powerful analytical techniques in the fields of genomics and proteomics is providing increasing opportunities to quickly screen and evaluate large amounts of data as we strive to characterize the underlying reasons for observed phenotypic variability in cell types (e.g., macro- vs. microvascular permeability), animal models, and patient populations. Complementary DNA microarray studies combined with proteomic evaluation and confirmation of candidate genes and polymorphisms for their importance in pulmonary vascular permeability regulation provide an opportunity for rapid identification of novel and cell-specific targets for intervention as we continue to explore the complex mechanisms of Ca^{2+} signaling within the pulmonary vascular endothelium.

ACKNOWLEDGMENTS

We thank Troy Stevens and James Sham for their invaluable assistance in the production of this manuscript. Joe G. N. Garcia receives support from the Johns Hopkins University David Marine Professorship and Program Project Grant P01 HL58064. Steven Dudek is supported by K-08 Grant HL70013-01. Dolly Mehta receives NIH support under Grant HL071794. Further support for this work is provided by the Center for Translational Respiratory Medicine at the Johns Hopkins University School of Medicine.

REFERENCES

1. Dudek SM, Garcia JG. Cytoskeletal regulation of pulmonary vascular permeability. J Appl Physiol 2001; 91:1487–1500.
2. Sandoval R, Malik AB, Naqvi T, Mehta D, Tiruppathi C. Requirement for Ca^{2+} signaling in the mechanism of thrombin-induced increase in endothelial permeability. Am J Physiol Lung Cell Mol Physiol 2001; 280:L239–L247.
3. Nilius B, Droogmans G. Ion channels and their functional role in vascular endothelium. Physiol Rev 2001; 81:1415–1459.
4. Tran Q-K, Ohashi K, Watanabe H. Calcium signalling in endothelial cells. Cardiovasc Res 2000; 48:13–22.
5. Siflinger-Birnboim A, Lum H, Del Vecchio PJ, Malik AB. Involvement of Ca^{2+} in the H_2O_2-induced increase in endothelial permeability. Am J Physiol 1996; 270(6 Pt 1):L973–L978.
6. Moore TM, Norwood NR, Creighton JR, Babal P, Brough GH, Shasby DM, Stevens T. Receptor-dependent activation of store-operated calcium entry increases endothelial cell permeability. Am J Physiol Lung Cell Mol Physiol 2000; 279:L691–L698.
7. Tiruppathi C, Freichel M, Vogel SM, Paria BC, Mehta D, Flockerzi V, Malik AB. Impairment of store-operated Ca^{2+} entry in $TRPC4^{-/-}$ mice interferes with increase in lung microvascular permeability. Circ Res 2002; 91:70–76.

8. Isshiki M, Anderson RGW. Calcium signal transduction from caveolae. Cell Calcium 1999; 26:201–208.
9. Ichimura H, Parthasarathi K, Quadri S, Issekutz AC, Bhattacharya J. Mechano-oxidative coupling by mitochondria induces proinflammatory responses in lung venular capillaries. J Clin Invest 2003; 111:691–699.
10. Parthasarathi K, Ichimura H, Quadri S, Issekutz A, Bhattacharya J. Mitochondrial reactive oxygen species regulate spatial profile of proinflammatory responses in lung venular capillaries. J Immunol 2002; 169:7078–7086.
11. Stevens T, Garcia JGN, Shasby DM, Bhattacharya J, Malik AB. Mechanisms regulating endothelial cell barrier function. Am J Physiol Lung Cell Mol Physiol 2000; 279:L419–L422.
12. Cioffi DL, Moore TM, Schaack J, Creighton JR, Cooper DM, Stevens T. Dominant regulation of interendothelial cell gap formation by calcium-inhibited type 6 adenylyl cyclase. J Cell Biol 2002; 157:1267–1278.
13. Moore TM, Chetham PM, Kelly JJ, Stevens T. Signal transduction and regulation of lung endothelial cell permeability. Interaction between calcium and cAMP. Am J Physiol 1998; 275(2 Pt 1):L203–L222.
14. Kelly JJ, Moore TM, Babal P, Diwan AH, Stevens T, Thompson WJ. Pulmonary microvascular and macrovascular endothelial cells: differential regulation of Ca^{2+} and permeability. Am J Physiol 1998; 274(5 Pt 1):L810–L819.
15. Hofmann T, Schaefer M, Schultz G, Gudermann T. Transient receptor potential channels as molecular substrates of receptor-mediated cation entry. J Mol Med 2000; 78:14–25.
16. Brough G, Wu S, Cioffi DL, Moore TM, Li M, Dean N, Stevens T. Contribution of endogenously expressed Trp1 to a Ca^{2+}-selective, store-operated Ca^{2+} entry pathway. FASEB J 2001; 15:1727–1738.
17. Moore TM, Brough GH, Babal P, Kelly JJ, Li M, Stevens T. Store-operated calcium entry promotes shape change in pulmonary endothelial cells expressing Trp1. Am J Physiol 1998; 275:L574–L582.
18. Holda JR, Blatter LA. Capacitative calcium entry is inhibited in vascular endothelial cells by disruption of cytoskeletal microfilaments. FEBS Lett 1997; 403:191–196.
19. Patterson R, van Rossum D, Gill D. Store-operated Ca^{2+} entry: evidence for a secretion-like coupling model. Cell 1999; 98:487–499.
20. van Rossum DB, Patterson RL, Ma H-T, Gill DL. Ca^{2+} entry mediated by store depletion, S-nitrosylation, and Trp3 channels comparison of coupling and function. J Biol Chem 2000; 275:28562–28568.
21. Putney JW Jr, Broad LM, Braun F-J, Lievremont J-P, Bird GSJ. Mechanisms of capacitative calcium entry. J Cell Sci 2001; 114:2223–2229.
22. Norwood N, Moore TM, Dean DA, Bhattacharjee R, Li M, Stevens T. Store-operated calcium entry and increased endothelial cell permeability. Am J Physiol Lung Cell Mol Physiol 2000; 279:L815–L824.
23. Carbajal JM, Schaeffer RC Jr. RhoA inactivation enhances endothelial barrier function. Am J Physiol 1999; 277:C955–C964.
24. Watanabe H, Takahashi R, Zhang X-X, Kakizawa H, Hayashi H, Ohno R. Inhibition of agonist-induced Ca^{2+} entry in endothelial cells by myosin light-chain kinase inhibitor. Biochem Biophys Res Commun 1996; 225:777–784.

25. Watanabe H, Takahashi R, Zhang X-x, Goto Y, Hayashi H, Ando J, Isshiki M, Seto M, Hidaka H, Niki I, Ohno R. An essential role of myosin light-chain kinase in the regulation of agonist- and fluid flow-stimulated Ca^{2+} influx in endothelial cells. FASEB J 1998; 12:341–348.
26. Watanabe H, Tran QK, Takeuchi K, Fukao M, Liu MY, Kanno M, Hayashi T, Iguchi A, Seto M, Ohashi K. Myosin light-chain kinase regulates endothelial calcium entry and endothelium-dependent vasodilation. FASEB J 2001; 15:282–284.
27. Wu S, Sangerman J, Li M, Brough GH, Goodman SR, Stevens T. Essential control of an endothelial cell ISOC by the spectrin membrane skeleton. J Cell Biol 2001; 154:1225–1234.
28. Garcia, JG, Davis HW, Patterson CE. Regulation of endothelial cell gap formation and barrier dysfunction: role of myosin light chain phosphorylation. J Cell Physiol 1995; 163:510–522.
29. Garcia JG, Lazar V, Gilbert-McClain LI, Gallagher PJ, Verin AD. Myosin light chain kinase in endothelium: molecular cloning and regulation. Am J Respir Cell Mol Biol 1997; 16:489–494.
30. Zhao X, Alexander JS, Zhang S, Zhu Y, Sieber NJ, Aw TY, Carden DL. Redox regulation of endothelial barrier integrity. Am J Physiol Lung Cell Mol Physiol 2001; 281:L879–L886.
31. Birukov KG, Jacobson JR, Flores AA, Ye SQ, Birukova AA, Verin AD, Garcia JGN. Magnitude-dependent regulation of pulmonary endothelial cell barrier function by cyclic stretch. Am J Physiol Lung Cell Mol Physiol 2003; 285(4):L785–797.
32. Garcia JG, Schaphorst KL, Shi S, Verin AD, Hart CM, Callahan KS, Patterson CE. Mechanisms of ionomycin-induced endothelial cell barrier dysfunction. Am J Physiol 1997; 273(1 Pt 1):L172–L184.
33. Borbiev T, Verin AD, Shi S, Liu F, Garcia JGN. Regulation of endothelial cell barrier function by calcium/calmodulin-dependent protein kinase II. Am J Physiol Lung Cell Mol Physiol 2001; 280:L983–L990.
34. Patterson CE, Lum H, Schaphorst KL, Verin AD, Garcia JG. Regulation of endothelial barrier function by the cAMP-dependent protein kinase. Endothelium 2000; 7:287–308.
35. Liu F, Verin AD, Borbiev T, Garcia JGN. Role of cAMP-dependent protein kinase A activity in endothelial cell cytoskeleton rearrangement. Am J Physiol Lung Cell Mol Physiol 2001; 280:L1309–L1317.
36. Stevens T, Nakahashi Y, Cornfield DN, McMurtry IF, Cooper DM, Rodman DM. Ca^{2+}-inhibitable adenylyl cyclase modulates pulmonary artery endothelial cell cAMP content and barrier function. Proc Natl Acad Sci USA 1995; 92:2696–2700.
37. Fagan KA, Smith KE, Cooper DM. Regulation of the Ca^{2+}-inhibitable adenylyl cyclase type VI by capacitative Ca^{2+} entry requires localization in cholesterol-rich domains. J Biol Chem 2000; 275:26530–26537.
38. Fagan KA, Mahey R, Cooper DM. Functional co-localization of transfected Ca^{2+}-stimulable adenylyl cyclases with capacitative Ca^{2+} entry sites. J Biol Chem 1996; 271:12438–12444.

39. Sun HQ, Yamamoto M, Mejillano M, Yin HL. Gelsolin, a multifunctional actin regulatory protein. J Biol Chem 1999; 274:33179–33182.
40. Becker PM, Kazi AA, Wadgaonkar R, Pearse DB, Kwiatkowski D, Garcia JGN. Pulmonary vascular permeability and ischemic injury in gelsolin-deficient mice. Am J Respir Cell Mol Biol 2003; 28:478–484.
41. Sun H-q, Lin K-m, Yin HL. Gelsolin modulates phospholipase C activity in vivo through phospholipid binding. J Cell Biol 1997; 138:811–820.
42. Dudek SM, Wang P, Birukov KG, Garcia JG. Cortactin and myosin light chain kinase regulate sphingosine-1-phosphate-induced pulmonary vascular barrier enhancement. Am J Respir and Crit Care Med 2003; 167:A563.
43. Kajimura M, Curry FE. Endothelial cell shrinkage increases permeability through a Ca^{2+}-dependent pathway in single frog mesenteric microvessels. J Physiol 1999; 518:227–238.
44. Verin AD, Patterson CE, Day MA, Garcia JG. Regulation of endothelial cell gap formation and barrier function by myosin-associated phosphatase activities. Am J Physiol 1995; 269(1 Pt 1):L99–L108.
45. Leung YM, Kwan TK, Kwan CY, Daniel EE. Calyculin A-induced endothelial cell shape changes are independent of $[Ca^{2+}]_i$ elevation and may involve actin polymerization. Biochim Biophys Acta 2002; 1589:93–103.
46. He P, Zeng M, Curry FE. cGMP modulates basal and activated microvessel permeability independently of $[Ca^{2+}]_i$. Am J Physiol 1998; 274(6 Pt 2): H1865–H1874.
47. Murray MA, Heistad DD, Mayhan WG. Role of protein kinase C in bradykinin-induced increases in microvascular permeability. Circ Res 1991; 68: 1340–1348.
48. Schnitzer JE, Siflingerbirnboim A, Delvecchio PJ, Malik AB. Segmental differentiation of permeability, protein glycosylation, and morphology of cultured bovine lung vascular endothelium. Biochem Biophys Res Commun 1994; 199:11–19.
49. Mehta D, Tiruppathi C, Sandoval R, Minshall RD, Holinstat M, Malik AB. Modulatory role of focal adhesion kinase in regulating human pulmonary arterial endothelial barrier function. J Physiol 2002; 539:779–789.
50. Stevens T, Fouty B, Hepler L, Richardson D, Brough G, McMurtry IF, Rodman DM. Cytosolic Ca^{2+} and adenylyl cyclase responses in phenotypically distinct pulmonary endothelial cells. Am J Physiol 1997; 272(1 Pt 1):L51–L59.
51. Stevens T, Creighton J, Thompson WJ. Control of cAMP in lung endothelial cell phenotypes. Implications for control of barrier function. Am J Physiol 1999; 277:L119–L126.
52. Qiao J, Huang F, Lum H. 2003. cAMP-dependent protein kinase inhibits RhoA activation: a protection mechanism against endothelial barrier dysfunction. Am J Physiol Lung Cell Mol Physiol 2003; 284:L978–L980.
53. Creighton JR, Masada N, Cooper DMF, Stevens T. Coordinate regulation of membrane cAMP by Ca^{2+}-inhibited adenylyl cyclase and phosphodiesterase activities. Am J Physiol Lung Cell Mol Physiol 2003; 284:L100–L107.
54. Chetham PM, Guldemeester HA, Mons N, Brough GH, Bridges JP, Thompson WJ, Stevens T. Ca^{2+}-inhibitable adenylyl cyclase and pulmonary microvascular permeability. Am J Physiol 1997; 273(1 Pt 1):L22–L30.

23

Role of Ca^{2+} Sparks in the Regulation of Pulmonary Vascular Tone

James S. K. Sham, Anita Umesh, Xiao-Ru Yang, and Mo-Jun Lin
Johns Hopkins School of Medicine, Baltimore, Maryland, U.S.A.

I. INTRODUCTION

In biological systems, intracellular Ca^{2+} ions serve as a ubiquitous messenger for numerous cellular functions ranging from muscle contraction to gene expression. Ca^{2+} signals are generated by multiple specific Ca^{2+} transporters, delivered globally or locally, and decoded by various effectors according to the signal amplitude and frequency in their immediate vicinities (1). In pulmonary vascular smooth muscle, major attention has been focused on the global elevation of $[Ca^{2+}]_i$, because it is responsible for the initiation of actin–myosin interactions during smooth muscle contraction. However, due to the spatial distribution of different Ca^{2+} transporters, the diffusion kinetics of Ca^{2+} ions, and the subcellular microarchitecture, heterogeneity in local $[Ca^{2+}]$ is expected. It has been estimated on theoretical grounds that $[Ca^{2+}]$ can exceed 100 μM in the vicinity (Ca^{2+} microdomain) of an open Ca^{2+} conducting channel (2). Such large local gradients of $[Ca^{2+}]$ can provide fast and specific Ca^{2+} signals to neighboring effector molecules to trigger Ca^{2+}-dependent processes that may not be responsive to global submicromolar increase in $[Ca^{2+}]_i$.

Local Ca^{2+} release events, or "Ca^{2+} sparks," were first visualized in cardiac myocytes by the use of laser scanning confocal microscopy (3). They originate from clusters of ryanodine receptors (RyRs) and are considered to be the elementary Ca^{2+} release events underlying excitation–contraction coupling in cardiac and skeletal muscles. During an action potential, thousands of Ca^{2+} sparks are evoked to generate global Ca^{2+} transients for muscle contraction. Ca^{2+} sparks have also been identified in various types of vascular and nonvascular smooth muscle cells. However, they appear to modulate, rather than directly activate, smooth muscle contraction. Recently, we identified and characterized Ca^{2+} sparks in rat intralobar pulmonary arterial smooth muscle cells (PASMCs) (4,5). Emerging evidence suggests that Ca^{2+} sparks of PASMCs regulate pulmonary vascular reactivity in a unique tissue specific manner (4,6–8). In this chapter, we provide a brief review on the structure and functions of the RyR Ca^{2+} release channel and Ca^{2+} sparks of systemic vascular smooth muscle (for details see reviews in Refs. 9 and 10), and discuss the physiological and functional properties of Ca^{2+} sparks of PASMCs. We hope this review will arouse interest for future investigations on the local Ca^{2+} signaling in pulmonary vasculature.

II. RYANODINE RECEPTOR: THE MEDIATOR OF Ca^{2+} SPARKS

A. Molecular Structure of Ryanodine Receptor

The sarcoplasmic Ca^{2+} release channel, ryanodine receptor, is the mediator of Ca^{2+} sparks. In mammals, three different isoforms of RyRs, namely RyR1, RyR2, and RyR3, have been isolated, cloned, and characterized, originally in skeletal muscle, cardiac muscle, and brain, respectively (11–13). RyR1 is predominantly expressed in skeletal muscle, and RyR2 is the major isoform expressed in cardiac muscle. However, coexpression of multiple RyR isoforms has been reported in various types of tissues. The three RyR isoforms are each about 5000 amino acids in length and tetramerize to form the functional RyR calcium release channel of over 2000 kDa. They are approximately 66–70% identical in amino acid sequence. The RyR monomer consists of a long cytoplasmic N-terminal accounting for 80% of the total protein, a transmembrane domain region, and a cytoplasmic tail (Fig. 1). The long cytoplasmic N-terminal region consists of 10 or more loosely packed domains. It represents the modulatory region of RyR, containing the high- and low-affinity Ca^{2+}-binding sites, the phosphorylation sites, and binding sites for mucleotide, calmodulin, and FKBP. The C-terminal membrane-spanning region forms the Ca^{2+} release channel. Hydropathic analysis suggests that the number of transmembrane-spanning domains ranges between four and twelve (12–14). A recent study examining the topology of RyR1 using trunctated RyR1-EGFP fusion constructs suggests that RyR1 contains eight transmembrane helices, with a pore-forming sequence between the last two transmembrane domains (15). In spite of the high level of homology between the three RyR

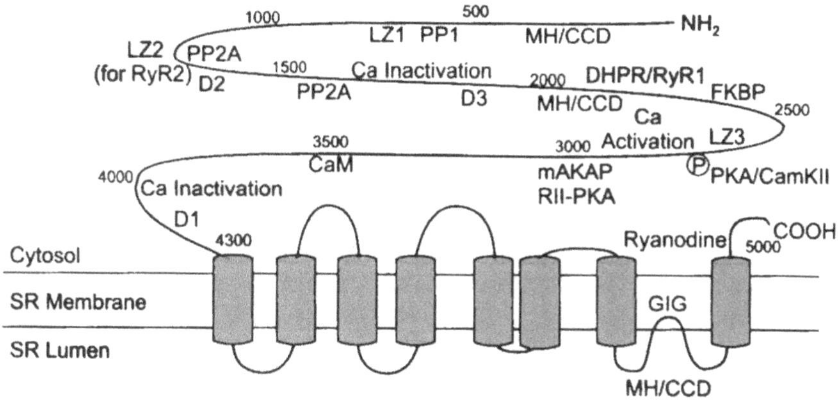

Figure 1 Schematic of structural domains of ryanodine receptor. Eight transmembrane domains are adopted according to Du et al. (15). Locations of putative interaction sites for phosphatases 1 and 2, PP1 and PP2; kinase anchoring protein, mAKAP; PKA/CaMKII phosphorylation site, ⓟCa^{2+} activation and inactivation sites; pore region (GIG); mutation sites associated with malignant hyperthermia or central core disease (MH/CCD); dihydropyridine receptors and RyR1 interaction site; divergence regions 1, 2 and 3, D1, D2, and D3; and leucine zippers, LZ1 and LZ2, are marked based on diagrams of Bers (128).

isoforms, the amino acid sequences also show three divergence-conferring regions, namely, D1, D2, and D3, of which D2 is entirely absent from RyR3 (11).

Three-dimensional reconstruction of RyR based on cryoelectron microscopic images showed that RyR1 has a fourfold symmetry, with 28 nm along each side and 14 nm above the SR membrane. The RyR channel has two distinct domains: the large cytoplasmic assembly, which corresponds to the junctional "feet" observed by electron microscopy, and the small transmembrane assembly, which has an apparent central hole occluded by a plug like mass, presumably representing the ion-selective pore and its gate (16). Similar studies also revealed sites where calmodulin, FKBP, imperatoxin, and dihydropyridine receptor interact with the RyR channel (17,18). In fact, the RyR is a megacomplex in which multiple proteins, including FKBP, calmodulin, anchoring protein of PKA, phosphatases (PP1 and PP2A), junctin/triadin, and sorcin, are closely packed together (19). The 3D structures of RyR2 and RyR3 have also been reconstructed (20,21). The shape of the RyR2 channel is similar to that of RyR1, except for some specific differences in the corner regions that are thought to be the interacting sites for dihydropyridine receptors in RyR1 (20). Specific differences were also observed in RyR3, corresponding to the absence of the D2 region (21).

B. Subcellular Organization of RyRs

Substantial evidence indicates that RyRs are organized in groups or clusters and operate in a highly coordinated manner. In skeletal muscle, discrete domains of SR containing RyR1 interact with specialized domains of surface membranes or t-tubules, containing dihydropyridine receptors, to form the dyadic, triadic, or peripheral junctions. Ultrastructural studies show that the cytoplasmic "foot" processes of RyR1 span the 10–12 nm junctional cleft, with dozens of RyRs packing tightly together on a junctional SR to form a matrix of parallel arrays of RyRs. Moreover, each alternating RyR in the array is overlaid by exactly four dihydropyridine receptors (22), which contact physically with the RyR1 channel and act as the voltage sensors for depolarization-induced Ca^{2+} release" (23,24). The physical coupling between RyR and dihydropyridine receptors is specific for RyR1, because neither RyR2 nor RyR3 can substitute for RyR1 in the depolarization-induced Ca^{2+} release. In cardiac muscle, a similar clustering of RyR2 channels is present in the dyadic and peripheral junctions. Sarcolemmal L-type Ca^{2+} channels are also spatially associated and functionally coupled to these RyR clusters (25,26). However, the spatial arrangement of RyR is less regular, and L-type Ca^{2+} channels are scattered instead of aligned as tetrads in the t-tubular or sarcolemmal side of the dyadic junctions (27). In contrast with the direct physical coupling of RyR1-DHPR, RyR2 is activated by the Ca^{2+} influx via the L-type Ca^{2+} channels by a mechanism known as Ca^{2+}-induced Ca^{2+} release (28). Electron micrographs showed that an average of 17–38 RyR1 channels are present in each skeletal junction complex and 60–300 RyR2 channels are present in each cardiac junctional complex, depending on the species (29). It has been proposed that all or most of the RyRs within a junctional complex operate in a concerted manner as a single Ca^{2+} release unit, or "couplon", to generate Ca^{2+} sparks (30).

Similar junctional complexes are present in smooth muscle cells, in which junctional SR with "foot" processes dock to sarcolemmal invaginations known as caveolae (10,31,32). It has been suggested that, at least in one type of smooth muscle cells, L-type Ca^{2+} channels are also present in caveolae, forming the cardiac type of Ca^{2+} release units (31–33). In addition to the peripheral coupling, some smooth muscle cells also have a major component of central SR (or nonjunctional SR) (34,35). These two distinct populations of SR each containing RyRs may be involved in different physiological functions and activated by different mechanisms. Moreover, coexpression of the three isoforms of RyR has been demonstrated in vascular smooth muscle cells (36–39). Recent studies have shown heteromerization of RyR2 with RyR1 and RyR3 (40). Smooth muscles express alternatively spliced variants of RyR3, which can heteromerize with wild-type RyR3 and RyR2 monomers to form functional RyR channels (41). This raises the intriguing possibility that RyR heterotetramerization may occur in smooth muscle to generate distinctive RyR heterotetrameric channels in specific vascular beds.

The subcellular organization of RyRs plays a major role in determining the physical characteristics of Ca^{2+} sparks. It dictates the local interactions between RyRs within and between clusters. In fact, a hierarchy of local Ca^{2+} release events consisting of quarks, sparks, macrosparks, waves, and global transients has been proposed (42,43). These events represent Ca^{2+} release generated by the recruitment of a single RyR, a cluster of RyRs, several neighboring RyR clusters, and the majority of RyR Ca^{2+} release units, respectively. Depending on the nature of the stimuli and the physiological conditions of the cells, Ca^{2+} release events may manifest in one or more forms. Nevertheless, Ca^{2+} sparks are the predominant local Ca^{2+} events activated by the L-type Ca^{2+} channels in the couplons of striated muscles.

C. Physiological Properties and Regulation of RyRs

Lipid bilayer single-channel recording showed that the permeation properties of different RyR isoforms are quite similar. They exhibit very little selectivity between different monovalent cations or between different divalent cations but have a modest selectivity for divalents over monovalents, e.g., $P_{Ca}/P_K \sim 6.5$ (44). When monovalent cations are used as the charge carrier, RyR has a high single-channel conductance of several hundred picosiemens (45). However, when Ca^{2+} is used as the charge carrier under conditions approaching physiological (2 mM $[Ca^{2+}]_{SR}$, 150 mM $[K]_{cyto}$, and 1 mM $[Mg]_{cyto}$), the conductance is much lower, with a single-channel current of only about 0.3 pA (46). The typical mean open time for RyR1 and RyR2 is ~3 ms (47), whereas RyR3 has a longer mean open time of ~5 ms (48). RyR channel activity is regulated by many physiological factors or modulators. They can be activated by cytosolic and luminal Ca^{2+}, ATP, adenine nucleotides, caffeine, halothane, submicromolar ryanodine, sulfhydryl reagents, and cyclic adenosine dephosphoribose (cADPR); inhibited by millimolar Mg^{2+}, $>10\,\mu M$ ryanodine, procaine, and ruthenium red; and modulated by FK506-binding protein (FKBP), calmodulin, sorcin, and phosphorylation.

Cytosolic and Luminal Ca^{2+}

Cytosolic $[Ca^{2+}]$ is the most important activator of RyR channels, causing Ca^{2+}-induced activation and inactivation of RyRs (28). The Ca^{2+} dependence of RyR activation is biphasic, such that low (micromolar) cytosolic $[Ca^{2+}]$ activates the channels and high (millimolar) cytosolic $[Ca^{2+}]$ inhibits them. It has been proposed that RyR possesses high-and low-affinity Ca^{2+} binding sites, which are thought to participate in the biphasic modulation of channel activity. For cardiac RyR2 channels, activity begins to increase at 0.2–0.3 μM Ca^{2+}, reaching the maximum activity ($P_o \sim 1$) near 100 μM, and declines at supramaximal concentrations (1–10 mM) (49–51). Skeletal muscle RyR1 channels are less strongly activated by Ca^{2+} alone. They exhibit two distinct modes of low and high P_o, the latter of which reaches a maximal activity ($P_o \sim 0.2$–0.3) near 10 μM Ca^{2+} and is completely inactivated by 1 mM Ca^{2+} (48,49). The Ca^{2+} dependence of RyR3 channels is similar to that of RyR2 (52,53); therefore, they are both considered "Ca^{2+}-induced Ca^{2+} release" channels. In addition to cytosolic Ca^{2+}, intra-SR luminal Ca^{2+} also regulates RyR activity. Activity of RyR channels and their sensitivity to certain agonists appear to increase at high luminal [Ca^{2+}]. Studies using trypsin digestion of the luminal side of RyR channels suggest the presence of both activating and inactivating sites (54). However, it is also possible that the luminal SR Ca^{2+} effects are mediated in part by associated proteins in the SR.

Magnesium

Cytosolic free Mg^{2+} concentration (~1 mM in most cells) is known to inhibit RyR by interfering with Ca^{2+} binding to its high- and low-affinity sites. At low [Ca^{2+}], Mg^{2+} competes for binding at the Ca^{2+} activation site; and at high [Ca^{2+}], Mg^{2+} competes for the low-affinity Ca^{2+} inhibition site to inhibit RyR. In fact, the low-affinity Ca^{2+} inhibitory site does not discriminate between different divalent ions; hence, inhibition of RyRs by Ca^{2+} or Mg^{2+} is dependent on the total concentration of divalent cations (i.e., Ca^{2+} and Mg^{2+}) rather than on the nature of the divalent cation involved (55,56).

ATP and cADP-Ribose

Adenosine triphosphate and other adenine nucleotides are effective endogenous activators of RyR channels. The cytosolic total ATP in most cells is ~5 mM and largely bound by Mg^{2+}. Only free ATP (~300 μM) is the active species, which binds and activates RyRs in an isoform-specific manner. For example, RyR1 is more sensitive, responding to ATP even in the absence of Ca^{2+} or Mg^{2+} (57). In contrast, RyR2 and RyR3 are less ATP-sensitive, requiring high enough Ca^{2+} for partial activation of RyRs (52,53,58). Cyclic ADP-ribose (cADPR), another endogenous mediator, also plays an important role in the regulation of RyRs (59). It is generated from β-nicotinamide adenine dinucleotide (NAD) by ADP-ribosyl cyclase and degraded by cyclic ADP-ribose hydrolase. It is certain that cADPR appears to induce Ca^{2+} release from RyR-gated Ca^{2+} stores in a wide variety of cells, because the Ca^{2+} response can be effectively blocked by ryanodine and ruthenium red and potentiated by caffeine. However, its action mechanism is still controversial. Single-channel experiments failed to find any consistent effect of cADPR in reconstituted RyR1, RyR2, or RyR3. It is proposed that accessory proteins such as FKBP or calmodulin or phosphorylation states of RyRs may be important in conferring the cADPR sensitivity (60,61).

Redox Regulation

A ryanodine receptor contains many cysteine residues (80–100 in each RyR monomer), which are convenient targets for redox modifications. It has been proposed that RyRs may function as a redox or O_2 sensor (62,63), a notion that is supported by evidence that oxidants enhance and reducing agents attenuate the RyR activity by modifying the sensitivity to Ca^{2+}, Mg^{2+}, and other channel modulators (62,64,65). Moreover, there is evidence for NO modulation of RyR channel activity through S-nitrosylation (51,63), which may interact with pO_2-dependent and other oxidation-dependent RyR activation mechanisms (63,66).

FK506 Binding Protein

FK506 binding proteins, FKBP12 (MW 12,000) and FKBP-12.6 (MW 12,600), are cis–trans peptidylprolyl isomerases that act as receptors for immunosuppressant drugs such as FK506 and rapamycin. They associate with RyR1, RyR2, and RyR3 in a stoichiometry of four FKBPs to one RyR tetramer. In skeletal muscle, RyR1 and RyR3 bind predominantly to FKBP12 because of its abundance, whereas RyR2 in cardiac muscle binds almost exclusively to FKBP12.6 because of its much higher affinity (~600 times higher than FKBP12) to RyR2 (67,68). Dissociation of FKBP from RyRs with FK506 or rapamycin modify the gating behavior of RyRs, showing clearly the appearance of subconductance states, an increase in overall channel open probability, and alleviation of RyR adaptation (69,70). It has been proposed that the binding of FKBP to RyRs physically stabilizes the gating of RyR channels by facilitating "coupled gating," such that the four RyR monomers in one homotetrameric complex are coordinated to proceed simultaneously from the fully closed to the fully open state (19).

Circumstantial evidence shows that PKA-dependent phosphorylation of RyR2 causes dissociation of FKBP, and there are speculations that such a mechanism is involved in heart failure (19).

Calmodulin

Calmodulin (CaM) binds to the cytoplasmic sites of RyR channel close to the entrance of the transmembrane pore (71), with a ratio of four CaM molecules to one RyR homotetramer (72,73). Both apoCaM (Ca^{2+}-free) and CaCaM (Ca^{2+}-bound) bind the same CaM-binding sites (72). Application of CaM to RyR1 and RyR3 causes channel activation at low $[Ca^{2+}]$ (<100 nM) and channel inhibition at high $[Ca^{2+}]$ (>1 μM) (53,73). In constrast, CaM causes only inhibition of RyR2, irrespective of $[Ca^{2+}]$, and only one molecule of CaM binds to a RyR2 tetramer at low $[Ca^{2+}]$ (73). It has been suggested that oxidation of RyRs may modify their interactions with CaM, and CaM binding may protect RyRs from oxidative modifications (74).

Sorcin

Sorcin is another accessory protein associated with RyR2 (75). It is a 22 kDa penta-EF-hand Ca^{2+}-binding protein that localizes to the dyadic junctions and coimmunoprecipitates with RyRs in the heart. Application of sorcin to the cytosolic side of RyR inhibits channel activity over a wide range of $[Ca^{2+}]$, independent of calmodulin and calpain (76). PKA-dependent phosphorylation of sorcin reduces its inhibitory effect on RyR. Moreover, myocytes from transgenic mice with sorcin overexpression exhibit reduced Ca^{2+} release; and myocytes from rats with heart failure show disruption in the colocalization of sorcin and RyR (75,76).

Phosphorylation and Dephosphorylation

Ryanodine receptor channel activity is modulated by phosphorylation. Protein sequence analysis reveals that RyR contains multiple consensus phosphorylation sites, of which Ser-2809 of RyR2 in particular is phosphorylated by both endogenous PKA and CaMKII with one phosphate per RyR tetramer (19,77).

Hyperphosphorylation of RyR2 (four phosphates per tetramer) has been reported in exogenous CaMKII-dependent phosphorylation experiments (77) as well as during heart failure due to less phosphatase (PP1 and PP2A) binding to RyR2 (19). PKA-dependent phosphorylation increases P_o of RyR1 and RyR2 (78,79). Additionally, it alters the gating behavior of RyRs such that PKA-dependent phosphorylation of RyR2 enhances the instantaneous increase in P_o induced by a rapid photolytic increase in local $[Ca^{2+}]$ and accelerates the subsequent decline in P_o at the maintained $[Ca^{2+}]$ (a phenomenon known as the adaptation of RyR) (79). Phosphorylation may also destabilize RyR2 to promote a subconductance state by binding to FKBP (19). The effect of CaMKII-dependent phosphorylation is less consistent, with reports showing either an increase or a decrease in P_o of RyR2 (77,78).

Caffeine and Ryanodine

Caffeine and ryanodine are the most commonly used agents for probing RyR function. Caffeine at concentrations of 1–5 mM activates all three types of RyRs. It acts on the cytosolic side of RyR, shifting the apparent Ca^{2+} dependence of RyR activation to the lower $[Ca^{2+}]$, and increases both the open frequency and duration of RyR channels. In intact cells, submillimolar caffeine sensitizes RyRs for Ca^{2+}-induced Ca^{2+} release, whereas millimolar caffeine causes regenerative Ca^{2+} release leading to the depletion of SR Ca^{2+} (80).

Ryanodine has a very complex action on RyR channels. It activates open events of long duration with subconductance at concentration of

10 μM or less, and locks the RyR channel in the closed state at very high concentrations (e.g., 100 μM or higher) (81,82). A RyR homotetramer has one high-affinity and three low-affinity ryanodine-binding sites (82) located close to the C-terminus of the RyR monomer, and ryanodine binds to the high-affinity site when the RyR channel is in the open conformation (83).

The above-mentioned physiological factors and pharmacological agents have been shown to have significant modulatory effects on the Ca^{2+} spark activity in striated and smooth muscles. The major molecular and functional properties of the three RyR isoforms are tabulated in Table 1 for comparison.

Table 1 Molecular and Functional Properties of RyR1, RyR2, and RyR3

Subtype	RyR1	RyR2	RyR3
Number of amino acids	5032	4967	4866
Mol wt (KDa)	564	564	551
Gene locus	19q13.1	1q42.1–1q43	15q14–15
Stimulus	Voltage, CICR	CICR	CICR
Major localization	Skeletal muscle	Heart	Brain
K_D for ryanodine (nM)			
High-affinity site	8	2	3–12
Low-affinity sites	53, 555, 2800	36, 681, 4320	?
Activation			
Ca^{2+}(μM)	+	++	++
Caffeine	++	++	++
ATP	++	+	+
Inhibition			
Ca^{2+}(mM)	++	+	++
Mg^{2+}	++	++	++
Ruthenium red	++	++	++
Calmodulin	Inhibition (low Ca^{2+}) Activation (high Ca^{2+})	Inhibition	Inhibition (low Ca^{2+}) Activation (high Ca^{2+})
Kinase modulation			
PKA	Yes (S2843)	Yes (S2809)	?
CaMKII	Yes	Yes	?
Phosphatase modulation			
PP1	Yes	Yes	?
PP2A	No	Yes	?
FKBP subtype	FKBP12	FKBP12.6	FKBP12

III. Ca^{2+} SPARKS OF SYSTEMIC VASCULAR SMOOTH MUSCLE

A. Characteristics of Systemic Ca^{2+} Sparks

Calcium Ton sparks of smooth muscle were first identified in cerebral arterial myocytes (84) and subsequently in different types of vascular smooth muscle cells from coronary and mesenteric arteries and portal vein, and in nonvascular smooth muscle cells from the trachea, ileum, and urinary bladder. Resting spontaneous spark frequency is generally low in vascular smooth muscle cells, ranging between 0.1 and 0.4 spark/s when measured using linescan (a length of about 35 μm) or between 0.1 and 0.7 spark per cell per second when recorded using high-speed frame scanning (6,7,85–89). Spark amplitude varies from 30 nM in rat portal veins to 200–300 nM in rat cerebral arteries (38,84,85,87–90). Average spark duration ranges from 30 to 65 ms, with a typical rise time of ~20 ms and a decay half-time of 48–56 ms, and the spatial spread [full-width, half-maximum (FWHM)] usually ranges from 1.5 to 2.4 μm. However, there are reports of Ca^{2+} sparks of much longer duration (100–600 ms) and much larger size (3–4 μm). The variability in the amplitude and size of Ca^{2+} sparks in different vascular smooth muscle cells may reflect heterogeneities in the size of RyR clusters and the content of ryanodine-sensitive Ca^{2+} stores in different smooth muscles.

B. Physiological Functions of Systemic Ca^{2+} Sparks

The physiological functions of Ca^{2+} sparks have been studied most thoroughly in cerebral arterial myocytes (84). In intact cerebral arteries, myogenic vasoconstriction is activated by elevation of intraluminal pressure, which causes membrane depolarization, activation of L-type Ca^{2+} channels, and vasoconstriction. This positive feedback mechanism is counterbalanced by a Ca^{2+} spark-mediated vasorelaxation process (33,84). There is substantial evidence suggesting that RyR clusters in these arterial myocytes are functionally coupled to Ca^{2+}-activated K^+ (K_{Ca}) channels in sarcolemmal invaginations of caveolae (10,31,32). A Ca^{2+} spark originating within these complexes causes a large local increase of $[Ca^{2+}]$ in the junctional cleft (~20 nm wide), activating a group of apposing K_{Ca} channels to generate spontaneous transient outward currents (STOCs) to cause membrane hyperpolarization, closure of L-type Ca^{2+} channels, and vasodilation (31,84). Because of the large conductance of K_{Ca} channels (80 pS at physiological $[K^+]$) and the number of channels (at least 15) being activated, a single Ca^{2+} spark can cause a substantial hyperpolarization of up to 20 mV (91). This robust Ca^{2+} spark–K_{Ca} channel interaction operates as a frequency-dependent braking mechanism for counteracting the myogenic tone. The importance of this feedback mechanism on vasomotor tone and blood pressure control has been confirmed in the K_{Ca} channel β1-subunit gene knockout mice, which show a decrease in calcium sensitivity of K_{Ca} channels, a reduction in functional coupling of calcium sparks to STOCs, an increase in arterial tone as well as an elevation in blood pressure and cardiac hypertrophy (92). Similar Ca^{2+} spark–K_{Ca} channel interaction has been reported in many other vascular and nonvascular smooth muscles. Because of the highly localized and transient nature of Ca^{2+} sparks, they are thought to contribute little to the direct activation of myofilaments and smooth muscle contraction.

In addition to K_{Ca} channels, some vascular smooth muscle cells express Ca^{2+}-activated Cl^- (Cl_{Ca}) channels. Simultaneous activation of a group of Cl_{Ca} channels generates spontaneous transient inward currents (STICs) (8,93), which cause membrane depolarization, increased Ca^{2+} influx, and cell contraction. For example, in tracheal myocytes it has been demonstrated that Ca^{2+} sparks activate STICs in a manner similar to STOCs (94). Hence, the net physiological effect of Ca^{2+} sparks is dependent on the relative activity of the counteracting Ca^{2+}-activated (K_{Ca} or Cl_{Ca}) channels and on the membrane potential (relative to the equilibrium potential of K^+ and Cl^-, E_K and E_{Cl}, respectively) at which the Ca^{2+} sparks are generated. However, only a few types of vascular smooth muscle cells exhibit STICs (8,93). Therefore, the default action of Ca^{2+} sparks in vascular myocytes is membrane hyperpolarization, and STICs may serve a special physiological function unique to the particular vascular bed.

In addition to the regulation of vascular tone, a recent study suggests that Ca^{2+} sparks may be involved in the regulation of gene expression. In cerebral arteries, uridine 5′-triphosphate (UTP) was found to enhance the Ca^{2+}-dependent translocation of the transcription factor nuclear factor of activated T-cells (NFAT3c) from the cytosol to the nucleus and to inhibit Ca^{2+} spark frequency (95,96). The nuclear translocation of NFAT3c was further enhanced by the inhibition of Ca^{2+} sparks with ryanodine, suggesting that UTP may act by inhibiting Ca^{2+} sparks to exert an inhibitory influence on NFATc3 nuclear accumulation. Because NFAT has been implicated in the pathogenesis of cardiac and skeletal muscle hypertrophy, it is possible that Ca^{2+} sparks may involved in vascular proliferative disease such as atherosclerosis.

C. Regulation of Systemic Ca^{2+} Sparks

As discussed earlier with reference to the regulation of RyRs, the activity of Ca^{2+} sparks in vascular smooth muscle is regulated by many different mechanisms. Among these mechanisms, L-type Ca^{2+} channel activity appears to play a pivotal role. Activation of Ca^{2+} channels either by membrane depolarization or by Ca^{2+} channel agonists increases spark frequency in all smooth muscle cell preparations. It has been postulated that L-type Ca^{2+} channels are colocalized with RyRs in the caveolae-junctional SR complexes (31,32,87), similar to those in the dyadic junctions in cardiac myocytes (26). The triumvirate of L-type Ca^{2+} channels, RyRs, and K_{Ca} channels operates as a functional unit to control $[Ca^{2+}]_i$ (31,32), as exemplified by the enhancement of Ca^{2+} sparks in cerebral arteries during pressurization (33). However, the association between Ca^{2+} channels and RyRs in vascular smooth muscle is likely tissue-specific. In fact, "loose" coupling or uncoupling of Ca^{2+} channels and RyRs has been implicated in a nonvascular smooth muscle (97).

In vascular smooth muscle, Ca^{2+} spark activity is modulated by agonist-dependent and -independent mechanisms. Vasodilators, such as nitric oxide (NO), carbon monoxide (CO), and cyclic nucleotides, enhance vasorelaxation by increasing spark frequency and/or the efficacy of the spark–STOC interaction (6,98,99). By contrast, vasoconstricting agonists, such as norepinephrine (NE) and UTP, decrease Ca^{2+} sparks through PKC activation (85,95), which may potentiate vasoconstriction by reducing the negative feedback imposed by K_{Ca} channels. It has been proposed that vasoconstrictors shift Ca^{2+} signaling modalities from Ca^{2+} sparks to Ca^{2+} waves through the concerted actions of PKC and IP_3, such that PKC inhibits RyRs to reduce Ca^{2+} sparks and IP_3 stimulates IP_3Rs to generate Ca^{2+} waves. However, modulation of Ca^{2+} sparks by neurohormonal factors may vary between vascular beds and agonists. For example, in rat portal vein myocytes, angiotensin II has been shown to trigger Ca^{2+} sparks at low concentrations but elicit Ca^{2+} waves at high concentrations (90).

Vasoactive agents can also modulate Ca^{2+} sparks indirectly through the regulation of SR Ca^{2+} content. Enhancing SR Ca^{2+} uptake through phosphorylation of phospholamban potentiates, whereas inhibiting SR Ca^{2+}-ATPase by thapsigargin reduces, Ca^{2+} spark frequency (100,101). Moreover, a recent study in cerebral arteries shows that a slight alkaline external pH increases the occurrence of Ca^{2+} sparks, and higher alkaline pH causes global regenerative activation of RyRs to generate Ca^{2+} waves (102).

IV. CA^{2+} SPARKS OF PASMCs

A. Identification of RyRs in PASMCs

In pulmonary arteries, the expression of RyR subtypes has not been reported. Ongoing studies in our laboratory have detected mRNA of all three RyR subtypes using reverse transcription polymerase chain reaction (RT-PCR) and expression of RyR1 and RyR2 proteins by Western blot and immunostaining techniques in rat intralobar PASMCs (Yang and Sham, unpublished data; (5)). Quantitative real-time RT-PCR analysis suggests that RyR2 mRNA is most abundantly expressed. The expression of multiple RyR subtypes in rat PASMCs is consistent with reports in systemic vascular myocytes (36–39). PASMCs double-stained with BODIPY TR-X ryanodine and $DiOC_6$, a fluorescent marker of sarcoplasmic reticulum (SR), revealed that RyRs and SR are colocalized in regions closely associated with the sarcolemma and in the perinuclear regions (Yang and Sham, unpublished data). These findings suggest that PASMCs contain two distinctive SR populations, peripheral and perinuclear SR, which contain multiple RyR subtypes. The expression of multiple RyR subtypes in PASMCs may have special physiological significance. In portal vein myocytes, studies using antisense oligonucleotides show that RyR1 and RyR2 are both required for Ca^{2+} spark generation, presumably because these channels participate in the formation of RyR clusters (37), whereas RyR3 channels appear to play a modulatory role in spark frequency or contribute to global $[Ca^{2+}]_i$ (38,39). Moreover, recent studies show that different RyR subtypes can form heterotetramers, and a smooth-muscle-specific dominant negative splice variant of RyR3 can form heteromeric channels with RyR2 and suppress the activities of RyR2 (40,41). Hence, it is possible that specific expression and heteromerization of different RyR subtypes may confer a unique RyR phenotype to PASMCs.

B. Biophysical Properties of Ca^{2+} Sparks in PASMCs

To date, only five papers have been published on pulmonary Ca^{2+} sparks (4–8), and information on these sparks is sparse. In rat intralobar PASMCs, the resting spontaneous spark frequency is ~0.4 spark/s or 0.01 spark/(μms), and averaged amplitude ($\Delta F/F_0$) is ~0.5 or 75 nM when expressed in $\Delta F/F_0$ or $\Delta[Ca^{2+}]_i$, respectively. The spatial spread (FWHM) is ~1.6 μm, and the duration [full-duration, half-maximum, (FDHM)] is ~35 ms (4). The spark frequency is comparable to those reported in canine PASMCs and other vascular myocytes (7,87,88), but the amplitude of Ca^{2+} sparks in rat PASMCs is smaller than the 200 nM recorded in cerebral arteries (32,84,85,87,88) and canine PASMCs (7). The difference in spark amplitude could be due to a smaller number of RyRs in a Ca^{2+} release unit and a lower SR Ca^{2+} content in rat PASMCs. It could also be due to a bias in spark detection, because spark selection in our rat PASMCs was guided by an automated algorithm (4) instead of by eye, which tends to select sparks of larger amplitudes. Nevertheless, the duration and size of Ca^{2+} sparks of PASMCs are similar to those of other vascular smooth muscle. Therefore, generally speaking, despite the smaller spark amplitude, the spatiotemporal properties are similar in PASMCs and systemic vascular smooth muscle cells. The major properties of Ca^{2+} sparks of PASMCs and systemic myocytes are listed in Table 2 for comparison.

In PASMCs, spontaneous Ca^{2+} sparks originate exclusively via RyRs. This is based on the observations that (1) ryanodine concentration-dependently abolishes Ca^{2+} sparks; (2) enhancement of RyR activity using a subthreshold concentration of caffeine increases spark frequency, an effect that can be reversed by ryanodine; and (3) IP_3 receptor antagonists, 2-aminoethoxy diphenylborate (2-APB) and xestospongin C, have no effect

Table 2 Properties of Ca^{2+} Spark in Systemic and Pulmonary Arterial Smooth Muscle Cells

	Systemic myocytes	Pulmonary myocytes
Unstimulated spark frequency	0.24 sparks/(cell s)	0.3 sparks/(cell s) 0.01 sparks/(μm s)
Amplitude	~1	0.5–1
($\Delta F/F_0$ nM)	110–200	75
Spread (FWHM), μm	1.5–2.4	1.6
Duration (half-time), ms	30–65	35–50
RyR subtypes	RyR1, RyR2, RyR3	RyR1, RyR2, RyR3
Effect on membrane potential	Hyperpolarization	Depolarization (rat distal PASMCs) Hyperpolarization (fetal PASMCs)
Activation	Local Ca^{2+} BAY K8644 Caffeine Nitric oxide Cyclic nucleotides	Local Ca^{2+} BAY K8644 Caffeine ET-1 IP_3
Inhibition	Ryanodine PKC NE	Ryanodine NE

on resting spark frequency (4,7). These observations are in agreement with most previous studies in other cell types.

C. Ca^{2+} Sparks and L-Type Ca^{2+} Channels in PASMCs

Similar to systemic vascular myocytes, the L-type Ca^{2+} channel is an important modulator of Ca^{2+} spark in PASMCs. Enhancing Ca^{2+} influx via Ca^{2+} channels either by direct channel activation with the Ca^{2+} channel agonist BAY K8644, by membrane depolarization with elevated $[K^+]_o$, or by increasing $[Ca^{2+}]_o$ unequivocally increases Ca^{2+} spark frequency, and these effects can be reversed by nifedipine (4). However, it is unclear if the Ca^{2+} influx via Ca^{2+} channels activates PASMC RyRs directly due to the close association of the two sets of channels, as in cerebral arterial myocytes (31,32), or indirectly by increasing SR Ca^{2+} load (101). Immunostaining shows that RyRs are located in sites close to the sarcolemma as well as deep in the cytoplasm (perinuclear), and both sites are capable of generating Ca^{2+} sparks (unpublished data, Yang and Sham). Hence, even if Ca^{2+} influx via L-type Ca^{2+} channels indeed activates the closely associated RyRs in the peripheral junctions to generate Ca^{2+} sparks, the RyRs in the uncoupled central SR are likely to be regulated by some other signaling pathway(s).

In addition, inhibition of L-type Ca^{2+} channels by nifedipine has no effect on resting spontaneous spark frequency, suggesting that the spontaneous Ca^{2+} sparks in resting PASMCs are not triggered by L-type Ca^{2+} channels (4) but are initiated by the intrinsic random stochastic activity of RyRs. This agrees with observations in cardiac and many other vascular smooth muscle cells (84,90,103).

D. Ca^{2+} Sparks and Membrane Potential in PASMCs

A major difference in physiological function between Ca^{2+} sparks of pulmonary and systemic myocytes is their role in regulating membrane potential. When measured using the perforated-patch techinque to avoid disturbing subcellular Ca^{2+} dynamics, the resting membrane potential of adult rat intralobar PASMCs is usually nonquiescent, interrupted by frequent small sporadic depolarizations. Activation of Ca^{2+} spark with a subthreshold concentration (0.5 mM) of caffeine causes immediate membrane depolarizations of about 10 mV that can be completely blocked by ryanodine (4). This is in sharp contrast to the hyperpolarization elicited by Ca^{2+} sparks in systemic myocytes and raises the possibility that Ca^{2+} sparks may contribute to vasoconstriction rather than vasorelaxation. The disparity from systemic myocytes is likely due to (1) a diminished influence of K_{Ca} channels, (2) a prominent expression of Cl_{Ca} channels, and (3) the activation of other Ca^{2+}-dependent membrane transporters in rat PASMCs. Developmental studies show that Ca^{2+} sparks and STOCs are very active in fetal rabbit PASMCs (104). However, the occurrence of STOCs, the expression of K_{Ca} protein and mRNA, and the response of $[Ca^{2+}]_i$ to K_{Ca} channel blockers in distal PASMCs diminish with maturation (104,105). The lower expression of K_{Ca} channels in adult PASMCs, and/or less effective coupling between RyRs and K_{Ca} channels may compromise the ability of Ca^{2+} sparks to induce hyperpolarization. On the other hand, prominent Cl_{Ca} channels and STICs are found in PASMCs of several species (106–108). A recent study shows that metabolic inhibition induced by a low concentration of cyanide (1 mM), which has no effect on global $[Ca^{2+}]_i$, activates Ca^{2+} sparks and elicits STICs in rat PASMCs (8). This finding suggests that the Cl_{Ca} channel of PASMCs is a major physiological target of Ca^{2+} sparks. Moreover, ion channels are differentially expressed in PASMCs, such that Cl_{Ca} and voltage-gated K^+ (K_V) channels are more abundant and K_{Ca} channels are much reduced in PASMCs of distal arteries (109,110). The specific distribution of ion channels allows Ca^{2+} spark to preferentially exert its depolarizing influence in distal resistant arteries. In addition, Ca^{2+} sparks may cause further membrane depolarization by inhibiting K_V channels (111) and by activating electrogenic forward Na^+–Ca^{2+} exchange. Schematic diagrams comparing the modulation of membrane potential by Ca^{2+} sparks of systemic and pulmonary arterial smooth muscle cells are presented in Fig. 2.

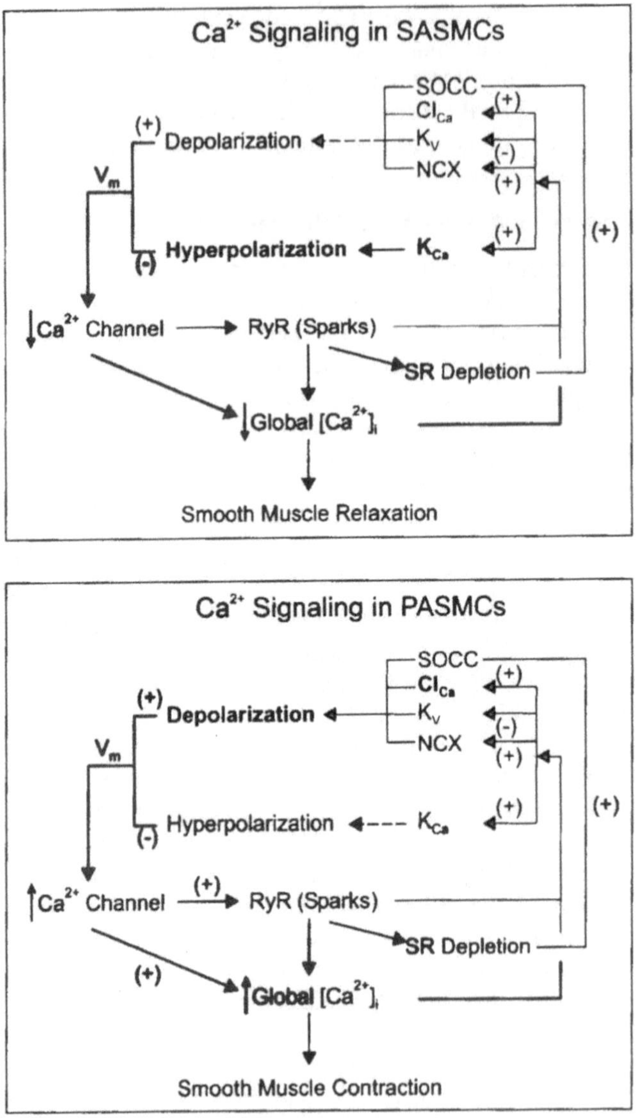

Figure 2 Schematic diagrams depicting the possible Ca^{2+} signaling pathways in PASMCs (bottom) and systemic arterial smooth muscle cells (SASMCs) (top). SOCC, store-operated Ca^{2+} channels; NCX, Na^+–Ca^{2+} exchanger; RyR, ryanodine receptors; Cl_{Ca}, Ca^{2+}-activated Cl^- channels; K_{Ca}, Ca^{2+}-activated K^+ channels; K_v, voltage-gated K^+ channels; V_m, membrane potential.

E. ET-1 and Ca^{2+} Sparks in PASMCs

Under basal conditions, Ca^{2+} sparks of PASMCs are unlikely to elicit vasoconstriction, because resting spark frequency is low. However, depending on the physiological states, PASMCs are subjected to the influence of a wide variety of vasoactive factors, some of which may exert their effects by modulating Ca^{2+} sparks. Endothelin-1 (ET-1), one of the most potent vasoconstrictors, has been implicated as an important modulator/mediator of acute and chronic hypoxic pulmonary vasoconstriction. When applied exogenously to rat intralobar PASMCs, ET-1 elicits a dramatic global Ca^{2+} mobilization, involving Ca^{2+} release from RyR-gated Ca^{2+} stores (112). At the subcellular level, ET-1 at concentrations of 10^{-10}–10^{-8} M causes a concentration-dependent increase in spark frequency, with a two fold increase at the lowest, to a four- to fivefold increase at the highest concentration (5). The increase in spark frequency is associated with increases in spark amplitude and duration. The ET-1-induced increase in spark frequency can be inhibited by BQ-123, an ET_A receptor antagonist; by U-73122, a PLC inhibitor; and by xestospongin C and 2-APB, antagonists of IP_3Rs, indicating that the effect of ET-1 is mediated through ET_A-receptor activation of phospholipase C, leading to IP_3 generation, Ca^{2+} release from IP_3Rs, and activation of RyRs. Further experiments show that the effect of ET-1 is unrelated to SR Ca^{2+} content, activation of L-type Ca^{2+} channel activation, protein kinase C, or cyclic ADP-ribose production (5). A schematic depicting the signaling pathways for ET-1-induced Ca^{2+} sparks is presented in Fig. 3. More important, Ca^{2+} sparks contribute to ET-1-induced pulmonary vasoconstriction, as demonstrated by the fact that inhibition of Ca^{2+} sparks with ryanodine causes a significant rightward shift in the ET-1 concentration–tension relationship in endothelium-denuded intralobar pulmonary arteries. The shift in the concentration–tension curve without an apparent change in the maximal developed tension suggests that Ca^{2+} sparks play a more important role in vasoconstriction at the lower ET-1 concentrations.

It is worthwhile to note that Ca^{2+} spark activation is agonist-specific and independent of the global increase in $[Ca^{2+}]_i$. Norepinephrine (NE) in fact reduces Ca^{2+} spark frequency at a concentration that elicits global Ca^{2+} transients comparable to those of ET-1 (4). This is similar to several previous studies on systemic vascular smooth muscles showing that vasoconstrictors typically reduce Ca^{2+} spark frequency via a PKC-dependent mechanism (85,95). The agonist-specific activation of Ca^{2+} sparks by ET-1 may provide a special mechanism for the unique physiological function of intralobar PASMCs.

F. Local Ca^{2+} Signaling Between RyRs and IP_3Rs in PASMCs

Pharmacological experiments on ET-1-induced Ca^{2+} sparks reveal an important interaction between IP_3R and RyRs in rat PASMCs; as Ca^{2+}

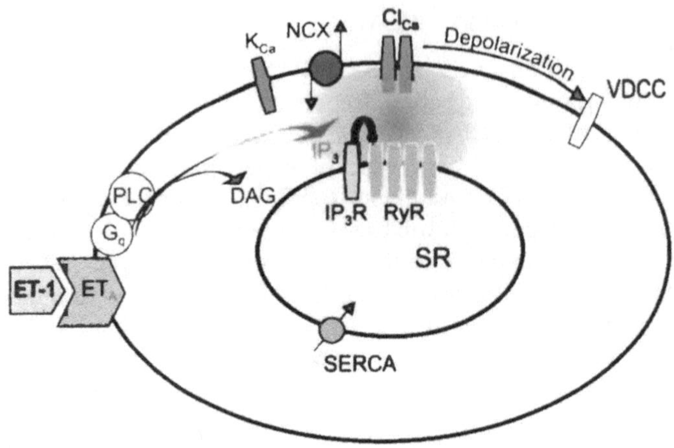

Figure 3 A schematic diagram depicting the signaling pathways for ET-1 induction of Ca^{2+} sparks in PASMCs. ET_A, ET-A receptor; Gq, G protein; PLC, phospholipase C, DAG, diacylglycerol; SERCA, sarcoplasmic/endoplasmic reticulum Ca^{2+}-ATPase; NCX, Na^+–Ca^{2+} exchanger; RyR, ryanodine receptor; Cl_{Ca}, Ca^{2+}-activated Cl^- channel, K_{Ca}, Ca^{2+}-activated K^+ channel; VDCC, voltage-gated Ca^{2+} channel.

sparks evoked by ET-1 can be effectively abolished by xestospongin C and 2-APB, which are antagonists of IP_3Rs (5). This interaction has been directly demonstrated by the photolysis of the membrane-permeant caged-IP_3 analog ci-IP_3/PM. Uncaging of IP_3 causes immediate activation of solitary Ca^{2+} sparks, which intensify and merge into larger clusters of Ca^{2+} events and subsequently transform into an avalanche of global Ca^{2+} release (Fig. 4). The IP_3-induced Ca^{2+} sparks can be abolished by ryanodine, and the residual global Ca^{2+} transient can be completely obliterated by 2-APB, suggesting that the IP_3-induced Ca^{2+} sparks originate from RyRs and are initiated by Ca^{2+} release from IP_3Rs. Ca^{2+} release from IP_3Rs appears to activate Ca^{2+} sparks through elevation of local $[Ca^{2+}]$ in the vicinity of RyRs, because there is no noticeable increase in global $[Ca^{2+}]$ before spark activation. Moreover, double-immunostaining experiments showed that RyRs and IP_3Rs exhibit similar distribution patterns, indicating close spatial association or colocalization of the two sets of release channels in PASMCs (5). Hence, it is likely that some IP_3Rs in PASMCs reside close to or within a cluster of RyRs, allowing the local Ca^{2+} microdomain of IP_3R to act as a trigger to ignite the Ca^{2+} release unit. This functional coupling between IP3Rs and RyRs may provide a highly efficient amplification mechanism for pharmacomechanical coupling in PASMCs to mobilize Ca^{2+} simultaneously from IP_3R- and RyR-gated

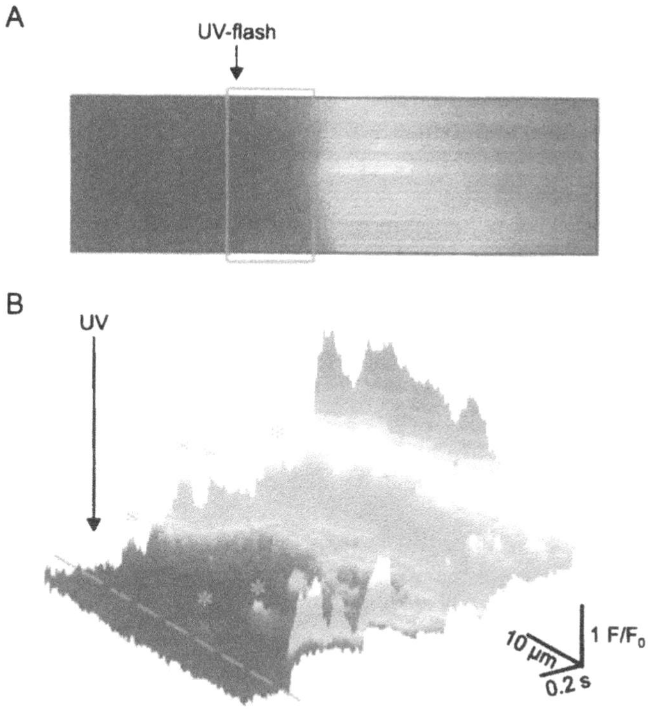

Figure 4 Effects of photorelease of caged IP_3 on the local and global changes in intracellular $[Ca^{2+}]$. (A) The linescan image recorded in a PASMC local with the membrane permeable caged IP_3 analog ci-IP_3/PM and IP_3 was photoreleased by a UV laser pulse. (B) The surface plot of the area inside the box in (A). Local Ca^{2+} sparks marked by asterisks were observed immediately after the UV pulse without prior noticeable increase in global $[Ca^{2+}]$, followed by larger clusters of Ca^{2+} events and global Ca^{2+} release. (Modified from Ref. 5.)

stores upon stimulation. Local interactions of IP_3R and RyR have also been proposed recently in portal vein myocytes (113) and in gastric and vas deferens smooth muscle cells.

In addition, the local Ca^{2+} cross-signaling indicates that a portion of IP_3Rs and RyRs are gating the same SR in PASMCs. This is consistent with a report on rat PASMCs that the activation of IP_3Rs and RyRs with norepinephrine and caffeine, respectively, are mutually exclusive and therefore use the same SR Ca^{2+} pool (8), but contrasts with the findings that in canine PASMCs Ca^{2+} stores gated by IP_3Rs and RyRs are functionally distinct and physically separate (7). Future studies are required to elucidate the species difference in the IP_3R and RyR interactions and their associated functional differences in PASMCs.

V. PHYSIOLOGICAL ROLES OF Ca^{2+} SPARK IN PASMCs

The above-mentioned evidence clearly shows that Ca^{2+} sparks of PASMCs play a significant role in pulmonary vasoconstriction by causing membrane depolarization and amplifying Ca^{2+} release induced by ET-1 and perhaps by some other vasoactive agonists. There is also strong evidence suggesting that RyRs play a central role in hypoxic pulmonary vasoconstriction. This notion is highlighted by the observations that inhibition of RyRs completely abolishes or partially inhibits hypoxia-induced Ca^{2+} responses in PASMCs (114) and hypoxia-induced vasoconstriction in isolated perfused lung (115) and pulmonary arteries (116,117). Currently, there are two hypotheses proposing RyR activation as an essential intermediate step for hypoxic pulmonary vasoconstriction. The first hypothesis proposes that hypoxia causes a reduction of the β-NAD^+/β-NADH ratio, which stimulates ADP-ribosyl cyclase and inhibits cyclic ADP-ribose hydrolase, leading to the accumulation of cADPR, an endogenous activator of RyRs, to activate Ca^{2+} release from the SR (118). The second hypothesis proposes that hypoxia increases the production of reactive oxygen species (perhaps H_2O_2) in the proximal sites of the electron transport chain in mitochondria, leading to Ca^{2+} release via RyRs (119). Because RyR activity is modulated by multiple mechanisms, superoxide may stimulate cADPR sysnthesis, and β-NADH may promote mitochondrial superoxide generation (118,120), detailed future studies are required to delineate the exact mechanism for RyR activation during hypoxia.

Irrespective of its activation mechanism, Ca^{2+} release from RyR-gated stores may contribute to the hypoxic response by (1) providing Ca^{2+} to directly activate myofilaments, (2) acting as a trigger to initiate a chain of Ca^{2+} events, or (3) acting synergistically with other mechanisms to generate pulmonary vasoconstriction. Application of a high concentration of caffeine is known to generate large Ca^{2+} transients and to cause contraction of pulmonary arteries (5,8), indicating that the RyR-gated store of PASMCs is capable of providing sufficient global Ca^{2+} for direct myofilament activation. In the case that hypoxia elicits a moderate activation of RyRs, the increase in Ca^{2+} spark frequency may cause a membrane depolarization exceeding the activation threshold (−40 mV) of L-type Ca^{2+} channels to increase Ca^{2+} influx. Activation of Ca^{2+} sparks may also lead to local SR Ca^{2+} depletion, resulting in the activation of store-operated Ca^{2+} channels and capacitative Ca^{2+} entry (121) to further promote vasocontraction. In addition, membrane depolarization may help to sustain a vasoconstriction by reducing the rate of Ca^{2+} removal through Na^+–Ca^{2+} exchange. In the case of a mild RyR activation by hypoxia, Ca^{2+} sparks may be insufficient to activate L-type Ca^{2+} channels. However, it may set the membrane potential close to the activation threshold, to potentiate other hypoxia-induced voltage-dependent mechanisms, such as K_V channel inhibition

(122) and Ca^{2+} channel activation (123). Indeed, it was shown previously that a "priming" depolarization is required for hypoxia-induced membrane depolarization and $[Ca^{2+}]_i$ elevation in PASMCs (124,125). A subthreshold concentration of ET-1 (10^{-10} M), which causes a twofold increase in spark frequency but by itself does not cause an increase in global $[Ca^{2+}]_i$ or contraction, potentiates hypoxia-induced contraction by sixfold in porcine PASMCs (5,126). The same concentration of ET-1 also restores acute hypoxic constriction in endothelium-denuded porcine distal pulmonary arteries, which are otherwise unresponsive to hypoxia (117,126).

In contrast to adult rat distal PASMCs, Ca^{2+} sparks of fetal PASMCs primarily activate K_{Ca} channels to generate STOCs, causing membrane hyperpolarization and vasorelaxation similarly to systemic arterial myocytes (104,105). Normoxia or high O_2 tension activates this Ca^{2+} spark/K_{Ca} channel mechanism to elicit O_2-dependent perinatal pulmonary vasodilation, which is critical for the transition to air breathing at birth. Malfunction of this mechanism, with a decrease in K_{Ca} channel expression, is associated with an experimental model of pulmonary hypertension of the newborn (127). These findings indicate that Ca^{2+} sparks have multiple physiological functions; their manifestation may vary in different developmental stages, species, and locations in the pulmonary vasculature, depending on the relative expression and activity of the various Ca^{2+}-activated channels in PASMCs.

VI. CONCLUDING REMARKS

Calcium ion signaling is a temporally and spatially complex process controlling numerous cellular processes. A Ca^{2+} spark from RyRs is only one of many local Ca^{2+} signaling events. Specific Ca^{2+} signaling processes mediated through various types of Ca^{2+}-conducting channels and specific long-range and short-range Ca^{2+}-dependent modulations have been described in various cell types. In the pulmonary circulation, the research on the function and regulation of local Ca^{2+} signals has just begun, and an enormous wealth of important information is awaiting discovery. As a bait for more future studies, we have described in this chapter the biophysical properties of Ca^{2+} sparks and their physiological roles in membrane potential regulation and ET-1-induced vasoconstriction as well as their interactions with IP_3Rs in adult rat intralobar PASMCs. We hope this information will serve as a starting point for future studies of local Ca^{2+} signaling in the pulmonary circulation.

ACKNOWLEDGMENTS

This work is supported in part by grants from the NIH (HL 071835 and HL63813) and AHA to J. S. K. Sham.

REFERENCES

1. Berridge MJ. The AM and FM of calcium signalling. Nature 1997; 386: 759–760.
2. Stern MD. Theory of excitation-contraction coupling in cardiac muscle. Biophys J 1992; 63:497–517.
3. Cheng H, Lederer WJ, Cannell MB. Calcium sparks: elementary events underlying excitation-contraction coupling in heart muscle. Science 1993; 262: 740–744.
4. Remillard CV, Zhang W-M, Shimoda LA, Sham JSK. Physiological properties and functions of Ca^{2+} sparks in rat intrapulmonary arterial smooth muscle cells. Am J Physiol Lung Cell Mol Physiol 2002; 283:L433–L444.
5. Zhang W-M, Yip K-P, Lin M-J, Shimoda LA, Li W-H, Sham JSK. Endothelin-1 activates Ca^{2+} sparks in pulmonary arterial smooth muscle cells: local Ca^{2+} signaling between inositol trisphosphate- and ryanodine-receptors. Am J Physiol Lung Cell Mol Physiol 2003; 285:L680–L690.
6. Porter VA, Bonev AD, Knot HJ, Heppner TJ, Stevenson AS, Kleppisch T, Lederer WJ, Nelson MT. Frequency modulation of Ca^{2+} sparks is involved in regulation of arterial diameters by cyclic nucleotides. Am J Physiol 1998; 274:C1346–C1355.
7. Janiak R, Wilson SM, Montague S, Hume JR. Heterogeneity of calcium stores and elementary release events in canine pulmonary arterial smooth muscle cells. Am J Physiol Cell Physiol 2001; 280:C22–C33.
8. Wang Y-X, Zheng Y-M, Abdullaev I, Kotlikoff MI. Metabolic inhibition with cyanide induces calcium release in pulmonary artery myocytes and *Xenopus* oocytes. Am J Physiol Cell Physiol 2003; 284:C378–C388.
9. Fill M, Copello JA. Ryanodine receptor calcium release channels. Physiol Rev 2002; 82:893–922.
10. Jaggar JH, Porter VA, Lederer WJ, Nelson MT. Calcium sparks in smooth muscle. Am J Physiol Cell Physiol 2000; 278:C235–C256.
11. Hakamata Y, Nakai J, Takeshima H, Imoto K. Primary structure and distribution of a novel ryanodine receptor/calcium release channel from rabbit brain. FEBS Lett 1992; 312:229–235.
12. Otsu K, Willard HF, Khanna VK, Zorzato F, Green NM, MacLennan DH. Molecular cloning of cDNA encoding the Ca^{2+} release channel (ryanodine receptor) of rabbit cardiac muscle sarcoplasmic reticulum. J Biol Chem 1990; 265:13472–13483.
13. Takeshima H, Nishimura S, Matsumoto T, Ishida H, Kangawa K, Minamino N, Matsuo H, Ueda M, Hanaoka M, Hirose T, Numa S. Primary structure and expression from complementary DNA of skeletal muscle ryanodine receptor. Nature 1989; 339:439–445.
14. Zorzato F, Fujii J, Otsu K, Phillips M, Green NM, Lai FA, Meissner G, MacLennan DH. Molecular cloning of cDNA encoding human and rabbit forms of the Ca^{2+} release channel (ryanodine receptor) of skeletal muscle sarcoplasmic reticulum. J Biol Chem 1990; 265:2244–2256.
15. Du GG, Sandhu B, Khanna VK, Guo XH, MacLennan DH. Topology of the Ca^{2+} release channel of skeletal muscle sarcoplasmic reticulum (RyR1). Proc Natl Acad Sci USA 2002; 99:16725–16730.

16. Orlova EV, Serysheva II, van Heel M, Hamilton SL, Chiu W. Two structural configurations of the skeletal muscle calcium release channel. Nat Struct Biol 1996; 3:547–552.
17. Samso M, Trujillo R, Gurrola GB, Valdivia HH, Wagenknecht T. Three-dimensional location of the imperatoxin A binding site on the ryanodine receptor. J Cell Biol 1999; 146:493–499.
18. Wagenknecht T, Radermacher M, Grassucci R, Berkowitz J, Xin H-B, Fleischer S. Locations of calmodulin and FK506-binding protein on the three-dimensional architecture of the skeletal muscle ryanodine receptor. J Biol Chem 1997; 272:32463–32471.
19. Marx SO, Reiken S, Hisamatsu Y, Jayaraman T, Burkhoff D, Rosemblit N, Marks AR. PKA phosphorylation dissociates FKBP12.6 from the calcium release channel (ryanodine receptor): defective regulation in failing hearts. Cell 2000; 101:365–376.
20. Sharma MR, Penczek P, Grassucci R, Xin H-B, Fleischer S, Wagenknecht T. Cryoelectron microscopy and image analysis of the cardiac ryanodine receptor. J Biol Chem 1998; 273:18429–18434.
21. Sharma MR, Jeyakumar LH, Fleischer S, Wagenknecht T. Three-dimensional structure of ryanodine receptor isoform three in two conformational states as visualized by cryoelectron microscopy. J Biol Chem 2000; 275:9485–9491.
22. Block BA, Imagawa T, Campbell KP, Franzini-Armstrong C. Structural evidence for direct interaction between the molecular components of the transverse tubule/sarcoplasmic reticulum junction in skeletal muscle. J Cell Biol 1988; 107:2587–2600.
23. Schneider MF, Chandler WK. Voltage dependent charge movement of skeletal muscle: a possible step in excitation-contraction coupling. Nature 1973; 242:244–246.
24. Tanabe T, Beam KG, Adams BA, Niidome T, Numa S. Regions of the skeletal muscle dihydropyridine receptor critical for excitation-contraction coupling. Nature 1990; 346:567–569.
25. Carl SL, Felix K, Caswell AH, Brandt NR, Ball WJ Jr, Vaghy PL, Meissner G, Ferguson DG. Immunolocalization of sarcolemmal dihydropyridine receptor and sarcoplasmic reticular triadin and ryanodine receptor in rabbit ventricle and atrium. J Cell Biol 1995; 129:672–682.
26. Sham JSK, Cleemann L, Morad M. Functional coupling of Ca^{2+} channels and ryanodine receptors in cardiac myocytes. Proc Natl Acad Sci USA 1995; 92:121–125.
27. Flucher BE, Franzini-Armstrong C. Formation of junctions involved in excitation-contraction coupling in skeletal and cardiac muscle. Proc Natl Acad Sci USA 1996; 93:8101–8106.
28. Fabiato A. Time and calcium dependence of activation and inactivation of calcium-induced release of calcium from the sarcoplasmic reticulum of a skinned canine cardiac Purkinje cell. J Gen Physiol 1985; 85:247–289.
29. Franzini-Armstrong C, Protasi F, Ramesh V. Shape, size, and distribution of Ca^{2+} release units and couplons in skeletal and cardiac muscles. Biophys J 1999; 77:1528–1539.

30. Stern MD, Pizarro G, Rios E. Local control model of excitation-contraction coupling in skeletal muscle. J Gen Physiol 1997; 110:415–440.
31. Jaggar JH, Wellman GC, Heppner TJ, Porter VA, Perez GJ, Gollasch M, Kleppisch T, Rubart M, Stevenson AS, Lederer WJ, Knot HJ, Bonev AD, Nelson MT. Ca^{2+} channels, ryanodine receptors and Ca^{2+}-activated K^+ channels: a functional unit for regulating arterial tone. Acta Physiol Scand 1998; 64:577–587.
32. Löhn M, Fürstenau M, Sagach V, Elger M, Schulze W, Luft FC, Haller H, Gollasch M. Ignition of calcium sparks in arterial and cardiac muscle through caveolae. Circ Res 2000; 81:1034–1039.
33. Jaggar JH. Intravascular pressure regulates local and global Ca^{2+} signaling in cerebral artery smooth muscle cells. Am J Physiol Cell Physiol 2001; 281:C439–C448.
34. Lesh RE, Nixon GF, Fleischer S, Airey JA, Somlyo AP, Somlyo AV. Localization of ryanodine receptors in smooth muscle. Circ Res 1998; 82:175–185.
35. Kowarski D, Shuman H, Somlyo AP, Somlyo AV. Calcium release by noradrenaline from central sarcoplasmic reticulum in rabbit main pulmonary artery smooth muscle. J Physiol 1985; 366:153–175.
36. Neylon CB, Richards SM, Larsen MA, Agrotis A, Bobik A. Multiple types of ryanodine receptor/Ca^{2+} release channels are expressed in vascular smooth muscle. Biochem Biophys Res Commun 1995; 215:814–821.
37. Coussin F, Macrez N, Morel J-L, Mironneau J. Requirement of ryanodine receptor subtypes 1 and 2 for Ca^{2+}-induced Ca^{2+} release in vascular myocytes. J Biol Chem 2000; 275:9596–9603.
38. Löhn M, Jessner W, Furstenau M, Wellner M, Sorrentino V, Haller H, Luft FC, Gollasch M. Regulation of calcium sparks and spontaneous transient outward currents by RyR3 in arterial vascular smooth muscle cells. Circ Res 2001; 89:1051–1057.
39. Mironneau J, Coussin F, Jeyakumar LH, Fleischer S, Mironneau C, Macrez N. Contribution of ryanodine receptor subtype 3 to Ca^{2+} responses in Ca^{2+}-overloaded cultured rat portal vein myocytes. J Biol Chem 2001; 276: 11257–11264.
40. Xiao B, Masumiya H, Jiang D, Wang R, Sei Y, Zhang L, Murayama T, Ogawa Y, Lai FA, Wagenknecht T, Chen SRW. Isoform-dependent formation of heteromeric Ca^{2+} release channels (ryanodine receptors). J Biol Chem 2002; 277:41778–41785.
41. Jiang D, Xiao B, Li X, Chen SR. Smooth muscle tissues express a major dominant negative splice variant of the type 3 Ca^{2+} release channel (ryanodine receptor). J Biol Chem 2003; 278:4763–4769.
42. Lipp P, Niggli E. Fundamental calcium release events revealed by two-photon excitation photolysis of caged calcium in guinea-pig cardiac myocytes. J Physiol 1998; 508:801–809.
43. Lipp P, Niggli E. A hierarchical concept of cellular and subcellular Ca^{2+}-signalling. Prog Biophys Mol Biol 1996; 65:265–296.
44. Smith JS, Imagawa T, Ma J, Fill M, Campbell KP, Coronado R. Purified ryanodine receptor from rabbit skeletal muscle is the calcium-release channel of sarcoplasmic reticulum. J Gen Physiol 1988; 92:1–26.

45. Williams AJ. Ion conduction and selectivity in the ryanodine receptor channel. Front Biosci 2002; 7:d1223–d1230.
46. Mejia-Alvarez R, Kettlun C, Rios E, Stern M, Fill M. Unitary Ca^{2+} current through cardiac ryanodine receptor channels under quasi-physiological ionic conditions. J Gen Physiol 1999; 113:177–186.
47. Tinker A, Lindsay AR, Williams AJ. Cation conduction in the calcium release channel of the cardiac sarcoplasmic reticulum under physiological and pathophysiological conditions. Cardiovasc Res 1993; 27:1820–1825.
48. Murayama T, Oba T, Katayama E, Oyamada H, Oguchi K, Kobayashi M, Otsuka K, Ogawa Y. Further characterization of the type 3 ryanodine receptor (RyR3) purified from rabbit diaphragm. J Biol Chem 1999; 274: 17297–17308.
49. Xu L, Meissner G. Regulation of cardiac muscle Ca^{2+} release channel by sarcoplasmic reticulum lumenal Ca^{2+}. Biophys J 1998; 75:2302–2312.
50. Rousseau E, Meissner G. Single cardiac sarcoplasmic reticulum Ca^{2+}-release channel: activation by caffeine. Am J Physiol 1989; 256:H328–H333.
51. Xu L, Eu JP, Meissner G, Stamler JS. Activation of the cardiac calcium release channel (ryanodine receptor) by poly-S-nitrosylation. Science 1998; 279:234–237.
52. Jeyakumar LH, Copello JA, O'Malley AM, Wu GM, Grassucci R, Wagenknecht T, Fleischer S. Purification and characterization of ryanodine receptor 3 from mammalian tissue. J Biol Chem 1998; 273:16011–16020.
53. Chen SRW, Li X, Ebisawa K, Zhang L. Functional characterization of the recombinant type 3 Ca^{2+} release channel (ryanodine receptor) expressed in HEK293 cells. J Biol Chem 1997; 272:24234–24246.
54. Ching LL, Williams AJ, Sitsapesan R. Evidence for Ca^{2+} activation and inactivation sites on the luminal side of the cardiac ryanodine receptor complex. Circ Res 2000; 87:201–206.
55. Laver DR, Baynes TM, Dulhunty AF. Magnesium inhibition of ryanodine-receptor calcium channels: evidence for two independent mechanisms. J Membr Biol 1997; 156:213–229.
56. Laver DR, Owen VJ, Junankar PR, Taske NL, Dulhunty AF, Lamb GD. Reduced inhibitory effect of Mg^{2+} on ryanodine receptor-Ca^{2+} release channels in malignant hyperthermia. Biophys J 1997; 73:1913–1924.
57. Xu L, Tripathy A, Pasek DA, Meissner G. Potential for pharmacology of ryanodine receptor/calcium release channels. Ann NY Acad Sci 1998; 853: 130–148.
58. Rousseau E, Smith JS, Henderson JS, Meissner G. Single channel and $^{45}Ca^{2+}$ flux measurements of the cardiac sarcoplasmic reticulum calcium channel. Biophys J 1986; 50:1009–1014.
59. Galione A, Churchill GC. Cyclic ADP ribose as a calcium-mobilizing messenger. Sci STKE 2000; 2000:PE1.
60. Lee HC, Aarhus R, Graeff R, Gurnack ME, Walseth TF. Cyclic ADP ribose activation of the ryanodine receptor is mediated by calmodulin. Nature 1994; 370:307–309.
61. Takasawa S, Ishida A, Nata K, Nakagawa K, Noguchi N, Tohgo A, Kato I, Yonekura H, Fujisawa H, Okamoto H. Requirement of calmodulin-

dependent protein kinase II in cyclic ADP-ribose-mediated intracellular Ca^{2+} mobilization. J Biol Chem 1995; 270:30257–30259.
62. Xia R, Stangler T, Abramson JJ. Skeletal muscle ryanodine receptor is a redox sensor with a well defined redox potential that is sensitive to channel modulators. J Biol Chem 2000; 275:36556–36561.
63. Eu JP, Sun J, Xu L, Stamler JS, Meissner G. The skeletal muscle calcium release channel: coupled O_2 sensor and NO signaling functions. Cell 2000; 102:499–509.
64. Oba T, Murayama T, Ogawa Y. Redox states of type 1 ryanodine receptor alter Ca^{2+} release channel response to modulators. Am J Physiol Cell Physiol 2002; 282:C684–C692.
65. Marengo JJ, Hidalgo C, Bull R. Sulfhydryl oxidation modifies the calcium dependence of ryanodine-sensitive calcium channels of excitable cells. Biophys J 1998; 74:1263–1277.
66. Aghdasi B, Reid MB, Hamilton SL. Nitric oxide protects the skeletal muscle Ca^{2+} release channel from oxidation induced activation. J Biol Chem 1997; 272:25462–25467.
67. Timerman AP, Onoue H, Xin H-B, Barg S, Copello J, Wiederrecht G, Fleischer S. Selective binding of FKBP12.6 by the cardiac ryanodine receptor. J Biol Chem 1996; 271:20385–20391.
68. Fessenden JD, Wang Y, Moore RA, Chen SR, Allen PD, Pessah IN. Divergent functional properties of ryanodine receptor types 1 and 3 expressed in a myogenic cell line. Biophys J 2000; 79:2509–2525.
69. Ahern GP, Junankar PR, Dulhunty AF. Subconductance states in single-channel activity of skeletal muscle ryanodine receptors after removal of FKBP12. Biophys J 1997; 72:146–162.
70. Xiao RP, Valdivia HH, Bogdanov K, Valdivia C, Lakatta EG, Cheng H. The immunophilin FK506-binding protein modulates Ca^{2+} release channel closure in rat heart. J Physiol 1997; 500:343–354.
71. Wagenknecht T, Grassucci R, Frank J, Saito A, Inui M, Fleischer S. Three-dimensional architecture of the calcium channel/foot structure of sarcoplasmic reticulum. Nature 1989; 338:167–170.
72. Moore CP, Rodney G, Zhang JZ, Santacruz-Toloza L, Strasburg G, Hamilton SL. Apocalmodulin and Ca^{2+} calmodulin bind to the same region on the skeletal muscle Ca^{2+} release channel. Biochemistry 1999; 38:8532–8537.
73. Fruen BR, Bardy JM, Byrem TM, Strasburg GM, Louis CF. Differential Ca^{2+} sensitivity of skeletal and cardiac muscle ryanodine receptors in the presence of calmodulin. Am J Physiol Cell Physiol 2000; 279:C724–C733.
74. Zhang J-Z, Wu Y, Williams BY, Rodney G, Mandel F, Strasburg GM, Hamilton SL. Oxidation of the skeletal muscle Ca^{2+} release channel alters calmodulin binding. Am J Physiol 1999; 276:C46–C53.
75. Meyers MB, Pickel VM, Sheu SS, Sharma VK, Scotto KW, Fishman GI. Association of sorcin with the cardiac ryanodine receptor. J Biol Chem 1995; 270:26411–26418.
76. Lokuta AJ, Meyers MB, Sander PR, Fishman GI, Valdivia HH. Modulation of cardiac ryanodine receptors by sorcin. J Biol Chem 1997; 272:25333–25338.

77. Witcher DR, Kovacs RJ, Schulman H, Cefali DC, Jones LR. Unique phosphorylation site on the cardiac ryanodine receptor regulates calcium channel activity. J Biol Chem 1991; 266:11144–11452.
78. Hain J, Onoue H, Mayrleitner M, Fleischer S, Schindler H. Phosphorylation modulates the function of the calcium release channel of sarcoplasmic reticulum from cardiac muscle. J Biol Chem 1995; 270:2074–2081.
79. Valdivia HH, Kaplan JH, Ellis-Davies GC, Lederer WJ. Rapid adaptation of cardiac ryanodine receptors: modulation by Mg^{2+} and phosphorylation. Science 1995; 267:1997–2000.
80. O'Neill SC, Eisner DA. A mechanism for the effects of caffeine on Ca^{2+} release during diastole and systole in isolated rat ventricular myocytes. J Physiol 1990; 430:519–536.
81. Rousseau E, Smith JS, Meissner G. Ryanodine modifies conductance and gating behavior of single Ca^{2+} release channel. Am J Physiol 1987; 253: C364–C368.
82. Lai FA, Misra M, Xu L, Smith HA, Meissner G. The ryanodine receptor-Ca^{2+} release channel complex of skeletal muscle sarcoplasmic reticulum. Evidence for a cooperatively coupled, negatively charged homotetramer. J Biol Chem 1989; 264:16776–16785.
83. Chu A, Diaz-Munoz M, Hawkes MJ, Brush K, Hamilton SL. Ryanodine as a probe for the functional state of the skeletal muscle sarcoplasmic reticulum calcium release channel. Mol Pharmacol 1990; 37:735–741.
84. Nelson MT, Cheng H, Rubart M, Santana LF, Bonev AD, Knot HJ, Lederer WJ. Relaxation of arterial smooth muscle by calcium sparks. Science 1995; 270:633–637.
85. Bonev AD, Jaggar JH, Rubart M, Nelson MT. Activators of protein kinase C decrease Ca^{2+} spark frequency in smooth muscle cells from cerebral arteries. Am J Physiol 1997; 273:C2090–C2095.
86. Gollasch M, Wellman GC, Knot HJ, Jaggar JH, Damon DH, Bonev AD, Nelson MT. Ontogeny of local sarcoplasmic reticulum Ca^{2+} signals in cerebral arteries: Ca^{2+} sparks as elementary physiological events. Circ Res 1998; 83:1104–1114.
87. Jaggar JH, Stevenson AS, Nelson MT. Voltage dependence of Ca^{2+} sparks in intact cerebral arteries. Am J Physiol 1998; 274:C1755–C1761.
88. Pérez GJ, Bonev AD, Patlak JB, Nelson MT. Functional coupling of ryanodine receptors to K_{Ca} channels in smooth muscle cells from rat cerebral arteries. J Gen Physiol 1999; 113:229–237.
89. Mironneau J, Arnaudeau S, Macrez-Leprêtre N, Boittin FX. Ca^{2+} sparks and Ca^{2+} waves activate different Ca^{2+}-dependent ion channels in single myocytes from rat portal vein. Cell Calcium 1996; 20:153–160.
90. Arnaudeau S, Macrez-Leprêtre N, Mironneau J. Activation of calcium sparks by angiotensin in vascular myocytes. Biochem Biophys Res Commun 1996; 222:809–815.
91. Ganitkevich V, Isenberg G. Isolated guinea pig coronary smooth muscle cells. Acetylcholine induces hyperpolarization due to sarcoplasmic reticulum calcium release activating potassium channels. Circ Res 1990; 67:525–528.

92. Brenner R, Perez GJ, Bonev AD, Eckman DM, Kosek JC, Wiler SW, Patterson AJ, Nelson MT, Aldrich RW. Vasoregulation by the β1 subunit of the calcium-activated potassium channel. Nature 2000; 407:870–876.
93. Hogg RC, Wang Q, Large WA. Effects of Cl channel blockers on Ca-activated chloride and potassium currents in smooth muscle cells from rabbit portal vein. Br J Pharmacol 1994; 111:1333–1341.
94. ZhuGe R, Sims SM, Tuft RA, Fogarty KE, Walsh JV. Ca^{2+} sparks activate K^+ and Cl^- channels, resulting in spontaneous transient currents in guinea-pig tracheal myocytes. J Physiol 1998; 513:711–718.
95. Jaggar JH, Nelson MT. Differential regulation of Ca^{2+} sparks and Ca^{2+} waves by UTP in rat cerebral artery smooth muscle cells. Am J Physiol Cell Physiol 2000; 279:C1528–C1539.
96. Gomez MF, Stevenson AS, Bonev AD, Hill-Eubanks DC, Nelson MT. Opposing actions of inositol 1,4,5-trisphosphate and ryanodine receptors on nuclear factor of activated T-cells regulation in smooth muscle. J Biol Chem 2002; 277:37756–37764.
97. Collier ML, Ji G, Wang Y-X, Kotlikoff MI. Calcium-induced calcium release in smooth muscle: loose coupling between the action potential and calcium release. J Gen Physiol 2000; 115:653–662.
98. Bychkov R, Gollasch M, Steinke T, Ried C, Luft FC, Haller H. Calcium-activated potassium channels and nitrate-induced vasodilation in human coronary arteries. J Pharmacol Exp Ther 1998; 285:293–298.
99. Jaggar JH, Leffler CW, Cheranov SY, Tcheranova D, Shuyu E, Cheng X. Carbon monoxide dilates cerebral arterioles by enhancing the coupling of Ca^{2+} sparks to Ca^{2+}-activated K^+ channels. Circ Res 2002; 91:610–617.
100. Cheranov SY, Jaggar JH. Sarcoplasmic reticulum calcium load regulates rat arterial smooth muscle calcium sparks and transient K_{Ca} currents. J Physiol 2002; 544:71–84.
101. Wellman GC, Santana LF, Bonev AD, Nelson MT. Role of phospholamban in the modulation of arterial Ca^{2+} sparks and Ca^{2+}-activated K^+ channels by cAMP. Am J Physiol Cell Physiol 2001; 281:C1029–C1037.
102. Heppner TJ, Bonev AD, Santana LF, Nelson MT. Alkaline pH shifts Ca^{2+} sparks to Ca^{2+} waves in smooth muscle cells of pressurized cerebral arteries. Am J Physiol Heart Circ Physiol 2002; 283:H2169–H2176.
103. Bolton TB, Gordienko DV. Confocal imaging of calcium release events in single smooth muscle cells. Acta Physiol Scand 1998; 164:567–575.
104. Porter VA, Reeve HL, Cornfield DN. Fetal rabbit pulmonary artery smooth muscle cell response to ryanodine is developmentally regulated. Am J Physiol Lung Cell Mol Physiol 2000; 279:L751–L757.
105. Rhodes MT, Porter VA, Saqueton CB, Herron JM, Resnik ER, Cornfield DN. Pulmonary vascular response to normoxia and K_{Ca} channel activity is developmentally regulated. Am J Physiol Lung Cell Mol Physiol 2001; 280:L1250–L1257.
106. Wang Q, Wang YX, Yu M, Kotlikoff MI. Ca^{2+}-activated Cl^- currents are activated by metabolic inhibition in rat pulmonary artery smooth muscle cells. Am J Physiol 1997; 273:C520–C530.

107. Yuan XJ. Role of calcium-activated chloride current in regulating pulmonary vasomotor tone. Am J Physiol 1997; 272:L959–L968.
108. Clapp LH, Turner JL, Kozlowski RZ. Ca^{2+}-activated Cl^- currents in pulmonary arterial myocytes. Am J Physiol 1996; 270: H1577–H1584.
109. Archer SL, Huang JMC, Reeve HL, Hampl V, Tolarová S, Michelakis E, Weir EK. Differential distribution of electrophysiologically distinct myocytes in conduit and resistance arteries determines their response to nitric oxide and hypoxia. Circ Res 1996; 78:431–442.
110. Smani T, Iwabuchi S, López-Barneo J, Ureña J. Differential segmental activation of Ca^{2+}-dependent $Cl^-$and K^+ channels in pulmonary arterial myocytes. Cell Calcium 2001; 29:369–377.
111. Gelband CH, Gelband H. Ca^{2+} release from intracellular stores is an initial step in hypoxic pulmonary vasoconstriction of rat pulmonary artery resistance vessels. Circulation 1997; 96:3647–3654.
112. Shimoda LA, Sylvester JT, Sham JSK. Mobilization of intracellular Ca^{2+} by endothelin-1 in rat intrapulmonary arterial smooth muscle cells. Am J Physiol Lung Cell Mol Physiol 2000; 278:L157–L164.
113. Gordienko DV, Bolton TB. Crosstalk between ryanodine receptors and IP_3 receptors as a factor shaping spontaneous Ca^{2+}-release events in rabbit portal vein myocytes. J Physiol 2002; 542:743–762.
114. Vadula MS, Kleinman JG, Madden JA. Effect of hypoxia and norepinephrine on cytoplasmic free Ca^{2+} in pulmonary and cerebral arterial myocytes. Am J Physiol 1993; 265:L591–L597.
115. Morio Y, McMurtry IF. Ca^{2+} release from ryanodine-sensitive store contributes to mechanism of hypoxic vasoconstriction in rat lungs. J Appl Physiol 2002; 92:527–534.
116. Jabr RI, Toland H, Gelband CH, Wang XX, Hume JR. Prominent role of intracellular Ca^{2+} release in hypoxic vasoconstriction of canine pulmonary artery. Br J Pharmacol 1997; 122:21–30.
117. Liu Q, Sham JSK, Shimoda LA, Sylvester JT. Hypoxic constriction of porcine distal pulmonary arteries: endothelium and endothelin dependence. Am J Physiol Lung Cell Mol Physiol 2001; 280:L856–L865.
118. Evans AM, Dipp M. Hypoxic pulmonary vasoconstriction: cyclic adenosine diphosphate-ribose, smooth muscle Ca^{2+} stores and the endothelium. Respir Physiol Neurobiol 2002; 132:3–15.
119. Waypa GB, Marks JD, Mack MM, Boriboun C, Mungai PT, Schumacker PT. Mitochondrial reactive oxygen species trigger calcium increases during hypoxia in pulmonary arterial myocytes. Circ Res 2002; 91:719–726.
120. Kumasaka S, Shoji H, Okabe E. Novel mechanisms involved in superoxide anion radical-triggered Ca^{2+} release from cardiac sarcoplasmic reticulum linked to cyclic ADP-ribose stimulation. Antioxid Redox Signal 1999; 1: 55–69.
121. Robertson TP, Hague D, Aaronson PI, Ward JPT. Voltage-independent calcium entry in hypoxic pulmonary vasoconstriction of intrapulmonary arteries of the rat. J Physiol 2000; 525:669–680.

122. Yuan XJ, Goldman WF, Tod ML, Rubin LJ, Blaustein MP. Hypoxia reduces potassium currents in cultured rat pulmonary but not mesenteric arterial myocytes. Am J Physiol 1993; 264:L116–L123.
123. Franco-Obregon A, Lopez-Barneo J. Differential oxygen sensitivity of calcium channels in rabbit smooth muscle cells of conduit and resistance pulmonary arteries. J Physiol 1996; 491:511–518.
124. Turner JL, Kozlowski RZ. Relationship between membrane potential, delayed rectifier K^+ currents and hypoxia in rat pulmonary arterial myocytes. Exp Physiol 1997; 82:629–645.
125. Bakhramov A, Evans AM, Kozlowski RZ. Differential effects of hypoxia on the intracellular Ca^{2+} concentration of myocytes isolated from different regions of the rat pulmonary arterial tree. Exp Physiol 1998; 83:337–347.
126. Sham JSK, Crenshaw BR Jr, Deng LH, Shimoda LA, Sylvester JT. Effects of hypoxia in porcine pulmonary arterial myocytes: roles of K_V channel and endothelin-1. Am J Physiol Lung Cell Mol Physiol 2000; 279:L262–L272.
127. Cornfield DN, Resnik ER, Herron JM, Abman SH. Chronic intrauterine pulmonary hypertension decreases calcium-sensitive potassium channel mRNA expression. Am J Physiol Lung Cell Mol Physiol 2000; 279:L857–L862.
128. Bers DM. Excitation–Contraction Coupling and Cardiac Contractile Force. Dordrecht: Kluwer Academic, 2001.

24

Ion Channels and Hypoxic Pulmonary Vasoconstriction

Vladimir A. Snetkov and Jeremy P. T. Ward
Guy's King's and St. Thomas' School of Medicine, King's College, London, U.K.

I. INTRODUCTION

Hypoxic pulmonary vasoconstriction (HPV) is a highly specialized response of the pulmonary circulation to hypoxic challenge. It manifests itself as a pressor response in vivo or in perfused lung and as a contraction in isolated small pulmonary arteries and pulmonary artery smooth muscle cells (PASMCs). At least a component of the mechanisms underlying HPV must reside in the PASMC itself, although there is considerable evidence that several exogenous factors derived from the endothelium play a facilitatory, permissive, and/or modulatory role for the full development of HPV. In particular, an intact endothelium appears to be essential for the development of sustained (>20 min) HPV, via a Rho-kinase-mediated increase in Ca^{2+} sensitivity of the underlying smooth muscle (see Ref. 1). Nevertheless, it is universally accepted that a rise in PASMC intracellular Ca^{2+} concentration ($[Ca^{2+}]_i$) is critical for HPV, and there is general consensus that this involves Ca^{2+} entry via one or several types of ion channels, although it has been suggested that release of Ca^{2+} from the sarcoplasmic reticulum alone may be sufficient (2). This chapter briefly reviews the potential role of the various types of ion channels that have been or could be implicated in the rise of intracellular $[Ca^{2+}]$ during HPV.

II. CA^{2+} ENTRY PATHWAYS

It is worth reiterating up front the main types of ion channels through which Ca^{2+} is able to enter the cell and that could contribute to the hypoxia-induced rise in $[Ca^{2+}]_i$. Most attention has focused on voltage-gated Ca^{2+} channels (VOCCs), specifically L-type, following the initial demonstration that the L-type blocker verapamil could inhibit HPV in perfused lungs (3). Although the most obvious method of activation of VOCCs is cellular depolarization subsequent to inhibition of K^+ channels, it is also conceivable that hypoxia could modulate their gating and activation either directly or indirectly via phosphorylation, redox, and/or reactive oxygen species (ROS). Additionally, there has recently been considerable interest in the role of a variety of voltage-independent ion channels that are permeable to Ca^{2+}. These are often also permeable to other cations, particularly Na^+ (and so could themselves cause depolarization), and the term nonselective cation channel (NSCC) is commonly used as an all-encompassing nomenclature. The mechanisms by which such channels are activated are not fully understood, but depending on type they may include direct activation by receptor-coupled G proteins [receptor-operated channels (ROCs)], store emptying [store-operated channels (SOCs)] leading to capacitative Ca^{2+} entry (CCE), and indirect activation by diacylglycerol (DAG) generated by PLC. It has been suggested that many of these channels may consist of members of the Trp family (see e.g., Ref. 4).

Loose criteria can be used to determine whether any of these various Ca^{2+} entry pathways has an indispensable role in HPV (i.e., whether, if they are blocked, HPV cannot be elicited under any circumstances). For voltage-gated Ca^{2+} channels, these would include the inability to elicit HPV under conditions such that depolarization does not or cannot occur and/or in the presence of L-type Ca^{2+} channel blockers. The situation is trickier for NSCCs, because there are no good selective blockers, although low micromolar concentrations of lanthanides have been shown to block CCE selectively in small pulmonary arteries (5). It must be noted, however, that HPV is a multifactorial system (6), and several mechanisms may contribute to the rise in $[Ca^{2+}]_i$. Thus, depending on the circumstances, HPV may still be apparent experimentally even though a mechanism that is normally an important component *in vivo* is lacking. This has contributed largely to the continuing controversy surrounding the mechanisms of HPV.

III. DEPOLARIZATION AND VOLTAGE-GATED CA^{2+} CHANNELS

It has long been known that resting smooth muscle cells have a high permeability to K^+ and that this results in a membrane potential of about -50 to $-60\,mV$. This permeability reflects background activity of various types of K^+ channels, and most authors have suggested that voltage-gated K^+ channels are major players in determining membrane potential of smooth muscle cells. A decrease in K^+ activity should therefore cause cell depolarization and thus activation of Ca^{2+} entry via VOCCs and subsequent contraction via the Ca^{2+}-calmodulin–MLCK pathway. Within the framework of this (quite simplistic) scheme, hypoxia could cause HPV either by decreasing the K^+ conductance of PASMCs or, possibly, by directly affecting VOCCs. Both hypotheses have been investigated; a great deal of attention has been focused on the types of VOCCs and K^+ channels that are involved in HPV and the mechanisms by which their activity may be modulated by hypoxia.

Voltage-gated Ca^{2+} channels mediate Ca^{2+} entry into cells in response to depolarization. According to their electrophysiological properties they are designated as L-, N-, P-, Q-, R-, and T-type. Molecularly, Ca^{2+} channels are built from an α_1 subunit, a complex of α_2 and δ subunits, and sometimes a γ subunit. The Ca_V1 family of α subunits is generally associated with the L-type current; the Ca_V2 family with N-, P/Q-, and R-type currents; and the Ca_V3 family with T-type currents (7). The main VOCC in all types of vascular smooth muscle is the L-type, for which there are a range of more or less selective blockers, including verapamil and the dihydropyridines.

There is a strong body of evidence suggesting that L-type Ca^{2+} channels are the main means of Ca^{2+} entry to PASMCs during HPV. This follows from the initial demonstration that HPV in perfused lung is inhibited by the L-type Ca^{2+} channel antagonists SK&F 525 and verapamil (3). In experiments on isolated pulmonary arteries, verapamil also inhibited hypoxia-induced depolarization and the associated contraction (8). Moreover, in PASMCs isolated from adult (9) and fetal (10) arteries, the rise of $[Ca^{2+}]_i$ caused by hypoxia was shown to be inhibited by verapamil. Although activation of these channels during hypoxia is generally believed to be due to depolarization secondary to inhibition of K^+ channels, there is also evidence that Ca^{2+} channels in vascular and other smooth muscle cells, glomus cell, and central neurons may be directly influenced by hypoxia (11). Although in systemic and large pulmonary arteries this modulation may take the form of inhibition, in small resistance pulmonary arteries the current has been shown to be potentiated (12). Nevertheless, L-type Ca^{2+} channels have a very low open-state probability at the resting potential of PASMCs, so it is likely that any direct effect of hypoxia on VOCCs is of secondary importance to that of hypoxia-induced depolarization.

IV. CHANNELS CAUSING DEPOLARIZATION: K^+ AND Cl^- CHANNELS

Because K^+ channels are the prime determinants of resting membrane potential, they are obvious candidates as effectors for inducing membrane depolarization during hypoxia. Inhibition of K^+ currents by hypoxia was first demonstrated in PASMCs by Post et al. (13). Although these results have since been confirmed and extended by numerous other studies (reviewed in Ref. 11), there is still uncertainty concerning the molecular identity of the K^+ channel or channels that are actually inhibited by hypoxia and the mechanisms by which this occurs. Apart from those channels that may act specifically as the effector for depolarization during hypoxia, other K^+ channels activated by secondary pathways may play an important role in modulating these effects and either potentiate or limit the depolarization depending on the degree of hypoxia. The characteristics of the main K^+ channel types found in PASMCs and implicated in some way with HPV are therefore briefly described below, before we return to a discussion of the pros and cons of the depolarization hypothesis of HPV per se.

A. Voltage-Gated K^+ Channels (K_V)

Voltage-gated K^+ channels are present in all smooth muscle types. Pharmacologically they can be isolated by relatively selective inhibition with 4-aminopyridine (4-AP) but not TEA, ChTX, or IbTx. In electrophysiological studies they are generally classified according to their kinetics as a delayed-rectifier, transient outward current, or noninactivating current. Molecularly mammalian K_V channels form nine subfamilies, four (K_V1–K_V4) related to known *Drosophila* genes (*Shaker*, *Shab*, *Shal*, and *Shaw*) and five additional subfamilies specific to mammals (K_V5–K_V9). These families encode over 30 α subunits that form channels with different biophysical properties when expressed in heterologous systems. Functional K_V channels are homo- or heterotetramers, though some subunits are not functional when expressed alone. This creates an additional level of complexity. For example, the $K_V9.3$ subunit has attracted significant attention recently in terms of HPV, but it does not form functional homomultimeric channels, instead affecting the voltage sensitivity and kinetics of heteromultimeric complexes (14). Additionally, three of the four accessory β subunits ($K_V\beta1$–$K_V\beta3$) that affect K_V channel properties have been shown to be expressed in PASMCs (15).

There is reasonable evidence that the membrane potential of PASMCs is controlled by a delayed rectifier K^+ current (e.g., Ref. 16, though see below). There is also a wide consensus that the K^+ current suppressed by hypoxia is voltage-gated and sensitive to 4-AP and therefore most probably a K_V channel (17–20). However, the identity of the oxygen-sensitive moiety that underlies HPV remains elusive. $K_V1.1$, 1.2, 1.3, 1.5, 1.6, 2.1, 3.1b, and 9.3 subunits have all been shown to be expressed in PASMCs (14,15,18,21). Although Kv1.2, 1.5, 2.1, 3.1, 3.3, 4.2, and 9.3 have all been reported to be oxygen-sensitive when expressed in heterologous systems (22), the literature is by no means consistent. Osipenko et al. (21) found that only recombinant

$K_V3.1b$ subunits were sensitive to hypoxia when expressed in L929 cells, and not K_V 1.1, 1.2 or 1.5. Hulme et al. (23) also showed no oxygen sensitivity for homomeric $K_V1.5$ and found oxygen sensitivity only for $K_V1.2$ and 2.1 at potentials more positive than 30 mV. In contrast, Archer et al. (18), using antibodies in native tissue, showed evidence for oxygen sensitivity of $K_V1.5$ but not $K_V2.1$, although the latter appeared to be the main determinant of resting membrane potential. It is notable that in recent studies from the same group $K_V1.5$ knockout mice showed reduced (but not abolished) HPV (24). A key role for $K_V2.1$ in HPV has, however, been suggested by others in similar recent studies (25). The apparent complexity and inconsistency of these and other reports suggests that no single K_V α subunit (or homomultimeric channel) is likely to be act as the sensor or effector for HPV. Moreover, doubt has been cast concerning whether such delayed-rectifier channels are actually open at PASMC resting membrane potentials, because most of them activate at potentials more positive than −40 mV (26). In contrast, heteromultimeric channels have characteristics different from those of either subunit individually, and several studies have provided evidence to suggest that it is more likely that heteromultimers such as $K_V1.2/K_V1.5$ or $K_V2.1/K_V9.3$, or possibly $K_V3.1b$, form the functional channels that are inhibited by hypoxia in PASMCs (14,23,27). There is also evidence implying that $K_V\beta1$ subunits confer oxygen sensitivity to such heteromultimers in pulmonary artery (28).

B. Twin-Pore-Domain K^+ Channels

Twin-pore-domain K^+ (K_2P) channels are voltage-insensitive and are expressed in many cell types, including mammalian lung. Members of the twin-pore-domain, acid-sensitive K^+ (TASK) channel family have also been shown to be oxygen-sensitive in carotid and neuroepithelial bodies (29,30). Osipenko et al. (20) provided evidence than an atypical low-threshold, non-inactivating K^+ current (K_n) plays an important role in regulating the membrane potential of PASMCs and is also oxygen-sensitive. This current has much in common with that carried via TASK, and PASMCs have been stained positively with antibody against TASK-1 (26). Gurney (31) therefore speculated that TASK-1 may not only be the prime determinant of resting membrane potential in PASMCs but may also act as the main oxygen sensor/effector for HPV. This interesting and thought-provoking proposal warrants further investigation.

C. K_{ATP} Channels

ATP-activated K^+ (K_{ATP}) channels are regulated by the ADP/ATP ratio and are thus linked to cell metabolism. They are sensitive to block with sulfonylureas such as glibenclamide, and there are several compounds that activate them directly (e.g., cromakalim). It has been suggested that a fall in ATP during hypoxia might cause activation of K_{ATP} channels, thereby limiting any depolarization due to inhibition of other K^+ channels. However, ATP has been shown not to fall significantly in pulmonary artery during moderate hypoxia (32), and most studies suggest that glibenclamide has little effect on HPV (e.g., Ref. 33) except when hypoxia is severe (<10 mmHg) (34). Conversely, Sato et al. (35), in a series of experiments on both conscious rats and perfused lungs, came to the conclusion that ET-1 enabled HPV by causing a subthreshold depolarization mediated by K_{ATP} channel inhibition. These latter experiments are of particular interest because they impinge on the well-known but little understood potentiating effect of small amounts of pretone on HPV (see Ref. 6); in most other studies where glibenclamide was ineffective, an exogenous preconstrictor such as angiotensin or $PGF_{2\alpha}$ was used. The role of permissive depolarization in HPV is further discussed below.

D. Large-Conductance, Ca^{2+}-Activated K^+ Channels

The open-state probability of large-conductance, Ca^{2+}-activated K^+, (BK_{Ca}) channels increases with depolarization and increased intracellular [Ca^{2+}]. They have a high single-channel conductance (150–250 pS in symmetrical KCl) and are sensitive to TEA, charybdotoxin, and iberiotoxin. Most studies on pulmonary vascular and other smooth muscle types suggest that BK_{Ca} channels are largely inactive at resting membrane potentials and levels of intracellular [Ca^{2+}] (~100 nM) and can thus play little or no role in maintenance of the resting membrane potential. This makes them very poor candidates as potential effectors for hypoxia-induced depolarization in PASMCs, even though this role was initially attributed to them (13). There is now general acceptance that they do not play a primary role in HPV, although it should be noted that depolarization and any subsequent rise in intracellular [Ca^{2+}] will increase BK_{Ca} channel activity and hence limit the extent of depolarization. Moreover, endothelium-derived NO and prostacyclin may act as physiological brakes to HPV, partially by activating BK_{Ca} channels. Notwithstanding the above, and in contrast to all other species studied, we have shown that BK_{Ca} channels in freshly isolated human smooth muscle cells from small pulmonary arteries have an important role in setting the resting membrane potential, even at 100 nM intracellular [Ca^{2+}]; moreover, iberiotoxin and TEA cause substantial depolarization (36). We have reported a similar situation in human airway smooth muscle and have shown that in this species and tissue BK_{Ca} channels have a particularly high sensitivity to [Ca^{2+}] (37). This raises potentially serious questions concerning the role of K_V channels and the depolarization hypothesis in HPV in humans, if only because any hypoxia-induced depolarization, particularly if coupled with a rise in $[Ca^{2+}]_i$, would be resisted by strong activation of BK_{Ca} channels.

E. Cl^- Channels

Although both Ca^{2+}-activated (Cl_{Ca}) and volume-regulated Cl^- channels are known to be present in PASMCs, comparatively little work has been done on their role in the regulation of pulmonary vascular tone in general and HPV in particular. Moderate increases in intracellular [Ca^{2+}] are sufficient to activate Cl_{Ca}, thereby causing a depolarizing inward current. It has been suggested that this depolarization may play an important contributory role in pulmonary artery vasoconstriction elicited by agonist-induced Ca^{2+} release from stores (38). Of particular interest is a report that the ratio of Cl_{Ca} to BK_{Ca} channels is increased in small resistance arteries compared to that in conduit pulmonary arteries, such that an increase in intracellular [Ca^{2+}] due to store release would favor depolarization in resistance arteries but hyperpolarization in large arteries (39). This reflects the well-known segmental pattern of HPV, and as it is also accepted that Ca^{2+} release is a primary event in HPV (for review see Ref. 6), this begs the question as to whether Cl_{Ca} channels play a significant role in the depolarization observed during HPV.

V. PROS AND CONS OF THE K^+ CHANNEL AND DEPOLARIZATION HYPOTHESIS

Whatever channel may be the primary hypoxic sensor or effector, the crucial point in this hypothesis is that pulmonary arterial vasoconstriction is caused by Ca^{2+} entry through L-type Ca^{2+} channels subsequent to depolarization. There is a large body of evidence that would appear to support this established and well-supported hypothesis, including the following findings: (1) Hypoxia does inhibit K^+ channels (see Sec. IV) and (2) cause depolarization in pulmonary artery and PASMCs; (3) L-type channel blockers suppress HPV (see Sec. III); and (4) inhibitors of K^+ channels such as 4-AP inhibit HPV (reviewed in Refs. 40 and 41).

However, not all the available evidence is supportive; for example, several studies have found that neither 4-AP (42) nor L-type Ca^{2+} channel blockers (e.g., Ref. 5) necessarily block HPV, and, more convincing perhaps, we have shown that HPV in small pulmonary arteries was essentially unaffected by prior full depolarization coupled with complete blockade of L-type channels (5). Moreover, several studies have failed to show significant or sufficient hypoxia-induced depolarization (i.e., to ~ -30 mV, to activate L-type channels) in PASMCs, except in the presence of some form of priming stimulus (19,20,42). It is notable in this regard that Archer et al. (18) found that antibodies to $K_V1.5$, their preference for the oxygen sensor, did not affect resting membrane potential but did inhibit HPV, again suggesting that some form of priming is required before hypoxia can elicit significant depolarization. We previously discussed possible roles and mechanisms for the well-known potentiating or facilitating effects of priming and preconstriction on HPV (6) and suggested that at least part of the inhibitory effects of agents such as L-type Ca^{2+} channel blockers may be due to suppression of priming, rather than HPV per se, because when priming was carefully matched, these agents failed to block HPV (5). This may be consistent with the proposal of Gurney (31) that turns the K^+ channel hypothesis on its head by suggesting that inhibition of K^+ channels might not be the principal mediator of HPV at all, but instead a facilitatory mechanism.

None of the above can be taken as hard evidence that inhibition of K^+ channels is not involved in the generation of HPV; indeed, we believe that it is. However, the data do strongly suggest that other mechanisms are of at least equal importance both for the rise in intracellular Ca^{2+} and for the subsequent sustained contraction. Although the latter seems to involve an endothelium-dependent increase in Ca^{2+} sensitivity (see Ref. 1), there is reasonable evidence that the former involves both release of Ca^{2+} from intracellular stores (e.g., Ref. 43) and Ca^{2+} entry via voltage-independent pathways (5), quite apart from the voltage-dependent mechanisms discussed above.

VI. VOLTAGE-INDEPENDENT Ca^{2+} ENTRY IN HPV

It has become clear in recent years that the membrane of many cell types, but specifically smooth muscle cells, contains a variety of voltage-independent Ca^{2+}-permeable ion channels. These have variable selectivity for Ca^{2+}, and many are equally as or more permeable to Na^+ and other small cations; such channels are commonly called by the unspecific term nonselective cation channels (NSCCs) and may be formed of homo- or heteromultimers of Trp proteins (see Sec. II). Members of the Trp family (Trp 1 and 4) have been associated with capacitative Ca^{2+} entry (CCE) mechanisms in a variety of native and model cell types (4) and have been found to be expressed in PASMCs (44). There is strong evidence that Ca^{2+} release from stores is a key initial element in the response to hypoxia in pulmonary arteries and PASMCs (9,43,45), suggesting that CCE could contribute to the hypoxia-induced rise in intracellular Ca^{2+}. Indeed, the subsequent sustained increase in $[Ca^{2+}]$ observed by Salvaterra and Goldman (9) was only partially blocked by verapamil or nifedipine, although it was dependent on external Ca^{2+}. We have shown that at least the initial transient component of HPV in small pulmonary arteries, in terms of both the rise in intracellular $[Ca^{2+}]$ and the subsequent increase in tension, is almost entirely related to CCE (5). Interestingly, we also recently found that although both small pulmonary and systemic arteries exhibit a large increase in intracellular $[Ca^{2+}]$ following store emptying that is due to CCE, it is only in the small pulmonary arteries that this is coupled to an increase in tension (46). This suggests that CCE may be of particular importance in regulating pulmonary vascular tone.

Although CCE may contribute to the sustained rise in intracellular $[Ca^{2+}]$ during HPV, the latter was only partially inhibited by concentrations of La^{3+} sufficient to block CCE completely, although it was completely abolished by 100 μM SK&F 96365 (a blocker of other NSCCs) or removal of external Ca^{2+} (5). This implies that an additional voltage-insensitive Ca^{2+} entry pathway involving NSCCs is activated during sustained HPV. The identity of this putative pathway remains to be elucidated.

VII. MECHANISMS OF OXYGEN SENSITIVITY OF ION CHANNELS

There is insufficient space to provide other than a very brief overview of the many and various potential oxygen-sensing mechanisms that may affect ion channel activity, and the reader is directed to the reviews in Refs. 11, 27, and 40. In general, the potential mechanisms by which ion channels can be affected by hypoxia fall into two main categories; those that involve a direct effect on a channel protein or chaperone, and those that require a second-messenger signaling pathway from a separate primary sensor or sensors. Neither exclude the existence of the other, and it is quite possible, if not likely, that several sensors are involved. However, there is considerable controversy concerning the nature of the second pathway, with, for example, two apparently mutually exclusive proposals, one suggesting that ROS formation is increased in hypoxia (e.g., Ref. 47) and the other that ROS is decreased (48).

Most early studies that suggested a direct oxygen-sensing mechanism for (primarily) K^+ channels suffered from the semi-intractable problem that some significant component of the cell [e.g., mitochondria, NAD(P)H oxidase] might remain adhered to excised patches. More recent approaches have circumvented this potential failing in a variety of ways. Although there is evidence that the sensing function of $K_V3.1b$ may be at least membrane-delimited (21), it is likely that most $K_V\alpha$ subunits do not sense oxygen directly but require K_V β subunits (27). These β subunits have similarities to NAD(P)H-sensitive oxidoreductases and could potentially link K_V channels to the cellular redox state (49). The redox state and ROS have also been implicated in activation of NSCCs and Trp channels and in cADPR-mediated Ca^{2+} release (43,50). A change in redox state has long been promoted as a potential signal between the primary oxygen sensors and their effectors (40). The two major systems that have been implicated in affecting redox state and ROS production are a membrane-associated NAD(P)H oxidase and the mitochondia (47). Recent support has tended to favor the latter, as knockout of the gp91 phox subunit of NAD(P)H oxidase did not affect HPV (51). However, it has recently been argued that another type of NAD(P)H oxidase with a different subunit is more important in PASMCs (52).

VIII. CONCLUSION

It is clear that many membrane ion channels may contribute in various ways to the rise in intracellular [Ca^{2+}] that is a predeterminant for HPV: this is summarized in Fig. 1. What is not yet clear is the relative or absolute importance of any of these channels to the response in vivo. Although current opinion is still very much in favor of a K_V-based delayed rectifier as the primary sensor or effector for hypoxia, there is a growing realization that several other channel types may be at least as important. Moreover, depolarization and Ca^{2+} entry via VOCCs have been shown to be nonessential for HPV; although it is highly likely that they do play a major role, it is apparent that voltage-independent systems are equally able to support full development of HPV. The relative importance of these various mechanisms leading to Ca^{2+} entry in hypoxia is currently unknown, but it would seem that HPV, apart from being multifactorial in origin, has a fair degree of redundancy in its underlying mechanisms.

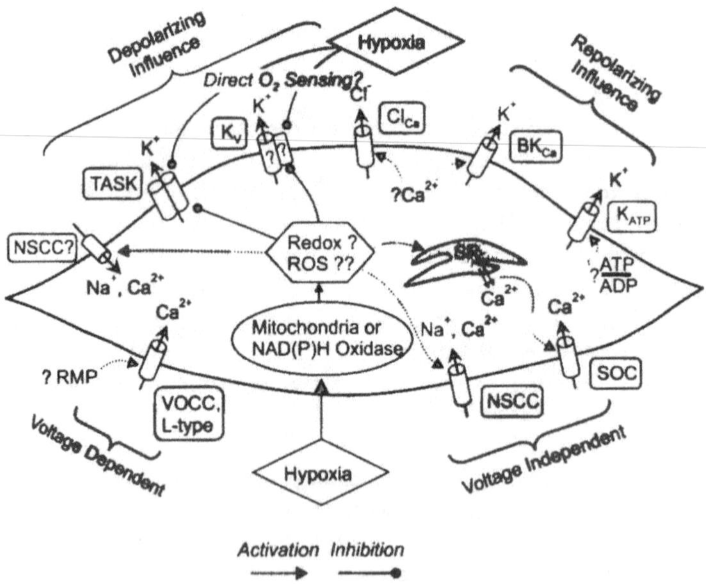

Figure 1 A summary diagram of the various ion channels and signaling pathways that have been associated with HPV. The top part of the figure shows channels that influence membrane potential and the effect of their inhibition or stimulation during hypoxia; the lower part shows Ca^{2+} entry pathways. Putative activation pathways are shown as dashed arrows, and inhibitory pathways as solid lines.

ACKNOWLEDGMENT

Work in our laboratory is funded by the Wellcome Trust.

REFERENCES

1. Aaronson PI, Robertson TP, Ward JP. Endothelium-derived mediators and hypoxic pulmonary vasoconstriction. Respir Physiol Neurobiol 2002; 132: 107–120.
2. Evans AM, Dipp M. Hypoxic pulmonary vasoconstriction: cyclic adenosine diphosphate-ribose, smooth muscle Ca^{2+} stores and the endothelium. Respir Physiol Neurobiol 2002; 132:3–15.
3. McMurtry IF, Davidson AB, Reeves JT, Grover RF. Inhibition of hypoxic pulmonary vasoconstriction by calcium antagonists in isolated rat lungs. Circ Res 1976; 38:99–104.
4. Birnbaumer L, Zhu X, Jiang M, Boulay G, Peyton M, Vannier B, Brown D, Platano D, Sadeghi H, Stefani E, Birnbaumer M. On the molecular basis and regulation of cellular capacitative calcium entry: roles for Trp proteins. Proc Natl Acad Sci USA 1996; 93:15195–15202.
5. Robertson TP, Hague DE, Aaronson PI, Ward JPT. Voltage-independent calcium entry in hypoxic pulmonary vasoconstriction of intrapulmonary arteries of the rat. J Physiol 2000; 525:669–680.
6. Ward JPT, Aaronson PI. Mechanisms of hypoxic pulmonary vasoconstriction: can anyone be right?. Respir Physiol 1999; 115:261–271.
7. Catterall WA. Structure and regulation of voltage-gated Ca^{2+} channels. Annu Rev Cell Dev Biol 2000; 16:521–555.
8. Harder DR, Madden JA, Dawson CA. A membrane electrical mechanism for hypoxic vasoconstriction of small pulmonary arteries from the cat. Chest 1985; 88:233–235.
9. Salvaterra CG, Goldman WF. Acute hypoxia increases cytosolic calcium in cultured pulmonary arterial myocytes. Am J Physiol 1993; 264:L323–L328.
10. Cornfield DN, Stevens T, McMurtry IF, Abman SH, Rodman DM. Acute hypoxia causes membrane depolarization and calcium influx in fetal pulmonary artery smooth muscle cells. Am J Physiol 1994; 266:L469–L475.
11. López-Barneo J, Pardal R, Ortega-Saenz P. Cellular mechanism of oxygen sensing. Annu Rev Physiol 2001; 63:259–287.
12. Smani T, Hernandez A, Urena J, Castellano AG, Franco-Obregon A, Ordonez A, López-Barneo J. Reduction of Ca^{2+} channel activity by hypoxia in human and porcine coronary myocytes. Cardiovasc Res 2002; 53:97–104.
13. Post JM, Hume JR, Archer SL, Weir EK. Direct role for potassium channel inhibition in hypoxic pulmonary vasoconstriction. Am J Physiol 1992; 262: C882–C890.
14. Patel AJ, Lazdunski M, Honore E. Kv2.1/Kv9.3, a novel ATP-dependent delayed-rectifier K^+ channel in oxygen-sensitive pulmonary artery myocytes. EMBO J 1997; 16:6615–6625.

15. Yuan XJ, Wang J, Juhaszova M, Golovina VA, Rubin LJ. Molecular basis and function of voltage-gated K^+ channels in pulmonary arterial smooth muscle cells. Am J Physiol 1998; 274:L621–L635.
16. Smirnov SV, Robertson TP, Ward JPT, Aaronson PI. Chronic hypoxia is associated with reduced delayed rectifier K^+ current in rat pulmonary artery muscle cells. Am J Physiol 1994; 266:H365–H370.
17. Post JM, Gelband CH, Hume JR. $[Ca^{2+}]_i$ inhibition of K^+ channels in canine pulmonary artery: novel mechanism for hypoxia-induced membrane depolarization. Circ Res 1995; 77:131–139.
18. Archer SL, Souil E, Dinh-Xuan AT, Schremmer B, Mercier JC, El Yaagoubi A, Nguyen-Huu L, Reeve HL, Hampl V. Molecular identification of the role of voltage-gated K^+ channels, Kv1.5 and Kv2.1, in hypoxic pulmonary vasoconstriction and control of resting membrane potential in rat pulmonary artery myocytes. J Clin Invest 1998; 101:2319–2330.
19. Turner JL, Kozlowski RZ. Relationship between membrane potential, delayed rectifier K^+ currents and hypoxia in rat pulmonary arterial myocytes. Exp Physiol 1997; 82:629–645.
20. Osipenko ON, Evans AM, Gurney AM. Regulation of the resting potential of rabbit pulmonary artery myocytes by a low threshold, O_2-sensing potassium current. Br J Pharmacol 1997; 120:1461–1470.
21. Osipenko ON, Tate RJ, Gurney AM. Potential role for Kv3.1b channels as oxygen sensors. Circ Res 2000; 86:534–540.
22. Patel AJ, Honore E. Molecular physiology of oxygen-sensitive potassium channels. Eur Respir J 2001; 18:221–227.
23. Hulme JT, Coppock EA, Felipe A, Martens JR, Tamkun MM. Oxygen sensitivity of cloned voltage-gated K^+ channels expressed in the pulmonary vasculature. Circ Res 1999; 85:489–497.
24. Archer SL, London B, Hampl V, Wu X, Nsair A, Puttagunta L, Hashimoto K, Waite RE, Michelakis E. Impairment of hypoxic pulmonary vasoconstriction in mice lacking the voltage-gated potassium channel Kv1.5. FASEB J 2001; 15:1801–1803.
25. Hogg DS, Davies AR, McMurray G, Kozlowski RZ. $K_V2.1$ channels mediate hypoxic inhibition of I_{KV} in native pulmonary arterial smooth muscle cells of the rat. Cardiovasc Res 2002; 55:349–360.
26. Gurney AM, Osipenko ON, MacMillan D, Kempsill FE. Potassium channels underlying the resting potential of pulmonary artery smooth muscle cells. Clin Exp Pharmacol Physiol 2002; 29:330–333.
27. Coppock EA, Martens JR, Tamkun MM. Molecular basis of hypoxia-induced pulmonary vasoconstriction: role of voltage-gated K^+ channels. Am J Physiol Lung Cell Mol Physiol 2001; 281:L1–L12.
28. Coppock EA, Tamkun MM. Differential expression of K_V channel α and β subunits in the bovine pulmonary arterial circulation. Am J Physiol Lung Cell Mol Physiol 2001; 281:L1350–L1360.
29. Hartness ME, Lewis A, Searle GJ, O'Kelly I, Peers C, Kemp PJ. Combined antisense and pharmacological approaches implicate hTASK as an airway O_2 sensing K^+ channel. J Biol Chem 2001; 276:26499–26508.

30. Buckler KJ, Williams BA, Honore E. An oxygen-, acid- and anaesthetic-sensitive TASK-like background potassium channel in rat arterial chemoreceptor cells. J Physiol 2000; 525:135–142.
31. Gurney AM. Multiple sites of oxygen sensing and their contributions to hypoxic pulmonary vasoconstriction. Respir Physiol Neurobiol 2002; 132: 43–53.
32. Leach RM, Sheehan DW, Chacko VP, Sylvester JT. Energy state, pH, and vasomotor tone during hypoxia in precontracted pulmonary and femoral arteries. Am J Physiol Lung Cell Mol Physiol 2000; 278:L294–L304.
33. Leach RM, Robertson TP, Twort CH, Ward JPT. Hypoxic vasoconstriction in rat pulmonary and mesenteric arteries. Am J Physiol 1994; 266:L223–L231.
34. Wiener CM, Dunn A, Sylvester JT. ATP-dependent K^+ channels modulate vasoconstrictor responses to severe hypoxia in isolated ferret lungs. J Clin Invest 1991; 88:500–504.
35. Sato K, Morio Y, Morris KG, Rodman DM, McMurtry IF. Mechanism of hypoxic pulmonary vasoconstriction involves ET_A. A receptor-mediated inhibition of K_{ATP} channel. Am J Physiol Lung Cell Mol Physiol 2000; 278: L434–L442.
36. Snetkov VA, Ward JPT. Large conductance potassium channels in freshly isolated human pulmonary artery. Am J Respir Crit Care 1998; 157:A210.
37. Snetkov VA, Hirst SJ, Twort CH, Ward JPT. Potassium currents in human freshly isolated bronchial smooth muscle cells. Br J Pharmacol 1995; 115: 1117–1125.
38. Yuan XJ. Role of calcium-activated chloride current in regulating pulmonary vasomotor tone. Am J Physiol 1997; 272:L959–L968.
39. Smani T, Iwabuchi S, Lopez-Barneo J, Urena J. Differential segmental activation of Ca^{2+}-dependent Cl^- and K^+ channels in pulmonary arterial myocytes. Cell Calcium 2001; 29:369–377.
40. Weir EK, Hong Z, Porter VA, Reeve HL. Redox signaling in oxygen sensing by vessels. Respir Physiol Neurobiol 2002; 132:121–130.
41. Sweeney M, Yuan JX-J. Hypoxic pulmonary vasoconstriction: role of voltage-gated potassium channels. Respir Res 2000; 1:40–48.
42. Sham JS, Crenshaw BR Jr, Deng LH, Shimoda LA, Sylvester JT. Effects of hypoxia in porcine pulmonary arterial myocytes: roles of K_V channel and endothelin-1. Am J Physiol Lung Cell Mol Physiol 2000; 279:L262–L272.
43. Wilson HL, Dipp M, Thomas JM, Lad C, Galione A, Evans AM. ADP-ribosyl cyclase and cyclic ADP-ribose hydrolase act as a redox sensor: a primary role for cADPR in hypoxic pulmonary vasoconstriction. J Biol Chem 2001; 276: 11180–11188.
44. Ng LC, Gurney AM. Store-operated channels mediate Ca^{2+} influx and contraction in rat pulmonary artery. Circ Res 2001; 89:923–929.
45. Jabr RI, Toland H, Gelband CH, Wang XX, Hume JR. Prominent role of intracellular Ca^{2+} release in hypoxic vasoconstriction of canine pulmonary artery. Br J Pharmacol 1997; 122:21–30.
46. Snetkov VA, Aaronson PI, Ward JP, Knock G, Robertson TP. Capacitative calcium entry as a pulmonary specific vasoconstrictor mechanism in small muscular arteries of the rat. Br J Pharmacol 2003; 140:97–106.

47. Chandel NS, Schumacker PT. Cellular oxygen sensing by mitochondria: old questions, new insight. J Appl Physiol 2000; 88:1880–1889.
48. Michelakis ED, Hampl V, Nsair A, Wu X, Harry G, Haromy A, Gurtu R, Archer SL. Diversity in mitochondrial function explains differences in vascular oxygen sensing. Circ Res 2002; 90:1307–1315.
49. Gulbis JM. The β subunit of Kv1 channels: voltage-gated enzyme or safety switch? Novartis Found Symp 2002; 245:127–141
50. Balzer M, Lintschinger B, Groschner K. Evidence for a role of Trp proteins in the oxidative stress- induced membrane conductances of porcine aortic endothelial cells. Cardiovasc Res 1999; 42:543–549.
51. Archer SL, Reeve HL, Michelakis E, Puttagunta L, Waite, Nelson DP, Dinauer MC, Weir EK. O_2 sensing is preserved in mice lacking the gp91 phox subunit of NADPH oxidase. Proc Natl Acad Sci USA 1999; 96:7944–7949.
52. So I, Earm YE. Is K_v channel inhibition a common path to hypoxic pulmonary vasoconstriction? Cardiovasc Res 2002; 55:233–235.

25

Essential Role of Anion Channels in Induction of Apoptotic and Necrotic Cell Death

Yasunobu Okada, Emi Maeno, Takashi Nabekura, and Shin-ichiro Mori

National Institute for Physiological Sciences, Okazaki, Japan

I. INTRODUCTION

In excitable cells in which the intracellular Cl concentration is maintained at a level lower than that at equilibrium, anion channels stabilize the membrane by shifting the membrane potential toward the equilibrium potential for Cl (E_{Cl}). In this way, ligand-gated anion channels coupled to GABA or glycine receptors exert an inhibitory effect on neuronal excitation. The resting membrane potential in skeletal muscle is maintained at a very negative level by the activity of a particular type of anion channel, CLC1. To play such an electrogenic role, anion channel operation produces a simple charge separation but does not necessarily result in net Cl transport across the plasma membrane. In nonexcitable epithelial cells, in contrast, anion channels are involved in substantial Cl^- transport, which eventually results in the absorption or secretion of isotonic NaCl fluids. The best-known anion channel functioning in a variety of Cl^--secreting epithelial cells is the cystic fibrosis transmembrane conductance regulator (CFTR), which is activated by cAMP/PKA.

Recent studies have demonstrated additional roles for anion channels in more general cell functions including cell volume regulation (1,2), cell proliferation (3), mitosis (4), and cell death (2). In this chapter, we summarize the current understanding of the essential role of anion channels in the induction of apoptotic and necrotic cell death.

II. VOLUME REGULATION DYSFUNCTION ASSOCIATED WITH THE CELL DEATH PROCESS

Under normal physiological conditions, the volume of individual cells is maintained at a constant level. It is maintained despite an osmotic imbalance produced across the cell membrane by colloidal osmotic pressure due to intracellular membrane-impermeable anionic macromolecules and by the fluctuation in the intracellular osmolyte concentration associated with cell metabolism and the transport of osmolytes. Even under anisotonic conditions, animal cells can regulate their volume by responding to osmotic cell swelling and shrinkage with regulatory volume decrease (RVD) and increase (RVI), respectively (5,6). However, it appears that volume-regulatory mechanisms are impaired during cell death processes, because persistent cell swelling and shrinkage occur in and are major hallmarks of the early phases of necrotic and apoptotic cell death, respectively.

Necrotic cells exhibit a progressive swelling termed the necrotic volume increase (NVI) (2) until death by cell rupture, which results in tissue injury and inflammation. On the other hand, apoptotic cells show a persistent shrinkage. The apoptotic cell shrinkage consists of two phases: the early-phase whole-cell shrinkage termed apoptotic volume decrease (AVD) (7) and the late-phase cell fragmentation, namely the formation of apoptotic bodies that are cleared by phagocytes. To elucidate the mechanisms of cell death initiation, it is therefore important to investigate the early-phase hallmarks of cell death, AVD and NVI.

III. ROLES OF K^+ AND Cl^- CHANNELS IN THE INDUCTION OF AVD

Inducers of receptor-mediated apoptosis, Fas ligand and TNFα, as well as an inducer of mitochondrion-mediated apoptosis, staurosporine (STS), were found to induce shrinkage within 1 h in HeLa, U937, PC12, and NG108–15 cells before cell fragmentation (apoptotic body formation), which started around 2 h after stimulation (7). As shown in Fig. 1A, significant AVD was readily observed 30 min after stimulation with STS or TNFα in PC12 cells. Furthermore, the induction of AVD was coupled to a facilitation of the RVD (Fig. 1B), which is known to occur through activation of volume-regulatory K^+ and Cl^- channels (5,6), for all four cell types under hypotonic conditions after stimulation with STS (7), TNFα (7), or Fas ligand (2). This suggests that K^+ and Cl^- channels are activated in cells undergoing apoptosis even though the cells have not undergone swelling. As seen in Fig. 1, in fact, both the induction of AVD and the facilitation

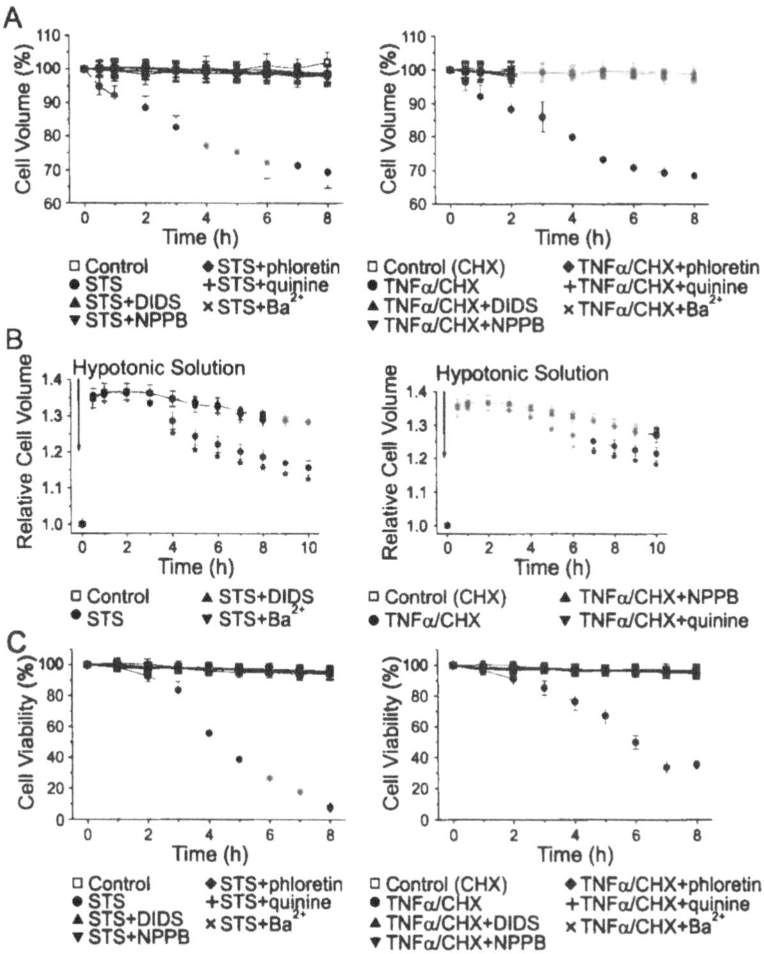

Figure 1 Induction of AVD (A), facilitation of RVD (B), and induction of cell death (C) by treatment with an apoptosis inducer, and their prevention by simultaneous treatment with a channel blocker in PC12 cells. Treatment with the apoptosis inducer STS or TNFα plus CHX was for varying time periods (A, C) or for 2 h (B). The channel blocker was 0.5 mM DIDS, 0.5 mM NPPB, 30 μM phloretin, 0.5 mM quinine, or 5 mM Ba^{2+}. (A, B): Mean cell volume were measured by an electronic sizing technique after washing out any drugs, and the data were normalized with measurements taken immediately before treatment with the apoptosis inducer (A) or hypotonic challenge (65% osmolality) (B). (C) Cell viability was assessed by MTT assay, and the data were normalized with measurements taken immediately before treatment with the apoptosis inducer. Each data point represents the mean ± SEM (vertical bar) of 16 observations. (*) $P < 0.05$ vs. corresponding control.

of RVD were abolished by broad-spectrum blockers of K^+ channels (quinine and Ba^{2+}) and of Cl^- channels (DIDS and NPPB) (7). Phloretin, which is a blocker relatively selective for volume-sensitive outwardly rectifying (VSOR) Cl^- channels (8), was also effective in blocking the induction of AVD and the facilitation of RVD (7). Similarly, a number of K^+ channel blockers, such as 4-aminopyridine, quinine, and TEA and its analog, have been observed to block apoptotic cell shrinkage induced by a variety of stimuli (9–13). Also, apoptotic cell shrinkage was found to be inhibited by the conventional Cl^- channel blockers DIDS and SITS in neuroblastoma cells (14).

Patch-clamp studies have demonstrated that a variety of apoptotic stimuli give rise to augmentation of currents via voltage-gated K^+ channels (K_v) or Ca^{2+}-activated K^+ channels (K_{Ca}) in a number of cell types (15–21) including pulmonary artery smooth muscle cells (22–24). In addition, apoptosis induction has been observed to be coupled to activation of outwardly rectifying Cl^- currents in liver cells (19,25), Jurkat cells (26), *Xenopus* oocytes (27) and HeLa cells (28) as well as to activation of Ca^{2+}-dependent Cl^- currents in human neutrophils (29). Taken together, these results suggest that parallel activation of K^+ and Cl^- channels that occurs upon stimulation by apoptosis inducers is responsible for the induction of AVD, which starts prior to the formation of apoptotic bodies.

IV. CASPASE-INDEPENDENT INDUCTION OF AVD

The cytoskeleton is known to be involved in the regulation of ion channels (30,31). The activation of VSOR Cl^- channels, for example, has been shown to depend on cytoskeletal components (1,32). During apoptosis, proteolytic cleavage of a number of cytoskeletal proteins is induced by activation of caspases (33,34). It is therefore natural to assume that the activity of ion channels involved in the induction of AVD is dependent on the activity of caspases. However, our previous studies showed that the onset of AVD preceded the activation of caspase-3 in HeLa, U937, PC12, and NG108-15 cells stimulated with STS or TNFα (7). Furthermore, the broad-spectrum caspase blockers zVAD-fmk and zD-dcb failed to abrogate the induction of AVD, which was clearly detected within 1 h in U937 cells, although these pan-caspase blockers inhibited apoptotic body formation, which started 2 h after stimulation with STS (7,35). A similar insensitivity of apoptotic cell shrinkage to caspase blockers has been observed in Jurkat T cells stimulated with a Ca^{2+} ionophore (36), thapsigargin (36), or UV irradiation (37).

On the other hand, pan-caspase inhibitors have been reported to inhibit apoptotic cell shrinkage in Jurkat T cells stimulated with glucocorticoids (38) or Fas ligand (36). Sensitivity of apoptotic cell shrinkage to caspase blockers has also been reported in other leukemic cells stimulated with etoposide, TGFβ, or methylprednisolone (39–41). However, it should be noted that in these studies sensitivity to caspase blockers was observed 4–48 h after apoptotic stimulation, and such late-phase shrinkage may have been caused mainly by apoptotic body formation that is sensitive to the activity of caspases.

Because AVD is an early event upstream of caspase activation, some (non-caspase) signals that trigger the activation of volume-regulatory K^+ and/or Cl^- channels must exist. In some instances, cytosolic Ca^{2+} may serve as the signal for the AVD induction that takes place upon activation of Ca^{2+}-dependent K^+ channels (13,22) and/or Ca^{2+}-dependent Cl^- channels (29). However, some other signals must be involved in the AVD induction that is caused by operation of Ca^{2+}-independent K^+ channels (such as K_v) and Cl^- channels (such as VSOR).

V. RESCUE FROM APOPTOTIC CELL DEATH BY ANION CHANNEL BLOCK

As shown in Fig. 1C, when the induction of AVD was blocked by a K^+ or Cl^- channel blocker, PC12 cells stimulated with STS or TNFα were rescued from apoptotic cell death. Results obtained using HeLa, U937 and NG108–15 cells stimulated with STS or TNFα were identical (7). At the same time, cytochrome c release, caspase-3 activation, and DNA laddering were all abrogated by channel blocker-induced inhibition of AVD (7). Thus, it appears that AVD is an early prerequisite for apoptosis (2,35), as schematically illustrated in Fig. 2. Recently, Hortelano et al. (42) reported a similar dependence on AVD in HeLa and Jurkat cells stimulated with STS or NO. The same authors also reported an exception in which block of apoptotic cell shrinkage by a Cl channel blocker, SITS or phloretin, did not rescue cells of a macrophage cell line, RAW264.7, from NO-induced apoptotic cell death (42). However, there is a possibility that the NO-induced macrophage death was due, at least in part, to necrosis, judging from the degree of caspase activation and the smearlike DNA degradation. Alternatively, it is possible that NO or its downstream signal is the same as a signal downstream from the AVD event triggered by STS in macrophages.

The AVD event appears to be a prerequisite to apoptotic cell death in all, or at least most, cell types. Thus, it is understandable that a large variety of cell types could be rescued from apoptotic cell death by blockers of K^+ channels (9–13,16–18,23,43,44) and by blockers of Cl^- channels (14,26, 45–49). Under normal conditions, K^+ channels function ceaselessly in the basal resting state of most cell types, whereas Cl channels often have a scanty basal activity in most cell types except for specific Cl^- conductance-dominant cell types such as skeletal muscle cells. Thus, Cl^- channels may provide a safer and more promising target for drugs protective against apoptotic cell death associated with pathological insults such as ischemia/reperfusion.

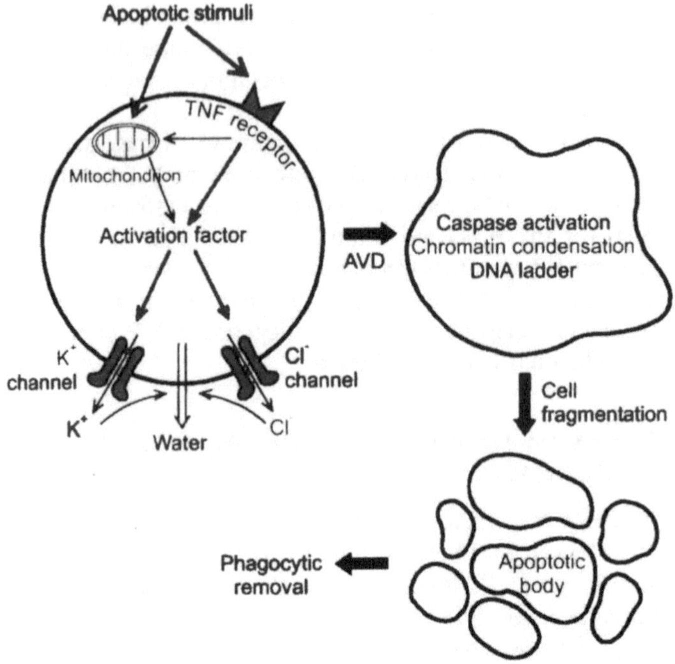

Figure 2 Schematic illustration of the role of ion channels in the induction of AVD and the relation between AVD and other apoptotic processes.

VI. ROLES OF ION CHANNELS AND TRANSPORTERS IN THE INDUCTION OF NVI

Necrosis occurs as a result of ATP depletion under severe ischemia or hypoxia conditions, exposure to a variety of toxins and poisons, lytic viral infection, complement attack, hyperthermia, lactacidosis, and excitotoxicity. Necrotic cell death is associated with persistent swelling that eventually results in cell membrane rupture. Such cytolytic swelling, called necrotic volume increase (NVI) (2), has actually been shown in vitro to be induced by a variety of cytotoxic agents, including glutamate (50,51), kainate (52), oxidants (53), and arachidonic acid (54), as well as by anoxia (55) and lactacidosis (56) in neurons (50,51,55), retinal cells, (52), liver cells (53), and astrocytes (54).

Glutamate neurotoxicity, called excitotoxicity (57), is triggered by activation of the ligand-gated cation channel coupled to the NMDA receptor (NMDAR) and is associated with either apoptosis or necrosis, depending on the intensity and duration of the insult (58,59). Both Ca^{2+} influx and Na^+ influx through the NMDAR play causative roles in excitotoxicity (60,61). Reactive oxygen species (ROS) were also shown to induce Na^+

and Ca^{2+} influx by activating nonselective cation channels (NSCCs), thereby bringing about the NVI (53,62). The molecular identity of the ROS-activated NSCCs was recently determined to be TRPM2, a member of the TRP family (63). Depolarization caused by the activation of NMDAR or NSCCs may drive Cl^- influx, resulting in an NaCl inflow that brings about NVI, as schematically depicted in Fig. 3.

In neurons, depolarization should also trigger activation of voltage-gated Na^+ channels (Na_v), which are a direct pathway for Na^+ influx, and voltage-gated Ca^{2+} channels (Ca_v), which may indirectly increase Na^+ influx by stimulating Na^+/Ca^{2+} antiporters (NCX) (Fig. 3). Under ATP-depleting conditions such as in ischemia or hypoxia, inhibition of the Na^+,K^+-ATPase is known to lead to depolarization, thereby activating Na_v and Ca_v (12). Hypoxia by itself has been reported to activate persistent Na^+ currents that in turn induce depolarization and activation of both Ca_v and NCX, leading to neuronal damage in the hippocampus (64). ATP depletion has been shown to stimulate the ATP-sensitive NSCCs and hence induce swelling in brain astrocytes (65).

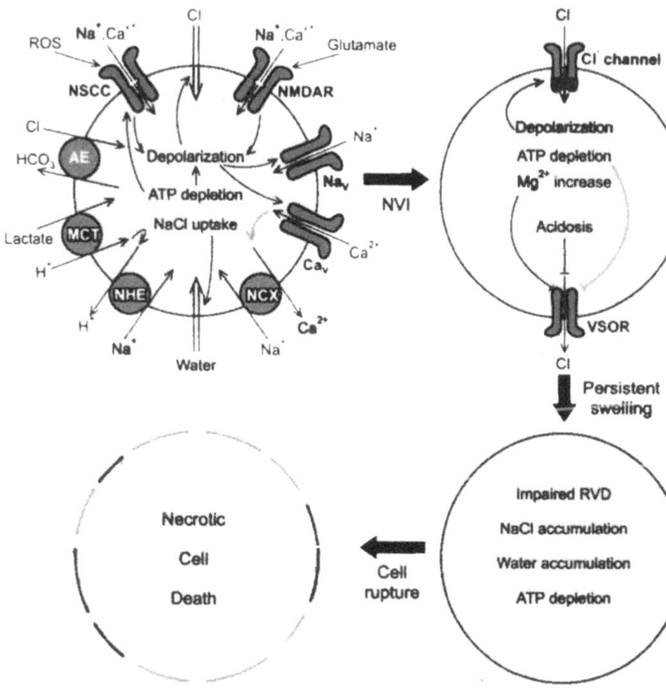

Figure 3 Schematic illustration of the role of ion channels and transporters in the induction of NVI and the dysfunction of RVD during necrosis.

Hypoxia, ischemia, seizure, and spreading depression in the brain are associated with lactate accumulation due to enhanced anaerobic glycolysis (66). Cerebral ischemia or trauma results in acidosis due to proton liberation from ATP hydrolysis, which occurs at a rate greater than that of ATP synthesis (67,68). The degree of acidosis is known to be proportional to the amount of lactate accumulated (69). Acidosis coupled to lactate accumulation, called lactacidosis, causes cytotoxic brain edema and the necrotic death of nerve and glial cells (70,71). In vitro, lactacidosis was indeed demonstrated to lead to NVI in neuronal (71,72) and glial (56,73–79) cells. Studies up until now (see Refs. 56, 72, 76, 78, and 79) have shown that mechanisms of lactacidosis-induced NVI involve lactate and proton influx via the monocarboxylate transporter (MCT), Na^+ influx via the Na^+/H^+ antiporter (NHE), and Cl^- influx via the Cl^-/HCO_3^- antiporter (AE), as schematically illustrated in Fig. 3.

VII. PROTECTION AGAINST NECROTIC CELL DEATH BY MANIPULATION OF ANION CHANNELS

In necrotic cell death, swelling persists until the rupture of the cell, and volume regulation does not occur. This suggests that dysfunction of the RVD mechanism is associated with situations that cause necrosis. The RVD was, in fact, demonstrated to be impaired in cerebellar granule neurons subjected to hypoxic conditions (80) as well as in neuronal (72) and glial (79) cells subjected to lactacidosis conditions.

VSOR Cl^- channels, which serve as the Cl^- efflux pathway during the RVD process in most cell types (1), are known to be dependent on intracellular ATP and to be sensitive to intracellular free Mg^{2+} (1,81). The activity of a VSOR channel should therefore be inhibited by ATP depletion and the resultant increase in the cytosolic free Mg^{2+} concentration. Actually, hypoxia and chemical metabolic inhibition were both shown to inhibit the VSOR current in endothelial cells (82) and cerebellar granule neurons (80). It is known that arachidonic acid is accumulated during cerebral ischemia, injury, or seizure (83–86). Because arachidonic acid is the most potent known blocker of VSOR Cl^- channels (87), its effect should also contribute to the dysfunction of RVD. Our recent studies (72,79) demonstrated that VSOR Cl^- channels are suppressed by cytosolic acidification in neuronal cells (Fig. 4A) and glial cells (Fig. 4B) subjected to lactacidosis, but not in cells subjected to acidosis alone. Thus, as illustrated in Fig. 3, the dysfunction of RVD resulting from impaired VSOR Cl^- channel activity prevents recovery from the NVI.

Preactivation or introduction of the volume-regulatory anion conductance may be a promising treatment to protect cells from necrotic injury. Diaz et al. (88) provided evidence, in fact, that preactivation of the volume-sensitive Cl^- channel is involved in ischemic preconditioning in

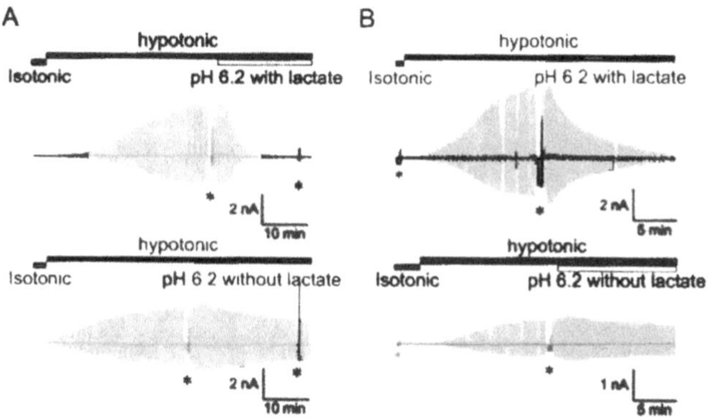

Figure 4 Effects of lactacidosis (top traces) and acidosis (bottom traces) on VSOR Cl channels in neuronally differentiated NG108–15 cells (A) and astrocytic C6 cells (B). The current was monitored by applying alternating step pulses to ± 40 mV every 15 s from a holding potential of 0 mV. Step pulses from -100 to $+120$ mV (A) or from -60 to $+100$ mV (B) in 20 mV increments were applied at asterisks. (Modified from data presented in Refs. 72 and 79.)

rabbit ventricular myocytes. Stimulation of the glycine receptor, which is coupled to an anion channel, was reported to protect against necrotic cell death in epithelial cells of rabbit renal proximal tubules (89). A recent study of ours demonstrated that the introduction of a toxin protein from *Helicobacter pylori*, VacA, which forms an acid-resistant anion-selective channel, results in complete recovery from lactacidosis-induced swelling in glial cells (79). Thus, we believe that the introduction of an exogenous anion channel activity might be a novel approach for treating cerebral edema associated with lactacidosis. An alternative approach would be to restore endogenous anion channel activity. However, it should be kept in mind that neither restoration of, nor introduction of, anion channels can ameliorate the NVI in cells in which prominent depolarization drives Cl influx (Fig. 3).

ACKNOWLEDGMENTS

We thank E. L. Lee, M. Ohara, and T. Okayasu for manuscript preparation, technical assistance, and secretarial assistance. This work was supported by a Grant-in-Aid for Scientific Research (A) from the Ministry of Education, Culture, Sports, Science and Technology of Japan.

REFERENCES

1. Okada Y. Volume expansion-sensing outward-rectifier Cl^- channel: fresh start to the molecular identity and volume sensor. Am J Physiol 1997; 273: C755–C789.

2. Okada Y, Maeno E, Shimizu T, Dezaki K, Wang J, Morishima S. Receptor-mediated control of regulatory volume decrease (RVD) and apoptotic volume decrease (AVD). J Physiol 2001; 532:3–16.
3. Wondergem R, Gong W, Monen SH, Dooley SN, Gonce JL, Conner TD, Houser M, Ecay TW, Ferslew KE. Blocking swelling-activated chloride current inhibits mouse liver cell proliferation. J Physiol 2001; 532:661–672.
4. Shen M-R, Droogmans G, Eggermont J, Voets T, Ellory JC, Nilius B. Differential expression of volume-regulated anion channels during cell cycle progression of human cervical cancer cells. J Physiol 2000; 529:385–394.
5. Hoffmann EK, Simonsen LO. Membrane mechanisms in volume and pH regulation in vertebrate cells. Physiol Rev 1989; 69:315–382.
6. Okada Y, Hazama A. Volume-regulatory ion channels in epithelial cells. News Physiol Sci 1989; 4:238–242.
7. Maeno E, Ishizaki Y, Kanaseki T, Hazama A, Okada Y. Normotonic cell shrinkage because of disordered volume regulation is an early prerequisite to apoptosis. Proc Natl Acad Sci USA 2000; 97:9487–9492.
8. Fan H-T, Morishima S, Kida H, Okada Y. Phloretin differentially inhibits volume-sensitive and cyclic AMP-activated, but not Ca-activated, Cl^- channels. Br J Pharmacol 2001; 133:1096–1106.
9. Beauvais F, Michel L, Dubertret L. Human eosinophils in culture undergo a striking and rapid shrinkage during apoptosis. Role of K^+ channels. J Leuko Biol 1995; 57:851–855.
10. McCarthy JV, Cotter TG. Cell shrinkage and apoptosis: a role for potassium and sodium ion efflux. Cell Death Differ 1997; 4:756–770.
11. Trimarchi JR, Liu L, Smith PJ, Keefe DL. Apoptosis recruits two-pore domain potassium channels used for homeostatic volume regulation. Am J Physiol Cell Physiol 2002; 282:C588–C594.
12. Xiao AY, Wei L, Xia S, Rothman S, Yu SP. Ionic mechanism of ouabain-induced concurrent apoptosis and necrosis in individual cultured cortical neurons. J Neurosci 2002; 22:1350–1362.
13. Elliott JI, Higgins CF. IKCa1 activity is required for cell shrinkage, phosphatidylserine translocation and death in T lymphocyte apoptosis. EMBO Rep 2003; 4:189–194.
14. O'Reilly N, Xia Z, Fiander H, Tauskela J, Small DL. Disparity between ionic mediators of volume regulation and apoptosis in N1E 115 mouse neuroblastoma cells. Brain Res 2002; 943:245–256.
15. Houzen H, Kikuchi S, Kanno M, Shinpo K, Tashiro K. Tumor necrosis factor enhancement of transient outward potassium currents in cultured rat cortical neurons. J Neurosci Res 1997; 50:990–999.
16. Yu SP, Yeh C-H, Sensi SL, Gwag BJ, Canzoniero LMT, Farhangrazi ZS, Ying HS, Tian M, Dugan LL, Choi DW. Mediation of neuronal apoptosis by enhancement of outward potassium current. Science 1997; 278:114–117.
17. Colom LV, Diaz ME, Beers DR, Neely A, Xie W, Appel SH. Role of potassium channels in amyloid-induced cell death. J Neurochem 1998; 70:1925–1934.
18. Wang L, Xu D, Dai W, Lu L. An ultraviolet-activated K^+ channel mediates apoptosis of myeloblastic leukemia cells. J Biol Chem 1999; 274:3678–3685.

19. Nietsch HH, Roe MW, Fiekers JF, Moore AL, Lidofsky SD. Activation of potassium and chloride channels by tumor necrosis factor α. Role in liver cell death. J Biol Chem 2000; 275:20556–20561.
20. McLaughlin B, Pal S, Tran MP, Parsons AA, Barone FC, Erhardt JA, Aizenman E. p38 activation is required upstream of potassium current enhancement and caspase cleavage in thiol oxidant-induced neuronal apoptosis. J Neurosci 2001; 21:3303–3311.
21. Bock J, Szabo I, Jekle A, Gulbins E. Actinomycin D-induced apoptosis involves the potassium channel Kv1.3. Biochem Biophys Res Commun 2002; 295:526–531.
22. Krick S, Platoshyn O, Sweeney M, Kim H, Yuan JX-J. Activation of K^+ channels induces apoptosis in vascular smooth muscle cells. Am J Physiol Cell Physiol 2001; 280:C970–C979.
23. Ekhterae D, Platoshyn O, Krick S, Yu Y, McDaniel SS, Yuan JX-J. Bcl-2 decreases voltage-gated K^+ channel activity and enhances survival in vascular smooth muscle cells. Am J Physiol Cell Physiol 2001; 281:C157–C165.
24. Platoshyn O, Zhang S, McDaniel SS, Yuan JX-J. Cytochrome c activates K^+ channels before inducing apoptosis. Am J Physiol Cell Physiol 2002; 283:C1298–C1305.
25. Meng X-J, Carruth MW, Weinman SA. Leukotriene D_4 activates a chloride conductance in hepatocytes from lipopolysaccharide-treated rats. J Clin Invest 1997; 99:2915–2922.
26. Szabo I, Lepple-Wienhues A, Kaba KN, Zoratti M, Gulbins E, Lang F. Tyrosine kinase-dependent activation of a chloride channel in CD95-induced apoptosis in T lymphocytes. Proc Natl Acad Sci USA 1998; 95:6169–6174.
27. Souktani R, Berdeaux A, Ghaleh B, Giudicelli JF, Guize L, Le Heuzey JY, Henry P. Induction of apoptosis using sphingolipids activates a chloride current in *Xenopus laevis* oocytes. Am J Physiol Cell Physiol 2000; 279:C158–C165.
28. Shimizu T, Okada Y. Electrophysiological characteristics of Cl channel currents activated by apoptosis inducers. Jpn J Physiol 2003; 53(Suppl.):S145.
29. Schumann MA, Gardner P, Raffin TA. Recombinant human tumor necrosis factor α induces calcium oscillation and calcium-activated chloride current in human neutrophils. The role of calcium/calmodulin-dependent protein kinase. J Biol Chem 1993; 268:2134–2140.
30. Ordway RW, Singer JJ, Walsh JV Jr. Direct regulation of ion channels by fatty acids. Trends Neurosci 1991; 14:96–100.
31. Meves H. Modulation of ion channels by arachidonic acid. Prog Neurobiol 1994; 43:175–186.
32. Morishima S, Shimizu T, Kida H, Okada Y. Volume expansion sensitivity of swelling-activated Cl channel in human epithelial cells. Jpn J Physiol 2000; 50:277–280.
33. Nicholson D, Thornberry, NA. Caspases: killer proteases. Trends Biochem Sci 1997; 22:299–306.
34. Tan X, Wang JYJ. The caspase-RB connection in cell death. Trends Cell Biol 1998; 8:116–120.
35. Okada Y, Maeno E. Apoptosis, cell volume regulation and volume-regulatory chloride channels. Comp Biochem Physiol A 2001; 130:377–383.

36. Bortner CD, Cidlowski JA. Caspase independent/dependent regulation of K^+, cell shrinkage, and mitochondrial membrane potential during lymphocyte apoptosis. J Biol Chem 1999; 274:21953–21962.
37. Vu CCQ, Bortner CD, Cidlowski JA. Differential involvement of initiator caspases in apoptotic volume decrease and potassium efflux during Fas- and UV-induced cell death. J Biol Chem 2001; 276:37602–37611.
38. Hughes FM Jr, Cidlowski JA. Glucocorticoid-induced thymocyte apoptosis: protease-dependent activation of cell shrinkage and DNA degradation. J Steroid Biochem Mol Biol 1998; 65:207–217.
39. Zhivotovsky B, Gahm A, Ankarcrona M, Nicotera P, Orrenius S. Multiple proteases are involved in thymocyte apoptosis. Exp Cell Res 1995; 221:404–412.
40. Wolf CM, Reynolds JE, Morana SJ, Eastman A. The temporal relationship between protein phosphatase, ICE/CED-3 proteases, intracellular acidification, and DNA fragmentation in apoptosis. Exp Cell Res 1997; 230:22–27.
41. Schrantz N, Blanchard DA, Auffredou M-T, Sharma S, Leca G, Vazquez A. Role of caspases and possible involvement of retinoblastoma protein during TGFβ-mediated apoptosis of human B lymphocytes. Oncogene 1999; 18:3511–3519.
42. Hortelano S, Zeini M, Castrillo A, Alvarez AM, Bosca L. Induction of apoptosis by nitric oxide in macrophages is independent of apoptotic volume decrease. Cell Death Differ 2002; 9:643–650.
43. Dallaporta B, Marchetti P, de Pablo MA, Maisse C, Duc H-T, Metivier D, Zamzami N, Geuskens M, Kroemer G. Plasma membrane potential in thymocyte apoptosis. J Immunol 1999; 162:6534–6542.
44. Wang X, Xiao AY, Ichinose T, Yu SP. Effects of tetraethylammonium analogs on apoptosis and membrane currents in cultured cortical neurons. J Pharmacol Exp Therap 2000; 295:524–530.
45. Fujita H, Yanagisawa A, Ishikawa K. Suppressive effect of a chloride bicarbonate exchanger inhibitor on staurosporine-induced apoptosis of endothelial cells. Heart Vessels 1997; Suppl 12:84–88.
46. Rasola A, Farahi Far D, Hofman P, Rossi B. Lack of internucleosomal DNA fragmentation is related to Cl^- efflux impairment in hematopoietic cell apoptosis. FASEB J 1999; 13:1711–1723.
47. Barriere H, Poujeol C, Tauc M, Blasi JM, Counillon L, Poujeol P. CFTR modulates programmed cell death by decreasing intracellular pH in Chinese hamster lung fibroblasts. Am J Physiol Cell Physiol 2001; 281:C810–C824.
48. Small DL, Tauskela J, Xia Z. Role for chloride but not potassium channels in apoptosis in primary rat cortical cultures. Neurosci Lett 2002; 334:95–98.
49. Araki T, Hayashi M, Watanabe N, Kanuka H, Yoshino J, Miura M, Saruta T. Down-regulation of Mcl-1 by inhibition of the PI3-K/Akt pathway is required for cell shrinkage-dependent cell death. Biochem Biophys Res Commun 2002; 290:1275–1281.
50. Sohn S, Kim EY, Gwag BJ. Glutamate neurotoxicity in mouse cortical neurons: atypical necrosis with DNA ladders and chromatin condensation. Neurosci Lett 1998; 240:147–150.

51. Sun DA, Sombati S, DeLorenzo RJ. Glutamate injury-induced epileptogenesis in hippocampal neurons: an in vitro model of stroke-induced "epilepsy." Stroke 2001; 32:2344–2350.
52. Chen Q, Moulder K, Tenkova T, Hardy K, Olney JW, Romano C. Excitotoxic cell death dependent on inhibitory receptor activation. Exp Neurol 1999; 160:215–225.
53. Barros LF, Stutzin A, Calixto A, Catalan M, Castro J, Hetz C, Hermosilla T. Nonselective cation channels as effectors of free radical-induced rat liver cell necrosis. Hepatology 2001; 33:114–122.
54. Staub F, Winkler A, Haberstok J, Plesnila N, Peters J, Chang RCC, Kempski O, Baethmann A. Swelling, intracellular acidosis, and damage of glial cells. Acta Neurochir 1996; Suppl 66:56–62.
55. Friedman JE, Haddad GG. Major differences in $Ca^{2+}{}_i$ response to anoxia between neonatal and adult rat CA1 neurons: role of $Ca^{2+}{}_i$ and $Na^{+}{}_i$. J Neurosci 1993; 13:63–72.
56. Staub F, Baethmann A, Peters J, Kempski O. Effects of lactacidosis on volume and viability of glial cells. Acta Neurochir 1990; Suppl 51:3–6.
57. Olney JW. Inciting excitotoxic cytocide among central neurons. Adv Exp Med Biol 1986; 203:631–645.
58. Bonfoco E, Krainc D, Ankarcrona M, Nicotera P, Lipton SA. Apoptosis and necrosis: two distinct events induced, respectively, by mild and intense insults with *N*-methyl-D-aspartate or nitric oxide/superoxide in cortical cell cultures. Proc Natl Acad Sci USA 1995; 92:7162–7166.
59. Grammatopoulos T, Morris K, Ferguson P, Weyhenmeyer J. Angiotensin protects cortical neurons from hypoxic-induced apoptosis via the angiotensin type 2 receptor. Mol Brain Res 2002; 99:114–124.
60. Choi DW. Ionic dependence of glutamate neurotoxicity. J Neurosci 1987; 7: 369–379.
61. Olney JW, Price MT, Samson L, Labruyere J. The role of specific ions in glutamate neurotoxicity. Neurosci Lett 1986; 28:65–71.
62. Barros LF, Hermosilla T, Castro J. Necrotic volume increase and the early physiology of necrosis. Comp Biochem Physiol A 2001; 130:401–409.
63. Hara Y, Wakamori M, Ishii M, Maeno E, Nishida M, Yoshida T, Yamada H, Shimizu S, Mori E, Kudoh J, Shimizu N, Kurose H, Okada Y, Imoto K, Mori Y. LTRPC2 Ca^{2+}-permeable channel activated by changes in redox status confers susceptibility to cell death. Mol Cell 2002; 9:163–173.
64. Hammarstrom AK, Gage PW. Oxygen-sensing persistent sodium channels in rat hippocampus. J Physiol 2000; 529:107–118.
65. Chen M, Simard JM. Cell swelling and a nonselective cation channel regulated by internal Ca^{2+} and ATP in native reactive astrocytes from adult rat brain. J Neurosci 2001; 21:6512–6521.
66. Paschen W, Djuricic B, Mies G, Schmidt-Kastner R, Linn F. Lactate and pH in the brain association and dissociation in different pathophysiological states. J Neurochem 1987; 48:154–159.
67. Marmarou A. Intracellular acidosis in human and experimental brain injury. J Neurotrauma 1992; 9:S551–S562.

68. Siesjö BK. Acidosis and ischemic brain damage. Neurochem Pathol 1988; 9: 31–88.
69. Paschen W, Siesjo BK, Ingvar M, Hossmann KA. Regional differences in brain glucose content in graded hypoglycemia. Neurochem Pathol 1986; 5:131–142.
70. Kraig RP, Petito CK, Plum F, Pulsinelli WA. Hydrogen ions kill brain at concentrations reached in ischemia. J Cereb Blood Flow Metab 1987; 7:379–386.
71. Staub F, Mackert B, Kempski O, Peters J, Baethmann A. Swelling and death of neuronal cells by lactic acid. J Neurol Sci 1993; 119:79–84.
72. Mori S, Morishima S, Takasaki M, Okada Y. Impaired activity of volume-sensitive anion channel during lactacidosis-induced swelling in neuronally differentiated NG108–15 cells. Brain Res 2002; 957:1–11.
73. Jakubovicz DE, Klip A. Lactic acid-induced swelling in C6 glial cells via Na^+/H^+ exchange. Brain Res 1989; 485:215–224.
74. Jakubovicz DE, Grinstein S, Klip A. Cell swelling following recovery from acidification in C6 glioma cells: an in vitro model of postischemic brain edema. Brain Res 1987; 435:138–146.
75. Kempski O, Staub F, Jansen M, Schödel F, Baethmann A. Glial swelling during extracellular acidosis in vitro. Stroke 1988; 19:385–392.
76. Lomneth R, Medrano S, Gruenstein EI. The role of transmembrane pH gradients in the lactic acid induced swelling of astrocytes. Brain Res 1990; 523:69–77.
77. Plesnila N, Haberstok J, Peters J, Kölbl I, Baethmann A, Staub F. Effect of lactacidosis on cell volume and intracellular pH of astrocytes. J Neurotrauma 1999; 16:831–841.
78. Ringel F, Plesnila N, Chang RCC, Peters J, Staub F, Baethmann A. Role of calcium ions in acidosis-induced glial swelling. Acta Neurochir 1997; Suppl 70:144–147.
79. Nabekura T, Morishima S, Cover TL, Mori S, Kannan H, Komune S, Okada Y. Recovery from lactacidosis-induced glial cell swelling with the aid of exogenous anion channels. Glia 2003; 41:247–259.
80. Patel AJ, Lauritzen I, Lazdunski M, Honoré E. Disruption of mitochondrial respiration inhibits volume-regulated anion channels and provokes neuronal cell swelling. J Neurosci 1998; 18:3117–3123.
81. Oiki S, Kubo M, Okada Y. Mg^{2+} and ATP-dependence of volume-sensitive Cl^- channels in human epithelial cells. Jpn J Physiol 1995; 44:S77–S79.
82. Oike M, Droogmans G, Nilius B. The volume-activated chloride current in human endothelial cells depends on intracellular ATP. Pflügers Arch 1994; 427:184–186.
83. Bazan NGJ. Effects of ischemia and electroconvulsive shock on free fatty acid pool in the brain. Biochim Biophys Acta 1970; 218:1–10.
84. Siesjö BK, Ingvar M, Westerberg E. The influence of bicuculline-induced seizures on free fatty acid concentrations in cerebral cortex, hippocampus, and cerebellum. J Neurochem 1982; 39:796–802.
85. Baethmann A, Maier Hauff K, Schürer L, Lange M, Guggenbichler C, Vogt W, Jacob K, Kempski O. Release of glutamate and of free fatty acids in vasogenic brain edema. J Neurosurg 1989; 70:578–591.

86. Kinouchi H, Imaizumi S, Yoshimoto T, Motomiya M. Phenytoin affects metabolism of free fatty acids and nucleotides in rat cerebral ischemia. Stroke 1990; 21:1326–1332.
87. Kubo M, Okada Y. Volume-regulatory Cl^- channel currents in cultured human epithelial cells. J Physiol 1992; 456:351–371.
88. Diaz RJ, Losito VA, Mao GD, Ford MK, Backx PH, Wilson GJ. Chloride channel inhibition blocks the protection of ischemic preconditioning and hypo-osmotic stress in rabbit ventricular myocardium. Circ Res 1999; 84: 763–775.
89. Miller GW, Lock EA, Schnellmann RG. Strychnine and glycine protect renal proximal tubules from various nephrotoxicants and act in the late phase of necrotic cell injury. Toxicol Appl Pharmacol 1994; 125:192–197.

26

Downregulated K_V Channels and Upregulated TRPC Channels in Primary Pulmonary Hypertension

Donna D. Tigno, Mehran Mandegar, Carmelle V. Remillard, and Jason X.-J. Yuan

Department of Medicine, University of California, San Diego, California, U.S.A.

I. INTRODUCTION

Primary pulmonary hypertension (PPH) is a progressive, fatal disease of unknown cause. It is characterized by elevation of pulmonary arterial pressure (PAP) and pulmonary vascular resistance (PVR), leading progressively to right heart failure and, eventually, death. Incidence of this disease is rare, occurring in one or two per million in the general population, and predominantly affects women. The time from diagnosis to right heart failure and death is short (median of 2.8 years) (1,2).

Pulmonary arterial pressure is the product of PVR and cardiac output. In healthy subjects, maintenance of a normal PAP at rest depends on low vascular resistance to blood flow. Pulmonary hypertension, which is due to a sustained elevation of PAP, develops mainly from an increase in PVR. In patients with PPH, increased PVR occurs through several mechanisms: vasoconstriction, vascular wall remodeling (medial and intimal proliferation), vascular injury, and in situ thrombosis (1–3). Other factors contributing to the elevated PVR in patients with PPH include an increased excretion of endothelium-derived constricting factors (e.g., thromboxane A_2 and endothelin-1) and a decreased excretion of endothelium-derived relaxing factors (e.g., prostacyclin and nitric oxide) (4–7). The imbalance of excretion of vasodilating and vasoconstricting factors has been implicated in both PPH and secondary pulmonary hypertension (SPH).

There is ample evidence suggesting that the mechanisms contributing to pulmonary vascular medial hypertrophy, which is the most consistent pathological finding in PPH, are mainly due to the presence of intrinsic abnormalities in pulmonary artery smooth muscle cells (PASMCs). However, SPH can be associated with and/or a direct consequence of other ailments such as chronic pulmonary thromboembolic disease, collagen vascular disorders, congenital cardiac abnormalities, sarcoidosis, and infection with human immunodeficiency virus type 1 (HIV-1), all of which share the histological features manifested by complex lumen-occluding vascular lesions (plexiform lesions) and in situ thrombosis. Pulmonary arteries from patients with PPH seem to exhibit more smooth muscle hypertrophy than vessels from patients with SPH (8). Pulmonary vascular rings from PPH patients are more sensitive to vasoconstrictor agents than those from normal subjects (9).

II. ROLE OF Ca^{2+} IN PULMONARY VASOCONSTRICTION AND PASMC PROLIFERATION

Calcium ions (Ca^{2+}) play a pivotal role in many cellular processes, including muscle contraction, neurotransmitter release, cell proliferation, and migration (10). An increase in cytoplasmic free Ca^{2+} concentration ($[Ca^{2+}]_{cyt}$) in PASMCs is a major trigger for pulmonary vasoconstriction and also an important stimulus for cell proliferation and migration. Additionally, pulmonary vasoconstriction increases pressure in the lumen of the vessel and leads to the elastic stretch of the smooth muscle cell membrane. Interestingly, the mechanical stretch of the smooth muscle cells can independently stimulate PASMC growth and synthetic activity, further contributing to smooth muscle cell hypertrophy and hyperplasia and, ultimately, to vascular remodeling (14,15). Therefore, pulmonary vasoconstriction not only directly causes the elevation of PVR and PAP but also indirectly increases PVR and PAP through stimulation of pulmonary vascular remodeling, contributing to the obliterative process that is often seen in severe pulmonary hypertension.

Regulation of $[Ca^{2+}]_{cyt}$ in PASMCs is achieved by two mechanisms: (1) trans-sarcolemmal influx of Ca^{2+} through Ca^{2+} channels or extrusion of Ca^{2+} through the Ca^{2+}-Mg^{2+} ATPase and (2) the mobilization (or release) of Ca^{2+} from the intercellular stores such as the sarcoplasmic reticulum (SR) through Ca^{2+} release channels or sequestration of Ca^{2+} into the SR by the SR Ca^{2+}-Mg^{2+} ATPase (Fig. 1). The influx of extracellular

Ca^{2+} into the cells occurs through at least three types of Ca^{2+} channels in the plasma membrane: (1) voltage-dependent Ca^{2+} channels (VDCCs), which are regulated by changes in the membrane potential (E_m); (2) receptor-operated Ca^{2+} channels (ROCs), which are regulated by agonist–receptor interactions and the downstream signal transduction proteins (11); and (3) store-operated Ca^{2+} channels (SOCs), which are activated by depletion of Ca^{2+} from the SR (12). All three types of channels participate in the excitation–contraction coupling processes in pulmonary vascular smooth muscle. Generally, change in E_m regulates the activity of VDCCs, which is required for the electromechanical coupling that alters the vascular tone. VDCCs are opened by membrane depolarization and closed by membrane hyperpolarization. Membrane depolarization not only opens VDCCs to elevate $[Ca^{2+}]_{cyt}$ but also (1) facilitates the production of inositol 1,4,5-trisphosphate (IP_3), which stimulates the release of SR Ca^{2+} into the cytoplasm, and (2) promotes Ca^{2+} entry via reverse-mode Na^+–Ca^{2+} exchange. Sustained elevation of $[Ca^{2+}]_{cyt}$ induces sustained vasoconstriction and mechanical stretch of the PASMC membrane, which indirectly contributes to smooth muscle cell hypertrophy and vascular remodeling. Membrane hyperpolarization, on the other hand, closes the VDCC, reduces $[Ca^{2+}]_{cyt}$, and leads to vasodilation.

A. Extracellular Ca^{2+} Influx is Required for Pulmonary Vasoconstriction

The fact that Ca^{2+} is necessary for pulmonary vasoconstriction is further illustrated by induction of pulmonary vasoconstriction by either raising extracellular K^+ concentration from 5 to 40 mM (which shifts the equilibrium potential for K^+ and causes membrane depolarization) or applying phenylephrine, an α-adrenoceptor agonist, to rat pulmonary arterial rings (Fig. 2A). The 40 mM K^+-induced pulmonary vasoconstriction is mainly attributed to membrane depolarization-mediated opening of VDCCs and Ca^{2+} influx, whereas the phenylephrine-induced constriction is caused by both Ca^{2+} release from the SR and Ca^{2+} influx through ROCs and SOCs (also see Fig. 1). Removal of extracellular Ca^{2+} abolishes the 40 mM K^+-induced pulmonary vasoconstriction and significantly inhibits the agonist-mediated sustained contraction in isolated PA rings (Fig. 2A), suggesting that a rise in $[Ca^{2+}]_{cyt}$ due to Ca^{2+} influx plays a pivotal role in mediating pulmonary vasoconstriction (13).

B. Extracellular Ca^{2+} Influx is Necessary for Mitogen-Mediated PASMC Growth

Pulmonary vascular medial hypertrophy is mainly due to excessive PASMC proliferation. In addition to causing smooth muscle cell contraction, Ca^{2+} also participates in regulating PASMC growth through its intimate involvement with the cell cycle. A rise in cytoplasmic and nuclear $[Ca^{2+}]$ is required for the transition (1) from the G_0 (resting state) phase to the G_1 (beginning of DNA synthesis) phase, (2) from G_1 to S phase (DNA synthesis), and (3) from G_2 to the M (mitosis) phase, as well as for the whole mitotic process (Fig. 1) (16). In addition to facilitating cell passage through the cell cycle, a rise in $[Ca^{2+}]_{cyt}$ also activates mitogen-activated protein II kinase (MAP II kinase), an enzyme involved in the phosphorylation cascade that leads to upregulating DNA synthesis-promoting factors (17,18). Furthermore, activation and expression of the early responsive gene *c-fos* is also dependent on intracellular Ca^{2+} and calmodulin (19). As shown in Fig. 2B, human PASMC proliferation is significantly inhibited by chelation of extracellular free Ca^{2+} with EGTA in the presence of 5% fetal bovine

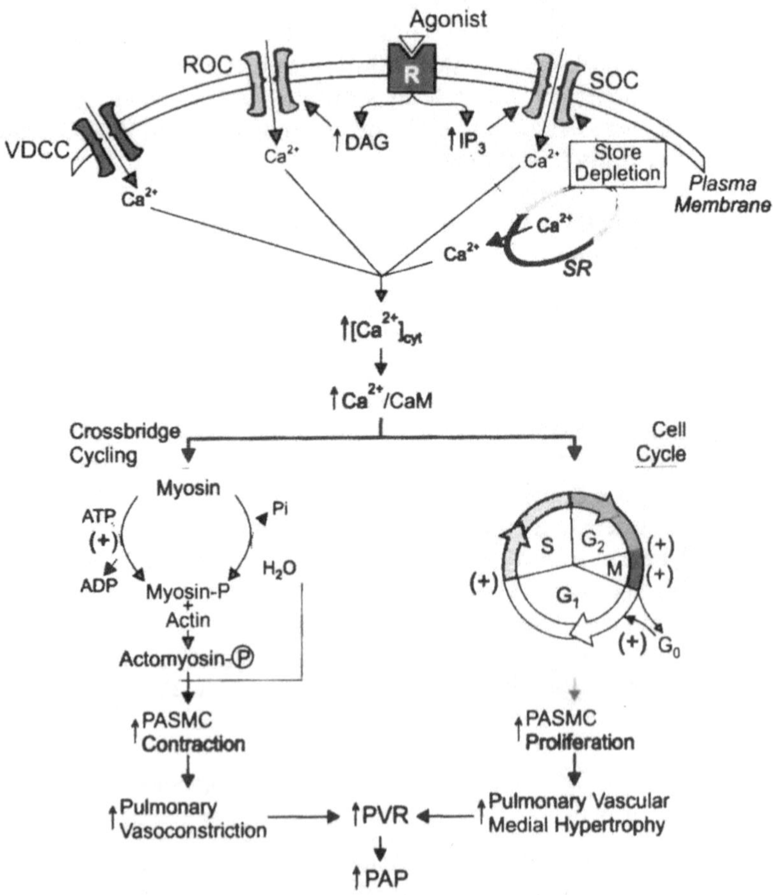

Figure 1 (*Caption on facing page.*)

serum and growth factors, suggesting that a constant influx of Ca^{2+} is necessary for PASMC proliferation.

Intracellular Ca^{2+} stores or levels of Ca^{2+} in the SR also influence cell growth. Depletion of Ca^{2+} from intracellular stores, such as the SR, causes smooth muscle cell growth arrest and, conversely, increases in Ca^{2+} cause the resumption of the S phase of the cell cycle, leading to mitosis (20,21). These observations demonstrate that sustained Ca^{2+} influx through sarcolemmal Ca^{2+} channels and sufficient Ca^{2+} maintained within the SR are both required for PASMC growth.

C. Cytoplasmic $[Ca^{2+}]$ is Increased in PASMCs from PPH Patients

An increase in $[Ca^{2+}]_{cyt}$ in PASMCs contributes to initiating and maintaining vasoconstriction and cell growth, two processes that are enhanced in PPH. It is therefore not unexpected that the resting $[Ca^{2+}]_{cyt}$ is much higher in PASMCs from patients with PPH than in cells from patients with nonpulmonary hypertension (NPH), cardiopulmonary disease, or SPH (Fig. 3A), even though PPH and SPH patients both have pulmonary vascular medial hypertrophy (Fig. 3B) and often have similar PAP (22). Because the resting $[Ca^{2+}]_{cyt}$ levels are higher in PPH-PASMCs, the $[Ca^{2+}]$ in the SR ($[Ca^{2+}]_{SR}$)

Figure 1 *(Facing page)* Regulation of $[Ca^{2+}]_{cyt}$ and the role of intracellular Ca^{2+} in the development of pulmonary hypertension. $[Ca^{2+}]_{cyt}$ is increased by Ca^{2+} release from the sarcoplasmic reticulum (SR) and Ca^{2+} influx through voltage-dependent Ca^{2+} channels (VDCCs), receptor-operated Ca^{2+} channel (ROC), and store-operated Ca^{2+} (SOCs) channels. Activity of VDCCs is controlled by membrane potential; membrane depolarization (i.e., due to inhibition of K^+ channel function) opens VDCCs and increases Ca^{2+} entry. Upon activation of membrane receptors, increased diacylglycerol (DAG) and inositol 1,4,5-trisphosphate (IP_3) activate ROCs in the plasma membrane and IP_3 receptors in the SR, respectively, and cause Ca^{2+} influx and release. The IP_3-mediated Ca^{2+} mobilization leads to store depletion that then opens SOCs to trigger capacitative Ca^{2+} entry (CCE) for refilling Ca^{2+} into the SR and for maintaining a high level of $[Ca^{2+}]_{cyt}$. When $[Ca^{2+}]_{cyt}$ rises, Ca^{2+} binds to calmodulin (CaM) to form a Ca^{2+}/CaM complex, which stimulates the activity of myosin ATPase [shown as (+)], hydrolyzing ATP to generate energy for the cycling of the myosin cross-bridges with the actin filament. The formation of these cross-bridges underlies smooth muscle cell contraction, prompting vasoconstriction. Furthermore, elevated $[Ca^{2+}]_{cyt}$ is responsible for propelling the quiescent cells into the cell cycle and mitosis and eventually stimulating cell proliferation. The Ca^{2+}/CaM complex activates at least four steps in the cell cycle, shown as (+). Pulmonary vasoconstriction and vascular remodeling lead to chronic and sustained elevation of pulmonary vascular resistance (PVR) and pulmonary arterial pressure (PAP) and cause pulmonary hypertension.

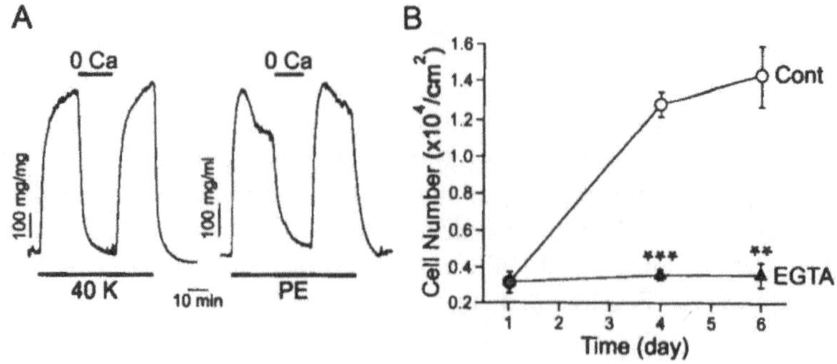

Figure 2 Extracellular Ca^{2+} is required for pulmonary vasoconstriction and PASMC proliferation. (A) Isometric tension in an isolated rat pulmonary arterial ring was measured before, during, and after application of 40 mM K^+ (40 K) or 2 μM phenylephrine (PE). Extracellular Ca^{2+} was removed when 40 K- and PE-mediated contractions reached plateaus. (B) Cell numbers were determined in PASMCs cultured (for 1–6 days) in serum-containing media with (EGTA) or without (Cont) 2 mM EGTA, a chelator of free Ca^{2+}. (***) $P < 0.001$; (**) $P < 0.01$ vs. Cont. (Reproduced with permission from Refs. 13 and 59.)

may also be significantly higher due to Ca^{2+} sequestration mediated by the Ca^{2+}-ATPase in the SR membrane (23). Indeed, the increase in $[Ca^{2+}]_{cyt}$ due to Ca^{2+} mobilization from intracellular stores by cyclopiazonic acid (CPA) is significantly greater in PASMCs from PPH patients than in those from SPH patients (see Sec. IV) (24). This supports the hypothesis that there is

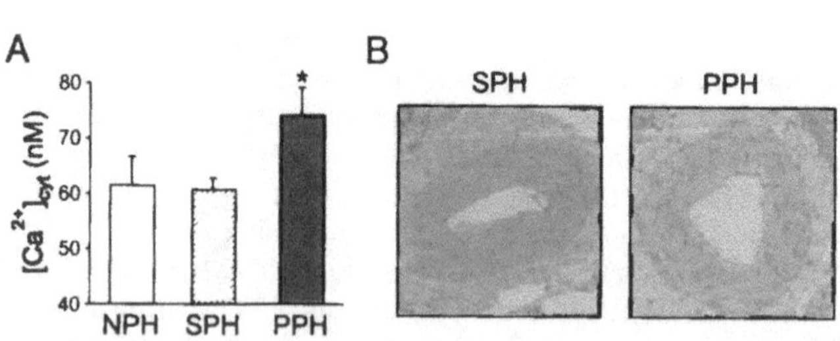

Figure 3 Resting $[Ca^{2+}]_{cyt}$ in PASMCs is increased in patients with primary pulmonary hypertension (PPH). (A) Summarized data showing resting $[Ca^{2+}]_{cyt}$ in PASMCs from patients with normotensive (NPH) disease, secondary pulmonary hypertension (SPH), and PPH. (*) $P < 0.05$ vs. NPH and SPH. (B) Histological examination of muscular pulmonary arteries in lung tissues isolated from patients with SPH (right) and PPH (left) demonstrates a similar degree of medial hypertrophy. Hematoxylin eosin stain, original magnification ×200. (Reproduced with permission from Refs. 22 and 45.)

a unique "defect" within the PASMCs of PPH patients that results in increased $[Ca^{2+}]_{cyt}$.

III. ROLE OF DYSFUNCTIONAL OR DOWNREGULATED K_V CHANNELS IN THE DEVELOPMENT OF PPH

A. Activity of K_V Channels Regulates Resting E_m

Because of the voltage dependence of VDCCs, E_m is a key determinant of $[Ca^{2+}]_{cyt}$. As stated earlier, membrane depolarization results in a sustained increase in $[Ca^{2+}]_{cyt}$ via extracellular Ca^{2+} influx through VDCCs (11,25) and triggers the release of Ca^{2+} from the SR into the cytoplasm by facilitating the production of IP_3 (26). The E_m in vascular smooth muscle cells is determined by the concentration gradients of electrically charged ions across the plasma membrane and the membrane permeability of the ions. The transmembrane K^+ current, generated by K^+ efflux through K^+ channels, plays a significant role in regulating the resting E_m in PASMCs (27,28).

In vascular smooth muscles, there are at least five types of K^+ channels: (1) voltage-gated K^+ (K_V) channels (27,29), (2) Ca^{2+}-activated K^+ (K_{Ca}) channels (30), (3) ATP-sensitive K^+ (K_{ATP}) channels (31), (4) inward-rectifier K^+ (K_{IR}) channels (32), and (5) tandem-pore K^+ (K_T) channels (33). K^+ currents through K_V channels (and K_T channels) are predominantly responsible for the resting E_m in PASMCs (27,28). The amplitude of whole-cell K_V currents ($I_{K(V)}$) not only depends on the conductance and open probability of single K_V channels but also relies on the number of K_V channels that are expressed in the plasma membrane. Therefore, inhibition of K_V channel conductance or open probability and downregulation of K_V channel expression can both cause membrane depolarization by decreasing whole-cell $I_{K(V)}$, which subsequently increases $[Ca^{2+}]_{cyt}$ by promoting Ca^{2+} influx through VDCCs and by facilitating Ca^{2+} release via increasing IP_3 production (Fig. 4A).

B. Dysfunction and Downregulation of K_V Channels are Involved in the Elevation of $[Ca^{2+}]_{cyt}$ in PASMCs from PPH Patients

In native cells, functional K_V channels are heteromultimeric tetramers composed of two subunits, the pore forming α subunit and the regulatory β subunit (34). In PASMCs from PPH patients, we observed that whole-cell $I_{K(V)}$ was significantly decreased in comparison to PASMCs from patients with non pulmonary hypertension (NPH), cardiopulmonary diseases, and SPH (Fig. 4B) (22). The decreased $I_{K(V)}$ was associated with a more depolarized E_m in PPH-PASMCs [Fig. 4B(c)]. Furthermore, the mRNA expression of some K_V channel α subunits, such as Kv1.5 (Fig. 4C) and Kv1.2, was also significantly downregulated in PASMCs from PPH patients compared to cells from normal subjects and NPH and SPH patients (35). The

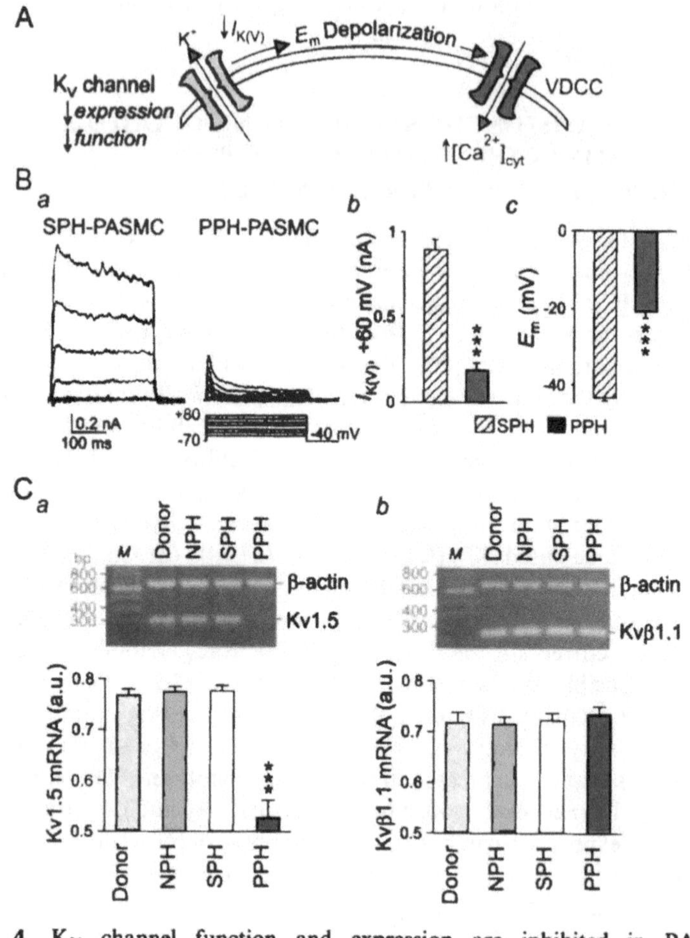

Figure 4 K_V channel function and expression are inhibited in PASMCs from patients with PPH. (A) Schematic diagram depicting that decreased K_V currents ($I_{K(V)}$), due to inhibited K_V channel function and expression, cause membrane depolarization and promote Ca^{2+} influx by opening voltage-dependent Ca^{2+} channels (VDCCs). E_m, membrane potential. (B) Representative whole-cell $I_{K(V)}$ (a), elicited by depolarization to test potentials ranging from −40 to +80 mV (holding potential, −70 mV), in PASMCs from patients with secondary pulmonary hypertension (SPH) and PPH. Averaged current amplitude at +60 mV (b) and resting E_m (c) are expressed as mean ± SE. (***) $P < 0.001$ vs. SPH. (C) RT-PCR-amplified products are displayed in agarose gels for Kv1.5 (a) and Kvβ1.1 (b) in PASMCs from normal subjects (Donors) and patients with normotensive (NPH) cardiopulmonary disease, SPH, and PPH. β-Actin was used as a positive control. "*M*" represents DNA ladder. Data normalized to the amount of *β*-actin are expressed as means ± SE (lower panels). (***) $P < 0.001$ vs. Donors, NPH and SPH. (Reproduced with permission from Refs. 22 and 35.)

downregulation of K_V channel mRNA expression would cause a decrease in the number of functional K_V channels, resulting in a reduced whole-cell $I_{K(V)}$ and membrane depolarization (Fig. 4B).

In smooth muscle cells, the voltage window for activation of plasmalemmal L-type VDCCs and sustained elevation of $[Ca^{2+}]_{cyt}$ ranges between −40 and −15 mV (25). Therefore, the membrane depolarization that occurs in PASMCs from PPH patients would cause a sustained increase in $[Ca^{2+}]_{cyt}$ (Fig. 3A) by promoting Ca^{2+} entry through opened VDCCs (11,22,25,27). Indeed, in PASMCs from PPH patients, the resting $[Ca^{2+}]_{cyt}$ is much higher than in PASMCs from patients with NPH or SPH (Fig. 3A). In addition, the more depolarized E_m in PPH-PASMCs may also promote Ca^{2+} mobilization due to increased production of IP_3, further contributing to the elevated $[Ca^{2+}]_{cyt}$.

In summary, downregulated K_V channel expression and decreased whole-cell $I_{K(V)}$ in PASMCs from PPH patients may be important for elevating $[Ca^{2+}]_{cyt}$ by activating VDCCs. The increased $[Ca^{2+}]_{cyt}$ in PASMCs, as mentioned earlier, not only causes pulmonary vasoconstriction but also stimulates PASMCs proliferation, ultimately contributing to the development of pulmonary vascular remodeling.

C. Decreased K_V Channel Activity Leads to Inhibition of Apoptotic Volume Decrease and Apoptosis

Apoptosis is a physiological mode of cell death that is triggered by diverse external and internal signals. Dysfunction of the programmed cell death process contributes to the pathogenesis of cancer, atherosclerosis, and pulmonary vascular disease. Although apoptosis has long been recognized as a principal mechanism for the elimination of redundant, autoreactive, or neoplastic cells, it may also be a mechanism for the elimination of "abnormally" proliferative or hypertrophied PASMCs in the remodeled pulmonary vasculature (36–38). Indeed, regression of medial hypertrophy has been attributed to apoptosis of hypertrophied PASMCs, whereas inhibition of apoptosis is related to progression of pulmonary vascular medial thickening in animal models (38). Therefore, precise control of the balance between PASMC proliferation and apoptosis is important in maintaining the structural and functional integrity of the pulmonary vasculature. Disturbance of this balance seems to be an important anomaly that leads to increased proliferation and decreased apoptosis of PASMCs, contributing to vessel wall thickening and vascular remodeling (36–38).

Cell shrinkage or volume loss is an early characteristic feature of cells undergoing apoptosis. This process is called apoptotic volume decrease (AVD). Potassium (K^+), a dominant cation in the cytosol at a concentration of 140–150 mM, plays a critical role in maintaining intracellular ion homeostasis and cell volume. Loss of intracellular K^+ ($[K^+]_i$) is in part responsible for AVD (39). K^+ channels thus play an important role in regulating apoptosis by modulating the K^+ flux across the plasma membrane. Activation of K^+ channels leads to efflux or loss of K^+, which induces or accelerates AVD and apoptosis (Fig. 5A). Conversely, inhibition or decreased activity of K^+ channels has been shown to cause accumulation of K^+ in the cells, maintaining $[K^+]_i$ sufficiently high to decelerate AVD and inhibit apoptosis. Furthermore, maintenance of sufficient $[K^+]_i$ appears to suppress the activity of caspases and nucleases (40–44). In short, diminished $[K^+]_i$ due to increased K^+ efflux through plasmalemmal K^+ channels results in cell shrinkage and the activation of cytoplasmic caspases, whereas maintenance of sufficient K^+ in the cytosol due to decreased activity of K^+ channels inhibits apoptosis.

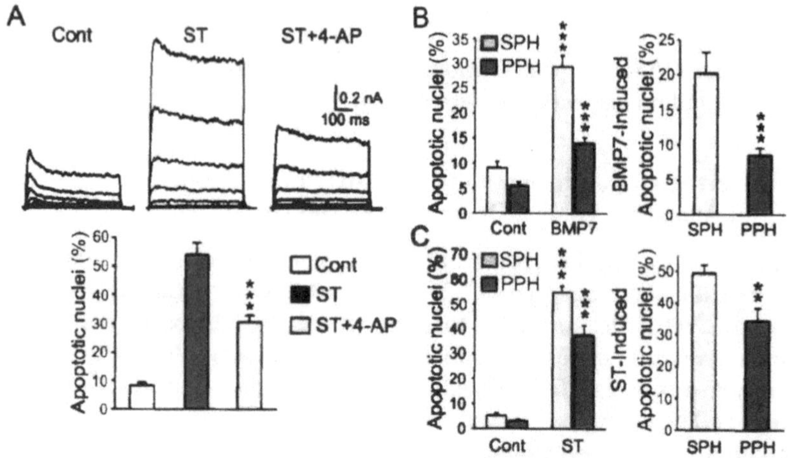

Figure 5 Decreased $I_{K(V)}$ is associated with inhibited apoptosis in PASMCs from patients with PPH. (A) Representative families of currents (upper panels) elicited by depolarization to test potentials ranging from −40 to +80 mV (holding potential, −70 mV) in a normal PASMC before (Cont) and during treatment with staurosporine (ST, 20 nM), an apoptosis inducer, in the absence (ST) or presence (ST+4-AP) of 4-aminopyridine (4-AP, 5 mM), a potent blocker of K_V channels. Summarized data showing the percentage of apoptotic nuclei in PASMCs cultured in control medium and media containing ST or ST+4-AP are shown in the accompanying bar graph. (***) $P<0.001$ vs. ST. (B, C) Comparison of apoptotic effects of BMP7 (200 nM) and ST (20 nM) on PASMCs isolated from patients with SPH and PPH. Cells were cultured in media that included vehicle (Cont), BMP7 (B), or ST (C). Data are expressed as means ± SE from 14–15 experiments. Normalized apoptotic effects of BMP7 and ST to baseline control levels of apoptosis before treatment are shown in the right-hand panels. (***) $P<0.001$; (**) $P<0.01$ vs. Cont or SPH. (Reproduced with permission from Refs. 45 and 60.)

We previously reported that apoptosis induced in PASMCs from PPH patients, by bone morphogenetic proteins (BMPs) and staurosporine was significantly inhibited in comparison to cells isolated from SPH patients (Figs. 5B and C) (45). Furthermore, overexpression of the $K_V1.5$ gene in PASMCs increased whole-cell $I_{K(V)}$, markedly accelerated staurosporine-mediated apoptotic cell shrinkage, and enhanced apoptosis (46). These data suggest that the inhibited apoptosis in PPH-PASMCs may be related to decreased K_V channel activity.

D. K_V Channels are Regulated by Pro- and Antiapoptotic Agents

Further evidence that K_V channels may play a significant role in the apoptotic pathway comes from experiments involving staurosporine and Bcl-2 (47). Staurosporine is a potent apoptosis inducer that increases whole-cell $I_{K(V)}$ (Fig. 5A), leading to the loss of $[K^+]_i$ and, ultimately, initiation of AVD and apoptosis. Bcl-2, on the other hand, is an antiapoptotic protein. Overexpression of Bcl-2 decreases whole-cell $I_{K(V)}$, leading to maintenance of a healthy $[K^+]_i$ level and prevention of AVD (47). When K^+ efflux through K_V channels is pharmacologically blocked by 4-AP, the staurosporine-induced apoptosis is attenuated (Fig. 5A). Additionally, the staurosporine-mediated apoptosis is inhibited in PASMCs transfected with the Bcl-2 gene in comparison to those cells transfected with an empty vector (47). These experiments show that the antiapoptotic protein-mediated decrease in $I_{K(V)}$, similar to functional blockade of K_V channels (e.g., by 4-AP), is an important mechanism by which Bcl-2 (and other antiapoptotic proteins) enhances cell survival in human and rat PASMCs. Dysfunctional apoptotic pathways, due partially to downregulated K_V channels, in PASMCs from PPH patients may play a role in the development of pulmonary vascular medial hypertrophy.

IV. ROLE OF UPREGULATED TRPC CHANNELS AND ENHANCED CAPACITATIVE Ca^{2+} ENTRY IN THE DEVELOPMENT OF PPH

In addition to Ca^{2+} influx through VDCCs, $[Ca^{2+}]_{cyt}$ can also be increased by promoting Ca^{2+} influx through receptor-operated Ca^{2+} channels (ROCs) and store-operated Ca^{2+} channels (SOCs) (Fig. 1). Therefore, the elevated $[Ca^{2+}]_{cyt}$ in PPH-PASMCs may be caused by multiple mechanisms; i.e., enhanced Ca^{2+} entry through VDCCs opened by membrane depolarization due to inhibited K_V channels is only one of the important pathways for elevated $[Ca^{2+}]_{cyt}$ and its resultant sequelae in the development of pulmonary vasoconstriction and vascular remodeling in PPH. Activation of SOCs by depletion of intracellular Ca^{2+} stores has been implicated in the elevation of $[Ca^{2+}]_{cyt}$ in PASMCs from PPH patients.

Calcium-mediated stimulation of cell proliferation involves increases in cytoplasmic and nuclear [Ca^{2+}] and maintenance of sufficient Ca^{2+} in the SR. Upon activation of membrane receptors (e.g., G-protein coupled receptors and tyrosine kinase receptors) by mitogenic agonists (e.g., ET-1, 5-HT, ATP, PDGF, EGF), an initial transient increase in $[Ca^{2+}]_{cyt}$ is usually due to Ca^{2+} release from the SR, which is then followed by a sustained increase in $[Ca^{2+}]_{cyt}$ stemming from Ca^{2+} influx through sarcolemmal Ca^{2+} channels (by opening both ROCs and SOCs). Both components (i.e., agonist-mediated Ca^{2+} mobilization and Ca^{2+} influx) contribute to promoting cell proliferation by stimulating quiescent cells to enter the cell cycle as well as by driving proliferating cells through the cell cycle and mitosis (Fig. 1). Beyond signal transduction, an adequate level of Ca^{2+} in the SR is crucial for normal cellular functions including posttranslational modifications (e.g., correct folding, assembly, and glycosylation) of recombinant proteins. Therefore, maintenance of a high $[Ca^{2+}]_{SR}$ also plays an important role in optimizing protein and lipid synthesis and sorting.

A. TRP Channels are Involved in Forming SOCs Responsible for Capacitative Ca^{2+} Entry

Influx of Ca^{2+} through SOCs plays an important role in refilling the depleted SR stores and in maintaining a sustained increase in $[Ca^{2+}]_{cyt}$ during agonist stimulation via a mechanism known as capacitative Ca^{2+} entry (CCE) (48,49). Therefore, CCE is a mechanism that links $[Ca^{2+}]_{SR}$ to plasma membrane Ca^{2+} permeability and allows for the refilling of intracellular Ca^{2+} stores and maintenance of Ca^{2+} influx. It is important to understand that SOC channels are not selectively permeable for Ca^{2+}; they also allow for the passage of other cations such as Na^{+}.

The molecular composition of functional SOCs, which are responsible for CCE, in vascular smooth muscle cells is not fully understood. However, numerous reports have indicated that the transient receptor potential (TRP) channels participate in forming functional SOCs (and ROCs) in native cells (excitable and nonexcitable cells). This is based on observations that expression of *TRP* genes in the heterologous transfection system leads to the formation of Ca^{2+}-permeable channels activated by store depletion and receptor activation (48–52). Each *TRP*-encoded subunit contains six transmembrane domains (S1–S6) with a pore-forming loop between S5 and S6, and both the N- and C-termini are located in the cytoplasm (52).

The mammalian TRP family can be divided into three subfamilies: (1) the TRP-canonical (TRPC) family (or short TRP channels), which comprises seven members, TRPC1–7; (2) the TRP-vanilloid (TRPV) family (or Osm-9-like TRP channels), which consists of six members, TRPV1–6; and (3) the TRP-melastatin (TRPM) family (or long TRP channels), which has eight members, TRPM1–8 (52). There are three or more ankyrin domains in the N-terminal cytosolic region of the short (TRPC) and Osm-9-like (TRPV) TRP channels, a proline-rich cytosolic motif in the cytosolic C-terminal region in the vicinity of S6 of the short and long (TRPM) TRP channels (52). It has been demonstrated that native SOCs are mainly hetero-tetramers consisting of different TRP isoforms (48–52). Sensitivity to store depletion may be mediated by the cytosolic C-terminal tail connected to the S6 transmembrane domain, but the mechanism linking store depletion to SOC activation is still unclear. The greatest homology between the subfamilies is seen in the S6 transmembrane domain, and the greatest variance is found in the carboxyl terminus. The subfamily members differ in their distribution throughout the body as well as in their mode of regulation (49).

Of the known TRP channels, TRPC1, 2, 4, 5, and 6 are expressed in human PASMCs. Additionally, TRPC1, 3, and 5 are expressed in pulmonary artery endothelial cells (50,51,53–55). Inhibition of TRPC1 and TRPC6 with antisense oligonucleotides specifically targeting on these channels' mRNA attenuates CCE in PASMCs induced by passive depletion of the SR Ca^{2+} using cyclopiazonic acid (CPA), a blocker of the Ca^{2+}, Mg^{2+}-ATPase in the SR membrane (50,51,53). Furthermore, inhibition of TRPC4 with small interfering RNA (siRNA) specifically for TRPC4 mRNA also attenuates CPA-mediated CCE in pulmonary artery endothelial cells (54). These observations suggest that TRPC1, 4, and 6 are potentially involved in forming functional SOCs in PASMCs and pulmonary artery endothelial cells that are activated by store depletion.

B. CCE is Important in Pulmonary Vasoconstriction

Store-operated Ca^{2+} channels play an important physiological role in contributing to agonist-mediated pulmonary vasoconstriction, distinct from that of VDCCs or ROCs. Ca^{2+} influx induced by activation of membrane receptors involves both ROCs and SOCs. In isolated rat pulmonary artery rings, as shown in Fig. 6, the contraction induced by CCE can be distinguished from the contraction induced by Ca^{2+} through SOCs. In the absence of extracellular Ca^{2+}, application of phenylephrine (PE), an α-adrenoceptor agonist, causes a transient contraction (or increase in tension) due apparently to Ca^{2+} mobilization from the SR, eventually depleting the SR Ca^{2+} stores. When the transient contraction (or increase in tension) returns to the baseline level, indicative of store depletion, the α-adrenoceptor blocker phentolamine is applied to terminate the receptor-coupled signaling cascade (e.g., production of IP_3 and diacylglycerol and activation of PKCs) that is required to open ROCs. Restoration of extracellular Ca^{2+} in the presence of the α-receptor blocker phentolamine and the VDCC blocker verapamil induces a similar contraction that is selectively due to CCE triggered by PE-induced store depletion (Fig. 6B). Washout of phentolamine in the presence of extracellular Ca^{2+} and the agonist phenylephrine induces a

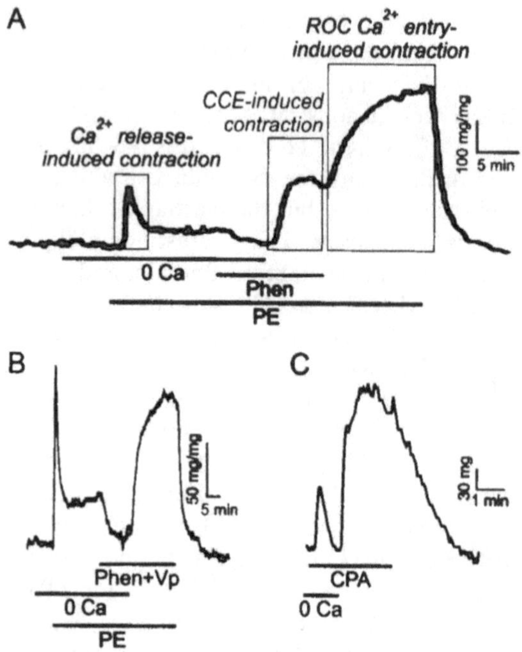

Figure 6 Capacitative Ca^{2+} entry mediates vasoconstriction in isolated rat pulmonary arterial rings. (A) Phenylephrine (PE) (2 μM) was first applied to the vessel in the absence of extracellular Ca^{2+}, which induced contraction due to Ca^{2+} mobilization from the SR. Phentolamine (Phen) (1 μM), an α-adrenoceptor blocker, was then applied to the vessel when the PE-induced transient contraction returned to the baseline. In the presence of Phen, restoration of extracellular Ca^{2+} induced a contraction, which was mostly likely due to CCE. Removal of Phen in the presence of PE further enhanced the contraction, likely due to Ca^{2+} influx via receptor-operated Ca^{2+} channels (ROC). (B) Addition of verapamil (Vp) (0.5 μM), a dihydropyridine blocker of voltage-dependent Ca^{2+} channels, did not affect the CCE-mediated contraction. (C) Depletion of stored Ca^{2+} by cyclopiazonic acid (CPA) (50 μM), an inhibitor of the Ca^{2+}, Mg^{2+}-ATPase in the SR, causes pulmonary vasoconstriction. CPA applied to the vessel in the absence of extracellular Ca^{2+} caused a transient contraction, which was likely due to a transient rise in $[Ca^{2+}]_{cyt}$ resulting from leakage of Ca^{2+} from the SR to the cytosol. Restoration of extracellular Ca^{2+} caused a large contraction, likely due to CCE. (Reproduced with permission from Ref. 13.)

further contraction, which is potentially due to Ca^{2+} influx through ROCs (Fig. 6A). The CCE-mediated pulmonary artery contraction in the presence of phentolamine and verapamil accounts for approximately 23% of the total peak contraction induced by PE in the presence of extracellular Ca^{2+} (13). Furthermore, CPA-mediated passive depletion of Ca^{2+} also induces a sustained contraction in isolated pulmonary arteries with (Fig. 6C) and without endothelium. Furthermore, blockade of SOCs with Ni^{2+}, La^{3+}, or SK&F 96365 markedly reduces the amplitude of I_{SOC} and CCE in PASMCs and significantly attenuates the CCE-mediated pulmonary vasoconstriction (Kunichika, Yu, and Yuan, unpublished data). These results provide evidence that in addition to Ca^{2+} entry through VDCCs and ROCs, CCE is also involved in mediating pulmonary artery contraction in response to vasoconstricting agonists.

C. CCE is Enhanced and TRP Channels are Upregulated in Proliferating PASMCs

During cell division, the chromosomes must be duplicated and segregated into the daughter cells. Eukaryotic cells duplicate and segregate their chromosomes at distinct times during cell division. The events required for a single round of cell division, collectively known as the cell cycle, can be divided into four phases: G_1, S, G_2, and M. DNA synthesis occurs during the S phase of the cell cycle, resulting in the duplication of each chromosome. Chromosome segregation occurs during mitosis, or the M phase of the cell cycle. Ca^{2+}/CaM is required for both chromosome duplication and segregation (16–21).

In comparison to growth-arrested cells (cultured in media without serum and growth factors), proliferating human PASMCs (cultured in media containing serum and growth factors) exhibit a high level of resting $[Ca^{2+}]_{cyt}$ potentially maintained by a constant Ca^{2+} influx. Removal or chelation of extracellular free Ca^{2+} significantly inhibits PASMC proliferation, determined by cell number, [^{3}H]thymidine incorporation, BrdU uptake, and protein and DNA content (50). Interestingly, PASMC proliferation is associated with a significant increase in mRNA and protein expression of TRPC channels such as TRPC1 (Fig. 7A) (50). After incubation of previously growth-arrested PASMCs in media containing serum and growth factors for 6 days, the time course of changes in TRPC1 mRNA level and cell number indicates that the increase in TRPC1 mRNA expression precedes the increase in cell number [Fig. 7A(c)]. In other words, upregulation of TRPC channel gene expression may be prerequisite for cell division or chromosome duplication and segregation. Consistent with the upregulated TRPC channel expression, the amplitude of CCE is also significantly greater in proliferating PASMCs than in growth-arrested cells (Fig. 7B) (50,53). Inhibition of TRPC1 expression (53) with antisense oligonucleotides specifically targeting on the TRPC1 gene markedly decreases the amplitude of CCE (Fig. 8A) and significantly inhibits PASMC proliferation in the presence of serum and growth factors (Fig. 8B).

In addition to TRPC1, TRPC6, a TRPC isoform that is preferentially expressed in lung tissues and pulmonary arteries, is also upregulated when

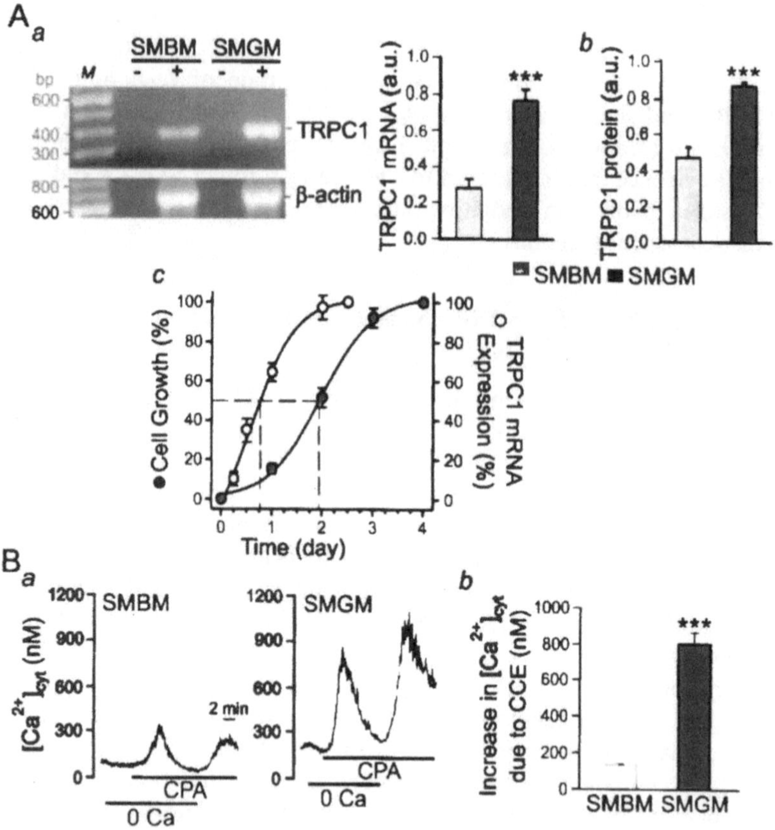

Figure 7 TRPC1 expression is upregulated in PASMCs during proliferation. (A) RT-PCR-amplified products on agarose gel (a) for TRPC1 (372 bp) and β-actin (661 bp) in growth-arrested (cultured in SMBM) and proliferating (cultured in SMGM) cells. The RT-PCR was performed in the presence (+) or absence (−) of reverse transcriptase. *M*, 100 bp DNA ladder. Summarized data (mean ± SE) showing the mRNA (*a*, right panel) and protein (b) levels of TRPC1, normalized to the amount of β-actin, in growth-arrested (SMBM) and proliferating (SMGM) cells. The time course (*c*) shows the relative changes in (•) cell number and (○) TRPC1 mRNA expression in proliferating PASMCs (cultured in SMGM for up to 4 days). Vertical broken lines indicate the time required for a 50% increase in cell growth or TRPC1 mRNA expression. (B) Representative records (*a*) showing the time course of $[Ca^{2+}]_{cyt}$ changes induced by CPA (10 μM) in the absence (0 Ca) or presence of extracellular Ca^{2+} in growth-arrested (SMBM) and proliferating (SMGM) PASMCs. Summarized data (*b*) showing the increase in $[Ca^{2+}]_{cyt}$ due to CCE in growth-arrested (SMBM) and proliferating (SMGM) cells. (***) $P < 0.001$ vs. SMBM. (Reproduced with permission from Refs. 50 and 53.)

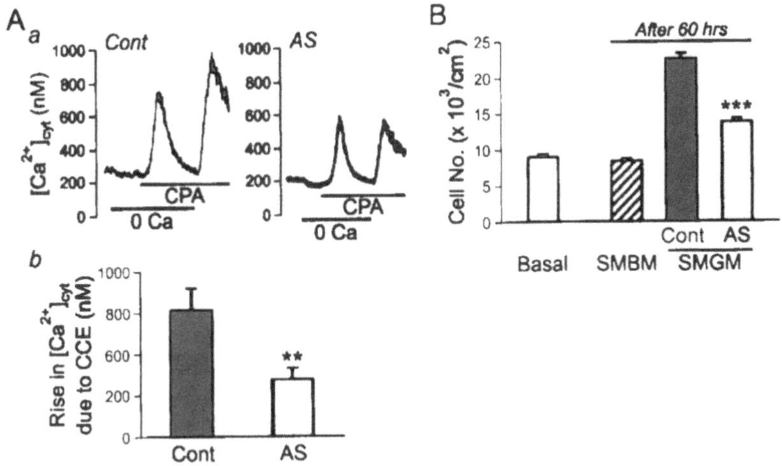

Figure 8 Downregulation of human TRPC1 gene expression with antisense oligonucleotides (AS) attenuates CCE and inhibits PASMC proliferation. (A) Representative records (*a*) showing the time course of $[Ca^{2+}]_{cyt}$ changes in cells treated with control (Cont) or AS oligonucleotides (specifically targeting TRPC1 mRNA). CPA (10 μM) was applied to the cells in the absence (0 Ca) and presence of 1.8 mM extracellular Ca^{2+}. Summarized data (*b*) showing the CCE amplitudes in cells treated with control or AS oligonucleotides. (B) Cell numbers were determined before (basal) and after 60 h incubation in SMBM and in SMGM containing control or AS oligonucleotides. (**) $P<0.01$; (***) $P<0.001$ vs. Cont. (Reproduced with permission from Ref. 53.)

PASMCs proliferate in response to platelet-derived growth factor (PDGF) (55). The PDGF-mediated upregulation of TRPC6 expression is also associated with an increase in CCE, whereas pharmacological blockade of SOCs (e.g., with Ni^{2+} of La^{3+}) significantly decreases CCE, resulting in the inhibition of PDGF-mediated PASMC proliferation (55). PDGF levels are noted to be higher in lung tissues of patients with severe pulmonary hypertension, and PDGF is implicated in the development of pulmonary hypertension (56–58). Therefore, PDGF appears to mediate cell proliferation in part by upregulating TRPC6 expression and increasing CCE in PASMCs.

D. TRPC Channels are Upregulated in PASMCs from PPH Patients

In normal PASMCs, functional expression of TRPC channels (e.g., TRPC1 and TRPC6) is involved in agonist-mediated pulmonary vasoconstriction and mitogen-mediated cell proliferation. In addition to its essential role in normal pulmonary artery contraction and PASMC proliferation, increased CCE, secondary to increased formation of SOCs by upregulated TRPC genes, may be important in the development of pulmonary vascular remodeling in patients with PPH. Using PASMCs isolated from patients undergoing lung transplant for either PPH or SPH, our laboratory has been able to compare the magnitude of CCE between PPH-PASMCs and SPH-PASMCs. When matched for pulmonary arterial pressure and pulmonary vascular resistance, growth-arrested PASMCs from PPH patients demonstrate significantly higher resting $[Ca^{2+}]_{cyt}$ compared to cells from SPH patients (Fig. 9). In addition, the magnitude of CCE evoked by passive store depletion with CPA is significantly greater in PASMCs from PPH patients than in cells from SPH patients (Fig. 9) (50). PPH is a heterogeneous disorder with abnormal PASMC proliferation as its central theme. These data suggest that CCE is essential in maintaining the adequate cytoplasmic, nuclear, and SR Ca^{2+} required for PASMC proliferation. Enhanced CCE, possibly via upregulation of TRPC channels such as TRPC1, TRPC3, and TRPC6 (Yu, Remillard, Landsberg, and Yuan, unpublished data) may represent another critical downstream pathogenic event or mechanism involved in the development of severe pulmonary hypertension. Accordingly, interruption of CCE at any point, by agents ranging from those that downregulate TRPC gene expression to specific blockers for SOCs in

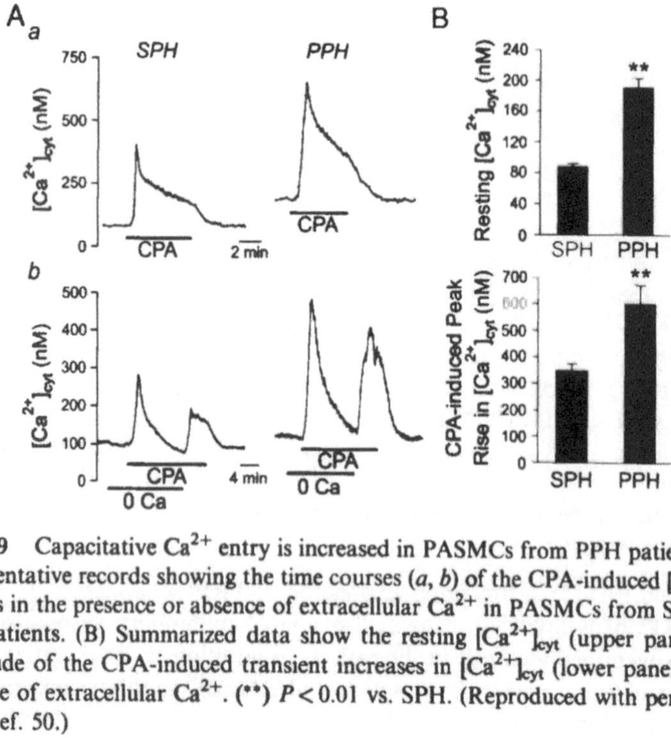

Figure 9 Capacitative Ca^{2+} entry is increased in PASMCs from PPH patients. (A) Representative records showing the time courses (*a*, *b*) of the CPA-induced $[Ca^{2+}]_{cyt}$ changes in the presence or absence of extracellular Ca^{2+} in PASMCs from SPH and PPH patients. (B) Summarized data show the resting $[Ca^{2+}]_{cyt}$ (upper panel) and amplitude of the CPA-induced transient increases in $[Ca^{2+}]_{cyt}$ (lower panel) in the presence of extracellular Ca^{2+}. (**) $P < 0.01$ vs. SPH. (Reproduced with permission from Ref. 50.)

PASMCs, may prove beneficial in the development of therapeutic approaches for treatment of severe pulmonary hypertension.

V. SUMMARY

The predominant pathological findings in PPH include pulmonary vasoconstriction, vascular wall remodeling (intimal and medial hypertrophy), vascular injury, and in situ thrombosis. A sustained increase in $[Ca^{2+}]_{cyt}$, which is involved in regulating many cell functions (e.g., smooth muscle contraction and cell growth), plays an important role in the pathogenesis of PPH. Intracellular $[Ca^{2+}]$ (e.g., $[Ca^{2+}]_{cyt}$ and $[Ca^{2+}]_{SR}$) is much higher in PASMCs from PPH patients than in PASMCs isolated from normal subjects and patients with nonpulmonary hypertension disease and SPH, suggesting

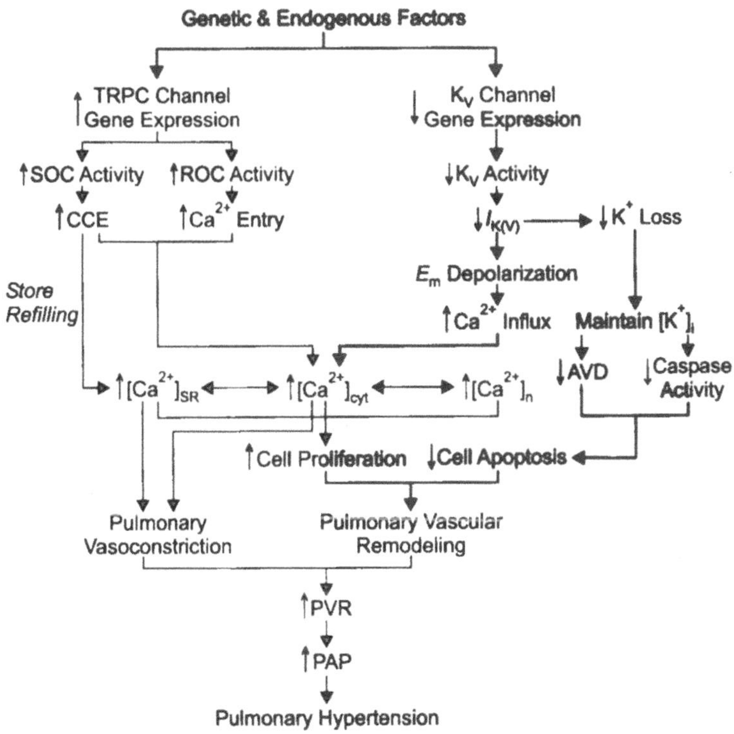

Figure 10 Schematic diagram depicting the potential roles of upregulated TRPC channels and downregulated K_V channels in the development of pulmonary hypertension. SOC, store-operated Ca^{2+} channel; ROC, receptor-operated Ca^{2+} channel; CCE, capacitative Ca^{2+} entry; $[Ca^{2+}]_{SR}$, $[Ca^{2+}]$ in the SR; $[Ca^{2+}]_n$, nuclear $[Ca^{2+}]$; AVD, apoptotic volume decrease; PVR, pulmonary vascular resistance; PAP, pulmonary arterial pressure.

a unique role of increased $[Ca^{2+}]_{cyt}$ in mediating pulmonary vasoconstriction and vascular medial hypertrophy in PPH. Membrane depolarization-mediated increase in $[Ca^{2+}]_{cyt}$ due to opening of VDCCs is not only an important mechanism in excitation–contraction coupling in vascular smooth muscle but also a pathway involved in stimulating PASMC hypertrophy and proliferation (59). Owing to its dependence on K^+ permeability across the plasma membrane, E_m is regulated by the activity of K^+ channels. The downregulated or dysfunctional K_V channels in PASMCs from PPH patients may be a critical cause of the elevated $[Ca^{2+}]_{cyt}$ in PPH-PASMCs via activation of VDCCs (Fig. 10). Clinical studies, however, demonstrate that only 15–20% of PPH patients respond to conventional VDCC blockers (e.g., nifedipine and diltiazem), suggesting that other mechanisms (or Ca^{2+}-permeable channels) may be involved in augmenting Ca^{2+} influx in PASMCs from PPH patients.

In addition to VDCCs, PASMCs also express functional SOCs, putatively formed by TRPC channel subunits, which represents another important pathway for extracellular Ca^{2+} entry. CCE, potentially through heterotetrameric TRPC channels in PASMCs, is an important process for cell proliferation and for vasoconstriction (50,51,53–55). Upregulation of TRPC channels and augmentation of the amplitude of CCE in PASMCs may be another cause of the elevated $[Ca^{2+}]_{cyt}$ in some PPH patients (Fig. 10). Accordingly, TRPC channel subunits may serve as a novel pharmacological target for treatment of PPH in the future, especially for patients who do not respond to Ca^{2+} channel blockers. Currently, the optimal treatment for PPH is a multitargeted approach consisting of one or more combinations of prostacyclin, endothelin receptor blocker, Ca^{2+} channel blocker, and nitric oxide. Agents targeted on activating K^+ channels or blocking TRPC channels may be a promising alternative or an additional therapeutic measure on the horizon.

ACKNOWLEDGMENTS

We thank L. J. Rubin, O. Platoshyn, S. Zhang, Y. Yu, I. Fantozzi, N. Kunichika, D. Ekhterae, S. Krick, J. Kriett, and P. A. Thistlethwaite for their contributions to and assistance in this work. The work is supported by grants from the National Institutes of Health (HL54043, HL64945, HL66012, HL69758, and HL66941).

REFERENCES

1. Rubin LJ. Primary pulmonary hypertension. N Engl J Med 1997; 336:111–117.
2. Runo JR, Loyd JE. Primary pulmonary hypertension. Lancet 2003; 361: 1533–1544.

3. Davies PF, Tripathi S. Mechanical stress mechanisms and the cell. Circ Res 1993; 72:239–245.
4. Christman BW, McPherson CD, Newman JH, King GA, Bernard GR, Groves BM, Loyd JE. An imbalance between the excretion of thromboxane and prostacyclin metabolites in pulmonary hypertension. N Engl J Med 1992; 327: 70–75.
5. Dinh-Xuan AT, Higenbottam TW, Clelland CA, Pepke-Zaba J, Cremona G, Butt AY, Large SR, Wells FC, Wallwork, J. Impairment of endothelium dependent pulmonary artery relaxation in chronic obstructive lung disease. N Engl J Med 1991; 324:1539–1547.
6. Giaid A, Yanagisawa M, Langleben D, Michel RP, Levy R, Shennib H, Kimura S, Masaki T, Duguid WP, Stewart DJ. Expression of endothelin-1 in the lungs of patients with pulmonary hypertension. N Engl J Med 1993; 328:1732–1739.
7. Giaid A, Saleh D. Reduced expression of endothelial nitric oxide synthase in the lungs of patients with pulmonary hypertension. N Engl J Med 1995; 333:214–221.
8. Pietra GG. The pathology of primary pulmonary hypertension. In: Rubin LJ, Rich S, eds. Primary Pulmonary Hypertension. New York: Marcel Dekker, 1997:19–61.
9. Brink C, Cerrina C, Labat C, Verley J, Benveniste J. The effects of contractile agonists on isolated pulmonary arterial and venous muscle preparations derived from patients with primary pulmonary hypertension. Am Rev Respir Dis 1988; 137:A106 (Abstract).
10. Berridge MJ, Lipp P, Bootman MD. The versatility and universality of calcium signaling. Nat Rev Mol Cell Biol 2000; 1:11–21.
11. Nelson MT, Patlak JB, Worley JF, Standen NB. Calcium channels, potassium channels and voltage dependence of arterial smooth muscle tone. Am J Physiol 1990; 259:C3–C18.
12. Parekh AB, Penner R. Store depletion and calcium influx. Physiol Rev 1997; 77:901–930.
13. McDaniel SS, Platoshyn O, Wang J, Yu Y, Sweeney M, Krick S, Rubin LJ, Yuan JX-J. Capacitative Ca^{2+} entry in agonist induced pulmonary vasoconstriction. Am J Physiol Lung Cell Mol Physiol 2001; 280:L870–L880.
14. Hishikawa K, Nakaki T, Maruno T, Hayashi M, Suzuki H, Kato R, Saruta T. Pressure promotes DNA synthesis in rat cultured vascular smooth muscle cells. J Clin Invest 1994; 93:1975–1980.
15. Kolpakov V, Rekhtar MD, Gordon D, Wang WH, Kulik, TJ. Effects of mechanical forces on growth and matrix protein synthesis in the in vivo pulmonary artery, analysis of the role of individual cell types. Circ Res 1995; 77:823–831.
16. Means AR. Calcium calmodulin and cell cycle regulation. FEBS Lett 1994; 347:1–4.
17. Berridge MJ. Inositol triphosphate and calcium signaling. Nature 1993; 361:315–325.
18. Chao TS, Byron KL, Lee KM, Villereal M, Rosner MR. Activation of MAP kinases by calcium dependent and calcium independent pathways: stimulation

by thapsigargin and epidermal growth factor. J Biol Chem 1992; 267: 19876–19883.

19. Hardingham GE, Chawala S, Johnson CM, Bading H. Distinct functions of nuclear and cytoplasmic calcium in the control of gene expression. Nature 1997; 385:260–265.
20. Mogami H, Kojima I. Stimulation of calcium entry is a prerequisite for DNA synthesis induced by platelet derived growth factor in vascular smooth muscle cells. Biochem Biophys Res Commun 1993; 196:650–658.
21. Short AD, Bian J, Ghosh TK, Waldron RT, Rybak SL, Gill DL. Intracellular Ca^{2+} pool content is linked to control of cell growth. Proc Natl Acad Sci USA 1993; 90:4986–4990.
22. Yuan JX-J, Aldinger AM, Juhaszova M, Wang J, Conte JV, Gaine SP, Orens JB, Rubin LJ. Dysfunctional voltage-gated K^+ channels in pulmonary artery smooth muscle cells of patients with primary pulmonary hypertension. Circulation 1998; 98:1400–1406.
23. Blaustein MP. Physiological effects of endogenous ouabain: control of intracellular Ca^{2+} stores and cell responsiveness. Am J Physiol 1993; 264: C1367–C1389.
24. Yuan JX-J, Rubin LJ. Altered expression and function of Kv channels in primary pulmonary hypertension. In: Archer and, Rusch, eds. Potassium Channels in Cardiovascular Biology. New York: Kluwer Academic/Plenum, 2000:821–836.
25. Fleischmann BK, Murray RK, Kotlikoff MI. Voltage window for sustained elevation of cytosolic calcium in smooth muscle cells. Proc Natl Acad Sci USA 1994; 91:11914–11918.
26. Ganitkevich VY, Isenberg G. Membrane potential modulates inositol 1,4,5-triphosphate-mediated Ca^{2+} transients in guinea pig coronary myocytes. J Physiol 1993; 470:35–44.
27. Yuan JX-J. Voltage gated K^+ currents regulate resting membrane potential and $[Ca^{2+}]_i$ in pulmonary arterial myocytes. Circ Res 1995; 77:370–378.
28. Evans AM, Osipenko ON, Gurney AM. Properties of a novel K^+ current that is active at resting potential in rabbit pulmonary artery smooth muscle cells. J Physiol 1996; 496:407–420.
29. Chandy KG, Gutman GA. Voltage gated K^+ channels. In: North RA, ed. Ligand and Voltage Gated Ion Channels. Boca Raton, FL: CRC Press, 1995:1–31.
30. Bae YM, Park MK, Lee SH, Ho WK, Earm YE. Contribution of Ca^{2+} activated K^+ channels and nonselective cation channels to membrane potential of pulmonary arterial smooth muscle cells of the rabbit. J Physiol 1999; 514:747–758.
31. Clapp LH, Gurney AM. ATP sensitive K^+ channels regulate resting potential of pulmonary arterial smooth muscle cells. Am J Physiol 1992; 262: H916–H920.
32. Nelson MT, Quayle JM. Physiological roles and properties of potassium channels in arterial smooth muscle. Am J Physiol 1995; 268:C799–C822.
33. Lesage F, Lazdunski M. Molecular and functional properties of two-pore-domain potassium channels. Am J Physiol Renal Physiol 2000; 279:F793–F801.

34. Isom LL, De Jongh KS, Catterall WA. Auxiliary subunits of voltage gated ion channels. Neuron 1994; 12:1183–1194.
35. Yuan JX-J, Wang J, Juhaszova M, Gaine SP, Rubin LJ. Attenuated K^+ channel gene transcription in primary pulmonary hypertension. Lancet 1998; 351:726–727.
36. Durmowicz AG, Stenmark KR. Mechanisms of structure remodeling in chronic pulmonary hypertension. Pediatr Rev 1999; 20:e91–e102.
37. Haunstetter A, Izumo S. Apoptosis: basic mechanisms and implications for cardiovascular disease. Circ Res 1998; 82:1111–1129.
38. Rabinovitch M. Elastase and pathobiology of unexplained pulmonary hypertension. Chest 1998; 114:213–224.
39. Yu SP, Choi DW. Ions, cell volume and apoptosis. Proc Natl Acad Sci USA 2000; 97:9360–9362.
40. Bortner CD, Cidlowski JA. Caspase independent/dependent regulation of K^+ cell shrinkage and mitochondrial membrane potential during lymphocyte apoptosis. J Biol Chem 1999; 274:21953–21962.
41. Bortner CD, Hughes FM Jr, Cidlowski JA. A primary role for K^+ and Na^+ efflux in the activation of apoptosis. J Biol Chem 1997; 272:32436–32442.
42. Dallaporta B, Hirsch T, Susin SA, Zamzami N, Larochette N, Brenner C, Marzo I, Kroemer G. Potassium leakage during the apoptotic degradation phase. J Immunol 1998; 160:5605–5615.
43. Hoffman EK, Simonsen LO. Membrane mechanisms in volume and pH regulation in vertebrate cells. Physiol Rev 1989; 69:315–382.
44. Hughes FM Jr, Bortner CD, Purdy GD, Cidlowski JA. Intracellular K^+ suppresses the activation of apoptosis in lymphocytes. J Biol Chem 1997; 272: 30567–30576.
45. Zhang S, Fantozzi I, Tigno DD, Yi ES, Platoshyn O, Thistlethwaite PA, Kriett JM, Yung G, Rubin LJ, Yuan JX-J. Bone morphogenetic proteins induce apoptosis in human pulmonary vascular smooth muscle cells. Am J Physiol Lung Cell Mol Physiol 2003; 285:L740–L754.
46. Brevnova EE, Platoshyn O, Zhang S, Yuan JX-J. Overexpression of human increases $I_{K(V)}$ and enhances apoptosis. *KCNA5* Am J Physiol cell physiol 2004; 287: C715-C722.
47. Ekhterae D, Platoshyn O, Krick S, Yu Y, McDaniel SS, Yuan JX-J. Bcl-2 decreases voltage gated K^+ channel activity and enhances survival in vascular smooth muscle cells. Am J Physiol Cell Physiol 2001; 281:C157–C165.
48. Hoth M, Penner R. Depletion of intracellular calcium stores activates a calcium current in mast cells. Nature 1992; 355:353–356.
49. Putney JW Jr. Capacitative Calcium Entry. Georgetown, TX: Landes, 1997.
50. Golovina VA, Platoshyn O, Bailey CL, Wang J, Limsuwan A, Sweeney M, Rubin LJ, Yuan JX-J. Upregulated TRP and enhanced capacitative Ca^{2+} entry in human pulmonary artery myocytes during proliferation. Am J Physiol Heart Circ Physiol 2001; 280:H746–H755.
51. Ng LC, Gurney AM. Store operated channel mediate Ca^{2+} influx and contraction in rat pulmonary artery. Circ Res 2001; 89:923–929.
52. Clapham DE, Runnels LW, Strubing C. The TRP ion channel family. Nature Rev Neurosci 2001:387–396.

53. Sweeney M, Yu Y, Platoshyn O, Zhang S, McDaniel SS, Yuan JX-J. Inhibition of endogenous TRP1 decreases capacitative Ca^{2+} entry and attenuates pulmonary artery smooth muscle cell proliferation. Am J Physiol Lung Cell Mol Physiol 2002; 283:L144–L155.
54. Fantozzi I, Zhang S, Platoshyn O, Remillard CV, Cowling RT, Yuan JX-J. Hypoxia increases AP-1 binding activity by enhancing capacitative Ca^{2+} entry in human pulmonary artery endothelial cells. Am J Physiol Lung Cell Mol Physiol 2003; 285:L1233–L1245.
55. Yu Y, Sweeney M, Zhang S, Platoshyn O, Landsberg J, Rothman A, Yuan JX-J. PDGF stimulates pulmonary vascular smooth muscle cell proliferation by upregulating TRPC6 expression. Am J Physiol Cell Physiol 2003; 284: C316–C330.
56. Berg JT, Breen EC, Fu Z, Mathieu-Costello O, West JB. Alveolar hypoxia increases gene expression of extracellular matrix proteins and platelet derived growth factor B in lung parenchyma. Am J Respir Crit Care Med 1998; 156:1920–1928.
57. Stenmark KR, Mecham RP. Cellular and molecular mechanisms of pulmonary vascular remodeling. Annu Rev Physiol 1997; 59:89–144.
58. Tanabe Y, Saito M, Ueno A, Nakamura M, Takeishi K, Nakayama K. Mechanical stretch augments PDGF receptor-β expression and protein tyrosine phosphorylation in pulmonary artery tissue and smooth muscle cells. Mol Cell Biochem 2000; 215:103–113.
59. Platoshyn O, Golovina VA, Bailey CL, Limsuwan A, Krick S, Juhaszova M, Seiden JE, Rubin LJ, Yuan JX-J. Sustained membrane depolarization and pulmonary artery smooth muscle cell proliferation. Am J Physiol Cell Physiol 2000; 279:C1540–C1549.
60. Krick S, Platoshyn O, McDaniel SS, Rubin LJ, Yuan JX-J. Augmented K^+ currents and mitochondrial membrane depolarization in pulmonary artery myocyte apoptosis. Am J Physiol Lung Cell Mol Physiol 2001; 281:L887–L894.

27

Developmental Regulation of Ion Channel Function and Expression in the Pulmonary Vasculature

David N. Cornfield

University of Minnesota Medical School, Minneapolis, Minnesota, U.S.A.

I. INTRODUCTION

During fetal development, gas exchange is accomplished at the placenta. Fetal pulmonary blood flow is less than 10% of biventricular output, and pulmonary arterial blood pressure exceeds systemic blood pressure. Closely regulated pulmonary blood flow is necessary for optimal lung development (1). Recent evidence suggests that branching morphogenesis and alveolarization is contingent, to a significant degree, on carefully regulated blood flow in the fetal lung (2–4).

Although fetal pulmonary blood flow is closely circumscribed, at birth the pulmonary vasculature must accommodate an exponential increase in pulmonary blood flow (1). Within moments after birth, pulmonary blood flow increases 8–10-fold while pulmonary artery pressure decreases by 50% over the first 24 h of life. The increase is both essential and unique, because pulmonary vasodilation is imperative at, and only at, parturition. Although the mechanisms whereby the pulmonary vasculature respond to an acute increase in oxygen tension remain incompletely understood, emerging evidence suggests a role for pulmonary vascular K^+ channels both in limiting fetal pulmonary blood flow and in mediating the response to perinatal pulmonary vasodilator stimuli.

In 1953, Dawes et al. (5) published a seminal manuscript demonstrating that ventilation and establishment of an air/liquid interface caused an immediate increase in pulmonary blood flow and a decrease in PA blood pressure. Evidence for an integral role for O_2 in the postnatal adaptation of the pulmonary circulation came first with the finding that whereas ventilation with nitrogen caused pulmonary vasodilation, ventilation with O_2 caused even greater pulmonary vasodilation (6). The demonstration that fetal blood flow increased more than threefold when pregnant ewes with chronically instrumented fetal lambs were placed in a hyperbaric chamber provided clear evidence that an increase in fetal oxygen tension, absent any other physiological stimulus, could cause fetal pulmonary vasodilation (7). Interestingly, the capacity of oxygen to cause fetal pulmonary vasodilation appears late in gestation. Morin et al. (8) demonstrated that an acute increase in fetal oxygen tension increases fetal pulmonary blood flow only in fetal lambs after more than 125 days gestation.

Among the first evidence that implicated a role for the pulmonary endothelium in the transition of the pulmonary circulation were data demonstrating an increase in prostaglandin production immediately following birth (9). Blockade of prostaglandin production did not prevent either postnatal adaptation of the pulmonary circulation (10) or fetal pulmonary vasodilation caused by an increase in fetal O_2 tension alone (8). The observation that pharmacological blockade of endothelium-derived relaxing factor (EDRF), later identified as nitric oxide (NO) (11,12), prevented the postnatal adaptation of the pulmonary circulation in lambs ventilated with 100% O_2 (13) demonstrated the critical importance of the pulmonary endothelium in the postnatal adaptation of the pulmonary circulation.

The observation that pharmacological blockade of NO production attenuated the decrease in pulmonary vascular resistance both with ventilation alone and with ventilation with 100% O_2 provided direct evidence that NO production played a key role in O_2-induced fetal pulmonary vasodilation (14). Two separate studies found that O_2-induced pulmonary vasodilation was either attenuated or prevented by pharmacological blockade of NO in the chronically instrumented fetal lamb (15,16). These findings, in concert with the observation that O_2 tension is capable of modulating NO production in fetal PA endothelial cells (17), implied that the increase in O_2 tension that occurs at birth may contribute to sustained and progressive pulmonary vasodilation by providing a stimulus for augmented NO production by the pulmonary endothelium.

Concomitant with the emergence of data demonstrating a critically important role for NO in the transition of the perinatal pulmonary circulation were studies indicating a link between the vasodilation caused by NO and K^+ channel activation in vascular smooth muscle cells (SMCs). Robertson et al. (18) demonstrated that in cerebral artery smooth muscle cells, cyclic guanosine 3′,5′-monophosphate (cGMP)-dependent protein kinase

(PK) acts to phosphorylate the large conductance K_{Ca} channel. In PA SMCs, NO-induced increases in intracellular levels of cGMP cause activation of a cGMP-sensitive kinase, and this in turn activates a K_{Ca} channel, resulting in vasodilation (19). NO has also been shown to directly activate K_{Ca} channels (20). Thus, if NO caused pulmonary vasodilation through K^+ channel activation, then blockade of K^+ channel activation would prevent perinatal pulmonary vasodilation associated with the physiological stimuli that occur at birth.

II. K^+ CHANNEL PHYSIOLOGY IN THE PERINATAL PULMONARY CIRCULATION

The initial evidence that K^+ channels were present in the fetal lung derived from reports indicating that ATP-sensitive K^+ channel agonists cause pulmonary vasodilation. Although there was consensus surrounding the ability of activation of ATP-sensitive K^+ channels to cause fetal and neonatal pulmonary vasodilation, there was controversy surrounding the mechanism whereby these agents might work. Two separate groups of investigators reported that the perinatal pulmonary vasodilation associated with activation of the ATP-sensitive K^+ channel was endothelium-independent (21,22), while another group indicated that an antagonist of nitric oxide blocked the ATP-sensitive K^+ channel activation and induced perinatal pulmonary vasodilation (23). In vitro work suggests that a component of ATP-sensitive K^+ channel activation may derive from the endothelium. Moreover, there do not seem to be maturational differences in the response to ATP-sensitive K^+ channel activators (24). Experiments in chronically instrumented fetal lambs demonstrated that inhibition of the channel resulted in an increase in systemic, but not pulmonary, vascular tone (22). The implication of this observation is that in the low oxygen tension environment of the normal fetus, ATP-sensitive K^+ channel activity plays a role in determining systemic but not pulmonary vascular tone.

Definitive evidence for the importance of K_{Ca} channel activation in O_2-induced fetal pulmonary vasodilation came from studies in acutely instrumented late-gestation ovine fetuses. In this series of experiments, O_2-induced fetal pulmonary vasodilation is blocked by tetraethylammonium, a K^+ channel blocker (25), and iberiotoxin, a specific K_{Ca} channel antagonist (26), but is unaffected by glibenclamide, a blocker of the ATP-sensitive K^+ channel blocker (26). These data suggested that O_2 caused fetal pulmonary vasodilation through K_{Ca} channel activation. The mechanism was further characterized through pharmacological inhibition of either guanylate cyclase or cyclic nucleotide-dependent kinases. Combined use of these inhibitors attenuated O_2-dependent fetal pulmonary vasodilation, implying that elevated fetal O_2 acts to increase cyclic nucleotide-dependent cyclase activity and cGMP concentration and activate cyclic nucleotide-dependent kinases, causing K_{Ca} channel activation and vasodilation (27).

To further characterize the effect of an acute increase in O_2 tension on the fetal pulmonary artery smooth muscle cells, electrophysiological studies were performed on freshly dispersed pulmonary artery smooth muscle cells obtained from the distal pulmonary vasculature. In these studies, whole-cell K^+ current increased dramatically concomitant with an increase in O_2 tension. Application of nitric oxide activated K_{Ca} channels, increasing I_K by $253 \pm 28\%$ (at +40 mV) (27). The increase in K^+ current was attenuated in the presence of either charybdotoxin or tetraethylammonium but unaffected by treatment with 4-aminopyridine. Moreover, the K^+ current demonstrated high, spiking, transient increases in current. The pattern was consistent with spontaneous transient outward K^+ current or STOCs, a pattern that is consistent with K^+ current trafficking through the high-conductance calcium-sensitive K^+ channel.

Physical factors and vasoactive products elaborated by the pulmonary vascular endothelium are involved in the regulation of perinatal pulmonary vascular tone (13). To determine whether sustained and progressive perinatal pulmonary vasodilation requires pulmonary vascular K^+ channel activation, experiments were performed in acutely instrumented late-gestation fetal lambs. In the experimental series, the separate and interactive effects of ventilation and ventilation combined with oxygenation were evaluated. K^+ channel inhibition with TEA, but not glibenclamide, attenuated both ventilation-induced and ventilation-with-oxygen-induced perinatal pulmonary vasodilation. The data argued compellingly that sustained and progressive perinatal pulmonary vasodilation requires K^+ channel activation (see Fig. 1) (28).

To determine whether K^+channel activation mediates shear-stress-induced pulmonary vasodilation in the fetus, Storme and coworkers (28a) studied the hemodynamic effects of K^+ channel blockers on basal pulmonary vascular resistance and on the pulmonary vascular response to partial compression of the ductus arteriosus (DA) in chronically prepared late-gestation fetal lambs (128–132 days gestation). Study drugs included tetraethylammonium (TEA), a Ca^{2+}-dependent K^+ channel blocker; glibenclamide (Glib), an ATP-dependent K^+ channel blocker; charybdotoxin (CTX), a preferential high-conductance Ca^{2+}-dependent K^+ channel blocker; apamin (Apa), a low-conductance Ca^{2+}-dependent K^+ channel blocker; and 4-aminopyridine (4-AP), a voltage-dependent K^+ channel blocker. Pharmacological probes were selectively infused into the left pulmonary artery. An inflatable vascular occluder was placed around the DA. LPA flow was measured with an ultrasonic flow transducer. Compression of the ductus arteriosus caused a time-related decrease in pulmonary vascular resistance in the control, glibencalmide, apamine, and charybdotoxin groups, but not in the high-dose tetraethylammonium and 4-aminopyridine

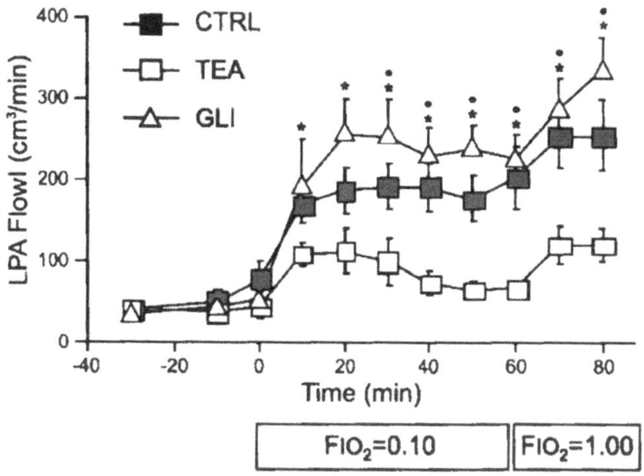

Figure 1 Effect of K^+ channel inhibition with either tetraethylammonium (TEA) or glibenclamide (GLI) on left pulmonary artery blood flow (LPA flow) in response to sequential ventilation with low and high O_2. LPA flow in the TEA group was attenuated compared to control (CTRL) in response to both low and high O_2. There was no difference in LPA flow between CTRL and GLI groups. (*) $p < 0.01$ all groups compared to baseline value. (•) $p < 0.01$ CTRL vs. TEA. (From Ref. 28.)

groups. These data indicate that shear stress causes perinatal pulmonary vasodilation through activation of Ca^{2+}-sensitive and voltage-dependent K^+ channels, but via activation of either low-conductance Ca^{2+}- and ATP-sensitive K^+ channels.

As outlined above, data from studies performed in the early 1990s clearly demonstrated that nitric oxide mediates the transition of the perinatal pulmonary circulation. Both nitric oxide and oxygen stimulate perinatal pulmonary vasodilation via a guanylate cyclase-sensitive route (8,16). However, how an NO-induced increase in cytosolic cGMP levels leads to perinatal pulmonary vasodilation had not been outlined.

Given data suggesting that NO causes vasodilation via either direct or indirect effects on the K_{Ca} channel, the hypothesis that in the perinatal pulmonary circulation NO causes vasodilation through K_{Ca} channel activation was tested. Previous data from our laboratory demonstrated that NO activated K_{Ca} channels, increasing I_K by $253 \pm 28\%$ (at +40 mV) (27). To determine whether NO causes perinatal pulmonary vasodilation through K_{Ca} channel activation through release of Ca^{2+} from ryanodine-sensitive stores, endogenous nitric oxide production was pharmacologically blocked in acutely instrumented, late-gestation fetal lambs. Lambs were ventilated, and inhaled NO was administered in the presence and absence of either

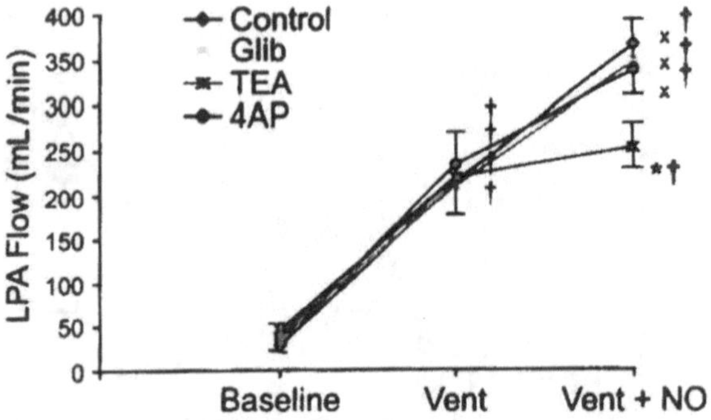

Figure 2 Effect of K^+ channel inhibition on sequential vent with FIO_2 of 1.00 and vent with FIO_2 of 1.00 and 20 ppm inhaled nitric oxide (NO). In the presence of pharmacological blockade of endogenous NO production with nitro-L-arginine, left pulmonary artery (LPA) flow increased in each experimental group during vent with FIO_2 of 1.00 and was not affected by K^+ channel inhibition. Vent with FIO_2 of 1.00 and 20 ppm inhaled NO caused a significant increase in LPA flow in each study group. Compared with control group, treatment with TEA, a preferential Ca^{2+}-activated K^+ channel blocker, attenuated the increase in LPA blood flow associated with vent and inhaled NO ($P < 0.0001$). Glibenclamide (Glib), an ATP-sensitive K^+ channel blocker, and 4-AP, a voltage-dependent K^+ channel blocker, had no effect on NO-induced pulmonary vasodilation. Significant difference ($P < 0.05$) from: (*) control group; (†) preventilation value. (From Ref. 29.)

pharmacological blockade of the K_{Ca} channel, ryanodine, or cGMP-kinase. In that series of experiments, TEA and ryanodine, but not 4-aminopyridine, a blocker of the voltage-sensitive K^+ (Kv) channel, attenuated the perinatal pulmonary vasodilation caused by NO (Fig. 2). The authors concluded that K_{Ca}, but not Kv, channel activation plays a key role in NO-induced perinatal pulmonary vasodilation and requires release of Ca^{2+} from ryanodine-sensitive stores (29).

Considered together, the above data support the notion that the pulmonary vascular SMC K_{Ca} channel plays a critically important role in mediating pulmonary vasodilation at a biologically critical point in development. The most essential perinatal pulmonary vasodilator stimuli—ventilation, oxygenation, shear stress, and nitric oxide—cause vasodilation through activation of PA SMC K_{Ca} channels. Activation of the PA SMC K_{Ca} channel leads to membrane hypolarization, closure of voltage-operated calcium channels, a decrease in PA SMC $[Ca^{2+}]_i$, and vasodilation. Thus, data are available that suggest that the K_{Ca} channel is a legitimate molecular target for a novel therapeutic approach to the abnormal perinatal pulmonary vasoreactivity that characterizes persistent pulmonary hypertension of the newborn (PPHN).

III. ONTOGENY OF PULMONARY VASCULAR K⁺ CHANNELS

Given the observation that the fetal and neonatal pulmonary circulation are uniquely well adapted to respond to an acute increase in oxygen tension, it follows that both K_{Ca} channel expression and activity diminish with maturation. Data from both pulmonary arteries and pulmonary artery smooth muscle cells in primary culture indicate that K_{Ca} α-subunit channel gene expression is greatest in the fetal lung and decreases with maturation (30) (Fig. 2). Indeed, the physiology of pulmonary vascular SMCs is consistent with the molecular biology (31). In fetal PA SMCs, resting membrane potential is determined by the K_{Ca} channel, whereas in adult PA SMCs Kv channel activity determines resting membrane potential (32). In fetal PA SMCs, an acute increase in oxygen tension results in membrane hyperpolarization and a decrease in PA SMC $[Ca^{2+}]_i$ and has no effect on adult PA SMC membrane potential or $[Ca^{2+}]_i$ (30). Taken together, these observations indicate that the developmental regulation of K_{Ca} channel expression allows for the fetal PA SMCs to be uniquely well adapted to respond to an acute increase in oxygen tension with a decrease in $[Ca^{2+}]_i$ and vasorelaxation. The molecular mechanisms whereby a maturation-related decrease in K_{Ca} and increase in Kv channel activity occurs remain unknown.

Further support for the hypothesis that K_{Ca} channel activity decreases with maturation derives from the observation that protein levels of the α K_{Ca} channel decrease with maturation. K_{Ca} channel protein levels in isolated vascular structures from the lungs of fetal and adult sheep demonstrate a clear increase in fetal K_{Ca} protein levels with maturation (Fig. 3) (30), suggesting that K_{Ca} activity might be modulated at the transcriptional level.

To demonstrate the physiological relevance of the maturation-related decreases in K_{Ca} channel expression, Rhodes and coworkers (30) tested the overall hypothesis that PA SMCs from the fetal, but not the adult, pulmonary circulation respond to an acute increase in O_2 tension. Using fluorescence microscopy, Rhodes et al. studied the effect of an acute increase in O_2 tension on cytosolic Ca^{2+} ($[Ca^{2+}]_i$) of SMCs isolated from adult and fetal PA. Fetal, but not adult, PA SMCs responded to an acute increase in O_2 tension with a decrease in $[Ca^{2+}]_i$, thereby providing data that maturation-related changes in the ability of the pulmonary vasculature to respond to an acute increase in O_2 tension are intrinsic to the PA SMCs (30) (Fig. 4). The O_2-induced decrease in fetal PA SMC $[Ca^{2+}]_i$ was blocked by iberiotoxin, a specific blocker of the K_{Ca} channel (30). Further support for a developmental role for the K_{Ca} channel comes from the observation that fetal, but not adult, PA SMCs respond to iberiotoxin with an increase in basal $[Ca^{2+}]_i$, suggesting that the K_{Ca} channel determines basal $[Ca^{2+}]_i$ in fetal PA SMCs (33).

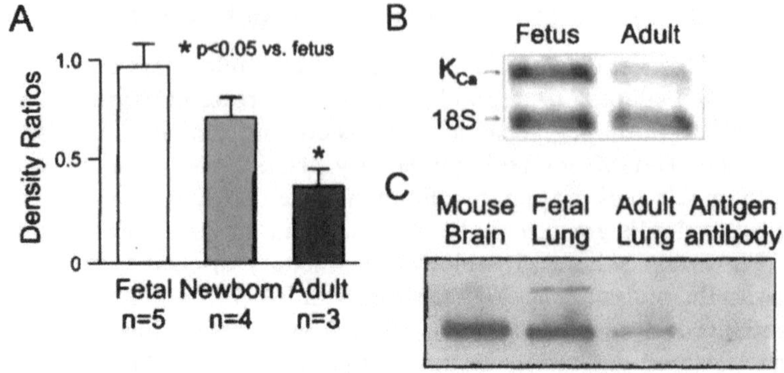

Figure 3 (A) K_{Ca} channel mRNA levels in the distal pulmonary vasculature decreases with maturation. Band intensities were determined by densitometry. K_{Ca} band intensity was normalized to that of the 18S band. mRNA was extracted directly from pulmonary arteries isolated from three fetal ($n = 3$ animals; 9 gels) and three adult ($n = 3$ animals; 9 gels) sheep. RT-PCR was performed four times for each mRNA sample. (B) Representative gel of a reverse transcriptase polymerase chain reaction (RT-PCR) analysis of K_{Ca} channel mRNA expression during development. The K_{Ca} band (~313 base pairs) was compared to the control 18S band (~480 base pairs) in fetal and adult samples. K_{Ca} channel band intensity was determined by densitometry and normalized to that of the 18S band. K_{Ca} channel mRNA levels decrease with maturation. (C) Western blot of adult and fetal samples from the distal pulmonary artery obtained with anti-K_{Ca} channel polyclonal antibody. Each lane was loaded with 20 μg of immunoprecipitated protein. The predicted bands of approximately 125 kDa were observed in both adult and fetal samples. Intensity of the band indicates decreasing K_{Ca} channel protein levels with postnatal maturation. The 125 kDa band is consistent with previously published reports. In the fetal samples an additional band of approximately 180 kDa is consistently observed. The band is absent from samples from the adult pulmonary circulation and the adult mouse brain. Protein extracted from the adult mouse brain served as the positive control. Coincubation with both the antigen and antibody served as the negative control (From Ref. 30.)

In coordination with a maturation-related decrease in K_{Ca} channel expression and activation, the Kv channel increases with maturation. There is relatively more Kv 2.1 channel protein and message in the adult than in the fetal and neonatal pulmonary circulation (34). The increase in Kv 2.1 channel protein parallels the increasing capacity of PA SMCs to sense and respond to acute decreases in O_2 tension, because in response to acute hypoxia $[Ca^{2+}]_i$ increases more rapidly and to a greater degree in adult, as compared to fetal, PA SMCs (34). Thus, the maturation-related increase in hypoxic pulmonary vasoconstriction that was previously reported (35,36) might derive from the parallel increases in Kv 2.1 channel activity, protein, and message with maturation (Fig. 5).

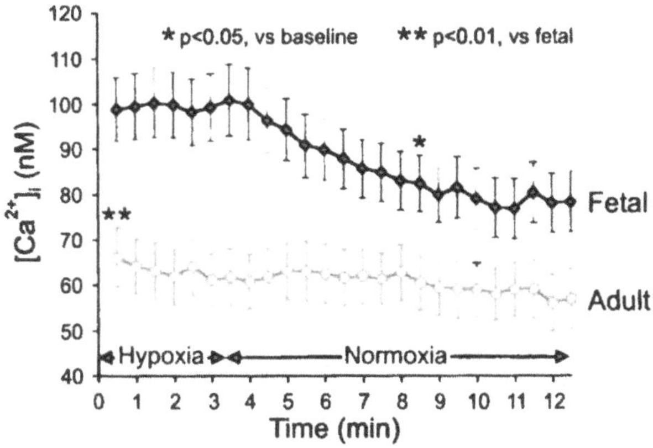

Figure 4 Comparison of cytosolic Ca^{2+} concentration ($[Ca^{2+}]_i$) in fetal (113 cells; six animals) and adult (99 cells; four animals) pulmonary artery smooth muscle cells (PA SMCs) maintained in hypoxia. Under hypoxic conditions, basal $[Ca^{2+}]_i$ was significantly higher in fetal than in adult PA SMCs. In response to an acute increase in O_2 tension, fetal, but not adult, PA SMCs demonstrate a decrease in $[Ca^{2+}]_i$. (From Ref. 30.)

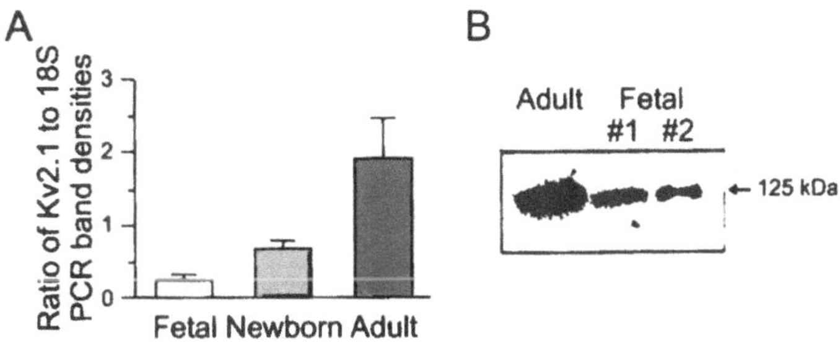

Figure 5 Kv2.1 expression increases with maturation. Using quantitative, internally controlled RT-PCR, relative levels of mRNA expression were determined in tissue derived from the distal pulmonary arteries of fetal or adult lambs. Band intensities were determined by densitometry. Kv2.1 band intensity was normalized to that of the 18S band. Results are from PAs obtained from three fetal, three newborn, and three adult sheep. Values are means ± SE. PA SMC, pulmonary artery smooth muscle cell. (B) Western blot of adult and fetal samples from distal PAs obtained with anti-voltage-gated K 1 (Kv2.1) polyclonal antibody. Each lane was loaded with 80 μg of protein. Predicted bands of 130 kDa were observed in both adult and fetal samples. Intensities were subsequently assessed by densitometry. Intensity of the band indicates increasing channel protein levels of Kv2.1 channel with postnatal maturation. The 125 kDa band is consistent with previously published reports. (Data from Ref. 34.)

IV. DEVELOPMENTAL REGULATION OF RYANODINE-SENSITIVE STORES

Given the developmental regulation of O_2-induced decreases in PA SMC $[Ca^{2+}]_i$, Porter et al. reasoned that ryanodine sensitivity may be developmentally regulated. To test this hypothesis, PA SMCs were freshly dispersed from the proximal and distal pulmonary arteries of fetal (0.9 term), neonatal (< 24 h old), and juvenile rabbits. In this model, ryanodine caused a substantial increase in $[Ca^{2+}]_i$ in PA SMCs isolated from the distal fetal, but not neonatal or juvenile, pulmonary arteries (37) (Fig. 6). Given the evidence of developmental regulation of ryanodine-sensitive stores, the investigators sought to determine the mechanism whereby ryanodine causes an increase in $[Ca^{2+}]_i$. Removal of external calcium or application of diltiazem, a blocker of the voltage-operated calcium channels (VOCCs), suppressed the ryanodine-induced increase in $[Ca^{2+}]_i$, providing evidence that ryanodine causes an increase in $[Ca^{2+}]_i$ through an influx of extracellular calcium via VOCCs (37).

Given the similar pattern of developmental regulation of the K_{Ca} channel and the ryanodine-sensitive stores in PA SMCs, it seemed possible that quantal release of calcium from ryanodine-sensitive stores, termed calcium sparks, and K_{Ca} channels work in a coordinated fashion to control PA SMCs $[Ca^{2+}]_i$. To this end, confocal microscopy was used to demonstrate the presence of calcium sparks in fetal PA SMCs (38). Although calcium sparks had been demonstrated in other vascular structures (39–41), the

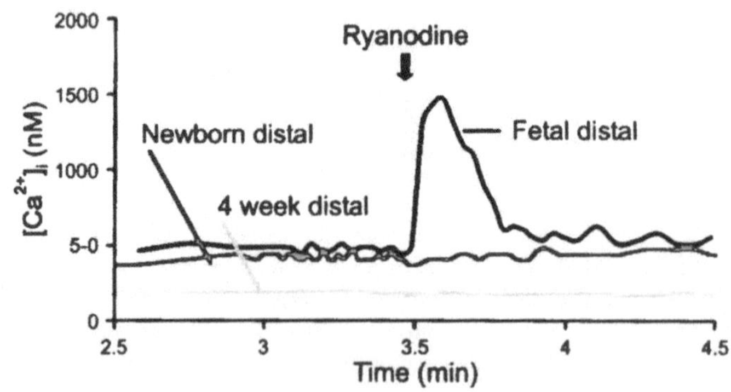

Figure 6 Developmental regulation of ryanodine release as illustrated by the response of isolated pulmonary artery smooth muscle cells (PASMCs) to ryanodine. Representative traces showing intracellular calcium concentration (in nanomoles) measured in single smooth muscle cells isolated from fetal, newborn, and juvenile distal rabbit pulmonary arteries. Ryanodine (50 mM) was added at the arrow. Only the fetal distal pulmonary artery cell responded to ryanodine with an increase in calcium. (From Ref. 38.)

report of Porter et al. represents the first evidence of calcium sparks in the fetal pulmonary circulation. The observations that pretreatment with iberiotoxin, a specific blocker of the K_{Ca} channel, blocked the ryanodine-induced increase in $[Ca^{2+}]_i$, whereas pretreatment with ryanodine blocked the increase in $[Ca^{2+}]_i$ caused by iberiotoxin demonstrate a link between release of calcium from ryanodine-sensitive stores and K_{Ca} channel activity (37,38). Taken together, these data suggest that quantal release of calcium from ryanodine-sensitive stores exerts a tonic stimulus on K_{Ca} channels, thereby limiting tone. With the stimulus of oxygen, the frequency of calcium sparks increases, leading to activation of the K_{Ca} channels, membrane hyperpolarization, closure of VOCCs, a decrease in PA SMC $[Ca^{2+}]_i$, and vasodilation.

To further characterize the subcellular mechanism whereby oxygen causes fetal pulmonary vasodilation, the investigators performed both in vivo and in vitro experiments. In vivo studies were performed in acutely instrumented fetal sheep. The results from both experimental systems were consistent. In the whole-animal studies, acutely instrumented late-gestation fetal lambs were studied. The pregnant ewe was administered 100% oxygen for 30 min, with a resulting increase in fetal oxygen tension from 18 ± 2 to 28 ± 3 torr. Left pulmonary artery (LPA) blood flow increased from 27.9 ± 8.9 to 241.5 ± 71 cm^3/min. After a 1 h recovery period, ryanodine (100 μg) was administered to the fetus via the LPA over 10 min. Despite a similar increase in fetal arterial oxygen tension, ryanodine attentuated the O_2-induced increase in LPA blood, increasing from 37.6 ± 12 to 118 ± 42.6 cm^3/min ($n = 5$; $p < 0.05$, versus control period) (38) (Fig. 7).

In vitro studies were performed both in freshly dispersed late-gestation ovine PA SMCs and in fetal ovine PA SMCs maintained in primary culture. In vitro, ryanodine prevented the O_2-induced decrease in PA SMC $[Ca^{2+}]_i$ (38). To detail the relationship between release of calcium from the ryanodine-sensitive intracellular stores and K_{Ca} channel activation, electrophysiological experiments were performed in freshly dispersed PA SMCs. In several experimental systems a key step between calcium sparks and membrane hyperpolarization has been spontaneous transient outward currents, (STOCs). Calcium sparks have been shown to cause activation of the K_{Ca} channel, leading to a short-lived increase in K^+ efflux or STOCs. The initial demonstration of STOCs in fetal PA SMCs came in 1996. The report in 2001 that an acute increase in oxygen tension increased both calcium sparks and STOCs provided critical information for the link between calcium sparks and membrane hyperpolarization. This led to the conclusion that Ca^{2+} release from the ryanodine-sensitive store mediates the O_2-induced decrease in PA SMC $[Ca^{2+}]_i$ by increasing STOC activity, which sums to cause membrane hyperpolarization.

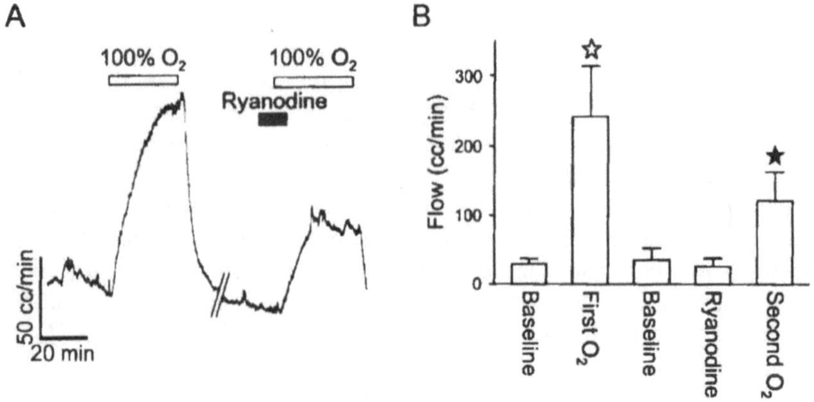

Figure 7 Ryanodine attenuates oxygen-induced increase in fetal pulmonary blood flow in late-gestation fetal lambs. (A) Representative trace shows left pulmonary artery (LPA) flow vs. time from an acutely instrumented fetal sheep. Fetal LPA flow increased when inspired air to the pregnant ewe was switched to 100% O_2. Ryanodine (100 mg total) was infused into the LPA at a rate of 1 mL/min over a 10 min period. (B) Values are averages ± standard error from measurements of five animals taken from traces like those shown in (A). Time points are immediately before first O_2 increase; after exposure to O_2; recovery; after administration of ryanodine before initiation of second exposure to O_2; and during the second exposure to O_2(☆) < 0.05 vs. baseline. ★ < 0.05 vs. control. (From Ref. 38.)

V. CONCLUSION

Ion channel expression and activity in the pulmonary artery smooth muscle cells change with development. The predominance of the calcium-sensitive K^+ channel as the primary determinant of resting membrane potential in fetal PA SMCs is in contrast to the voltage-gated K^+ channel as the determinant of the resting membrane potential in PA SMCs derived from the adult circulation. Developmental differences in PA SMCs transcend plasma membrane K^+ channel expression, because intracellular calcium homeostasis and stores differ between fetal and adult PA SMCs. The implications of these differences is that fetal and neonatal PA SMCs are well adapted to respond to physiological signals that are at the same time crucial for and unique to the perinatal time period. Conversely, PA SMCs derived from the adult pulmonary circulation are adapted to respond to hypoxia, thereby ensuring optimal ventilation–perfusion relationships and minimizing intrapulmonary shunting. The underlying molecular mechanisms responsible for these teleologically essential adaptations remain unknown. Insight into these mechanisms likely has significant implications for novel approaches to difficult and to this point insoluble disease states.

REFERENCES

1. Rudolph A. Distribution and regulation of blood flow in the fetal and neonatal lamb. Circ Res 1985; 57:811–821.
2. Bhatt AJ, Pryhuber GS, Huyck H, Watkins RH, Metlay LA, Maniscalco WM. Disrupted pulmonary vasculature and decreased vascular endothelial growth factor, Flt-1, and TIE-2 in human infants dying with bronchopulmonary dysplasia. Am J Respir Critic Care Med 2001; 164:1971–1980.
3. Lassus P, Turanlahti M, Heikkila P, Andersson LC, Nupponen I, Sarnesto A, Andersson S. Pulmonary vascular endothelial growth factor and Flt-1 in fetuses, in acute and chronic lung disease, and in persistent pulmonary hypertension of the newborn. Am J Respir Crit Care Med 2001; 164: 1755–1756.
4. Jakkula M, Le Cras TD, Gebb S, Hirth KP, Tuder RM, Voelkel NF, Abman SH. Inhibition of angiogenesis decreases alveolarization in the developing rat lung. Am J Physiol Lung Cell Mol Physiol 2000; 279: L600–L607.
5. Dawes GS, Mott JC, Widdicombe JG, Wyatt DG. Changes in the lungs of the newborn lamb. J Physiol 1953; 121:141–162.
6. Cassin S, Dawes GS, Mott JC, Ross BB, Strang LB. The vascular resistance of the fetal and newly ventilated lung of the lamb. J Physiol 1964; 171:61–79.
7. Assali NS, Kirchbaum TH, Dilts PV. Effects of hyperbaric oxygen on in utero placental and fetal circulation. Circ Res 1968; 22:573–588.
8. Morin F, Eagan E, Ferguson W, Lundgren CEG. Development of pulmonary vascular response to oxygen. Am J Physiol 1988; 254:H542–H546.
9. Leffler CW, Hessler JR, Green RS. The onset of breathing at birth stimulates pulmonary vascular prostacyclin synthesis. Pediatr Res 1984; 18:938–942.
10. Leffler CW, Tyler TL, Cassin S. Effect of indomethacin on pulmonary vascular response to ventilation of fetal goats. Am J Physiol 1978; 235: H346–H351.
11. Furchgott RF. Studies on relaxation of rabbit aorta by sodium nitrite: the basis for the proposal that the acid-activatable inhibitory factor from bovine retractor penis is inorganic nitrite and the endothelium-derived relaxing factor is nitric oxide. Vanhoutte PM, ed. Vasodilatation. New York: Raven Press, 1988:410–414.
12. Ignarro LJ, Buga GM, Wood KS, Byrns RE, Chaudhuri G. Endothelium-derived relaxing factor produced and released from artery and vein is nitric oxide. Proc Natl Acad Sci USA 1987; 84:9265–9269.
13. Abman SH, Chatfield BA, Hall SL, McMurtry IF. Role of endothelium-derived relaxing factor during transition of pulmonary circulation at birth. Am J Physiol 1990; 259:H1921–H1927.
14. Cornfield D, Chatfield B, McQueston J, McMurtry I, Abman S. Effects of birth-related stimuli on L-arginine-dependent pulmonary vasodilation in ovine fetus. Am J Physiol 1992; 262:H1474–H1481.
15. McQueston JA, Cornfield DN, McMurtry IF, Abman SH. Effects of oxygen and exogenous L-arginine on EDRF activity in fetal pulmonary circulation. Am J Physol 1993; 264.

16. Tiktinsky MH, Morin FCd. Increasing oxygen tension dilates fetal pulmonary circulation via endothelium-derived relaxing factor. Am J Physiol 1993; 265: H376–H380.
17. Shaul PW, Wells LB. Oxygen modulates nitric oxide production selectively in fetal pulmonary endothelial cells. Am J Respir Cell Mol Biol 1994; 11:432–438.
18. Robertson BE, Schubert R, Hescheler J, Nelson M. cGMP-dependent protein kinase activates Ca-activated K channels in cerebral artery smooth muscle cells. Am J Physiol 1993; 265:C299–C303.
19. Archer SL, Huang JMC, Hampl V, Nelson DP, Shultz PJ, Weir EK. Nitric oxide and cGMP cause vasorelaxation by activation of a charybdotoxin-sensitive K channel by cGMP-dependent protein kinase. Proc Natl Acad Sci USA 1994; 91:7583–7587.
20. Bolotina VM, Najibi S, Palacino JJ, Pagano PJ, Cohen RA. Nitric oxide directly activates calcium-dependent potassium channels in vascular smooth muscle. Nature 1994; 368:850–853.
21. Pinheiro JM, Malik AB. K^+ATP-channel activation causes marked vasodilation in the hypertensive neonatal pig lung. Am J Physiol 1992; 263: H1532–H1536.
22. Cornfield DN, McQueston JA, McMurtry IF, Rodman DM, Abman SH. Role of ATP-sensitive potassium channels in ovine fetal pulmonary vascular tone. Am J Physiol 1992; 263:H1363–H1368.
23. Chang J-K, Moore P, Fineman JR, Soifer SJ, Heymann MA. K^+ channel pulmonary vasodilation in fetal lambs: role of endothelium-derived nitric oxide. J Appl Physiol 1992; 73:188–194.
24. Boels PJ, Gao B, Deutsch J, Haworth SG. ATP-dependent K^+ channel activation in isolated normal and hypertensive newborn and adult porcine pulmonary vessels. Pediatr Res 1997; 42:317–326.
25. Nelson MT, Quayle JM. Physiological roles and properties of potassium channels in arterial smooth muscle. Am J Physiol 1995; 268:C799–C822.
26. Cook NS. Potassium Channels: Structure, Classification, Function, and Therapeutic Potential. Chichester, England: Ellis Horwood, 1990.
27. Cornfield DN, Reeve HL, Tolarova S, Weir EK, Archer SL. Oxygen causes fetal pulmonary vasodilation through activation of a calcium-dependent potassium channel. Proc Natl Acad Sci USA 1996; 93:8089–8094.
28. Tristani-Firouzi M, Martin EB, Tolarova S, Weir EK, Archer SL, Cornfield DN. Ventilation-induced pulmonary vasodilation at birth is modulated by potassium channel activity. Am J Physiol 1996; 271:H2353–H2359.
28a. Storme L, Rairigh RL, Parker TA, Cornfield DN, Kinsella JP, Abman SH. K^+ channel blockade inhibits shear stress-induced pulmonary vasodilation in the ovine fetus. Am J Physiol 1999; 276:L220–L228.
29. Saqueton CB, Miller RM, Porter VA, Millla CM, Cornfield DN. Nitric oxide causes perinatal pulmonary vasodilation through K^+ channel activation and requires intracellular calcium release. Am J Physiol 1999; 276:L925–L932.
30. Rhodes MT, Porter VA, Saqueton CB, Herron JM, Resnik ER, Cornfield DN. Pulmonary vascular response to normoxia and K_{Ca} channel activity is developmentally regulated. Am J Physiol Lung Cell Mol Physiol 2001; 280: L1250–L1257.

31. Evans AM, Osipenko ON, Haworth SG, Gurney AM. Resting potentials and potassium currents during development of pulmonary artery smooth muscle cells. Am J Physiol 1998; 275:H887–H899.
32. Reeve HL, Archer SL, Weir EK, Cornfield DN. Maturational changes in K^+ channel activity and oxygen sensing in the ovine pulmonary vasculature. Am J Physiol 1998; 275:L2019–L2025.
33. Cornfield DN, Stevens T, McMurtry IF, Abman SH, Rodman DM. Acute hypoxia causes membrane depolarization and calcium influx in fetal pulmonary artery smooth muscle cells. Am J Physiol 1994; 266:L469–L475.
34. Cornfield DN, Saqueton CB, Porter VA, Herron JM, Resnik ER, Haddad IY, Reeve HL. Voltage-gated K^+ channel activity in the ovine pulmonary vasculature is developmentally regulated. Am J Physiol Lung Cell Mol Physiol 2000; 278:L1297–L1304.
35. Gordon JB, Hartup J, Hakim A. Developmental effects of hypoxia and indomethacin on distribution of vascular responses in lamb lungs. Pediatr Res 1989; 26:325–329.
36. Rendas A, Reid L. Response of the pulmonary circulation to acute hypoxia in the growing pig. J Appl Physiol 1982; 52:811–814.
37. Porter VA, Reeve HL, Cornfield DN. Fetal rabbit pulmonary artery smooth muscle cell response to ryanodine is developmentally regulated. Am J Physiol Lung Cell Mol Physiol 2000; 279:L751–L757.
38. Porter VA, Rhodes MT, Reeve HL, Cornfield DN. Oxygen-induced perinatal pulmonary vasodilation is mediated by ryanodine-sensitive activation of a calcium-sensitive K^+ channel. Am J Physiol Lung Cell Mol Physiol 2001; 281:L1379–L1385.
39. Nelson MT, Cheng H, Rubart M, Santana LF, Bonev AD, Knot HJ, Lederer WJ. Relaxation of arterial smooth muscle by arterial sparks. Science 1995; 270:633–637.
40. Gomez AM, Valdivia HH, Cheng H, Lederer MR, Santana LF, Cannell MB, McCune SA, Altschuld RA, Lederer WJ. Defective excitation-contraction coupling in experimental cardiac hypertrophy and heart failure. Science 1997; 276:800–806.
41. Porter VA, Bonev AD, Knot HJ, Heppner TJ, Stevenson AS, Kleppisch T, Lederer WJ, Nelson MT. Frequency modulation of Ca^{2+} sparks is involved in regulation of arterial diameter by cyclic nucleotides. Am J Physiol 1998; 274:C1346–C1355.

28

Anorexigens and Pulmonary Arterial Hypertension

The Role of Potassium Channels

Sean McMurtry and Evangelos D. Michelakis[†]
University of Alberta, Edmonton, Alberta, Canada

I. INTRODUCTION

Anorexigens are drugs that suppress appetite mainly bymodulating the serotonin [5-hydroxytryptamine (5-HT)] signaling pathway in the brain. It was always obvious that the efficacy of anorexigens was at most modest, leading to sustained weight reductions of only 5–10% more than placebo and diet alone. A significant group of anorexigen users had been minimally above the ideal body weight, and thus one can see these compounds as examples of "image-enhancing drugs" rather than tools against the battle of obesity. The industry of image-enhancing drugs has always been powerful and has repeatedly won over common sense and independent scientific thinking. The anorexigen story is an interesting example of the failure of Poincaré's principle:

> *The method of the physical sciences is based upon the induction which leads us to expect recurrence of a phenomenon when the circumstances which give rise to it are repeated.* (H. Poincaré, Science and Hypothesis, 1905.)

SM is a CIHR Strategic Fellow (TORCH program) and a Fellow in the University of Alberta Clinician Investigator Program.
[†] EM is a CIHR New Investigator and AHFMR Scholar.

Over the past 30 years and despite the experience and several warnings, various anorexigens kept getting approved, leading repeatedly to pulmonary arterial hypertension (PAH) epidemics (1,2).

Following a brief review of the history linking anorexigens with PAH over the past 30 years, the potential mechanisms of action of these drugs in the pulmonarycirculation will be presented and a unifying hypothesis will be proposed. Although several of these drugs have been withdrawn from the market, the interest of the scientific community remains high. This is because, despite recent progress, the etiology of PAH remains unknown (3). This is in part due to the lack of appropriate animal models for this devastating disease. Anorexigens might have offered us a human model of the disease, and thus their mechanism of action might lead to important clues in the pathogenesis of PAH. In addition to the better-studied effects of anorexigens on the 5-HT axis in the vasculature, this review will focus on a newly discovered mechanism of these drugs, i.e., their ability to potently inhibit potassium (K^+) channels (4). The K^+ channel-inhibiting properties of anorexigens might explain many of their effects and might further strengthen the theory suggesting that vascular K^+ channel inhibition is etiologically related to the development of PAH (3).

II. HISTORY

A. Aminorex

One year after the first anorexigen, aminorex, was released in central Europe in 1965, the first cases of PAH were reported, and a strong association was quickly established (5,6). A few years later, a retrospective study revealed a ten-fold increase in the incidence of PAH in central Europe (7). There was an odds ratio of >1000 for the development of PAH among patients exposed to aminorex (7). Interestingly, about half of the patients with aminorex-induced PAH weighed only 10% above the ideal body weight (7). Within a few years from the drug's discontinuation, the prevalence of PAH in central Europe returned to baseline (8,9). Follow-up studies showed an unpredictable course: whereas in some patients PAH was progressive, others showed almost normalization of their pulmonary artery pressures, at least at rest (8,9). This suggested that although aminorex might have been the initiating factor, progression of PAH perhaps depended on the presence of additional predisposing factors.

B. The Fenfluramines

The first case reports linking fenfluramine with PAH were published in 1981, and many others followed (10–13). The first large retrospective study that showed a strong association between fenfluramine and PAH was published in 1993 (14). In an effort to eliminate fenfluramine's sympathomimetic side effects, the D-isomer dexfenfluramine was introduced in the market in the

1990s. Dexfenfluramine was approved by the FDA despite the association of aminorex and fenfluramine with PAH and soon became the most commonly used anorectic drug (15). The reports linking fenfluramine and PAH triggered the International Primary Pulmonary Hypertension Study (IPPHS), which was sponsored by the Medical Research Council of Canada and funded by Servier, the manufacturer of dexfenfluramine (16). This was a case-controlled study and assessed 95 patients with PAH from 35 European centers and sex- and age-matched controls recruited from general practice (16). The study showed that any use of anorectic drugs (the most common of which was dexfenfluramine) was associated with an increased risk of PAH (odds ratio 6.3, 95% confidence interval 3.0–13.2). For the use of anorectic drugs within the preceding year for more than 3 months the odds ratio was 23.1 (16). At the same time, the weight loss achieved with dexfenfluramine, even with prolonged use, was not significant. In one study, the group of patients using dexfenfluramine lost no more than one body mass index unit compared to the group on placebo (17). There were no morbidity or long-term follow-up data from the IPPHS, becuase less than one year after the publication of the study the drug was discontinued. However, there were reports of rapidly progressing and fatal cases from dexfenfluramine-induced pulmonary hypertension (18,19). Interestingly, the reason for dexfenfluramine's discontinuation was not the IPPHS but the findings of a small study reporting that up to 30% of its users develop left heart valvular abnormalities (20).

C. Fen-Phen

Although the most common way of prescribing dexfenfluramine was in the form of Fen-Phen (dexfenfluramine plus phentermine), the IPPHS did not assess possible differential effects of the two drugs on the pulmonary circulation, and data on the side effects of phentermine alone are generally lacking. Phentermine can inhibit monoamine oxidase B, an action that could potentially inhibit the metabolism of 5-HT, hence increasing local and plasma levels of 5-HT. Phentermine has also been shown to prolong the vasoconstrictor effects of 5-HT in rat lung (21). As in the aminorex case, the IPPHS was not able to identify possible predisposing factors for the development of anorectic-induced PAH. Now we know that such potential predisposing factors might have been polymorphisms in the 5-HT transporter, abnormalities in the voltage-gated K^+ channels in the pulmonary artery smooth muscle cells, as well as functional mutations in the bone morphogenetic factor receptor II (for review see Ref. 3).

The argument used in the approval of fenfluramine, dexfenfluramine, and Fen-Phen (following the PAH epidemics) was that these drugs are different enough to have different peripheral effects and that the benefits of treating obesity might outweigh the risk for PAH. The unfortunate truth is

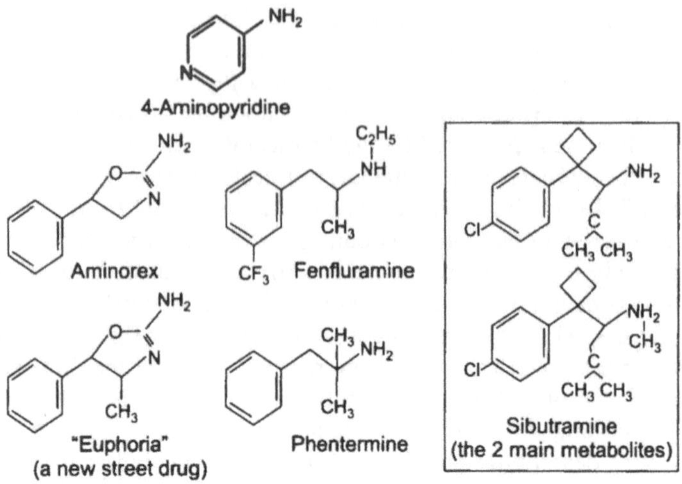

Figure 1 Structure may predict function in anorexigens. Interesting similarities in the structure of withdrawn and currently used anorexigens. Euphoria (U-4-E-uh or "ice") is a new street drug (a stimulant) that has been associated with PAH (22). Note the similarities in the $NH_2$and CH_3 groups. Structural similarity between these drugs and the Kv channel inhibitor 4-aminopyridine can also be seen; this might predict the potent Kv channel inhibitory properties of these drugs (see Fig. 4).

that these drugs do have very similar mechanisms of action on the 5-HT axis and, as we will discuss below, on K^+ channels. Interestingly, even looking at their structure, one can recognize intriguing similarities among them and compared to the common K^+ channel blocker 4-aminopyridine (Fig. 1). It is intriguing that a common street drug (U-4-E-Uh, pronounced "euphoria," also known as "ice") was recently associated with the development of PAH (22). Its structural similarity to aminorex is striking (Fig. 1). Therefore the fact that all of these agents are associated with the development of PAH is not surprising at all. It is important that the structure of these drugs is also similar to a very recently approved and widely used anorexigen, sibutramine (23,24) (Fig. 1). As will be discussed below, sibutramine is also a very potent K^+ channel blocker. Although no association has been made yet between the use of sibutramine and PAH, as we discuss below, PAH might need more time before it is detectable. Also, PAH is a very challenging disease to diagnose clinically and certainly one has to "look" in order to "see."

III. THE 5-HT STORY

A. Anorexigens and 5-HT

The fenfluramines cause 5-HT release and inhibit 5-HT reuptake in central nervous system synapses (15). In addition to the effects on 5-HT release and uptake (25), aminorex (a catechol derivative) increases brain norepinephrine levels (26). Although the inhibition of 5-HT *reuptake* is clearly due to the inhibition of the 5-HT transporter (5-HTT), the mechanism by which anorexigens cause *release* of 5-HT is unclear. Ninety-eight percent of free plasma 5-HT is cleared by the pulmonary endothelium in a single circulation (27). This process in the endothelium is 5-HTT-mediated and is similar to 5-HT uptake from nerve endings and platelets, the main carriers of 5-HT in the blood (27). Within the pulmonary endothelium, 5-HT is deaminated by monoamine oxidase.

In the same way that anorexigens increase synaptic 5-HT levels in the brain, they also appear to cause release of 5-HT from platelets (28) and perhaps from endothelial cells. However, although it is likely that the anorexigens increase 5-HT levels locally in microenvironments within the vasculature, it is not clear whether long-term treatment with anorexigens increases the 5-HT levels in the plasma. For example, the fenfluramines increase 5-HT levels in the CSF but not in the plasma (29).

B. 5-HT and PAH

Multiple lines of evidence suggest that 5-HT is very important in the pathogenesis of PAH (30), in addition to several other mechanisms, including pulmonary vascular K^+ channels (31,32), imbalance of endogenous vasodilators (33,34) and vasoconstrictors (35,36), endogenous proteases (37), dysregulated angiogenesis (38), and abnormal bone morphogenetic protein signaling (39). For example, treatment with 5-HT can potentiate the development of chronic hypoxic pulmonary hypertension in rats, supporting an etiological or contributory role for 5-HT in the vascular remodeling of PAH (40). Also, patients with PAH have elevated plasma 5-HT levels compared to controls ($30.1 \pm 9.2 \times 10^{-9}$ mol/L versus $0.6 \pm 0.1 \times 10^{-9}$ mol/L), and 5-HT levels remain high even after heart-lung transplantation (41), suggesting that this is not a secondary effect due to the plexogenic lesions and endothelial dysfunction seen in PAH. However, a direct causative role of increased 5-HT levels in the plasma and PAH is still missing. The fawn-hooded rat, which has a genetic deficiency in platelet 5-HT handling, develops pulmonary hypertension spontaneously when exposed to mild hypoxia or high altitude (42). Furthermore, PAH has been described in patients with platelet storage pool disease, a rare condition where platelets have defective 5-HT uptake (43). On the other hand, patients with metastatic carcinoid tumors that have elevated plasma 5-HT levels do not develop PAH.

The mechanisms by which 5-HT might cause PAH have started to be elucidated. 5-HT is a vasoconstrictor and a well-known vascular smooth muscle cell (VSMC) mitogen (44). It exerts its cellular effects by binding to several types of 5-HT receptors in the cell membrane. In addition, 5-HT can exert some of its effects inside the cell, internalized by the

5-HTT. It is not clear whether the effects of anorexigens leading to PAH are mediated by the 5-HT receptor, the 5-HTT, or both.

In an elegant recent study, Launay et al. (45) showed that 5-HT receptor 2B ($5\text{-}HT_{2B}$) is critical in the development of 5-HT-induced PAH, at least in mice. The pulmonary vascular remodeling effects that chronic hypoxia induces in mice are potentiated by dexfenfluramine. The effects of both chronic hypoxia and dexfenfluramine are absent from $5\text{-}HT_{2B}{}^{-/-}$ mice. It is interesting that the dexfenfluramine metabolite nordexfenfluramine acts as a high-affinity ligand for $5\text{-}HT_{2B}$ receptors. This suggests that, in addition to the effects mediated by the dexfenfluramine-induced release in 5-HT, there might be direct effects mediated by the activation of $5\text{-}HT_{2B}$ by nordexfenfluramine.

Other studies have provided evidence suggesting that the long-term effects of anorexigens on the pulmonary vasculature are mediated by 5-HTT (46). The mechanism of 5-HT signaling for the growth of pulmonary artery smooth muscle cells (PASMCs) through 5-HTT has been shown to involve internalization of 5-HT and tyrosine phosphorylation of a GTPase-activating protein (46), the production of activated oxygen species, and the activation of the redox-sensitive MEK-ERK pathway (47). More recently, the downstream components of the pathway activated by ERK were characterized. Suzuki et al. (48) showed that 5-HT regulates PASMC proliferation by activation of GATA-4. The GATA family of transcription factors includes six genes with a conserved zinc finger DNA-binding domain that interacts with DNA regulatory elements containing the consensus (A/T) GATA (A/G) sequence. Interestingly, in systemic VSMCs, the GATA-6 has been shown to maintain cells in the quiescent state and mitogens downregulate GATA-6 to induce proliferation (48). In contrast, in PASMCs, 5-HT and other mitogens such as endothelin-1 increase growth by upregulating GATA-4, which in turn regulates the expression of cyclin D2 (49). This is a fascinating difference between the pulmonary and systemic VSMCs that might be involved in the different responses of the pulmonary and systemic circulations to injury, hypoxia, etc. Another recently described fundamental difference is that the mitochondria, critical oxygen sensors and regulators of apoptosis, between pulmonary and systemic VSMCs are different (50).

The 5-HTT is upregulated by hypoxia, with concomitant mitogenic effects on PASMCs (51). Mice lacking the 5-HTT are protected from chronic hypoxic pulmonary hypertension (52). 5-HTT overexpression has been found in patients with PAH (53), and there is an association between PAH and the L-allelic variant of the 5-HTT that may contribute to susceptibility to the PAH phenotype (53,54).

C. Summary

Although an increase in plasma 5-HT levels has not been described in anorexigen users, these drugs might cause PAH in part by increasing 5-HT levels in microenvironments in the vasculature. This is achieved first by inhibiting the 5-HTT in the platelets and endothelial cells and second by increasing the release of 5-HT from platelets and neurons. Some anorexigens, such as nordexfenfluramine, might also have direct effects on the 5-HT_{2B} receptors. The mechanism of the increased release is not known, but, as we discuss below, this might be mediated by inhibition of K^+ channels in platelets and neurons. In addition, the K^+ channel inhibitory effects of anorexigens in VSMCs might directly cause pulmonary (and systemic) vasoconstriction and remodeling, independent of the 5-HT axis.

IV. THE K^+ CHANNEL STORY

A. K^+ Channels and Vascular Disease

Potassium ion channels are critical for the development of vascular disease because they control vascular tone as well as VSMC proliferation and apoptosis. Vasoconstriction, increased VSMC proliferation, and decreased VSMC apoptosis rates lead to medial hypertrophy, a hallmark of vascular disease in many vascular beds. K^+ channels control membrane potential (E_m) in many cells including VSMCs. Downregulation or inhibition of K^+ channels leads to a decreased efflux of K^+ down the normal concentration gradient (140 meq intracellular, 5 meq extracellular), whereas the influx of K^+ through energy-dependent pumps continues. This leads to a shift of the E_m from approximately −60 mV toward more positive potentials (depolarization). When E_m becomes more positive than −30 mV, the open probability of the voltage-gated L-type Ca^{2+} channels increases, resulting in influx and increase in the intracellular Ca^{2+} and vasoconstriction. In addition, the depolarization-induced increase of PASMC intracellular Ca^{2+} concentration may contribute to SMC proliferation (55). Furthermore, the decreased K^+ channels lead to decreased efflux and an increase in the intracellular K^+. Intracellular K^+ has been shown to tonically inhibit the function of several caspases, suppressing apoptosis in a variety of cell types, including PASMCs (56,57).

There are several K^+ channel families, the most important being the inward rectifier K^+ channels (K_{ir}), which include the ATP-sensitive K^+ channels; the calcium-activated K^+ channels (K_{Ca}); and the voltage-gated K^+ channels (Kv). The Kv family has several subfamilies, and specific Kv channels such as Kv1.5 and Kv2.1 have been shown to control E_m in resistance PASMCs (58).

In summary, a K^+ channel deficiency state in the vasculature is associated with vasoconstriction, increased VSMC proliferation rates, and suppressed apoptosis, eventually leading to medial hypertrophy and vascular remodeling. It is therefore not surprising that PAH in a variety of animal models and in humans is indeed a Kv channel deficiency state.

B. K^+ Channels and PAH

Patients with PAH have been shown to have a selective transcriptional reduction of specific Kv channels (i.e., Kv1.5) in PASMCs (31,32). Both Kv1.5 and Kv2.1 are decreased in the PASMCs from rats with chronic hypoxic pulmonary hypertension (CH-PHT) (59). Exogenous restoration of Kv1.5 expression with gene therapy (inhaled replication-deficient adenovirus carrying the gene for green fluorescence protein and Kv1.5) improves pulmonary hypertension and right ventricular hypertrophy in rats with CH-PHT (60). These data suggest that Kv1.5 and perhaps other selective Kv channels (such as Kv2.1) are important in the control of pulmonary vascular tone and the development of PAH. The selective deficiency of these channels might lead to PAH in a manner similar to cystic fibrosis, where a selective loss of Cl^- channels leads to the development of the disease. In other words, PAH might be a form of vascular "channelopathy" (3). Thus, it is not surprising that all anorexigens are potent Kv channel inhibitors, as will be discussed below. This recently discovered property of anorexigens not only provides a novel mechanism by which these drugs cause PAH but also further strengthens the hypothesis that the function and expression of Kv channels is etiologically related to the development of PAH (3).

C. Anorexigens and Kv Channels

Weir et al. (61) first showed that both aminorex and the fenfluramines rapidly inhibit K^+ currents in freshly isolated rat resistance PASMCs. These currents are sensitive to 4-aminopyridine (4-AP), a relatively specific inhibitor of Kv channels, suggesting that they are Kv currents (61) (Fig. 2A). This inhibition is physiologically significant becuase it leads to PASMC depolarization and a rise in pulmonary vascular resistance, measured in the isolated perfused rat lung model using clinically relevant doses (61) (Fig. 2B).

Since then, anorexigens have been shown to acutely inhibit 4-AP-sensitive currents in several tissues, including smooth muscle cells from rat systemic arteries (62), human ductus arteriosus (63), rat ventricular myocytes (64), and rabbit megakaryocytes (65). Of importance, incubation of cultured human PASMCs with dexfenfluramine ($200\,\mu M \times 73\,h$) leads to a decrease in Kv1.5 mRNA and expressed protein level (66) (Fig 3A). The effects of anorexigens on isolated PASMCs and in isolated perfused organs strongly suggest that the effects of these drugs in K^+ channels are direct and independent of 5-HT.

However, the most direct evidence that anorexigens inhibit Kv channels independent of 5-HT comes from electrophysiological experiments on cloned Kv channels in expression systems. Dexfenfluramine significantly inhibits cloned Kv2.1 expressed in *Xenopus* oocytes (67). Very recently, a number of different anorectic agents, including aminorex, dexfenfluramine, phentermine, and sibutramine were shown to inhibit Kv1.5

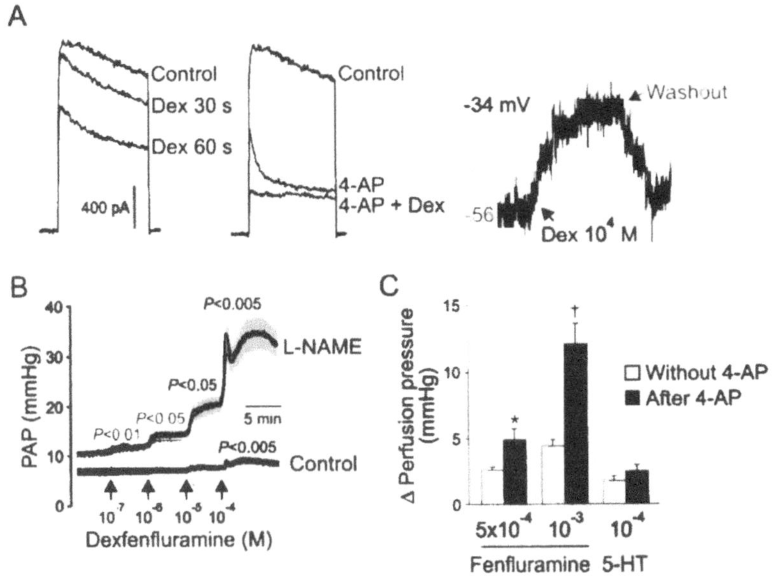

Figure 2 Anorexigens inhibit Kv channels in the rat pulmonary circulation. (A) Dexfenfluramine rapidly (within 30 s) inhibits outward potassium current (I_K) in rat resistance pulmonary arterial smooth muscle cells (left, the current resulting from a depolarizing step from −70 to +50 mV is shown), causing depolarization (right). Standard whole-cell patch-clamp recordings are shown. Addition of dexfenfluramine (Dex) with 4-aminopyridine (4-AP) does not cause further I_K inhibition, suggesting that Dex and 4-AP work through the same mechanism, i.e., Kv channel inhibition. (B) Clinically relevant (10^{-7} and 10 ^{6} M) doses of dexfenfluramine increase pulmonary vascular resistance in the isolated rat lung model only when L-NAME is added to the perfusate to inhibit nitric oxide synthase. Because the flow is kept constant in this model, increases in pulmonary artery pressure reflect increases in total pulmonary vascular resistance. Deficiency in the NO axis might be an important predisposing factor for the development of anorexigen-induced PAH. (C) Using the same perfused rat lung model as in (B) Bèlohlávková et al. (72) showed that pretreatment with 4-AP potentiates the constrictor effects of fenfluramine but not of 5-HT. This suggests that deficiencies in PASMC Kv channels might be another important predisposing factor for the development of anorexigen-induced PAH. (A and B are reprinted from Ref. 61 and C from Ref. 72, with permission.)

expressed in CHO cells (68) (Fig. 4). Fluoxetine (Prozac®), a 5-HT reuptake inhibitor that is being used as both an antidepressant and an anorectic, was also found to inhibit expressed Kv1.5 (68). Interestingly, sibutramine and fluoxetine are more potent Kv1.5 inhibitors than aminorex and dexfenfluramine at positive membrane potentials. However, both sibutramine's and fluoxetine's inhibitory effects are strongly mem-

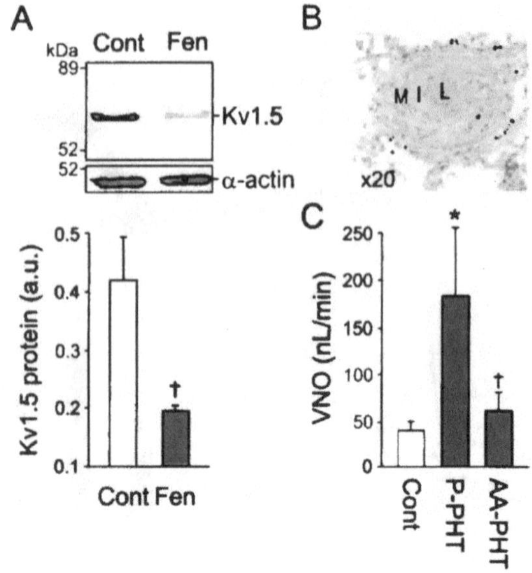

Figure 3 Anorexigen-induced PAH in humans. (A) Exposure of human cultured PASMCs to fenfluramine causes a decrease in the mRNA and expressed protein of Kv1.5. (B) Severe remodeling (intimal hyperplasia and medial hypertrophy) in a pulmonary artery from a young woman who developed severe PAH and died after short-term use of fenfluramine. M, media; I, intima; L, lumen. (C) Patients with anorectic-induced pulmonary hypertension (AA-PHT) have decreased breath nitric oxide (NO) levels compared with patients with primary pulmonary hypertension (P-PHT). Patients with P-PHT have increased breath NO levels compared to normal controls. This suggests that NO production might be a defensive mechanism in the development of PHT and that its deficiency might predispose to the development of AA-PHT (also see Fig. 2B). Breath NO was measured by chemiluminescence and was controlled for ventilation (VNO). The amount of VNO also correlates with the severity of pulmonary hypertension, invasively studied in patients with AA-PPH (not shown). (A was reprinted from Ref. 66, B from Ref. 19, and C from Ref. 71, with permission.)

brane potential dependent; i.e., the more depolarized the cell, the higher their potency (68). This confirms earlier findings by Reeve et al. (69), who showed that fluoxetine inhibits PASMC Kv currents but causes depolarization only if the cell is already depolarized by current injection. Elegant single-channel analysis in expressed Kv1.5 has shown that at least sibutramine and fluoxetine bind to the channel in the open state (68). This explains their stronger effects in depolarized potentials because Kv channels open as the cell membrane depolarizes. This could potentially, at least in part, explain why fluoxetine has not so far been associated with vascular complications, although there is some evidence that sibutramine

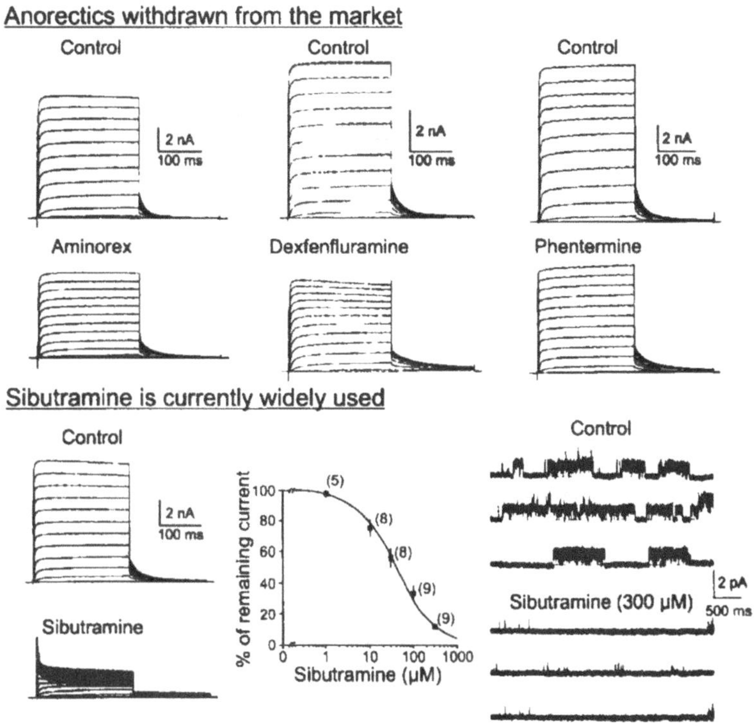

Figure 4 Anorexigens are potent Kv1.5 inhibitors. (A) Aminorex (1 mM), dexfenfluramine (1 mM), and phentermine (300 μM) inhibit Kv1.5 expressed in CHO cells (250 ms pulses in 10 mV steps from a holding potential of −70 mV to +70 mV). These three drugs were withdrawn from the market. (B) Sibutramine, currently widely used, is a more potent Kv1.5 blocker, and its potency increases as the membrane depolarizes. A dose response is shown as mean data ($n = 5$–9). A cell-attached single-channel recording is shown at the bottom. Sibutramine (300 μM) decreases the open probability but not the amplitude of expressed Kv1.5 (recording at +60 mV). (Reprinted with permission from Ref. 68.)

is associated with systemic hypertension (70). In other words, these drugs might not have any effects in normal PASMCs because at normal E_m (i.e., < -60 mV), the relevant Kv channels will be closed. However, in diseased or depolarized PASMCs, Kv channels will be open (they are called voltage-gated because they are activated by depolarization) and therefore subject to inhibition. Examples of these scenarios include PASMC depolarization due to endothelial dysfunction (and lack of the tonic hyperpolarizing effects of NO or prostacyclin) or PASMC depolarization because of genetic Kv channel deficiency.

D. Predisposing Factors for Anorexigen-Induced PAH

Although the pressor effects of several anorexigens in the perfused rat lung were only modest in clinically relevant doses, in lungs pretreated with inhibitors of the NO synthase (NOS) the pressor effects were greatly potentiated (61) (Fig. 2B). Becuase Kv channels are also present in systemic blood vessels, it is not surprising that dexfenfluramine constricts several systemic vessels as well, including cerebral and renal arteries of the rat (62). Interestingly, there are several case reports of systemic vascular events associated with anorexigen use (for review see Ref. 4). Once again, although the effects of intravenous dexfenfluramine on rat systemic arterial pressure is only modest at clinically relevant doses, these effects are potentiated in rats pretreated with NOS inhibitors (62).

That NO insufficiency might be a permissive mechanism in the development of anorexigen-induced PAH was later supported by the findings of a small case-control study (71). In this study exhaled NO was compared in patients with primary versus anorexigen-induced PAH. Exhaled NO was significantly lower in the latter. Interestingly, the primary PAH group had increased levels of exhaled NO compared to normal controls (Fig. 3C) (71). Furthermore, exhaled NO levels correlated inversely with pulmonary vascular resistance (71). These data suggest that an increase in NO production might be a defensive mechanism that limits the extent of PAH.

In addition to endothelial dysfunction (prevalent in obese patients) or NO deficiency, another factor predisposing patients to develop anorexigen-induced PAH is a genetic deficiency in Kv channels. This hypothesis is supported by the observation that in the isolated perfused rat lung model, 4-AP (mimicking a Kv channel deficiency state) potentiates the pressor response to dexfenfluramine but not to 5-HT (72) (Fig. 2C). As discussed above, the inhibition by dexfenfluramine is enhanced because the inhibition of Kv channels in PASMCs effectively depolarizes the cell, activating the remaining Kv channels and thus making them "available" for inhibition by dexfenfluramine.

The anorectic drugs inhibit Kv channels at micromolar doses, which are higher than the therapeutic levels of these drugs in the serum. However, the levels of these drugs in the serum of patients developing complications are not known, and it is possible that predisposed individuals might have higher serum levels. In addition, the concentration of the drug within the vascular wall is not known in treated patients. For example, it is possible that some patients metabolize the drugs abnormally, although this has not been proven.

Dexfenfluramine has been shown to raise pulmonary vascular resistance in dogs (73,74) and also to cause human and porcine pulmonary arterial rings in tissue baths to constrict (75). On the other hand, dexfenfluramine does not potentiate the development of pulmonary hypertension in rats due to either chronic hypoxia (76) or monocrotaline (77), in contrast to the potentiation of chronic hypoxic pulmonary hypertension in mice (45). The mechanistic implications of these species differences in the response to anorexigens are not well understood.

V. A PROPOSED UNIFYING MECHANISM

Piecing the various mechanisms together into a coherent theory for the development of anorexigen-related PAH is a challenge. The studies on the effects of anorexigens on expressed Kv channels and on isolated cells and organs show that the Kv channel blocking properties of anorexigens are primary and not mediated by 5-HT. They further raise the provocative possibility that, at least in some tissues such as neurons or platelets, the increase in 5-HT release caused by anorexigens is due to Kv channel inhibition.

The release of 5-HT from neurons is dependent on E_m and $[Ca^{2+}]_i$ (78), and 4-AP causes 5-HT release in brain slices (79). This suggests that Kv channels might regulate the release of neuronal 5-HT. Therefore, anorexigens may indirectly cause the release of 5-HT in neurons by inhibiting Kv channels. Similarly, both anorexigens and 4-AP increase the release of 5-HT from human platelets (28), and dexfenfluramine directly inhibits Kv currents in freshly isolated megakaryocytes (the precursors of platelets) (65) (Fig. 5). In other words, the Kv channel blocking properties of anorexigens might be important in both their primary effect (i.e., effects in the brain and appetite suppression) and their vascular complications. Furthermore, 5-HT itself has recently been shown to inhibit a variety of K^+ channels (including Kv channels), via mechanisms involving 5-HT receptor-mediated phosphorylation (80–84).

In summary (Fig. 6), the anorexigen effects on 5-HT reuptake are clearly mediated by the anorexigen inhibition of the 5-HTT activity. A mechanism for the anorexigen-induced release of 5-HT from membrane-bound vesicles, however, is not clear; we propose that this might be mediated by the anorexigen-induced Kv channel inhibition and depolarization, with the resultant increase in intracellular Ca^{2+} and exocytosis of the 5-HT vesicles. Therefore, the anorexigen-induced Kv channel inhibition in neurons and platelets will contribute to 5-HT release. At the same time the anorexigen-induced Kv channel inhibition in VSMCs will cause depolarization, an increase in intracellular Ca^{2+} levels, constriction, increased proliferation, and suppressed apoptosis levels, i.e., medial hypertrophy and vascular remodeling (Fig. 3B). The direct effects of anorexigens on VSMCs will be greatly potentiated in already depolarized cells, as might be found in endothelial dysfunction or in genetic deficiency of Kv channels (Figs. 2B and 3C). The locally increased 5-HT levels might potentiate the vascular effects of the anorexigens by further inhibiting Kv channels in a positive feedback loop manner.

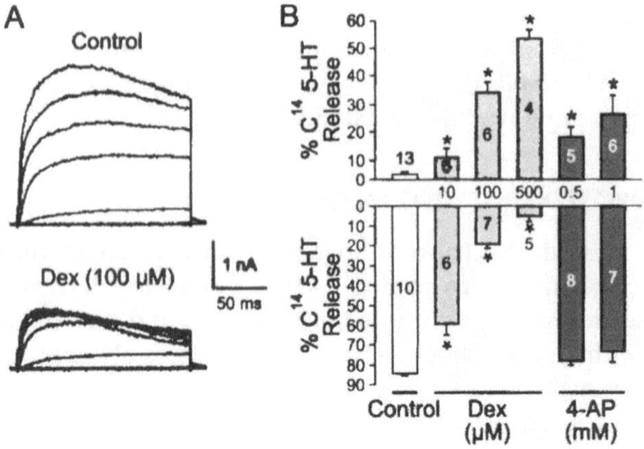

Figure 5 Anorexigens inhibit K^+ channels and cause 5-HT release from platelets. (A) Dexfenfluramine (Dex) inhibits K^+ current in rat megakaryocytes. A family of currents in response to depolarizing steps from −70 mV to +50 mV are shown (whole-cell patch clamp). (Reprinted from Ref. 65 with permission.) (B) The Kv channel blocker 4-aminopyridine (4-AP), like dexfenfluramine (Dex), increases 5-HT release. Whereas Dex decreases 5-HT reuptake, 4-AP does not. Fresh platelets from human volunteers were studied using C^{14}-labeled 5-HT. The decrease in 5-HT reuptake by Dex is due to inhibition of the 5-HT transporter and thus is 4-AP insensitive. Release of 5-HT from platelets, on the other hand, as in neurons, might be membrane-potential-sensitive, and these data suggest that it might be specifically due to Kv channel inhibition.

VI. LESSONS FOR THE FUTURE

Sibutramine is a novel weight loss drug that was approved for clinical use in the United States in 1997. It has combined serotonergic and noradrenergic properties (23), which are both thought to contribute to its weight loss effects. To date there are only short-term safety data for sibutramine (26,85), and it has been found to be generally well tolerated.

As can be seen in Fig. 4, sibutramine is a very potent Kv channel inhibitor (in expression systems). PAH has not yet been reported in sibutramine users (although one has to "look" for PAH in order to "see" it), but very concerning reports for sibutramine-related systemic hypertension have started to appear. In a trial of sibutramine in obese hypertensive patients, diastolic blood pressure was increased despite a modest weight reduction (70). In another trial involving healthy volunteers, sibutramine increased the blood pressure significantly, although at the same time it decreased systemic norepinephrine levels (86). Long-term safety data are necessary to further define its safety profile. Interestingly, AHA published a warning for the use of sibutramine. The following is a quote from the American Heart Association web site:

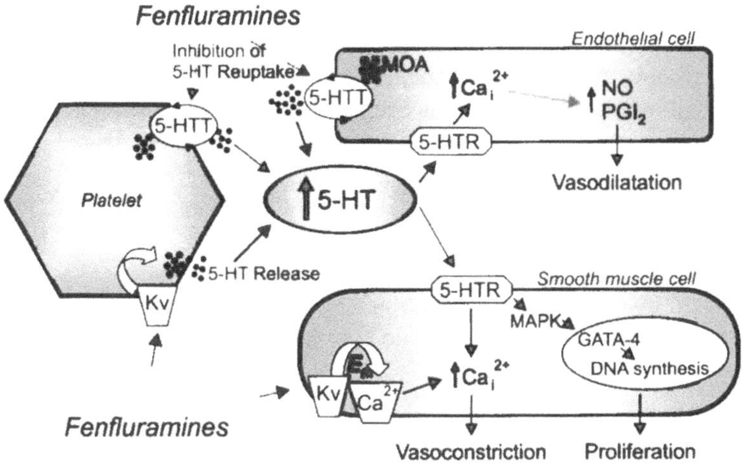

Figure 6 A schematic diagram summarizing the vascular effects of the anorectic drugs. Vascular smooth muscle cells, endothelial cells, and platelets are all involved in the proposed mechanism of anorexigen-induced PAH. The two primary mechanisms of anorexigens (such as the recently commonly used fenfluramine) are shown: (1) Inhibition of the 5-HT transporter (5-HTT) in platelets and endothelial cells, leading to increase in the extracellular 5-HT, which will in turn cause PASMC contraction and proliferation. (2) Inhibition of platelet and PASMC Kv channels leading to release of 5-HT from platelets (and neurons) and PASMC contraction and proliferation independent of 5-HT. Abnormal endothelium will decrease the counterbalance of the vasodilators produced in response to the rise in intracellular $[Ca^{2+}]$ caused by the binding of 5-HT on the endothelial 5-HT receptors (5-HTR). Also, the lack of these hyperpolarizing factors would depolarize VSMCs, activating Kv channels and making them "available for inhibition" by the fenfluramines, in a positive feedback loop manner.

> Sibutramine increases the blood pressure in some people... We urge caution when considering the use of sibutramine (Meridia). Before definitive data are available, patients and their physicians should carefully weigh the benefits vs. the risks of using this new medication. It's especially important that this drug be considered only for people for whom obesity poses a health risk. (http://www.americanheart.org/presenter.html?identifier=4530).

Given the enormous burden of obesity in western societies (87), it is certain that weight loss medications will remain an attractive goal of drug development. Indeed, there are additional weight loss medications currently on the market, and likely more will follow (88). It is imperative that the possibility of future epidemics of PAH be minimized, and therefore it is essential that lessons be learned from the previous experiences with anorexigen-related PAH (1,17). Fast screening of candidate anorexigens in expressed Kv channels might identify patients at higher risk for vascular complications. Such Kv-blocking drugs would have to be aggressively tested in a variety of cell and organ models before approval for clinical use.

ACKNOWLEDGMENTS

Supported by The Canadian Institutes of Health Research, The Heart and Stroke Foundation of Canada, and the Alberta Heritage Foundation for Medical Research.

REFERENCES

1. Fishman AP. Aminorex to Fen/phen: an epidemic foretold. Circulation 1999; 99:156–161.
2. Voelkel NF, Clarke WR, Higenbottam T. Obesity, dexfenfluramine, and pulmonary hypertension A lesson not learned? Am J Respir Crit Care Med 1997; 155:786–788.
3. Archer S, Rich S. Primary pulmonary hypertension: a vascular biology and translational research "Work in progress". Circulation 2000; 102:2781–2791.
4. Michelakis E. Anorectic drugs and vascular disease: the role of voltage-gated K^+ channels. Vascul Pharmacol 2002; 38:51–59.
5. Stuhlinger W, Raberger G, Kraupp O. Effect of Aminorex (Menocil) on pulmonary hemodynamics. (In German.) Naunyn Schmiedebergs Arch Pharmakol 1969; 264:314–315.
6. Kay JM, Smith P, Heath D. Aminorex and the pulmonary circulation. Thorax 1971; 26:262–270.
7. Greiser E. Epidemiologic studies on the relation between use of appetite depressants and primary vascular pulmonary hypertension. (In German.) Internist (Berl) 1973; 14:437–442.
8. Mlczoch J, Weir E, Reeves JT, Grover RF. Long term effects of the anorectic agent fenfluramine alone and in combination with aminorex on pulmonary and systemic circulation of the pig. Basic Res Cardiol 1979; 74:313–320.
9. Mlczoch J. Drug and Dietary Induced Pulmonary Hypertension. New York: Futura, 1984.
10. Douglas JG, Munro JF, Kitchin AH, Muir AL, Proudfoot AT. Pulmonary hypertension and fenfluramine. Br Med J (Clin Res Ed) 1981; 283:881–883.
11. Gaul G, Blazek E, Deutsch E, Heeger H. Ein Fall von chronischer pulmonaler hypertonie nach Fenfluramineinnahme. Wiener Klin. Wschr 1982; 22:618–621.
12. McMurray J, Bloomfield P, Miller HC. Irreversible pulmonary hypertension after treatment with fenfluramine. Br Med J (Clin Res Ed) 1986; 293:51–52.
13. Pouwels HM, Smeets JL, Cheriex EC, Wouters EF. Pulmo-nary hypertension and fenfluramine. Eur Respir J 1990; 3:606–607.

14. Brenot F, Herve P, Petitpretz P, Parent F, Duroux P, Simonneau G. Primary pulmonary hypertension and fenfluramine use. Br Heart J 1993; 70: 537–541.
15. McTavish D, Heel R. Dexfenfluramine: a review of its pharmacologic properties and therapeutic potential in obesity. Drugs 1992; 43:713–733.
16. Abenhaim L, Moride Y, Brenot F, Rich S, Benichou J, Kurz X, Higenbottam T, Oakley C, Wouters E, Aubier M, Simonneau G, Begaud B. Appetite-suppressant drugs and the risk of primary pulmonary hypertension. International Primary Pulmonary Hypertension Study Group. N Engl J Med 1996; 335:609–616.
17. Voelkel NF. Appetite suppressants and pulmonary hypertension. Thorax 1997; 52:S63–S67.
18. Strother J, Fedullo P, Yi ES, Masliah E. Complex vascular lesions at autopsy in a patient with phentermine-fenfluramine use and rapidly progressing pulmonary hypertension. Arch Pathol Lab Med 1999; 123:539–540.
19. Mark EJ, Patalas ED, Chang HT, Evans RJ, Kessler SC. Fatal pulmonary hypertension associated with short-term use of fenfluramine and phentermine. N Engl J Med 1997; 337:602–606.
20. Connolly HM, Crary JL, McGoon MD, Hensrud DD, Edwards BS, Edwards WD, Schaff HV.· Valvular heart disease associated with fenfluramine-phentermine. N Engl J Med 1997; 337:581–588.
21. Seiler KU, Wassermann O, Wensky H. On the role of serotonin in the pathogenesis of pulmonary hypertension induced by anorectic drugs; an experimental study in the isolated perfused rat lung, II. Fenfluramine, mazindol, mefenorex, phentermine and R 800. Clin Exp Pharmacol Physiol 1976; 3:323–330.
22. Gaine SP, Rubin LJ, Kmetzo JJ, Palevsky HL, Traill TA. Recreational use of aminorex and pulmonary hypertension. Chest 2000; 118:1496–1497.
23. Luque CA, Rey JA. Sibutramine: a serotonin-norepinephrine reuptake-inhibitor for the treatment of obesity. Ann Pharmacother 1999; 33:968–978.
24. Ryan DH. Use of sibutramine and other noradrenergic and serotonergic drugs in the management of obesity. Endocrine 2000; 13:193–199.
25. Fristrom S, Airaksinen MM, Halmekoski J. Release of platelet 5-hydroxytryptamine by some anorexic and other sympathomimetics and their acetyl derivatives. Acta Pharmacol Toxicol (Copenh) 1977; 41:218–224.
26. Glazer G. Long-term pharmacotherapy of obesity 2000: a review of efficacy and safety. Arch Intern Med 2001; 161:1814–1824.
27. Frishman WH, Huberfeld S, Okin S, Wang YH, Kumar A, Shareef B. Serotonin and serotonin antagonism in cardiovascular and non-cardiovascular disease. J Clin Pharmacol 1995; 35:541–572.
28. Michelakis E, Johnson G, Leis LA, Archer SL, Weir EK. Dexfenfluramine and 4-aminopyridine (an inhibitor of voltage gated potassium channels) increase serotonin release from human platelets. Am J Respir Crit Care Med 1998; 157:A588.
29. Martin F, Artigas F. Simultaneous effects of p-chloroamphetamine, d-fenfluramine, and reserpine on free and stored 5-hydroxytryptamine in brain and blood. J Neurochem 1992; 59:1138–1114.

30. MacLean MR, Herve P, Eddahibi S, Adnot S. 5-Hydroxytryptamine and the pulmonary circulation: receptors, transporters and relevance to pulmonary arterial hypertension. Br J Pharmacol 2000; 131:161–168.
31. Yuan XJ, Wang J, Juhaszova M, Gaine SP, Rubin LJ. Attenuated K^+ channel gene transcription in primary pulmonary hypertension. Lancet 1998; 351: 726–727.
32. Yuan JX-J, Aldinger AM, Juhaszova M, Wang J, Conte JV Jr, Gaine SP, Orens JB, Rubin LJ. Dysfunctional voltage-gated K^+ channels in pulmonary artery smooth muscle cells of patients with primary pulmonary hypertension. Circulation 1998; 98:1400–1406.
33. Tuder RM, Cool CD, Geraci MW, Wang J, Abman SH, Wright L, Badesch D, Voelkel NF. Prostacyclin synthase expression is decreased in lungs from patients with severe pulmonary hypertension. Am J Respir Crit Care Med 1999; 159:1925–1932.
34. Giaid A, Saleh D. Reduced expression of endothelial nitric oxide synthase in the lungs of patients with pulmonary hypertension. N Engl J Med 1995; 333: 214–221.
35. Stewart DJ, Levy RD, Cernacek P, Langleben D. Increased plasma endothelin-1 in pulmonary hypertension: marker or mediator of disease? Ann Intern Med 1991; 114:464–469.
36. Christman BW. Lipid mediator dysregulation in primary pulmonary hypertension. Chest 1998; 114:205S–207S.
37. Cowan KN, Heilbut A, Humpl T, Lam C, Ito S, Rabinovitch M. Complete reversal of fatal pulmonary hypertension in rats by a serine elastase inhibitor. Nat Med 2000; 6:698–702.
38. Voelkel NF, Cool C, Lee SD, Wright L, Geraci MW, Tuder RM. Primary pulmonary hypertension between inflammation and cancer. Chest 1998; 114: 225S–230S.
39. Du L, Sullivan CC, Chu D, Cho AJ, Kido M, Wolf PL, Yuan JX-J, Deutsch R, Jamieson SW, Thistlethwaite PA. Signaling molecules in nonfamilial pulmonary hypertension. N Engl J Med 2003; 348:500–509.
40. Eddahibi S, Raffestin B, Pham I, Launay JM, Aegerter P, Sitbon M, Adnot S. Treatment with 5-HT potentiates development of pulmonary hypertension in chronically hypoxic rats. Am J Physiol 1997; 272:H1173–H1181.
41. Herve P, Launay J-M, Scrobohaci M-L, Brenot F, Simonneau G, Petitpretz P, Poubeau P, Cerrina J, Duroux P, Drouet L. Increased plasma serotonin in primary pulmonary hypertension. Am J Med 1995; 99:249–254.
42. Sato K, Webb S, Tucker A, Rabinovitch M, O'Brien RF, McMurtry IF, Stelzner TJ. Factors influencing the idiopathic development of pulmonary hypertension in the fawn-hooded rat. Am Rev Respir Dis 1992; 145:793–797.
43. Herve P, Drouet L, Dosquet C, Launay J-M, Rain B, Simmoneau G, Caen J, Duroux P. Primary pulmonary hypertension in a patient with a familial platelet storage pool disease: role of serotonin. Am J Med 1990; 89:117–120.
44. Lee SL, Wang WW, Moore BJ, Fanburg BL. Dual effect of serotonin on growth of bovine pulmonary artery smooth muscle cells in culture. Circ Res 1991; 68:1362–1368.

45. Launay J-M, Herve P, Peoc'h K, Tournois C, Callebert J, Nebigil CG, Etienne N, Drouet L, Humbert M, Simonneau G, Maroteaux L. Function of the serotonin 5-hydroxytryptamine 2B receptor in pulmonary hypertension. Nat Med 2002; 8:1129–1135.
46. Lee SL, Wang WW, Fanburg BL. Association of Tyr phosphorylation of GTPase-activating protein with mitogenic action of serotonin. Am J Physiol 1997; 272:C223–C230.
47. Lee SL, Wang WW, Finlay GA, Fanburg BL. Serotonin stimulates mitogen-activated protein kinase activity through the formation of superoxide anion. Am J Physiol 1999; 277:L282–L291.
48. Suzuki E, Evans T, Lowry J, Truong L, Bell DW, Testa JR, Walsh K. The human GATA-6 gene: structure, chromosomal location, and regulation of expression by tissue-specific and mitogen-responsive signals. Genomics 1996; 38:283–290.
49. Suzuki YJ, Day RM, Tan CC, Sandven TJ, Liang Q, Molkentin JD, Fanburg BL. Activation of GATA-4 by serotonin in pulmonary artery smooth muscle cells. J Biol Chem 2003; 278:17525 17531.
50. Michelakis ED, Hampl V, Nsair A, Wu X, Harry G, Haromy A, Gurtu R, Archer SL. Diversity in mitochondrial function explains differences in vascular oxygen sensing. Circ Res 2002; 90:1307–1315.
51. Eddahibi S, Fabre V, Boni C, Martres MP, Raffestin B, Hamon M, Adnot S. Induction of serotonin transporter by hypoxia in pulmonary vascular smooth muscle cells. Relationship with the mitogenic action of serotonin. Circ Res 1999; 84:329–336.
52. Eddahibi S, Hanoun N, Lanfumey L, Lesch KP, Raffestin B, Hamon M, Adnot S. Attenuated hypoxic pulmonary hypertension in mice lacking the 5-hydroxytryptamine transporter gene. J Clin Invest 2000; 105:1555–1562.
53. Eddahibi S, Humbert M, Fadel E, Raffestin B, Darmon M, Capron F, Simonneau G, Dartevelle P, Hamon M, Adnot S. Serotonin transporter over-expression is responsible for pulmonary artery smooth muscle hyperplasia in primary pulmonary hypertension. J Clin Invest 2001; 108:1141–1150.
54. Rabinovitch M. Linking a serotonin transporter polymorphism to vascular smooth muscle proliferation in patients with primary pulmonary hypertension. J Clin Invest 2001; 108:1109–1111.
55. Platoshyn O, Golovina VA, Bailey CL, Limsuwan A, Krick S, Juhaszova M, Seiden JE, Rubin LJ, Yuan JX-J. Sustained membrane depolarization and pulmonary artery smooth muscle cell proliferation. Am J Physiol Cell Physiol 2000; 279:C1540–C1549.
56. Krick S, Platoshyn O, Sweeney M, Kim H, Yuan JX-J. Activation of K^+ channels induces apoptosis in vascular smooth muscle cells. Am J Physiol Cell Physiol 2001; 280:C970–C979.
57. Krick S, Platoshyn O, McDaniel SS, Rubin LJ, Yuan JX-J. Augmented K^+ currents and mitochondrial membrane depolarization in pulmonary artery myocyte apoptosis. Am J Physiol Lung Cell Mol Physiol 2001; 281:L887–L894.
58. Archer SL, Souil E, Dinh-Xuan AT, Schremmer B, Mercier JC, El Yaagoubi A, Nguyen-Huu L, Reeve HL, Hampl V. Molecular identification of the role of voltage-gated K^+ channels, Kv1.5 and Kv2.1, in hypoxic pulmonary

vasoconstriction and control of resting membrane potential in rat pulmonary artery myocytes. J Clin Invest 1998; 101:2319–2330.
59. Michelakis ED, McMurtry MS, Wu X-C, Dyck JRB, Moudgil R, Hopkins TA, Lopaschuk GD, Puttagunta L, Waite R, Archer SL. Dichloroacetate, a metabolic modulator, prevents and reverses chronic hypoxic pulmonary hypertension in rats: role of increased expression and activity of voltage-gated potassium channels. Circulation 2002; 105:244–250.
60. Pozeg ZI, Michelakis ED, McMurtry MS, Thébaud B, Wu X-C, Dyck JRB, Hashimoto K, Wang S, Moudgil R, Harry G, Sultanian R, Koshal A, Archer SL. In vivo gene transfer of the O_2-sensitive potassium channel Kv1.5 reduces pulmonary hypertension and restores hypoxic pulmonary vasoconstriction in chronically hypoxic rats. Circulation 2003; 107:2037–2044.
61. Weir EK, Reeve HL, Huang JMC, Michelakis E, Nelson DP, Hampl V, Archer SL. Anorexic agents aminorex, fenfluramine, and dexfenfluramine inhibit potassium current in rat pulmonary vascular smooth muscle and cause pulmonary vasoconstriction. Circulation 1996; 94:2216–2220.
62. Michelakis ED, Weir EK, Nelson DP, Reeve HL, Tolarova S, Archer SL. Dexfenfluramine elevates systemic blood pressure by inhibiting potassium currents in vascular smooth muscle cells. J Pharmacol Exp Ther 1999; 291: 1143–1149.
63. Reeve H, Tolarova S, Michelakis E, Archer S, Weir EK. Effects of the anorectic agent dexfenfluramine and 4-aminopyridine of the ductus arteriosus during development. Circulation 1997; 96:1–245.
64. Hu S, Wang S, Gibson J, Gilbertson TA. Inhibition of delayed rectifier K^+ channels by dexfenfluramine (Redux). J Pharmacol Exp Ther 1998; 287: 480–486.
65. Weir EK, Reeve HL, Johnson G, Michelakis ED, Nelson DP, Archer SL. A role for potassium channels in smooth muscle cells and platelets in the etiology of primary pulmonary hypertension. Chest 1998; 114:200S–204S.
66. Wang J, Juhaszova M, Conte JV Jr, Gaine SP, Rubin LJ, Yuan JX-J. Action of fenfluramine on voltage-gated K^+ channels in human pulmonary-artery smooth-muscle cells. Lancet 1998; 352:290.
67. Patel AJ, Lazdunski M, Honoré E. Kv2.1/Kv9.3, a novel ATP-dependent delayed-rectifier K^+ channel in oxygen-sensitive pulmonary artery myocytes. EMBO J 1997; 16:6615–6625.
68. Perchenet L, Hilfiger L, Mizrahi J, Clément-Chomienne O. Effects of anorexinogen agents on cloned voltage-gated K^+ channel hKv1.5. J Pharmacol Exp Ther 2001; 298:1108–1119.
69. Reeve HL, Nelson DP, Archer SL, Weir EK. Effects of fluoxetine, phentermine, and venlafaxine on pulmonary arterial pressure and electrophysiology. Am J Physiol 1999; 276:L213–L219.
70. McMahon FG, Fujioka K, Singh BN, Mendel CM, Rowe E, Rolston K, Johnson F, Mooradian AD. Efficacy and safety of sibutramine in obese white and African American patients with hypertension: a 1-year, double-blind, placebo-controlled, multicenter trial. Arch Intern Med 2000; 160:2185–2191.
71. Archer SL, Djaballah K, Humbert M, Weir EK, Fartoukh M, Dall'ava-Santucci J, Mercier J-C, Simonneau G, Dinh-Xuan AT. Nitric oxide deficiency

in fenfluramine- and dexfenfluramine-induced pulmonary hypertension. Am J Respir Crit Care Med 1998; 158:1061–1067.
72. Bèlohlávková S, Šimák J, Kokešsová A, Hniličková O, Hampl V. Fenfluramine-induced pulmonary vasoconstriction: role of serotonin receptors and potassium channels. J Appl Physiol 2001; 91:755–761.
73. Naeije R, Maggiorini M, Delcroix M, Leeman M, Melot C. Effects of chronic dexfenfluramine treatment on pulmonary hemodynamics in dogs. Am J Respir Crit Care Med 1996; 154:1347–1350.
74. Barman SA, Isales CM. Fenfluramine potentiates canine pulmonary vasoreactivity to endothelin-1. Pulm Pharmacol Ther 1998; 11:183–7.
75. Higenbottam T, Marriott H, Cremona G, Laude E, Bee D. The acute effects of dexfenfluramine on human and porcine pulmonary vascular tone and resistance. Chest 1999; 116:921–930.
76. Eddahibi S, Raffestin B, Launay J-M, Sitbon M, Adnot S. Effect of dexfenfluramine treatment in rats exposed to acute and chronic hypoxia. Am J Respir Crit Care Med 1998; 157:1111–1119.
77. Mitani Y, Mutlu A, Russell JC, Brindley DN, DeAlmeida J, Rabinovitch M. Dexfenfluramine protects against pulmonary hypertension in rats. J Appl Physiol 2002; 93:1770–1778.
78. Miyamoto JK, Uezu E, Yusa T, Terashima S. Efflux of 5-HIAA from 5-HT neurons: a membrane potential dependent process. Physiol Behav 1990; 47: 767–772.
79. Pei Q, Leslie RA, Grahame-Smith DG, Zetterstrom TS. 5-HT efflux from rat hippocampus in vivo produced by 4-aminopyridine is increased by chronic lithium administration. Neuroreport 1995; 6:716–720.
80. Imbrici P, Tucker SJ, D'Adamo MC, Pessia M. Role of receptor protein tyrosine phosphatase α (RPTP) and tyrosine phosphorylation in the serotonergic inhibition of voltage-dependent potassium channels. Pflügers Arch 2000; 441:257–262.
81. Lambe EK, Aghajanian GK. The role of Kv1.2-containing potassium channels in serotonin-induced glutamate release from thalamocortical terminals in rat frontal cortex. J Neurosci 2001; 21:9955–9963.
82. Perrier JF, Alaburda A, Hounsgaard J. 5-HT1A receptors increase excitability of spinal motoneurons by inhibiting a TASK-1-like K^+ current in the adult turtle. J Physiol 2003; 548:485–492.
83. Alshuaib WB, Mathew MV, Hasan MY, Fahim MA. Serotonin reduces potassium current in rutabaga and wild-type *Drosophila* neurons. Int J Neurosci 2003; 113:1413–1425.
84. Jeong H-S, Lim YC, Kim TS, Heo T, Jung S-M, Cho YB, Jun JY, Park J-S. Excitatory effects of 5-hydroxytryptamine on the medial vestibular nuclear neuron via the 5-HT2 receptor. Neuroreport 2003; 14:2001–2004.
85. Gokcel A, Gumurdulu Y, Karakose H, Melek Ertorrer E, Tanaci N, Bascil Tutuncu N, Guvener N. Evaluation of the safety and efficacy of sibutramine, orlistat and metformin in the treatment of obesity. Diabetes Obes Metab 2002; 4:49–55.

86. Birkenfeld AL, Schroeder C, Boschmann M, Tank J, Franke G, Luft FC, Biaggioni I, Sharma AM, Jordan J. Paradoxical effect of sibutramine on autonomic cardiovascular regulation. Circulation 2002; 106:2459–2465.
87. Hill JO, Wyatt HR, Reed GW, Peters JC. Obesity and the environment: where do we go from here? Science 2003; 299:853–855.
88. Halpern A, Mancini MC. Treatment of obesity: an update on anti-obesity medications. Obes Rev 2003; 4:25–42.

29

Isolation and Culture of Pulmonary Artery Smooth Muscle Cells

Shen Zhang, Carmelle V. Remillard, Oleksandr Platoshyn, and Jason X.-J. Yuan

University of California, San Diego, California, U.S.A.

I. INTRODUCTION

Cell isolation is perhaps the most important part of the cell experimentation process. If cell quality is bad, either the experiments do not work or the results are quirky. Although it is now possible to purchase cells from various sources, such as Cambrex and ATCC, most research groups have developed their own techniques for isolating cells from tissues, techniques that can be adapted relatively from one tissue type to another. In addition, although some prefer to use freshly isolated cells (<8 h postisolation), many are now turning to cell culture as a viable alternative to freshly dissociated cells. The following sections deal with the isolation of pulmonary artery smooth muscle cells (PASMCs), particularly those from humans and rats. Generally speaking, the methods we outline can also be applied to PASMCs from other species, although some slight modifications may be required. Although this discussion is beyond the scope of the current chapter, similar techniques have also been used extensively to isolate smooth muscle cells from other vascular beds. Readers are advised to consult the extensive literature to identify the technique most applicable to their needs. There are also monographs and review articles dealing specifically with smooth muscle cell isolation that may prove invaluable to many readers (1–4).

II. ISOLATION OF PASMCs FROM RATS AND HUMANS

A. Preparation of Primary Culture PASMCs

There are two general methods for the preparation of primary cultures of vascular smooth muscle cells. One is the direct isolation of cells from enzymatically digested vessels (enzymatic isolation method), and the other involves isolating cells that migrate out from small tissue samples. Because enzyme dissociation is the most commonly used approach, we will describe the procedure we have used successfully for human and rat PASMC isolation.

Collection of Human and Rat Tissue Samples

Human lung tissue samples can be obtained from patients undergoing lung transplantation and biopsy. Typically, a small (~1 cm long) piece of the peripheral lung tissues is removed from the lung and placed in cold (4°C) saline until dissection can be performed (within 3 h of transplantation). For rats, following euthanasia (decapitation or cervical dislocation are ideal to reduce trauma to the lungs), lungs and heart are removed *en bloc* and placed in warm HEPES-buffered saline solution (HBSS). Once the tissues are obtained, fat, blood, and connective tissue are removed using aseptic techniques so that PASMCs can be dissociated.

Enzyme Dissociation of PASMCs

The vascular wall is organized into three layers: an inner layer composed of endothelial cells (intima), a middle layer of smooth muscle cells (SMCs) (media), and an outer layer composed of fibroblasts, connective tissues, and nerve endings (adventitia) (Fig. 1, inset). The smooth muscle cells that make up the media are involved in processes relating to vascular growth and repair, response to injury, and vascular contraction.

In order for the enzymes to reach the medial PASMCs and to isolate pure smooth muscle cells, the first steps of PASMC isolation involve removing the adventitia and intima (Fig. 1a–c). The vessel is placed in fresh HBSS, carefully stretched, and pinned onto a dissecting dish. The adventitia (which mainly contains fibroblasts) can be peeled away from the media with forceps. After removal of the adventitia, the vessel is cut open longitudinally so the endothelial layer can be gently scraped away.

The pulmonary artery, now mostly vascular media, is then cut into pieces and placed in an enzyme solution composed of collagenase (typically 2–3 mg/mL) (Fig. 1d) in HBSS at 37°C for 20 min, after which the tissue is allowed to recover overnight for 10–12 h at 37°C in Dulbecco's modification of Eagle's medium (DMEM) supplemented with fetal bovine serum, penicillin or streptomycin, and L-glutamine (200 mM). The vessel is then transferred to a fresh enzyme solution containing collagenase, elastase, and albumin and is incubated at 37°C for ~50 min (Fig. 1e). Finally, the tissue

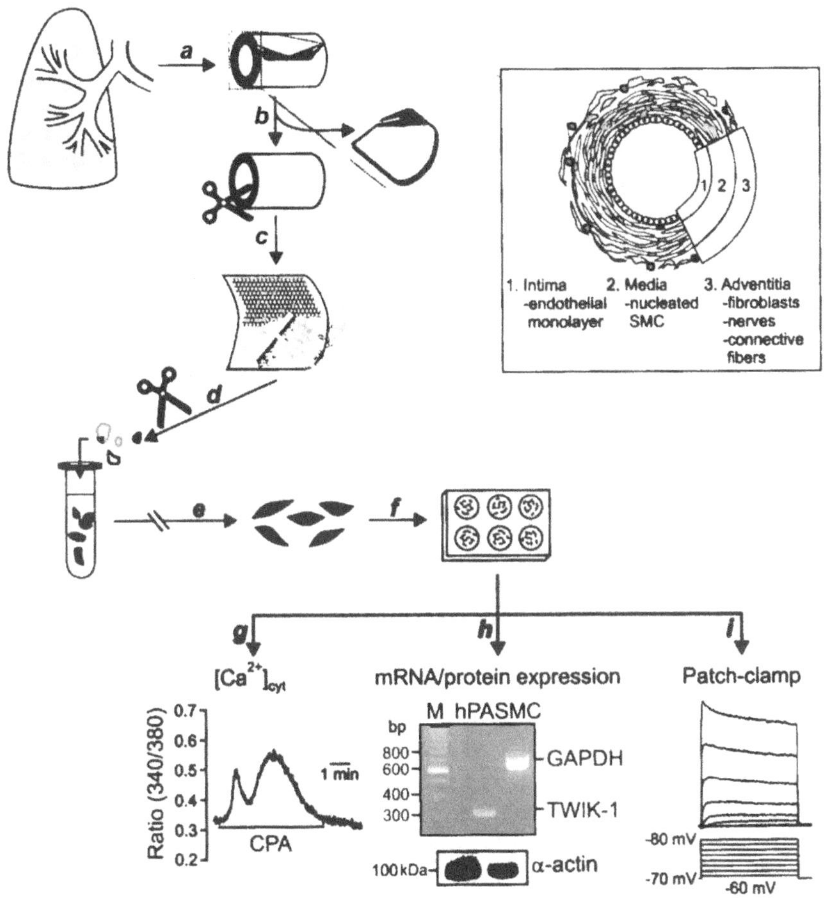

Figure 1 Overview of rat and human PASMC isolation. (a) Pulmonary arteries are removed from the lung, and the adventitia is stripped using forceps. *Inset*: Cross section of an artery showing the intima, media, and adventia layers. (b) The arterial ring is cut open, and the endothelium is removed with gentle rubbing (c). (d) The tissue is cut into small pieces for initial digestion by collagenase. (e) Following an overnight rest period in enzyme-free solution, new enzymes are added, the tissue is digested, and trituration releases isolated cells. (f) Cells are plated for later use to measure Ca^{2+} (g), mRNA or protein (h, top and bottom, respectively) expression, or ion (K^+) currents (i).

is gently triturated to release cells; DMEM (containing 20% FBS) halts digestion. The enzyme-containing cell suspension is then centrifuged, and the pellet containing the PASMCs is resuspended in fresh 10% FBS-DMEM. Dissociated cells can now be refrigerated for immediate use or plated in tissue culture dishes (Fig. 1f) containing prewarmed growth medium.

For rat PASMCs, we use 10% FBS-DMEM. For human PASMCs, we use a smooth muscle growth medium (SMGM, Cambrex Corporation) that contains 10% FBS and is supplemented with insulin, hEGF, hFGF-B, gentamicin, and amphotericin-B. Cells are incubated at 37°C for further growth. Cell media should be changed initially after 24 h and every 48 h subsequently.

Although we have placed emphasis on DMEM and SMGM, several media are available to support smooth muscle cell (SMC) growth, including MEM (Eagle's Minimal Essential Medium), Medium 199 with Earle's or Hank's salt (M199), and Ham's F12. Many researchers now use plastic, rather than glass, dishes to plate SMCs. Cell attachment to plastic dishes or cover slips may be enhanced by coating the surface with fibronectin, vitronectin, laminin, collagen, or lysine (1,5,6).

B. Cell Subculture and Storage

Subculturing Cells

Because large quantities of primary tissues can be difficult to obtain, it is useful to subculture cells in order to amplify the cell sample for future experiments. Cultured cells should be passaged when they are approximately 70–80% confluent. Passaging of PASMCs is quite straightforward. After aspirating the medium from the culture dishes containing the cells, prewarmed HBSS is used to wash the cells. HBSS is then replaced by prewarmed trypsin/EDTA to detach the cells. Cell detachment, monitored on a microscope, usually takes approximately 5 min, although this will vary according to temperature, cell confluence, cell type, and trypsin concentration. A trypsin-neutralizing solution is added to the solution when the majority of cells are floating freely in order to halt trypsinization. The cell solution is then centrifuged, the supernatant is discarded, and the pellet containing cells is resuspended in warm medium for renewed plating. As with freshly isolated and plated cells, media should be changed initially after 24 h and every 48 h thereafter following each cell passage.

Optimal cell density for passaging and plating is dependent on the surface area of the plating dish. When cells are purchased, the supplier normally provides an estimate of the basal cell density. For those using freshly dissociated cells, the cells must be counted to approximate cell number. For PASMCs, cells are plated initially at an average density of 3500 cells/cm^2.

Cell proliferation is multiphasic. In the initial lag phase, cell growth is minimal. Within a few days, cell growth increases exponentially during the logarithmic growth phase until confluence is attained, at which point growth is maximal and cells may begin to differentiate. In the presence of the required growth factors to stimulate cell proliferation, initial seeding density and seeding efficiency regulate the rate of cell proliferation. Cells seeded at higher initial density begin to proliferate earlier than those at low density. Optimal seeding density is also dependent on cell type.

Cell Storage

Cell storage in liquid nitrogen is the most efficient way to keep cells for long-term storage or for later use, especially those cells originating from a rare tissue source. When the cultured cells are ~70–80% confluent, they are passaged as described above. However, instead of using media, the final cell pellet is resuspended in a freezing solution consisting of dimethyl sulfoxide (DMSO, 5–10%) and medium (FBS/DMEM for rat PASMCs, FBS/SMGM for human PASMCs). Cells in the freezing solution should be aliquoted in cryogenic tubes and gradually frozen until they can be placed in liquid nitrogen. This can be done by placing the cells first in the refrigerator (at 4°C), then at 0°C, −20°C, and −80°C, sequentially, before being placed in liquid nitrogen (−196°C). Many core cell facilities have equipment that can gradually freeze samples by decreasing the freezer temperature by 1°C/min down to −196°C before the samples are placed in liquid nitrogen.

Cell Thawing and Reseeding

After cells have been frozen, they can be thawed and plated for later use. Cells should be thawed quickly (< 3min) in a 37°C water bath. The vial should be sterilized with ethanol before opening to avoid contamination of this cell stock. The cell solution should be gently aspirated to evenly distribute the cells in their medium. Culture dishes containing prewarmed medium are then seeded, gently rocked to disperse the cells, and incubated at 37°C. As always, after the initial seeding, cell media should be changed initially after 24 h and subsequently every 48 h.

III. MORPHOLOGICAL CHARACTERISTICS OF PRIMARY AND SUBCULTURED CELLS

A. Phase-Contrast Photomicrographs

Two morphological phenotypes of vascular SMCs are usually defined, epithelioid cells and spindle-shaped cells (7). Functionally these phenotypes have been suggested to correlate with the synthetic and contractile cell types, respectively. Contractile vascular SMCs express high levels of contractile proteins including myosin and low levels of α-actin. In contrast, synthetic vascular SMCs express high levels of α-actin, extracellular matrix proteins, and low levels of myosin. In general, the spindle-shaped, contractile vascular SMCs are not proliferating or migrating, whereas the epithelioid, synthetic vascular SMCs have entered the cell cycle and are proliferating (8).

With phase-contrast microscopy, SMCs appear flattened and spindle-shaped with central oval nuclei and long cytoplasmic extensions. Freshly

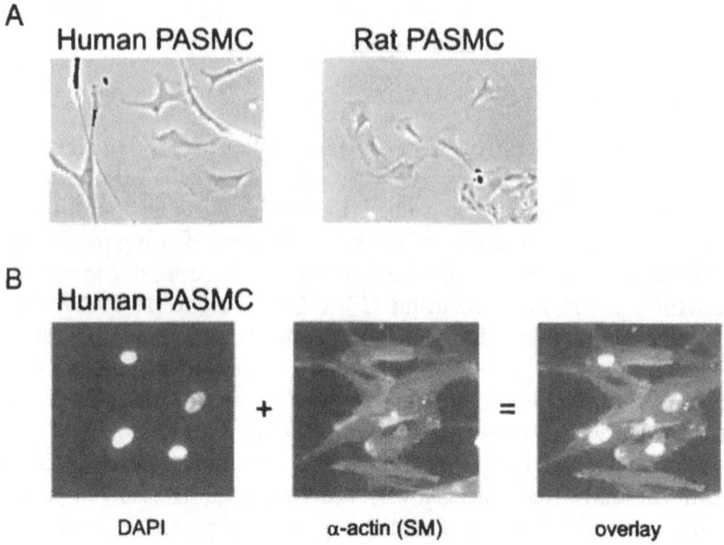

Figure 2 PASMC appearance and identification. (A) Phase-contrast micrographs of subcultured human PASMCs (left) and primary cultured rat PASMCs (right). (B) Identification of PASMCs by α-actin staining. DAPI staining identifies nucleated cells (left). Smooth muscle (SM) α-actin antibody attaches to α-actin, which is highly expressed in contractile SMCs (middle). An overlay of the DAPI and α-actin fluorescence images identifies the nucleated SMCs.

dissociated cells, although smaller and thicker, have a similar appearance. Confluent cells appear to be aligned in parallel so that the broad nuclear region of one cell lies adjacent to the thin cytoplasmic area of another, forming a "hill-and-valley" appearance. Unlike endothelial cells, SMCs do not show contact inhibition and will therefore grow as multilayers (1). The time of phenotypic change (i.e., from synthetic to contractile phenotypes) is dependent on the tissue type, donor age, and species. It is not dependent on the presence or absence of serum or serum components in the culture medium (9). Figure 2A shows a photomicrograph of subcultured human PASMCs and primary cultured rat PASMCs.

B. Identification of SMC by α-Actin Expression

α-Actin is produced from a smooth muscle specific gene. During development, when vascular SMCs exhibit a "synthetic" phenotype, the main actin isoform expressed is β-actin (10,11). As the vessel matures, there is a decrease in β-actin and an increase in smooth-muscle-specific α-actin expression (11). Smooth muscle α-actin expression persists in SMCs even after extensive passaging in culture (3). Figure 2B shows fluorescent images of human PASMCs stained with the membrane-permeable nucleic acid stain 4′,6′-diamidino-2-phenylindole (DAPI) (5 μmol/L). The blue fluorescence emitted at 461 nm by this dye can be used to estimate total cell number in the cultures because DAPI will stain each nucleated SMC. A specific monoclonal antibody raised against smooth muscle α-actin can be used to evaluate cellular purity of the cultures, and the secondary antibody FITC-conjugated anti-mouse IgG can be used to display the fluorescent image (emitted at 529 nm). Only SMCs (not fibroblasts) will be marked by the α-actin antibody. An overlay of the DAPI and smooth muscle α-actin identifies the SMCs in the field.

IV. SAMPLE USES OF CULTURED PASMCs

Cultured PASMCs can be used for a wide range of experimental, techniques including fluorescence microscopy, electrophysiology, biochemistry, and molecular biology. Many of these approaches have been described in preceding chapters and are therefore beyond the scope of this chapter. We have, however, provided some representative data obtained in our lab using rat and human PASMCs. In Fig. 1g, a time course of cytosolic Ca^{2+} concentration ($[Ca^{2+}]_{cyt}$) is shown for a cell stimulated with cyclopiazonic acid (CPA), an inhibitor of the sarcoplasmic reticulum Ca^{2+}-ATPase reuptake pump. In this experiment, $[Ca^{2+}]_{cyt}$ is expressed as a function of the 340/380 ratio for Fura-2, the fluorescent Ca^{2+} indicator used in this experiment. Figure 1h shows sample PCR and Western blots for TWIK-1 (a tandem-pore K^+ channel) and α-actin, respectively, from human PASMCs. Finally, patch-clamp electrophysiology can be used to measure ion currents in isolated cells. Figure 1i shows representative K^+ currents recorded from human PASMCs during repetitive incremental depolarizations.

V. SUMMARY

Smooth muscle cell culture has been in use since 1913 (4), but it has undergone some significant changes over the decades. As can be attested to by the scope of this monograph, the use of cultured and freshly dissociated PASMCs has allowed for a thorough examination of the physiology and pathology of HPV and pulmonary hypertension. Mechanisms ranging from heterogeneity of cell phenotype and function (12–14) to the role of K^+ channel activity and gene expression (15,16) have already been elucidated, which may explain, at least in part, the physiological basis of HPV. Because heterogeneity of cell expression and function is rapidly becoming an important concept, especially as it relates to HPV (13,14), further emphasis may be placed on the role of autocrine (a cell synthesizes and/or secretes a substance that stimulates that same cell type to undergo a growth response)

(17) and paracrine (cells responding to the growth factor synthesize and/or secrete a substance that stimulates neighboring cells of another cell type) growth factors in vascular SMC growth (8). Therefore, further modifications in current cell isolation and growth techniques may hold the key to elucidating the physiological basis of HPV.

ACKNOWLEDGMENTS

We thank N. Elliott for her contribution to this manuscript. This work was supported by grants HL 64945, HL 54043, HL 69758, HL66012, and HL 66941, from the National Heart, Lung, and Blood Institute of the National Institutes of Health.

REFERENCES

1. Gallicchio MA. Culture of human smooth muscle cells In: Drew AF, ed. Atherosclerosis: Experimental Methods and Protocols. Totowa: Humana Press 2001; 52:137–146.
2. Pang SC, Venance SL. Cultured smooth muscle approach in the study of hypertension. Can J Physiol Pharmacol 1992; 70:573–579.
3. Pauly RR, Bilato C, Cheng L, Monticone R, Crow MT. Vascular smooth muscle cell cultures. Methods Cell Biol 1997; 52:133–154.
4. Champey C. Quelques résultats de la méthode de culture des tissus. Arch Zool Exp Gen 1913/14; 53:42–51.
5. Wagner RC, Matthews MA. The isolation and culture of capillary endothelium from epididymal fat. Microvasc Res 1975; 10:286–297.
6. MacPhee MJ, Wiltrout RH, McCormick KL, Sayers TJ, Pilaro AM. A method for obtaining and culturing large numbers of purified organ-derived murine endothelial cells. J Leukoc Biol 1994; 55:467–475.
7. Bochaton-Piallat ML, Ropraz P, Gabbiani F, Gabbiani G. Phenotypic heterogeneity of rat arterial smooth muscle cell clones. Implications for the development of experimental intimal thickening. Arterioscler Thromb Vasc Biol 1996; 16:815–820.
8. Berk BC. Vascular smooth muscle growth: autocrine growth mechanisms. Physiol Rev 2001; 81:999–1030.
9. Chamley-Campbell JH, Campbell GR. What controls smooth muscle phenotype? Atherosclerosis 1981; 40:347–357.
10. Gabbiani G, Kocher O, Bloom WS, Vandekerckhove J, Weber K. Actin expression in smooth muscle cells of rat aortic intimal thickening, human atheromatous plaque, and cultured rat aortic media. J Clin Invest 1984; 73:148–152.
11. Kocher O, Gabbiani G. Analysis of α-smooth-muscle actin mRNA expression in rat aortic smooth-muscle cells using a specific cDNA probe. Differentiation 1987; 34:201–209.
12. Stenmark KR, Frid M, Nemenoff R, Dempsey EC, Das M. Hypoxia induces cell-specific changes in gene expression in vascular wall cells: implications for pulmonary hypertension. Adv Exp Med Biol 1999; 474:231–258.

13. Frid MG, Aldashev AA, Dempsey EC, Stenmark KR. Smooth muscle cells isolated from discrete compartments of the mature vascular media exhibit unique phenotypes and distinct growth capabilities. Circ Res 1997; 81:940–952.
14. Benzakour O, Kanthou C, Kanse SM, Scully MF, Kakkar VV, Cooper DN. Evidence for cultured human vascular smooth muscle cell heterogeneity: isolation of clonal cells and study of their growth characteristics. Thromb Haemost 1996; 75:854–858.
15. Platoshyn O, Yu Y, Golovina VA, McDaniel SS, Krick S, Li L, Wang JY, Rubin LJ, Yuan JX-J. Chronic hypoxia decreases K_V channel expression and function in pulmonary artery myocytes. Am J Physiol Lung Cell Mol Physiol 2001; 280:L801–L812.
16. Yuan JX-J, Aldinger AM, Juhaszova M, Wang J, Conte JV Jr, Gaine SP, Orens JB, Rubin LJ. Dysfunctional voltage-gated K^+ channels in pulmonary artery smooth muscle cells of patients with primary pulmonary hypertension. Circulation 1998; 98:1400–1406.
17. Frid MG, Aldashev AA, Nemenoff RA, Higashito R, Westcott JY, Stenmark KR. Subendothelial cells from normal bovine arteries exhibit autonomous growth and constitutively activated intracellular signaling. Arterioscler Thromb Vasc Biol 1999; 19:2884–2893.

30

Measurement of Ion Channel Function Using Conventional Patch-Clamp Techniques

Carmelle V. Remillard and Jason X.-J. Yuan
University of California, San Diego, California, U.S.A.

I. INTRODUCTION

Transmembrane ion flux plays an important role in the control of membrane potential (E_m) and contractility of pulmonary vascular smooth muscle, the end effector in the regulation of pulmonary vasomotor activity. Ion channels are integral membrane proteins possessing selective permeability for monovalent and divalent ions. The activity of ion channels is dependent on their biophysical characteristics, molecular composition, and physiological function. This chapter confronts the more practical aspects of determining ion channel activity and expression, including the direct measurement of transmembrane current flow in intact cells.

Although E_m may be measured with fluorescent dyes, patch-clamp electrophysiology has proven itself to be the preeminent tool for the study of ion transport via ion channels, pumps, and exchangers. Use of patch-clamp techniques has allowed scientists to measure both E_m and membrane ionic currents that contribute to the regulation of E_m. This chapter will focus on the application of patch-clamp electrophysiology in understanding the role played by transmembrane and intracellular ion movement in the regulation of pulmonary vascular tone, proliferation, and cellular volume.

II. BRIEF HISTORICAL PERSPECTIVE OF PATCH-CLAMP ELECTROPHYSIOLOGY

As early as the 1950s, scientists believed that positive and negative ions flowed according to their electrochemical gradients across the biological membrane via hydrophilic pores formed by integral transmembrane proteins. A decade later, discrete electrical events were recorded from bacterial membrane proteins embedded in artificial lipid bilayers (1). Similar recordings could not be done in isolated cells or tissues because of the low-resolution capabilities of the amplifiers available at that time.

In 1976, Neher and Sakmann (2) published the first report of unitary currents from cation channels recorded from an intact 1 μm^2 denervated frog muscle fiber membrane patch using glass micropipettes. Over the next five years, these scientists optimized cell isolation techniques, pipette fabrication techniques (to control pipette geometry, size, and composition), and electronic component designs. The major breakthrough in the advent of modern-day patch clamping occurred when Hamill et al. (3) found that applying suction to the membrane patch via the glass pipette increased seal resistance into the gigaohm (GΩ) range. In combination with the improved electronic detection and acquisition components, the gigaohm seal allowed for (1) an improved signal-to-noise ratio, thereby improving resolution and reproducibility, (2) the application of voltage or current pulses directly to the membrane proteins within the patched membrane area; and (3) mechanical stability of the patch during excision. Today, patch-clamp electrophysiologists use the improved technology to measure subpicoampere unitary (single-channel) currents, and macroscopic (whole-cell) currents, and membrane and action potentials (current clamp). The development of different membrane patch configurations has also enabled the users to fully investigate the cellular environment and, therefore, channel modulation.

III. DESCRIPTION OF THE PATCH-CLAMP TECHNIQUE

Successful patch clamping depends on many factors, including good hand–eye coordination, cell quality, pipette geometry, and solution composition. This section introduces the basic elements of patch clamping that should enable the reader to understand the concepts. Those interested in furthering their knowledge of the more practical aspects (pipette fabrication, microcircuitry, electronics, voltage-clamp protocols) of patch clamping should consult other textbooks and monographs on these subjects (4–6).

A. Forming the Gigaohm Seal

A pipette with a tip resistance ranging from 3 to 6 MΩ is maneuvered toward the cells, typically using a motorized micromanipulator (Fig. 1).

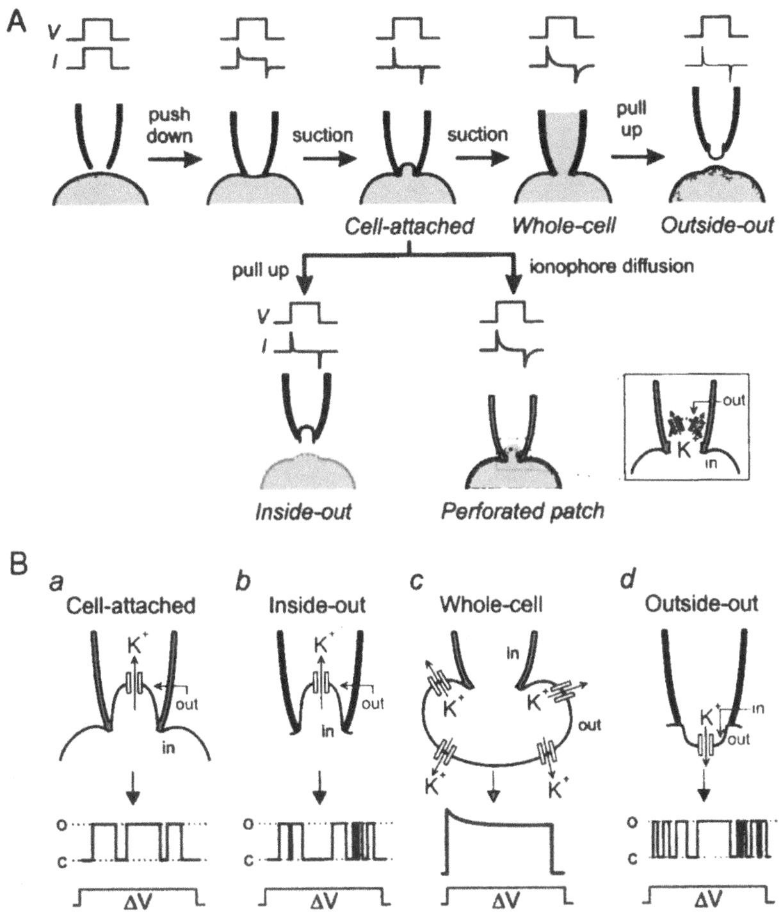

Figure 1 Patch-clamp configurations. (A) Schematic diagram of the steps involved in the formation of a gigaohm seal on a cell with a pipette. The steps involved in achieving the various configurations of the patch clamp are also shown (described in the text). V is a repetitive low-amplitude ($<5\,\mathrm{mV}$) command pulse applied to the patch during formation of the seal to monitor pipette current (I). Note that I decreases as the pipette touches the membrane and the gigaohm seal is formed. Capacitative currents also become apparent when the membrane is ruptured or perforated due to charging and discharging of membrane capacitance. Inset: Magnified view of perforated patch membrane. (B) Magnified view of pipette and cell membranes (only K^+ channel proteins shown here) for the various configurations (*a–d*: cell-attached, inside-out, whole-cell, and outside-out, respectively) as well as the appearance of the currents during a voltage pulse.

When the pipette filled with electrolyte solution is immersed in the bathing medium, a junction potential is created that must be nulled prior to touching the cell membrane. As the pipette is further approached to the cell, tip resistance (R) is increased, making the square-wave voltage pulse (V) seem smaller according to Ohm's law,

$$V = \frac{I}{R} \tag{1}$$

where I is the amount of current injected via the pipette. With the tip of the pipette firmly pressed down on the cell (near the center of the cell to satisfy the "space clamp" criterion), negative pressure (suction) is applied via a port in the pipette holder, and tip resistance increases gradually into the gigaohm range. At this point, the current record at the voltage pulse should be seen as a flat line, with capacitance spikes apparent at its right and left edges.

B. Patch-Clamp Configurations

The patch is said to be in the *cell-attached* configuration once the gigaohm seal has been formed on the intact cell membrane. Voltage pulses applied via the pipette can modulate the activity of channels located within the patched membrane area. In this configuration, one can control channel activity via alterations of voltage or ionic composition of the solutions. It is possible to measure current activity [unitary (Fig. 1B(*a*)) or macroscopic] while controlling both the intra- and extracellular environments by employing other patch-clamp configurations (see Fig. 1 for schematic diagrams).

1. In the *inside-out* configuration, the outer face of the membrane patch is sealed within the pipette while the previously inner membrane is exposed to the perfusing solution [Fig. 1B(*b*)]. This configuration is achieved by rapidly pulling up the pipette from the attached cell without breaking the gigaohm seal.
2. The *perforated-patch* configuration allows for the diffusion of small molecules such as ions, but not of cytoplasmic proteins and larger molecules. To achieve this configuration, an antibiotic ionophore (e.g., nystatin, amphotericin B) is added to the pipette solution and allowed to diffuse toward the membrane. Over time, the ionophore molecules embed themselves in the membrane, thereby permeabilizing the patched membrane.
3. Following stabilization of the gigaohm seal, additional suction or a strong and fast voltage surge ("zap") can be applied via the pipette to rupture the membrane patch, giving the user access to the intracellular medium (*whole-cell* configuration). In this mode, the user can easily control ion flow across the sarcolemmal membrane by modifying ionic composition and ion concentration in both the

pipette and bath solutions. Macroscopic currents recorded from cells represent the cumulative activity of all the ion channels contained within the cell membrane [Fig. 1B(*c*)].

4. The *outside-out* configuration is achieved after the whole-cell configuration has been attained by gently pulling up the pipette, thereby stretching the membrane outside the pipette until it reseals itself, forming a miniature cell [Fig. 1B(*d*)].

Each of these patch-clamp configurations has its experimental applications, as evidenced by the sheer volume of articles published on work using the patch-clamp technique as the tool of choice. Single-channel current recordings from cell-attached patches provide vital information about the gating and kinetics of individual channel proteins and allow biophysicists to distinguish between currents flowing through related channels (e.g., K^+ ions flowing through maxi-K_{Ca} vs. K_V channel proteins) based on their single-channel conductance. Unfortunately, successful single-channel recordings require that at least one (preferably, only one) channel protein be present within the membrane patch, not always possible, depending on the overall protein density of certain channels. The ability to simultaneously record the activity of a whole population of the same channel (e.g., L-type Ca^{2+} channels) on the entire cell membrane is the greatest advantage provided by the whole-cell configuration. More specifically, whole-cell patch clamping allows for the recording of currents generated by ion channels with either a small individual conductance or low density and of currents that may be difficult to resolve in cell-attached patches. On the other hand, the large pipette volume also acts as a "sink" into which normally intracellular metabolic factors can dissolve, potentially causing channel rundown during an experiment. The advantage of the inside-out and outside-out excised-patch configurations is the ability to precisely control the cellular environment, i.e., the user controls the ionic compositions of solutions on either side of the membrane. This total control of the membrane environment allows for a better understanding of the permeation processes (pore selectivity and conductance), gating properties (channel opening and closure), and regulation (e.g., by cytosolic proteins) of the channels.

The flexibility of the patch-clamp configurations provides the researcher with a selection of tools available to study current activity. Because they have been used most extensively, subsequent sections of this chapter discuss in further detail the practical applications of the cell-attached and whole-cell configurations in measuring and characterizing channel activity.

C. Troubleshooting and Limitations

Perhaps the most serious limitation of the patch-clamp technique is the relative inability to control the cellular environment without modifying the cell's physiological properties. Because we can only speculate as to the exact composition of the intra- and extracellular media, the ionic composition of the solutions used in patch-clamp experiments becomes a determining factor in isolating and identifying currents. Currents can be identified using ion-selective solutions. For example, in studying voltage-dependent Na^+ currents in vascular smooth muscle cells, K^+ may be replaced by cesium (Cs^+) in both the pipette and bath solution to minimize K^+ channel activity. This experiment might also be performed using a Ca^{2+}-free bath solution to prevent Ca^{2+} influx into the cells via Ca^{2+} channels, Na^+ channels (permeable to Ca^{2+} ions as well as Na^+ ions in cardiac cells (7)), or Na^+–Ca^{2+} exchange proteins (8). Patch-clamp electrophysiologists also distinguish currents using selective pharmacological tools. For example, replacing external Na^+ with *N*-methyl-D-glucamine (which will not permeate through Na^+ channels) or applying tetrodotoxin, a selective blocker of Na^+ channels (9), to these cells should abolish the aforementioned rapid voltage-dependent Na^+ currents.

In a more physiological environment, the ability to control E_m can also allow the user to selectively regulate channel activation. For example, rapidly inactivating Na^+ currents are elicited by membrane depolarizations from very negative potentials (−80 to −60 mV), whereas activation of these channels can be minimized by using a holding potential of −40 mV, because many of the channels are inactivated at this relatively negative E_m. Similarly, L-type and T-type Ca^{2+} channels can be differentiated from each other by using different holding potentials (−70 and −100 mV, respectively). However, the ability to regulate channel activity by modifying the holding potential does not alleviate the need to minimize the activity of other "contaminating" currents. Therefore, ion replacement and pharmacological approaches must still be applied.

As all electrophysiologists well understand, the optimal cellular environment and cell quality, although critical, are not the only limiting factors in completing an experiment. Successful patch clamping is highly dependent on the technical ability of the user, effective cancelation of external electrical noise, attenuation of vibration within the system, and pipette reliability. Conventional patch-clamp electrophysiology relies on the use of glass microelectrodes maneuvered onto a cell to form a gigaohm seal on its membrane. In a typical experiment, the cell is sandwiched between a 150 μm thick cover glass and a pipette attached to a mechanical micromanipulator positioned inches away (a light year away as far as a cell is concerned!) in order to obtain the gigaohm seal. The number of things that can go wrong is amazingly high.

1. Vibration in the system can reduce the success and longevity of an experiment; most patch-clamp setups are mounted on air tables that absorb floor vibration and allow maintenance of the seal.

2. Most setups are housed within a Faraday cage to insulate against random external electrical noise. The electrode being held high above a cell is an effective antenna for electrical noise. Therefore, all components connecting to electrical supply systems must be effectively grounded to allow for the resolution of small currents.
3. Approaching the pipette to the cell membrane and forming a seal requires an operator with a high level of training. Because the cell is relatively flat on the cover glass, a few extra micrometers down onto the cell may transform a potential gigaohm seal into cell impalement or shattering of the pipette tip.
4. Finally, the fabrication of glass microelectrodes is not entirely reliable despite the vast improvements in pipette puller technology. As a result, the size and geometry of the pipettes vary from one glass tube to the next and between pulls on the same day. Correcting for this variation is a time-consuming and tedious process that must be addressed constantly.

IV. VOLTAGE- AND CURRENT-CLAMP MODES

Most commercially available patch-clamp amplifiers allow the user to select between the voltage-clamp and current-clamp modes. Ion current measurement is done in the voltage-clamp mode, where the user specifies the desired voltage to be clamped by the amplifier. In this mode, the amplifier measures E_m, then injects or removes electrons (current) to deflect the E_m toward the desired (clamp) potential. The amplitude of the current that is applied by the amplifier is measured by the acquisition software and is assumed to be equal to, but opposite in direction to, the amount of current generated by the channel proteins at that membrane voltage. Voltage-clamp studies are useful for studying the kinetics of specific ion channels at specified voltages.

In the current-clamp mode, the amplifier simply reports E_m while applying a desired current to the cell membrane. This mode is useful to study the natural response of a cell to stimuli, such as the membrane depolarization induced by chronic hypoxia or by K_V channel inhibition in pulmonary artery smooth muscle cells (PASMCs) (10,11).

V. CHARACTERIZING ION CHANNEL CURRENTS

The flux of ions through the transmembrane channel pores is controlled by two mechanisms: permeation and gating (12). The pore region of a channel protein contains amino acid sequences that determine the size, geometry, and charge within the channel pore, thereby acting as a filter to select which ions can be conducted and controlling the net rate of ion flux through the channel pore. The opening and closing of the channel protein, or "gating," occurs randomly between the open (allowing ion flux) and closed (preventing ion flux) states. What follows is a description of how patch configurations can be applied to study the passive membrane properties, and the permeability and gating characteristics of ion channels.

A. Characterizing Unitary Currents

Following the laws of probability, ion channels open and close in a stochastic fashion. However, the probability of finding the channel closed or open is not a fixed number but can be modified or modulated by an external stimulus such as the voltage (for voltage-gated channels), stretch (for mechanosensitive channels), or an agonist (for ligand-gated channels). Use of the patch-clamp technique can provide information on the open probability and channel conductance of ion channels. However, this is difficult to do using macroscopic currents (I) recorded in the whole-cell configuration, because the latter is a function of the single-channel current (i), the number of channels (N), and the probability of the channel being in the open state (P_o):

$$I = iNP_o \tag{2}$$

These elements are difficult to distinguish for individual channels in whole-cell patches. Therefore, single-channel current recordings from cell-attached patches provide information about the gating and kinetics of individual channel proteins that cannot be elucidated as easily by studying macroscopic currents. Single-channel recordings are typically obtained from cell-attached patches, although they can also be obtained from inside-out or outside-out membrane patches as described earlier. In the simplest scenario, the small membrane patch surrounded by the walls of the glass pipette contains a single channel protein (Fig. 2A); nature rarely cooperates this readily. As a result, a typical single-channel recording shows the opening of multiple channel proteins located within the same patch. Figure 2B shows a sample 400 ms recording obtained in human PASMCs where three channel openings of similar amplitude (o_1, o_2, and o_3) are apparent when the patch potential is +50 mV. Computer analysis allows the user to characterize the unitary channels according to three important criteria as outlined below.

Channel Conductance and Selectivity and Current Amplitude

Each opening of a channel allows for the flow of ions through the protein, generating a current. The ease of flow of current across the membrane via the channel, the *conductance* (measured in siemens, S), cannot be directly measured. However, it can be approximated from the *amplitude* of the channel openings at different voltages. Amplitude, the differential amplitude between the maximum open level of one channel (o_1) and the closed level (c), can be determined manually, using a ruler and a reference scale. Most will agree that this approach lacks a certain element of elegance and preci-

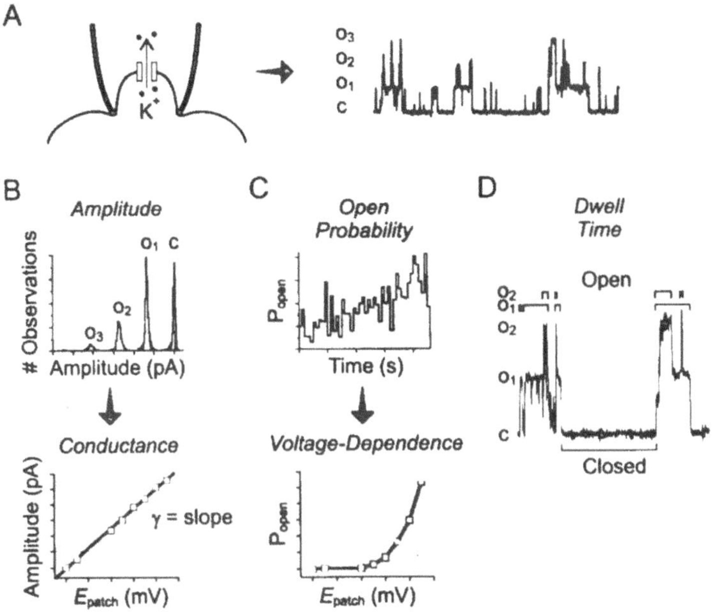

Figure 2 Single-channel recordings and analysis. (A) Left panel: Cartoon view of the cell-attached configuration. Although many channel proteins are likely present within the patched area, a single channel is represented here. Right: Sample single-channel current recording from a human PASMC at a patch potential (E_{patch}) of +50 mV. Note that up to three channels (o_1, o_2, o_3) are present within the patch; "c" represents the closed level. Unitary channel openings are characterized by their amplitude [(B), Top panel] with peaks for open levels 1–3 indicated; conductance [(B), bottom panel], derived from current amplitude); open probability (C); and open-and closed-time durations (D). Voltage dependence of single-channel gating can be established as shown in (C), lower panel.

sion, not to mention that it is time-consuming. The more conventional approach involves using computer software to create a histogram, based on the raw data, and report the number of events (i.e., openings) as a function of their amplitude. The upper panel of Fig. 2B depicts the amplitude histogram based on a 30 s recording, part of which is shown in Fig. 2A. Fitting the histogram peaks with Gaussian distributions provides the mean amplitude of each open level (o_1–o_3). In this example, the amplitudes of the multiple openings were multiples of each other, suggesting that the responsible channel proteins were of the same type. The determined amplitude values are then plotted as a function of the applied patch potential [$E_{patch} = -(E_{applied}) - |E_m|$, where E_m is −40 mV] (Fig. 2B, bottom panel). A linear fit of the data results in a calculated slope (γ), which approximates the conductance of the channel, as described above. For the example shown, the slope conductance was 189 pS, a value typically associated with smooth muscle large-conductance Ca^{2+}-activated K^+ channels (K_{Ca}, BK_{Ca}, maxi-K_{Ca}). As mentioned earlier, single-channel conductance is unique for each channel type.

The current–voltage relationship can also provide some indication as to the selectivity of the channel. Using outside-out patches, one can control the ion content of both the internal and external milieus of the cell patches. For each concentration gradient, the reversal potential (E_X, as defined by the Nernst equation,

$$E_X = \frac{RT}{zF} \log \frac{[X]_o}{[X]_i} \tag{3}$$

where R is the gas constant, T is the absolute temperature (Kelvin), z is the valence of the ion, F is the Faraday constant, and $[X]_o/[X]_i$ is the ratio of extracellular to intracellular concentrations of the ion. E_X can be determined by measuring the voltage at which the unitary current changes direction, i.e., amplitude goes from positive to negative (or vice versa) on the current–voltage curve.

Channel-Open Probability

Assuming that single-channel conductance is independent of E_m, the measured current can also be described by the equation

$$i(t) = N\gamma P_o(E,t)(E - E_X) \tag{4}$$

where $i(t)$ is the time-dependent ionic current measured, N is the number of channels in the patch, γ is the single-channel conductance, $P_o(E,t)$ is the probability that a channel is in the open state, E is the membrane potential (controlled by the patch-clamp system), and E_X is the reversal potential of the current, determined using a double-pulse protocol (13) or the Nernst equation. As suggested by Eq. (4), the open probability of a channel protein is a function of time and membrane potential. For each patch, total single-channel open probability (NP_o) is calculated as

$$NP_o = \frac{\Sigma(O_n n)}{T} \tag{5}$$

where n is the number of channels in the patch (1, 2, 3, ...), O_n is the time spent at the open level for each channel (i.e., 1–n), and T is the total recording time. The fraction of channels in the open state varies between 0 (closed) and 1 (open) depending on the nature of the channel and the stimulus. Figure 2D shows the NP_o histogram generated at a patch potential of +50 mV for the full recording (part of which is shown in Fig. 2B). At +50 mV, calculated NP_o was 0.27; in the same patch, NP_o values of 0.15, 0.08, 0.03, 0.01, and 0.003 were calculated at patch potentials of +40,

+30, +20, +10, and +0 mV, respectively. Therefore, the channel shown in Fig. 2 possesses voltage-dependent and high-conductance properties, even more suggestive of a large-conductance K_{Ca} channel.

Channel Gating

Finally, single-channel recordings can provide information regarding the behavior of the channel protein(s). *Dwell times* reflect the amount of time channels spend in the open or closed states. Like amplitude measurements, the durations of the channel transitions from the closed to open states can be measured and sorted into histogram bins. From these histograms, one can estimate the number of closed and open states and their respective time constants. Typically, dwell times are plotted as a function of the number of observations. Alternatively, one may wish to plot dwell times as a function of time, i.e., a time course, in order to monitor the behavior of a channel over time, such as during drug application or in response to an external stimulus. Dwell-time analysis should be performed only in patches with a single open level to better approximate channel behavior, simply because channel closure may be masked by the simultaneous opening of another channel. In some cases, the openings are "flickery," as shown by the left-side openings in Fig. 2D. Dwell-time analysis of these recordings should be done using burst analysis. The latter applies to recordings where consecutive channel openings are separated by a dwell time less than the interburst (definite channel closure) interval. Only the durations of events (openings or closings), not their amplitude, are measured in this mode; therefore, burst analysis cannot be performed on data with more than one amplitude level.

B. Macroscopic Currents

As mentioned earlier, the whole-cell configuration provides a certain degree of experimental flexibility because the user can simultaneously control both intra- and extracellular ion content and voltage. Another advantage to measuring whole-cell currents is that it allows for the determination of the function of a channel type as a whole family. Therefore, it can be used to successfully characterize a channel protein type in terms of both its permeability and gating characteristics.

Passive Cell Membrane Properties

Likening the whole-cell configuration to an electrical circuit (Fig. 3) allows electrophysiologists to determine passive cell membrane properties, i.e., membrane capacitance, membrane resistance, and cell surface area. A capacitor is composed of two charged surfaces separated by a dielectric substance. The pipette, with its two charged surfaces, is a dielectric substance and therefore is represented by a capacitor in the circuit. Pipette capacitance [C_p, measured in farads (F)] is complicated in character, but

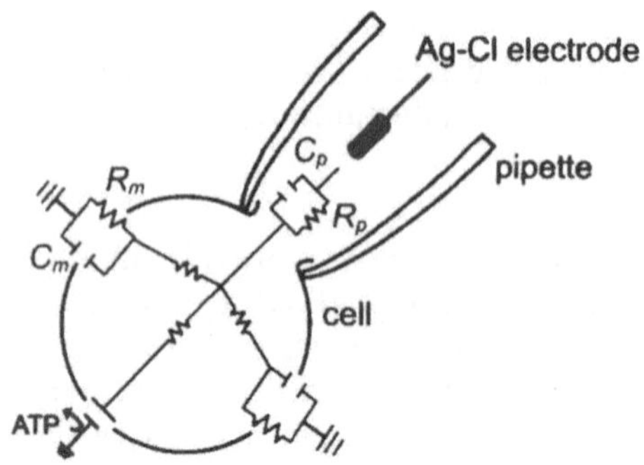

Figure 3 Cartoon representation of the electric circuit formed by the cell and pipette in the whole-cell patch-clamp configuration. Membrane capacitance (C_m) and resistance (R_m) are indicators of cell size and transmembrane ion flux, respectively. Pipette capacitance (C_p) is compensated for by injecting current to charge the pipette surface, and pipette resistance (R_p) can be measured once whole-cell access is attained.

its contribution to the overall circuit is usually minimized electronically by injecting a current transient designed to precharge the glass surface to the desired potential. The pore of the pipette presents a resistance to current flow that can be easily measured before seal formation (R_p, measured in ohms). During whole-cell access, however, this resistance is increased by further resistance to current flow due to the contents or geometry of the cell itself ("series resistance" or "access resistance"), i.e., resistance to filling the entire cytosolic space with the desired amount of charge, or potential due to interaction of charges with proteins or to limited flux through long cell processes or narrow cell geometry.

Once the cytosolic space of the cell is voltage-clamped, the cell membrane also presents its own capacitance. Unlike the pipette, the cell membrane is of relatively uniform thickness and uniform dielectric content (lipids); therefore in most cells the specific membrane capacitance (C_m), which is normalized by the area of the plasma membrane, is $\sim 1\ \mu F/cm^2$ (12); cell capacitance is a good indicator of cell size (i.e., the surface area of a cell). The cell membrane itself is a very good dielectric, presenting a resistance of several gigaohms, in effect stopping the flow of charge across the membrane. However, the membrane resistance (R_m) is strongly influenced by the presence of ion conductances through membrane ion channels.

Ion channels are selectively permeable to specific cations and have a gating mechanism that can be controlled by voltage or other methods. Ion channels produce a conductance (g, inverse of R) that is dependent on the transmembrane electrical potential energy [ΔE, measured in volts (V)] and defined by Ohm's law [Eq. (1)], which can be alternatively expressed as

$$I_x = g\,\Delta E \tag{6}$$

where I_x is the current through a channel. The overall membrane resistance is the inverse of the sum of all the conductances present on the membrane (simplified in Fig. 3 to show just two conductances). The simple measurement of overall membrane resistance is therefore a good indicator of the amount of current carried through all the open channels on the membrane. Because many membrane channels are voltage-dependent, the membrane resistance likewise varies with changes in E_m.

Experimentally, cell membrane capacitance (C_m) is determined by software based on the equation

$$C_m = \frac{\int I_{tr}}{\Delta V_{comm}} \tag{7}$$

where ΔV_{comm} is the amplitude of a small hyperpolarization applied to induce a current transient (I_{tr}). Similarly, membrane input resistance (R_m) can be calculated from the equation

$$R_m = \frac{R_{total} \times R_{seal}}{R_{seal} - R_{total}} \tag{8}$$

where R_{seal} and R_{total} are the resistances determined, respectively, from the steady-state currents of I_{tr} in response to ΔV_{comm} (-5 mV) before and after break-in. In human PASMCs, we have measured average C_m and R_m values of 35 pF and 5 GΩ, respectively (Platoshyn, Remillard, and Yuan, unpublished observations).

The resting membrane potential (RMP) is also a very important property of quiescent cells. Although other techniques may also be used, RMP can be measured in the current-clamp mode once whole-cell access has been established. In vascular smooth muscle, RMP ranges between −75 and −40 mV, typically close to the reversal potential for potassium ions (E_K). Coincidentally, as has been discussed in earlier chapters, the activity of K^+-permeable channels is the main determinant of RMP in many excitable cells. In PASMCs, RMP is approximately −45 mV, although it can vary depending on species and cell isolation technique (14,15).

Channel Permeation and Ion Selectivity

Channel selectivity can be studied by using the relative permeability (P_x/P_y) of a channel to different permeant ions. Because the driving force for ions in a cell membrane is dependent on voltage, a simplified voltage form of the

Goldman–Hodgkin–Katz equation,

$$E_{rev} = \frac{RT}{zF} \log \frac{P_x[X]_o}{P_y[Y]_i} \tag{9}$$

can be used to approximate P_x/P_y. Using either the outside-out or whole-cell patch-clamp configurations to fix the ionic gradients, this ratio can be easily determined and the reversal potential of a current (E_{rev}) can be measured, providing that ions X and Y are the only permeating ions on the external and internal sides of the membrane.

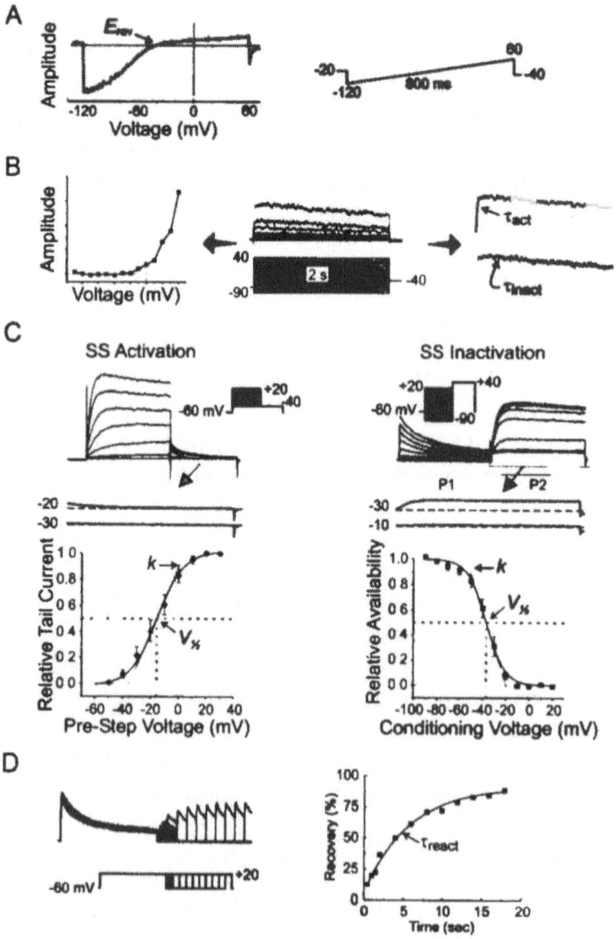

Figure 4 *(Caption on facing page.)*

Under whole-cell conditions, reversal potential (therefore ion selectivity) can be established in two different ways. First, rapid current–voltage (I–V) relationships can be established by using ramp protocols under whole-cell conditions. In this scenario, the reversal potential is determined in similar fashion to that using single-channel analysis (Fig. 4A). Second, a double-pulse protocol can be used whereby cells are depolarized to a single potential, then hyperpolarized to a range of potentials in which the voltage dependence and E_{rev} of the current overlap. A current–voltage relationship generated by plotting the amplitude of the tail current (deactivating current induced by the hyperpolarizing step) as a function of its voltage can clearly reveal the E_{rev} and selectivity of a particular channel.

Channel Gating Properties

The stochastic behavior of a channel dictates that it oscillate between its open (O) and closed (C) states, with a jump of an energy barrier required

---

Figure 4 (*Facing page*) Examples of protocols used and typical macroscopic current recordings providing information on the permeation and gating mechanisms of channels. Reversal potential (E_{rev}) can be determined using I–V relationships generated by ramp protocols (A), as shown for the typical cardiac inward rectifier current (I_{K1}) depicted here. (B) Step protocols can be used to generate I–V relationships. Currents were elicited by 2 s steps ranging between −90 and +40 mV (10 mV increments) from a holding potential of 70 mV applied to human PASMCs. Peak amplitude plotted as a function of voltage generates the I–V curve shown to the left. Activation (τ_{act}) and inactivation (τ_{inact}) kinetics can be determined by mathematical fits of the current recordings (right panels, superimposed black lines represent fits). (C). Double-pulse protocols are used to determine voltage dependence of channel activation and inactivation. Examples provided are from rabbit coronary artery cells. (Modified with permission from Ref. 16.) Left: Example of a steady-state (SS) activation curve generated by stepping the cell membrane for 250 ms to potentials between −60 and +20 mV, followed by repolarization to −40 mV to record tail currents. Sample tail currents after steps to −20 and −30 mV are magnified below. Their relative amplitudes are plotted as a function of the prestep voltage. Right: The membrane was stepped (P1) between −90 and +20 mV for 10 s (from −60 mV) and depolarized further to +40 mV (P2) for 250 ms before being allowed to repolarize. Tail currents (P2) recorded at −10 and −30 mV are magnified below. The relative amplitude of the currents recorded during P2 (I/I_{max}) is plotted vs. the conditioning voltage (P1) to generate the SS inactivation curve. Mathematical fits for the SS activation ($n = 10$) and inactivation ($n = 11$) curves as well as the derived properties are described in the text. (D) Sample recording from a rabbit coronary artery cell using a typical recovery protocol where the membrane was depolarized from −60 to +20 mV for 20 s, repolarized to −60 mV for a variable duration (0.5–18 s), and depolarized again to +20 mV for 2 s. Current recovery is plotted as a function of the time interval between P1 and P2, and points are fitted by mathematical function to derive τ_{react}.

for each state transition. In some cases, the channels may also be found in intermediate inactivated (I) or subconductance states (O′).

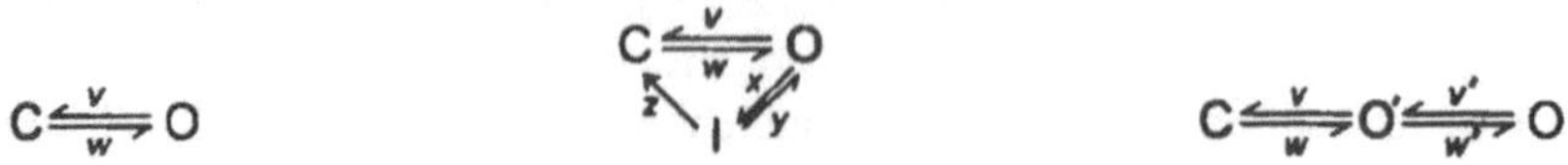

Transitions between these conformational states can be dependent on time, voltage, or the binding of ligands, hormones, and/or drugs; the speed of these transitions is given by rate constants (v, v', w,w', x, and z). Establishing a channel's voltage dependence is typically achieved by a simple step protocol by which the cell membrane is depolarized to a range of potentials before repolarization to a common negative potential near the cell's resting E_m. Plotting current amplitude as a function of the test potential establishes the current–voltage relationship for a current (Fig. 4B). Analysis of the shape of the currents also provides some information as to the activation (time to peak, τ_{act}) and inactivation (peak to steady state, τ_{inact}) kinetics, at least for time-dependent currents, which can be used to derive the rate constants for the channel state transitions.

One problem associated with using simple I–V protocols to study the gating properties of a channel is that one cannot dissociate the combined effect of the gating mechanisms from the electrochemical driving force for the ion on channel gating. The simplest way to bypass this issue is to use a double-pulse protocol (Fig. 4C). An initial voltage step (P1) is applied to activate the channels, followed by a step down to a negative potential (P2) to allow time-dependent channel closure. Plotting the relative amplitude of the tail current as a function of the step voltage provides an indication of the voltage sensitivity and activation thresholds (Fig. 4C, left) of the current in question. Relative availability of the channels following current inactivation can also be determined using a similar double-pulse protocol (Fig. 4C, right). The slope of the mathematical fit (Boltzmann function) to the activation curve as written in the equation

$$Y = \left[1 + \exp\left(\frac{V_{1/2} - V}{k}\right)\right]^{-1} \tag{10}$$

and the inactivation curve (replace $V_{1/2}$–V with V–$V_{1/2}$) provides an indication of how voltage controls the gating mechanisms, information that is particularly useful when one is studying the functional effect of a drug on channel activity. In this equation, $V_{1/2}$ represents the half-maximal activation or inactivation potential and k is the slope factor, which, in the examples shown in Fig. 4, is a good indicator of the steepness of the voltage dependence of channel opening and closing. In the case of the K_V current recorded in rabbit coronary myocytes depicted here, activation of the channel became apparent at potentials less negative than −30 mV and was maximal at +20 mV. Conversely, currents were completely inactivated at potentials less negative than −10 mV. Many channel-modulating compounds shift or alter $V_{1/2}$ and/or k values, to produce their physiological effects. In the case of rabbit coronary artery K_V currents, inhibition of K_V currents by 4-aminopyridine (4-AP) shifted the steady-state activation curve to more positive potentials ($V_{1/2}$ shifted from −16 mV in control to −7 mV with 2 mM 4-AP) and steepened the Voltage dependence (k) of activation (16). Similarly, channel availability was also shifted to more positive potentials ($V_{1/2}$ shifted from −37 to −21 mV) by 4-AP (16), rendering more channels available for activation at more positive potentials.

Finally, one property of inactivating currents remains to be investigated: the recovery from inactivation (I→C transition). The protocol to study recovery also employs a double-pulse strategy, with the determining factor being the delay between P1 and P2 (the latter two being of similar amplitude and duration). In the example shown in Fig. 4D, the membrane is depolarized from the holding potential to a positive membrane potential for 20 s (P1, to allow for full channel inactivation), repolarized to the holding level (~RMP), and depolarized again (P2) to the same potential as P1 for a shorter time. The pulses are repeated, with the time delay between P1 and P2 varying for each episode of the stimulus train. Percentage recovery (P2/P1 × 100) is then plotted as a function of the time delay between P1 and P2. A recovery time constant (τ_{react}) derived from a mathematical fit of the resulting data points describes the recovery kinetics of the current. Repeating this protocol using different holding potentials can be useful in interpreting the voltage dependence of the transition between the inactivated and closed states; i.e., the change in τ_{react} may be dependent on voltage.

VI. SUMMARY

The ions transported through transmembrane ion channels are involved in a plethora of cell functions, including the modulation of cell volume by Cl^-, the maintenance of E_m by K^+, the regulation of action potentials by Na^+, and transcriptional regulation by Ca^{2+}, to name only a few. Patch-clamp electrophysiology has proven to be an essential tool not only in the identification of the channels involved in the maintenance of the normal physiological state, but also in (1) the development of pharmacological tools against diseases (e.g., systemic and pulmonary hypertension, stroke, cardiac disease, diabetes), (2) the identification of the molecular composition of ion channels, and, most recently, (3) the development of K^+ channel gene transfer as a treatment for pulmonary hypertension (17).

The main goal of this chapter was to provide a simple yet comprehensive description of the patch-clamp technique and how the information generated provides insight into the permeation and gating properties of ion currents in freshly dissociated and cultured cells as well as in intact tissues. Advanced molecular biological techniques, as described in upcoming chapters, have provided much information about the molecular composition of ion channels. However, patch-clamp electrophysiology has proven to be an important tool in ascribing biological and physiological properties to the channel subunits and in differentiating between their contributions to the overall physiological state. The conjunction of ion channel electrophysiology with biochemical, molecular, and transgenic technologies will no doubt improve the ongoing progress in the treatment of disease.

ACKNOWLEDGMENTS

This work was supported by grants from the National Institutes of Health (HL 64945, HL54043, HL 66012, HL 69758, and HL 66941).

REFERENCES

1. Bean RC, Shepherd WC, Chan H, Eichner J. Discrete conductance fluctuations in lipid bilayer protein membranes. J Gen Physiol 1969; 53:741–757.
2. Neher E, Sakmann B. Single-channel currents recorded from membrane of denervated frog muscle fibers. Nature 1976; 260:799–802.
3. Hamill OP, Marty A, Neher E, Sakmann B, Sigworth FJ. Improved patch-clamp techniques for high-resolution current recording from cells and cell-free membrane patches. Pflügers Arch 1981; 391:85–100.
4. Guia A, Remillard CV, Leblanc N. Concepts for patch clamp recording of whole-cell and single-channel K^+ currents in cardiac and vascular myocytes. In: Archer SL, Rusch NJ, eds. Potassium Channels in Cardiovascular Biology. Vol. 1. New York, NY: Kluwer Academic/Plenum, 2001:119–142.
5. Purves RD. Microelectrode Methods for Intracellular Recording and Ionophoresis. Biological Technique Series. London; New York: Academic Press, 1981:146.
6. Sakmann B, Neher E, eds. Single-Channel Recording. New York: Plenum Press, 1995.
7. Santana LF, Gómez AM, Lederer WJ. Ca^{2+} flux through promiscuous cardiac Na^+ channels: slip-mode conductance. Science 1998; 279:1027–1033.
8. Leblanc N, Hume JR. Sodium current induced release of calcium from cardiac sarcoplasmic reticulum. Science 1990; 248:372–376.
9. Fozzard HA, January CT, Makielski JC. New studies of the excitatory sodium currents in heart muscle. Circ Res 1985; 56:475–485.
10. Smirnov SV, Robertson TP, Ward JPT, Aaronson PI. Chronic hypoxia is associated with reduced delayed rectifier K^+ current in rat pulmonary artery muscle cells. Am J Physiol 1994; 266:H365–H370.
11. Yuan XJ. Voltage-gated K^+ currents regulate resting membrane potential and $[Ca^{2+}]_i$ in pulmonary arterial myocytes. Circ Res 1995; 77:370–378.

12. Hille B. Ionic Channels of Excitable Membranes. Sunderland, MA: Sinauer Associates, 1992.
13. Alvarez O, Gonzalez C, Latorre R. Counting channels: a tutorial guide on ion channel fluctuation analysis. Adv Physiol Educ 2002; 26:327–341.
14. Post JM, Gelband CH, Hume JR. $[Ca^{2+}]_i$ inhibition of K^+ channels in canine pulmonary artery. Novel mechanism for hypoxia-induced membrane depolarization. Circ Res 1995; 77:131–139.
15. Post JM, Hume JR, Archer SL, Weir EK. Direct role for potassium channel inhibition in hypoxic pulmonary vasoconstriction. Am J Physiol 1992; 262:C882–C890.
16. Remillard CV, Leblanc N. Mechanism of inhibition of delayed rectifier K^+ current by 4-aminopyridine in rabbit coronary myocytes. J Physiol 1996; 491: 383–400.
17. Pozeg ZI, Michelakis E, McMurtry S, Thébaud B, Wu X-C, Dyck JRB, Hashimoto K, Wang S, Moudgil R, Harry G, Sultanian R, Koshal A, Archer SL. In vivo gene transfer of the O_2-sensitive potassium channel Kv1.5 reduces pulmonary hypertension and restores hypoxic pulmonary vasoconstriction in chronically hypoxic rats. Circulation 2003; 107:2037–2044.

31

Planar Electrodes

The Future of Voltage Clamp

António Guia and Jia Xu
AVIVA Biosciences Corp., San Diego, California, U.S.A.

I. INTRODUCTION

The study of electrical signaling and excitability of tissues can be traced back to the 19th century [Höber, 1905 (1) as quoted by Hille (2)]. It took more than 50 years of study to develop a comprehensive model to describe membrane electrical circuits,(2–5) and another 20 years to voltage-clamp a loose patch (6). Ten years after the invention of the voltage-clamp technique, a gigaohm seal was finally achieved, which allowed high-fidelity recordings of the activity of a single molecule in a patch of cell membrane: single-channel currents (7,8). After more than a century of study, the invention of the microchip-based electrode finally enabled automation of the voltage-clamp technique, thus bringing about a new revolution in the study of ion channels.

In most major jumps in technology, timing is no accident. For example, membrane potential measurement required the invention of the electronics components necessary to construct a low-noise voltage amplifier. Such components were themselves developed in response to other events in history that made them possible and necessary. Likewise, the gigaohm seal could not have been achieved without the development of proper pipette fabrication techniques. Finally, even if the technology had existed over 100 years ago, the lack of understanding of ion channels would have failed to provide a driving force to develop voltage-clamp technology. Indeed, planar voltage-clamp electrodes were attempted in 1975 (9) but at the time could not be developed further due to the unavailability of the necessary technologies or driving forces. Presently both the driving force and the technology are in place to develop new techniques in electrophysiology.

A. Driving Forces

In the mid- to late-1990s many electrophysiologists shifted their focus from the 20–30 major channel phenotypes (2) to the channel genotypes. The NIH Human Genome Project has identified at least 300 and possibly more than 400 different genes that are likely to code for ion channels (10). In the pharmaceutical industry, ion channels are considered to be relatively accessible drug targets by virtue of their being located on the plasma membrane. It is estimated that ion channels represent at least 25% of the available drug targets, yet, despite this, presently only 5–7% of compounds on the market are targeted against ion channels (11,12). Hence there is great pressure in both academia and the pharmaceutical industry to accelerate their efforts in the study of and screening against ion channels. The need for higher throughput has outgrown the technologies of the past.

The genotypic approach to ion channel study has provided considerable insight into the interactions between and within ion channels and has given rise to a new field that describes pathologies linked to ion channel disturbances: channelopathy. One particular channelopathy is a defect in the hERG channel that results in the *torsade des pointes* type of cardiac arrhythmia and causes sudden death in a subset of the population with Long Q-T Syndrome (13) when exposed to certain drugs. The normal hERG channel also proved susceptible when the patient's cardiac repolarization reserve was reduced by compounding factors. Subsequently many established drugs (e.g., antihistamines, antihypertensives) and many emerging pharmaceutical compounds that unexpectely block this channel had to be withdrawn from the market. As a result, clinical candidate compounds must now be excluded from any human testing if they are found to inhibit the hERG channel (a recommendation from the various regulatory agencies). This has generated a great need for high-throughput assays for ion channel activity, and voltage clamping is the standard to which any other method must be compared and with which it must be confirmed.

Indeed, *torsade des pointes* was only the first channelopathy of clinical relevance. Many others have already been identified (14), and yet more are in the pipeline (a few examples are shown in Table 1). The pharmaceutical industry needs to screen hundreds to thousands of compounds per week, but an electrophysiologist can perform only 10–15 experiments per day. In response to the demand, other techniques have been developed that estimate ion channel activity without having to voltage clamp the cells, such as fluorescence techniques or radioisotope uptake assays. These secondary techniques are less accurate and pose a higher risk of false positives and false

Table 1 Examples of Channelopathies and the Specific Ion Channels Involved

Channel	Channelopathy
KCNQ1, hERG, SCNA5	Long QT syndrome
KCNQ4	Tinnitus
ClC7	Osteoporosis
CHRNA4, KCNQ	Epilepsy
ClC5	Kidney stones
ClC1	Myotonia
KCNQ1, KCNQ4	Deafness
CACN1A	Migraine
Cl channel	Diarrhea

negatives. The availability of a higher-throughput voltage-clamp method would resolve this impasse.

B. Technological Readiness

Four significant advances in technology have provided the stepping-stones for the advent of planar electrodes: computation, microfabrication and micromanufacturing, transgenic cell lines, and synergy with other high-throughput screening technologies.

First, recent computational advances have enabled the level of multitasking, speed, and storage space that are necessary to automate high-throughput data handling and analysis. For example, high-speed data acquisition in parallel across 16–48 channels requires a data throughput of 800 kbytes/s, with a storage capacity of 1–5 Gbytes/day. Also, analog-to-digital signal conversion with the small cells that are typically used for ion channel screening requires a 500 kHz sampling rate to capture the short capacitative transient (6–20 pF) during a voltage step (time constant less than 100 μs) in 16 data channels (~30 kHz per channel). This is required to successfully detect a transition from a gigaohm seal to a whole-cell access configuration. These data throughput and storage requirements have only recently become achievable.

The second significant advance is the development of new micro fabrication technologies with submicrometer resolution. Advances in microfabrication techniques such as ion beam milling, etching, and laser processing as well as advances in substrate technologies such as silicon, fused silica or quartz, SiO_2, glass, and plastics have enabled the production of a 1 μm "feature" (hole) on a planar substrate. Also, low-resistance substrates may be converted into high-resistance dielectrics suitable for voltage-clamp recordings. For example, silicon (a semiconductor) can be drilled and then converted (e.g., by high-temperature oxidation) into SiO_2, a high-resistance dielectric that is suitable for performing high-quality electrophysiological measurements across the aperture. Finally, to enable gigaohm seals, some companies, such as AVIVA Biosciences, chemically engineer the surface of the substrate to favor the formation of a gigaohm seal with cell membranes.

A third recent advance that has enabled the development of a high-throughput device is the availability of transgenic cell lines expressing ion channels of interest. The greatest advantage of planar electrodes is the ability to automate and miniaturize the voltage-clamp technique. This is possible only because of recent advances in cell engineering that enable stable expression of target ion channel genes in otherwise electrically quiescent cells that have been immortalized as a perpetual cell line. These cell lines can then be used to provide a continuous supply of isolated and uniform cells for automated processing.

The final advance is the synergy among high-throughput screening tools being developed. The need for high-throughput screening technologies has brought about prepackaged automation components such as robotic fluidic handling systems, high-precision robots, standardized multiwell plate formats, and automation software. The emergence of such component technologies under a high-throughput screening paradigm has facilitated the growth of new technologies, including planar electrode voltage-clamp technology, by providing the design concepts, reducing the development time for instrumentation, and making available interfacing technologies and commercial products. The availability of ready-made components for high-throughput screening has significantly reduced the financial burden of developing the instrumentation necessary to interface with the newly developed biochips.

II. PIONEERS AND THEIR METHODS

Any electrophysiological apparatus must contain six elements: (1) an intracellular chamber, (2) an intracellular electrode, (3) an extracellular chamber, (4) an extracellular electrode, (5) a hole between the two chambers that can form a high-resistance seal with a cell, and (6) a conductive medium in each chamber and within the hole. The following sections offer descriptions of recent inventions that allow automation of the voltage-clamp technique.

As a generalization, automated electrophysiological technologies, presently available or in development, rely on the quality of cells that are isolated and delivered to the electrode in suspension. The cells must be relatively uniform in size, and the medium must be free of debris that could contaminate or occlude the aperture during the cell positioning, a step that is usually accomplished by negative pressure. However, there are two exceptions worth noting. Sophion's Apatchi-1® moves the pipette to a cell that is already settled onto a surface; therefore, negative pressure is not required to locate the cell onto the electrode. Cytocentrics's CytoPatch® places the aperture within a larger hole so that positive pressure can be applied to the recording aperture while attracting a cell with negative pressure in the larger hole.

A. Pipette-Based Automation

Even in its infancy, planar electrode technology has already been included in or been the subject of a handful of reviews (10,15–18), although the evolution of electrophysiology has really occurred in two discrete-steps. The first is automation. Since the voltage-clamp technique came into prominence, the level of technical competence required to carry out experiments attracted the same talent that is good at and interested in automating the techniques. In striving for automation, a few companies have come out with fully automated pipette-based platforms.

CeNeS (Cambridge, UK, www.cenes.com) developed AutoPatch AP1®, which uses a technique called interface patch clamping (Fig. 1A) (18). In this technique, a small number of cells in suspension are added to a hanging droplet of solution and allowed to settle to the bottom, at the interface of solution and air. The pipette is then advanced blindly from below to the lowest point of the droplet, where there should be a high density of cells. This technique achieves a rate of 50–60% successful whole-cell recordings. The technology was sold to Xention (Cambridge, UK, www.xention.com), where it is used for internal development.

Sophion Biosciences (Ballerup, Denmark, www.sophion.dk) developed Apatchi-1®, which uses a computer with machine vision to identify a cell and guide a micromanipulator to pick up a pipette tip and deliver it

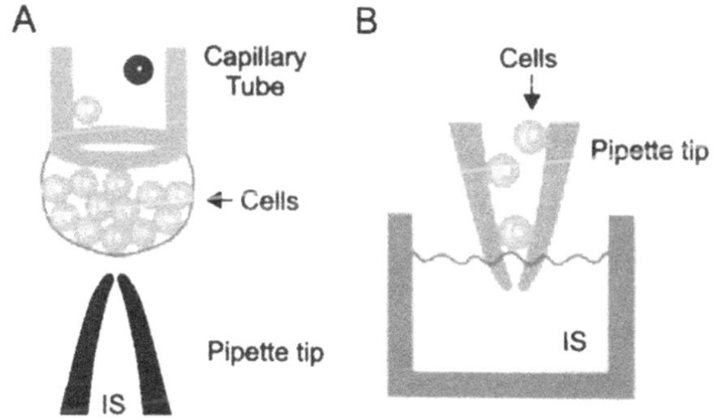

Figure 1 Automation technologies based on glass pipettes. (A) Interface clamping technique where the pipette is raised to the liquid interface of a hanging drop. Note that the cells collect at the air/liquid interface at the lowest point of the hanging drop. (B) Inverted clamping technique where cells are added to the inside of the pipette. Note that cells drop by gravity to the pipette tip and may reduce drug access to the clamped cell. IS, intracellular solution.

to the cell membrane, gain whole-cell access, and perfuse drugs (19). The technology is designed to step sequentially through multiple pipettes and up to eight cell chambers unattended. This technology has been replaced by their planar patch system, QPatch®.

Other companies (e.g., Bristol-Myers-Squibb) have experimented with automated voltage clamp for their internal use, and there are a handful of automated systems for use with oocytes [e.g., Abbott Labs (20), Axon Instruments OpusXpress®, Multi Channel Systems Robocyte® (21), Scion Pharmaceuticals]. In general, however, pipette-based systems have only modestly improved throughput over manual techniques. Recently, Flyion (Tübingen, Germany, www.flyion.com) developed Flyscreen®, which uses a pipette embedded in a plastic disposable cartridge, and the cell suspension is added to the inside of the pipette instead of approaching the cells with its tip (Fig. 1B) (22). This technology does not require coordination of the pipette, and it allows for three to eight experiments to be performed in parallel. Additionally, Flyion claims a 60–80% whole-cell success rate with gigaohm seals and only 3–5 MΩ access resistance. Because the limited space within the pipette can result in slow compound addition and removal, this technique precludes the measurement of rapidly inactivating receptor-operated channels. The addition of cells to the inside of the pipette instead of outside (a technique that Flyion calls "flip the tip") has been demonstrated in the past, but a marketable product was not achieved, likely because of the lack of the appropriate driving forces and other enabling technologies.

B. Planar Electrode Pioneers

Although planar structures have been in use for electrophysiology since the 1970s (9), it was not until the mid- to late-1990s that all the prerequisite technologies were ready. Moreover, there was a big push for miniaturization and for finding alternatives to the patch pipette. By 2001, at least five companies and one academic laboratory had demonstrated their planar chips with real data (see Table 2) and a few others had announced their own planar electrode development programs.

Affymax (Palo Alto, CA; www.affymax.com) claimed that they could produce micrometer-sized conical holes in glass. A laser-machined through-hole on the surface of the substrate could produce gigaohm seals after being painted with a "molecular glue." Very few data are available on the Affymax technology.

AVIVA Biosciences (San Diego, CA; www.avivabio.com) demonstrated over 90% success rate of achieving gigaohm seals, usually within 15 s, and better than 75% success rate (overall) of maintaining subsequent whole-cell access for 15 min with a good membrane resistance ($R_m >$ 200 MΩ) as well as access resistance ($R_a <$ 10 MΩ) (23,24). Their glass-based planar electrodes have been incorporated into the disposable *Seal*Chip$_{16}$®

Table 2 Early Pioneers of Planar Electrode Technology

Company	Electrode design
AVIVA Biosciences, San Diego, CA, U.S.A.	Chips from multiple substrates with chemically engineered surface to promote seals
Cytocentrics CCS, Reutlingen, Germany	Chips with small recording aperture and larger concentric cell-positioning aperture
Cytion, Lausanne, Switzerland	Silicon-based chips, with modified surface to generate either SiO_2 or SiN
Essen Instruments, Ann Arbor, MI, U.S.A.	Plastic sheet with holes, then coated with a glass surface
Nanion Technologies, Münich, Germany	Quartz or glass chips, wet-etched to thin out small area and again then to generate apertures
Sophion Biosciences, Ballerup, Denmark	Chip fitted into a cartridge with microfluidic channels
Sigworth, Yale University, New Haven, CT, U.S.A.	Molded Sylgard chip, modified with oxygen plasma to create SiO_2 surface

(Figs. 2A and 2B), which allows 16 parallel recordings in an instrument, PatchXpress®, developed by Axon Instruments (Union City, CA; www.axon.com). At the time of this writing, AVIVA's partnership with Axon Instruments has allowed AVIVA to focus entirely on producing quality chips and Axon to focus entirely on producing quality instruments. As a result, the AVIVA/Axon product is one of only two planar electrode systems commercially available and is currently the quality leader of the market.

Cytocentrics CCS (Reutlingen, Germany; www.cytocentrics.com) has produced a prototype planar chip, CytoPatch®, that draws the cell into an aperture containing a microfabricated (with a focused ion beam) pipette-tip-like structure and then presses it onto the tip while holding positive pressure within that tip (Figs. 2C, 2D, and 2E) (25). This technique, which they term "cytocentering," approximates techniques used in conventional electrophysiology. Very few functional data have been released on their technology, and the date of product release is still unknown.

Cytion SA (Lausanne, Switzerland) developed a silicon-based chip with a high-resistance Si_3N_4 thin membrane containing a micrometer-sized hole, which is then coated with SiO_2 and positively charged to facilitate gigaohm seals with negatively charged vesicles and cells (Fig. 2F) (26). The membrane is sufficiently thin to allow electrophoretic attraction and positioning of cells from up to 20 μm from the hole. Although this

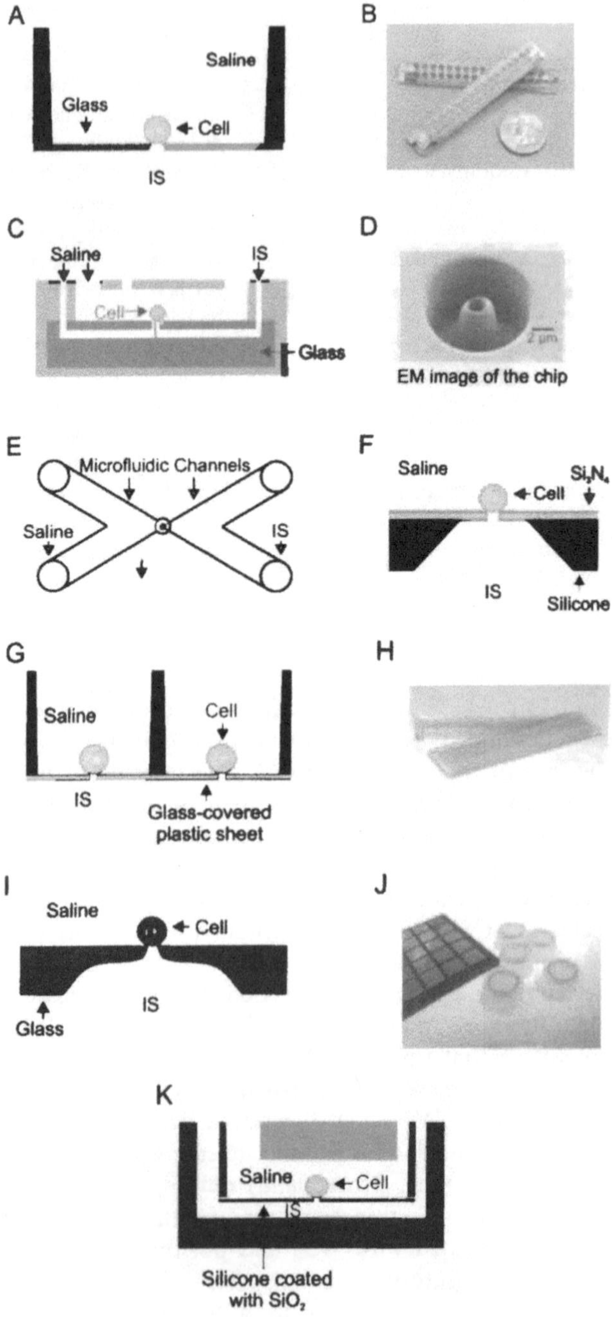

Figure 2 (*Caption on facing page*)

technology has been demonstrated with membrane vesicles, there is no evidence of its success rate with cells. It has been suggested that the membrane is too thin to provide sufficient binding area for a gigaohm seal with a cell (17). Molecular Devices acquired Cytion in 2001, and no further development has been released since.

Essen Instruments (Ann Arbor, MI; www.essen-instruments.com) has developed a planar electrode based on a plastic sheet on the bottom of a multiwell plate, called PatchPlate® (Figs. 2G and 2H) (27,28). Each well contains one laser-drilled hole on the plastic sheet, which is then coated with SiO_2 to enable seals of 20–250 MΩ (averaging 100 MΩ) on cells. This arrangement allows for a 60–80% success rate for up to 6 min. Additionally, their approach to achieving whole-cell access is the perforated-patch technique. Whereas a purist may argue that without a gigaohm seal it is difficult to measure absolute membrane currents, Essen relies on monitoring changes in membrane current (differential data) during voltage ramp protocols to

---

Figure 2 (*Facing page*) Automation technologies based on planar electrodes. (A). AVIVA's *Seal*Chip$_{16}$® design. A glass chip with 16 recording apertures is bound to the bottom of a plastic 16-well chamber. The 16 chambers in the plastic act as the extracellular chamber. The disposable does not contain bottom chambers but instead is sealed onto individual bottom chambers on the instrument. (B) Image of *Seal*-Chip$_{16}$, as shown at http://patchxpress.com/cs_PatchXpress.html. (C) Cytocentrics's CytoPatch® design: a simplified section of the chip demonstrating the fluidic channel for cells and microfluidic channels for "cytocentering" and for intracellular solution (IS). (D) Scanning microscopic image of CytoPatch showing the top view of the recording aperture, as shown at http://cytocentrics.com/technology/chip.html. (E) Schematic view of the microfluidic channels embedded in the CytoPatch chip. The fluidic channel on the left opens to the cytocentering hole (the larger hole). Once filled it is used to locate the cells onto the central intracellular aperture, which is continuous with the channel on the right. Pressure is independently controlled for each channel. (F) Cytion's chip design. The chip is based on silicon nitride on silicon technology. Once the counterbore and aperture are formed, the structure is coated with SiO_2. No information was available about the design of the disposable. (G) Essen's PatchPlate® design. Two chambers are included to emphasize that the intracellular solution (IS) is common for all test chambers. The hole on the plastic sheet is drilled before coating with glass. (H) Image of a PatchPlate showing a disposable with 384 wells in a 1536-well spacing, as shown at http://www.molecular devices.com/pages/instruments/ionworks.html. (I) Nanion's NPC-1® design. The chips are wet-etched to produce smooth surfaces. Cells are patched on the exit-hole side of the chips. (J) Image showing the NPC-1 disposable and some individual unmounted chips, as shown on http://www.nanion.de /products_npc1.htm. (K) Sophion's QPatch® design. Fluidic channels are used for both intracellular and extracellular chambers. One side of the extracellular chamber is open and available for cell and drug delivery.

determine qualitative drug effects. Molecular Devices (Sunnyvale, CA; www.moleculardevices.com) is the exclusive marketer for this technology, distributed for the IonWorks® HT instrument. It is currently one of only two products available on the market. The device is distributed as a 384-well disposable, and measurements are made in parallel, sequentially 48 wells at a time.

Nanion Technologies (Munich, Germany; www.nanion.de) produces a glass-based planar electrode (Figs. 2I and 2J) (29–31). Their technique is to first wet-etch concavities onto the glass or quartz to reduce the glass thickness to ~20 µm, then shoot a single heavy metal ion (gold) through the thinned segment of glass to create a weakened track in the glass, and finally, to wet-etch once again to open up the weakened track into a conical aperture onto the opposite side of the glass. Although Nanion was the first to demonstrate gigaohm seals with glass chips, the success rate achieved was only 30–50%. Nanion has released a single-chip miniaturized product, NPC-1®, that is intended for basic researchers. This product will automate only the voltage-clamping process with very little hardware overhead. A high-throughput product is also in development, with which 16 cells may be patched simultaneously.

In addition to their pipette-based Apatchi-1® system, Sophion Biosciences (Ballerup, Denmark; www.sophion.dk) is currently developing a silicon-based chip to provide 16 simultaneous recordings, called QPatch 16® (19). The chips are coated with a high-resistance dielectric substance and then mounted onto a cartridge that contains microfluidic channels (Fig. 2K). Although these complex structures simplify the performance of multiple experiments in parallel, they also increase the costs of the disposable electrode. Very few data are available on the success rate of the QPatch chips.

The Sigworth group from Yale University (New Haven, CT) developed a PDMS-based chip from Sylgard® that is made by a molding process (32). After curing, PDMS is a very good dielectric substance that can be converted into SiO_2 by treatment with O_2 plasma. This technology was not feasible for commercialization because of poor manufacturability and because experiments needed to be performed immediately after plasma treatment.

C. Access Resistance

Whereas the minimum current amplitude to allow resolution of 50% inhibition by a drug is dictated by background noise (signal-to-noise ratio should be >20 for $>95\%$ accuracy), the maximum current amplitude is dictated by access resistance. Access resistance, or series resistance, represents the ability to voltage clamp a membrane. Specifically, it is the amount of restriction to flow of current that exists across the aperture in whole-cell configuration; it must be significantly lower than membrane resistance to keep the cell voltage-clamped. Voltage escape results from high access resistance preventing proper clamping of the membrane voltage and may be calculated using Ohm's law (Voltage escape = whole-cell current × access resistance). With a typical current amplitude of 1 nA, an access resistance of less than 10 MΩ is desired to keep the variability of the voltage less than its variability due to other experimental conditions, including electrode drift, solution evaporation, and uncertainty in the measurement of liquid junction potential. Hence the chip should provide less than 10 MΩ of access resistance to clamp currents up to 1 nA in amplitude.

Access resistance also determines the speed of the voltage-clamping process (corner frequency = $1/2\pi RC$, where R is access resistance and C is cell capacitance). With an average 10 pF cell and 10 MΩ access resistance, the speed of the voltage clamp is 1.5 kHz (0.6 ms response time). Clamp speed is therefore not as much of a concern as voltage escape with a 10 pF cell.

III. DEVICES CURRENTLY AVAILABLE

This section deals with the second factor necessary for electrophysiological measurements: the procedure and its automation. At the time of this writing, two technologies had already emerged on the market. The first was the IonWorks® HT system from Molecular Devices (Fig. 3A), which was

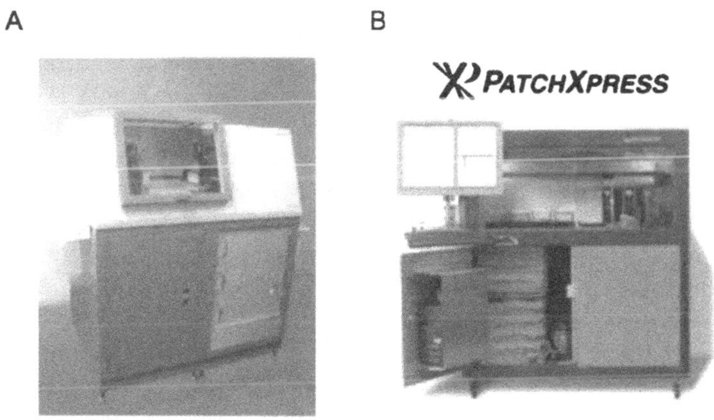

Figure 3 Automated high-throughput voltage-clamp systems available on the market. (A) The IonWorks® HT system is from Molecular Devices. Image available at http://www.moleculardevices.com/pages/instruments/ionworks.html. (B) The PatchXpress® system is from Axon Instruments. Image available at http://patchx-/patchxpress.com/cs_PatchXpress.html.

developed by Essen Instruments. The second system available on the market was the result of a collaborative effort between AVIVA Biosciences, focused on providing the planar electrode technology *Seal*Chip$_{16}$®, and Axon Instruments (Fig. 3B), focused on providing the automation hardware PatchXpress®.

The IonWorks® HT product (Fig. 3A) uses the PatchPlate® disposable electrode (Figs. 2G and 2H). The disposable electrode contains only the top chamber that receives the cells and the drug candidate compounds; there is no bottom chamber. The disposable is pressed onto a receptacle on the machine that, once sealed to the disposable, forms a common bottom chamber. The chambers are then filled with buffer before cells are added to the top chamber. Vacuum pressure is applied from the common bottom chamber to attract a cell onto each hole. Many cells (60–80%) achieve an average of 100 MΩ seals with this method. Whole-cell access is approximated by exchanging the buffer in the common bottom chamber with buffer containing ionophores (e.g., amphotericin) to produce a perforated patch with 10–15 MΩ access resistance. Because a gigaohm seal is not achieved, the currents must be leak-corrected by subtracting a linear component. This method does not provide sufficient precision to measure absolute values of whole-cell currents; it focuses instead on monitoring difference currents when drugs are added. Up to 48 currents are measured simultaneously with electrodes that are mounted on a robotic arm and moved sequentially through all 384 wells. The headstages clamp the extracellular compartment. The reference electrode is below in the intracellular compartment. This inverted clamp technique is necessary because all cells share a common bottom chamber. The recording electrodes must be removed from the extracellular medium to add buffer, cells, or drugs. Reintroduction of the electrodes, the presence of drug, or changes in fluid levels can result in ambiguous junction nulls or offset potentials. The IonWorks HT method also eliminates the possibility of measuring transient receptor-activated currents. Full fluid perfusion, monitoring during drug addition, and washout are not available on this instrument; it provides only a "mix-and-read" mode of drug delivery. Furthermore, the fixed-head electrode array and fluidics design cannot prevent compound consumption on unsuccessful wells, and consequently a quadruplicate screen is necessary to avoid missing compounds. In spite of the serious limitations imposed by its very low membrane resistance seals (10–100 MΩ), the IonWorks HT product has received some market acceptance due to the low cost of its consumable PatchPlate. Each 384-well PatchPlate is capable of patching 150–200 cells for up to 6 min, at approximately US$200 per plate.

The PatchXpress product from Axon Instruments (Union City, CA; http://PatchXpress.com) uses AVIVA's *Seal*Chip$_{16}$, a 16-well disposable, listed at about US$130, that is capable of patching more than 12 cells simultaneously for more than 15 min, for a cost of less than US$10 per cell. The elevated cost is compensated for by the longevity of the cells (15–30 min), allowing more drugs to be tested on each cell and allowing more complicated protocols to be applied. Furthermore, the *Seal*Chip$_{16}$ achieves true gigaohm seals and stable whole-cell accesses with high-quality voltage-clamp parameters, which ensures fidelity of the data. An added benefit of the PatchXpress system is that its fluidics function independently of the test electrodes, allowing for gap-free recording during drug application and hence allowing for recordings of transient currents from receptor-activated channels.

The *Seal*Chip$_{16}$ product also contains only a top chamber that receives the cells and the drug candidate compounds. Independent bottom chambers have been built in to the PatchXpress system, allowing for individual pneumatic control for cell landing, sealing, rupture to whole-cell access, and access resistance optimization and maintenance. The disposables are loaded automatically into the machine, allowing for unattended operation of the instrument. After insertion of the *Seal*Chip$_{16}$, the bottom chambers are filled individually with intracellular medium, then placed onto 16 independent voltage-clamp electrode tubes that also serve to transfer automatic pneumatic pressure control to the bottom (intracellular) chambers. The top chambers are connected to the reference electrodes via perfusion nozzles that are lowered into each well. The perfusion nozzles together with the robotic compound and cell-dispensing system enable complete washout and wash-in fluidics. Using automated suction protocols, many gigaohm seals ($>$90%) are achieved within 2 min of cell addition. Whole-cell access is obtained by rupturing the membrane patch within the chip aperture with stronger suction. An overall $>$75% success rate is achieved in maintaining stable whole-cell access for 15 min with membrane resistance above 200 MΩ, and access resistance below 10 MΩ (23). Sufficient space is left in each well that cells or compounds can be added by a separate robotic fluidic system. This provides the advantage of continuous recordings during addition or washout of a compound. Another important feature is the ability to avoid adding compound to unusable cells and instead add to the next successful cell. This intelligent screening method greatly reduces the chance of missing data points. The increased throughput places a strong demand for improved data analysis tools that are capable of performing repeated analyses over multiple files. Axon Instruments has ported their own analysis tools into a scripting-based tool that performs analyses on data contained in an SQL database (DataXpress).

The technologies presently on the market, though capable of achieving much higher throughput than would be possible with conventional techniques, are still far from being true high-throughput devices for primary screening. They achieve neither the throughput nor the cost per data point of currently marketed fluorescence-based systems. The companies discussed are therefore also developing higher throughput stations for automated electrophysiology. Additionally, both Molecular Devices and Axon/AVIVA have announced that they will provide a one- or two-well design for academic research and assay development. The Axon/AVIVA device will be based on their present planar electrode. It is unknown which technology will be used by Molecular Devices for their low-throughput academic version, but it is likely they will switch to the Cytion technology, because a low-throughput device will demand higher data quality and fidelity.

IV. SUMMARY AND FUTURE DIRECTIONS

The discovery of the channelopathies and the identification of ion-channel-related liabilities have placed a heavy burden on pharmaceutical companies to increase their safety screening efforts to ensure that their compounds do not interfere with ion channels. Genotypic ion channel research with fast-growing cell lines has also placed a great burden on electrophysiologists to keep up with the molecular biologists. The new demand for high-throughput and high-content data on ion channels has fueled the deve-lopment of high-throughput voltage-clamp technologies. A new generation of planar voltage-clamp biochips is now available, providing high-content, low-throughput screening one to two orders faster than conventional methods. Miniaturization has made it economical to perform multiple experiments in parallel, with simpler shielding from background noise, improved speed of solution exchange, reduced consumption, and increased efficiency. Planar substrates also offer immunity from vibration, which enables faster, more robust experiments. The sealing and voltage-clamp parameters may be equal to or better than those of the pipette, enabling reproducible, high-quality automated recordings.

At the time of this writing there were three products already on the market. Molecular Devices markets a 48-electrode disposable electrode that achieves 100–200 MΩ seals with 50–80% success rate, and Axon Instruments/AVIVA Biosciences employs a 16-electrode disposable that achieves > 1 GΩ seals with a success rate of 75–90%. The Molecular Devices instrument is ideal for quick experiments designed to probe for the presence or absence of effect of the test compounds. The Axon/AVIVA instrument is ideal for describing drug effects on absolute current amplitudes and on channel kinetics. Nanion Technologies released a miniaturized, portable, low-throughput single-electrode unit that automates only the patching process and leaves the fluidics to the user.

Both AVIVA/Axon and Molecular Devices have also committed to release a lower throughput, high-functionality product in the near future, using the high consumption rate of the pharmaceutical industry to keep the consumables economical and feasible for academia. The lower throughput devices may additionally allow optical observation and/or measurement of whole-cell fluorescence.

Future incarnations of the technology will produce higher throughput devices for pharmaceutical screening and lower throughput devices with expanded functionality, including more complicated optical observation for visual or automated selection of rare cells. Extracellular and intracellular buffer solutions will each be exchangeable in real time during an experiment. Cell positioning may be aided by the generation of alternating current electric charge fields to allow the use of primary or freshly dispersed cells that are isolated from tissue samples and do not immediately lose their shape. For example, smooth muscle cells that may remain spindle-shaped for days after isolation may become easily electronically manipulated to position the cells correctly onto a recording aperture. Future versions will allow the study of cell–cell interactions by simultaneously voltage-clamping two cells in very close proximity, or they may allow multiple parameters to be measured or clamped simultaneously. The long, laborious voltage-clamp experiment involving lengthy pipette preparation, tedious stabilization of vibration sources, searching for cells and pipette tips under a microscope, and so on, will all soon be a technique of the past.

ACKNOWLEDGMENTS

We thank Drs. Lei Wu, Xiaobo Wang, Mingxian Yang, and David Rothwarf for their assistance and technical discussions during research and development of this technology at AVIVA Biosciences.

REFERENCES

1. Höber R. Über den Einfluss der Salze auf den Ruhestrom des Froschmuskels. Pflügers Arch 1905; 106:599–635.
2. Hille B. Ionic Channels of Excitable Membranes. Sunderland, MA: Sinauer Associates Inc., 1992.
3. Hodgkin AL, Huxley AF. Movement of sodium and potassium ions during nervous activity. Cold Spring Harbor Symp Quant Biol 1952; 17:43–52.
4. Hodgkin AL, Huxley AF. A quantitative description of membrane current and its application to conduction and excitation in nerve. J Physiol 1952; 117: 500–544.
5. Hodgkin AL, Huxley AF. Propagation of electrical signals along giant nerve fibers. Proc Roy Soc Lond B Biol Sci 1952; 140:177–183.
6. Noble D, Tsien RW. The kinetics and rectifier properties of the slow potassium current in cardiac Purkinje fibres. J Physiol 1968; 195:185–214.
7. Hamill OP, Marty A, Neher E, Sakmann B, Sigworth FJ. Improved patch-clamp techniques for high-resolution current recording from cells and cell-free membrane patches. Pflügers Arch 1981; 391:85–100.
8. Neher E, Sakmann B. Single-channel currents recorded from membrane of denervated frog muscle fibers. Nature 1976; 260:799–802.

9. Kostyuk PG, Krishtal OA, Pidoplichko VI. Effect of internal fluoride and phosphate on membrane currents during intracellular dialysis of nerve cells. Nature 1975; 257:691–693.
10. Worley JF. Guest Editor's Introduction: An evolution of electrophysiology. Receptors Channels 2003; 9:1–2.
11. Drews J. Drug discovery: a historical perspective. Science 2000; 287:1960–1964.
12. http://www.windhover.com/contents/monthly/exex/e_2003900085.htm
13. Nattel S. The molecular and ionic specificity of antiarrhythmic drug actions. J Cardiovasc Electrophysiol 1999; 10:272–282.
14. Ashcroft FM. Ion Channels and Disease. New York: Academic Press, 2000:481.
15. Xu J, Wang X, Ensign B, Li M, Wu L, Guia A. Ion-channel assay technologies: quo vadis? Drug Discov Today 2001; 6:1278–1287.
16. Mattheakis LC, Savchenko A. Assay technologies for screening ion channel targets. Curr Opin Drug Discov Dev 2001; 4:124–134.
17. Sigworth FJ, Klemic KG. Patch clamp on a chip. Biophys J 2002; 82: 2831–2832.
18. Owen D, Silverthorne A. Channelling drug discovery—current trends in ion channel drug discovery research. Drug Discov World 2002; Spring:48–61.
19. Asmild M, Oswald N, Krzywkowski KM, Friis S, Jacobsen RB, Reuter D, Taboryski R, Kutchinsky J, Vestergaard RK, Schroder RL, Sorensen CB, Bech M, Korsgaard MP, Willumsen NJ. Upscaling and automation of electrophysiology: toward high throughput screening in ion channel drug discovery. Receptors Channels 2003; 9:49–58.
20. Trumbull JD, Maslana ES, McKenna DG, Nemcek TA, Niforatos W, Pan JY, Parihar AS, Shieh CC, Wilkins JA, Briggs CA, Bertrand D. High throughput electrophysiology using a fully automated, multiplexed recording system. Receptors Channels 2003; 9:19–28.
21. Schnizler K, Kuster M, Methfessel C, Fejtl M. The roboocyte: automated cDNA/mRNA injection and subsequent TEVC recording on *Xenopus* oocytes in 96-well microtiter plates. Receptors Channels 2003; 9:41–48.
22. Lepple-Wienhues A, Ferlinz K, Seeger A, Schafer A. Flip the tip: an automated, high quality, cost-effective patch clamp screen. Receptors Channels 2003; 9:13–17.
23. Xu J, Guia A, Rothwarf D, Huang M, Sithiphong K, Ouang J, Tao G, Wang X, Wu L. A benchmark study with *Seal*Chip® planar patch-clamp technology. Assay Drug Dev Technol 2003; 1:675–684.
24. Xu J, Guia A, Wang X, Koblan KS, Rothwarf D, Huang M, Yand Z, Xu J-Q, Sithiphong K, Wu L, Zhu Y. A microchip-based high quality patch clamp platform for high throughput automation. 2002, Society for Neurosciences Conference, Abstract. Program No. 312.1.
25. Stett A, Burkhardt C, Weber U, van Stiphout P, Knott T. Cytocentering: a novel technique enabling automated cell-by-cell patch clamping with the CytoPatch chip. Receptors Channels 2003; 9:59–66.
26. Schmidt C, Mayer M, Vogel H. A chip-based biosensor for the functional analysis of single ion channels. Angew Chem (Int Ed, Engl) 2000; 39: 3137–3140.

27. Schroeder K, Neagle B, Trezise DJ, Worley J. Ionworks HT: a new high-throughput electrophysiology measurement platform. J Biomol Screening 2003; 8:50–64.
28. Kiss L, Bennett PB, Uebele VN, Koblan KS, Kane SA, Neagle B, Schroeder K. High throughput ion-channel pharmacology: planar-array-based voltage clamp. Assay Drug Dev Technol 2003; 1:127–135.
29. Fertig N, Blick RH, Behrends JC. Whole cell patch clamp recording performed on a planar glass chip. Biophys J 2002; 82:3056–3062.
30. Fertig N, George M, Klau M, Meyer C, Tilke A, Sobotte C, Blick RH, Behrends JC. Microstructured apertures in planar glass substrates for ion channel research. Receptors Channels 2003; 9:29–40.
31. Fertig N, Meyer C, Blick RH, Trautmann C, Behrends JC. Microstructured glass chip for ion-channel electrophysiology. Physiol Rev E Stat Nonlin Soft Matter Phys 2001; 64:040901.
32. Klemic KG, Klemic JF, Reed MA, Sigworth FJ. Micromolded PDMS planar electrode allows patch clamp electrical recordings from cells. Biosens Bioelectron 2002; 17:597–604.

32

Correlation of Ion Channel Activity with Gene Expression Using Single-Cell RT-PCR and Patch-Clamp Techniques

Ying Yu, Oleksandr Platoshyn, and Jason X.-J. Yuan
Department of Medicine, University of California, San Diego, California, U.S.A.

I. INTRODUCTION

Ion channels are important for the regulation of cellular activity in a great variety of cell types from both simple and complex organisms (1). In the last two decades, technological advances in electrophysiology and molecular biology have led to great progress in ion channel research. As discussed in previous chapters in this monograph, the use of the patch-clamp method to record single-channel and whole-cell currents makes it possible to characterize the electrophysiological and pharmacological properties of ion channels and the mechanisms by which receptors and second messengers modulate ion channels (2,3). However, this technique is obviously restricted by (1) the specificity of the pharmacological tools available, (2) heterogeneity of ion channel expression and function in different cells, and (3) the extent of available knowledge about the receptor or ion channel family in question. In addition, genes and proteins do not act in isolation; i.e., physiological function of a cell is the result of the combined interactive action of many gene products. Techniques are required that can simultaneously assess the expression of genes and their relationship with the function of ion channels in single cells.

Evaluation of gene expression at the transcriptional level mainly involves techniques such as Northern blot analysis and nuclease protection assays (4). However, gene expression (especially of genes that express at a low level) in a single cell or a small population of cells is extremely difficult to determine using these techniques. Introduction of reverse transcription–polymerase chain reaction (RT-PCR) has led to a substantial increase in the sensitivity of gene expression analysis (5). RT-PCR consists of two elements: (1) synthesis of cDNA from RNA by reverse transcription (RT) and (2) amplification of a specific cDNA by PCR. RT-PCR has been shown to be an effective tool for amplifying very small quantities of cDNA reversely transcribed from cellular RNA. Whereas flow cytometry and microscopic technologies have allowed for cells to be sorted on the basis of cell-surface markers and morphological characteristics, the combination of patch-clamp electrophysiology and single-cell RT-PCR can sort cells according to their ion channel activity and gene expression. A combined patch-clamp and RT-PCR approach has been used successfully to sort cells both in culture and in situ in brain slices in vitro (6,7) based on their expression of ion channel genes (8–13).

This chapter focuses on the principles and technical processes of simple multiplex single-cell RT-PCR methods, followed by a brief description of the electrophysiological characterization of ion channels. Specific examples are provided from pulmonary artery smooth muscle cells (PASMCs) where patch-clamp and RT-PCR techniques have been used to establish a correlation between voltage-gated K^+ (Kv) channel activity and gene expression.

II. COMBINATION OF PATCH-CLAMP RECORDING AND SINGLE-CELL RT-PCR ANALYSIS

The combination of patch-clamp recording and single-cell RT-PCR requires some modifications to the standard procedures of both techniques. The major steps to achieve the combined analysis include (1) patch-clamp recording, (2) aspiration of the cell from which ion channel currents are recorded by a collection pipette, (3) reverse transcription without RNA isolation, (4) multiplex first-round PCR and specific nested PCR to detect gene expression, and (5) unique PCR primer design.

A. Patch-Clamp Recording and Sterile Technique

Patch-clamp recording is conducted using standard whole-cell voltage- or current-clamp configurations (3). It is important to create an RNase-free environment in order to protect the cellular RNA from the deleterious action of ubiquitous RNases and to avoid contamination of the solutions with previously amplified cDNAs. Both of these issues can be addressed by employing sterile laboratory practice as described below. The modifications in patch-clamp recording include the use of oven-heated (180°C for 2 h) thin-walled borosilicate glass for the manufacture of the patch and collection pipettes to prevent RNA loss. In addition, the experimenter must wear latex gloves during the preparation of solutions and the execution of the experiments in order to avoid contamination with RNases. Only dedicated stocks of chemicals and ultrafiltered double-distilled water of the highest purity (i.e., free of contaminating nucleases) should be used (7).

B. Aspiration of the Patched Cell for Single-Cell RT-PCR

Isolation and transfer of a single cell to a reaction tube is crucial to the success of single-cell RT-PCR. It has been reported that isolation of the cytoplasmic contents of a cell through direct suction applied to the interior of the patch pipette can increase the probability of RNA isolation (6). Nonetheless, aspiration of the patched cell by a collection pipette (described below) is used predominantly to collect the cell of interest for RT-PCR.

Collection pipettes (tip diameter 3–4 μm) are prepared with an electrode puller from heat-sterilized thin-walled borosilicate glass tubes and are fire polished. The collection pipette contains a solution that includes 10 μmol/L dNTP and 0.5 U/μL RNase inhibitor. The cells in the recording or tissue chamber are continuously superperfused with fresh physiological salt solution to remove debris from the cell before collection, thereby avoiding uptake of cell debris into the collection pipette. Cells are aspirated into the collection pipette in two stages (Fig. 1A). First, gentle suction attaches the cell to the collection pipette, allowing for the cell to be lifted from the bottom of the chamber. Second, further suction aspirates the entire cell into the collection pipette (14). The contents of the pipette are then expelled into a thin-walled silicon-coated PCR tube, frozen on dry ice, and stored at −80°C. Single cells usually are stable for up to 1 year under this condition (15). The cell-free samples collected during the patch-clamp experiment are used as negative controls.

C. RT Without RNA Isolation

Reverse transcription-PCR consists of two steps: (1) synthesis of cDNA from RNA by reverse transcriptase and (2) amplification of specific cDNA by PCR. For mRNA analysis using RT-PCR, isolation of pure RNA is critical; the RNA should be free of genomic DNA contamination. To isolate RNA from a single cell, however, is difficult because the sample can be lost during cell lysis, RNA extraction, or RNA recovery (16). To solve these problems, the simplest and most efficient approach is to integrate all cell lysis, RNA isolation, genomic DNA degradation, reverse transcription, and first-round PCR in a single PCR tube (Fig. 1B). Recently, several kits (e.g., Takara's One-step RNA RT-PCR kit, Ambion's Cell-to-cDNA™ kit, and Qiagen's OneStep RT-PCR kit) designed for the isolation of RNA from a single cell or a small cell population have become commercially available.

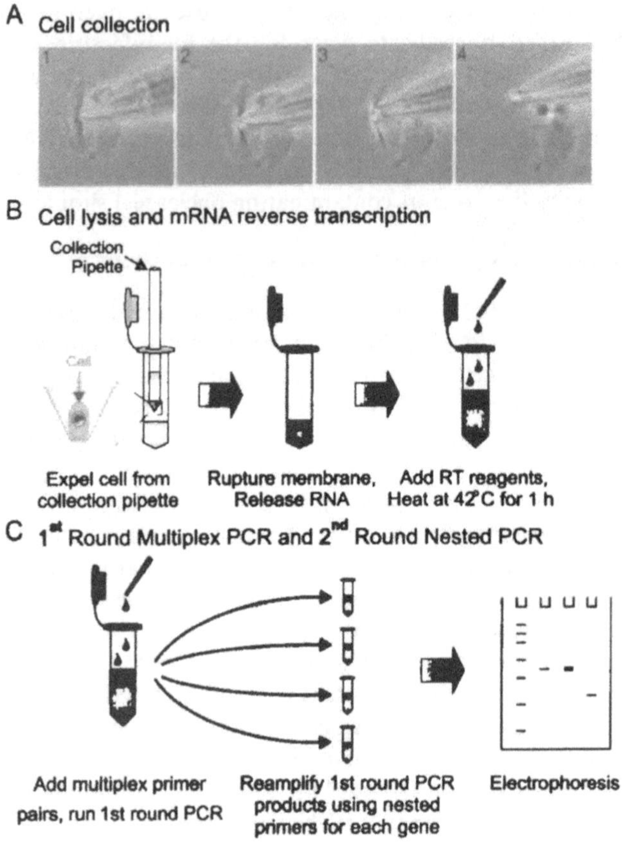

Figure 1 Schematic diagram depicting patch-clamp recording coupled with single-cell RT-PCR. (A) The patch pipette is placed on the cell surface and currents are recorded (step 1). After recording currents, further suction attaches the cell to the pipette, and it is gently lifted from the cover slip (steps 2 and 3). Finally, further suction aspirates the cell into the pipette (step 4). In this experiment, we used the recording pipette as the collection pipette. (B) The cell is expelled from the collection pipette into a PCR tube. The cell membrane is ruptured, and reverse transcription is initiated by adding the RT reagents. (C) Primer pairs for multiple genes are added to the isolated RNA samples and first round PCR is performed to target the genes of interest. PCR products for these genes are amplified using second round nested PCR. Nested PCR products are separated by electrophoresis on an agarose gel.

The first step in our procedure involves thawing the PCR tubes containing single cells, adding diluted nonionic surfactant NP-40 (to a final concentration of 0.4%), and then keeping the PCR tubes on ice so that the cell membranes are ruptured and RNA is released. Because the nucleus is aspirated as part of the cell, it is important to ensure that single-cell RT-PCR does not amplify genomic DNA, which may generate false positive results. This problem can be addressed by first treating the lysate with RNase-free DNase and then heating the sample to inactivate the DNase I. It has been reported that single cell RT-PCR followed by patch-clamp recording carries no risk of genomic DNA amplification because the genomic alleles are not exposed during this approach (17).

The second step is the reverse transcription of the RNA into cDNA. Reverse transcriptases from Moloney murine leukemia virus (MMLV) or avian myeloblastosis virus (AMV) appear to work equally well in single-cell based RT (7). The reverse transcriptase enzyme also requires a primer in order to make a cDNA copy of the template RNA. Three types of primers—oligo-dT primers, hexamer primers, and specific antisense primers—have been used successfully in single-cell RT-PCR (7,18–23). In our experiments, first strand cDNA synthesis is performed for 60 min at 42°C after adding a small volume of solution containing 10 mM Tris-HCl, 50 mM KCl, 2.5 mM $MgCl_2$, 10 mM DTT, 1.25 mM oligo(dT), 0.5 mM dNTPs, and 5 U AMV reverse transcriptase XL (Takara), followed by a 10 min heating cycle at 70°C to inactivate the enzyme.

D. Multiplex First-Round PCR and Specific Nested PCR to Detect Multiple Gene Expression

Multiplex PCR is a useful and effective technique for genetic screening and for other applications where it is necessary to amplify several products in a single reaction. To accurately quantify and identify the expression of multiple genes (such as several ion channel subunits in a single cell), multiplex PCR is used in first-round PCR. In a typical experiment, up to five different genes can be detected in a single cell.

The PCR tube containing a cell of interest is filled with a premixed PCR buffer containing 10 mM Tris-HCl, 50 mM KCl, 2.5 mM $MgCl_2$, 5 U *Taq* DNA polymerase (RNA PCR kit, Takara), and 20 nM of each sense and antisense primer (one set of multiple primer pairs for each gene of interest). The amplification protocol involves a denaturation step at 94°C for 3 min, followed by 40–45 cycles at 94°C for 30, at 55°C for 45, and at 72°C for 45, and a final extension stage at 72°C for 10 min.

To increase the sensitivity and specificity of the single-cell RT-PCR amplification for the target genes, a nested PCR strategy is used for a second round of PCR. In this approach, aliquots of the first-round PCR products are reamplified by 25–30 cycles in the thermal cycler, carried out separately with fully nested gene-specific primers (nested primers) for each target gene. Nested PCR-amplified products are then separated on a 1.5% agarose gel and visualized with gel staining (Fig. 1C). To semiquantify the PCR products, an invariant housekeeping gene such as glyceraldehyde-3-phosphate

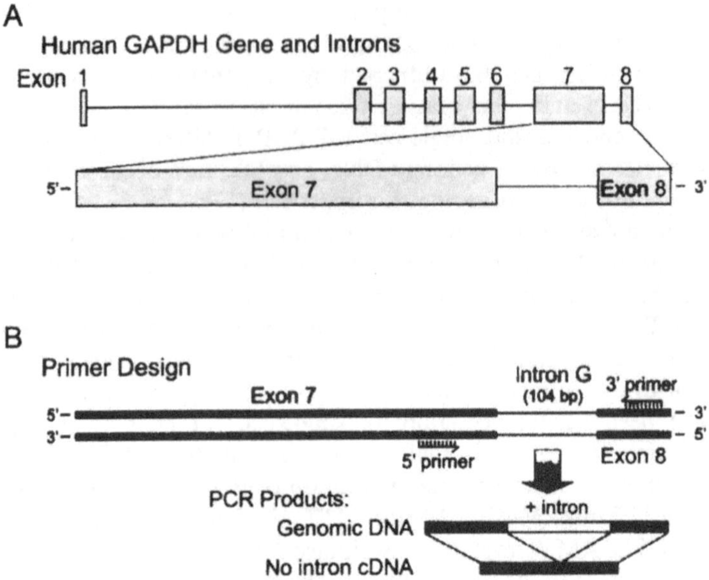

Predicted mRNA Size	Primer Sequence Sense/Antisense	Location (nt.)	Exon
First primers (404 bp)	5'-CCGGGAAACTGTGGCGTGATG-3'/ 5'-GTCCACCACCCTGTTGCTGTA-3'	4255-4275 4742-4762	7 8
Nested primers (198 bp)	5'-GATGACATCAAGAAGGTGGTG-3'/ 5'-GCTGTAGCCAAATTCGTTGTC-3'	4446-4466 4727-4747	7 8

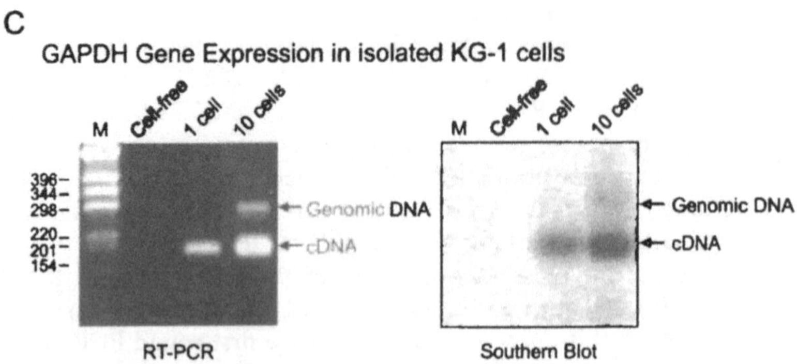

Figure 2 (*Caption on facing page*)

dehydrogenase (GAPDH) or β-actin is often used as an internal control. Further confirmation of the identity of the amplified products requires Southern blot analysis or PCR product sequencing.

E. Unique PCR Primers Design

The most critical parameter for successful PCR is the design of appropriate primers. Primer length, percent G-C content, melting temperature (T_m), and the 3′-end sequence need to be optimized for successful PCR (24,25). Ideally, the multiple primer pairs to be used in the first-round PCR should have approximately the same G-C content, similar T_m, and no complementary sequences in order to prevent the formation of hairpins or dimers. The amplification of contaminating genomic DNA often yields PCR products of a larger size than the amplification of cDNA, or no product at all if the intron is of sufficient size (Fig. 2). To avoid possible contamination due to the amplification of genomic DNA, primer design strategies should ensure that the sequences of the 5′ and 3′ primers of each pair target different exons of the genes to be detected. Because GAPDH or β-actin contains several introns, unique PCR primer pairs of GAPDH or β-actin are also useful controls for single-cell RT-PCR (sequences for GAPDH primers are shown in Fig. 2B). Nonetheless, although computer programs specialized for primer design are useful, the best primers and optimal conditions for the reactions must be determined experimentally (25).

III. APPLICATION OF PATCH-CLAMP AND SINGLE-CELL RT-PCR ASSAY IN PASMCs

The combination of patch-clamp recording and single-cell RT-PCR has proven to be a useful tool for the accurate identification of the ion channel

Figure 2 (*Facing page*) Primer design strategy for the human GAPDH gene. (A) The human GAPDH gene (Genbank #J04038) contains seven introns and eight exons (exons 7 and 8 magnified in bottom panel). (B) Primers designed against exons 7 (sense, 5′ primer) and 8 (antisense, 3′ primer). The amplification of contaminating genomic DNA will yield PCR products of a larger size (exons 7 and 8 and intron G) compared with the amplification of cDNA (bottom panel). Examples of the sequences of first-round and nested PCR primers for GAPDH are shown in the table. (C) GAPDH expression in KG-1 (human acute myeloid leukemia) cells. After cell lysis, RT-PCR is performed without DNase I treatment for a single cell or a sample from 10 KG-1 cells (left panel). A 198 bp intron-free (cDNA) fragment of the GAPDH gene is amplified from the single KG-1 cell. Both genomic DNA-derived 302 bp (containing introns) and 198 bp intron-free cDNA fragments were amplified from the sample containing 10 cells. The results were confirmed by Southern blot analysis (right panel).

subunits involved in a wide range of physiological responses. For example, we used the combined patch-clamp recording and single-cell RT-PCR approach to investigate whether overexpression of Bcl-2 affects voltage-gated K^+ (Kv) channel activity and which Kv channel subunits are affected by Bcl-2 in PASMCs (26,27).

The Bcl-2 protein superfamily has members that exert contrasting effects on apoptosis (28). One Bcl-2 family member also called Bcl-2 is an oncoprotein that acts as a suppressor of programmed cell death (28,29). To examine whether overexpression of Bcl-2 inhibits apoptosis in PASMCs by diminishing the activity of Kv channels, a human *bcl-2* gene was transfected into a primary cultured rat PASMC using an adenoviral vector. The effects of overexpression of *bcl-2* on Kv channel activity and expression were examined by recording Kv currents and determining mRNA expression of different Kv channel subunits in the same cell (26).

Whole-cell Kv currents ($I_{K(V)}$) were recorded in physiological $[K^+]$ (140 mM in the pipette; 5.4 mM in the bath) and nominally Ca^{2+} -free conditions (EGTA-buffered) to minimize the activity of Ca^{2+}-permeable

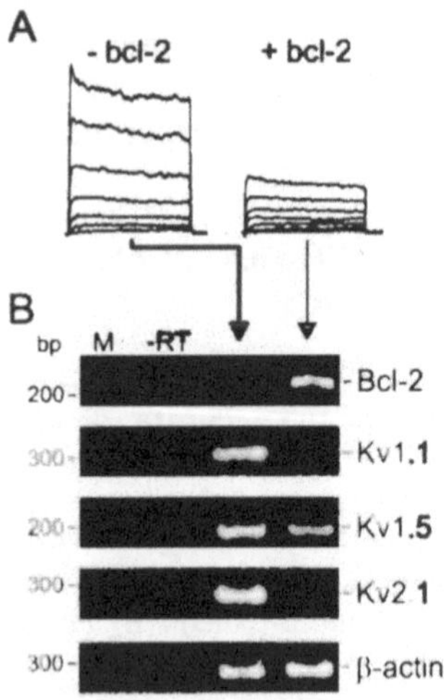

Figure 3 Overexpression of Bcl-2 downregulates Kv channel α subunits and reduces the amplitude of Kv currents in isolated rat PASMCs. (A) Representative whole-cell I_{Kv}, elicited by test potentials ranging from −40 to +80 mV, in a control cell (− *bcl-2*) and a *bcl-2*-infected cell (+ *bcl-2*). (B) Single-cell RT-PCR amplified products for the human Bcl-2 (267 bp) as well as rat Kv1.1 (298 bp), Kv1.5 (196 bp), Kv2.1 (269 bp), and β-actin (244 bp) transcripts in the control cell (−*bcl-2*; adenoviral vector without *bcl-2* gene) and the *bcl-2*-infected cell (+ *bcl-2*). M, molecular weight marker. -RT, RT performed in the absence of reverse transcriptase (i.e., cDNA alone). (Reproduced with permission from Ref. 26.)

and Ca^{2+}-sensitive channels (Fig. 3A). $I_{K(V)}$ was significantly decreased in *bcl-2*-transfected cells compared to cells infected with the empty vector. RT-PCR was then performed in the same cell from which $I_{K(V)}$ was recorded to determine the mRNA expression of Kv1.1, Kv1.5, Kv2.1, and Bcl-2. As expected, the mRNA level of Bcl-2 in the *bcl-2*-infected cell was much greater than in the control cell. Conversely, the mRNA levels of Kv1.1, Kv1.5, and Kv2.1 α subunits were significantly decreased in the *bcl-2*-infected cell in comparison to the control cell infected with an empty vector. The mRNA level of β-actin in the control cell was similar to that in the *bcl-2*-infected cells. These results provide compelling evidence that overexpression of Bcl-2 decreases $I_{K(V)}$ by downregulating the mRNA expression of the pore-forming Kv channel α subunits (Kv1.1, Kv1.5, and Kv2.1) in rat PASMCs.

IV. SUMMARY

A fundamental challenge in biology is to correlate physiological function with gene expression. This can be achieved only by understanding gene expression at the level of the single cell (30). The use of electrophysiological recordings coupled with single-cell RT-PCR techniques can provide valuable information to help us identify possible correlations between ion channel function and expression and to define the modulatory mechanisms of ion channels in an isolated cell.

ACKNOWLEDGMENTS

This work was supported by grants from the National Heart, Lung, and Blood Institute of the National Institutes of Health (HL 64945, HL 54043, HL 66012, HL 69758, HL 66941). Dr. Ying Yu was supported by a fellowship from the Pulmonary Hypertension Association. We thank Dr. Ando Kiyoshi, Tokai University School of Medicine, Japan for providing technical guidance.

REFERENCES

1. Hille B. Ion Channels of Excitable Membranes. 3rd Ed., Sunderland MA: Sinauer 2001.
2. Sakmann B, Neher E. Single-Channel Recording. Vol. 1, 2nd Ed., New York: Plenum Press, 1995.
3. Boulton AA, Baker GB, Walz W. Patch-Clamp Applications and Protocols. Neuromethods, Vol. 26. Totowa, NJ: Humana Press, 1995.
4. Davis LG, Kuehl WM, Battey JF. Basic Methods in Molecular Biology, 2nd Ed. Norwalk, CT: Appleton & Lange, 1994.

5. Siebert PD, Larrick JW. Gene cloning and analysis by RT-PCR. BioTechniques Mol Lab Methods Ser 1. Natick, MA: BioTechniques Books, 1998:14:350.
6. Sucher NJ, Deitcher DL. PCR and patch-clamp analysis of single neurons. Neuron 1995; 14:1095–1100.
7. Sucher NJ, Deitcher DL, Baro DJ, Warrick RM, Guenther E. Genes and channels: patch/voltage-clamp analysis and single-cell RT-PCR. Cell Tissue Res 2000; 302:295–307.
8. Gurantz D, Lautermilch NJ, Watt SD, Spitzer NC. Sustained upregulation in embryonic spinal neurons of a Kv3.1 potassium channel gene encoding a delayed rectifier current. J Neurobiol 2000; 42:347–356.
9. Baro DJ, Harris-Warrick RM. Differential expression and targeting of K^+ channel genes in the lobster pyloric central pattern generator. Ann NY Acad Sci 1998; 860:281–295.
10. Massengill JL, Smith MA, Son DI, O'Dowd DK. Differential expression of K_{4-AP} currents and Kv3.1 potassium channel transcripts in cortical neurons that develop distinct firing phenotypes. J Neurosci 1997; 17:3136–3147.
11. Martina M, Schultz JH, Ehmke H, Monyer H, Jonas P. Functional and molecular differences between voltage-gated K^+ channels of fast-spiking interneurons and pyramidal neurons of rat hippocampus. J Neurosci 1998; 18: 8111–8125.
12. Lien CC, Martina M, Schultz JH, Ehmke H, Jonas P. Gating, modulation and subunit composition of voltage-gated K^+ channels in dendritic inhibitory interneurones of rat hippocampus. J Physiol 2002; 538:405–419.
13. Song WJ. Genes responsible for native depolarization-activated K^+ currents in neurons. Neurosci Res 2002; 42:7–14.
14. Comer AM, Gibbons HM, Qi J, Kawai Y, Win J, Lipski J. Detection of mRNA species in bulbospinal neurons isolated from the rostral ventrolateral medulla using single-cell RT-PCR. Brain Res Brain Res Protoc 1999; 4: 367–377.
15. Wang X, Stollar BD. Human immunoglobulin variable region gene analysis by single cell RT-PCR. J Immunol Methods 2000; 244:217–225.
16. O'Connell J. RT-PCR PROTOCOLS. Totowa, NJ: Humana Press, 2002.
17. Johansen FF, Lambolez B, Audinat E, Bochet P, Rossier J. Single cell RT-PCR proceeds without the risk of genomic DNA amplification. Neurochem Int 1995; 26:239–243.
18. Lambolez B, Audinat E, Bochet P, Crepel F, Rossier J. AMPA receptor subunits expressed by single Purkinje cells. Neuron 1992; 9:247–258.
19. Bochet P, Audinat E, Lambolez B, Crepel F, Rossier J, Iino M, Tsuzuki K, Ozawa S. Subunit composition at the single-cell level explains functional properties of a glutamate-gated channel. Neuron 1994; 12:383–388.
20. Jonas P, Racca C, Sakmann B, Seeburg PH, Monyer H. Differences in Ca^{2+} permeability of AMPA-type glutamate receptor channels in neocortical neurons caused by differential GluR-B subunit expression. Neuron 1994; 12: 1281–1289.
21. Deitcher DL, Fekete DM, Cepko CL. Asymmetric expression of a novel homeobox gene in vertebrate sensory organs. J Neurosci 1994; 14:486–498.

22. Lee K, Dixon AK, Gonzalez I, Stevens EB, McNulty S, Oles R, Richardson PJ, Pinnock RD, Singh L. Bombesin-like peptides depolarize rat hippocampal interneurones through interaction with subtype 2 bombesin receptors. J Physiol 1999; 518:791–802.
23. Dixon AK, Richardson PJ, Pinnock RD, Lee K. Gene-expression analysis at the single-cell level. Trends Pharmacol Sci 2000; 21:65–70.
24. Dieffenbach CW, Dveksler GS. Setting up a PCR laboratory. PCR Methods Appl 1993; 3:S2–S7.
25. Dieffenbach CW, Lowe TM, Dveksler GS. General concepts for PCR primer design. PCR Methods Appl 1993; 3:S30–S37.
26. Ekhterae D, Platoshyn O, Krick S, Yu Y, McDaniel SS, Yuan JX-J. Bcl-2 decreases voltage-gated K^+ channel activity and enhances survival in vascular smooth muscle cells. Am J Physiol Cell Physiol 2001; 281:C157–C165.
27. Yu Y, Platoshyn O, Zhang J, Krick S, Zhao Y, Rubin LJ, Rothman A, Yuan JX-J. c-Jun decreases voltage-gated K^+ channel activity in pulmonary artery smooth muscle cells. Circulation 2001; 104:1557–1563.
28. Strasser A, O'Connor L, Dixit VM. Apoptosis signaling. Annu Rev Biochem 2000; 69:217–245.
29. Adams JM, Cory S. The Bcl-2 protein family: arbiters of cell survival. Science 1998; 281:1322–1326.
30. Dixon AK, Lee K, Richardson PJ, Bell MI, Skynner MJ. Single cell expression analysis—pharmacogenomic potential. Pharmacogenomics 2002; 3:809–822.

33

Ion Channel Trafficking

Steve H. Keller, Bethany H. Parker, and Jason X.-J. Yuan
Department of Medicine, University of California, San Diego, California, U.S.A.

I. INTRODUCTION

A. Ion Channel Biogenesis

Ion channels are complexly folded and assembled multipass transmembrane proteins that undergo biogenesis in the endoplasmic reticulum (ER) and traffic through the secretory pathway to the cell surface (1–3). Folding and assembly of the domains and subunits of ion channels take place in the ER and involve addition of disulfide bonds and conjugation of oligosaccharides that ultimately influence the correct conformation required to maintain the physical characteristics of the ion channel (4,5). Assembly of accessory subunits and modifications such as glycosylation, myristylation, and phosphorylation further modify the polypeptide backbone conformation and influence the activation and opening and closing characteristics of the channel. A cellular "quality control" is involved in detecting whether the ion channel is appropriately folded and assembled in the ER and is thought to operate by detecting exposed sequence and structural features in the protein (6). As the channel folds and assembles, these structural features are sterically occluded, buried within the polypeptide chains of the channel, and are no longer exposed to the cellular machinery that is involved in sequestering the channel in the ER (6–9). Forward directing targeting signals also appear to be present in ion channels and might– become exposed and accessible to the forward-targeting machinery when the channel is fully folded and assembled (10,11). Presumably, as the channel folds and assembles, the signals involved in sequestering are buried and those involved in forward targeting become exposed to the trafficking machinery that directs proteins upstream in the secretory pathway (12,13).

The procession in the secretory pathway can be thought of as a balance between the retrieval of incompletely folded and unassembled proteins and the forward progression of maturely folded and assembled proteins. The quality control mechanisms therefore attenuate the chance of misfolded or unassembled ion channels reaching the cell surface, where they might perform dysregulated and deleterious physiological roles. Misfolded, partially assembled, and unassembled subunits of an ion channel can be shuttled into a degradative pathway leading from the ER to the proteasome (discussed below) (14,15). These mechanisms therefore assist in directing fully operational ion channels to the cell surface where regulated and coordinated action is important.

B. Trafficking Beyond the Endoplasmic Reticulum

In addition to ER quality control, relatively uncharacterized mechanisms located upstream of the ER, and positioned at the Golgi apparatus, trans-Golgi network (TGN), and cell surface also detect the folding and assembly state of the channel and serve as further checkpoints that modulate the surface expression (16,17). For example, the cystic fibrosis transmembrane regulator (ΔF508 CFTR), the mutant chloride channel involved in cystic fibrosis, can be brought to the cell surface by reducing temperature or adding glycerol to the cell culture medium (18,19). However, at the cell surface ΔF508 CFTR is subjected to a significantly elevated rate of internalization and targeting into a degradative pathway relative to wild-type CFTR (18). Both lysosomal and proteasomal targeting can occur from the cell surface, providing an upstream quality control pathway as a further point of interception of a misfolded channel (20).

C. Targeting into a Degradative Pathway

Targeting into degradative pathways leading to the proteasome or lysosome is an opposing trafficking pathway that directs proteins away from the cell surface. In the ER, transmembrane proteins can be tagged with ubiquitin in their cytoplasmic loops and tails and then processed through a reverse translocation route out of the ER into the cytoplasm, where they are degraded in the proteasome (21). This process has been characterized for CFTR and other ion channel proteins (22). Although the details of why proteins are targeted into this degradative route when residing in the ER are poorly understood, it is thought that chaperone and heat shock protein recognition and the binding of scaffold proteins involved in recruiting the ubiquitin conjugating machinery recognize exposed hydrophobic patches or structures that initiate the process of degradative targeting. For an ion channel protein, expressed following transfection it appears that most of the synthesized nascent chain is targeted into the ubiquitin–proteasome pathway and degraded in the proteasome, as opposed to being expressed at the cell surface (22). Only a relatively small fraction of the nascent chain actually makes it to the cell surface as a functional ion channel.

Upstream of the ER, transmembrane proteins embedded in lipid vesicles can be targeted into additional degradative pathways involving trafficking from endosomes to the lysosomes. The lipid vesicles fuse with the assistance of an elaborate membrane fusion machinery, eventually leading to fusion with the lysosome. Multiple lysosomal hydrolases are then involved in degrading the protein. Several amino acid sequences have been identified that are involved in targeting proteins to lysosomal hydrolysis, such as the tyrosine-based and dileucine-based motifs (23). Presumably, these targeting signals become exposed in misfolded proteins, which are then targeted into this pathway. Proteasomal degradation of transmembrane proteins also appears to occur upstream of the ER, although the lysosome is believed to be the primary organelle involved in degradation that ultimately modulates the surface expression of the ion channel beyond the ER (24). Thus, the cell-surface expression of an ion channel is modulated by multiple points of interception and by independent mechanisms that operate at separate compartments of the secretory pathway. The last quantitative ion channel protein that finally makes it to the cell surface has proceeded through all of these checkpoints of the quality control machinery and thus consists of a small fraction of the original nascent protein that was synthesized.

D. Synthesis, Threading in the ER Membrane, Chain Elongation, and Membrane Topology

Synthesis of polytypic transmembrane proteins such as ion channels includes chain elongation in the rough endoplasmic reticulum and threading through the ER membrane to construct multiple loops and transmembrane domains (Fig. 1). Concomitant with chain elongation, ion channel proteins acquire disulfide bonds and carbohydrate chains and fold and assemble into the configuration that eventually constitutes the mature channel. ER and cytosolic chaperone proteins appear to assist in the biogenesis process, primarily by protecting subunits from degradation prior to assembly (25–28). ER-embedded proteins are subjected to degradative pathways that are mediated by the ubiquitin–proteasome pathway while they are still located in the ER membrane (Fig. 2) and also by degradative pathways located upstream in the secretory pathway (18,22).

E. The Secretory Pathway

When appropriately folded and assembled, the transmembrane protein traffics to the medial-trans-Golgi compartment and undergoes further

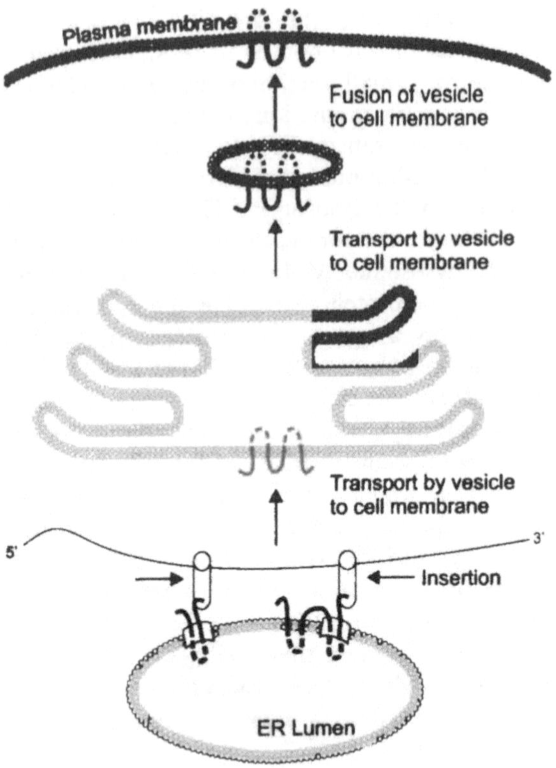

Figure 1 Elongation and membrane topology of a polytypic transmembrane protein. As the polypeptide chain is threaded through the ER, loops extending into the ER lumen and cytoplasmic domains are developed. The lumenal domains maintain the same topology in the Golgi and the budding vesicles but become inverted at the cell surface. Luminal domains then become extracellular at the cell surface.

modifications that include sialylation and complex oligosaccharide conjugation (Fig. 3). Ion channel proteins are embedded with an inside-out topology in lipid vesicles that bud and fuse with compartments of the secretory pathway in a pathway leading to the cell surface (Fig. 4). The lipid vesicles are carried along microtubules and molecular motors as they proceed in the trafficking route. The cell-surface expression of an ion channel can be modulated further by endocytosis or redirected into a degradative pathway leading to the lysosomes. Various techniques are available that enable detection of a protein at individual compartments of the secretory pathway, including multiple labeling and confocal microscopy using cellular markers for the compartments, and separately by cell fractionation protocols.

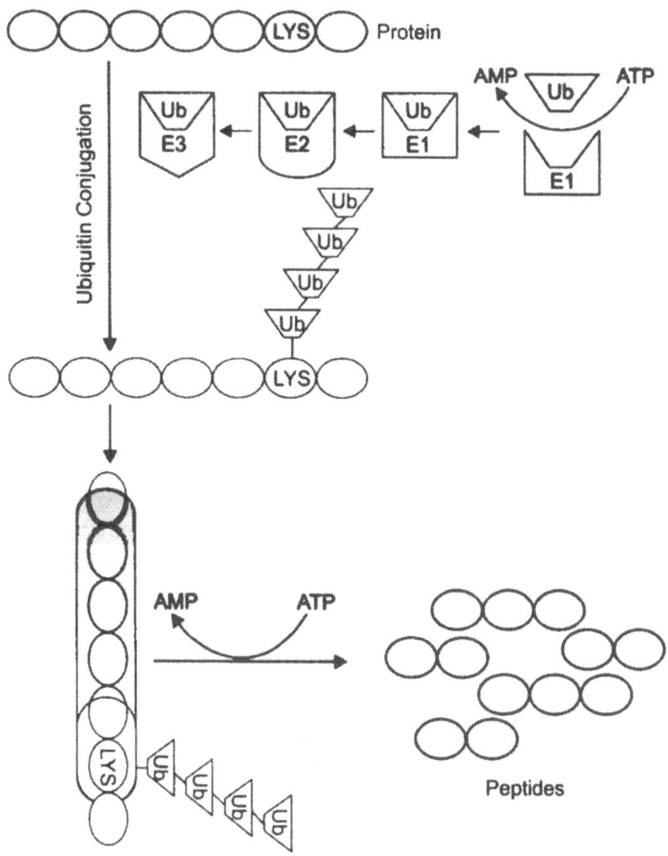

Figure 2 Ubiquitin–proteasome degradation pathway. Degradation by the ubiquitin–proteasome pathway is a major targeting route that ultimately influences the cell-surface expression of an ion channel. Degradation of ion channels in this pathway is best characterized when the channel is embedded in the ER and loops and C- and N-terminal tails extend into the cytoplasm. Proteins embedded in the ER membrane are susceptible to ubiquitin (Ub) tagging at lysine residues with the assistance of a three-enzyme system complex (E1, ubiquitin-activating enzyme; E2, ubiquitin-conjugating enzyme; E3, ubiquitin ligase). Once tagged, the transmembrane protein is thought to undergo retrotranslocation through a translocon pore and to be shuttled to the proteasome for hydrolysis into smaller peptides.

Several diseases associated with mutations in genes encoding ion channels and their associated trafficking deficits have been identified and characterized, with cystic fibrosis being the best known of these. Other well-known ion channel abnormalities associated with mutations in the channels include long QT syndrome associated with mutations in sodium and potassium

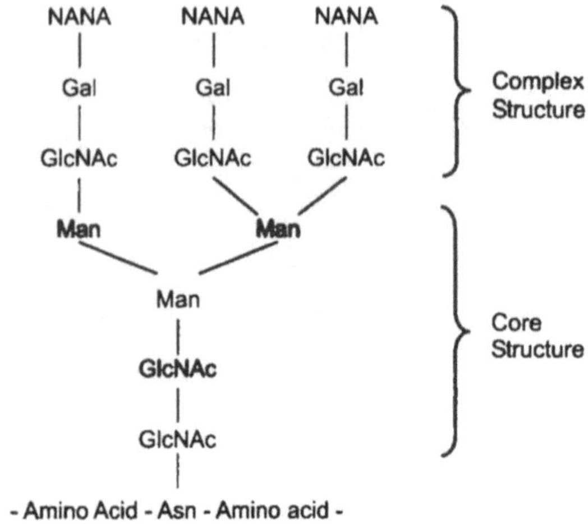

Figure 3 Complex oligosaccharide structure. Oligosaccharide structures linked to asparagines (Asn), coined N-linked oligosaccharides, consist of a core structure that is a result of conjugation of a larger structure consisting of two *N*-acetylglucosamines (GlcNac), nine mannose (Man) residues, and three glucoses. Trimming occurs in the ER, eliminating the glucose residues and one of the mannoses. This results in a core-glycosylated high–mannose structure found in the ER that is susceptible to endo-H cleavage. When the glycoprotein proceeds from the ER to the Golgi, it is trimmed further, with three more mannose residues subsequently removed. This structure then becomes substituted with additional monosaccharides, potentially including, but limited to, GlcNac, galactose (Gal), and *N*-acetylneuraminic acid (NANA; same as sialic acid). The complex oligosaccharide structure is generally greater in molecular weight than the core-glycosylated structure and is resistant to endo-H cleavage. Larger size and resistance to endo-H cleavage can serve as an indicator for trafficking to the Golgi.

channels (29–31), forms of epilepsy associated with mutations in potassium channels (9), and rare forms of myasthenia gravis, correlated with mutations in the acetylcholine receptor, for example (32).

F. Cystic Fibrosis Is the Most Commonly Inherited Disorder Associated with a Trafficking-Impaired Channel

Cystic fibrosis is the most commonly inherited autosomal disorder afflicting the newborn. Approximately 1 out of 29 individuals is a carrier of cystic fibrosis alleles and approximately 1 out of 2500 exhibits symptoms of the disease (33). The severity of cystic fibrosis is manifested primarily in the lung, although other organs are also targeted (33). Individuals afflicted with cystic fibrosis develop airway infection, inflammation, and obstruction that increase morbidity and mortality. A major component of the

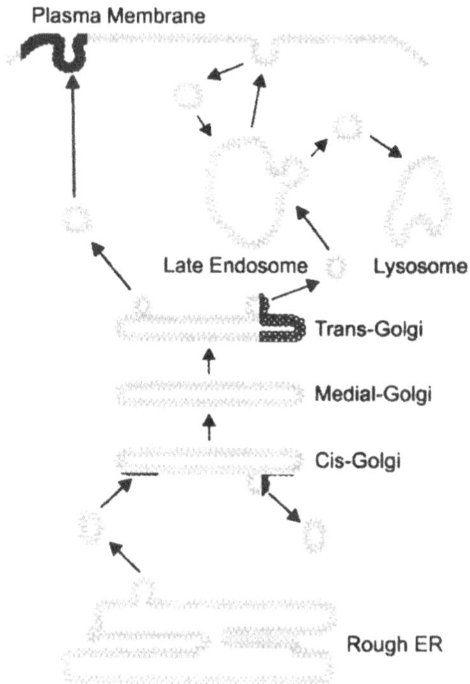

Figure 4 Secretory pathway. Transmembrane proteins synthesized and threaded in the rough ER incorporate in budding vesicles that traffic from the ER to the Golgi and then to the cell surface. Retrieval pathways are also manifested that bring proteins from the cis-Golgi back to the ER. A cellular quality control machinery is thought to operate by retrieving misfolded or unassembled proteins back into this pathway. The process of endocytosis internalizes transmembrane proteins and targets these proteins to endosomes and then to lysosomes. Ubiquitin tagging of transmembrane proteins at the cell surface can also send proteins into a degradative route to the lysosomes.

morbidity and mortality appears be due to inflammation and airway obstruction (33). Individuals expressing the ΔF508 CFTR allele are also more subject to bacterial infection, a major contributor to illness in the disease. Cystic fibrosis is associated with mutations in the chloride channel CFTR, a member of the ABC transported family, with the most prevalent mutation being an in-frame deletion of a phenylalanine residue at position 508 (designated as ΔF508 CFTR) (34). The etiological basis connecting the expression of the ΔF508 allele and cystic fibrosis is not understood, although numerous theories have been proposed that are supported, in part, by some experimental evidence. Reviews of this topic include Refs. 11 and 33–35.

ΔF508 CFTR is a misfolded channel with attenuated activation relative to wild-type CFTR (36,37). Approximately 95% of nascent ΔF508 CFTR channels fail to traffic to the cell surface in transfected cells, indicating that ΔF508 CFTR is trafficking-deficient. Individuals harboring this mutation with gene copies express reduced amounts of functional CFTR chloride channel in their epithelium (33). Lack of cell-surface expression of mutant CFTR was first discovered by electrophysiological methods and later characterized biochemically after the CFTR gene was identified, cloned, and sequenced. In transfected cells, ΔF508 CFTR fails to develop an upper complex glycosylated band owing to its confinement in the ER (38). Furthermore, in confocal microscopic images of transfected cells, a surface stain is evident in cells expressing wild-type CFTR but not ΔF508 CFTR (Fig. 5), suggesting that mutant CFTR is trafficking-deficient. As with a lack of understanding of the physiological bases of the disease, it is unclear why ΔF508 fails to traffic, although numerous hypotheses have been proposed and extensive experimental studies have taken place. Some of the hypotheses include interception by chaperones and heat shock proteins acting to confine the channel in the ER, aggregation preventing trafficking, enhanced degradation, ER calcium levels, and abnormal exposure of trafficking signals (39). Several of these factors are likely to act together in interfering with the surface expression of CFTR.

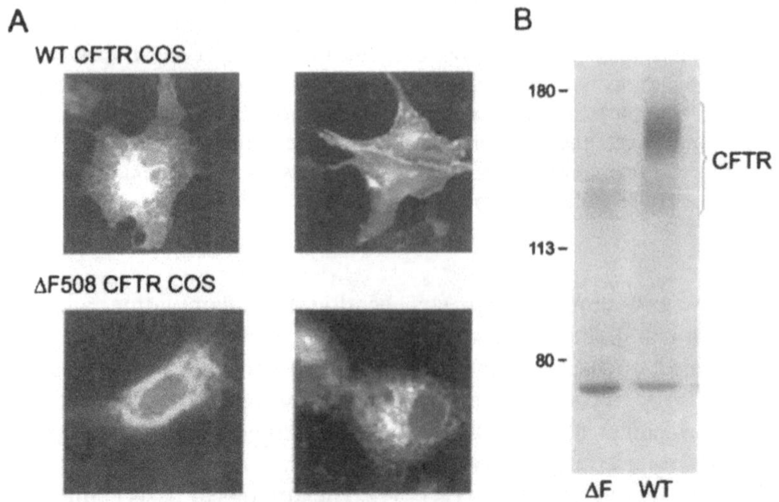

Figure 5 Wild-type and ΔF508 CFTR displayed in confocal immunofluorescent pictures (A) and on Western blot (B). Plasmids encoding wild-type (WT) and ΔF508 CFTR were transfected in HEK-293 cells that were processed for immunofluorescent microscopy or Western blotting, as detailed in this chapter.

II. METHODS TO STUDY ION CHANNEL TRAFFICKING

A. Trafficking from the ER to the Golgi, Detected by Complex Oligosaccharide Conjugation

The peptide chains of transmembrane proteins are threaded in the ER membrane through ribosomes associated with pores in the ER membrane. The peptide segments that that are located within the ER lumen have oligosaccharide conjugation sites. If sterically accessible to the oligosaccharde conjugation machinery, the sequence Asn-X-Ser/Thr becomes conjugated with oligosaccharide structures that are trimmed to produce the high-mannose configuration (Fig. 3). These oligosaccharides are categorized as N-linked oligosaccharides because they are conjugated to asparagine in the lumen of the ER and are distinguished from O-linked oligosaccharides that are conjugated to serine or threonine in the Golgi. Because N-linked oligosaccharide conjugation occurs in the lumen of the ER, N-linked oligosaccharides are positioned in the extracellular domain of the mature cell-suface glycoprotein.

As the transmembrane glycoprotein proceeds from the ER to the Golgi, domains that become extracellular are located within the lumen of the Golgi (Fig. 4). In the medial- and trans-Golgi, further monosaccharide addition occurs, producing a fairly large and complex oligosaccharide structure (Fig. 3) that can usually be detected by an increased mobility in gels. Often, glycoproteins that have proceeded to the Golgi resolve as doublets in gels that display a lower molecular weight band corresponding to the core-glycosylated form and an upper band corresponding to the glycoprotein that has proceeded to the Golgi and contains complex glycosylation. CFTR expressed in transfected cells is a notable example of this, as displayed in Fig 5. The mutant ΔF508 CFTR expressed by transfection in HEK cells shows only the core-glycosylated band, whereas wild-type CFTR reveals a doublet, with the upper band corresponding to the complex glycoform that proceeds to the Golgi (Fig. 5).

B. Detecting Trafficking to the Golgi by Endo-H/PNGase-F Cleavage

Glycosidase enzymes, such as endo-H, can be used to distinguish whether core or complex glycosylated structures are attached to the glycoprotein and can be employed to detect trafficking upstream of the ER. Endo-H cleaves high-mannose N-linked oligosaccharide structures conjugated to glycoproteins in the ER, but complex structures conjugated in the Golgi are resistant to this enzyme. Resistance to endo-H cleavage can therefore be employed as a tool to determine whether a glycoprotein has proceeded to the Golgi from the ER. PNGase-F cleaves N-linked oligosaccharides irrespective of substitution, and observing this cleavage demonstrates that an oligosaccharide resistant to endo-H is, in fact, conjugated to the glycoprotein.

For glycosidase cleavages, cells are lysed in a detergent buffer compatible with the glycosidase enzymes. A Triton-containing buffer is often suitable for this. A denaturing buffer is often also employed to unfold the protein chain and increase the accessibility of the oligosaccharides to cleavage. Cleavage is allowed to proceed at the temperature appropriate for the enzyme. The samples are then aliquoted and processed for SDS-PAGE. Samples with and without enzyme application are resolved in neighboring lanes in gels, and the proteins of interest are detected by either protein stain or Western blot. Susceptibility to enzyme cleavage is revealed by a downshifted protein band in the gel. Often the smeary appearance of a glycoprotein band is narrow and better defined by the glycosidase cleavages owing to the removal of attached oligosaccharides of heterogeneous size. Glycoproteins with N-linked oligosaccharides can be purchased as positive controls for glycosidase cleavage and cleaved and resolved in gels together with the protein of interest to verify the activity of the glycosidase reactions. A glycoprotein that is resistant to endo-H cleavage but susceptible to PNGase-F has conjugated complex oligosaccharides, indicating trafficking to the Golgi.

C. Microscopic Techniques

High-resolution microscopic techniques enable the detection of proteins located in compartments of the secretory pathway and allow for examination of the trafficking characteristics of an ion channel. Two techniques commonly employed to examine protein trafficking characteristics include confocal immunofluorescent microscopy and immunogold-EM microscopy. In confocal microscopy, a protein of interest can be detected either by epitope tag or by antibody. The antibody is added to permeabilized cells to recognize an internal epitope or to nonpermeabilized cells if it is directed to an extracellular epitope. A fluorophore-conjugated antibody, often used as a secondary antibody, is employed for fluorescence detection.

In immunogold labeling, the protein of interest is labeled with gold particles conjugated to an antibody. A primary antibody directed to the protein of interest can be incubated first with the samples, followed by addition of secondary antibody conjugated with gold particles. The cells are grown on a grid appropriate for EM microscopy, which then images the structures. The EM microscopic image reveals the cellular compartments, and the immunogold label is then used to identify the protein of interest (40–42). A more detailed discussion of these techniques is provided below.

D. Confocal Microscopy

Laser scanning confocal microscopy is a widely employed and valuable tool to examine the trafficking characteristics of a protein because it enables identification of specific cellular compartments of the secretory pathway (2,43,44). Cellular compartments such as ER, Golgi, TGN, lysosomes, endosomes, cytosol, and the cell surface are readily identified by this technique. Confocal microscopy has the ability to locate objects in a restricted three-dimensional space of a sample and can detect up to three separately labeled proteins or objects within the focal plane of the image. Overlap in the three-dimensional field is then determined by observing color mixes, such as the overlap of red and green fluorescence that produces a yellow coloration.

To follow ion channel trafficking, the gene encoding the channel of interest can be epitope-tagged with GFP and transfected into culture cells. Alternatively, native channels can be identified with specific antibodies. Generally, cells are fixed in paraformaldehyde or methanol and then permeabilized prior to antibody exposure. Cellular compartments can be identified by employing antibodies specific to proteins confined to these compartments. For example, the endoplasmic reticulum can be identified by exposing cells to an antibody that recognizes the ER-resident protein calnexin (8,45). Cells can also be loaded with fluorescent dyes and other molecules that accumulate in a specific compartment such as "lysotracker" or "mitotracker" (46,47). The primary antibody is then detected with a secondary antibody conjugated to a fluorophore such as FITC or rhodamine.

When planning multiple labeling, it should be kept in mind that each protein will be labeled with a separate fluorophore. Thus, if two proteins are labeled by antibodies, each primary antibody must be derived from a separate host so that distinct secondary antibodies can be employed for detection. For antibody labeling, first, permeabilized cells are exposed to a primary antibody, then a secondary antibody is conjugated with the fluorophore. Dyes emiting three distinct wavelengths can be employed to detect protein inside the cells. After completion of the staining procedure, an antifade preservative such as gelvatol is added to the cover slip, and the slide is stored in the dark. The sample is then ready for confocal microscopic imaging.

E. Labeling of Cell-Surface Proteins in Intact Cells

Antibodies recognizing epitopes in extracellular domains and lectins are also available to label proteins residing on the cell surface. Fluorescent microscopic imaging can then be employed to detect these reagents. In these techniques, cells are fixed and nonspecific binding sites are blocked with a nonspecific protein-containing buffer that lacks a permeabilizing detergent. The antibody is then incubated with the cells, followed by washes and exposure to the secondary antibody conjugated to a fluorophore. Limitations of this technique mainly concern nonspecific binding and fluorescence emission. An appropriate control to distinguish nonspecific from specific fluorescence displaying the correct epitope exposes cells to a nonspecific IgG antibody as a substitute for the primary antibody. Using a confocal microscope, the stain of cell-surface proteins should show a circular halo around the exterior of the cell (48).

F. Cell-Surface Biotinylation

Lysines, diols on carbohydrates, and cysteine residues positioned in extracellular domains can be tagged with reactive derivatives of biotin to examine whether proteins are expressed at the cell surface (Fig. 6) (48,49).

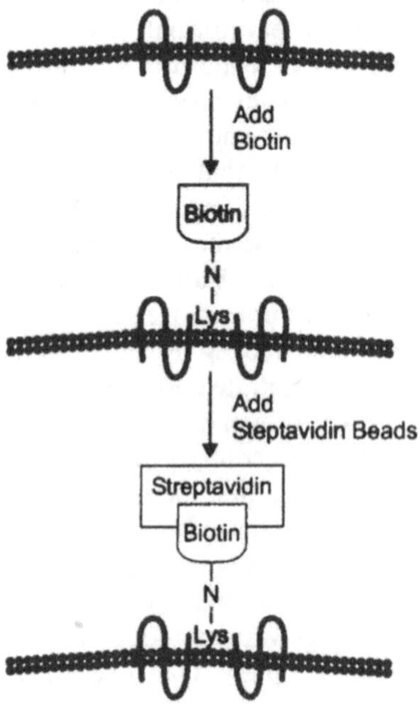

Figure 6 Tagging of cell-surface proteins with biotin. Extracellular domains of proteins can be labeled with biotin derivatives to demonstrate the surface expression and characterize the inside-out transmembrane topology of an ion channel protein. Because ion channels typically have a multitransmembrane-spanning configuration, extracellular domains and loops are available for labeling. The biotin moiety is linked to a reactive ester group that reacts with primary amines, attaching biotin to the extracellular domain of the protein of interest. The cell membrane is solubilized with a detergent buffer, releasing biotinylated proteins into the mixture. Streptavidin-linked beads are then added and employed as a solid support to concentrate and pull down the biotinylated proteins. Samples are resolved in SDS-PAGE gels, which are transferred with nitrocellulose for Western blotting. The protein of interest is then identified in the biotinylated fraction by immunoblotting.

Derivatized biotin does not traverse through the cell membrane, allowing only for surface tagging at the reactive structural feature of the cell-surface protein. The biotin technique can be detected either by developing nitrocellulose membranes with a secondary antibody conjugated with streptavidin or by binding directly to streptavidin, which is covalently linked to a resin.

Conjugation of extracellular lysines with biotin linked to a reactive ester is the most commonly employed technique to biotinylate ion channel proteins. In this technique, cells are prewashed in a PBS buffer adjusted to pH 8.0. The reagent sulfo-NHS-biotin is added to the cells for approximately 1 h with gentle shaking to prevent breakage of cells. A buffer without primary amines is employed for this reaction. The cells are then washed, and the reaction is quenched with a buffer containing free primary amines or a surplus of nonspecific protein such as BSA. After quenching, the cells are lysed in a detergent buffer. The biotinylated proteins can be resolved in gels and transferred to nitrocellulose. Immunoblotting is then employed to detect the protein of interest.

A common complication with these approaches is that the cells can inadvertently be lysed and lysine residues positioned in cytoplasmic domains can become tagged. To examine whether there is accidental cell breakage prior to quenching of the biotinylation reaction, Western blots of the biotinylated streptavidin-bound fraction can also be developed with an antibody to a protein confined to the inside of the cell, such as the ER-resident protein calnexin.

G. Fluorescence Recovery After Photobleaching (FRAP)

Movement of nascent protein into a compartment of the trafficking pathway can also be examined by photobleaching the light emission of a GFP-tagged protein and examining whether the tagged protein remigrates into this location by the appearance of new fluorescence (43,50,51). Usually, a GFP epitope-tagged protein is expressed by transfection and is allowed to traffic to and accumulate in the cell. GFP can be photobleached with intense localized light, removing fluorescence emission at a specific cellular location. This region thus becomes dark in the fluorescent microscopic image. The intense light beam is removed, and the cell is then allowed to recover from photobleaching. Nascent GFP-labeled protein then migrates into the photobleached cellular location, which can be visualized in a fluorescence microscope, potentially providing insight into the trafficking route. In living cells, the rate of reappearance of fluorescence corresponds to the rate trafficking into this region and can be used to estimate the trafficking kinetics.

H. Methods to Investigate Protein Ubiquitinylation and Proteasomal Hydrolysis

Degradation of ion channels in the ubiquitin–proteasome pathway is generally detected by examining whether degradation rates are attenuated when proteasome inhibitors are added to cells (22,24,52). Conjugation of polyubiquitin can also be detected by adding proteasomal inhibitors to cells and identifying a high molecular weight ladder pattern indicative of heterogeneous polyubiquitin chains attached to proteins (22,27). Commonly employed proteasome inhibitors used for this purpose include lactacystin, MG-132, and ALLN. Lactacystin is thought to be the most specific for proteasomal hydrolysis (22), whereas the other inhibitors may also inhibit nonproteasomal proteases.

Generally, cell-permeable inhibitors or inhibitors solubilized in DMSO are added to cells and the degradation rate of the protein of interest is examined, often by quantifying the kinetics of disappearance after pulse labeling. The protein of interest is immunoprecipitated, resolved in gels, and exposed to film. Gel bands are scanned, densities quantified, and the disappearance rate compared to cells not treated with proteasome inhibitors.

I. Subcellular Fractionation Markers

Because of the general availability of confocal microscopes, subcellular fractionation techniques using sucrose gradient ultracentrifugation to isolate proteins in compartments of the secretory pathway are not currently employed as extensively as they once were. Subcellular fractionation requires a much larger input of labor than confocal microscopy and is thus a less desirable approach to examine the trafficking characteristics. We include a brief description of this technique here for completeness.

In this technique, cells are sonicated in buffer without detergent, large debris is removed, and the sonicate, which contains subcellular organelles and cytoplasm, is placed on top of a tube preloaded with a sucrose gradient. The sucrose gradient is generated with a gradient maker, placing denser sucrose at the bottom of the tube. Samples are applied to the top of the centrifuge tube, and the components are sedimented by ultracentrifugation. After centrifugation, a hole is punched in the bottom of the tube and fractions are collected using devices designed for this purpose. The fractions are then analyzed to identify markers for cellular compartments and to locate the protein of interest among the fractionated samples.

J. Trafficking Kinetics

The rate of progression from the ER to the Golgi, or the kinetics of endocytosis, can be measured by metabolic labeling and pulse-chase techniques (18,53). For measurements of the kinetics of ER-to-Golgi trafficking, the rate of appearance of the more substituted complex oligosaccharide band can be employed to estimate the trafficking kinetics. Cells are subjected to a pulse chase as the start point and lysed at specific time points to solubilize and remove proteins from the membrane; then the proteins are immunoprecipitated. Samples are resolved in consecutive lanes in gels that are exposed to film. The densities of the gel bands corresponding to the protein of interest are quantified and plotted relative to the initiation of the chase. Particular emphasis is given to the locations of the core glycosylated and complex glycosylated bands of the protein of interest. The resulting plots therefore reveal the rate of appearance of the complex glycosylated band, which corresponds to the trafficking rate to the Golgi.

Alternatively, samples can be subjected to endo-H cleavage to resolve the glycoproteins conjugated with complex oligosaccharides relative to those conjugated with the core-glycosylated oligosaccharides. The complex-glycosylated bands should not show mobility changes following endo-H cleavage. After exposure to enzyme cleavage, the proteins are immunoprecipitated, resolved in gels, and characterized and quantified in the manner described above.

K. Brief Outline to Study Whether a Mutant Ion Channel is Trafficking-Deficient

Cell transfection provides an effective means to identify the trafficking characteristics of a mutant ion channel protein. The cDNA encoding the channel can be subcloned into an expression vector with a high-yield promoter. This expression vector with the cDNA inserts encoding the channel can be transfected into culture cells, with the assumption that the channel in the culture cell model retains the properties of the channel expressed endogenously in native cells. Although ion channels endogenously expressed in cells can also be employed to study trafficking by methods similar to those described below, cell transfection provides for higher expression yields, which facilitates biochemical detection. (One possible shortcoming of the use of transfection is that overexpression might lead to saturation of the cellular trafficking machinery and artifactual trafficking.)

Overall, the appropriate starting point is to identify whether there is a functional channel expressed in the membrane in native cells, which is usually screened by current measurements in the absence and presence of channel blockers. Reduced current amplitude might be indicative of impaired trafficking or function, or both. This observation then warrants further exploration of the mechanisms that modulate the deficiency: that is, is the channel trafficking-deficient or functionally deficient? Site-directed mutagenesis of cDNA encoding the gene can be performed to alter the sequence of the ion channel of interest to model the gene mutation. With the gene inserted into an expression vector, transfection of the gene into culture cells can be employed to follow the acquired trafficking characteristics.

It is critical to identify the protein expression of the transfected gene. Western blot analysis and immunofluorescence are employed to demonstrate transfection and expression of the introduced gene. Cells transfected with the complete cDNA can be compared to those transfected with empty vector to clarify that the antibody specifically identifies the correct protein on the Western blot or immunofluorescent image. Following the transfection period (typically 48 h for transient expression), cells are lysed, aliquots of the lysate are resolved in gels, and Western blots are developed with the appropriate antibodies. As with Western blot, immunofluorescence can also be employed to detect expression of transfected genes. Specificity for the immunofluorescence of the transfected gene can be determined in a similar manner. In transiently transfected cells not subjected to clonal selection, a mosaic of transfected and untransfected cells typically appears, as revealed by a bright stain of the transfected cells and a faint background stain corresponding to the untransfected cells.

A Western blot analysis can be employed first to identify whether the protein of interest is confined to the ER or has trafficked to upstream compartments of the secretory pathway. Conjugation of complex oligosaccharides, which can be detected on Western blots by observing high molecular weight diffuse bands, provides evidence for trafficking to the Golgi. The trafficking-impaired ion channel that contains the mutant may migrate in a lower position in a gel or show a singlet band instead of the diffuse and sometimes thick upper band indicative of complex oligosaccharide conjugation that corresponds with expression of the wild-type glycoprotein. Thus, comparing the banding characteristics between the wild-type and mutant proteins provides an initial indication of the trafficking characteristics. It should be noted that this test for trafficking to the Golgi is not universally applicable, and some proteins that reach the cell membrane still possess high-mannose oligosaccharides that are not processed further.

Further confirmation of trafficking can be determined by examining oligosaccharide substitution using endo-H and PNGase-F cleavages. The cells are lysed, and aliquots of lysate are diluted in appropriate buffers and subjected to enzyme cleavage. Samples are resolved in gels and detected in Western blots to examine whether shifts in the molecular weights have occurred. Enhanced mobility in the gel is indicative of cleavage. To verify the capacity for oligosaccharide cleavage, PNGase-F is also applied to aliquots and digestion is allowed to occur under similar conditions. Again the proteins are resolved in adjoining lanes, and the mobilities of the proteins of interest are compared with and without enzyme treatment. These data therefore make it possible to identify whether molecular weight shifts following glycosidase treatment are due to carbohydrate removal.

Cell-surface biotinylation can be employed to further identify cell-surface expression. Cells with the transfected gene and those transfected with empty vector can be employed for comparisons. Samples representing total-cell lysate, the bound biotinylated fraction, and the unbound fraction can be resolved in gels for comparison. If volume stoichiometries are maintained and it is assumed that the biotinylation reaction proceeded to completion, then a relatively quantitative assessment of cell-surface expression can be made.

Multiple-labeling confocal microscopy is an additional method that can be employed to examine trafficking characteristics. The protein of interest can be detected directly by a specific antibody or by epitope-tagging of the gene that will be transfected. Cellular compartments can be detected by labeling with antibody directed to proteins confined to these compartments. Overlap in the three-dimensional field of the confocal microscopic image provides an indication that the protein has trafficked to a specified compartment.

III. SUMMARY AND CONCLUSION

Because mutations in ion channels associated with disease have the propensity to create trafficking-deficient channels, studies aimed at identifying the mechanistic basis of a disease are likely to encounter the issue of protein trafficking. The role of impaired trafficking causing a loss in function can be identified by the biochemical techniques described in this section. Understanding the cellular and physiological bases of an ion channel deficiency by distinguishing reduced trafficking from impaired gating could lead to rationally designed pharmaceutical interventions aimed at directly treating a channel disease associated with an inherited mutation. As new mutations in ion channels are discovered that appear to correlate with a disease condition, it will become important to identify whether impaired trafficking has a role in the deficiency.

ACKNOWLEDGMENTS

This work was supported by an AHA Scientist Development Grant and a UCSD MERF Scholarship to S. H. Keller and by grants from the National Heart, Lung, and Blood Institute of the National Institutes of Health (HL 64945, HL 54043, HL 69758, HL 66012) to J. X.-J. Yuan. The imaging experiments used facilities at the National Center of Microscopy and Imaging Research at UCSD, which are supported by NIH grant RR04050 to M. Ellisman.

REFERENCES

1. Meacham GC, Patterson C, Zhang W, Younger JM, Cyr DM. The Hsc70 co-chaperone CHIP targets immature CFTR for proteasomal degradation. Nat Cell Biol 2001; 3:100–105.
2. Paulussen A, Raes A, Matthijs G, Snyders DJ, Cohen N, Aerssens J. A novel mutation (T65P) in the PAS domain of the human potassium channel HERG results in the long QT syndrome by trafficking deficiency. J Biol Chem 2002; 277:48610–48616.
3. Kosolapov A, Deutsch C. Folding of the voltage-gated K^+ channel T1 recognition domain. J Biol Chem 2003; 278:4305–4313.

4. Ryu EJ, Harding HP, Angelastro JM, Vitolo OV, Ron D, Greene LA. Endoplasmic reticulum stress and the unfolded protein response in cellular models of Parkinson's disease. J Neurosci 2002; 22:10690–10698.
5. Chapple JP, Cheetham ME. The chaperone environment at the cytoplasmic face of the endoplasmic reticulum can modulate rhodopsin processing and inclusion formation. J Biol Chem 2003; 278:19087–19094.
6. Hammond C, Helenius A. Folding of VSV G protein: sequential interaction with BiP and calnexin. Science 1994; 266:456–458.
7. Vashist S, Kim W, Belden WJ, Spear ED, Barlowe C, Ng DT. Distinct retrieval and retention mechanisms are required for the quality control of endoplasmic reticulum protein folding. J Cell Biol 2001; 155:355–368.
8. Cabral CM, Liu Y, Sifers RN. Dissecting glycoprotein quality control in the secretory pathway. Trends Biochem Sci 2001; 26:619–624.
9. Luzikov VN. Quality control: proteins and organelles. Biochemistry 2002; 67:171–183.
10. Nishimura N, Balch WE. A di-acidic signal required for selective export from the endoplasmic reticulum. Science 1997; 277:556–558.
11. Davies JC. *Pseudomonas aeruginosa* in cystic fibrosis: pathogenesis and persistence. Paediatr Respir Rev 2002; 3:128–134.
12. Grabenhorst E, Conradt HS. The cytoplasmic, transmembrane, and stem regions of glycosyltransferases specify their in vivo functional sublocalization and stability in the Golgi. J Biol Chem 1999; 274:36107–36116.
13. Mezzacasa A, Helenius A. The transitional ER defines a boundary for quality control in the secretion of tsO45 VSV glycoprotein. Traffic 2002; 3:833–849.
14. Demand J, Alberti S, Patterson C, Hohfeld J. Cooperation of a ubiquitin domain protein and an E3 ubiquitin ligase during chaperone/proteasome coupling. Curr Biol 2001; 11:1569–1577.
15. Hohfeld J, Cyr DM, Patterson C. From the cradle to the grave: molecular chaperones that may choose between folding and degradation. EMBO Rep 2001; 2:885–890.
16. Yoo JS, Moyer BD, Bannykh S, Yoo HM, Riordan JR, Balch WE. Nonconventional trafficking of the cystic fibrosis transmembrane conductance regulator through the early secretory pathway. J Biol Chem 2002; 277: 11401–11409.
17. Maitra R, Shaw CM, Stanton BA, Hamilton JW. Increased functional cell surface expression of CFTR and deltaF508-CFTR by the anthracycline doxorubicin. Am J Physiol Cell Physiol 2001; 280:C1031–C1037.
18. Sharma M, Benharouga M, Hu W, Lukacs GL. Conformational and temperature-sensitive stability defects of the ΔF508 cystic fibrosis transmembrane conductance regulator in post-endoplasmic reticulum compartments. J Biol Chem 2001; 276:8942–8950.
19. Brown CR, Hong-Brown LQ, Welch WJ. Strategies for correcting the AF508 CFTR protein-folding defect. J Bioenerg Biomembr 1997; 29:491–502.
20. Bross P, Corydon TJ, Andresen BS, Jorgensen MM, Bolund L, Gregersen N. Protein misfolding and degradation in genetic diseases. Hum Mutat 1999; 14: 186–198.

21. Ciechanover A. The ubiquitin proteolytic system and pathogenesis of human diseases: a novel platform for mechanism-based drug targeting. Biochem Soc Trans 2003; 31:474–481.
22. Fenteany G, Standaert RF, Lane WS, Choi S, Corey EJ, Schreiber SL. Inhibition of proteasome activities and subunit-specific amino-terminal threonine modification by lactacystin. Science 1995; 268:726–731.
23. Bonifacino JS, Traub LM. Signals for sorting of transmembrane proteins to endosomes and lysosomes. Annu Rev Biochem 2003; 72:395–447.
24. Staub O, Gautschi I, Ishikawa T, et al. Regulation of stability and function of the epithelial Na^+ channel (ENaC) by ubiquitination. EMBO J 1997; 16:6325–6336.
25. Pind S, Riordan JR, Williams DB. Participation of the endoplasmic reticulum chaperone calnexin (p88, IP90) in the biogenesis of the cystic fibrosis transmembrane conductance regulator. J Biol Chem 1994; 269:12784–12788.
26. Keller SH, Lindstrom J, Taylor P. Involvement of the chaperone protein calnexin and the acetylcholine receptor β-subunit in the assembly and cell surface expression of the receptor. J Biol Chem 1996; 271:22871–22877.
27. Keller SH, Lindstrom J, Taylor P. Inhibition of glucose trimming with castanospermine reduces calnexin association and promotes proteasome degradation of the α-subunit of the nicotinic acetylcholine receptor. J Biol Chem 1998; 273:17064–17072.
28. Okiyoneda T, Wada I, Jono H, Shuto T, Yoshitake K, Nakano N, Nagayama SI, Harada K, Isohama Y, Miyata T, Kai H. Calnexin Δ185–520 partially reverses the misprocessing of the ΔF508 cystic fibrosis transmembrane conductance regulator. FEBS Lett 2002; 526:87–92.
29. Priori SG, Bloise R, Crotti L. The long QT syndrome. Europace 2001; 3:16–27.
30. Groenewegen WA, Bezzina CR, van Tintelen JP, Hoorntje TM, Mannens MMAM, Wilde AAM, Jongsma HJ, Rook MB. A novel LQT3 mutation implicates the human cardiac sodium channel domain IVS6 in inactivation kinetics. Cardiovasc Res 2003; 57:1072–1078.
31. Veldkamp MW, Wilders R, Baartscheer A, Zegers JG, Bezzina CR, Wilde AAM. Contribution of sodium channel mutations to bradycardia and sinus node dysfunction in LQT3 families. Circ Res 2003; 92:976–983.
32. Quiram PA, Ohno K, Milone M, Patterson MC, Pruitt NJ, Brengman JM, Sine SM, Engel AG. Mutation causing congenital myasthenia reveals acetylcholine receptor β/δ subunit interaction essential for assembly. J Clin Invest 1999; 104:1403–1410.
33. Ratjen F, Doring G. Cystic fibrosis. Lancet 2003; 361:681–689.
34. Welsh MJ, Smith AE. Molecular mechanisms of CFTR chloride channel dysfunction in cystic fibrosis. Cell 1993; 73:1251–1254.
35. Doring G, Conway SP, Heijerman HG, Hodson ME, Hoiby N, Smyth A, Touw DJ. Antibiotic therapy against *Pseudomonas aeruginosa* in cystic fibrosis: a European consensus. Eur Respir J 2000; 16:749–767.
36. Haws CM, Nepomuceno IB, Krouse ME, Wakelee H, Law T, Xia Y, Nguyen H, Wine JJ. Delta F508-CFTR channels: kinetics, activation by forskolin, and potentiation by xanthines. Am J Physiol 1996; 270:C1544-C1555.
37. Schultz BD, Frizzell RA, Bridges RJ. Rescue of dysfunctional ΔF508-CFTR chloride channel activity by IBMX. J Membr Biol 1999; 170:51–66.

38. Cheng SH, Gregory RJ, Marshall J, Paul S, Souza DW, White GA, O'Riordan CR, Smith AE. Defective intracellular transport and processing of CFTR is the molecular basis of most cystic fibrosis. Cell 1990; 63:827–834.
39. Gelman MS, Kannegaard ES, Kopito RR. A principal role for the proteasome in endoplasmic reticulum-associated degradation of misfolded intracellular cystic fibrosis transmembrane conductance regulator. J Biol Chem 2002; 277:11709–11714.
40. Vorbrodt AW, Dobrogowska DH, Tarnawski M. Immunogold study of interendothelial junction-associated and glucose transporter proteins during postnatal maturation of the mouse blood-brain barrier. J Neurocytol 2001; 30:705–716.
41. Ye J, Yao K, Zeng Q, Lu D. Changes in gap junctional intercellular communication in rabbit lens epithelial cells induced by low power density microwave radiation. Chin Med J 2002; 115:1873–1876.
42. Inoue M, Wakayama Y, Liu JW, Murahashi M, Shibuya S, Oniki H. Ultrastructural localization of aquaporin 4 and alpha1-syntrophin in the vascular feet of brain astrocytes. Tohoku J Exp Med 2002; 197:87–93.
43. Massensini AR, Suckling J, Brammer MJ, Moraes-Santos T, Gomez MV, Romano-Silva MA. Tracking sodium channels in live cells: confocal imaging using fluorescently labeled toxins. J Neurosci Methods 2002; 116:189–196.
44. Hofmann T, Schaefer M, Schultz G, Gudermann T. Subunit composition of mammalian transient receptor potential channels in living cells. Proc Natl Acad Sci USA 2002; 99:7461–7466.
45. Penque D, Mendes F, Beck S, Farinha C, Pacheco P, Nogueira P, Lavinha J, Malho R, Arnaral MD. Cystic fibrosis F508del patients have apically localized CFTR in a reduced number of airway cells. Lab Invest 2000; 80:857–868.
46. McIntosh AL, Gallegos AM, Atshaves BP, Storey SM, Kannoju D, Schroeder F. Fluorescence and multiphoton imaging resolve unique structural forms of sterol in membranes of living cells. J Biol Chem 2003; 278:6384–6403.
47. Fossati, G, Moulding DA, Spiller DG, Moots RJ, White MR, Edwards SW. The mitochondrial network of human neutrophils: role in chemotaxis, phagocytosis, respiratory burst activation, and commitment to apoptosis. J Immunol 2003:1964–1972.
48. Luo Y, Vassilev PM, Li X, Kawanabe Y, Zhou J. Native polycystin 2 functions as a plasma membrane Ca^{2+}-permeable cation channel in renal epithelia. Mol Cell Biol 2003; 23:2600–2607.
49. Giblin JP, Quinn K, Tinker A. The cytoplasmic C-terminus of the sulfonylurea receptor is important for K_{ATP} channel function but is not key for complex assembly or trafficking. Eur J Biochem 2002; 269:5303–5313.
50. Haggie PM, Stanton BA, Verkman AS. Diffusional mobility of the cystic fibrosis transmembrane conductance regulator mutant, ΔF508-CFTR, in the endoplasmic reticulum measured by photobleaching of GFP-CFTR chimeras. J Biol Chem 2002; 277:16419–16425.
51. Johnson ML, Redmer DA, Reynolds LP, Bilski JJ, Grazul-Bilska AT. Gap junctional intercellular communication of bovine granulosa and thecal cells from antral follicles: effects of luteinizing hormone and follicle-stimulating hormone. Endocrine 2002; 18:261–270.

52. Malik B, Schlanger L, Al-Khalili O, Bao H-F, Yue G, Price SR, Mitch WE, Eaton DC. ENaC degradation in A6 cells by the ubiquitin-proteosome proteolytic pathway. J Biol Chem 2001; 276:12903–12910.
53. Chang XB, Cui L, Hou Y-X, Jensen TJ, Aleksandrov AA, Mengos A, Riordan JR. Removal of multiple arginine-framed trafficking signals overcomes misprocessing of ΔF508 CFTR present in most patients with cystic fibrosis. Mol Cell 1999; 4:137–142.

34

Functional Study of Cloned Ion Channels in Mammalian Transfection Systems Using Site-Directed Mutagenesis

Elena E. Brevnova, Bethany H. Parker, Oleksandr Platoshyn, and Jason X.-J. Yuan

Department of Medicine, University of California, San Diego, California, U.S.A.

I. INTRODUCTION

The function of ion channels is essential for many cell processes. Functional studies of a particular type of ion channel in native cells are sometimes rather complicated because of the diversity of native channel types. Certain mammalian cell lines developed with very low expression of endogenous ion channels have been used as convenient heterologous expression systems for the functional study of particular ion channels. These systems provide machinery and pathways similar to those of native mammalian cells with normal ion channel expression levels. Furthermore, the heterologous expression approach together with in vitro (or site-directed) mutagenesis allows investigation into protein structure and function targeted to the specific area of interest in an ion channel. The aim of this chapter is to describe the technique of site-directed mutagenesis and to illustrate how it is applied in functional studies of cloned ion channels heterologously expressed in mammalian cell lines.

II. OVERVIEW OF THE MUTAGENESIS APPROACH

Mutations, specific changes in a DNA sequence (such as nucleotide bases or DNA fragment substitutions, insertions, or deletions) of genetic elements (genes, promoters, etc.), can affect the functions of these elements or their protein products. DNA mutagenesis has long been used to provide insights into various aspects of biological functions, such as protein structure (1), trafficking (2), and physiological function (3); protein–protein or nuclear acid–protein interactions (4); gene expression and regulation (5); and pathological gene polymorphism (6).

Historically, mutants were obtained by selecting for organisms having new properties. Mutations were performed in vivo by spontaneous mutagenesis using X-rays or chemical mutagenic treatment. Then the mutant and relevant wild-type genes were isolated and sequenced. However, this classical approach had some disadvantages and limitations. First, in vivo mutagenesis constrained the mutations that were obtained; it was practically impossible to create specific mutations of interest, and mutations that did occur in the gene of interest were relatively rare. Second, because these mutations were identified by their phenotype, it was impossible to study the effect of mutations that did not cause a change in phenotype. Third, the entire organism was subjected to mutagenesis, so there was always a chance of getting multiple mutations (throughout the entire genome), and it could not be guaranteed that the effect of the mutation in the gene of interest was not influenced or even caused by other spontaneous mutations.

Development of the in vitro mutagenesis process has made it possible to reverse the procedure and logic of classical mutagenesis (Fig. 1). According to the modern approach, the DNA sequence containing the gene of interest is first identified and subcloned into an expression vector. This allows the gene of interest to be subjected to any kind of in vitro alterations. This new expression construct containing either the mutated or wild-type gene of interest can be used for transfection of mammalian cells. Transfection is the common strategy for introducing foreign genes into eukaryotic cells (see Sec. III). The resulting mutant protein produced by the mutated gene of interest can then be functionally analyzed and compared to the wild-type protein.

III. EXPRESSION OF FOREIGN GENES USING MAMMALIAN EXPRESSION SYSTEMS

As stated before, the gene of interest to be expressed must first be identified, isolated and cloned (Fig. 1). The gene may be isolated from either genomic DNA selected from chromosomal gene libraries or complementary DNA (cDNA) amplified from cellular mRNA by reverse transcription. A disadvantage of using the genomic DNA of most eukaryotic organisms is that the protein coding sequences, exons, are interrupted by non-coding

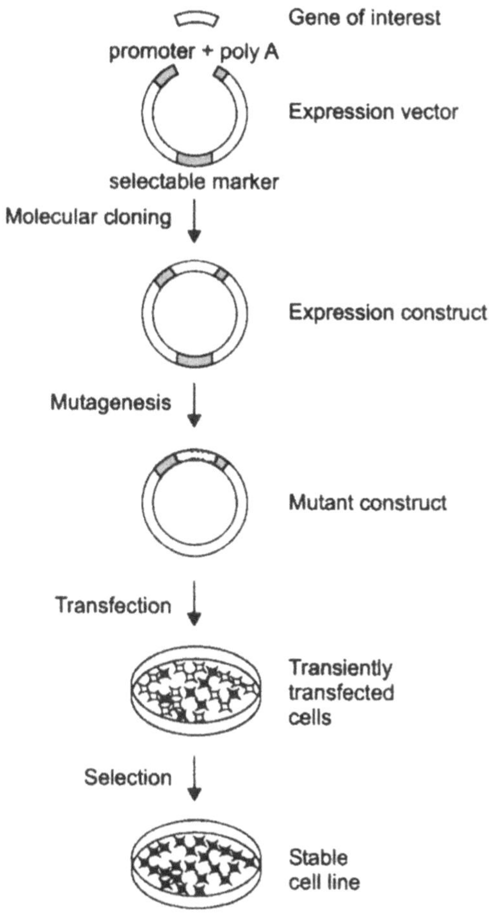

Figure 1 Cloning, mutagenesis, and expression of the gene of interest in mammalian cell lines. The DNA coding for the protein of interest is identified, isolated, and subcloned into an expression vector. The expression vector usually contains a promoter, a polyadenylation site, and a selectable marker that will allow for stable transfection. The gene of interest could then be subjected to in vitro mutagenesis. The expression construct containing either the mutated or wild-type gene of interest can be used for transient or stable transfection of mammalian cells. During the first few days after transfection, only a fraction of the cells carry the gene of interest (black cells). In a few cells, the gene of interest and the selectable marker are incorporated into the genome due to spontaneous recombination. These cells survive the application of the appropriate drug against which the selection marker gene confers resistance. The cells that do not integrate the transfected DNA lose the transiently transfected plasmid DNA and are killed by this drug, and only stably transfected cells propagate in culture (see details in text).

sequences, introns. Consequently, cDNA is the more commonly used source of heterologous genes because cDNA is amplified from mRNA and therefore does not include introns. The altered or wild-type gene of interest (see Sec. IV) can then be subcloned into an expression vector. The choice of expression vector depends on the cell line that is going to be used as a host for the heterologous expression of the gene of interest, and on the proposed strategy for introducing foreign genes into host cells.

Mammalian cells are popular as hosts for the expression of genes obtained from higher eukaryotes because the signals for protein synthesis, processing, and secretion are usually recognized. Various mammalian cell lines have been used for the expression of ion channels. These include fibroblast-type cells (NIH/3T3), COS-7, L, BHK, epithelial (HeLa), epithelial-like [Chinese hamster ovary (CHO)], human embryonic kidney (HEK-293), and lymphoblast cells (RBL-1) (7–14). The choice of host cells is critical and depends on the type of endogenous channels present and the type of channels to be expressed.

The introduction of the foreign DNA into the host cells (transfection) can be performed by various techniques. The most commonly used techniques are calcium phosphate precipitation (15), lipofection (15), electroporation (15), and virus-mediated infection (16). The calcium phosphate precipitation technique uses a HEPES-buffered solution, which, in the presence of $CaCl_2$, allows the formation of a DNA–calcium phosphate precipitate that adheres to the cell surface, allowing for the DNA to be endocytosed into the cells. The lipofection method uses cationic liposomes to introduce the DNA into the host cells. Though it is still not clear how it works, it is presumed that the negatively charged phosphate groups on the DNA bind to the positively charged surface of the liposome, creating a DNA–liposome complex. The residual positive charge then mediates binding of the complex to negatively charged sialic acid residues on the cell membrane. The electroporation method uses a high-voltage electric shock to perforate the cell membrane. The DNA can than enter the cells through these pores. Finally, the viral method uses viruses such as SV40 recombinant adenoviruses, retroviruses, and vaccinia viruses. In comparison to other expression strategies, very efficient transfections have been obtained using viruses. This technique, however, involves constructing and packaging a recombinant virus, which takes tremendous effort and is time-consuming.

There are two ways to transfect mammalian cells transiently and stably (Fig. 1). In a transient transfection, the transfected DNA is taken up by the nucleus but not incorporated in the genome. In this case, only a fraction of the cells express the foreign DNA, and eventually (approximately 2–6 days after transfection) the foreign DNA is lost through successive generations because the plasmids are not replicated when the cells divide. Expression of the transiently transfected gene can usually be analyzed 1–4 days after introduction of DNA, generally by harvesting the transfected cells. During the transient transfection stage, a few cells usually incorporate the foreign DNA into their genome due to spontaneous DNA recombination. These cells can be selected for if the vector used contains a selectable marker, i.e., a gene encoding resistance to a particular drug. The cells can be selected by cultivating them in growth media containing the appropriate drug. Only the cells with the marker gene that confers drug resistance will survive. When these cells divide and replicate and there are no cells left that do not carry the foreign DNA, a stable line has been established. The establishment of a stable cell line in which all the cells express the marker gene and the protein of interest usually takes 2–6 weeks. The most commonly used selectable marker is the Tn5 aminoglycoside phosphotransferase (*neo*^{r}) gene that confers resistance to neomycin, kanamycin, and G418 (17).

The choice of the transfection type (transient or stable) depends on the purpose of the experiment. When large quantities of identical cells are necessary for immunological or biochemical studies, stable transfection is preferable. However, transient transfection experiments take much less time, with the limitation that only a fraction of the cells are actually transfected. For some experiments, such as gene regulation analysis, this disadvantage is usually not that critical. For functional studies, such as electrophysiological patch-clamp recording, this disadvantage has now been overcome by introducing transfection markers into expression vectors. The most popular transfection marker is the green fluorescent protein (GFP) (or its derivatives), a protein from *Aequorea victoria* jellyfish that emits green light when excited with light in the blue range of the spectrum (18). The transfection marker can be cotransfected with the gene of interest in a separate expression vector or in the same vector as a separate protein, or it can be fused to the protein of interest.

Today the most commonly used mammalian cell expression vectors contain multiple elements, including (1) an SV40 origin of replication allowing for plasmid amplification to high copy number in mammalian cells; (2) a bacterial plasmid origin of replication allowing propagation in bacterial cells, which are used for plasmid DNA amplification; (3) an efficient promoter sequence for high-level transcription initiation; (4) mRNA processing signals, such as cleavage, polyadenylation, and transcription termination sequences; (5) polylinkers containing multiple restriction endonuclease sites for insertion of the gene of interest; and (6) selectable markers for selection of stably transfected mammalian cells and for selection of transformed bacterial cells (these could be the same or different genes).

IV. DNA SEQUENCE ALTERATIONS

A variety of enzymatic and chemical methods are available for recombining DNA sequences in vitro. In the past, to produce extended deletions or insertions, the subcloning approach was usually applied. This method was based on using specific restriction endonuclease sites in a gene of interest and in vitro DNA recombination and ligation (15). For point mutations or even short fragment mutations (several nucleotides), the most common methods use specific oligonucleotides as mutagens. Because oligonucleotides of any desired sequence can be chemically synthesized, oligonucleotide-directed mutagenesis can generate a precisely designed mutation in a DNA sequence. Historically, mutagenesis was usually performed on single-stranded cloning vectors, such as the M13 (19) or fd (20) bacteriophages. In oligonucleotide-based mutagenesis, a synthesized mutagenic oligonucleotide is hybridized to a single-stranded template containing the wild-type sequence and extended with T4 DNA polymerase (21). Using single-stranded DNA templates is labor intensive and technically difficult. Development of the polymerase chain reaction (PCR), a simple, generally applicable technique, now allows the single-stranded construct step to be skipped, and the oligonucleotide-based mutagenesis is performed directly on double-stranded expression vectors (22). The PCR method is based on the repeated serial reaction involving the use of oligonucleotide primers and DNA polymerase, which is used to amplify a particular DNA sequence of interest (15). Use of the PCR and gene splicing by overlap extension (gene SOEing) technique (22) provides a powerful tool for creating practically any kind of DNA sequence alterations without depending on particular restriction sites. This strategy is based on the fact that the ends of a PCR-generated DNA fragment can incorporate new, custom-designed sequences that were not present in the original template. The primers must match their template sequences well enough to prime, but they do not have to match precisely, especially toward the 5′ end of the sequence. Mismatches will then be incorporated into the final PCR product. This idea, originally called "mispriming" (23), provides a simple way to perform site-directed mutagenesis. However, simple mismatching is limited in that the mutations can be created only at the ends of a PCR product. Gene splicing by the overlap extension technique (gene SOEing) (24) has overcome this limitation. Originally this technique was devised as a way of introducing mutations in the center of PCR-generated DNA fragments in order to make PCR mutagenesis more universally applicable. However, now DNA SOEing also has other applications, such as creating gene hybrids.

After the DNA sequence alterations have been performed, verification that the desired mutation has been introduced is usually accomplished by DNA sequencing. Currently several techniques can be used to perform DNA sequencing (15). For instance, the most common procedure is called dideoxy or Sanger sequencing (25). For multiple screening of the mutants, some researchers use restriction analysis before sequencing. This includes introduction of a restriction site into the mutagenic primer along with the desired mutation. The restriction analysis mutation screening could be useful in primary mutant selection, especially when the mutation yield is very low. However, for further functional studies of the mutant, it is important to sequence the entire gene and not only the newly mutated region, because random errors can be introduced into the sequence of interest during the site-directed mutagenesis process owing to polymerase mistakes (26).

Several of the most commonly used mutagenesis methods based on using PCR are described below. Combining these techniques allows any kind of possible DNA sequence alteration on double-stranded vectors to be performed.

A. Generation of Point Mutations Using Site-Directed Mutagenesis

Currently, there are two commonly used approaches to create single (point) or several nucleotide mutations: oligonucleotide-directed mutagenesis (20,21) and mutagenesis by overlap extension (22). The oligonucleotide-directed mutagenesis method is the more popular of the two, most likely for historical reasons. Figure 2 illustrates the use of this strategy to produce a point or several-nucleotide mutation. The basic procedure uses a DNA vector with an inserted sequence of interest and a synthetic oligonucleotide containing the desired mutation near the center. The double-stranded template mutagenesis procedure uses two complementary strands of mutagenic oligonucleotides. The synthetic oligonucleotide primers, each complementary to the opposite strand of the target template except for a region of mismatch, hybridize to the gene of interest. During temperature cycling the primers are extended with a DNA polymerase (such as T4), creating a second complementary strand. The resulting product is a heteroduplex molecule containing the mismatch due to the mutation in the primer and a nick in the newly synthesized mutated strand due to the inability of the DNA polymerase to bind the 3′ end of the elongating DNA strand to the 5′ end of the primer. The duplex structure is then transformed into an *E. coli* host using any standard bacterial transformation technique (15). The nick in the new strand is sealed either in vitro (before *E. coli* transformation) or in vivo (in *E. coli*) with DNA ligase.

As already mentioned, oligonucleotide-based mutagenesis can be performed using either a double-stranded or single-stranded DNA template. The double-stranded procedure is faster and simpler and is consequently preferred for most situations. However, the single-stranded procedure may sometimes be more useful when trying to maximize the total number of transformants (for example, when generating mutant libraries or when the mutagenic primer is expected to have difficulty annealing to the template). Annealing problems can be caused by (1) multiple mismatches in the primer, (2) low annealing temperature (T_m) of the oligonucleotide, or (3) complicated secondary structure of the primer.

If *E. coli* transformants are not subjected to any selection after mutagenesis, the theoretical yield of mutants among transformants is 50% due to the semiconservative mode of DNA replication (Fig. 2). However,

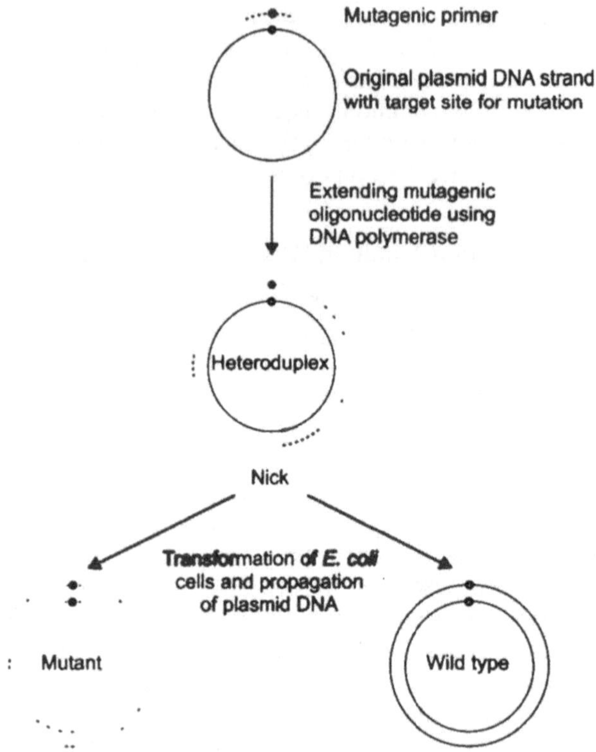

Figure 2 Basic steps in a common oligonucleotide-directed mutagenesis procedure. Synthesized mutagenic primer has to be complementary to the target site except for a mismatching mutation near the center of the primer. The single-stranded template approach uses one primer, but for a double-stranded template two complementary primers are needed. The primers, each complementary to the opposite strand of the target template, hybridize to the gene of interest. During temperature cycling the primers are extended with DNA polymerase, creating a second complementary strand. The resulting product is a heteroduplex molecule containing mismatch and a nick in the newly synthesized mutated strand. The duplex structure is then transformed into an *E. coli* host. The nick in the new strand is sealed in vitro (before *E. coli* transformation) or in vivo (in *E. coli*) with DNA ligase. The mismatches are repaired upon replication in *E. coli* cells. Theoretically, there has to be 50:50 proportion of mutated (gray) and parental (black) molecules owing to the semiconservative mode of DNA replication if no mutant selection was applied.

in practice, the mutant yield without selection may be much lower (sometimes down to only a few percent). Several possible factors may decrease the mutant yield; examples include incomplete in vitro polymerization, primer displacement by DNA polymerase, or in vivo mismatch repair mechanisms that preferably repair the unmethylated newly synthesized DNA strand.

There are different ways to significantly increase the mutant yield by applying selection to the transformants. The most common method of mutant selection treats the DNA duplex with endonucleases, which selectively digest only the parental unmutated DNA template. These endonucleases can distinguish the strands due to different DNA modifications (27). For instance, DNA isolated from almost all *E. coli* strains is *dam*-methylated and therefore susceptible to DpnI endonuclease digestion, while the new in vitro-synthesized strand is not methylated and is therefore not susceptible to digestion by DpnI. If DpnI is applied to treat the DNA duplex before the *E. coli* transformation step, most of the wild-type DNA is degraded, leaving mostly mutated DNA to be amplified in *E. coli*. This procedure can increase the mutant yield to 70–90% (27). Another mutant selection approach is based on incorporating a novel antibiotic resistance gene into the mutant strand to allow for selection (28). This type of selection involves altering the substrate specificity of TEM-1 β-lactamase, the enzyme responsible for bacterial resistance to β-lactam antibiotics such as ampicillin. The β-lactamase gene (selectable marker for plasmid amplification in bacterial cells) is commonly found in vectors used for molecular biology. Amino acid substitutions in several residues of β-lactamase result in increased hydrolytic activity against extended-spectrum penicillins and cephalosporins. This increased activity confers a novel resistance specific to the mutant and thus provides the basis of this selection strategy. This approach can be used only for templates containing the β-lactamase gene and involves simultaneous use of two couples of oligonucleotides during the mutagenesis procedure—mutagenic primers and selection primers.

Recently, another mutagenesis approach, DNA splicing by overlap extension (SOEing), has become popular. This technique provides a powerful mutagenesis method by combining PCR and in vitro recombination techniques (22). The concept is illustrated in Fig. 3. Four oligonucleotides must be synthesized: two complementary mutagenic primers (C and B in Fig. 3), a forward primer complementary to the 5′ end of the insert of interest (A), and a reverse primer complementary to the 3′ end of the insert (D). First, two fragments are amplified separately from the original double-stranded template. One fragment (AB) is amplified with primers A and B. The mutagenic primer B introduces a mutation at the right end of the AB product. Similarly, the second fragment (CD) is amplified with primers C and D, with primer C introducing the same mutation, but at the left end of product CD. The products AB and CD share a segment of identical sequence called the overlap region. The AB and CD intermediate products have to be purified, mixed together, melted, reannealed, and used as a template for a second PCR with the primers A and D. The top strand of AB can anneal to the bottom strand of CD in such a way that the two strands act as primers to one another. DNA polymerase can extend both of these strands, creating the full-length mutant molecule, AD product, in which AB and CD

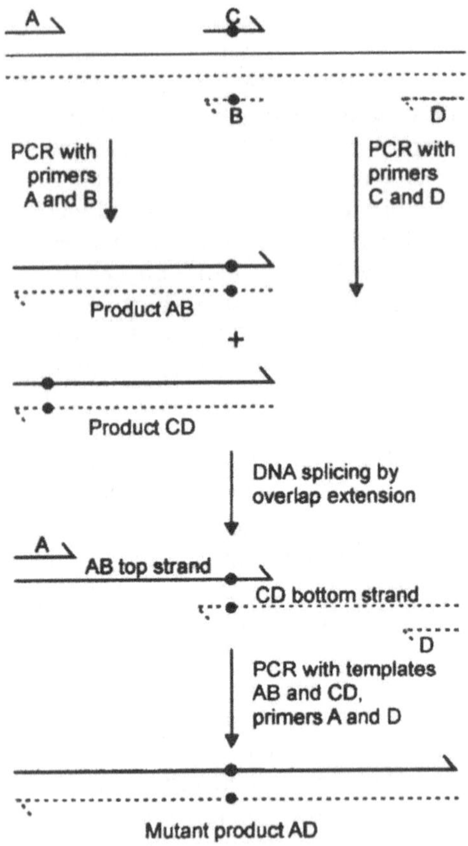

Figure 3 Site-directed mutagenesis by overlap extension. Two fragments are amplified separately from the same original double-stranded template. One fragment, AB, is amplified with primers A and B. The forward primer A, complementary to the 5′ end of the insert of interest, and the mutagenic primer B introduce a mutation at the right end of the AB product. The second fragment, CD, is amplified with primers C and D, with primer C introducing the same mutation, but at the left end of product CD, and the reverse primer D complementary to the 3′ end of the insert. The products AB and CD share a segment of identical sequence called the overlap region. The AB and CD intermediate products have to be purified, mixed together, melted, reannealed, and used as a template for a second PCR with the primers A and D. The top strand of AB (solid line) can anneal to the bottom strand of CD (dashed) in such a way that the two strands act as primers to one another. DNA polymerase can extend both of these strands, creating the full-length mutant molecule, AD product, in which AB and CD sequences are joined together. The AD product is then amplified with A and D primers during the same PCR.

sequences are joined together. The AD product is then amplified with A and D primers during the same PCR. To insert the mutated PCR product into an expression vector, any convenient endonuclease restriction site can be introduced in the 5′ ends of the forward (A) and reverse (D) primers.

Site-directed mutagenesis by overlap extension is simple and has many advantages over other methods. For example, essentially all of the product molecules are mutated (24), meaning 100% mutation yield. Consequently, this technique does not need any mutant selection. Also, the mutated product is produced in vitro without the need to propagate it as part of a plasmid or phage, and it may be used directly in experiments (29). Furthermore, recombination of different DNA sequences (see next subsection) and mutagenesis can be performed simultaneously. The only drawback of DNA recombination by SOEing is that occasionally, if intermediate PCR products are longer then 1500 bp, they may have difficulty annealing to each other during the second PCR, most likely due to the complicated secondary structure of the long DNA segments. This problem can be overcome by decreasing the length of the insert of interest by subcloning (unpublished observations).

B. Creating Gene Hybrids and DNA Deletions and Insertions

The DNA splicing by overlap extension technique can be used not only to produce point mutations in one gene but also to recombine sequences from different genes, creating hybrid constructs. As a method of DNA recombination, gene SOEing is tremendously useful in situations where no leeway can be given to use nearby restriction sites. There are many impressive examples of the use of this technique in protein engineering projects (30).

Figure 4 illustrates the concept of PCR-mediated DNA recombination by SOEing. Four primers must be designed: primers A and B complementary to the 5′ and 3′ ends, respectively, of the first gene (template 1), and primers C and D complementary to the 5′ and 3′ ends, respectively, of the second gene (template 2). An extra sequence is added to the 5′ end of primer B. This sequence is complementary to the 3′ end of template 2 (the beginning of primer C). During the first PCR, two products are amplified from separate templates. Product AB is amplified from template 1 with primers A and B, and product CD is amplified from template 2 with primers C and D. The AB and CD intermediate products have an overlap region of common sequence. In a second PCR, AB and CD are mixed together and used as a template with primers A and D. The top strand of AB product can anneal with the bottom strand of the CD product. These strands act as primers for each other and produce a giant "primer dimer," which is a recombinant molecule. Analogously to DNA SOEing mutagenesis (Fig. 3), the products AB and CD are extended by DNA polymerase and amplified with primers A and D. As was mentioned above, restriction sites can be

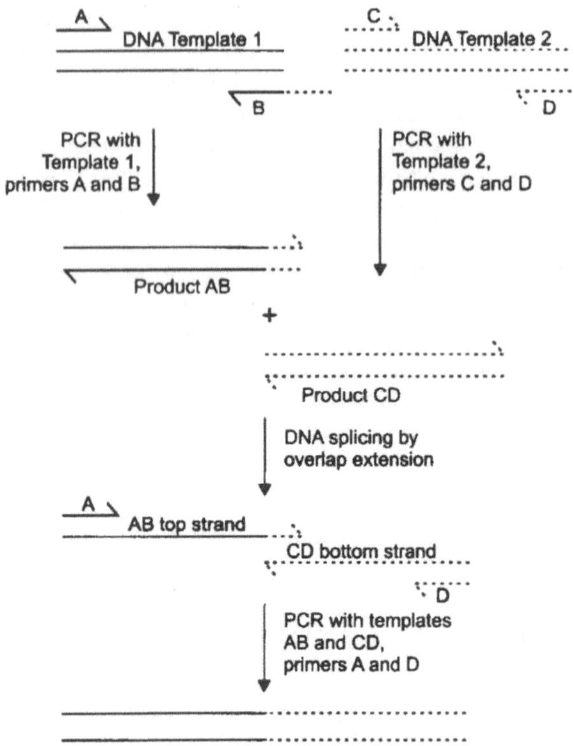

Figure 4 DNA recombination by SOEing. Two fragments are amplified from separate templates. One fragment, AB, is amplified from template 1 (soild) with primers A and B complementary to the 5′ and 3′ ends, respectively, of template 1. The second fragment, CD, is amplified from template 2 (dashed) with primers C and D complementary to the 5′ and 3′ ends, respectively, of template 2. The products AB and CD share a segment of identical sequence called the overlap region due to the extra sequence added to the 5′ end of primer B. This sequence is complementary to the 3′ end of template 2, i.e., to primer C. When AB and CD are mixed together and used as a template for PCR with primers A and D, the top strand of AB product can anneal with the bottom strand of CD product. These two strands act as primers to one another, producing a recombinant molecule. The AB and CD strands can be extended by DNA polymerase to create a full-length hybrid molecule and amplified with primers A and D.

introduced in the 5′ ends of the forward (A) and reverse (D) primers to insert the hybrid product into the multiple cloning site of an expression vector.

Figure 5 illustrates the use of PCR or PCR combined with DNA SOEing to create all possible deletion variants. To delete 5′ or 3′ DNA segments (Fig. 5A and 5B), a simple PCR strategy is sufficient. For 5′ deletions

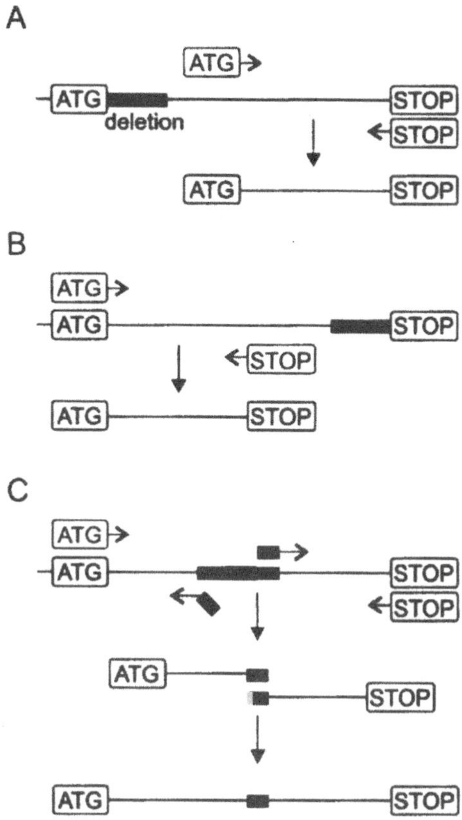

Figure 5 Deletion of 5′ (A), 3′ (B) or internal (C) DNA segments using PCR and DNA overlap extension. The fragments in A, B, and C indicated by heavier lines are the DNA segments to be deleted. (A) The forward primer, which is complementary to an internal segment of the gene of interest, contains a transcription start codon (ATG) and is used to amplify the 5′ deletion variant. (B) The reverse primer, which is complementary to an internal segment of the gene of interest, contains a transcription stop codon and is used to amplify the 3′ deletion variant. (C) Internal DNA deletion is performed by a combination of PCR and DNA SOEing (see Figs. 3 and 4). In the first PCR, the intermediate DNA fragments to be spliced together are amplified from different segments of the same template with the internal primers that have a common sequence, the overlap region (gray boxes). These fragments are reannealed to each other, extended, and amplified during the second PCR.

(Fig. 5A), the forward primer containing a transcription start codon (ATG) has to be complementary to the new beginning of the potential deletion variant. Analogously, for 3′ deletions (Fig. 5B), the reverse primer, complementary to the desired end of the gene of interest, has to introduce the stop codon at a new position.

The easiest way to perform internal DNA sequence deletions is to use restriction endonucleases and ligases (15). However, if there are no convenient restriction sites present near the desired sequence, or the deletion has to be made at a precise position, a combination of PCR with DNA SOEing can be applied to get the desired deletion (Fig. 5C). The idea is the same as in vitro DNA recombination (Fig. 4) or DNA SOEing site-directed mutagenesis (Fig. 3) described earlier. The only difference is that here, intermediate PCR products are amplified from different segments of the same template.

Figure 6 illustrates another example of using SOEing for DNA sequence recombination. The figure demonstrates the strategy for inserting the DNA fragment into a gene of interest. However, the same procedure can be applied to combine DNA segments from any number of different genes

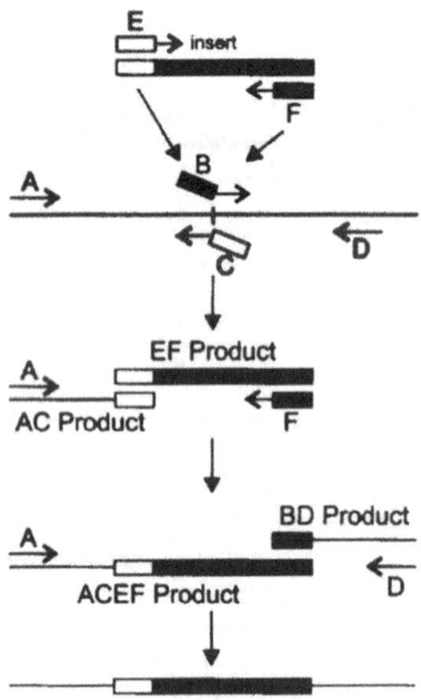

Figure 6 Insertion of internal DNA segments using PCR and DNA overlap extension. The procedure uses the sequential SOEing (see Figs. 3–5) of DNA fragments. The initial DNA fragments have to be amplified separately: AC product amplified with primers A and C, BD product amplified with primers B and D, and EF insert amplified with primers E and F. The AC and EF fragments have an overlap region (white boxes), due to the shared sequence of the C and E primers, and can be linked together by SOEing. The ACEF segment, product of the AC and EF SOEing, can then be linked to the BD segment due to a common sequence in the B and F primers (black boxes). The 5′ end of the primer B (black box), complementary to primer F, does not have to be complementary to the original template. Primer B anneals to the template due to the 3′ end, complementary to the template. The same applies to the 5′ end of primer C (white box), complementary to primer E.

or other DNA elements. The procedure involves the sequential SOEing of DNA fragments. First, every DNA fragment has to be amplified separately. AC (A and C primers) and BD (B and D primers) products are amplified from the template into which the DNA fragment has to be inserted. EF (E and F primers) is amplified from the template that contains the insert. Second, two fragments (AC and EF) that have an overlap region are bound together by SOEing. The product of this SOEing (ACEF) can then be linked to the next DNA fragment (BD), which shares a common sequence with the ACEF. Sequential SOEing can be continued by adding more and more DNA segments that share common sequences. The only limitation of this approach is that doing multiple PCR results in an accumulation of DNA polymerase errors in the final hybrid product.

V. ANALYSIS OF EXPRESSION AND FUNCTION OF HETEROLOGOUS ION CHANNELS

After ion channel genes are expressed in mammalian cells, the expression level, protein location, and function of these heterologous channels can be characterized. There are many approaches currently used to study ion channels expressed in mammalian cells, such as reverse transcription PCR (RT-PCR), Western blot analysis, electrophysiological recording (patch clamp), immunocytochemistry, immunoprecipitation, and crystallography.

Figure 7 illustrates an example of using some of these techniques to characterize expression and function of the human Kv1.5 potassium channel (31) in HEK-293 cells. Several techniques are available to characterize the gene expression on a transcription level, i.e., to evaluate the relative amount of mRNA transcripted from the gene of interest. The most commonly used techniques are RT-PCR (see Chapter 35) and Northern blot analysis. The RT-PCR method uses reverse transcriptase, an enzyme that can use mRNA as a template to synthesize complementary DNA (cDNA). The cDNA, obtained from the reverse transcription of the total cell mRNA, is then used as a template for regular PCR with the primers specific for the expressed gene of interest. The PCR product can be analyzed by a DNA gel electrophoresis technique. RT-PCR performed on mRNA isolated from an individual cell is called single-cell RT-PCR (see Chapter 32). If a dynamic of the PCR process is monitored, i.e., if the amount of PCR product can be measured at any particular PCR cycle, it is called real-time RT-PCR (32). Regular PT-PCR is useful for a quick evaluation of the gene transcription level; however, the real time RT-PCR technique can give more precise quantitative data. Figure 7A shows the products of regular and single-cell RT-PCR performed with mRNA isolated from native HEK-293 (W) cells and from HEK-293 cells transfected with the human Kv1.5 potassium channel expression construct (Kv1.5).

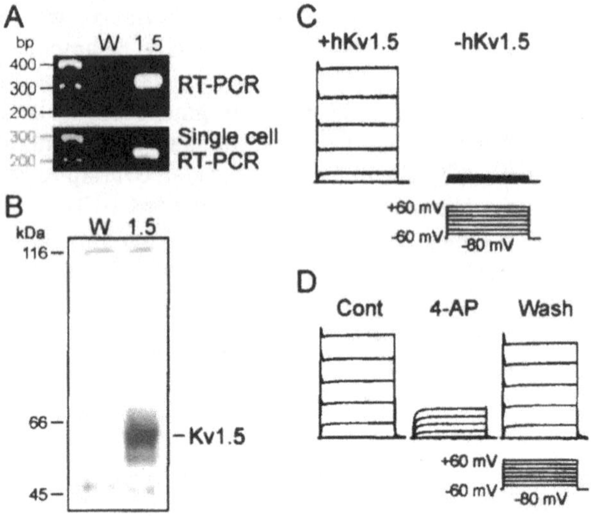

Figure 7 Characterization of expression and function of the human Kv1.5 potassium channel heterologously expressed in HEK-293 cells. The human Kv1.5 expression construct was obtained from Dr. Tamkun (Vanderbilt University, Nashville, TN). The construct includes human Kv1.5 encoding sequence (nucleotides −22 to +1895) subcloned into *Xba*I and *Kpn*I sites of the pBK-CMV expression vector (Stratagene, San Diego, CA). (A) DNA products of regular (upper) and single-cell (lower) RT-PCR performed with mRNA isolated from native HEK-293 cells (W) and from HEK-293 cells transfected with the hKv1.5 expression construct (1.5). The PCR products were separated in a 1% agarose gel. The amount of PCR product reflects the Kv1.5 expression at the mRNA level. The Kv1.5 transcription level in Kv1.5-transfected cells is much higher than in wild-type cells. (B) Western blots of the total-cell protein samples prepared from native HEK-293 cells (W) and from HEK-293 cells transfected with the hKv1.5 expression construct (1.5) with the Kv1.5-specific antibodies (Alomone Labs, Israel). Western blot analysis detected that the amount of Kv1.5 protein product heterologically expressed in Kv1.5 transfected cells is also very high compared to the nontransfected cells. (C) Patch-clamp-recorded whole-cell currents from HEK-293 cells transfected with empty pBK-CMV vector (−hKv1.5) and from HEK-293 cells transfected with hKv1.5 expression construct (+hKv1.5). In this experiment, whole-cell current amplitude reflects the ion channel protein expression level. The amplitude of whole-cell currents recorded from Kv1.5-transfected cells is almost 25 times bigger than in nontransfected cells. (D) Reversible inhibition of the function of the Kv1.5 channels heterologously expressed in HEK-293 cells by 4-aminopyridine (4-AP) (61), the specific blocker of the voltage-dependent potassium channels. The significant and reversible decrease of the whole-cell current amplitude in Kv1.5-transfected cells treated with 4-AP reflects a reversible inhibition of expressed ion channels by the voltage-dependent potassium channel blocker and shows the specificity of these channels.

Western blot analysis is the most commonly used technique for analysis of the ion channel expression at the protein level. Western blotting has an advantage over the other techniques currently used for protein analysis in that it is highly specific and can be applied for relatively small protein amounts (as little as 1 ng). The procedure includes electrophoretically separating proteins in a polyacrylamide gel, transferring proteins from the gel to a nitrocellulose membrane, and blotting the membrane with the antigen (protein of interest)-specific antibodies (primary antibodies). The protein–antibody complex on the membrane is then treated with species-specific anti-Ig secondary antibodies that can recognize and bind to the type of primary antibodies used. The protein–primary antibody–secondary antibody complex can be visualized by activation of enzymatic, fluorescent, or other kind of conjugates linked to the secondary antibodies. Figure 7B shows the Western blots of the total cell protein samples prepared from native HEK-293 (W) cells and from HEK-293 cells transfected with hKv1.5 expression construct (Kv1.5) that have been treated with Kv1.5-specific antibodies.

For characterization of ion channel function, the patch-clamp technique has been extremely useful (see Chapters 30 and 31). This technique allows recording of the electrical behavior of all channels present in the cell membrane (whole-cell recording) or just one or several ion channel proteins (single-channel recording). Figure 7C shows the patch-clamp-recorded whole-cell currents from native HEK-293 (-hKv1.5) cells and from HEK-293 cells transfected with the hKv1.5 expression construct (+Kv1.5). To confirm the specificity of the currents in the transfected cells, known blockers or other specific channel function modulators can be applied. Figure 7D shows that 4-aminopyridine (4-AP), a specific blocker of the voltage-dependent potassium channels, can reversibly inhibit the function of the heterologous Kv1.5 channels.

The immunocytochemistry (33) and biotinylation (34) methods are useful tools for studying ion channel trafficking machinery (see Chapter 33). The biotinylation technique tags proteins located on the cell surface, using biotin–streptavidin binding. An immunocytochemical approach allows detection of intracellular or cell-surface protein localization. Transfected cells are fixed to a glass surface and treated with antibodies specific for the protein of interest. The proteins are visualized with species-specific anti-Ig secondary antibodies linked to a fluorescent marker. The fluorescent-labeled proteins are observed using florescent or confocal microscopy.

Many approaches are available to study the binding properties of the transfected ion channels, such as two-hybrid methods, in vitro binding assays, and immunoprecipitation (35). Structural studies of ion channels have been successfully carried out using the protein the crystallographic technique (1).

VI. APPLICATION OF SITE-DIRECTED MUTAGENESIS FOR STUDY OF ION CHANNEL FUNCTIONS

The choice of mutagenic strategy depends on the purpose of the experiment. When studying the pathological mechanism of natively acquired mutations, the mutations of interest can be generated in vitro (36). To find out what region of the ion channel protein is responsible for a particular functional property, deletion or chimeric ion channels (ion channels containing segments from different proteins) can be generated (37). To clarify which amino acids play a key role in the ion channel function, certain amino acids (thought to be important to the functioning of the channel) can be mutated. The choice of amino acids to be mutated is usually based on the ion channel protein structure or other information from previous experiments (1).

There are numerous examples of the use of site-directed mutagenesis for ion channel studies. The following subsections illustrate just some of the possible applications of this powerful technique for studying ion channels expressed in mammalian cells.

A. Pharmacological Properties of Ion Channels

Mutagenic analysis is broadly used to study pharmacological properties of ion channels and to analyze ion channel interactions with endogenous modulators. For instance, with the site-directed mutagenesis approach, an ion channel chimeric construct is created (37). This construct contains a segment of the P-region of M-*eag* channel inserted into the human *ether-a-go-go*-related (HERG) channel (Fig. 8). Figure 8 demonstrates that this chimeric channel (HMH) abolished the inhibitory effect of the ergtoxin (ErgTx), a specific blocker of the HERG channels (ErgTx does not affect the function of either M-*eag* or M-*elk* channels). Chimeras of the P-region of the HERG channel into M-*eag* channels recovered the inhibitory effect. Point mutagenesis experiments revealed that the N598Q mutant of the HERG channel P-region shows about a 25% decrease of the ErgTx inhibitory effect.

Another example showing how just a single nucleotide mutation at the-functional region of an ion channel can significantly change the electrophysiologically recorded properties of the channel is ClC-3, a mammalian volume-regulated chloride channel. Site-specific mutational studies of the ClC-3 channel indicate that a serine residue (serine 51) within a consensus PKC-phosphorylation site in the intracellular amino terminus of the ClC-3 channel protein represents an important volume sensor of the channel(38).

B. Processing and Trafficking of Ion Channel Proteins

Another field in which the mutagenesis approach is actively applied is the study of ion channel trafficking mechanisms (2,34,36). For example, mutations in the KCNH2 gene of the HERG channel can cause a reduction

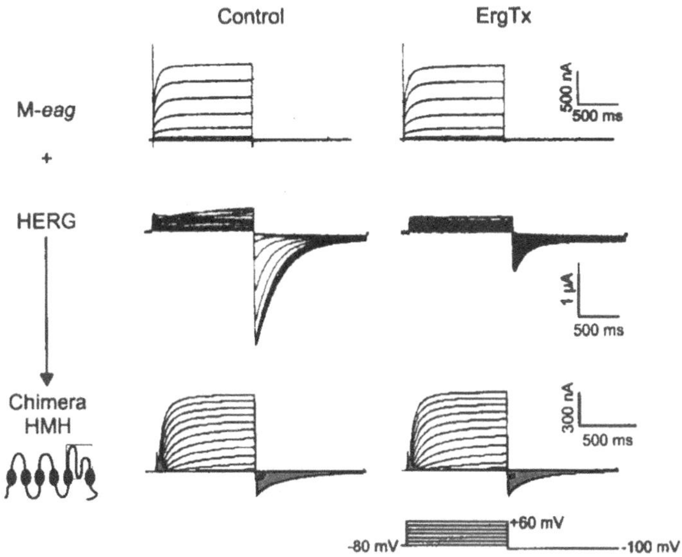

Figure 8 Effect of the substitution of the HERG channel P-region by M-*eag* channel P-region on the channel sensitivity to the ergtoxin (ErgTx). Outward K^+ currents were measured in oocytes expressing M-*eag* (top), HERG (middle), and HMH (bottom) channels. HMH is a chimeric channel containing a segment of the P-region of the M-*eag* channel (box) inserted into the HERG channel. Current records in the absence (control) or presence of ErgTx (100 nM for the M-*eag* and HERG channels, 200 nM for the HMH). Currents were elicited by step depolarizations (10 mV increments) ranging between −80 and +60 mV from a holding potential of −80 mV. (Reproduced from Ref. 37 with permission from Elsevier.)

in I_{Kr}, one of the currents responsible for cardiac repolarization. Delayed repolarization results in prolongation of the QT interval, which is the clinical hallmark of the congenital long QT syndrome, a cardiac disease characterized by an increased susceptibility to ventricular arrhythmias. The mechanism by which these mutations cause the problem is currently being studied. In particular, it was shown that the in vitro generated missense mutation T65P in the PAS (Per-Arnt-Sim) domain of HERG resulted in defective trafficking of the protein to the cell membrane (36).

C. Molecular Transitions and Multimerization of Ion Channel Proteins

The extraordinary pleiotropy of Andersen's syndrome provides an example of how generation of pathological mutations can clarify the ion channel multimerization mechanism. This autosomal dominant disorder is related to mutations of the potassium channel Kir2.1 and is characterized by cardiac arrhythmia, periodic paralysis, and dysmorphic bone structure. Site-directed mutagenesis experiments with the Kir2.1 potassium channel showed that coexpression of Kir2.1 mutants related to Andersen's syndrome with wild-type Kir2.1, Kir2.2, and Kir2.3 channels showed a dominantly negative effect, the extent of which varied between mutants (4).

The next example demonstrates the use of the site-directed mutagenesis technique to study a mechanism of molecular transitions of ion channels. Experiments with HERG channel mutants showed that deletion of the HERG-specific proximal domain (HERG D138–373) accelerated all individual forward transitions between closed states of the channel. Alteration of the initial *eag*/PAS domain by introduction of a short amino acid sequence at the beginning of the amino terminus did not alter transitions between closed states but prevented the channels from reaching the farthest open states that determine slower deactivation rates. This demonstrates that both proximal and *eag*/PAS domains in the amino terminus contribute to set the gating characteristics of HERG channels (39).

D. Structural Study of Ion Channels

The combination of site-directed mutagenesis with X-ray crystallography allows clarification of the structure of ion channels and mechanisms of ion channel function. Mutagenic and structural experiments with the mammalian Kv1.2 channel showed that the channel gating depends critically on residues at complementary surfaces of the T1 domain (which shares a cytoplasmic assembly domain of Kv voltage-gated potassium channels) in a polar interface. An isosteric mutation in this interface causes little structural alteration while stabilizing the closed channel and increasing the stability of T1 tetramers. Replacing T1 with a tetrameric structurally unrelated domain destabilizes the closed channel. Together, these data suggest that structural changes involving the buried polar T1 surfaces play a key role in the conformational changes leading to channel opening (1).

VII. SUMMARY

The site-directed mutagenesis technique has proven useful for the functional study of ion channels heterologously expressed in mammalian cells. In vitro mutagenesis of ion channels has provided information regarding channel gene regulation, the pathological mechanisms of natively occurring mutations, the pharmacological properties of ion channels, ion channel protein processing and trafficking, molecular transition and multimerization mechanisms, and ion channel protein structure. Development of DNA SOEing, a simple yet powerful mutagenesis method that combines PCR and in vitro DNA recombination, has allowed for the creation of various DNA sequence alterations and has opened a wide spectrum of possibilities for future detailed studies of ion channels.

ACKNOWLEDGMENTS

This work was supported by NIH/NHLBI grants HL-64945, HL-54043, HL-69758, and HL-66012 awarded to J. X.-J. Yuan. The authors thank Dr. Carmelle Remillard for editing this chapter.

REFERENCES

1. Minor DL, Lin YF, Mobley BC, Avelar A, Jan YN, Jan LY, Berger JM. The polar T1 interface is linked to conformational changes that open the voltage-gated potassium channel. Cell 2000; 102:657–670.
2. Campomanes CR, Carroll KI, Manganas LN, Hershberger ME, Gong B, Antonucci DE, Rhodes KJ, Trimmer JS. Kvβ subunit oxidoreductase activity and Kv1 potassium channel trafficking. J Biol Chem 2002; 277:8298–8305.
3. Levin G, Peretz T, Chikvashvilli D, Jing J, Lotan I. Deletion of the N-terminus of a K^+ channel brings about short-term modulation by cAMP and β1-adrenergic receptor activation. J Mol Neurosci 1996; 7:269–276.
4. Preisig-Müller R, Schlichthörl G, Goerge T, Heinen S, Brüggemann A, Rajan S, Derst C, Veh RW, Daut J. Heteromerization of Kir2.x potassium channels contributes to the phenotype of Andersen's syndrome. Proc Natl Acad Sci USA 2002; 99:7774–7779.
5. Mikala G, Klöckners U, Varadi M, Eisfeld J, Schwartz A, Varadi G. cAMP-dependent phosphorylation sites and macroscopic activity of recombinant cardiac L-type calcium channels. Mol Cell Biochem 1998; 185:95–109.
6. Hayashi K, Shimizu M, Ino H, Yamaguchi M, Mabuchi H, Hoshi N, Higashida H. Characterization of a novel missense mutation E637K in the pore-S6 loop of HERG in a patient with long QT syndrome. Cardiovasc Res 2002; 54:67–76.
7. Stutts MJ, Gabriel SE, Olsen JC, Gatzy JT, O'Connell TL, Price EM, Boucher RC. Functional consequences of heterologous expression of the cystic fibrosis transmembrane conductance regulator in fibroblasts. J Biol Chem 1993; 268:20653–20658.
8. Murata M, Buckett PD, Zhou J, Brunner M, Folco E, Koren G. SAP97 interacts with Kv1.5 in heterologous expression systems. Am J Physiol Heart Circ Physiol 2001; 281:H2575–H2584.
9. Uebele VN, England SK, Chaudhary A, Tamkun MM, Snyders DJ. Functional differences in Kv1.5 currents expressed in mammalian cell lines are due to the presence of endogenous Kvβ2.1 subunits. J Biol Chem 1996; 271:2406–2412.
10. Ding S, Kuroki S, Kameyama A, Yoshimura A, Kameyama M. Cloning and expression of the Ca^{2+} channel alpha1C and beta2a subunits from guinea pig heart. J Biochem 1999; 125:750–759.
11. Rapizzi E, Pinton P, Szabadkai G, Wieckowski MR, Vandecasteele G, Baird G, Tuft RA, Fogarty KE, Rizzuto R. Recombinant expression of the

voltage-dependent anion channel enhances the transfer of Ca^{2+} microdomains to mitochondria. J Cell Biol 2002; 159:613–624.

12. Meadows LS, Chen YH, Powell AJ, Clare JJ, Ragsdale DS. Functional modulation of human brain $Na_v1.3$ sodium channels, expressed in mammalian cells, by auxiliary β1, β2 and β3 subunits. Neuroscience 2002; 114:745–753.
13. Burbidge SA, Dale TJ, Powell AJ, Whitaker WR, Xie XM, Romanos MA, Clare JJ. Molecular cloning, distribution and functional analysis of the $Na_V1.6$ voltage-gated sodium channel from human brain. Brain Res Mol Brain Res 2002; 103:80–90.
14. Ikeda SR, Soler F, Zuhlke RD, Joho RH, Lewis DL. Heterologous expression of the human potassium channel Kv2.1 in clonal mammalian cells by direct cytoplasmic microinjection of cRNA. Pflügers Arch 1992; 422:201–203.
15. Ausubel FM, Brent R, Kingston RE, Moore DD, Seidman JG, Smith JA, Struhl K. Short Protocols in Molecular Biology. 2nd ed. Brooklyn: Greene Publishing, 1992.
16. Graham FL, Preves L. Manipulation of adenovirus vectors. In: Murrey EJ, ed. Methods in Molecular Biology. Clifton NJ: Humana Press 1991;17:109–128.
17. Southern PJ, Berg P. Transformation of mammalian cells to antibiotic resistance with a bacterial gene under control of the SV40 early region promoter. J Mol Appl Genet 1982; 1:327–341.
18. Chalfie M, Tu Y, Euskirchen G, Ward WW, Prasher DC. Green fluorescent protein as a marker for gene expression. Science 1994; 263:802–805.
19. Messing J, Groneneborn B, Müller-Hill B, Hofschneider PH. Filamentous coliphage M13 as a cloning vehicle: insertion of a *Hin*dII fragment of the *lac* regulatory region in M13 replicative form in vitro. Proc Natl Acad Sci USA 1977; 74:3642–3646.
20. Wasylyk B, Derbyshire R, Guy A, Molko D, Roget A, Teoule R, Chambon P. Specific in vitro transcription of conalbumin gene is drastically decreased by single-point mutation in T-A-T-A box homology sequence. Proc Natl Acad Sci USA 1980; 77:7024–7028.
21. Kunkel TA. Rapid and efficient site-specific mutagenesis without phenotypic selection. Proc Natl Acad Sci USA 1985; 82:488–492.
22. Horton RM. In vitro recombination and mutagenesis of DNA. In: White BA, ed. Methods in Molecular Biology. PCR Protocols: Current Methods and Applications. Totowa NJ: Humana Press, 1993; 15:251–261.
23. Mullis KB, Faloona FA. Specific synthesis of DNA in vitro via a polymerase-catalyzed chain reaction. Methods Enzymol 1987; 155:335–350.
24. Ho SN, Hunt HD, Horton RM, Pullen JK, Pease LR. Site-directed mutagenesis by overlap extension using the polymerase chain reaction. Gene 1989; 77:51–59.
25. Sanger F, Nicklen S, Coulson AR. DNA sequencing with chain-terminating inhibitors. Proc Natl Acad Sci USA 1977; 74:5463–5467.
26. Osinga KA, Van der Bliek AM, Van der Horst G, Groot Koerkamp MJ, Tabak HF, Veeneman GH, Van Boom JH. In vitro site-directed mutagenesis with synthetic DNA oligonucleotides yields unexpected deletions and insertions at high frequency. Nucleic Acids Res 1983; 11:8595–8608.

27. Li F, Mullins JI. Site-directed mutagenesis facilitated by DpnI selection on hemimethylated DNA. Methods Mol Biol 2002; 182:19–27.
28. Andrews CA, Lesley SA. Selection strategy for site-directed mutagenesis based on altered beta-lactamase specificity. Biotechniques 1998; 24:972–974, 976, 978.
29. Kain KC, Orlandi PA, Lanar DE. Universal promoter for gene expression without cloning: expression-PCR. Biotechniques 1991; 10:366–374.
30. Horton RM, Cai ZL, Ho SN, Pease LR. Gene splicing by overlap extension: tailor-made genes using the polymerase chain reaction. Biotechniques 1990; 8:528–535.
31. Tamkun MM, Knoth KM, Walbridge JA, Kroemer H, Roden DM, Glover DM. Molecular cloning and characterization of two voltage-gated K^+ channel cDNAs from human ventricle. FASEB J 1991; 5:331–337.
32. Gibson UE, Heid CA, Williams PMA. Novel method for real time quantitative RT-PCR. Genome Res 1996; 6:995–1001.
33. Hager H, Kwon T-H, Vinnikova AK, Masilamani S, Brooks HL, Frokiaer J, Knepper MA, Nielsen S. Immunocytochemical and immunoelectron microscopic localization of α-, β-, and γ-ENaC in rat kidney. Am J Physiol Renal Physiol 2001; 280:1093–1106.
34. Keller SH, Lindstrom J, Ellisman M, Taylor P. Adjacent basic amino acid residues recognized by the COP I complex and ubiquitination govern endoplasmic reticulum to cell surface trafficking of the nicotinic acetylcholine receptor α-subunit. J Biol Chem 2001; 276:18384–18391.
35. Maximov A, Sudhof TC, Bezprozvanny I. Association of neuronal calcium channels with modular adaptor proteins. J Biol Chem 1999; 274:24453–24456.
36. Paulussen A, Raes A, Matthijs G, Snyders DJ, Cohen N, Aerssens J. A novel mutation (T65P) in the PAS domain of the human potassium channel HERG results in the long QT syndrome by trafficking deficiency. J Biol Chem 2002; 277:48610–48616.
37. Pardo-López L, Garcia-Valdeé J, Gurrola GB, Robertson GA, Possani LD. Mapping the receptor site for ergtoxin, a specific blocker of ERG channels. FEBS Lett 2002; 510:45–49.
38. Duan D, Cowley S, Horowitz B, Hume JR. A serine residue in ClC-3 links phosphorylation-dephosphorylation to chloride channel regulation by cell volume. J Gen Physiol 1999; 113:57–70.
39. Gómez-Varela D, de la Peña P, Garcia J, Giráldez T, Barros F. Influence of amino-terminal structures on kinetic transitions between several closed and open states in human *erg* K^+ channels. J Membr Biol 2002; 187:117–133.

35

Screening for mRNA Expression Using the Polymerase Chain Reaction

Ivana Fantozzi, Carmelle V. Remillard, Mehran Mandegar, and Jason X.-J. Yuan

Department of Medicine, University of California, San Diego, California, U.S.A.

I. INTRODUCTION

Polymerase chain reaction (PCR) is an in vitro technique for amplifying a target DNA sequence in a short time. This is because both strands of DNA are copied simultaneously during PCR; therefore, there is an exponential increase in the number of copies of the target DNA fragment or gene with each cycle (1,2). Three fundamental aspects make PCR such a powerful tool in determining the qualitative expression of target genes:

1. PCR is less expensive, less time-consuming, and simpler than previous DNA (and RNA) duplication techniques, making it possible for anyone, even one with no training in molecular biology, to do genetic and molecular biological research.
2. PCR has an enormous amplification capability. Therefore, starting from an extremely tiny biological sample, it is possible to obtain a nearly unlimited supply of genetic material to manipulate.
3. Perhaps the most important aspect is the specificity of PCR. The specificity comes from the specific hybridization of the primers with DNA target regions. The length of the target sequence, if limited to less than a few kilobases, has a beneficial effect on specificity (3).

One of the strengths of PCR is its versatility. Modifications in the technique can change its application such that it can be used to analyze and amplify cellular RNA. This particular application, referred to as "reverse transcription-PCR" (RT-PCR), highly increases the sensitivity of detection and enables sequence analysis of RNA using the low amount of RNA templates available within the cells. This technique can also be used to screen for the intensity of mRNA expression of known genes. This chapter will discuss in detail how the RT-PCR technique can be used to screen for mRNA expression of ion channels.

II. THE POLYMERASE CHAIN REACTION TECHNIQUE

A. Basic PCR

Duplication and amplification of specific regions of DNA by PCR can be done using specific oligonucleotide primers that are complementary to the 5′ and 3′ ends of a defined sequence of the DNA template. Designing these primers (See Section IV) requires that the target nucleotide sequence be known.

Each PCR cycle is composed of three basic steps: DNA denaturation, annealing of the primers, and extension by DNA polymerases (Fig. 1), all of which are performed using a thermal cycler. In the denaturation step, extreme heating (92–96°C) breaks the hydrogen bonds between the base pairs that make up the double-stranded DNA, producing two complementary single-stranded DNA molecules. The time necessary to denature DNA depends on the DNA complexity, tube geometry, the thermal cycler, and the volume of the reaction. DNA sequences rich in G-C nucleotides require a longer denaturation time and can be enhanced by the addition of glycerol to the reaction mixture. High temperatures, however, cause thermal damage to DNA and induce misincorporation of nucleotides by polymerase during the PCR process. Therefore, if high fidelity is desired, high temperatures are generally avoided (4).

Once the DNA is separated, oligonucleotide primers can be added. The thermal cycler cools the mixture to a predetermined annealing temperature, typically ~50–60°C, at which primers can rapidly hybridize with complementary sequences on the single-stranded DNA. Generally, the primers are present at a significantly greater concentration than the original target DNA and are short in length. Therefore, they stand a better chance of binding the DNA target sites before the DNA strands can reanneal. Although the speed of primer binding reflects the affinity of the primers for the target sequence, itself dependent on the composition of the oligonucleotides, temperature will also control the affinity and intensity of annealing to the correct target sites. The annealing temperature depends on the melting temperature (T_m) of the primers, i.e., the temperature at which the primers start

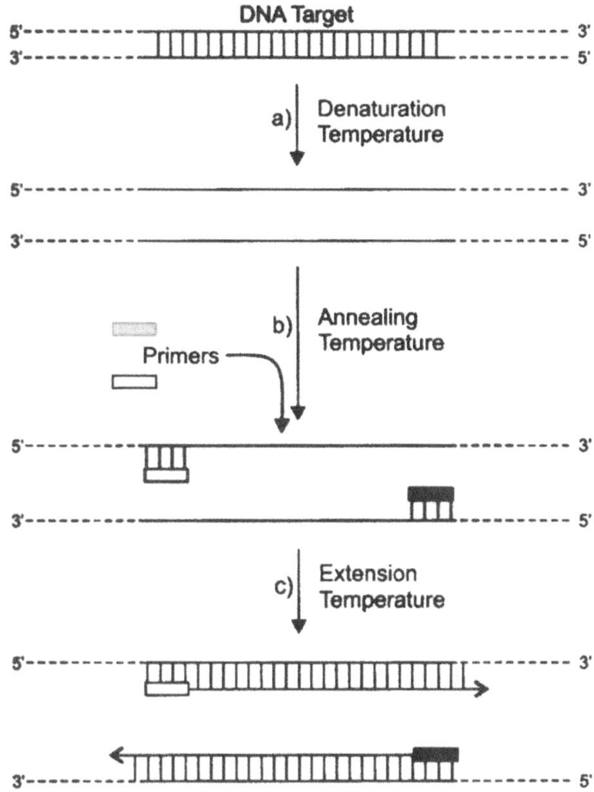

Figure 1 The first cycle in PCR. The double-stranded DNA template is denatured at high temperature, leaving two single-stranded DNA molecules. Cooling to the annealing temperature allows the primer to hybridize with the complementary target sequence. Temperature is raised for optimal polymerase activity, and the primers are extended from the 5′ end to the 3′ end.

dissociating from the binding sites. T_m varies according to the length of the primer, its G/C composition, and the presence of cations, as shown in Table 1 (5–7).

In the last step in PCR, the primer in extended by a DNA polymerase. Commonly used bacterial *Taq* DNA polymerases usually are optimally effective at temperatures between 72 and 75°C. The stability of *Taq* polymerase at higher temperature is advantageous in that DNA also tends to remain denatured during the extension step, making it easier for the polymerase to perform its task. Simply stated, the polymerase attaches the 3′ end of the primer and begins adding nucleotides (dNTPs are added in large quantities in the reaction mixture) to the primer from the 5′ to the 3′ direction while reading the template from the 3′ to the 5′ direction, until

Table 1 Three of the Most Commonly Used Formulas to Calculate T_m

1. For primers not longer than 20 nucleotides:
   T_m = [(number of A + T) × 2C + (number of G + C) × 4C] calculated in a 1 M salt concentration for oligonucleotide hybridization assay (5).
2. For oligonucleotides of 14–70 residues:
   $T_m = 81.5 + 16.6\,(\log_{10}[J^+]) + 0.41(\%C + G) - (600/l) - 0.63(\%FA)$ where $[J^+]$ = concentration of monovalent cations; l = oligonucleotide length, FA = formamide (6).
3. For oligonucleotides of 20–35 residues:
   $T_p = 22 + 1.46(l_n)$ where T_p = optimized annealing temperature ± 2–5°C, l_n = effective length of primer = 2 (number of G + C) + (number of A + T) (7).

eventually the end of the DNA strand is reached. Ultimately, a complementary copy of each DNA strand is generated. The time required to copy the template depends on the length of the PCR product. Although 2 min is usually sufficient to extend the DNA, the final cycle duration is normally ~10 min in order to ensure that DNA molecules are completely extended.

For each subsequent PCR cycle, the steps are exactly as described above. However, the products available at the beginning of the early cycles are more complex. After the denaturation step in the second cycle, there are three populations of single-stranded DNA present: the original genomic DNA and each of the complementary extended sequences produced during the first cycle. As a result of the primers and DNA polymerase action during the first cycle, the length of the DNA strands differs between the genomic DNA and the primer-extended sequences; i.e., the primer-extended sequences are truncated at their 5′ ends near the primer, whereas the genomic sequences are full length. Because the DNA polymerase reads from the 3′ to the 5′ end and "falls off" at the 3′ end of the DNA strand, after completion of the second PCR cycle all DNA copies are truncated at both ends (Fig. 2) and exactly correspond in length to the original target sequence. In subsequent cycles, the number of copies of this length increases exponentially, making up the bulk of the concentration in the mixture, whereas the number of the original strands with nonspecific length becomes small and almost negligible.

Therefore, after the *n*th amplification cycle, the reaction mixture would contain 2^n double-stranded DNA fragments confined between the two specific primers. The number of cycles necessary for best results depends mainly on the initial concentration of the target genetic sequence. A frequent mistake is to run too many cycles, because this increases the amount and complexity of nonspecific background products. Also, in running too many PCRs, one experiences a "plateau effect," where the exponential accumuation is attenuated once the concentration of PCR product reaches

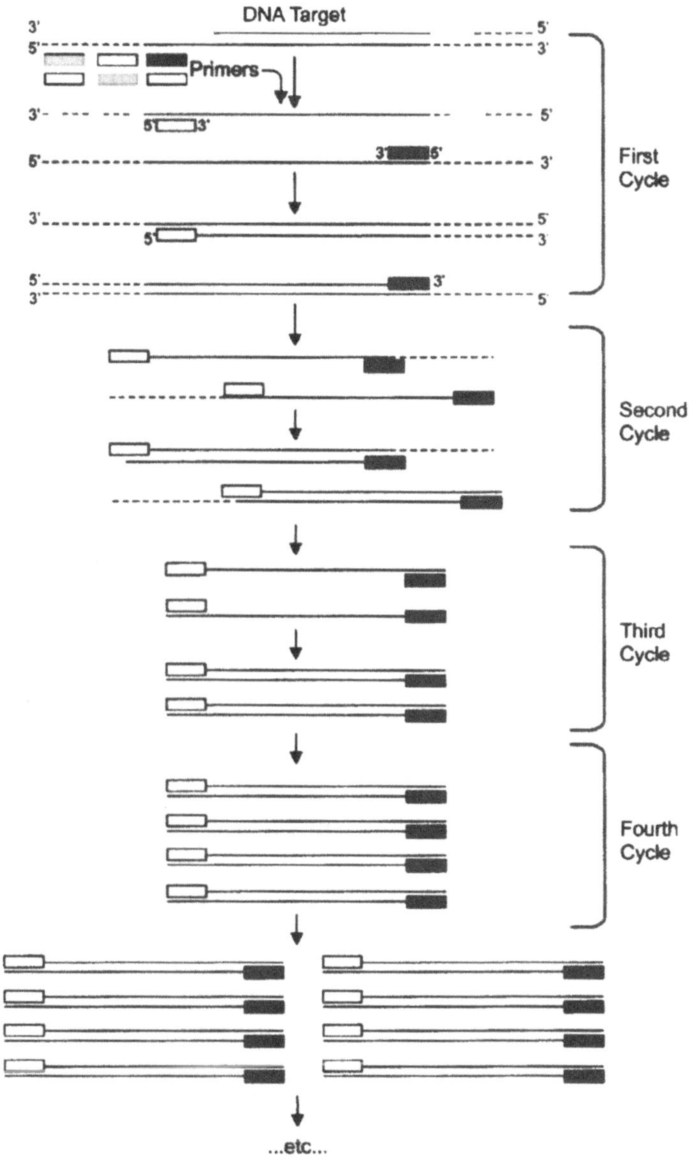

Figure 2 PCR amplification. Each PCR cycle consists of denaturation, annealing, and extension steps. Products of the first two cycles are more complex and of varying lengths (described in the text). After the third PCR cycle, the majority of the DNA copies are truncated at both ends. Amplification is exponential because the number of products doubles after each cycle is complete.

0.3–1 pM. This plateau may be influenced by several factors: availability of substrates (dNTP or primers), stability of reactants (enzymes, dNTP), end product inhibition due to pyrophosphate or duplex DNA formation, competition for reactants by nonspecific products (e.g., primer-dimer formations), reannealing of specific highly concentrated ($\geq 10^8$ M) complementary products, incomplete denaturation of products, and mispriming. In light of this information, it is essential to optimize the number of PCR cycles in order to limit the amplification of nonspecific and background products. On the other hand, running too few cycles gives a low product yield. As a rule, 25–30 cycles are recommended if the number of initial target DNA molecules is $\geq 3 \times 10^5$, 30–35 cycles for $\sim 1.5 \times 10^4$ initial molecules, and 40–45 cycles if the initial amount of DNA is less than 1×10^3. The products obtained at the end of the PCR run can be stored at −20°C until needed.

B. Increasing PCR Sensitivity and Specificity

Throughout the years, some modifications to the original PCR process have been devised to enhance its sensitivity and specificity. Touchdown PCR, designed to raise the sensitivity by using stringent conditions during the first cycles of PCR, is usually applied when the homology between the target sequence and the primers is unknown. In this technique the annealing temperature of the first cycle is set ~5°C above T_m. In subsequent cycles, this temperature is decreased by 1°C/cycle until the annealing temperature is ~5°C below T_m. This allows only targets with high homology to amplify in great numbers, because in the first few cycles only the primers with the highest homology can anneal and amplify owing to the high annealing temperature (8).

HOT START PCR increases PCR specificity (9). Although *Taq* polymerase is optimally active at 72°C, it may be mildly active at room temperature, making it possible to generate nonspecific products during experimental setup and at the beginning of thermal cycling when the temperature of the reaction mixture is below the annealing temperature. In Hot Start PCR, a key PCR element is retained until the last moment, thereby retarding DNA synthesis until conditions are optimal. Sometimes the PCR reaction mixture is set on ice and then placed into a preheated thermal cycler. Alternatively, the addition of *Taq* polymerase is delayed, sometimes until after the reaction mixture has reached the denaturation temperature, in order to limit the activity of *Taq* polymerase (10,11). Physical means such as a wax barrier can also be used to keep an important component (magnesium or polymerase) isolated or to keep reaction components (such as the template and buffer) separate.

C. PCR Reagents

In addition to the primers and the genetic material containing the target sequence, the PCR reaction mixture contains reagents that are essential for PCR. These reagents, with their associated buffers, include nucleotides (dNTP), magnesium, and the polymerase.

High-purity dNTPs (individual or mixed stocks) are commercially available. For PCR, the optimal dNTP concentration varies according to magnesium concentration, reaction stringency, primer concentration, length of the amplified products, and the number of PCR cycles. PCR is normally performed with a dNTP concentration of around 100 µM, resulting in an optimal balance among yield, specificity, and fidelity. The four dNTPs should be used at equivalent concentrations to avoid misincorporation errors. Usually, specificity and fidelity of PCR are increased by using lower dNTP concentrations than those recommended for Klenow-mediated PCR (12).

Magnesium plays a critical role in the process of DNA synthesis. Not only are magnesium ions (Mg^{2+}) essential for dNTP incorporation, but they also increase polymerase activity and the T_m of the double-stranded DNA (thereby affecting the primer–template interaction) and they affect primer annealing and the formation of primer-dimer and background products. It is therefore not surprising that too little Mg^{2+} results in low PCR product yields, whereas an excess of Mg^{2+} causes an accumulation of nonspecific products (13,14). The optimal [Mg^{2+}] depends on characteristics and concentrations of the primers and the template, but in a typical PCR containing 200 µM dNTP it falls between 1 and 1.5 mM.

Polymerases, like most other proteins, are generally thermolabile and become denatured at high temperatures. As described earlier, this rule does not apply to the commercially available *Taq* polymerase originally isolated from *Thermus aquaticus (Taq)*, a bacterium that naturally occurs in hot springs. The typical optimal concentration range for *Taq* polymerase is 1–2.5 units per 100 µL reaction when other parameters are optimized. If the enzyme concentration is too high, many nonspecific by-products can be accumulated in the reaction mixture. Too low a concentration leads to a low product yield.

III. REVERSE TRANSCRIPTION METHODOLOGY

A. Isolating Total RNA

The first step of RT-PCR is to isolate RNA from cells. To obtain optimal RNA yield, it is important to use an appropriate number of cells. If no information about RNA content for a specific cell type is available, it is recommended to start with no more than 3×10^6–4×10^6 cells. Depending on the RNA yield, it may be necessary to increase the number of cells used for RNA isolation. The cell sample to be used should be of the highest purity, i.e., no significant residual contaminants or other reagents present due to cell isolation and culture. RNA isolation is typically done using kits that contain all the necessary reagents and protocols. For human or rat PASMCs, we use the Qiagen RNeasy MiniKit® and follow the manufacturer's instructions.

The basic principles for RNA isolation briefly described here should apply for any cell type based on the kit specifications. First, a buffer added to the tube containing the cells disrupts the cell membranes. The mixture is incubated on ice for 5 min to allow cell lysis and release of cytoplasmic material. Cellular debris is concentrated by centrifugation and discarded. The supernatant containing cytoplasmic material, including mRNA, is collected into a microtube and treated with a premixed β-mercaptoethanol-supplemented Tris buffer solution and 96–100% ethanol before being applied to a RNeasy minicolumn. The minicolumn assembly is then centrifuged to allow RNA and DNA to bind the column's beads, and the solution that is ejected from the column is discarded. The column is washed again with a buffer, and a second centrifugation gets rid of impurities and proteins that may have been stuck among the column's beads. The column is then treated with DNase I, followed by a wash with an ethanol-supplemented buffer. The latter step eliminates DNA, and what remains will be pure RNA (including mRNA). RNase-free water added to the column releases the RNA from the beads, and this solution can be collected in a tube by centrifugation of the column. The RNA should be immediately stored at −70°C to prevent degradation.

The concentration of RNA (diluted with RNase-free water) is determined by measuring the absorbance at 260 nm (A_{260}) in a spectrophotometer. An absorbance of 1 unit at 260 nm is equivalent to 40 μg/mL of RNA described by the formula: Concentration of RNA sample = $A_{260} \times 40 \times$ dilution factor. The A_{260}/A_{280} ratio used to calculate the purity of RNA is influenced by pH. Therefore, RNA purity (absorbance at A_{260} and A_{280}) should be estimated using a Tris-HCl buffer (pH 7.5); the A_{260}/A_{280} ratio of pure RNA is ~1.9–2.1.

RNase is ubiquitous in nature. Therefore, care should be taken when handling RNA to avoid contamination of the sample with potential RNase-containing material, which can quickly degrade RNA products into a useless solution. One common mistake is to measure RNA concentration in contaminated cuvettes. The RNA in the cuvette is degraded rapidly before absorbance, giving a reading that is not representative of the true RNA concentration. Single-use, sterile, RNase-free, disposable cuvettes are best. If disposable cuvettes are not available, reusable cuvettes should be washed thoroughly with a solution containing 0.1 M NaOH and 1 mM EDTA in RNase-free water.

The RNA isolated with the above technique represents the total RNA of the cell. Generally, mRNA makes up only a small percentage of total RNA; significant amounts of other types of RNA (tRNA, rRNA) are also present and can therefore contaminate the sample. Because even the smallest contamination can alter or nullify the results of a study, other means must be applied to avoid the consequence of "non-mRNA" contaminants. These are discussed in greater detail in the following section.

B. Reverse Transcription

To screen for ion channel mRNA expression, the ability to detect and analyze mRNA is of critical importance. Because RNA is generally present in low abundance in the cells, the methods used for its detection and analysis must be extremely sensitive. Amplifying RNA would ease this limitation (15,16). However, because RNA cannot be directly amplified by PCR, a DNA surrogate for RNA is needed for this purpose. The concept of making a complementary DNA (cDNA) strand from RNA was introduced several years ago. This technique is the exact reverse of RNA transcription, hence the name "reverse transcription." The resulting cDNA from this process can be used in a process known as RT-PCR. RT-PCR is the most sensitive technique for mRNA detection and quantification currently available, being more sensitive and easier to perform than Northern blot, RNase protection assay, in situ hybridization, and S1 nuclease assay (17–19).

In addition to its use in detecting the transcription of a specific gene into mRNA, RT-PCR can also suggest how active the gene is in a cell population. RT-PCR of the unknown mRNA is performed alongside that of standardized samples with known mRNA amounts; comparing the results identifies how much mRNA is being produced by the gene. This technique is especially useful in determining how certain genetic manipulation or modification can up- or downregulate expression of a specific gene. RT-PCR is also used in obtaining full-length cDNA, homologous cDNA, and differentially expressed cDNA, and it has made possible in vitro cloning of DNA molecules. Furthermore, RT-PCR using cDNA allows for the elimination of introns, leaving only the functional or transcriptional parts of the genes for analysis.

As with RNA isolation, successful RT-PCR is dependent on purity of the sample. Contamination can occur during the production of the cDNA or during the collection of cDNA for subsequent PCR (only a fraction of the cDNA is used for PCR). Although sterile practice can help prevent contamination, performing the entire PCR (cDNA production and amplification) in one step is more efficient, especially when a large number of samples must be processed. Specially devised commercial kits are available for this purpose. The following section describes the steps involved in RT-PCR.

Generating cDNA from mRNA Using Reverse Transcription

Experimentally, reverse transcription is accomplished using a naturally occurring commercially available enzyme isolated from Moloney murine leukemia virus (MMLV) or avian myeloblastosis virus (AMV). This enzyme acts similarly to DNA polymerase, except that it uses RNA as a template instead of DNA. Reverse transcriptase (RTase) is an RNA-dependent DNA polymerase that uses single-stranded RNA as a template to synthesize cDNA. AMV reverse transcriptase possesses both DNA endonuclease and ribonuclease H (RNase H) activity and is therefore specific for RNA–DNA heteroduplexes. MMLV reverse transcriptase does not possess DNA endonuclease activity and presents lower RNase H activity, making it particularly useful in the production of full-length copies of large mRNA. Commercially modified RTase enzymes are now available that can serve specific purposes with more efficiency (20–23).

Like DNA polymerase, RTase needs an mRNA-complementary primer to extend the mRNA sequence. The primer that is used is generally a generic sequence or a random hexamer because most eukaryotic mRNAs share a poly-A sequence at their 3′ end. If any mRNA is present, the reverse transcriptase and primer will anneal to the mRNA and transcribe cDNA. The oligo(dT) primer first binds to the poly-A tail of the RNA that serves as the template (Fig. 3). Synthesis of a single-stranded cDNA proceeds to the 5′ end of the template. The resulting product is a DNA–RNA hybrid. Treatment with an alkali selectively degrades the RNA strand, leaving a single-stranded DNA with a hairpin loop at its 3′ end. The DNA polymerase uses this hairpin loop as primer to synthesize a double-stranded cDNA. The loop of the hairpin can subsequently be cleaved by a nuclease specific for single-stranded DNA. At this point, it is recommended that the cDNA samples be treated with RNase H to eliminate all residual RNA. The final cDNA product should be stored at −20°C until it is used for PCR-based amplification. Targeting specific sequences of this cDNA, PCR results will indicate if the mRNA for the targeted genes was present in the total RNA sample.

Primer-Specific cDNA Synthesis

As stated earlier, mRNA constitutes only a small percentage of the cytoplasmic total RNA, with the majority of the remainder of the RNA comprising either rRNA or tRNA. Performing RT-PCR on total RNA without the ability to target mRNA specifically would lead to crowding of the resulting cDNA library by cDNA derived from rRNA and tRNA. There are a few ways to resolve this issue (Fig. 4). The poly-A tail at the 3′ end ("polyadenylated") of most eukaryotic mRNAs can be used as a specifying tag for RT-PCR because a poly-T sequence [oligo(dT) primer] would be complementary to any poly-A region. Targeting the polyadenylated region, oligo(dT) primers bypasses all the other RNA types, and the resulting cDNA mainly represents mRNA. Random hexamers and gene-specific primers can also be used to prime cDNA synthesis. Random hexamers are nonspecific and prime the cDNA synthesis of nonpolyadenylated tRNA and rRNA. Random primers are the least specific, because they anneal to numerous positions along the whole transcript and generate short partial-length cDNA. This method is used to generate cDNA from RNA that reverse transcriptase cannot copy because of secondary structure or the presence of pause sites (2,15). In general, gene-specific primers are used to

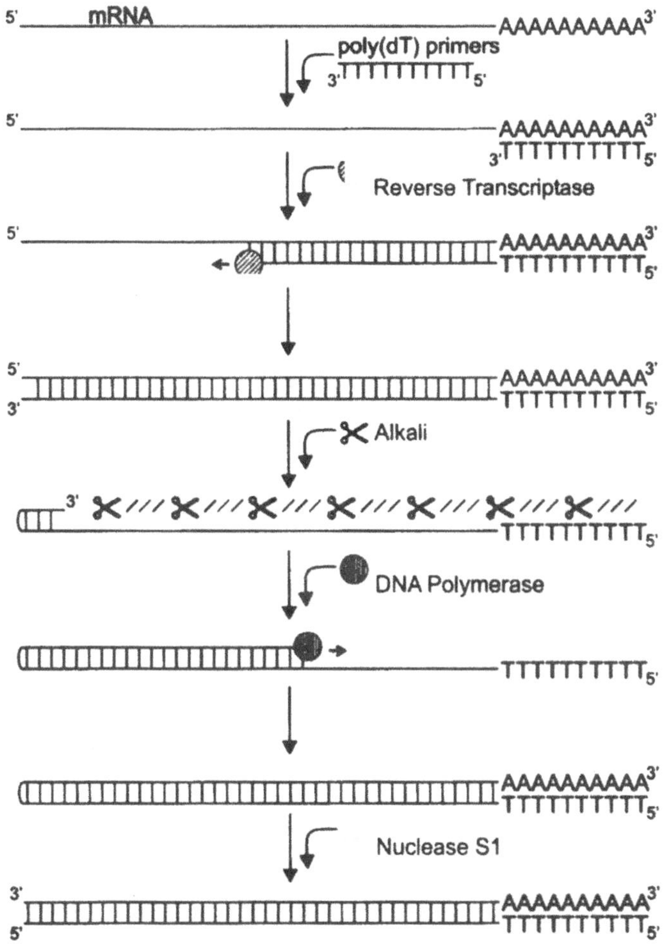

Figure 3 Synthesis of cDNA from mRNA. The oligo poly(dT) primer hybridizes to the poly-A tail of the mRNA. Reverse transcriptase attaches to the 3′ end of the poly(dT) and uses the mRNA molecule as a template to synthesize a cDNA copy. The resulting single-stranded complementary DNA chain terminates at the 5′ end of the template, producing a DNA–RNA hybrid. Alkali treatment of the hybrid selectively degrades the mRNA, leaving a single- stranded DNA with a 3′ hairpin loop. The DNA polymerase uses this hairpin loop as a primer in order to proceed with nucleotide incorporation. Single-stranded DNA specific nuclease S1 treatment cleaves the hairpin loop, leaving the double-stranded cDNA product.

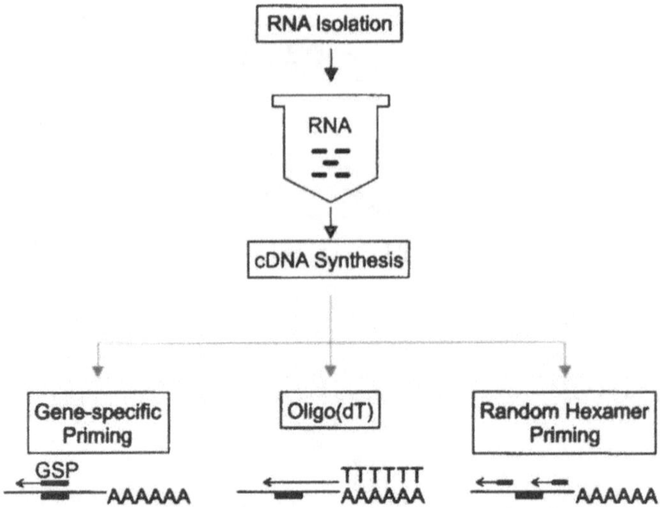

Figure 4 Priming cDNA synthesis in RT-PCR. The RT reaction can be primed with gene-specific primers (GSP), oligo(dT), or random hexamer primers. Advantages and disadvantages of each are provided in the text.

initiate the RT step. These primers are antisense oligonucleotides that anneal only to a specific target RNA sequence (usually an mRNA) (24) and are individually designed for each experiment to satisfy specific requirements.

The ratio of primers to RNA must be defined empirically for each RNA preparation to optimize cDNA production. In a 20 μL final volume, the initial concentration of random primers, oligo(dT) primers, and gene-specific primers used in the RT step should be 50–250 ng, 0.5 μg, and 1 pmol, respectively (25). Although these quantities may serve as guidelines, it is always appropriate for the user to determine the smallest amount of primers that can be used to give the best results, because primer excess can give more secondary amplified products, thereby confusing the results.

IV. PRIMERS

Primers are essential for polymerase attachment to the target DNA sequence and subsequent duplication. For each PCR reaction, generally one pair of primers complementary to the 3′ ends of the target sequences is used. Primers must be designed to flank the target sequence so that the full desired sequence is amplified. Ideally, primers should be designed so that they bind only to unique complementary sequences on the target DNA. In addition to the sequence, the proper annealing temperature is key to primer efficiency.

A. Characteristics of Primers

In general, the primers used in PCR are synthetic oligonucleotides 18–24 bases long, a size that allows for sequence distinctiveness, specificity of binding, and decreased mismatching (26). Primer specificity does not increase beyond the 24 nucleotide size. In fact, longer primers may anneal more slowly and can often hybridize with mismatches, leading to a lower PCR product yield.

The structural sequence of each primer is an important issue. Guanine (G) and cytosine (C) form three hydrogen bonds between them, making them more cohesive than adenine (A) and thymidine (T), which form only two. The triple G–C bonds are more stable than the double A–T bond. Also, a greater number of G–C bonds also affect the T_m of the primer, with more energy (heat) required to break three hydrogen bonds vs. two. Therefore, avoiding G–C combinations in the 3′ end of the primer but not at its 5′ terminus or near its center can increase primer stability with the DNA target (27).

Mismatches at the 3′ end of the primer also should be avoided. The last five nucleotides on the 3′ end should contain at least three consecutive A's (or T's), and the last 3′ nucleotide must anneal to the template for the polymerase to catalyze the extension (28). The primers should be designed to have an approximately equal number of each of the four bases (A, T, C, G), avoiding regions of unusual sequence homology such as stretches of polypurines, polypyrimidines, or repetitive motifs. Primers with significant secondary structure can destabilize primer annealing and should be avoided. Obviously, the primer sequence should be complementary to a reasonably unique region on the DNA target, because primers that anneal to multiple regions of the target will neither identify the targeted sequence nor extend correctly. Also, the primers should not be complementary, especially in their 3′ regions, in order to reduce the incidence of primer-dimer formation

For optimal PCR specificity, primer concentration should be between 0.1 and 0.5 μM. A higher concentration of primers may lead to amplification of nonspecific products (29). Commercially produced custom-lyophilized primers, when reconstituted in alkaline Tris-HCl/EDTA buffer to a final concentration of 10 μM, can be stored stably at −20°C for up to 6 months. Unreconstituted lyophilized primers can be stored for up to 1 year at the same temperature.

B. Degenerate and Nested Primers

A degenerate primer is a mixture of primers with a similar base sequence but with variation in at least one position. This type of primer may be used when its nucleotide sequence is deduced from a gene's amino acid sequence or when one is scanning for new members of a highly homologous gene family.

At sites where nucleotide identity can vary, deoxyinosine is used in the degenerate primer. However, because deoxyinosine can couple with all the bases and will lower the annealing temperature, it should not be included among the bases at the 3′ end of the primers, so as to prevent random annealing to other sites. Because annealing temperature is lowered by degenerate primers, the Hot Start PCR protocol is often recommended. In this protocol, the polymerase is added manually after the initial denaturation step has been completed, thereby preventing the extension of nonspecifically annealed primers.

Nested primers can be used to reduce the amplification of the wrong products. In this scenario, the products of an initial PCR amplification are used in a second PCR amplification in which one or both primers are located internally with respect to the primers of the first PCR. There is little chance that the wrong products contain sequences capable of hybridizing with a second primer set. This allows selective amplification of the sought-after DNA. As discussed in Chapter 32 of this monograph, nested primers can be used to more efficiently amplify specific target DNA when only a limited amount of genetic material is available at the start, as is the case for single-cell RT-PCR.

C. Data Mining and Primer Design

Designing primers requires knowledge of the sequence (either nucleotides or amino acids) of the gene of interest. Because many genes have been cloned, their sequences are available in databases. Although there are other sources, NIH-sponsored GenBank is likely the most comprehensive database of DNA and protein sequence information from various species, including humans, primates, and rodents.

Currently, computer software is used for primer design; Table 2 lists some of the most popular software programs. Most programs require the

Table 2 Computer Software Programs Available for Primer Design

Oligo (National Biosciences, Inc.)
RightPrimer (BioDisk Software)
PrimerGen
Primer (Stanford) Sun Sparcstation only
Primer (Whitehead) Unix, Vms
Primer 3 (http://www-genome.wi.mit.edu/cgi-bin/primer/primer3_www.cgi)
Amplify Bill Engels (Macintosh only)
PrimerDesign 1.04
PC-Rare by R.Griffais
Primer Design
CODEHOP
NetPrimer (PREMIER Biosoft International)

specification of various design criteria such as the minimum melting temperature, the desired length, and the GC content. Based on these criteria, the program evaluates all theoretically possible primers for the target sequence in question and identifies and eliminates those that have tendencies for self-complementarity, secondary priming sites, restriction sites, and formation of loops, secondary structures, or primer-dimers. It is important to remember that the resulting primers were designed without regard to other genes present in the organism's gene pool, i.e., the primers may not be unique to only the target gene, leading to a vast number of nonspecific PCR products. The specificity of these primers for all other genes must be confirmed before performing the PCR using BLAST software, which screens the complementarity of each resulting primer with all the genes registered in GenBank. For more technologically advanced users, virtual PCR software can run the resulting primers in a simulated PCR run to anticipate the resulting products. An example of the primers we have used to successfully identify Ca^{2+}-activated K^+ channel (K_{Ca}) channel subunits in human PASMCs [and its glyceraldehyde-3-phosphate dehydrogenase (GAPDH) control] is provided in Table 3. The full sequence for many genes, such as that encoding for the K_{Ca} α and β subunits, can be accessed using the gene-specific Genbank accession numbers.

V. VISUALIZATION AND QUANTIFICATION OF THE RT-PCR PRODUCTS

Once PCR is finished, microliter aliquots of PCR products are loaded onto agarose gels for electrophoresis. After electrophoretic migration, the amplified cDNA bands are visualized by ethidium bromide staining, and band size is determined using a standard DNA ladder marker. An invariant internal control mRNA (e.g., GAPDH) is used to semiquantify the PCR products. The net intensity of the cDNA bands can then be measured by a variety of electrophoresis documentation software systems. For quantification, the net intensity is normalized to the net intensity of the invariant control. A sample gel is shown in Fig. 5 for the human maxi-K_{Ca} channel α and β subunits. In this example from human PASMCs, we can clearly identify the mRNA corresponding to the sole pore-forming $\alpha 1$ subunit and two ($\beta 3$, $\beta 4$) of the four regulatory β subunits that form these channels. All subunits are present in human brain tissue. The GAPDH control bonds do not vary significantly in intensity, indicating that there were no problems with isolation of mRNA, PCR, or loading of the samples onto the gel, which could have resulted in altered sample yields.

To quantify the mRNA expression, the intensity of the band corresponding to the gene of interest is normalized to the intensity of the band of the internal control. This normalization can be done only if the intensity of the control is constant in all the samples. Normalization to the invariant

Table 3 Oligonucleotide Sequences of the Primers Used for Screening RT-PCR for Maxi-K_{Ca} Channel Subunits

Name (accession No.)[a]	Size (bp)	Sense/antisense sequence	Location (nt)	Chromosome
MaxiK$_{Ca}$-α1	444	5′-CTACTGGGATGTTTCACTGGTGT-3′	2210–2232	10q22
(NM-002247)		5′-TGCTGTCATCAAACTGCATA-3′	2634–2653	
MaxiK$_{Ca}$-β1	363	5′-TCTACTGCTTCTCCGCAC-3′	557–574	5q34
(NM-004137)		5′-GAGCAGGCAATGACTTCA-3′	902–919	
MaxiK$_{Ca}$-β2	449	5′-GGGACTGGCTATGATGGT-3′	502–519	3q26.2–q27.1
(NM-005832)		5′-GTGAATGGAACAGCACGTTG-3	931–950	
MaxiK$_{Ca}$-β3	351	5′-GCTCAACAGTGCTCTGGACA-3′	1013–1032	3q26.3–q27.1
(NM-014407)		5′-TGGCCACCGTCTTAAGATTT-3′	1344–1363	
MaxiK$_{Ca}$-β4	300	5′-CTGAGTCCAACTCTAGGGCG-3′	612–631	12q14.1–q15
(NM-014505)		5′-TGGTCAGGACCACAATGAGA-3′	892–911	
GAPDH[b]	714	5'-AGGGTCTCTCTCTTCCTCTT-3'	421–442	
		5′-GAGCCAAAAGGGTCATCATCTC-3′	1113–1134	

[a]GenBank accession numbers used to obtain mRNA sequences that were used for primer design.
[b]GAPDH used as positive internal control.

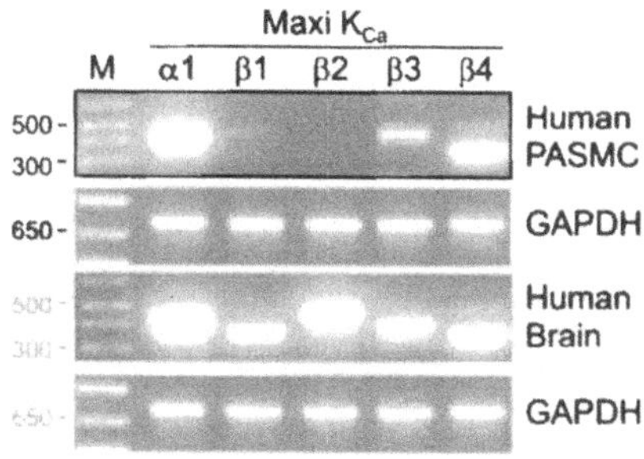

Figure 5 Expression of maxi-K_{Ca} channel subunit mRNA in human PASMCs and brain. Bands in a 1.5% agarose gel represent the mRNA transcription of α and β subunits of maxi-K_{Ca}. RT-PCR products from human brain cells, as well as GAPDH, were used as positive controls. M, 1 kb DNA ladder marker.

control nullifies any changes in band intensity that might be attributed to tube-to-tube variations caused by variable pipetting, enzymatic efficiency, or RNA quality. This gene/control ratio represents the relative mRNA expression for the gene(s) in question and can be used to compare samples for mRNA expression. This ratio does not, however, reflect the absolute number of mRNA copies present in each sample. Absolute quantification of mRNA expression can be done using competitive RT-PCR, where the target specimen is coamplified with known dilutions of a synthetic RNA (sRNA) with an identical but truncated sequence. The shorter sequence allows for it to be distinguished from the native mRNA by electrophoresis. An sRNA concentration–intensity curve is then generated from which one can deduce the concentration of native mRNA based on its band intensity.

VI. REAL-TIME PCR

Real-time PCR, although expensive, combines the best features of relative and competitive RT-PCR for easy yet precise quantification of mRNA expression (30). Real-time PCR allows for the quantification of the PCR products for each sample at the end of every cycle, a process that is laborious if basic RT-PCR is used (31,32). Automated real-time PCR systems take advantage of our ability to detect and quantify fluorescent or UV light. The basic PCR steps are still used for this process. The only difference is that the double-stranded DNA is conjugated with either a fluorescent agent (such as SYBR Green) or a UV transilluminator (such as ethidium bromide). Once bound to the DNA, these agents can be excited and their photonic emission during the transition from the excited to resting states can be detected and quantified. Using a thermal cycler coupled to an excitatory light source and an optical detection device, it is possible to measure the fluorescence in real time during each cycle of the PCR. However, because these agents can bind to any double-stranded DNA in the reaction mixture (not just the one of interest), it is a nonspecific approach that will result in overestimation of mRNA concentration unless well-designed primers are used.

For more complex experiments, even primer design may not suffice, and one must rely on fluorescence resonance energy transfer (FRET) properties of fluorophores. FRET is a distance-dependent interaction between the electronic excited states of two dye molecules in which excitation is transferred from a donor molecule to an acceptor molecule *without emission of a photon*. In one scenario, Taqman oligonucleotide probes labeled with a fluorescent dye and a quenching dye on the 5′ and 3′ ends, respectively, are allowed to hybridize to internal regions of the PCR products. As long as the probe containing the fluorescent and quenching dyes is intact, no light will be emitted upon light excitation. However, during PCR, the 5′ exonuclease of the DNA polymerase will cleave the probe as the latter travels along the DNA strand, destabilizing the probe and the resonance transfer between the dye molecules and causing fluorescence to be emitted by the fluorophore. This fluorescence is detected by the optical system and is reported as the production of one PCR product. As more and more PCR products are produced, the intensity of the fluorescent light will increase in proportion to the rate of probe cleavage. Molecular beacons are labeled like Taqman probes and are complementary to internal sequences of the PCR products. As long as they remain bound to the primers, these beacons will not fluoresce. However, during duplication, the beacons are displaced into solution, where they form hairpin structures (bringing the dyes closer together) and, due to FRET, they are nonfluorescent. Each time the beacon hairpins are broken during the PCR cycle, light is emitted because the dyes are no longer in close proximity, and they rebind the target sequences on the PCR product, thereby emitting light.

VII. USEFUL HINTS AND REMINDERS

1. Higher RT incubation temperatures increase product yield but should be adjusted according to the type of primer used.
2. Treating RNA samples with DNase-I before continuing with RT-PCR removes contaminating genomic DNA. After DNase I digestion, the RNA sample should be treated with EDTA to chelate Mg^{2+} and prevent RNA hydrolysis at high temperatures. Treatment of cDNA with RNase-H after the RT step and prior to performing PCR removes any contaminating RNA from the mixture that might interfere with primer annealing.

3. When working with eukaryotic mRNA, it is better to use primers derived from separate exons so that shorter PCR products derived from the target gene cDNA can be distinguished from larger products originating from contaminating genomic DNA.
4. RNase inhibitors added to RT mixtures improve cDNA yield by protecting RNA against degradation by bacterial RNase. Because they are ineffective for skin RNase, the user should wear gloves and a facial mask and use autoclaved tubes and solutions while working with RNA.
5. In RT-PCR, [dNTP] should not exceed 0.2 mM in order to decrease mutation frequency.
6. Because it plays a critical role in different PCR steps, the free [Mg^{2+}] in the final solution should be maintained at ~2 mM.
7. Never run more PCR cycles than necessary.

VIII. SUMMARY

RT-PCR is a powerful, convenient, and sensitive way to determine whether a gene is transcribed in a tissue or cell. Regular RT-PCR is an excellent tool for determining qualitative but not quantitative differences in gene transcription. However, real-time PCR can be used to determine quantitative differences. Although Western blotting and immunocytochemistry should be used to support PCR results in terms of gene expression, RT-PCR (including single-cell RT-PCR and real-time PCR) is an excellent approach in qualifying gene expression.

ACKNOWLEDGMENTS

This work was supported by grants HL 64945, HL 54043, HL 69758, HL 66012, and HL 66941 from the National Heart, Lung, and Blood Institute of the National Institutes of Health.

REFERENCES

1. Mullis KB, Faloona F. Specific synthesis of DNA in vitro via a polymerase-catalyzed chain reaction. Methods Enzymol 1987; 155:335–350.
2. Innis MA, Gelfand DH, Sinsky JJ, White TJ. PCR Protocols—A Guide to Methods and Applications. San Diego, CA: Academic Press, 1990.
3. Saiki RK, Gelfand DH, Stoffel S, Sharf SJ, Higuchi R, Horn GT, Mullis KB, Erlich HA. Primer-directed enzymatic amplification of DNA with a thermostable DNA polymerase. Science 1988; 239:487–491.
4. McPherson MJ, Quirke P and Taylor GR, PCR: A Pratical Approach. Oxford: Oxford University Press, 1991.

5. Suggs SV, Wallace RB, Hirose T, Kawashima EH, Itakura K. Use of synthetic oligonucleotides as hybridization probes: isolation of cloned cDNA sequences for human β_2-microglobulin. Proc Natl Acad Sci USA 1981; 76:6613–6617.
6. Sambrook J, Fritsch EF, Maniatis T. Molecular Cloning: A Laboratory Manual. 2nd ed. NY: Cold Spring Harbor, Laboratory Press., Cold Spring Harbor 1989.
7. Wu DY, Ugozzoli L, Pal BK, Qian J, Wallace RB. The effect of temperature and oligonucleotide primer length on the specificity and efficiency of amplification by the polymerase chain reaction. DNA Cell Biol 1991; 10:233–238.
8. Don RH, Cox PT, Wainwright BJ, Baker K, Mattick JS. 'Touchdown' PCR to circumvent spurious priming during gene amplification. Nucleic Acids Res 1991; 19:4008.
9. Chou Q, Russell M, Birch DE, Raymond J, Bloch W. Prevention of pre-PCR mispriming and primer dimerization improves low-copy-number amplifications. Nucleic Acids Res 1992; 20:1717–1723.
10. Li H, Cui X, Arnheim N. Direct electrophoretic detection of the allelic state of single DNA molecules in human sperm by using the polymerase chain reaction. Proc Natl Acad Sci USA 1990; 87:4580–4584.
11. Westfall B, Sitaraman K, Solus J, Hughes J, Rashtchian A. Improved PCR specificity and yield with Platinum® *Taq* DNA polymerase. Focus 1997; 19:46–47.
12. Cline J, Braman JC, Hogrefe HH. PCR fidelity of *Pfu* DNA polymerase and other thermostable DNA polymerases. Nucleic Acids Res 1996; 24:3546–3551.
13. Eckert KA, Kunkel TA. High fidelity DNA synthesis by the *Thermus aquaticus* DNA polymerase. Nucleic Acids Res 1990; 18:3739–3744.
14. Williams JF. Optimization strategies for the polymerase chain reaction. Biotechniques 1989; 7:762–769.
15. Dieffenbach CW, Dveksler GS. PCR Primers: A Laboratory Manual. NY: Cold Spring Harbor Laboratory Press, Cold Spring Harbor, 1995.
16. Siebert PD, Larrick JW. Competitive PCR. Nature 1992; 359:557–558.
17. Liang P, Pardee AB. Differential display. A general protocol. Mol Biotechnol 1998; 10:261–267.
18. Foley KP, Leonard MW, Engel JD. Quantization of RNA using the polymerase chain reaction. Trends Gen 1993; 9:380–385.
19. Mocharla H, Mocharla R, Hoges ME. Coupled reverse transcription-polymerase chain reaction (RT-PCR) as a sensitive and rapid method for isozyme genotyping. Gene 1990; 93:271–275.
20. Gerard GF, D'Alessio JM, Kotewicz ML. cDNA synthesis by cloned Moloney murine leukemia virus reverse transcriptase lacking RNase H activity. Focus 1989; 11:66–68.
21. Schwabe W, Lee JE, Nathan M, Xu RH, Sitaraman K, Smith M, Potter RJ, Rosenthal K, Rashtchian A, Gerard GF. Thermoscript® RT, a new avain reverse transcriptase for high-temperature cDNA synthesis to improve RT-PCR. Focus 1998; 20:30–33.
22. Schuster DM, Darfler M, Lee JE, Rashtchian A. Improved sensitivity and specificity of RT-PCR. Focus 1998; 20:34–35.
23. Nathan M, Mertz LM, Fox DK. Optimizing long RT-PCR. Focus 1995; 17: 78–80.

24. Lee EH, Sitaraman K, Schuster D, Rashtchian A. A highly sensitive method for one-step amplification of RNA by polymerase chain reaction. Focus 1997; 19:39–42.
25. Frohman MA, Dush MK, Martin GR. Rapid production of full-length cDNAs from rare transcripts: amplification using a single gene-specific oligonucleotide primer. Proc Natl Acad Sci USA 1988; 85:8998–9002.
26. Mullis KB. The unusual origin of the polymerase chain reaction. Sci Am 1990; 262:56–61, 64–65.
27. Lear W, McDonel M, Kashyap S, Boer P. Random primer p(dN)6-digoxigenin labeling for quantization of mRNA by Q-RT-PCR and ELISA. Biotechniques 1995; 18:78–84.
28. Kwok S, Kellogg DE, McKinney N, Spasic D, Goda L, Levenson C, Sinsky J. Effects of primer-template mismatches on the polymerase chain reaction: human immunodeficiency virus type 1 model studies. Nucleic Acids Res 1990; 18:999–1005.
29. White BA. PCR Protocols, Current Methods and Applications. Totowa, NJ: Humana Press, 1993.
30. Heid CA, Stevens J, Livak KJ, Williams PM. Real time quantitative PCR. Genome Res 1996; 6:986–994.
31. Holland PM, Abramson RD, Watson R, Gelfand DH. Detection of specific polymerase chain reaction product by utilizing the $5'\rightarrow3'$ exonuclease activity of *Thermus aquaticus* DNA polymerase. Proc Natl Acad Sci USA 1991; 88:7276–7280.
32. Tyagi S, Bratu DP, Kramer FR. Multicolor molecular beacons for allele discrimination. Nature Biotechnol 1998; 16:49–53.

36

Practical Aspects of Confocal Imaging of Ca^{2+} Sparks and Cytoplasmic Ca^{2+} Concentration

James S. K. Sham and Christopher Ian Spencer
Johns Hopkins School of Medicine, Baltimore, Maryland, U.S.A.

I. INTRODUCTION

In the past two decades, the understanding of intracellular Ca^{2+} homeostasis has advanced at an unprecedented pace, owing to the revolutionary discovery of Ca^{2+}-sensitive fluorescence indicator dyes and the tremendous progress in cell imaging techniques. Researchers are now able to study subcelullar Ca^{2+} regulation by resolving minute Ca^{2+} signals such as Ca^{2+} sparklets at the submicrometer level (1) as well as imaging $[Ca^{2+}]$ within intracellular organelles such as mitochondria and sarcoplasmic/endoplasmic reticulum (2–4). These technological breakthroughs allow us to begin to appreciate how the local $[Ca^{2+}]$ conveys target-specific messages in an amplitude- and frequency-dependent manner (5) and how these local processes blend into the mosaic of cytosolic Ca^{2+} regulation and gene expression (6–9). The local Ca^{2+} release event or "Ca^{2+} spark" that originates from a cluster of ryanodine receptors (RyRs) in the sarcoplasmic reticulum (SR) is one of the most thoroughly studied local Ca^{2+} events. It is the elementary event underlying global Ca^{2+} transients in striated muscles and an important modulator of membrane potential in smooth muscles. Ca^{2+} sparks have been recently identified and characterized in pulmonary arterial smooth muscle cells (10–14). However, most of their physiological functions in the regulation of pulmonary vascular reactivity are yet to be determined. In this chapter, we provide an introduction to Ca^{2+} spark measurement by discussing (1) the general aspects of Ca^{2+} fluorescent indicator dyes and their calibration, (2) the detection of Ca^{2+} sparks using laser scanning confocal microscopy, and (3) the basic analysis of Ca^{2+} spark properties. We hope this will lead to wider application of the technique in the field of pulmonary circulation.

II. GENERAL ASPECTS OF Ca^{2+} MEASUREMENT

A. Ca^{2+} Fluorescent Indicator Dyes

Since the creation of the archetypal indicator Quin-2 by Roger Tsien (15), more than 30 different Ca^{2+} fluorescent indicator dyes have become available. The synthetic approach that led to the present Ca^{2+} indicator dyes began with an effort to rationally design Ca^{2+} chelating molecules based on the tetracarboxylate structure of EGTA by eliminating its undesirable features of pH dependence and the slow on and off rate for Ca^{2+} ions and by incorporating fluorophores of different excitation and emission properties (15,16). The commonly used Ca^{2+} fluorescent indicator dyes can be divided into two classes, ratiometric indicators and single-wavelength indicators. Ratiometric indicators such as fura-2 and indo-1 have different specific absorption or emission spectra for the Ca^{2+}-free and Ca^{2+}-bound forms. For example, binding of Ca^{2+} ion by indo-1 causes a wavelength shift in the emission maximum from 485 nm to 410 nm when the dye is excited at 340 nm; whereas Ca^{2+} binding by fura-2 shifts the absorption maxima from 362 nm to 335 nm without significant change in the emission maxima at 510 nm. By measuring fluorescence intensity at the two emission wavelengths of indo-1 or the emission signals generated by the two excitation wavelengths of fura-2, a ratio can be obtained. The use of ratiometric measurement is reliable for calibration and minimizes many Ca^{2+}-independent artifacts such as photobleaching and leaking of dyes because most of these artifacts have an equivalent influence on both fluorescence signals. However, most ratiometric indicators require excitation in the UV range, which can cause significant autofluorescence and photodamage in some biological preparations, and they are also less popular for confocal imaging owing to the cost of UV lasers.

Single-wavelength indicators, such as fluo-3, fluo-4, rhod-2, Calcium Green, Calcium Orange, Calcium Crimson, and Oregon Green 488 BAPTA, use visible light for excitation, which is less liable to activate cellular autofluorescence and requires less stringent optical components. Binding of Ca^{2+} ions to these indicators causes an increase in the emission intensity without significant alteration in the spectral maxima. The emission intensity is proportional to the concentration of the Ca^{2+}-bound form of the indicator, which is in equilibrium with free Ca^{2+} according to the law of mass action. However, because measurement is made at a single wavelength, it is subject to Ca^{2+}-independent artifacts such as photobleaching or dye leakage, changes in cell thickness, and movement artifacts due to cell contraction. Some researchers circumvent this problem by simultaneously loading the cells with fluo-3 and another visible-light excitation indicator, fura-red. Because the fluorescence intensity of fura-red decreases with Ca^{2+} binding (excitation 488 nm and emission 660 nm), this double-dye procedure permits ratiometric measurement under laser scanning confocal microscopy (17). However, this application is limited by the much weaker fluorescence intensity of fura-red due to its low quantum efficiency and by the uncertainty of the distribution of indicators in the cellular compartments (18).

The selection of Ca^{2+} fluorescent indicators is usually based on practical considerations and physiological constraints. For example, fura-2 is most suitable for ratiometric Ca^{2+} imaging because a single wavelength of emitted light is collected through a single optical path, which guarantees exact spatial registration of the emission signals on the CCD camera. However, the temporal resolution is limited by the speed of the filter wheel or scanner for alternating excitation at two different wavelengths. On the other hand, indo-1 is more desirable for Ca^{2+} microfluorimetry because it is excited at one wavelength and two emission wavelengths can be recorded simultaneously with two photomultiplying tubes (PMTs). This provides continuous recording of Ca^{2+} transients essential for studying fast Ca^{2+} events such as cardiac excitation–contraction coupling. Special attention must also be paid to the binding affinity of fluorescent indicators and the $[Ca^{2+}]$ range of interest. As a general rule, the dissociation constant (K_D) of the indicator should approximately match the mean $[Ca^{2+}]$ that is going to be measured. This ensures a maximal dynamic range for the measurement. Ratiometric and single-wavelength indicators of high and low Ca^{2+} affinity with K_D ranging from 100 nM to 300 μM are available for different applications. High-affinity indicators such as indo-1 and fura-2, which have a K_D for Ca^{2+} of 200–300 nM, are most suitable for the measurement of resting $[Ca^{2+}]$ and Ca^{2+} transients of moderate amplitude but are not reliable for large Ca^{2+} transients above 1 μM because of dye saturation. Moreover, when used at a concentration > 200 μM, these Ca^{2+} indicators tend to buffer changes in $[Ca^{2+}]_i$ due to their high Ca^{2+} affinity. Indicators of very low Ca^{2+} affinity, such as Mag-Fura-2, Mag-Indo-1, Oregon Green 488 BAPTA-5N, Fluo-5N, and Rhod-5N, through unreliable for measuring resting $[Ca^{2+}]$, are extremely useful for the measurement of a large Ca^{2+} rise in localized microdomains and of high $[Ca^{2+}]$ within organelles such as the endoplasmic/sarcoplasmic reticulum and for tracking fast kinetics of rapid Ca^{2+} events (2,19,20). Generally speaking, the visible wavelength indicators fluo-3 and fluo-4 are the most popular dyes for both global and local Ca^{2+} measurements using confocal microscopy because they have a K_D of about 1 μM, which is right at the physiological range; a high quantum efficiency to produce bright emission; a large in situ dynamic range; and a low propensity of compartmentation, and they can be conveniently excited by the 488 nm line of an argon laser (18). However, they are more subsceptible to photobleaching and tend to leak at higher temperature.

B. Loading Indicators

The commonly used Ca^{2+} indicator dyes are polycarboxylate anions, which cannot diffuse freely through the lipid bilayer cell membrane. Direct loading of cells with indicator can be achieved by intracellular dialysis through patch pipettes during electrophysiological experiments, by microinjections, or by membrane permeabilization. These approaches have the advantage of controlling precisely the concentration of the indicator dye in the cytosol (typically 50–100 μM) and avoiding the complication of intracellular compartmentalization because the indicator cannot pass through the membrane of subcellular organelles. However, these techniques are invasive, causing disturbance to membrane integrity and cytoplasmic constitutents, and are sometimes very labor-intensive and technically demanding.

On the other hand, cells can be conveniently loaded with the membrane-permeant AM ester form of indicators, in which the acetoxymethyl (AM) group is added by esterification to mask the negative charges of carboxyl groups to render the indicator uncharged and membrane-permeant (21). The indicators are converted to the membrane-impermeant and Ca^{2+}-sensitive form after entering the cells through hydrolysis by endogenous esterases, a process known as "deesterification." However, AM esters have very low water solubility (e.g., 0.11 μM for fura-2 AM at 25°C) (22), which limits the dye concentration and the rate of loading. Their apparent solubility can be improved and effective loading can be achieved by dissolving the AM ester in a dimethyl sulfoxide (DMSO) stock solution containing a nonionic surfactant Pluronic F-127 as a dispersing agent. Pluronic F-127 promotes sequestration of AM ester in a micellar form to prevent precipitation in the physiological loading solution, and the sequestered ester serves as a steady source to replenish dyes taken up by the cells. Depending on the loading conditions and cell type, up to hundreds of micromoles of indicator can be trapped and accumulated inside the cells.

The AM esters present a complication, however, because they can penetrate membranous organelles, such as mitochondria, endoplasmic or sacroplasmic reticulum, and nuclei by passive diffusion and active endocytosis and subsequently accumulate in these subcellular compartments because of the presence of organellar esterases. Such compartmentalization of indicators may compromise Ca^{2+} measurement by (1) underestimating the amplitude of cytosolic Ca^{2+} transient because indicator dye within the organelles is not responsive to the change in cytosolic $[Ca^{2+}]$ and (2) overestimating the resting $[Ca^{2+}]$ due to the usually higher $[Ca^{2+}]$ within organelles such as the endoplasmic or sarcoplasmic reticulum. The degree of compartmentalization varies among indicators. For example, indo-1 shows less compartmentalization than fura-2, and fluo-3 shows the least compartmentalization among the visible-wavelength indicators (18,23,24). Moreover, indicator accumulation in subcellular organelles is temperature-dependent result from the effect on endocytosis. Compartmentalization is significantly less when cells are loaded at room temperature compared to loading at 37°C (25).

Loaded indicators can leak through the cell membrane via organic anion transporters in a temperature-sensitive manner. Fluorescence of cytosolic indicators such as fluo-3 disappears dramatically (complete loss within 30 min) at 37°C, even though it is relatively stable at room temperature (18). It has been shown that inhibition of anion transporters with probenecid or sulfinpyrazone can prevent the loss of indicator at body temperature (18,26–28). Therefore, special attention must be paid on the experimental temperature, which may have a large impact on indicator localization and retention. It is interesting to note that some researchers have exploited the temperature dependence of dye loading and leakage to load indicators preferentially into mitochondria to study mitochondrial Ca^{2+} regulation (3,4).

As a practical example, reasonable loading of indo-1 and fluo-3 AM in pulmonary arterial smooth muscle cells (PASMCs) can be achieved by using the following procedures: (1) preparing a fresh 2.5–5 mM stock solution in dry DMSO containing 20% Pluronic F-127, (2) dispersing the indicator (~1:1000) into a physiological loading solution (e.g., Tyrode's solution or culture medium) to a final concentration of 5 μM, (3) incubating the cells in loading solution for 30 min at 23°C (in cases where the loading solution contains bicarbonate buffer, loading should be carried out under 21% O_2 and 5% CO_2), (4) washing the cells thoroughly with fresh solution to remove the extracellular indicator and (5) equilibrating the cells at room temperature for 15–30 min for deesterification. For confocal imaging experiments, because a large portion of out-of-focus fluorescence is rejected by the pinhole and basal fluo-3 fluorescence is low, a higher loading concentration of 10 μM and a longer loading period of 45 min are required to obtain a better signal-to-noise ratio.

C. Calibration

Quantitative determination of intracellular $[Ca^{2+}]$ requires accurate calibration of fluorescence signals. Detailed descriptions of the theory and full derivations of the equations are available in the original papers (29,30). Calibration of the fluorescence signal relies on the fact that fluorescence emission intensity is a linear function of the concentration of indicator in either its Ca^{2+}-bound or Ca^{2+}-free forms at any given wavelength (l), except the isosbestic wavelength (where ratiometric indicators are Ca^{2+}-insensitive). Therefore, fluorescence intensity, $F_{(l)}$, is given by

$$F_{(l)} = S_{(l)}\ [I_{(f)}] \qquad (1)$$

where $S_{(I)}$ is the fluorescence proportionality constant and $[I_{(f)}]$ is the concentration of indicator in form "f" (i.e., Ca^{2+}-bound or free). $[Ca^{2+}]$ can be derived from the fraction of the indicator in the Ca^{2+}-bound form at any given $[Ca^{2+}]$ based on a knowledge of the intensity of fluorescence that is obtained when all of the indicator is either Ca^{2+}-free or Ca^{2+}-saturated. For a non-ratiometric (single-wavelength) indicator that increases fluorescence emission on binding Ca^{2+},

$$[Ca^{2+}] = \frac{K_D(F - F_{min})}{F_{max} - F} \tag{2}$$

where K_D is the dissociation constant of the Ca^{2+}–dye complex, F is fluorescence emission intensity, and the subscripts denote the minimal fluorescence of free dye and maximal fluorescence of fully complexed dye. For a ratiometric dye, with fluorescence intensities F_1 and F_2 measured at wavelengths λ_1 and λ_2, respectively, the equation becomes

$$[Ca^{2+}] = \frac{K_D\beta(R - R_{min})}{(R_{max} - R)} \tag{3}$$

where $R = F_1/F_2$, K_D is the dissociation constant of the Ca^{2+}–dye complex, and R_{min} and R_{max} are the minimal fluorescence ratio of free dye and maximal fluorescence ratio of fully complexed dye, respectively. The coefficient β, or $F_{2,free}/F_{2,bound}$, is the ratio of the measured intensity of F_2 when all the indicator is Ca^{2+}-free to that when all the indicators are bound.

The above-mentioned calibration equations for ratiometric and nonratiometric indicators require the determination of R_{min} and R_{max}, or F_{min} and F_{max}, respectively. These parameters differ in different experimental setups and are greatly affected by the physicochemical properties of the indicators in specific intracellular environments. Therefore, in situ determination of these parameters is essential for accurate calibration.

A typical calibration entails the following steps: (1) increasing Ca^{2+} permeability using 10 μM Br-A23187 in the presence of high extracellular $[Ca^{2+}]$ (10 mM) to saturate the indicator dye, (2) decreasing extracellular $[Ca^{2+}]$ to zero using EGTA or BAPTA in a nominally Ca^{2+} free medium, and (3) permeabilizing the cells with 10 μM digitonin to release cytosolic indicator or quenching the cytosolic indicator with a high concentration of Mn^{2+} to measure the background fluorescence signal.

Metabolic inhibitors such as FCCP are frequently included in the solution to inhibit active Ca^{2+} uptake and removal mechanisms. However, in situ calibration can be affected by the leak of indicators due to cell lysis at elevated $[Ca^{2+}]_i$ before R_{max} or F_{max} is attained and the slow Ca^{2+} diffusion via Br-A23187 at low submicromolar Ca^{2+} gradients, requiring long equilibration times to reach R_{min} or F_{min}. Under certain circumstances, such a determination is rather difficult. To circumvent these problems, an alternative approach is available for single-wavelength indicators, such as fluo-3, which has $F_{min} \approx 0$, whereby $[Ca^{2+}]$ can be calibrated using a fluorescence pseudo-ratio method (29) given by

$$[Ca^{2+}] = \frac{K_D R}{(K_D/[Ca^{2+}]_{rest}) + 1 - R} \tag{4}$$

where $R = F/F_0$ is the pseudo-ratio of fluorescence emissions calculated by dividing the fluorescence intensity (F) at any time during cell activation by the resting intensity (F_0), K_D is the dissociation constant of the Ca^{2+}–dye complex, and $[Ca^{2+}]_{rest}$ is the resting $[Ca^{2+}]$, which either is an assumed value or is obtained by an independent measurement. This pseudo-ratio method turns out to be a convenient alternative and has been used widely for the calibration of Ca^{2+} sparks and confocal Ca^{2+} imaging, despite the inherited disadvantages of single-wavelength indicators for Ca^{2+} calibration. A more generalized equation for the pseudo-ratio method using indicators with F_{min} not equal to 0 is also available (20).

In addition to F_{min} and F_{max}, determination of the Ca^{2+}-binding affinity of indicator dyes may change in situ due to the incomplete deesterification of the indicator (31,32), intracellular pH, and binding to protein and immobile sites in the cytoplasm (24,33–36). Hence, in situ determination of K_D is also required. This can be achieved by equilibrating Br-A23187-permeabilized cells with calibration solutions mixed from known quantities of EGTA and CaEGTA solutions (37) to generate a fluorescence intensity versus $[Ca^{2+}]$ relationship, and the K_D is obtained by fitting the data with the Hill equation. Generally speaking, fluorescent indicators chelate Ca^{2+} with lower affinity in situ, and Ca^{2+}-binding affinity can be different between cytoplasmic and nucleoplasmic compartments. A comparison of apparent in vitro and in situ K_D values of the common indicators used for confocal imaging is provided by Thomas et al. (18).

III. DETECTION OF Ca^{2+} SPARKS

The detection of Ca^{2+} sparks depends critically on the spatial resolution of the imaging system. In fluorescence light microscopy, an infinitely small luminous point object has a circular Airy diffraction image with a central bright disk and concentric dark and bright disks of progressively weaker intensity. The limit of lateral (x–y axis) resolution of the point object is given by the equation

$$r_{Airy} = 0.61\lambda_o/NA_{obj} \tag{5}$$

where r_{Airy} is the radius of the first dark ring around the central bright disk, λ_o is the wavelength of light in vacuum, and NA_{obj} is the numerical aperture of the objective. According to the Rayleigh criterion, the images of two equal point sources of light are said to be resolved if the distance between the sources is greater than or equal to r_{Airy}. For practical purposes, the lateral resolution is limited to approximately $\lambda_o/2$ with the use of high numerical aperture objectives (e.g., Nikon Neofluor 40X, NA = 1.3). The limit of z-axis resolution of an infinitely small point object is given by the equation

$$z_{min} = 2\lambda_o\eta/(NA_{obj})^2 \tag{6}$$

where η is the refractive index of the medium. For practical purposes, the axial resolution turns out to be about half of the lateral resolution [i.e., $z_{min} \approx (2\text{–}3)\ r_{Airy}$] with the use of high-NA objectives.

However, in a cell loaded with fluorescent indicator, dye within the cones of light above and below the plane of focus are also being excited, and emitted light from this out-of-focus area is also collected by the objective, therefore blurring the in-focus signal and greatly reducing the spatial resolution. This blurring effect precludes the detection of small local Ca^{2+} events in cells with thicknesses beyond a few micrometers without deconvolution. This problem can be overcome by the use of laser scanning confocal microscopy to reject the out-of-focus fluorescence, thereby improving spatial resolution of fluorescence signals generated from a diffraction-limited volume or a "voxel" within a living cell. With the use of a confocal microscope, a Ca^{2+} spark generated from virtually a point source can be detected with the least possible "dilution" by the basal fluorescence from the surrounding area. A schematic illustrating the discrimination of out-of-focus fluorescence in a laser scanning confocal microscope is shown in Fig. 1.

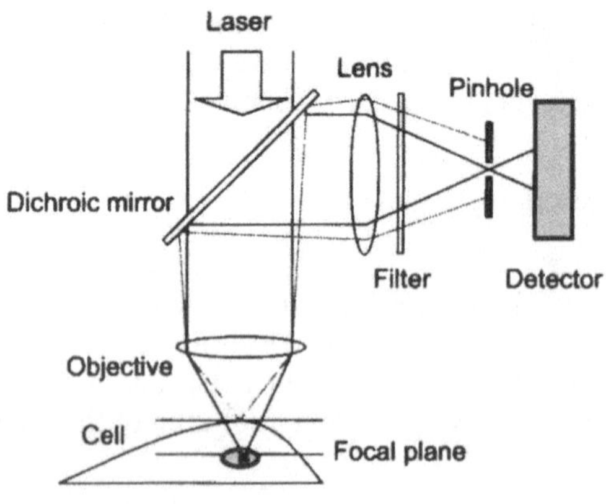

Figure 1 A schematic illustrating the discrimination of out-of-focus signals by the pinhole of a laser scanning confocal microscope. Solid lines indicate in-focus emission light passing through the pinhole aperture and detected by the PMT. Dotted lines indicate the out-of-focus emission light being rejected by the pinhole.

The pinhole in front of the PMT allows only the signal generated from the in-focus voxel to pass through and blocks the out-of-focus signal from being recorded by the detector. The optimal radius of the pinhole is 1 r_{Airy}. Increasing the aperture of the pinhole reduces axial resolution by allowing the detection of more out-of-focus light, whereas decreasing the aperture reduces the intensity of the signal by blocking part of the in-focus light. Opening the pinhole to a size not too much greater than the Airy disk diameter loses some advantage of high resolution but retains much of the capability for rejecting out-of-focus information while gaining in the fluorescence signal. However, for Ca^{2+} spark recording, increasing pinhole size generally reduces the spark amplitude.

Temporal resolution is also fundamentally important for Ca^{2+} spark detection. For the most commonly used laser scanning confocal microscopes, such as Zeiss LSM 410/510, Bio-Rad MRC 600/1000/1024, and Radiant2100, two-dimenional cell imaging is accomplished by scanning the laser beam spot across the specimen with a galvanometer mirror and recording the single-point output in a two-dimensional array. However, the speed of the galvanometer limits the rate of image acquisition such that scanning a typical 512 × 512 pixel image requires a minimum of 0.5 s per frame. Even though the frame rate can be improved somewhat by scanning a smaller area, two-dimensional imaging using these microscopes is inadequate for acquiring temporal information on a Ca^{2+} spark that has a half-duration of less than 50 ms. The limitation on temporal resolution is circumvented by using one-dimensional linescan, where a line across a cell is scanned repeatedly at a rate of about 2 ms/line (29). It must be noted that the information generated from a linescan image is a fair representation of that produced from two-dimensional imaging, on the assumption that Ca^{2+} sparks occur randomly or equally throughout the cell, such as in cardiac myocytes. However, in some cases where Ca^{2+} sparks occur preferentially in certain specific regions or hot spots (38), initial two-dimensional scans should be performed to guide the scan-line selection. Moreover, the orientation of the scan line—for example, transverse or longitudinal along a cell—may have an influence on the morphology of the Ca^{2+} spark depending on specific subcellular architecture (39). The temporal resolution of two-dimensional confocal imaging can be greatly improved by the acousto-optical deflector (AOD) systems used in the real-time confocal laser scanning microscopes such as Noran Odyssey or Oz. In these systems, a two-dimensional image of 225 × 99 pixels can be produced at a maximum rate of 240 Hz, or 4.6 ms/frame, a rate at which kinetic properties of cardiac Ca^{2+} sparks have been recorded (40,41). These systems have also been used to record Ca^{2+} sparks in vascular smooth muscle at a slower speed (42,43). However, because the linescan method is the most popular method for the detection and characterization of the spatiotemporal properties of Ca^{2+} spark, our discussion will remain focused on the information generated by linescan imaging.

Linescan imaging requires repeated illumination of the same line with a laser beam at a high rate, which inevitably introduces undesirable effects of photodamage of the living cells, generation of free radicals, and photobleaching or degradation of indicator dyes. It has been reported that photodegradation of indicators can generate fluorescent but Ca^{2+}-insensitive species (44), which may effectively reduce the apparent K_D of the indicator and affect the measurement of Ca^{2+} signal. Therefore, it is important to reduce the power of the excitation laser to the minimum while still allowing an acceptable baseline signal-to-noise ratio, to limit the duration of image acquisition, and to reposition the scan line during repeated Ca^{2+} spark detection. Using a Zeiss LSM 510 with the power of the argon laser (25 mW) reduced to 0.75%, we are able to linescan (2 ms/line) continuously for >10 s without noticeable cell damage or change in baseline Ca^{2+} fluorescence in cardiac myocytes and pulmonary arterial smooth muscle cells (12).

IV. ANALYSIS OF Ca^{2+} SPARKS

To extract quantitative information on Ca^{2+} sparks from linescan images, some image processing, such as normalization and filtering, is required. Normalization is necessary for generating the F/F_0 values required by the pseudo-ratio method of Ca^{2+} calibration and to eliminate the distortion of Ca^{2+} spark morphology resulting from the uneven distribution of fluorescent indicator along the scan line. A linescan image is a two-dimensional array, $A(m, n)$, with m elements in the time dimension and n elements in the space dimension. Normalization can be achieved by (1) subtracting the known background fluorescence from each element in the raw image to produce $A_1(m, n)$, (2) selecting a region in the time dimension from element m_i to m_j with no Ca^{2+} spark to generate a subarray of $A_1(m_{i,j}, n)$, (3) averaging the values in that region for each element in the space dimension to generate a one-dimensional array $A_0(n)$ of F_0 values, and (4) dividing F values of the array $A_1(m, n)$ by $A_0(n)$ for each element in the space dimension to produce a two-dimensional array of F/F_0 values. The effect of normalization on the linescan image of a cardiac Ca^{2+} spark is illustrated in Fig. 2. The horizontal line pattern in the raw image is due to dye accumulation in the t-tubule–SR junctional areas, the pattern is removed after normalization. Moreover, because of the high noise resulting from the low laser power and small pinhole aperture, some forms of filtering are usually required to improve the image quality. Smoothing procedures using boxcar pixel averaging or median filtering are most commonly used. For practical purposes, a 3×3 or 5×5 pixel averaging or median filtering has minimal effects on the amplitude, duration, and width of Ca^{2+} sparks. Several spatiotemporal parameters of Ca^{2+} sparks, including frequency, amplitude, rise time, half-duration, half-width, and half-decay time can be readily quantified from these linescan images, as depicted in Fig. 3. These

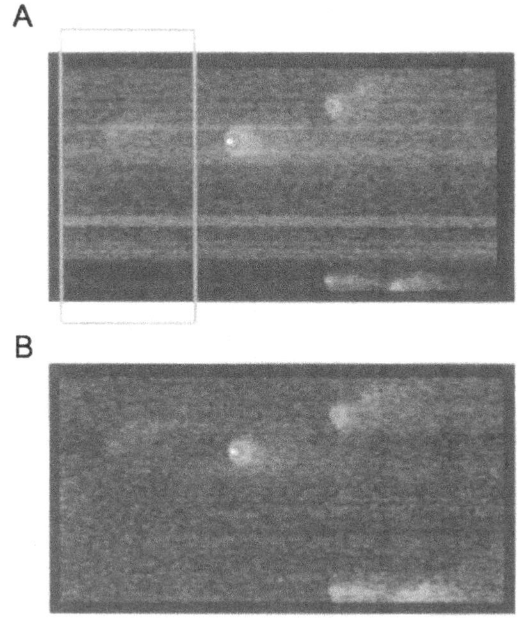

Figure 2 Linescan images (A) before and (B) after normalization. The box indicates the region used to generate the F_0 values. The images are filtered by 5×5 boxcar pixel averaging.

parameters provide specific information regarding the activities of Ca^{2+} release units, the magnitude of Ca^{2+} fluxes, Ca^{2+} diffusion, and buffering capacity.

A. Spark Frequency

The activity of RyR release units within a cell is indicated by spark frequency. It is usually expressed as the number of sparks per micrometer per second for linescan recording or the number of sparks per cell per second for high-speed two-dimensional imaging. In the early studies, Ca^{2+} sparks were detected by eye (29,45,46). In order to avoid selection bias, automated computer algorithms were developed based on a common strategy of identifying connected regions that are above a certain threshold defined by the noise level (40,47). In these algorithms, the mean m and standard deviation σ of baseline fluorescence of the normalized image are determined, and Ca^{2+} sparks are identified as regions above $m + Cri\ \sigma$, where Cri is a constant determining the "threshold" for event detection. Obviously, a spark of large amplitude has a high detectability, and the detectability improves as σ gets smaller. It is noteworthy that for a given signal-to-noise (m/σ) level, false detection (type I error) depends largely on Cri, and m/σ is a major determinant of erroneous

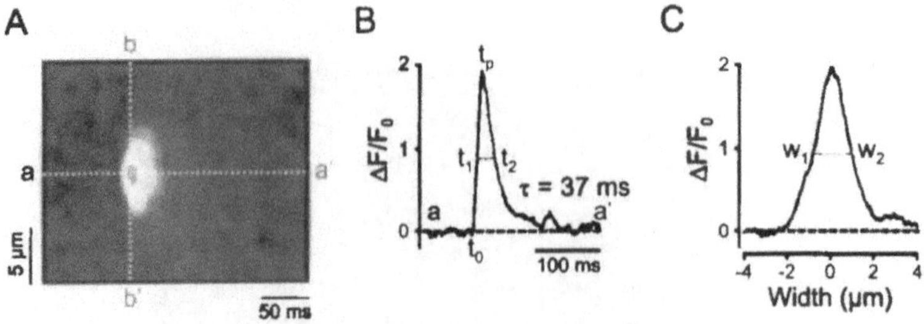

Figure 3 Spatiotemporal parameters of Ca^{2+} sparks. (A) Linescan image of a spark with fluorescence intensity F normalized by the basal fluorescence (F_0) scaled by pseudocolor. lines a to a' and b to b' refer to the temporal and spatial profiles, respectively. (B) Curve represents the temporal profile of a Ca^{2+} spark. The letters t_0, t_p, t_1, t_2 denote threshold, peak, half-rise, and half-decay time, respectively. The dashed line is the exponential fit of the declining phase, and τ is the time constant of decade. The dashed line denotes the full-duration half-maximum (FDHM). (C) The spatial profile of a Ca^{2+} spark. The line t_1-t_2 is a Gaussian function, and the solid line between w_1 and w_2 denotes full-width half-maximum (FWHM).

rejection (type II error). Therefore, increasing *Cri* decreases sensitivity but increases detection specificity, causing an underestimation of spark frequency by rejecting sparks of low amplitude. On the other hand, decreasing *Cri* causes an overestimation of spark frequency by including false detections. The optimal *Cri* value for different m/σ values can be determined by empirical methods (47).

B. Spark Amplitude

Spark amplitude is defined as the maximum increase in local $[Ca^{2+}]$ in a spark region. It is expressed in terms of either $\Delta F/F_0$ or $\Delta[Ca^{2+}]$ after calibration using the pseudo-ratio method [Eq. (4)]. Determination of the amplitude of a single spark is straightforward, but estimation of the average spark amplitude requires extra caution. The complication arises from the fact that spark amplitude distribution is non-Gaussian but highly left-skewed with monotonic decreasing amplitude. This results from an inherent sampling bias of confocal imaging, because most of the detected sparks do not originate precisely at the sampling spot but at a variable distance from the scan line (47–49). Therefore, sparks at a longer distance from the scan line are detected with lower amplitude. Because of the nonmodal distribution, spark amplitude should be described and compared using nonparametric statistics. Even so, the median of the apparent spark amplitude is not equivalent to the actual spark amplitude. This problem is managed in some studies by averaging the brightest sparks (e.g., the brightest 5%), because they are likely to originate at or near the scan line (50). On the other hand, a modal distribution can be obtained from repetitive Ca^{2+} sparks recorded at a fixed hyperactive site or hot spot, because the distance between the release site and the scan line stays constant (51,52). In addition, spark amplitude is biased toward a higher value owing to the presence of noise, a situation that is more serious for sparks of low amplitude; therefore, adequate filtering is necessary to reduce the overestimation.

C. Temporal Characteristics of Ca^{2+} Sparks

The temporal profile of Ca^{2+} spark consists of a rising phase and a declining phase, corresponding to the processes of Ca^{2+} release and dissipation, respectively. The rising phase is usually quantified by the rise time, which is the period between the times when the fluorescence transient exceeds a threshold level (e.g., 2σ) and when it reaches the peak amplitude, and by the rate of rise, which is the slope of the rising transient. Theoretical studies suggest that the rise time is determined primarily by the duration of Ca^{2+} release, and the rate of rise is a function of Ca^{2+} release flux or current (50,53,54). The declining phase is usually quantified by the half-decay time or by the time constant of decay (τ) estimated by fitting the declining transient with a single exponential. Experimental and theoretical studies indicate that the kinetics of the declining phase of Ca^{2+} sparks is mainly determined by the local Ca^{2+} diffusion from the source of Ca^{2+} release, with local SR Ca^{2+} uptake playing a lesser role (42,54,55). The duration of Ca^{2+} sparks can be represented by the half width or full-duration half-maximum (FDHM) (56), which is a combined function of both rising and declining phases of Ca^{2+} spark. Agents that modify RyR activity, such as ryanodine and FK-506, are known to affect spark duration (29,57).

D. Spatial Spread

The spatial spread or the size of Ca^{2+} spread is quantified by the full-width-half-maximum (FWHM), which is defined as the width of spark at half its amplitude. This parameter is mainly determined by the diffusion constant of Ca^{2+} and the endogenous Ca^{2+} buffers and to a much smaller extent by the amplitude of Ca^{2+} release and the rate of Ca^{2+} removal (42,54,55,58). Because Ca^{2+} spark originates virtually from a point source and Ca^{2+} buffering capacities are similar in muscle cells, solitary Ca^{2+} sparks typically have a width of $\leq 2\,\mu m$. However, in some cases, large Ca^{2+} sparks or macro sparks may arise from Ca^{2+} release from multiple neighboring sites recruited by Ca^{2+}-induced Ca^{2+} release (52). Similarly, large Ca^{2+} sparks are commonly observed when RyRs are sensitized with a low concentration of caffeine (12).

E. Signal Mass

The amount of Ca^{2+} released by a spark can be indexed by a parameter called the signal mass (M), which is defined as the integral of the change in the (normalized) fluorescence induced by a spark over space and time in a linescan image (53,59), given by

$$M = \int\int \frac{\Delta F}{F_0(x,t)\;dx\;dt} \tag{7}$$

where x and t are space and time, respectively. In addition to the determination of release source strength, this parameter has also been applied to estimate the number of sparks in a release cluster in which sparks are not discernible (59). This is achieved by dividing M of a cluster by the averaged M of solitary sparks recorded under the same experimental conditions.

V. CONCLUDING REMARKS

A major interest in the quantitative analysis of Ca^{2+} sparks is to decipher the kinetics of Ca^{2+} release fluxes generated from the Ca^{2+} release units. Major mathematical models, which take into account the diffusion of Ca^{2+} ions, endogenous Ca^{2+} buffers, Ca^{2+} removal processes, and subcellular microarchitecture, have been developed to reconstruct the SR Ca^{2+} release flux of sparks (J_{Spark}) (48,54,58,60,61). Recently, We developed a technique to measure directly the local Ca^{2+} release fluxes (Ca^{2+} spikes) and J_{Spark} in voltage-clamped cells using the strategy of minimizing the residence time of released Ca^{2+} in the cytoplasm with EGTA (4 mM 150 nM Ca^{2+}) and to optimize the detection of localized high [Ca^{2+}] in the release sites using a low-affinity, fast Ca^{2+} indicator, Oregon Green 488 BAPTA-5N (1 mM) (20,62). Using this technique, spatially and temporally resolved Ca^{2+} spikes can be recorded under conditions that Ca^{2+} sparks are usually indiscernible. This technique has been proven to be complementary to the Ca^{2+} spark measurement in muscle cells (51,63).

In conclusion, we have presented in this chapter information on cytosolic [Ca^{2+}] measurement and have discussed more specifically the detection and analysis of Ca^{2+} sparks. We hope this information will be useful for investigators who are contemplating joining the exciting journey of unraveling the fundamental mechanisms of local Ca^{2+} signaling in pulmonary circulation.

ACKNOWLEDGMENTS

This work is supported by grants from the NIH (HL 071835 and HL63813) and AHA to J. S. K. Sham.

REFERENCES

1. Wang S-Q, Song L-S, Lakatta EG, Cheng H. Ca^{2+} signalling between single L-type Ca^{2+} channels and ryanodine receptors in heart cells. Nature 2001; 410:592–596.

2. Golovina VA, Blaustein MP. Spatially and functionally distinct Ca^{2+} stores in sarcoplasmic and endoplasmic reticulum. Science 1997; 275:1643–1648.
3. Trollinger DR, Cascio WE, Lemasters JJ. Mitochondrial calcium transients in adult rabbit cardiac myocytes: inhibition by ruthenium red and artifacts caused by lysosomal loading of Ca^{2+}-indicating fluorophores. Biophys J 2000; 79: 39–50.
4. Trollinger DR, Cascio WE, Lemasters JJ. Selective loading of Rhod 2 into mitochondria shows mitochondrial Ca^{2+} transients during the contractile cycle in adult rabbit cardiac myocytes. Biochem Biophys Res Commun 1997; 236:738–742.
5. Berridge MJ. The AM and FM of calcium signalling. Nature 1997; 386: 759–760.
6. Dolmetsch RE, Lewis RS, Goodnow CC, Healy JI. Differential activation of transcription factors induced by Ca^{2+} response amplitude and duration. Nature 1997; 386:855–858.
7. Dolmetsch RE, Xu K, Lewis RS. Calcium oscillations increase the efficiency and specificity of gene expression. Nature 1998; 392:933–936.
8. Dolmetsch RE, Pajvani U, Fife K, Spotts JM, Greenberg ME. Signaling to the nucleus by an L-type calcium channel–calmodulin complex through the MAP kinase pathway. Science 2001; 294:333–339.
9. Dolmetsch R. Excitation–transcription coupling: signaling by ion channels to the nucleus. Sci STKE 2003; 2003:PE4.
10. Zhang W-M, Yip K-P, Lin M-J, Shimoda LA, Li W-H, Sham JSK. Endothelin-1 activates Ca^{2+} sparks in pulmonary arterial smooth muscle cells: local Ca^{2+} signaling between inositol trisphosphate- and ryanodine-receptors. Am J Physiol Lung Cell Mol Physiol 2003; 285:L680–L690.
11. Porter VA, Bonev AD, Knot HJ, Heppner TJ, Stevenson AS, Kleppisch T, Lederer WJ, Nelson MT. Frequency modulation of Ca^{2+} sparks is involved in regulation of arterial diameters by cyclic nucleotides. Am J Physiol 1998; 274:C1346–C1355.
12. Remillard CV, Zhang W-M, Shimoda LA, Sham JSK. Physiological properties and functions of Ca^{2+} sparks in rat intrapulmonary arterial smooth muscle cells. Am J Physiol Lung Cell Mol Physiol 2002; 283:L433–L444.
13. Janiak R, Wilson SM, Montague S, Hume JR. Heterogeneity of calcium stores and elementary release events in canine pulmonary arterial smooth muscle cells. Am J Physiol Cell Physiol 2001; 280:C22–C33.
14. Wang Y-X, Zheng Y-M, Abdullaev I, Kotlikoff MI. Metabolic inhibition with cyanide induces calcium release in pulmonary artery myocytes and *Xenopus* oocytes. Am J Physiol Cell Physiol 2003; 284:C378–C388.
15. Tsien RY. New calcium indicators and buffers with high selectivity against magnesium and protons: design, synthesis, and properties of prototype structures. Biochemistry 1980; 19:2396–2404.
16. Minta A, Kao JP, Tsien RY. Fluorescent indicators for cytosolic calcium based on rhodamine and fluorescein chromophores. J Biol Chem 1989; 264: 8171–8178.
17. Lipp P, Niggli E. Ratiometric confocal Ca^{2+}-measurements with visible wavelength indicators in isolated cardiac myocytes. Cell Calcium 1993; 14:359–372.

18. Thomas D, Tovey SC, Collins TJ, Bootman MD, Berridge MJ, Lipp P. A comparison of fluorescent Ca^{2+} indicator properties and their use in measuring elementary and global Ca^{2+} signals. Cell Calcium 2000; 28:213–223.
19. Escobar AL, Velez P, Kim AM, Cifuentes F, Fill M, Vergara JL. Kinetic properties of DM-nitrophen and calcium indicators: rapid transient response to flash photolysis. Pflügers Arch 1997; 434:615–631.
20. Song L-S, Sham JSK, Stern MD, Lakatta EG, Cheng H. Direct measurement of SR release flux by tracking "Ca^{2+} spikes" in rat cardiac myocytes. J Physiol 1998; 512:677–691.
21. Tsien RY. A non-disruptive technique for loading calcium buffers and indicators into cells. Nature 1981; 290:527–528.
22. Kao JP. Practical aspects of measuring [Ca^{2+}] with fluorescent indicators. Methods Cell Biol 1994; 40:155–181.
23. Wahl M, Lucherini MJ, Gruenstein E. Intracellular Ca^{2+} measurement with indo-1 in substrate-attached cells: advantages and special considerations. Cell Calcium 1990; 11:487–500.
24. Blatter LA, Wier WG. Intracellular diffusion, binding, and compartmentalization of the fluorescent calcium indicators indo-1 and fura-2. Biophys J 1990; 58:1491–1499.
25. Malgaroli A, Milani D, Meldolesi J, Pozzan T. Fura-2 measurement of cytosolic free Ca^{2+} in monolayers and suspensions of various types of animal cells. J Cell Biol 1987; 105:2145–2155.
26. Di Virgilio F, Steinberg TH, Silverstein SC. Inhibition of fura-2 sequestration and secretion with organic anion transport blockers. Cell Calcium 1990; 11: 57–62.
27. Di Virgilio F, Steinberg TH, Swanson JA, Silverstein SC. Fura-2 secretion and sequestration in macrophages. A blocker of organic anion transport reveals that these processes occur via a membrane transport system for organic anions. J Immunol 1988; 140:915–920.
28. Merritt JE, McCarthy SA, Davies MP, Moores KE. Use of fluo-3 to measure cytosolic Ca^{2+} in platelets and neutrophils. Loading cells with the dye, calibration of traces, measurements in the presence of plasma, and buffering of cytosolic Ca^{2+}. Biochem J 1990; 269:513–519.
29. Cheng H, Lederer WJ, Cannell MB. Calcium sparks: elementary events underlying excitation-contraction coupling in heart muscle. Science 1993; 262: 740–744.
30. Grynkiewicz G, Poenie M, Tsien RY. A new generation of Ca^{2+} indicators with greatly improved fluorescence properties. J Biol Chem 1985; 260:3440–3450.
31. Li Q, Altschuld RA, Stokes BT. Quantitation of intracellular free calcium in single adult cardiomyocytes by fura-2 fluorescence microscopy: calibration of fura-2 ratios. Biochem Biophys Res Commun 1987; 147:120–126.
32. Williams DA, Fay FS. Intracellular calibration of the fluorescent calcium indicator fura-2. Cell Calcium 1990; 11:75–83.
33. Konishi M, Olson A, Hollingworth S, Baylor SM. Myoplasmic binding of fura-2 investigated by steady-state fluorescence and absorbance measurements. Biophys J 1988; 54:1089–1104.

34. Baker AJ, Brandes R, Schreur JH, Camacho SA, Weiner MW. Protein and acidosis alter calcium-binding and fluorescence spectra of the calcium indicator indo-1. Biophys J 1994; 67:1646–1654.
35. Zhao M, Hollingworth S, Baylor SM. Properties of tri- and tetracarboxylate Ca^{2+} indicators in frog skeletal muscle fibers. Biophys J 1996; 70:896–916.
36. Owen CS, Shuler RL. Spectral evidence for non-calcium interactions of intracellular indo-1. Biochem Biophys Res Commun 1989; 163:328–333.
37. Bers DM. A simple method for the accurate determination of free [Ca] in Ca-EGTA solutions. Am J Physiol 1982; 242:C404-C408.
38. Gordienko DV, Greenwood IA, Bolton TB. Direct visualization of sarcoplasmic reticulum regions discharging Ca^{2+}sparks in vascular myocytes. Cell Calcium 2001; 29:13–28.
39. Parker I, Zang WJ, Wier WG. Ca^{2+} sparks involving multiple Ca^{2+} release sites along Z-lines in rat heart cells. J Physiol 1996; 497:31–38.
40. Goldhaber JI, Lamp ST, Walter DO, Garfinkel A, Fukumoto GH, Weiss JN. Local regulation of the threshold for calcium sparks in rat ventricular myocytes: role of sodium-calcium exchange. J Physiol 1999; 520:431–438.
41. Cleemann L, Wang W, Morad M. Two-dimensional confocal images of organization, density, and gating of focal Ca^{2+} release sites in rat cardiac myocytes. Proc Natl Acad Sci USA 1998; 95:10984–10989.
42. Gómez AM, Cheng H, Lederer WJ, Bers DM. Ca^{2+} diffusion and sarcoplasmic reticulum transport both contribute to $[Ca^{2+}]_i$ decline during Ca^{2+} sparks in rat ventricular myocytes. J Physiol 1996; 496:575–581.
43. Heppner TJ, Bonev AD, Santana LF, Nelson MT. Alkaline pH shifts Ca^{2+} sparks to Ca^{2+} waves in smooth muscle cells of pressurized cerebral arteries. Am J Physiol Heart Circ Physiol 2002; 283:H2169–H2176.
44. Scheenen WJ, Makings LR, Gross LR, Pozzan T, Tsien RY. Photodegradation of indo-1 and its effect on apparent Ca^{2+} concentrations. Chem Biol 1996; 3:765–774.
45. Santana LF, Cheng H, Gómez AM, Cannell MB, Lederer WJ. Relation between the sarcolemmal Ca^{2+} current and Ca^{2+} sparks and local control theories for cardiac excitation-contraction coupling. Circ Res 1996; 78:166–171.
46. López-López JR, Shacklock PS, Balke CW, Wier WG. Local calcium transients triggered by single L-type calcium channel currents in cardiac cells. Science 1995; 268:1042–1045.
47. Cheng H, Song LS, Shirokova N, González A, Lakatta EG, Ríos E, Stern MD. Amplitude distribution of calcium sparks in confocal images: theory and studies with an automatic detection method. Biophys J 1999; 76:606–617.
48. Pratusevich VR, Balke CW. Factors shaping the confocal image of the calcium spark in cardiac muscle cells. Biophys J 1996; 71:2942–2957.
49. Izu LT, Wier WG, Balke CW. Theoretical analysis of the Ca^{2+} spark amplitude distribution. Biophys. J. 1998; 75:1144–1162.
50. Terentyev D, Viatchenko-Karpinski S, Valdivia HH, Escobar AL, Gyorke S. Luminal Ca^{2+} controls termination and refractory behavior of Ca^{2+}-induced Ca^{2+} release in cardiac myocytes. Circ Res 2002; 91:414–420.
51. Wang S-Q, Song L-S, Xu L, Meissner G, Lakatta EG, Ríos E, Stern MD, Cheng H. Thermodynamically irreversible gating of ryanodine receptors in situ

revealed by stereotyped duration of release in Ca^{2+} sparks. Biophys J 2002; 83:242–251.
52. Gordienko DV, Bolton TB. Crosstalk between ryanodine receptors and IP_3 receptors as a factor shaping spontaneous Ca^{2+}-release events in rabbit portal vein myocytes. J Physiol 2002; 542:743–762.
53. ZhuGe R, Fogarty KE, Tuft RA, Lifshitz LM, Sayar K, Walsh JV. Dynamics of signaling between Ca^{2+} sparks and Ca^{2+}- activated K^+ channels studied with a novel image-based method for direct intracellular measurement of ryanodine receptor Ca^{2+} current. J Gen Physiol 2000; 116:845–864.
54. Smith GD, Keizer JE, Stern MD, Lederer WJ, Cheng H. A simple numerical model of calcium spark formation and detection in cardiac myocytes. Biophys J 1998; 75:15–32.
55. Santana LF, Kranias EG, Lederer WJ. Calcium sparks and excitation-contraction coupling in phospholamban-deficient mouse ventricular myocytes. J Physiol 1997; 503:21–29.
56. Song L-S, Stern MD, Lakatta EG, Cheng H. Partial depletion of sarcoplasmic reticulum calcium does not prevent calcium sparks in rat ventricular myocytes. J Physiol 1997; 505:665–675.
57. Xiao RP, Valdivia HH, Bogdanov K, Valdivia C, Lakatta EG, Cheng H. The immunophilin FK506-binding protein modulates Ca^{2+} release channel closure in rat heart. J Physiol 1997; 500:343–354.
58. Izu LT, Mauban JRH, Balke CW, Wier WG. Large currents generate cardiac Ca^{2+} sparks. Biophys J 2001; 80:88–102.
59. Zhou Y-Y, Song L-S, Lakatta EG, Xiao R-P, Cheng H. Constitutive β_2-adrenergic signalling enhances sarcoplasmic reticulum Ca^{2+} cycling to augment contraction in mouse heart. J Physiol 1999; 521:351–361.
60. Jiang Y-H, Klein MG, Schneider MF. Numerical simulation of Ca^{2+} "sparks" in skeletal muscle. Biophys J 1999; 77:2333–2357.
61. Chandler WK, Hollingworth S, Baylor SM. Simulation of calcium sparks in cut skeletal muscle fibers of the frog. J Gen Physiol 2003; 121:311–324.
62. Sham JSK, Song LS, Chen Y, Deng LH, Stern MD, Lakatta EG, Cheng H. Termination of Ca^{2+} release by a local inactivation of ryanodine receptors in cardiac myocytes. Proc Natl Acad Sci USA 1998; 95:15096–15101.
63. Song L-S, Wang S-Q, Xiao R-P, Spurgeon H, Lakatta EG, Cheng H. β-Adrenergic stimulation synchronizes intracellular Ca^{2+} release during excitation-contraction coupling in cardiac myocytes. Circ Res 2001; 88:794–801.

37

Use of Transgenic and Gene-Targeted Mice to Study Ion Channel Function in the Pulmonary Vasculature

Barry London and Maninder Singh Bedi
University of Pittsburgh, Pittsburgh, Pennsylvania, U.S.A.

I. INTRODUCTION

Transgenic and gene targeting technologies have led to marked advances in the understanding of the molecular basis of electrophysiology in the mouse (1,2). The ability to manipulate the genetic makeup of organisms by targeting selected genes has provided a novel means of investigating the mechanisms underlying ion channel function. As an increased number of research labs have used genetically altered mice in their studies, it has become clear that this technique offers novel opportunities but also raises questions specific to each field. Some concerns arise as a result of the genetic manipulation, which can (1) affect development and lead to compensatory changes in the organism or (2) affect multiple organs and lead to secondary effects. Other concerns derive from the use of the mouse as the model, whose physiology may differ radically from that of larger mammals.

This chapter will describe the application of transgenic and gene-targeted (knockout, knock-in, targeted gene replacement) mice to the study of the pathophysiology of ion channels in the pulmonary vasculature. Although still quite preliminary, the potential of these techniques for use in pulmonary vascular biology will be highlighted.

II. GENERATING TRANSGENIC AND GENE-TARGETED MICE

Two general techniques are used to engineer transgenic and gene-targeted mice (1). Genes can be added at random locations throughout the genome (transgenics), or specific genes can be manipulated (gene targeting). Both techniques can potentially be used to increase, decrease, or alter an individual gene product in a specific tissue (Fig. 1). The techniques and their advantages and disadvantages are discussed in more detail below.

A. Transgenic Overexpression

To overexpress a gene, foreign DNA is inserted into the host genome. DNA from the desired gene is amplified, cloned into a transgenic construct, and injected into the male pronucleus of fertilized mouse eggs (Fig. 1). These eggs are then implanted into the uterus of a pseudo-pregnant female, and a fraction of the live neonates carry the transgene randomly inserted into their chromosomes (F_o generation). These transgenic mice are then bred, and ~50% of the offspring will carry the transgene.

The spatial and temporal pattern of expression of the transgene depends largely on the promoter used and to a lesser extent on the site of integration of the transgene. For the heart, the α-myosin heavy-chain promoter effectively drives expression in adult ventricular myocytes (3). Unfortunately, there is no promoter that specifically drives expression in the pulmonary artery. Endothelial promoters such as TIE2 are not lung-specific, and smooth muscle cell promoters such as the smooth muscle α-actin promoter are not specific for pulmonary artery cells (4,5). A phenotype in mice using these promoters may relate, at least in part, to expression of the transgene in other organs. An alternative strategy for secreted proteins would be to use a lung-specific promoter such as the surfactant protein C promoter (SP-C) to drive expression in type II lung epithelial cells (6). Clearly, the potential effect of the expression of the transgene directly in the lung must be taken into account.

Transgenic mice have been used most often to study the effects of overexpression of proteins in various organs. Overexpression of dominant negative proteins has been used to create functional knockdown and knockout mice, however. In the ion channel field, this technique has been particularly useful for K^+ channels, where four α subunits coassemble to form a functional channel. A mutated or truncated subunit will coassemble with wild-type subunits to form nonfunctional channels. Overexpression of dominant negative subunits has been critical in determining the role of voltage-gated potassium channel genes in the heart and K_{ATP} channels in the pancreas (1,2,7).

Ideally, transgene expression could be turned on and off at will. A number of promoter-specific systems have been developed, some based on the use of tetracycline-responsive promoter elements (4,8). To date, low

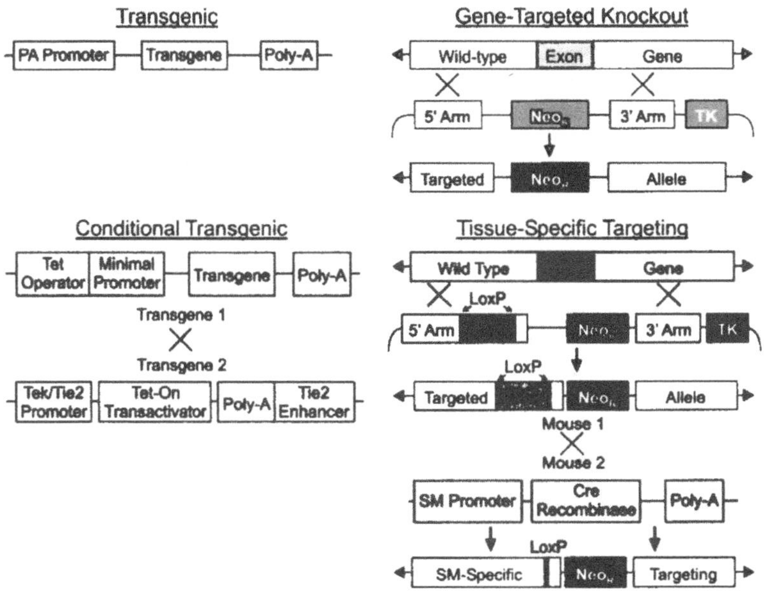

Figure 1 Comparison of the techniques used to engineer transgenic (upper left), conditional transgenic (lower left), gene-targeted (upper right), and tissue-specific gene-targeted mice (lower right). The transgenic constructs insert randomly into the mouse chromosome, and specificity depends on the presence of the promoter. In contrast, gene targeting requires homologous recombination at a specific chromosomal locus in embryonic stem cells in culture followed by generation of the mouse. The scheme shown here for the generation of a conditional transgenic mouse is the one used by Teng et al. (4). Transgene 2 expresses a transactivator protein in smooth muscle (Tie2 promoter) only in the presence of tetracycline compounds. Transgene 1 then expresses the transgene of interest only in the presence of that transactivator. Note also that the conditional transgenic mouse requires either coinjection of two transgenes during the engineering of the mouse (shown) or mating of the two independent transgenic lines. In addition, conditional transgenic mice can either be turned on by tetracycline compounds (as shown) or inhibited by them (tet-off transactivator). Tissue-specific gene targeting, on the other hand, always requires the mating of two genetically modified mice to achieve the desired specificity (see text). Neo_R, Neomycin resistance gene; TK, thymidine kinase gene; Tet, tetracycline; LoxP, 34 base pair element that undergoes internal recombination in the presence of cre recombinase.

expression levels and variable tissue specificity of the transgene (leakiness) have prevented widespread use of this technology.

It is important to note that a foreign DNA sequence is inserted at random locations in the host genome and that this process can disrupt genes at those loci. To definitively show that changes in phenotype are due to the inserted DNA sequence and not randomly disrupted host genes, multiple transgenic lines using the same construct must be tested. If different transgenic lines show the same change with different insertion sites, then the phenotype can be attributed to the foreign gene. It is difficult to know how many copies of the genes have been inserted, and copy number can alter the level of protein expression. This does allow for the examination of lines with varying amounts of transgene expression (dose effect). Expression levels can also be increased by mating two mice heterozygous for the transgene to obtain homozygotes. Phenotypic changes resulting from the insertion site of the transgene are more likely to occur in homozygous lines, however.

A potential problem with transgenic mice arises from the massive overexpression of a mutant protein. The protein may titrate away important factors such as β subunits or have direct toxic effects on cells. The dilated cardiomyopathy caused by overexpression of green fluorescent protein in the heart illustrates this problem (9).

B. Gene Targeting Using Homologous Recombination

Gene targeting involves the direct manipulation of a specific gene in the mouse (10). Embryonic stem (ES) cells are pluripotent stem cells derived from the inner cell mass of mouse blastocysts. Foreign DNA is inserted into ES cells in vitro by applying electric current to make the cell membrane porous to the DNA (electroporation). The altered DNA sequences of interest are then incorporated into the stem cell genome by homologous recombination, a process by which the wild-type sequence is replaced by the foreign electroporated DNA (Fig. 1). The foreign DNA is usually designed to make the gene completely inoperative so that the gene product is not expressed (knockout mice). Because homologous recombination is a rare event, the vector carrying the gene of interest also contains antibiotic resistance genes used for positive and negative selection. The Neo_R gene encodes an enzyme that provides resistance against aminoglycoside antibiotics, whereas the TK gene encodes thymidine kinase, which is lethal to the cell in the presence of gancyclovir. Thus, cells that have undergone homologous recombination at the appropriate locus and are heterozygous for the targeted allele will survive in the presence of both neomycin and gancyclovir.

Following confirmation of the stem cell genotype by Southern blot, targeted ES cells (SV129 line, male, derived from mice agouti in color) are injected into blastocysts (C57Black6 line, derived from mice black in color) and implanted into the uterus of pseudopregnant females. The offspring are chimeras containing cells derived from both the targeted ES cells and wild-type blastocysts. Male chimeras are then mated with female C57Black6 mice, and offspring from ES-cell-derived sperm will carry the dominant agouti coat color. Half of these agouti mice (F_1 generation) will be heterozygous for the targeted allele. These heterozygotes can then be mated with each other to generate homozygous targeted mice (F_2 generation).

The term knockout or targeted disruption refers to gene targeting where the endogenous gene is deleted in whole or in part and rendered nonfunctional. It is possible, using the same strategy, to replace one gene with another (targeted gene replacement) or to introduce subtle mutations into a gene (targeted mutagenesis) (11,12).

Gene targeting primarily affects a single gene and can be used to study gene function with specificity that is often not achievable by pharmacological means. Unlike the transgenic method described above, random insertion into the genome with accidental disruption of an unrelated gene is unlikely. Other uncertainties do remain, however. Related genes may be up- or downregulated to compensate for the targeted gene and can cloud the interpretation of the phenotype. The targeted mutation is present in all organs in which the gene is expressed, and an unknown role of the gene in another organ could contribute to the phenotype. Mutations are also present throughout embryonic development, and it can be difficult to determine whether the consequences of gene deletion are attributable to abnormal development or absence of the gene product in the adult animal.

The ability to engineer gene knockouts in a time- and tissue-restricted manner has been developed using the cre/lox system (Fig. 1). Here, gene targeting is used to surround the desired gene by two 34 bp loxP elements (10). Homozygous targeted mice are then mated with transgenic mice that express the cre recombinase enzyme in a tissue- and time-specific manner. In the presence of the cre recombinase protein, the part of the gene between the elements is removed and the conditional tissue-specific knockout is completed. This technique can also be used to remove the Neo_R gene inserted during the targeting process and to eliminate any phenotypic alterations resulting from this foreign gene.

The strain of the mouse can affect the phenotype produced by the genetic manipulations (13). When engineered as above using SV129 ES cells, the targeted mice are of mixed background (50% SV129; 50% C57BL/6). Mice of pure SV129 background can be engineered by mating male germ line chimeras with SV129 females. Mice of predominantly C57BL/6 background are usually produced by backcrossing heterozygous mice of mixed background with wild-type mice of C57BL/6 background. After 5–10 generations, most alleles will match those in the C57BL/6 strain, with the exception of genes linked to the targeted allele (in close proximity on the same chromosome) that cosegregate with that allele.

III. STUDYING TRANSGENIC AND GENE-TARGETED MICE

A number of techniques are available to study the pulmonary vasculature in genetically engineered mice. These include studies at the molecular, cellular, and organ levels.

A. Molecular Studies

Standard techniques for quantifying and localizing RNA expression of the modified gene include the Northern blot, ribonuclease protection assay (RPA), reverse transcription PCR, real-time PCR, and in situ hybridization. Techniques for quantifying and localizing protein include the Western blot, the enzyme-linked immunosorbent assay (ELISA), immunofluorescence, and immunohistochemistry. Pulmonary vasculature is complex (being composed of endothelial cells, smooth muscle cells, and fibroblasts), and expression can differ greatly among cell types. In situ hybridization and immunocytochemical techniques can be used to localize gene expression. Alternatively, individual cell types can be isolated and gene expression studies performed on the purified cells.

In transgenic models, the spatial localization of the transgene RNA and protein depends on the promoter. When gene targeting is used to mutate or replace a gene, expression levels and tissue specificity similar to those of the native gene are expected. In gene-targeted knockout models, the native gene product is usually decreased in heterozygous and absent from homozygous mice. Compensatory mechanisms can lead to normal protein levels in the heterozygotes, however.

RNA and protein expression of other genes are studied in transgenic and gene-targeted mice. Modification of one gene may lead to compensatory upregulation or downregulation of related genes at the RNA or protein levels (11,14). In addition, changes in physiology and/or pathophysiology in the transgenic animal may lead to secondary (or indirect) changes in gene expression.

B. Cellular Electrophysiology

Single murine pulmonary artery smooth muscle cells are isolated by enzymatic digestion and gentle trituration. These cells can then be studied using whole-cell voltage-clamp techniques (15). Pharmacological ion channel blockers, antibodies, signaling molecules, modulators of phosphorylation, and hypoxia can be used to probe ion channel function in this preparation.

C. Pulmonary Artery Physiology

An increasing array of physiological techniques have been adapted for the mouse. Right heart catheterization can be used to directly measure right ventricular and pulmonary artery pressure in the mouse (16). Transthoracic and transesophageal echocardiography allow the study of right ventricular function in vivo. Isolated lung models can be used to study pulmonary artery function, with direct control of pulmonary artery pressure, pulmonary venous pressure, oxygen, carbon dioxide, adrenergic stimulation, and other potential modifiers such as NO. In addition, pulmonary artery ring preparations with intact endothelium can be used to directly study developed tension in response to various stimuli.

IV. TARGETING ION CHANNELS IN THE PULMONARY VASCULATURE

Potassium and calcium channels play key roles in pulmonary artery function. K^+ channels maintain the resting membrane potential and oppose depolarization. When smooth muscle cells depolarize, Ca^{2+} enters via L-type Ca^{2+} channels and leads to vasoconstriction.

The mammalian genome contains more than 100 K^+ channel and 10 Ca^{2+} channel genes (including both α and β subunits), which are grouped into families based on homology and electrophysiological properties. Smooth muscle cells have been reported to express many voltage-gated K^+ channels (I_K: Kv1.1, Kv1.2, Kv1.3, Kv1.5, Kv1.6, Kv2.1, Kv2.2, Kv3.1, Kv3.2, Kv3.3, Kv9.3, erg; I_{to}: Kv4.3), inward rectifying channels (Kir3.1; I_{KATP}: Kir6.1/SUR2), and Ca^{2+}-activated K^+ channels (BK_{Ca}) (15,17–22). They also express L-type Ca^{2+} channels ($Ca_v1.2$ and $Ca_v1.3$) and Ca^{2+}-activated Cl^- channels (23,24).

The roles of individual gene products in the normal function of the pulmonary artery, in regulatory processes such as hypoxic pulmonary vasoconstriction (HPV), and in disease states such as pulmonary hypertension (PH) are unclear. Genetic modification of expression and/or function of these ion channels should provide insight into their physiological and pathophysiological roles. The following section describes the use of a Kv1.5-targeted mouse to explore the role of this gene in hypoxic pulmonary vasoconstriction.

A. Gene-Targeted Replacement of Kv1.5 with Kv1.1 Impairs Hypoxic Pulmonary Vasoconstriction

We engineered mice (SWAP mice) in which Kv1.5 was replaced with rat Kv1.1 by using gene targeting of embryonic stem cells (11). In the heart, Kv1.5 encodes a portion of the rapidly activating, slowly inactivating 4-aminopyridine (4-AP)-sensitive current $I_{K,slow}$. In the SWAP mice, the 4-AP-sensitive component of $I_{K,slow}$ was absent from cardiac myocytes, but total current was not altered due to upregulation at the protein level of Kv2.1, the gene that encodes the 4-AP-resistant component of $I_{K,slow}$ (25).

Prior studies suggested that Kv1.5 and/or Kv2.1 play a key role in the hypoxia-induced vasoconstriction of pulmonary arteries (HPV) that allows the matching of perfusion to ventilation (18). For this reason, HPV was compared in wild-type and SWAP mice (15). Pulmonary artery smooth muscle cells from SWAP mice were slightly depolarized and lacked a 4-AP- and hypoxia-sensitive component of the voltage-dependent K^+ current present in wild-type cells (Fig. 2). In addition, HPV was significantly reduced in both pulmonary artery rings and isolated lung preparations. Kv1.5 was absent from pulmonary arteries from SWAP mice, without overt

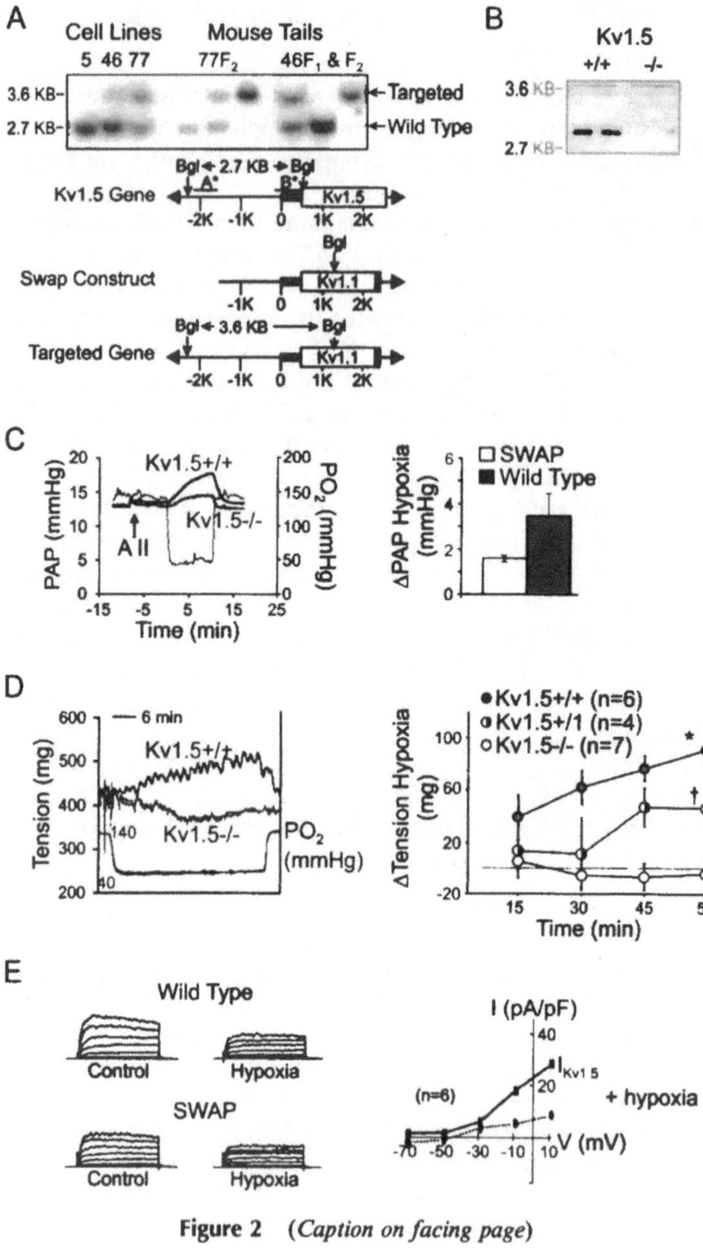

Figure 2 (*Caption on facing page*)

changes in expression in other ion channels. Thus, the findings from these mice confirm a role for Kv1.5 in HPV.

Significant questions regarding the role of Kv1.5 in HPV remain, however. It is not clear whether the loss of Kv1.5 from the endothelium plays a significant role in the phenotype. In addition, HPV was not completely abolished in the SWAP mice, and the role of other ion channels remains to be determined.

B. Gene-Targeted Mice

Table 1 includes a list of knockout and gene-targeted mice in which channels thought to be present in the pulmonary vasculature have been targeted. Characterization of pulmonary artery function remains largely unreported. This could be especially interesting in mice lacking K_{ATP} (Kir6.1 or SUR2), which have recently been shown to have coronary artery vasospasm (20,21). Mice lacking channel β subunits and channel chaperone proteins have also been engineered.

V. TRANSGENIC AND GENE-TARGETED MOUSE MODELS OF PULMONARY VASCULAR DISEASE

As the genes that cause or modify pulmonary vascular disease states become known, transgenic and gene-targeted models will be engineered and screened for abnormal pulmonary artery function. Analysis of transgenic and gene-targeted mice engineered for other reasons will also result in the identification of mice with abnormal pulmonary vascular function. Changes in pulmonary artery smooth muscle ion channels are likely to be present in these transgenic mice. Identification of these changes and correlation to the phenotype in the mice will help to elucidate the function of these channels. The ability to cross these mice with ion channel knockout and

---

Figure 2 (*Facing page*) Hypoxic pulmonary vasoconstriction is diminished in mice lacking Kv1.5. (A) Schematic representation of Kv1.5 gene and targeting construct (bottom), along with genomic Southern blots (top) showing cell lines heterozygous for the targeted allele (L46 and L77) and mice from each line heterozygous and homozygous for the targeted allele. The probe used for the Southern blot is designated as A*. (B) Western blot on lung tissue demonstrating the absence of Kv1.5 protein in the SWAP mice. (C) Hypoxic pulmonary vasoconstriction in an isolated perfused lung preparation with constant perfusate flow is impaired in SWAP mice. (D) Tension in response to hypoxia is diminished in fourth division PA rings from heterozygous and homozygous mice targeted mice. (E) Representative traces (left) and subtraction records (wild type minus SWAP, right) showing that the basal K^+ currents and hypoxia-induced K^+ currents are smaller in single voltage-clamped pulmonary artery smooth muscle cells from SWAP mice than in control mice. (From Ref. 15.)

Table 1 Smooth Muscle Ion Channel-Targeted Mice

Channel	Gene	Type	Current	Ref
Kv1.1	*Kcna1*	Knockout	I_K	37
Kv1.5	*Kcna5*	Targeted replacement, Kv1.5 → Kv1.1	I_K	11
Kv3.1	*Kcnc1*	Knockout	I_K	38
Kv3.2	*Kcnc2*	Knockout	I_K	39
Kv3.3	*Kcnc3*	Knockout	I_K	40
erg1	*Kcnh2*	Knockout	I_K	41
Kir3.1	*Kcnj3*	Knockout	I_{KACh}	42
Kir6.1	*Kcnj8*	Knockout	$I_{K,ATP}$	20
SUR2	*Sur2*	Knockout	$I_{K,ATP}$	21,43
$Ca_v1.2$	*Cacna1c*	Knockout	$I_{Ca,L}$ ($\alpha 1_C$)	44
$Ca_v1.3$	*Cacna1d*	Knockout	$I_{Ca,L}$ ($\alpha 1_D$)	45

gene-targeted mice may lead to additional insights. We will discuss mouse models of pulmonary hypertension as an example.

A. Mouse Models of Pulmonary Hypertension

The pathophysiology of primary pulmonary hypertension includes (1) cellular proliferation that reduces the lumen of small pulmonary vessels, (2) thrombosis in situ, and (3) vasoconstriction (26,27). Changes in ion channel expression and function have been documented in both familial and sporadic cases of primary pulmonary hypertension (28,29). The therapeutic role of Ca^{2+} channel blockers in treatment of pulmonary hypertension also supports a role for ion channels.

Vasoconstriction could result from an increased production of vasoconstrictors or decreased production of endogenous vasodilators. Endothelial dysfunction, primary or secondary, could be responsible for both increased endogenous vasoconstriction and decreased vasodilation. These vasoactive insults alter the vascular tone, which is determined mainly by smooth muscle cell membrane potential and calcium fluxes. Inflammation may enhance endothelial dysfunction and vasoconstriction. In addition, enhanced Ca^{2+} entry into smooth muscle cells may promote cellular proliferation. Thus, the mechanisms that contribute to pulmonary hypertension are complex.

Bone morphogenetic protein type II receptor (BMPR2) mutations cause a familial form of primary pulmonary hypertension linked to the PPH1 locus (30,31). Mutant alleles inhibit BMP/Smad-mediated signaling and upregulate p38(MAPK)-dependent proliferative pathways in vitro (32). Mice homozygous for null or hypomorphic alleles are embryonically lethal (33,34). Heterozygotes were reported to be phenotypically normal, but it is unknown whether changes occur in pulmonary artery smooth muscle ion channels.

Caveolin-1 knockout mice develop a dilated cardiomyopathy with pulmonary hypertension, despite markedly elevated systemic NO levels (16). Targeted overexpression of heme oxygenase-1 in the lung and the serine elastase inhibitor elafin in the cardiovascular system limits the development of pulmonary hypertension following hypoxia (35,36). An analysis of ion channel expression in these models would be interesting.

VI. SUMMARY/CONCLUSION

The explosion of cloned genes has led to an extraordinary accumulation of information on their functional diversity, gene organization, tissue-specific expression, and structure–function relationships. Transgenic and gene-targeted mice have contributed in a major way to our understanding of the molecular and genetic basis of human physiology.

Our knowledge of the mechanisms controlling pulmonary vascular tone and remodeling is still incomplete. In addition, the prognosis for many types of pulmonary vascular disease remains dismal. A better understanding of the pathobiology of these diseases is essential. This understanding may ultimately lead to novel pharmacological, gene-based, and stem-cell-based therapeutic options.

Genetically engineered mice can help us to understand the roles that ion channels play in the pulmonary vasculature. Many of the tools (including the mice) for these studies already exist. The key will be to exploit them in a logical, systematic, and cost-effective manner. The major challenge will then be to determine the relevance of the findings to humans.

REFERENCES

1. London B. Use of transgenic and gene-targeted mice to study K^+ channel function in the cardiovascular system. Archer SA, Rusch JF, eds. Potassium Channels in Cardiovascular Biology. New York: Plenum, 2001:177–191.
2. Nerbonne JM, Nichols CG, Schwarz TL, Escande D. Genetic manipulation of cardiac K^+ channel function in mice. What have we learned, and where do we go from here?. Circ Res 2001; 89:944–956.
3. Izumo S, Shioi T. Cardiac transgenic and gene-targeted mice as models of cardiac hypertrophy and failure: a problem of (new) riches. J Card Failure 1998; 4:349–361.
4. Teng PI, Dichiara MR, Komuves LG, Abe K, Quertermous T, Topper JN. Inducible and selective transgene expression in murine vascular endothelium. Physiol Genom 2002; 11:99–107.
5. Mack CP, Owens GK. Regulation of smooth muscle alpha-actin expression in vivo is dependent on CArG elements within the 5′ and first intron promoter regions. Circ Res 1999; 84:852–861.

6. Everett AD, Kamibayashi C, Brautigan DL. Transgenic expression of protein phosphatase 2A regulatory subunit B56gamma disrupts distal lung differentiation. Am J Physiol Lung Cell Mol Physiol 2002; 282:L1266–L1271.
7. Miki T, Tashiro F, Iwanaga T, Nagashima K, Yoshitomi H, Aihara H, Nitta Y, Gonoi T, Inagaki N, Miyazaki J, Seino S. Abnormalities of pancreatic islets by targeted expression of a dominant-negative KATP channel. Proc Natl Acad Sci USA 1997; 94:11969–11973.
8. Fishman GI. Timing is everything in life: conditional transgene expression in the cardiovascular system. Circ Res 1998; 82:837–844.
9. Huang WY, Aramburu J, Douglas PS, Izumo S. Transgenic expression of green fluorescence protein can cause dilated cardiomyopathy. Nat Med 2000; 6: 482–483.
10. Van der Weyden L, Adams DJ, Bradley A. Tools for targeted manipulation of the mouse genome. Physiol Genom 2002; 11:133–164.
11. London B, Guo W, Pan X-H, Lee JS, Shusterman V, Rocco CJ, Logothetis DA, Nerbonne JM, Hill JA. Targeted replacement of Kv1.5 in the mouse leads to loss of the 4-aminopyridine-sensitive component of $I_{K,slow}$ and resistance to drug-induced QT prolongation. Circ Res 2001; 88:940–946.
12. Geisterfer-Lowrance AA, Christe M, Conner DA, Ingwall JS, Schoen FJ, Seidman CE, Seidman JG. A mouse model of familial hypertrophic cardiomyopathy. Science 1996; 272:731–734.
13. Shusterman V, Usiene I, Harrigal C, Lee JS, Kubota T, Feldman AM, London B. Strain-specific patterns of cardiac rhythm and autonomic nervous system activity in mice. Am J Physiol Heart Circ Physiol 2002; 282:H2076–H2083.
14. Guo J, Li H, London B, Nerbonne JM. Functional consequences of elimination of $I_{to,f}$ and $I_{to,s}$: early afterdepolarizations, atrioventricular block and ventricular arrhythmias in mice lacking Kv1.4 and expressing a dominant-negative Kv4 α subunit. Circ Res 2000; 87:73–79.
15. Archer SL, London B, Hampl V, Wu X, Nsair A, Puttagunta L, Hashimoto K, Waite RE, Michelakis ED. Impairment of hypoxic pulmonary vasoconstriction in mice lacking the voltage-gated potassium channel Kv1.5. FASEB J 2001; 15: 1801–1803.
16. Zhao Y-Y, Liu Y, Stan R-V, Fan L, Gu Y, Dalton N, Chu P-H, Peterson K, Ross J, Chien KR. Defects in *caveolin-1* cause dilated cardiomyopathy and pulmonary hypertension in knockout mice. Proc Natl Acad Sci USA 2002; 99:11375–11380.
17. Reeve HL, Archer SL, Weir EK. Ion channels in the pulmonary vasculature. Pulm Pharmacol Ther 1997; 10:243–252.
18. Archer SL, Souil E, Dinh-Xuan AT, Schremmer B, Mercier JC, El Yaagoubi A, Nguyen-Huu L, Reeve HL, Hampl V. Molecular identification of the role of voltage-gated K^+ channels, Kv1.5 and Kv2.1, in hypoxic pulmonary vasoconstriction and control of resting membrane potential in rat pulmonary artery myocytes. J Clin Invest 1998; 101:2319–2330.
19. Patel AJ, Lazdunski M, Honore E. Kv2.1/Kv9.3, an ATP-dependent delayed-rectifier K^+ channel in pulmonary artery myocytes. Ann NY Acad Sci 1999; 868:438–441.

20. Miki T, Suzuki M, Shibasaki T, Uemura H, Sato T, Yamaguchi K, Koseki H, Iwanaga T, Nakaya H, Seino S. Mouse model of Prinzmetal angina by disruption of the inward rectifier Kir6.1. Nat Med 2002; 8:466–472.
21. Chutkow WA, Pu J, Wheeler MT, Tomoyuki W, Makielski JC, Burant CF, McNally EM. Episodic coronary artery vasospasm and hypertension develop in the absence of Sur2 K_{ATP} channels. J Clin Invest 2003; 110:203–208.
22. Bae YM, Park MK, Lee SH, Ho WK, Earm YE. Contribution of Ca^{2+}-activated K^+ channels and non-selective cation channels to membrane potential of pulmonary arterial smooth muscle cells of the rabbit. J Physiol 1999; 514:747–758.
23. Muth JN, Varadi G, Schwartz A. Use of transgenic mice to study voltage-dependent Ca^{2+} channels. Trends Pharm Sci 2001; 22:526–531.
24. Yuan XJ. Role of calcium-activated chloride current in regulating pulmonary vasomotor tone. Am J Physiol 1997; 272:L959–L968.
25. Xu H, Barry DM, Li H, Brunet S, Guo W, Nerbonne JM. Attenuation of the slow component of delayed rectification, action potential prolongation, and triggered activity in mice expressing a dominant-negative Kv2 α subunit. Circ Res 1999; 85:623–633.
26. Archer SL, Rich S. Primary pulmonary hypertension. A vascular biology and translational research "work in progress". Circulation 2000; 102:2781–2791.
27. Jeffery TK, Morrell NW. Molecular and cellular basis of pulmonary vascular remodeling in pulmonary hypertension. Prog Cardiovasc Dis 2002; 45:173–202.
28. Geraci MW, Moore M, Gesell T, Yeager ME, Alger L, Golpon H, Gao B, Loyd JE, Tuder RM, Voelkel NF. Gene expression patterns in the lungs of patients with primary pulmonary hypertension. A gene microarray analysis. Circ Res 2001; 88:555–562.
29. Yuan JX-J, Aldinger A, Juhaszova M, Wang J, Conte JV, Gaine SP, Orens J, Rubin LJ. Dysfunctional voltage-gated K^+ channels in pulmonary artery smooth muscle cells of patients with primary pulmonary hypertension. Circulation 1998; 98:1400–1406.
30. Deng Z, Morse JH, Slager SL, Cuervo N, Moore KJ, Venetos G, Kalachikov S, Cayanis E, Fischer SG, Barst RJ, Hodge SE, Knowles JA. Familial primary pulmonary hypertension (gene PPH1) is caused by mutations in the bone morphogenetic protein receptor-II gene. Am J Hum Genet 2000; 67:737–744.
31. Newman JH, Wheeler L, Lane KB, Loyd E, Gaddipati R, Phillips JA 3rd, Loyd JE. Mutation in the gene for bone morphogenetic protein receptor II as a cause of primary pulmonary hypertension in a large kindred. N Engl J Med 2001; 345:319–324.
32. Rudarakanchana N, Flanagan JA, Chen H, Upton PD, Machado R, Patel D, Trembath RC, Morrell NW. Functional analysis of bone morphogenetic protein type II receptor mutations underlying primary pulmonary hypertension. Hum Mol Genet 2002; 11:1517–1525.
33. Beppu H, Kawabata M, Hamamoto T, Chytil A, Minowa O, Noda T, Miyazono K. BMP type II receptor is required for gastrulation and early development of mouse embryos. Dev Biol 2000; 221:249–258.

34. Delot EC, Bahamonde ME, Zhao M, Lyons KM. BMP signaling is required for septation of the outflow tract of the mammalian heart. Development 2003; 130:209–220.
35. Minamino T, Christou H, Hsieh C-M, Liu Y, Dhawan V, Abraham NG, Perrella MA, Mitsialis SA, Kourembanas S. Targeted expression of heme oxygenase-1 prevents the pulmonary inflammatory and vascular responses to hypoxia. Proc Natl Acad Sci USA 2001; 98:8798–8803.
36. Zaidi SHE, You X-M, Ciura S, Husain M, Rabinovitch M. Overexpression of the serine elastase inhibitor elafin protects transgenic mice from hypoxic pulmonary hypertension. Circulation 2002; 105:516–521.
37. Smart SL, Lopantsev V, Zhang CL, Robbins CA, Wang H, Chiu SY, Schwartzkroin PA, Messing A, Tempel BL. Deletion of the K(V)1.1 potassium channel causes epilepsy in mice. Neuron 1998; 20:809–819.
38. Sanchez JA, Ho CS, Vaughan DM, Garcia MC, Grange RW, Joho RH. Muscle and motor-skill dysfunction in a K^+ channel-deficient mouse are not due to altered muscle excitability or fiber type but depend on the genetic background. Pflügers Arch 2000; 440:34–41.
39. Lau D, Vega-Saenz de Miera EC, Contreras D, Ozaita A, Harvey M, Chow A, Noebels JL, Paylor R, Morgan JI, Leonard CS, Rudy B. Impaired fast-spiking, suppressed cortical inhibition, and increased susceptibility to seizures in mice lacking Kv3.2 K^+ channel proteins. J Neurosci 2000; 20:9071–9085.
40. Espinosa F, McMahon A, Chan E, Wang S, Ho CS, Heintz N, Joho RH. Alcohol hypersensitivity, increased locomotion, and spontaneous myoclonus in mice lacking the potassium channels Kv3.1 and Kv3.3. J Neurosci 2001; 21: 6657–6665.
41. London B, Pan X-H, Lewarchik CM, Lee JS. QT interval prolongation and arrhythmias in heterozygous Merg1-targeted mice. Circulation 1998; 98:I-56 [Abstract].
42. Bettahi I, Marker CL, Roman MI, Wickman K. Contribution of the Kir3.1 subunit to the muscarinic-gated atrial potassium channel IKACH. J Biol Chem 2002; 277:48282–48288.
43. Chutkow WA, Samuel V, Hansen PA, Pu J, Valdivia CR, Makielski JC, Burant CF. Disruption of Sur2-containing KATP channels enhances insulin-stimulated glucose uptake in skeletal muscle. Proc Natl Acad Sci USA 2001; 98:11760–11764.
44. Seisenberger C, Specht V, Welling A, Platzer J, Pfeifer A, Kuhbandner S, Striessnig J, Klugbauer N, Feil R, Hofmann F. Functional embryonic cardiomyocytes after disruption of the L-type α_{1C} ($Ca_v1.2$) calcium channel gene in the mouse. J Biol Chem 2000; 275:39193–39199.
45. Platzer J, Engel J, Schrott-Fischer A, Stephan K, Bova S, Chen H, Zheng H, Striessnig J. Congenital deafness and sinoatrial node dysfunction in mice lacking class D L-type Ca^{2+} channels. Cell 2000; 102:89–97.

Index

T - #0229 - 101024 - C0 - 229/152/44 [46] - CB - 9780824759681 - Gloss Lamination